MW00845071

The Atlas of Emergency Radiology

To my dear friends
Cathie and Harvey –
a glimpse into what I do
all day when I am not
running around the neighborhood
with the boys.

Marty Jordanov
6-9-2013

Notice

Medicine is an ever-changing science. As new research and clinical experience broaden our knowledge, changes in treatment and drug therapy are required. The authors and the publisher of this work have checked with sources believed to be reliable in their efforts to provide information that is complete and generally in accord with the standards accepted at the time of publication. However, in view of the possibility of human error or changes in medical sciences, neither the authors nor the publisher nor any other party who has been involved in the preparation or publication of this work warrants that the information contained herein is in every respect accurate or complete, and they disclaim all responsibility for any errors or omissions or for the results obtained from use of the information contained in this work. Readers are encouraged to confirm the information contained herein with other sources. For example and in particular, readers are advised to check the product information sheet included in the package of each drug they plan to administer to be certain that the information contained in this work is accurate and that changes have not been made in the recommended dose or in the contraindications for administration. This recommendation is of particular importance in connection with new or infrequently used drugs.

The Atlas of Emergency Radiology

Editors

Jake Block, MD
Associate Professor of Radiology, Orthopaedic Surgery and Rehabilitation, and Emergency Medicine
Director of Musculoskeletal and Emergency Radiology
Department of Radiology and Radiological Sciences
Vanderbilt University Medical Center
Nashville, Tennessee

Martin I. Jordanov, MD
Assistant Professor of Radiology and Emergency Medicine
Department of Radiology and Radiological Sciences
Vanderbilt University Medical Center
Nashville, Tennessee

Lawrence B. Stack, MD
Associate Professor of Emergency Medicine and Pediatrics
Department of Emergency Medicine
Vanderbilt University Medical Center
Nashville, Tennessee

R. Jason Thurman, MD
Assistant Professor of Emergency Medicine
Associate Director, Residency Program
Department of Emergency Medicine
Vanderbilt University Medical Center
Nashville, Tennessee

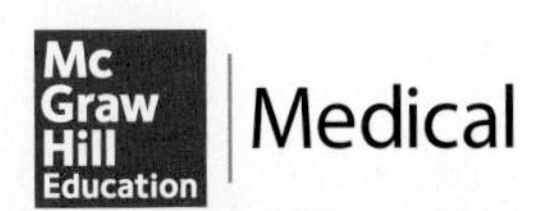

New York Chicago San Francisco Lisbon London Madrid Mexico City
Milan New Delhi San Juan Seoul Singapore Sydney Toronto

The Atlas of Emergency Radiology

1 2 3 4 5 6 7 8 9 0 CTP/CTP 18 17 16 15 14 13

ISBN 978-0-07-174442-3
MHID 0-07-174442-8

This book was set in Times Roman by Thomson Digital.
The editors were Anne M. Sydor and Robert Pancotti.
The production supervisor was Jeffrey Herzich.
Project management was provided by Charu Bansal, Thomson Digital.
The text designer was Janice Bielawa; the cover was by Pehrrsen Design.
Cover image of doctor holding a portable computer with MR scan of the human brain by Thomas Tolstrup/Getty Images.
China Translation & Printing Services, Ltd. was printer and binder.

Library of Congress Cataloging-in-Publication Data

The atlas of emergency radiology / editors, Jake Block ... [et al.].
p. ; cm.
Includes index.
ISBN 978-0-07-174442-3 (print book : alk. paper)
ISBN 0-07-174442-8 (print book : alk. paper)
ISBN 0-07-176044-X (ebook)
I. Block, Jake.
[DNLM: 1. Radiography—methods—Atlases. 2. Critical Care—methods—Atlases. 3. Emergency Treatment—methods—Atlases. 4. Wounds and Injuries—radiography—Atlases. WN 17]
616.07'572—dc23
2012035885

McGraw-Hill Education books are available at special quantity discounts to use as premiums and sales promotions, or for use in corporate training programs. To contact a representative please e-mail us at bulksales@mcgraw-hill.com.

To my amazing wife Melanie, with my love and gratitude for the unwavering support that she so generously gives.

To my sons Owen and Wyatt whose curiosity and wonderment bring me great inspiration. What a joy it is to rediscover the world with you both.

Jake Block, MD

To my wonderful wife Wendy. I couldn't have asked for a better partner in life. Thank you for being my best friend for the past 20 years.

To my precious boys Max and Alex. You are the fulfillment of my dreams and the magic in my world.

And to my parents Adriana and Ivan. I am forever grateful for your love and guidance.

Martin I. Jordanov, MD

To my Vanderbilt Emergency Medicine and Radiology colleagues, for inspiring me to provide excellence in patient care and medical education. To the patients of Vanderbilt University, Children's, and Veteran's Administration Hospitals, for the privilege and trust you have given us to care for you.

Lawrence B. Stack, MD

To my wife Lauren and children Kate and Ben. I am thankful for your patience, love, and understanding, and for bringing true joy into every day of my life. To the Emergency Medicine Residents of Vanderbilt, who are exceptionally talented and make every shift fun! To our Radiology colleagues, whose expertise teaches us daily and improves the care of our patients always. And finally, to all those who have generously provided mentoring, especially my mother and father, Drs. Slovis, Wrenn, Pancioli, Jauch, Jones, and Stack: all of whom have made a tremendous impact on my life.

R. Jason Thurman, MD

CONTENTS

CONTRIBUTORS

Joseph Blake, MD
Chief of MRI Services
Kettering Network Radiologists, Inc.
Kettering, Ohio

Jake Block, MD
Associate Professor of Radiology, Orthopaedic Surgery and Rehabilitation, and Emergency Medicine
Director of Musculoskeletal and Emergency Radiology
Department of Radiology and Radiological Sciences
Vanderbilt University Medical Center
Nashville, Tennessee

Allison D. Bollinger, MD
Emergency Physician
Department of Emergency Medicine
Vanderbilt University Medical Center
Nashville, Tennessee

Cari L. Buckingham, MD
Assistant Professor
Department of Radiology and Radiological Sciences
Vanderbilt University Medical Center
Nashville, Tennessee

Matthew D. Dobbs, MD
Fellow of Neuroradiology
Department of Radiology
Stanford University Hospital
Palo Alto, California

Jason Dowling, MD
Section Chief of Diagnostics
Kaiser Permanente Georgia
Atlanta, Georgia

Robinson M. Ferre, MD
Assistant Professor
Director, Emergency Ultrasound
Department of Emergency Medicine
Vanderbilt University Medical Center
Nashville, Tennessee

James F. Fiechtl, MD
Assistant Professor of Emergency Medicine, and Orthopaedics and Rehabilitation
Department of Emergency Medicine
Vanderbilt University Medical Center
Nashville, Tennessee

Robert Warne Fitch, MD
Assistant Professor of Emergency Medicine, and Orthopaedics and Rehabilitation
Department of Emergency Medicine
Vanderbilt University Medical Center
Nashville, Tennessee

Katherine G. Hartley, MD
Assistant Professor of Radiology and Emergency Medicine
Department of Radiology and Radiological Sciences
Vanderbilt University Medical Center
Nashville, Tennessee

Michael N. Johnston, MD
Assistant Professor
Department of Emergency Medicine
Vanderbilt University Medical Center
Nashville, Tennessee

Martin I. Jordanov, MD
Assistant Professor of Radiology and Emergency Medicine
Department of Radiology and Radiological Sciences
Vanderbilt University Medical Center
Nashville, Tennessee

J. Herman Kan, MD
Clinical Associate Professor of Radiology
Baylor College of Medicine
Chief of Musculoskeletal Radiology
Texas Children's Hospital
Houston, Texas

Christopher Kuzniewski, MD
Commander, Medical Corps United States Navy
Program Director, Diagnostic Radiology Residency
Academic Section Head, Cardiothoracic Radiology
Department of Radiology
Naval Medical Center
Portsmouth, Virginia

Laurie M. Lawrence, MD
Assistant Professor of Emergency Medicine
Department of Emergency Medicine
Vanderbilt University Medical Center
Nashville, Tennessee

Mark Meredith, MD
Assistant Professor of Pediatrics and Emergency Medicine
Clinical Director for Pediatric EMS
Division of Pediatric Emergency Medicine
Vanderbilt University Medical Center
Nashville, Tennessee

Marc Mickiewicz, MD
Assistant Professor
Department of Emergency Medicine
Vanderbilt University Medical Center
Nashville, Tennessee

Camiron L. Pfennig, MD
Assistant Professor and Director of Undergraduate Medical Education
Department of Emergency Medicine
Vanderbilt University Medical Center
Nashville, Tennessee

Dorris Elise Powell-Tyson, MD
Assistant Professor
Department of Emergency Medicine
Vanderbilt University Medical Center
Nashville, Tennessee

Gary Schwartz, MD
Assistant Professor of Emergency Medicine and Pediatrics
Department of Emergency Medicine
Vanderbilt University Medical Center
Nashville, Tennessee

Charles Seamens, MD
Assistant Professor
Department of Emergency Medicine
Vanderbilt University Medical Center
Nashville, Tennessee

Kurt A. Smith, MD
Assistant Professor
Department of Emergency Medicine
Vanderbilt University Medical Center
Nashville, Tennessee

Lawrence B. Stack, MD
Associate Professor of Emergency Medicine and Pediatrics
Department of Emergency Medicine
Vanderbilt University Medical Center
Nashville, Tennessee

Megan Kay Strother, MD
Associate Professor of Neuroradiology and Neurological Surgery
Department of Radiology and Radiological Sciences
Vanderbilt University Medical Center
Nashville, Tennessee

Christie Sullivan, MD
Emergency Medicine Physician
Department of Emergency Medicine
Vanderbilt University Medical Center
Nashville, Tennessee

David S. Taber, MD
Assistant Professor of Radiology and Emergency Medicine
Department of Radiology and Radiological Sciences
Vanderbilt University Medical Center
Nashville, Tennessee

R. Jason Thurman, MD
Assistant Professor of Emergency Medicine
Associate Director, Residency Program
Department of Emergency Medicine
Vanderbilt University Medical Center
Nashville, Tennessee

Almost all medical texts are collaborations, yet rarely are they partnerships between two distinct specialties. *The Atlas of Emergency Radiology* combines the radiographic expertise of radiologists with the clinical expertise of practicing emergency physicians. By teaming radiologists, who specialize in teaching others how to interpret films, with emergency physicians, who have devoted their careers to teaching the practice of emergency medicine, this book provides a truly unique way to learn the most important radiographic findings encountered in the emergency department.

This book's greatest strength is the presentation of each radiographic entity in three ways. First the radiologist provides a **Radiographic Summary**. This summary is a succinct explanation of the radiograph's findings. Then the emergency physician provides the **Clinical Implications**, which is a brief focused discussion on the mechanism of injury, related complications, or likely other clinical findings. Finally in the **Pearls Section**, both authors combine their expertise and many years of clinical experience to teach important related facts and "pearls" of wisdom. The book is organized into 12 chapters based on anatomic regions from head to toe and each chapter is divided into traumatic and non-traumatic conditions.

The authors learned from their successes in creating each of their three editions of *The Atlas of Emergency Medicine* and apply it to *The Atlas of Emergency Radiology*. In doing so, this book, like their prior text, can serve many purposes. It can be the initial source for students and residents to look up the classic findings of the diseases and fractures encountered in the emergency department on a trauma rotation or when doing orthopedics. It is also the perfect companion when studying for the in-service or board examination, allowing the user to quickly go from a written text to view classic radiologic findings, and it is the ideal reference text for the practicing emergency physician.

The chapters in this book cover all of the important radiological findings that the emergency medicine clinician needs to know. Radiographic findings in the emergency department are often subtle and difficult to master. Finally there is a book that is designed as the "go to source" to quickly look up any classic X-ray abnormality or fracture normally encountered within emergency medicine, allow rapid viewing of the key radiographic findings and their clinical implications, and provide clinical insights and pearls of wisdom related to the X-ray, CT, or MRI findings.

Corey M. Slovis, MD

PREFACE

Diagnostic images provide crucial information for the emergent care of the critically sick and injured. Effective clinical care requires expertise in the rapid and accurate interpretation of the many radiographic studies and their nuances used in the emergency department setting. *The Atlas of Emergency Radiology* provides nearly 1500 carefully selected diagnostic images combined with succinct descriptions of the radiographic features of over 330 emergent medical diagnoses to facilitate its readers in acquiring this expertise.

The Atlas of Emergency Radiology is modeled after *The Atlas of Emergency Medicine*, Third Edition, in which the chapters are organized by anatomic region with a variety of medical conditions presented in each chapter. Similarly, *The Atlas of Emergency Radiology* is divided into 12 chapters by anatomic region and further divided into traumatic or nontraumatic conditions. All chapters are co-written by practicing radiologists and emergency physicians to maximize the expertise in describing the radiographic findings of each diagnosis and then the clinical applications of these findings. One specialty chapter on pediatrics is included.

Each medical condition is presented in the following format: *radiographic summary, clinical implications*, and *radiographic pearls*. The *radiographic summary* succinctly describes the radiographic findings necessary to support the diagnosis. The *clinical implications* section provides a rationale to bridge the radiographic findings to the clinical findings. Each diagnosis concludes with 2-4 *radiographic pearls*, choice tips, or unique aspects about the condition.

The editors wish to thank our colleagues in the radiology and emergency medicine departments at Vanderbilt University Medical Center for their congenial collaboration and for providing their expertise and valuable time in the preparation of the content. We also wish to express our gratitude to Dr. Anne Sydor, Executive Editor at McGraw-Hill Medical, Amber Allen, Managing Editor of Integra-Chicago, and Charu Bansal, Production Manager of Thompson Digital for their tireless efforts to make this book an academic work of excellence. Finally, we want to thank the users of this book and trust that it will serve you well as you care for your patients.

Jake Block, MD
Martin I. Jordanov, MD
Lawrence B. Stack, MD
R. Jason Thurman, MD

Chapter 1

HEAD AND FACIAL TRAUMA

Megan Kay Strother
Matthew D. Dobbs
Lawrence B. Stack

Radiographic Summary

An acute epidural hematoma (EDH) is a hyperdense (higher Hounsfield unit number), extra-axial (outside the brain parenchyma) blood collection that occurs after a coup injury. The "classical" EDH occurs from a laceration of the middle meningeal artery after blunt trauma and is biconvex (lens-shaped) in appearance.

Hypodense blood within an EDH represents *acute unclotted* hemorrhage, while hyperdense blood corresponds to *acute clotted hemorrhage*. The mixed-density pattern, termed the "swirl sign," is caused by clotted and unclotted blood products.

EDH is confined by dural attachments to the cranium, which occur at cranial sutures. EDH will cross the sagittal suture at the midline but subdural hematomas (SDH) will not, because the dura does not invest the superior sagittal sinus.

EDH in the middle cranial fossa anterior to the temporal lobe tips is due to venous injury of the sphenoparietal sinus.

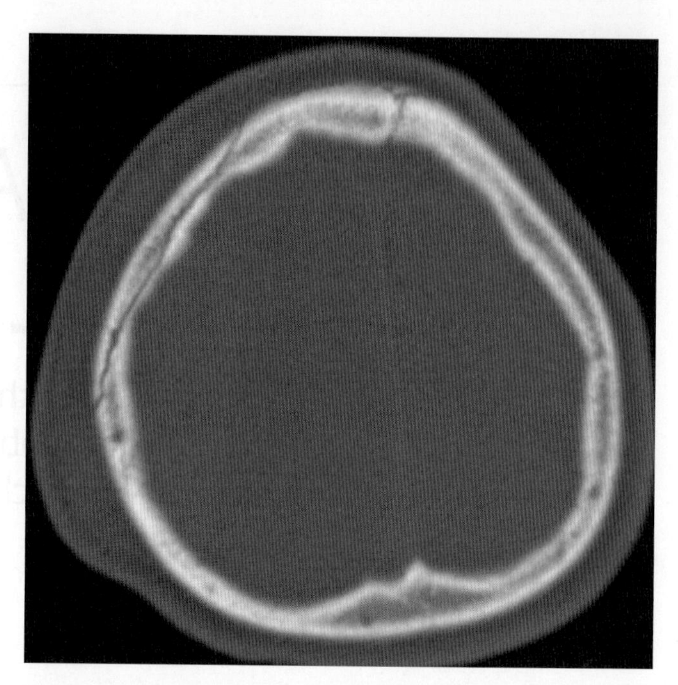

FIGURE 1.2 ■ Skull Fracture. NECT in bone windows shows a nondisplaced right parietal skull fracture that involves the right coronal suture (allowing blood to extend past the suture).

Clinical Implications

EDH comprise 1 to 4% of traumatic brain injury (TBI) and most often occur from falls less than 10 ft or from assault with an object (coup injury). The classical clinical scenario,

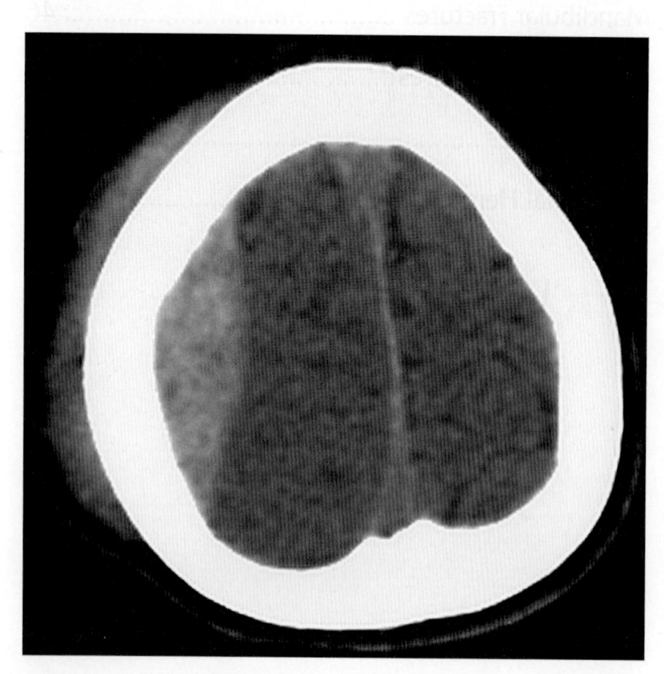

FIGURE 1.1 ■ Epidural Hematoma. NECT shows a lenticular (lens-shaped) hyperdense collection of blood along the high right parietal convexity with overlying scalp swelling.

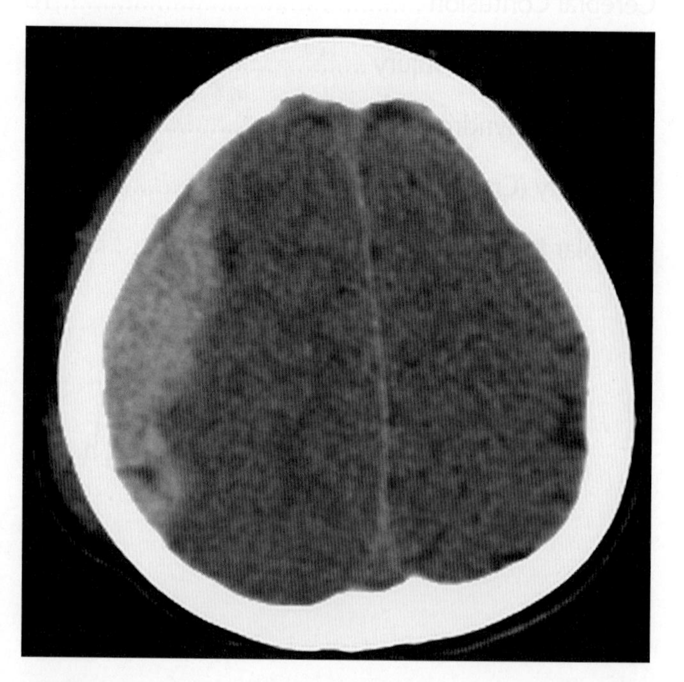

FIGURE 1.3 ■ Epidural Hematoma. NECT shows a large collection of hyperdense blood along the right parietal surface. Note the swelling of the subjacent sulci and mass effect on the normally midline falx cerebri.

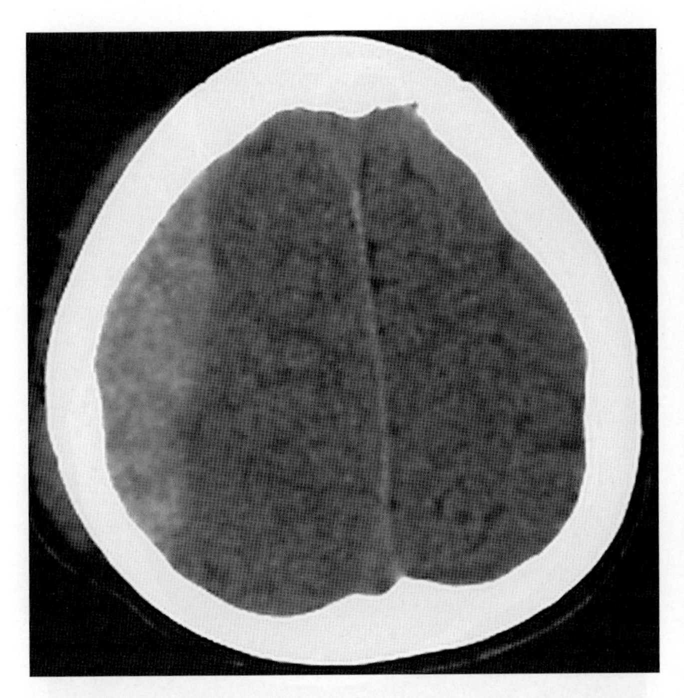

FIGURE 1.4 ■ Epidural Hematoma. NECT shows a collection of hyperdense blood along the right parietal convexity.

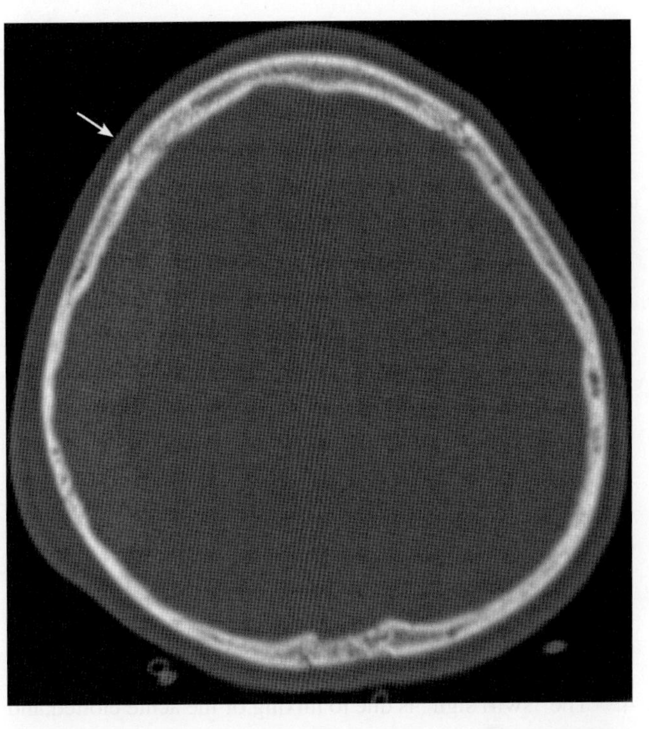

FIGURE 1.5 ■ Skull Fracture. NECT shows a faintly visible skull fracture extending to the right coronal suture (arrow). Although imaged in bone windows, underlying epidural hematoma and overlying scalp swelling is seen.

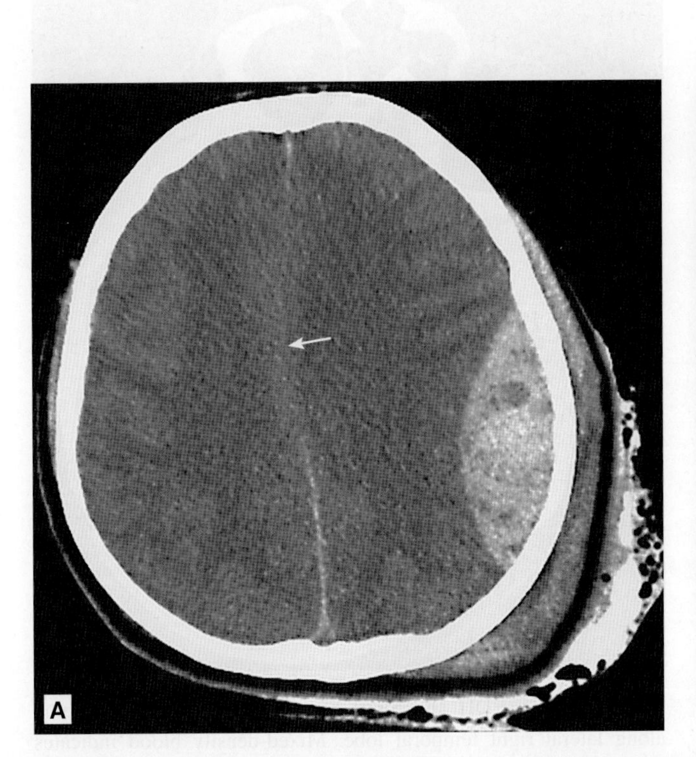

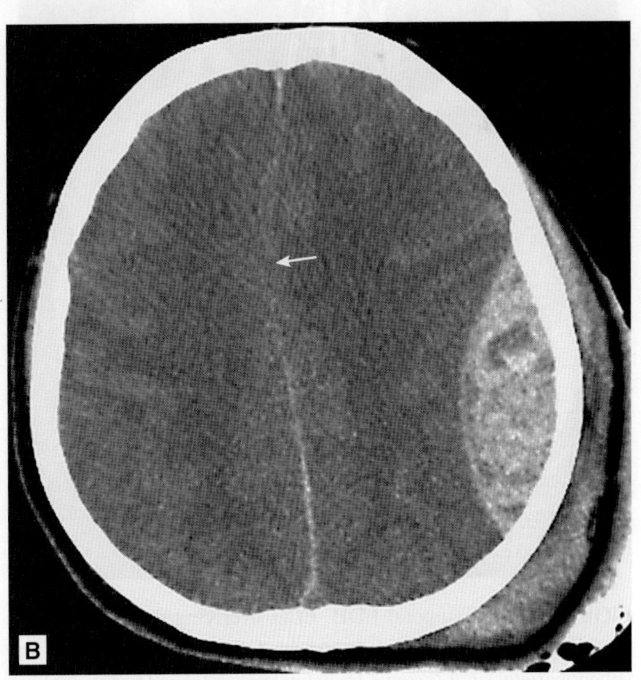

FIGURE 1.6 ■ Acute and Hyperacute EDH. **A, B:** NECT shows a large lenticular mixed-density collection of blood over the left parietal lobe. There is midline shift and transfalcine herniation (left cingulate gyrus pushed beneath the falx cerebri, arrows). Mixed density of the blood indicates both hyperacute and acute blood products that portends a worse prognosis.

which occurs in 10% of patients with EDH, presents with loss of consciousness, followed by a period of lucency. Patients then become progressively obtunded as the EDH enlarges. EDH may expand rapidly, causing mass effect that can lead to herniation. Decompressive craniectomy is required in most patients with rapidly expanding EDH. Despite the possibility for rapid expansion with EDH, patients with EDH generally have a better prognosis than patients with SDH. EDH of the anterior temporal lobes is venous rather than arterial, and typically has a benign course and frequently does not require surgical evacuation.

Pearls

1. Noncontrast head CT is the preferred study to evaluate all acute TBI.
2. Greater than 90% of EDH have overlying skull fractures.
3. EDH is a coup lesion, with 85% caused by arterial injury.
4. The "swirl sign" is due to mixing of the acute clotted and acute unclotted blood in an EDH or SDH and carries a worse clinical prognosis.

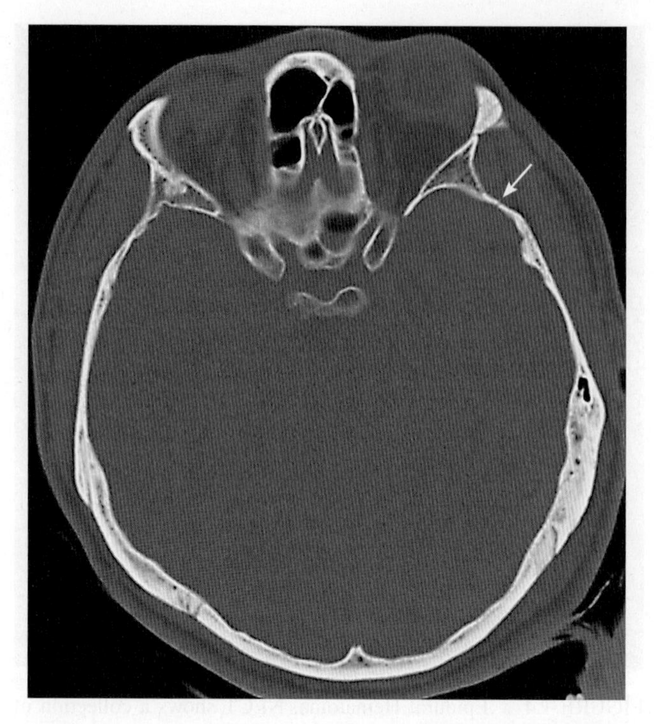

FIGURE 1.8 ■ Skull Fracture. Corresponding to Fig. 1.7, subtle fracture line is seen along the sphenoparietal suture on the left (arrow).

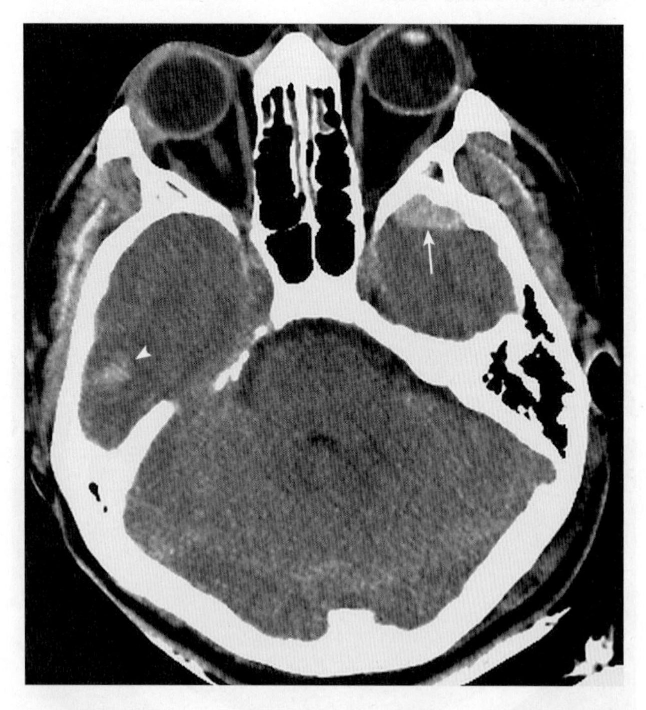

FIGURE 1.7 ■ Temporal EDH. EDH overlying the left temporal lobe is caused by venous hemorrhage following disruption of the sphenoparietal sinus (arrow). Ipsilateral preseptal soft tissue swelling is characteristic. EDH in this location (anterior temporal) typically has a benign course. A contrecoup injury to the right posterior temporal lobe, with hemorrhagic contusion, is also present (arrowhead).

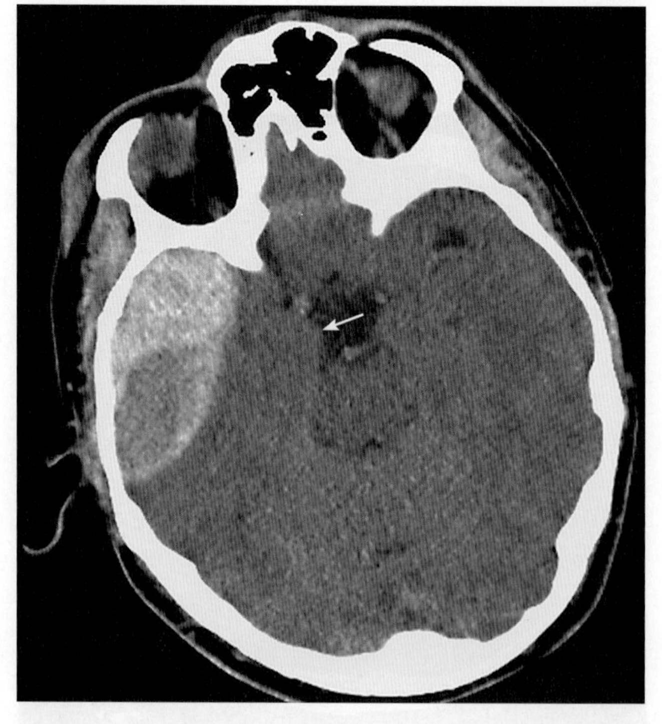

FIGURE 1.9 ■ EDH and Swirl Sign. Large epidural hematoma along lateral right temporal lobe. Mixed-density blood indicates hyperacute bleeding ("swirl sign"), which is a worse prognosis. The figure shows medial deviation of the uncus into the basilar cistern representing early transtentorial herniation (arrow).

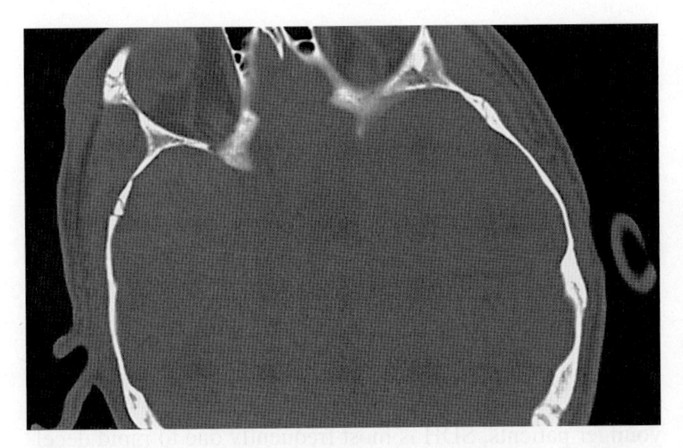

FIGURE 1.10 ■ Temporal Bone Fracture. Mildly displaced fracture of right squamosal temporal bone. The middle meningeal artery runs along this bone and is often lacerated due to the fracture.

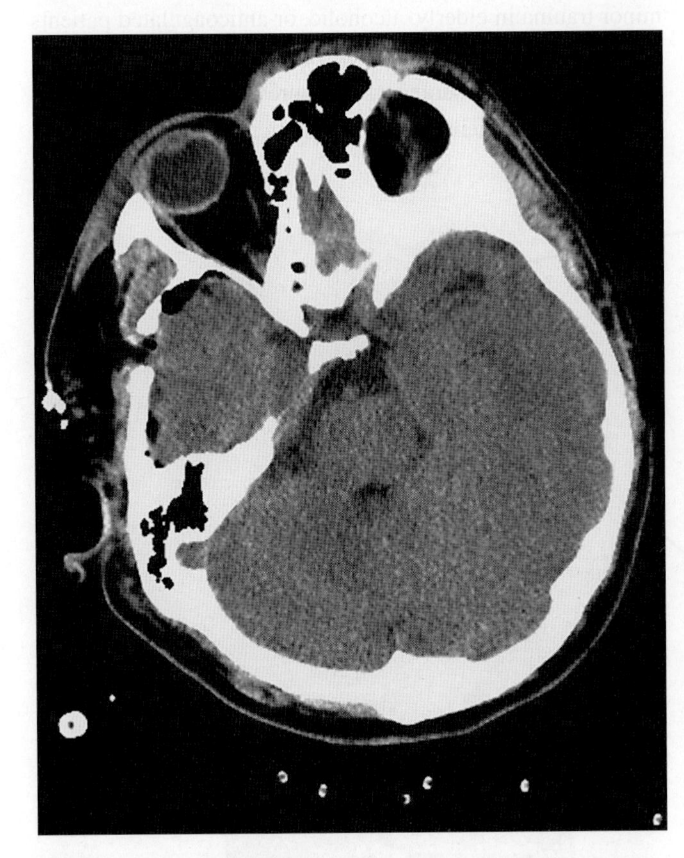

FIGURE 1.11 ■ EDH Postevacuation. Due to herniation and neurological decline, the epidural hematoma was urgently evacuated. Craniotomy defect is present.

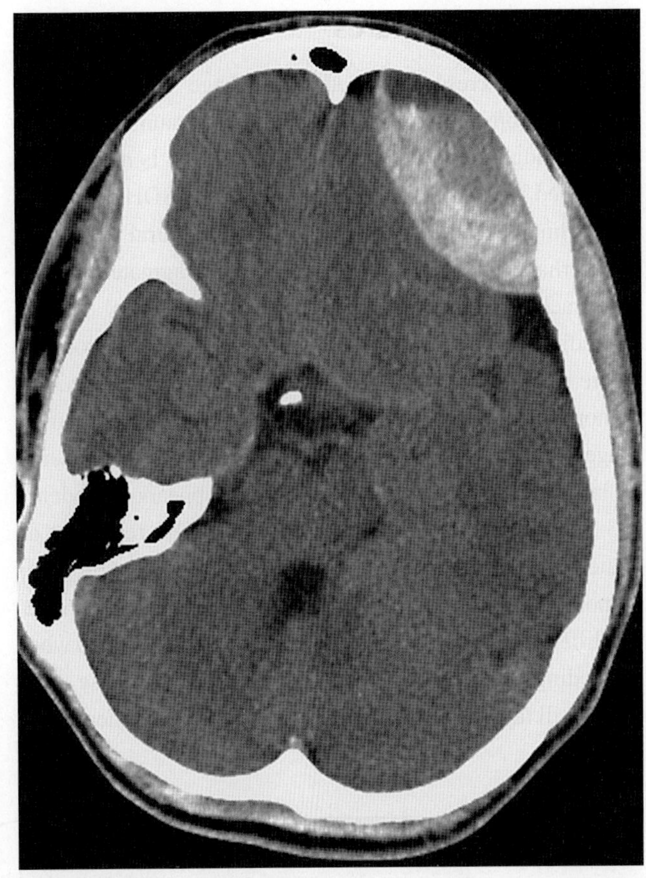

FIGURE 1.12 ■ EDH with Swirl Sign. An axial head CT image shows a large epidural hematoma along left frontal lobe with layering of blood products ("swirl sign") indicating active bleeding.

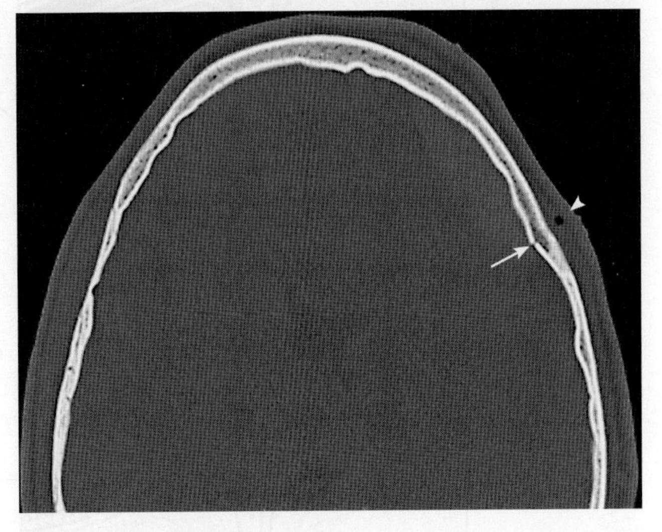

FIGURE 1.13 ■ Frontotemporal Fracture. Fracture seen over left frontotemporal bone (arrow) with small foci of air (arrowhead) in the subgaleal soft tissue at the fracture site.

Radiographic Features

A SDH is a crescent-shaped hemorrhage typically found along the convexities of the skull due to traumatic disruption of bridging cortical veins. In adults, SDH is not as often associated with overlying fracture as EDH. SDH will cross suture lines except at the falx, which is a dural reflection. Hemorrhage in the subdural space will invaginate with the falx, tracking between the frontal and parietal lobes.

Radiographic density varies with age of the blood products. Acute *unclotted* hemorrhage, also described as a *hyperacute* hemorrhage, is hypodense (0-2 hours); acute *clotted* hemorrhage is hyperdense (<1 week); a subacute SDH is isodense to brain (1-3 weeks); a chronic SDH appears hypodense (>3 weeks). Mixed densities within the SDH represent an acute bleed into a chronic SDH. The "hematocrit effect" is demonstrated when a sharp transition point is seen between the different densities in a SDH, which occurs most often when rebleeding occurs into a chronic SDH. The hyperdense acute blood will layer dependently. Patients with severe anemia can present with acute clotted SDH that appears hypodense. Septa within a SDH represent adhesions and make surgical drainage more difficult.

Detection of SDH is more sensitive with MRI than with CT, particularly for thin convexity SDH. The MRI appearance depends on age of the blood products.

Clinical Implications

SDH has much higher morbidity and mortality than EDH. In younger patients, SDH is most frequently due to rapid deceleration injury from a motor vehicle crash. While the slowly expanding hematoma can potentially contribute to secondary brain injury, it is the diffuse brain injury caused by the impact that creates the greatest morbidity. In contrast, seemingly minor trauma in elderly, alcoholic, or anticoagulated patients may cause SDH. Patients with SDH should be immediately evaluated by neurosurgery. Decompressive craniectomy may be required if patients are symptomatic.

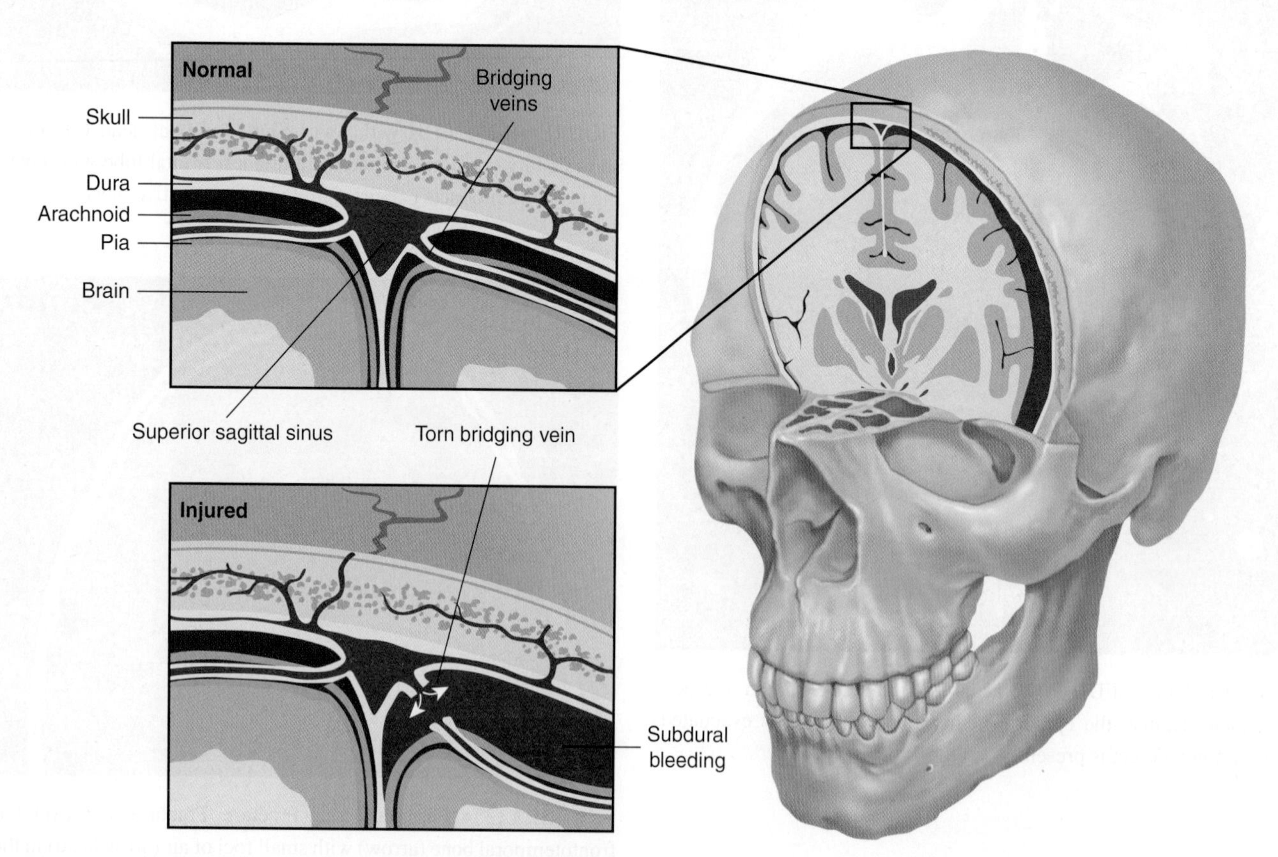

FIGURE 1.14 ■ Subdural Hematoma Anatomy. Normal and injured bridging vein anatomy demonstrating acute SDH mechanism of injury.

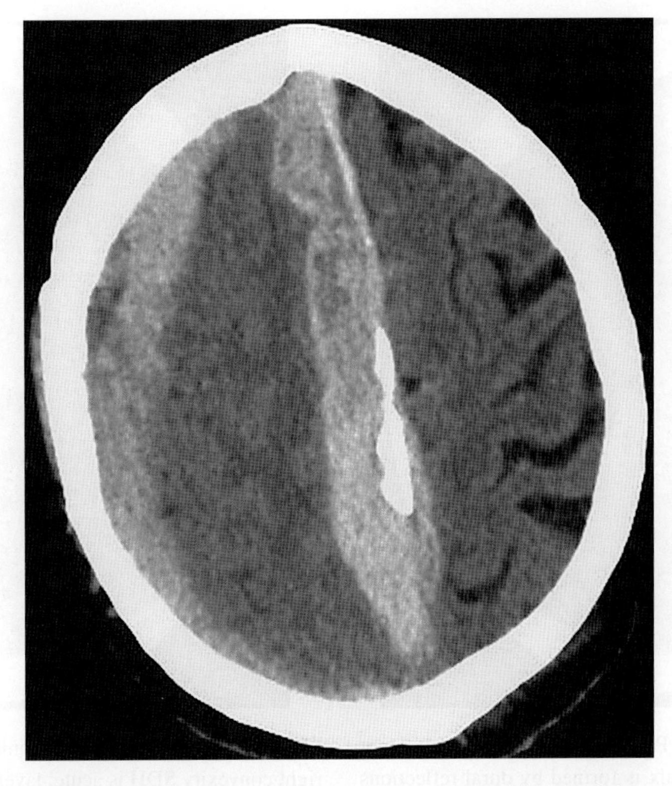

FIGURE 1.15 ■ Convexity and Parafalcine SDH. Along the right cerebral convexity and falx cerebri are hyperdense extra-axial fluid collections that cross cranial sutures. Areas of heterogeneity in the fluid represent varying ages of the blood products (very high-density structure along the midline falx is normal dural calcification). Mass effect on the right cerebral hemisphere causes loss of the normal sulcation as the cortical gyri are compressed.

Pearls

1. An MRI without contrast is better than CT at identifying hyperacute or chronic SDH. In these settings, SDH may be isodense to brain cortex on CT.
2. Radiographic features differentiating an EDH from SDH are seen in Table 1.1.
3. CT subdural window settings (window 150, level 5) are helpful for identifying subtle SDH. Subdural windows remove streak artifact that occurs from overlying bone.
4. Table 1.2 lists the CT window and level settings commonly used to evaluate the NECT of the traumatic brain.

TABLE 1.1 ■ RADIOGRAPHIC FEATURES OF EDH AND SDH

Feature	EDH	SDH
Shape	Lenticular	Crescentic
Origin	Arterial	Bridging vein
Crosses midline	Yes	No, except in posterior fossa
Coup injury	Yes	Yes
Contrecoup injury	No	Yes—more common
Associated fracture	>90%	Uncommon
Crosses sutures	No	Yes

TABLE 1.2 ■ CT WINDOW AND LEVEL SETTINGS FOR EVALUATION OF THE TRAUMATIC BRAIN

Setting	Window	Level	Utility
Parenchyma	80	40	Standard brain evaluation
Subdural	150	5	Improves detection of small SDH adjacent to bone
Bone	1500	450	Pneumocephalus, fractures, sinuses
Stroke	30	30	Ischemia/infarction

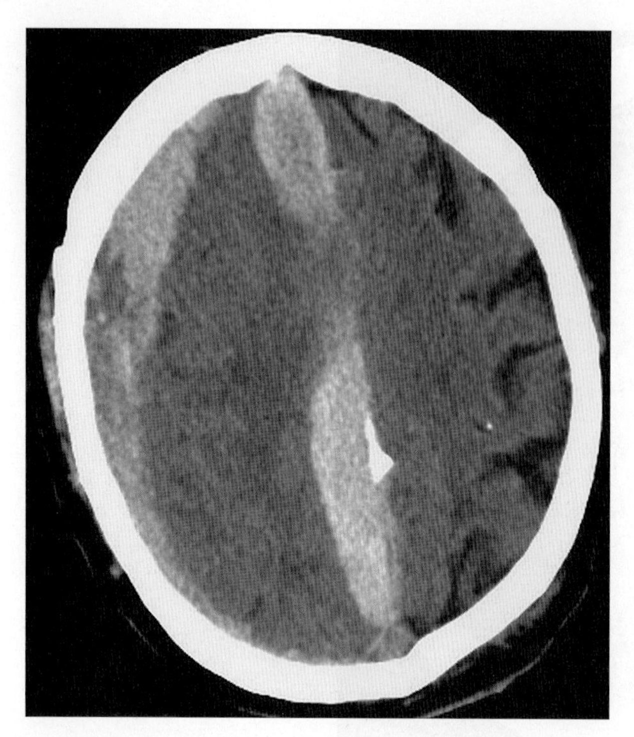

FIGURE 1.16 ■ Convexity and Parafalcine SDH. SDH will not cross the falx cerebri, since the falx is formed by dural reflections at the midline. In this patient, SDH overlies the frontal convexities and has an interhemispheric component. The high attenuation of this SDH will last for a week, and then begin to darken as the SDH ages.

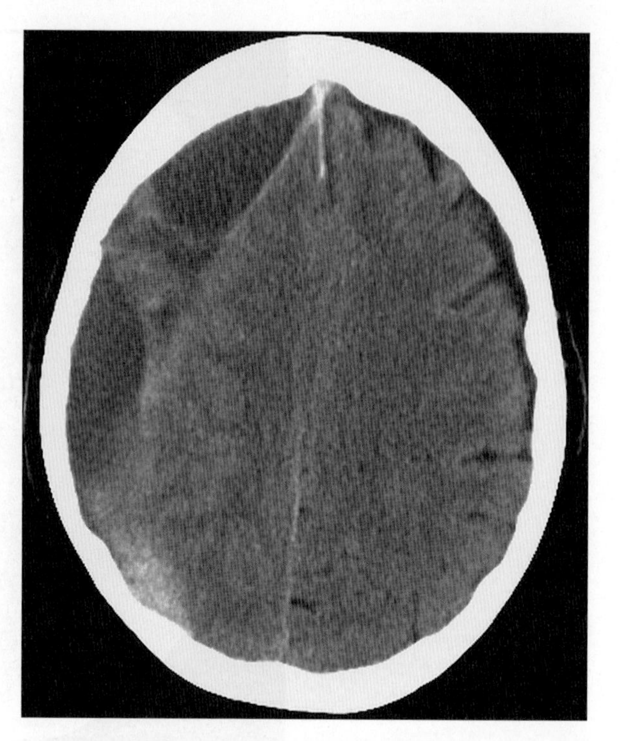

FIGURE 1.17 ■ Acute on Chronic SDH. The brighter blood in this right convexity SDH is acute, layering dependently within the SDH. The darker blood, which has the same attenuation on CT as CSF, is chronic (greater than 3 weeks) SDH. Chronic SDH are more likely to have adhesions.

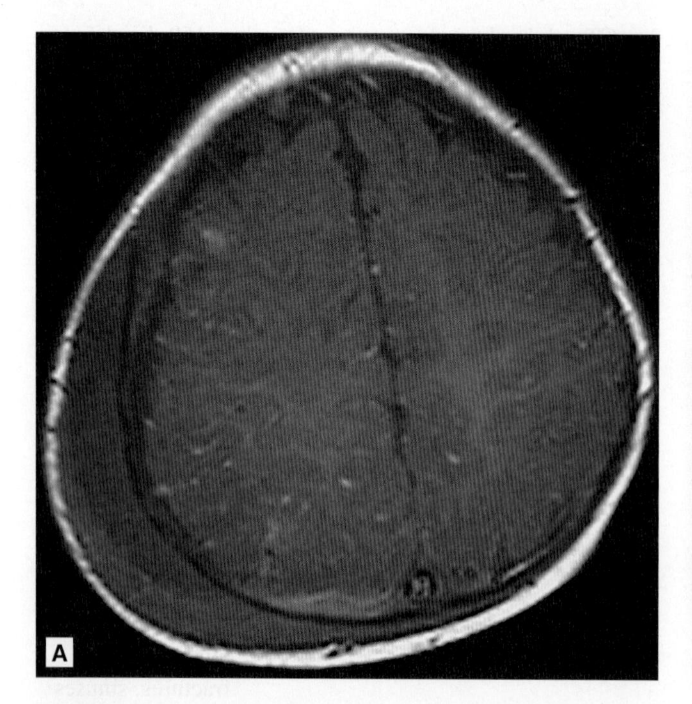

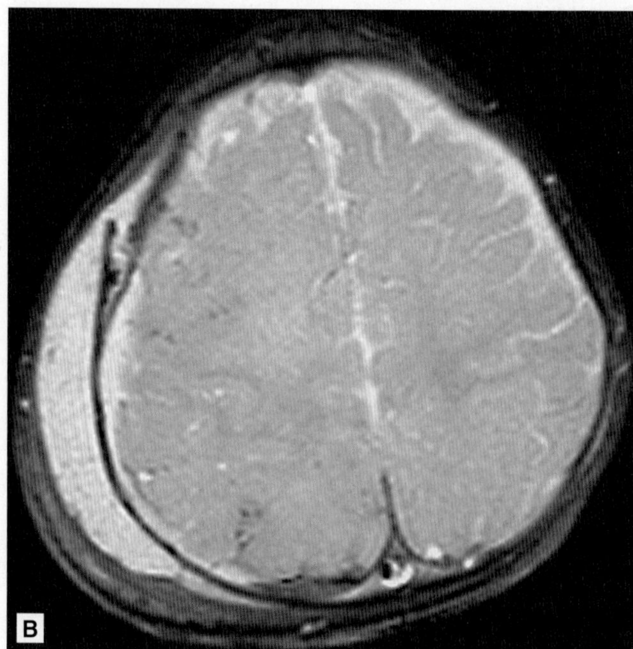

FIGURE 1.18 ■ Acute Subdural Hematoma. A 1-year-old female post injury. **A:** T1WI, **B:** T2*/GRE, **C:** FLAIR, and **D:** T2WI. On all images note the large right parietal scalp swelling. Best seen on the FLAIR and T1WI are bright fluid collections along the posterior and anterolateral right parietal lobe that represent blood. MRI is much more sensitive than CT for detection of SDH.

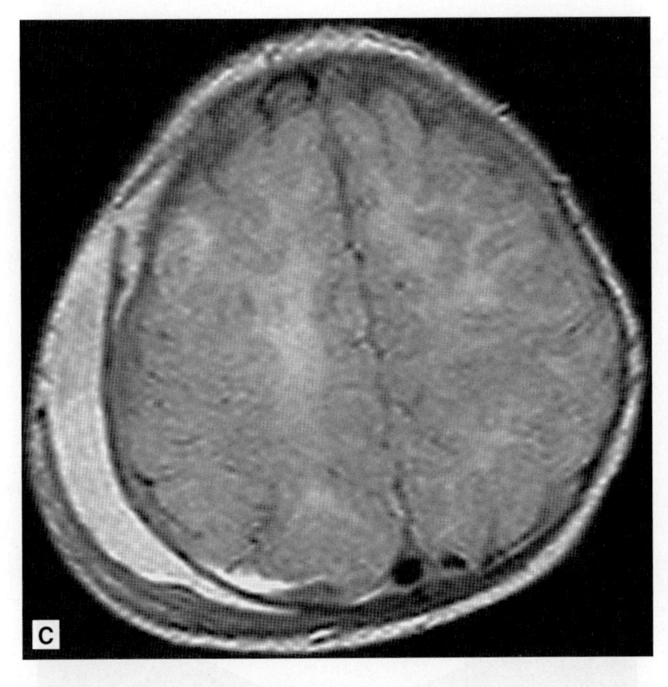

FIGURE 1.18 ■ *(Continued)*

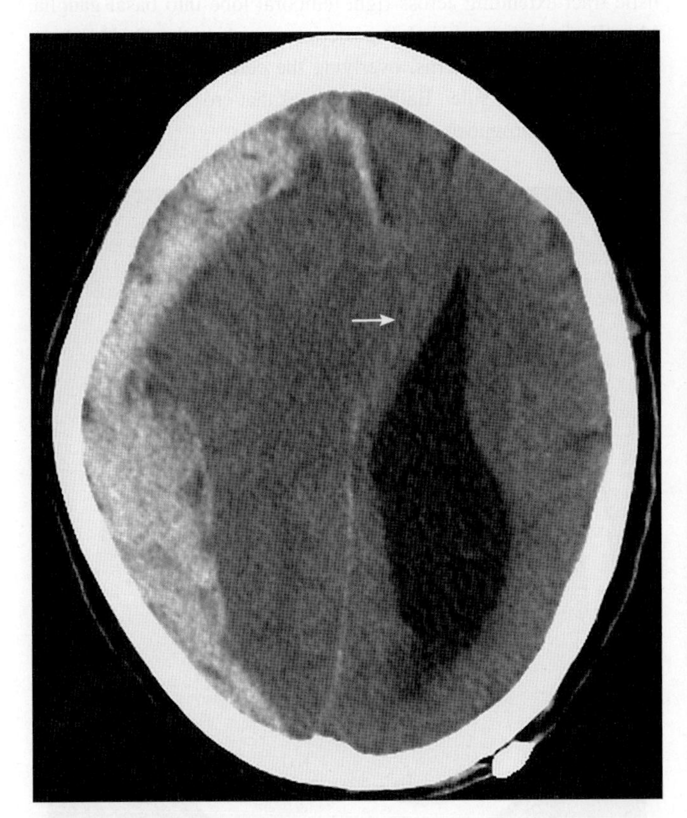

FIGURE 1.19 ■ Acute Subdural Hematoma. Large crescentic collection of acute blood along the right hemisphere representing an acute SDH. Note mass effect, dilation of the contralateral ventricle due to CSF outflow obstruction, and subfalcine herniation (arrow). Blood also extends into interhemispheric region.

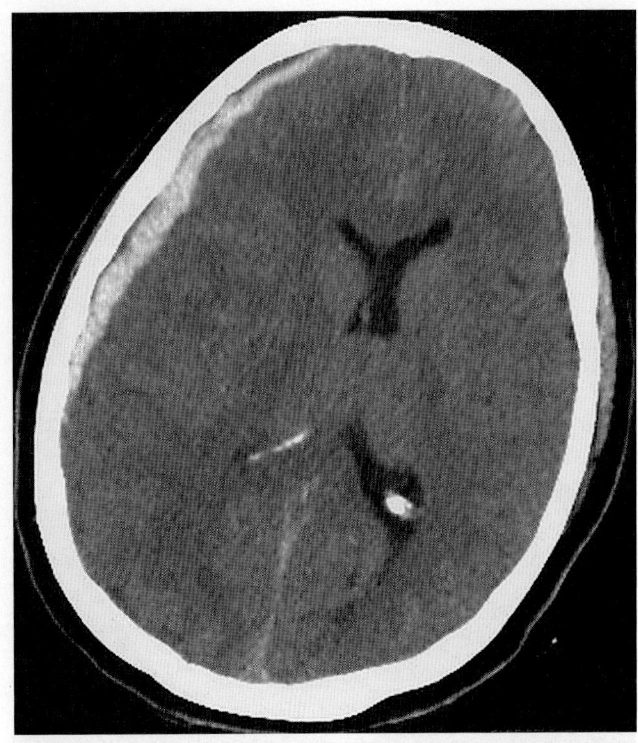

FIGURE 1.20 ■ Acute SDH with Mass Effect. Thin dense crescentic collection of blood along right side with mild mass effect (note smaller size of right lateral ventricle frontal horn).

Radiographic Features

tSAH is blood within the subarachnoid space that results from injury to small cortical vessels or as contiguous extension of a cerebral contusion, SDH, or EDH. Common locations for tSAH are basilar cisterns, the convexities, and the contre-coup Sylvian fissure. tSAH on unenhanced CT scan appears as curvilinear hyperdense areas that follow the cortical sulci. SAH is visible on CT for up to 1 week. tSAH of 1 to 2 mL, however, may only be picked up by MRI FLAIR, which is much more sensitive than conventional T2-weighted imaging for SAH. Patients with SAH are at risk for communicating hydrocephalus due to blocked arachnoid granulations (which absorb CSF).

Clinical Implications

tSAH is the most common CT abnormality in patients with moderate to severe TBI and is seen in 11% of TBI patients. Small-volume tSAH is inconsequential if confined to sulci of

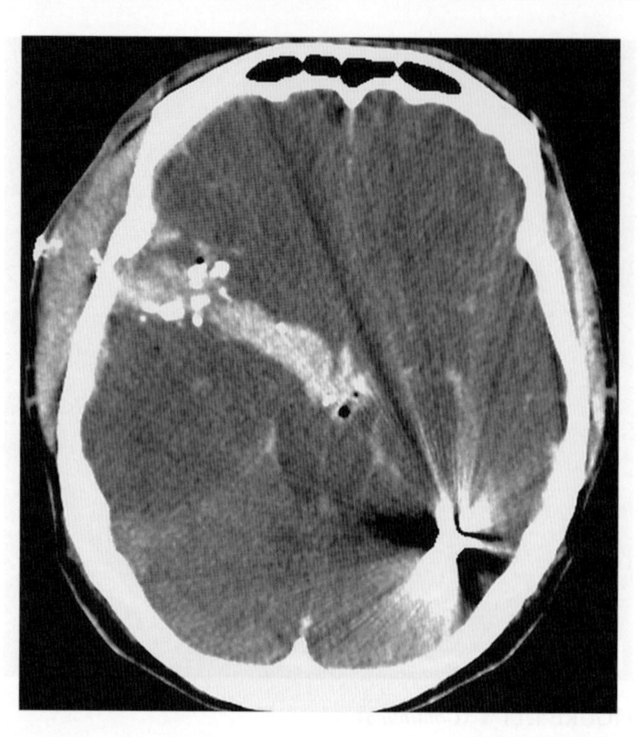

FIGURE 1.22 ■ Ballistic Injury with tSAH. NECT shows ballistic tract extending across right temporal lobe into basal ganglia. Metallic fragment seen in left posterior temporal lobe. SAH is present in the basilar cisterns, overlying the cerebellar tentorium, and scattered over the sulci. Ballistic injuries that cross the hemispheres have a worse prognosis.

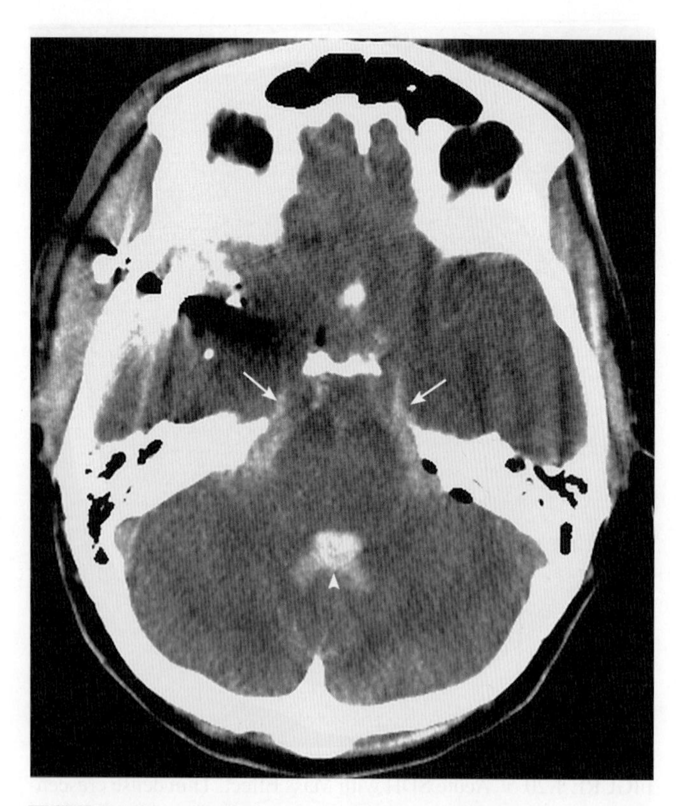

FIGURE 1.21 ■ Ballistic Injury with tSAH. NECT shows ballistic injury in right temporal lobe and bone. Dense blood (SAH) is present surrounding the basilar cisterns (arrows) as well as blood in the fourth ventricular cavity (arrowhead).

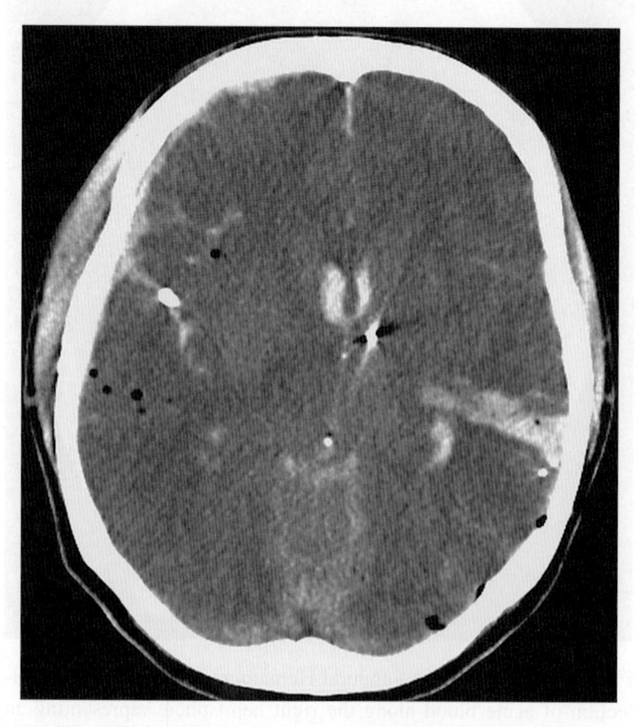

FIGURE 1.23 ■ tSAH with Intraventricular Blood. NECT shows SAH over the sulci, blood in the lateral and third ventricles, pneumocephalus, and ballistic injury.

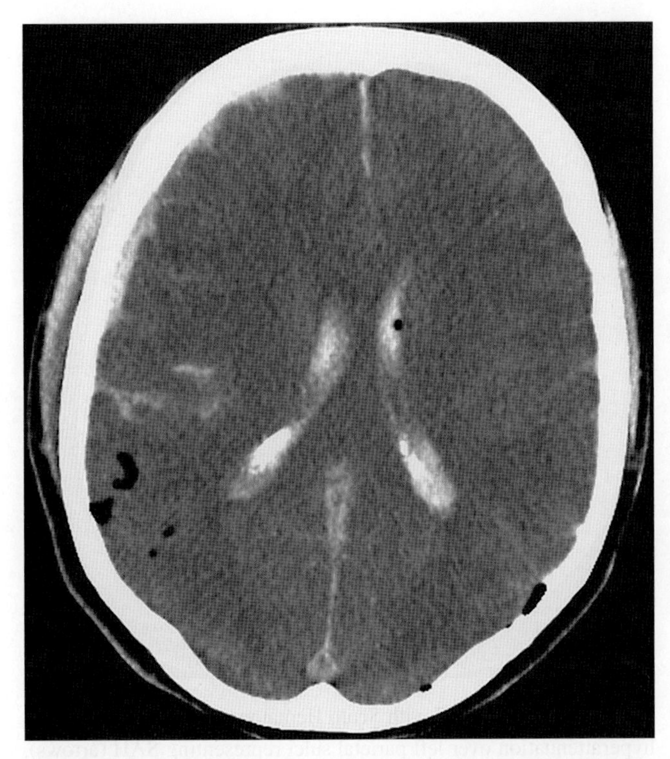

FIGURE 1.24 ▪ tSAH with Intraventricular Blood. NECT shows blood filling both lateral ventricles, pneumocephalus, and SAH within the sulci bilaterally.

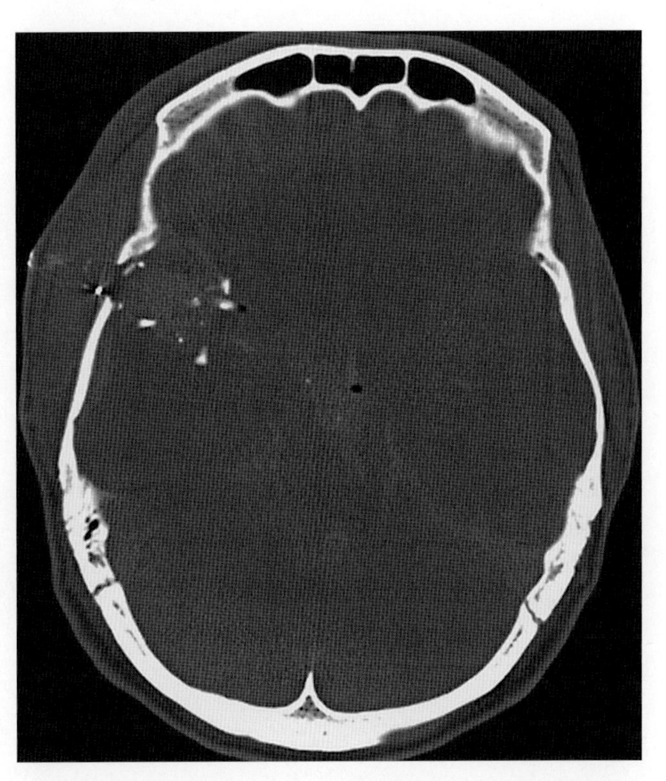

FIGURE 1.25 ▪ Ballistic Temporal Bone Fracture. Bone windows CT better shows the ballistic injury along right temporal bone with bony debris scattered along the entry site.

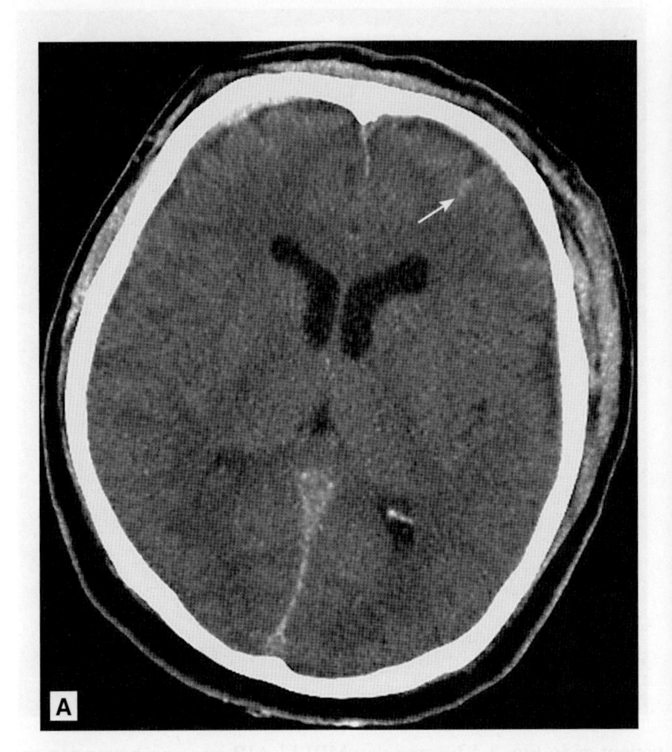

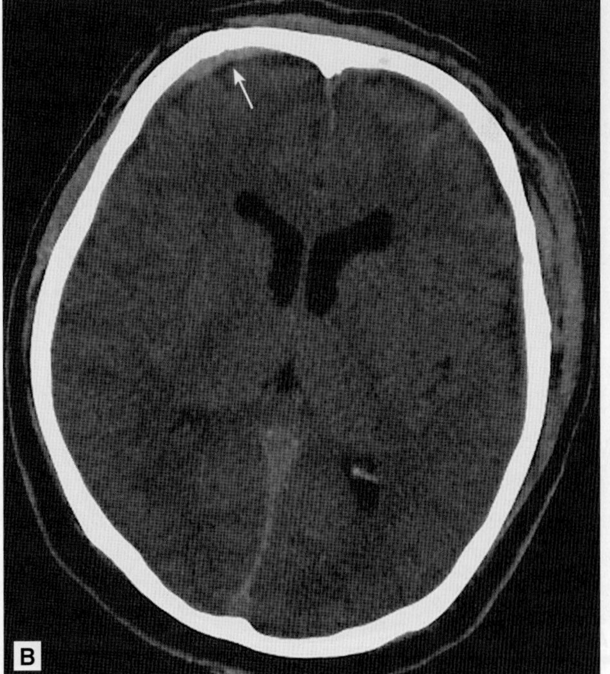

FIGURE 1.26 ▪ Traumatic Subarachnoid Hemorrhage. **A, B:** Faint hyperdensity over left frontal sulci represents SAH (arrow). Interesting to note is that these 2 images are exactly the same, except the second image is windowed differently with "subdural windows," which accentuates discovery of the small subdural hematoma along the right frontal bone (arrow).

the convexities. If the tSAH involves ventricular system, mortality and morbidity substantially increases.

Once identified, tSAH requires neurosurgical consultation for definitive management.

Pearls

1. tSAH can dissipate in 1 to 2 days due to high CSF turnover.
2. MRI FLAIR sequences suppress the T2 bright signal from CSF. Bright SAH will be contrasted against the darker surrounding cortex.
3. CT terminology describes acute clotted blood as hyperdense, high attenuation, or higher Hounsfield units. MRI terminology describes acute clotted blood as hyperintense or bright.

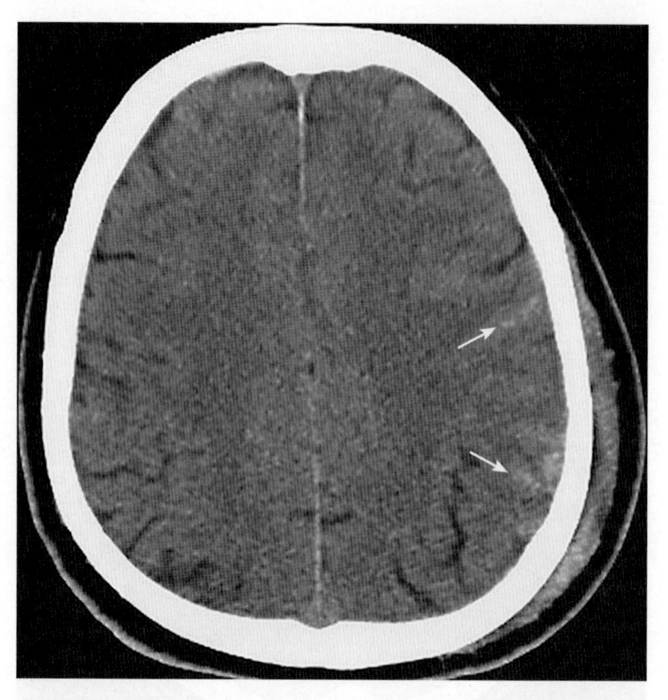

FIGURE 1.27 ■ tSAH with Scalp Hematoma. NECT shows subtle hyperattenuation over left parietal sulci representing SAH (arrows). Note overlying scalp hematoma.

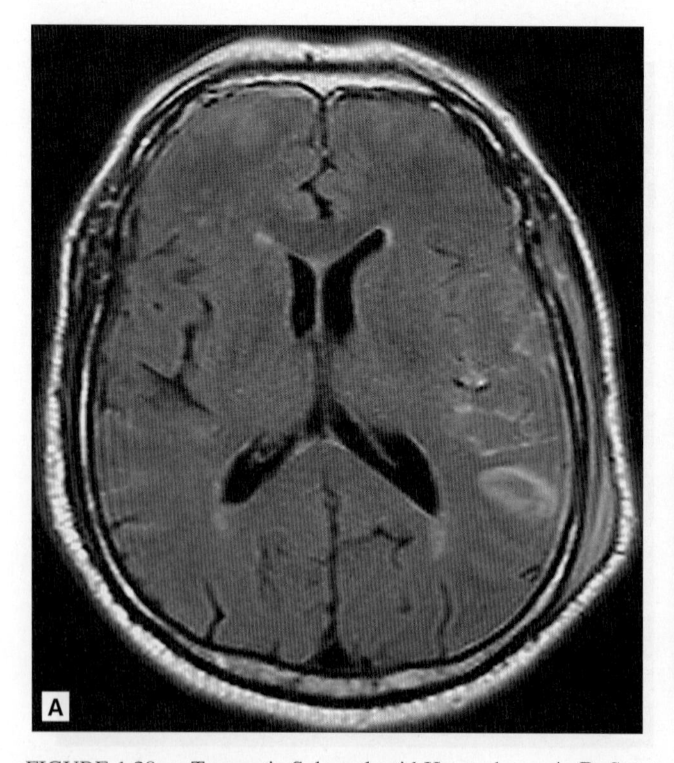

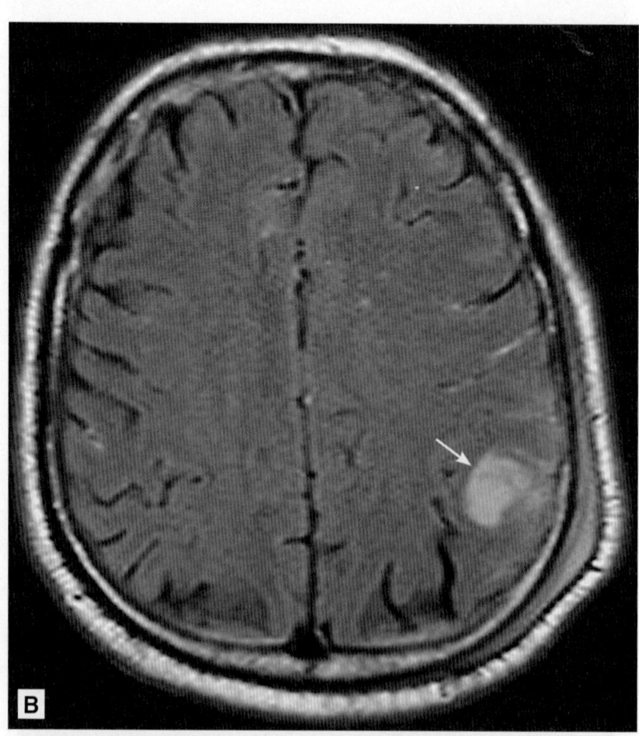

FIGURE 1.28 ■ Traumatic Subarachnoid Hemorrhage. **A, B:** Same patient as in Fig. 1.12: same-day MRI FLAIR imaging better demonstrates the SAH scattered over the left parietal lobe and a small parenchymal contusion (arrow). MRI (especially the FLAIR sequence) is much more sensitive than CT for SAH detection.

Radiographic Features

Increased cerebral volume results from increased cerebral blood volume (hyperemia) or increased tissue fluid (cerebral edema). Cerebral hyperemia is due to loss of cerebral autoregulation, and may progress to cerebral edema. Cerebral edema may be diffuse or focal. CT findings of diffuse cerebral edema include loss of gray-white attenuation and effacement of ventricles, sulci, or basilar cisterns.

Clinical Implications

Cerebral edema can occur from trauma, metabolic conditions such as DKA and hyponatremia, ischemic brain injury, tumors, rapid ascent to high altitudes, and intraparenchymal or extra-axial bleeding. Cerebral edema requires neurosurgical or neurological management of the underlying cause.

Cerebral edema may be vasogenic or cytotoxic. Vasogenic edema is primarily caused by increase in extracellular water from disruption of the blood–brain barrier, and is usually reversible. It primarily involves the white matter. Cytotoxic edema is due to cellular swelling with malfunction of ATP Na^+/K^+ pumps and classically seen with cerebral infarction. Cytotoxic edema is typically irreversible.

Pearls

1. Traumatic cerebral edema tends to be diffuse. Focal edema tends to occur around areas of ischemia or tumor.
2. MRI is more sensitive than CT in detecting small areas of focal edema.

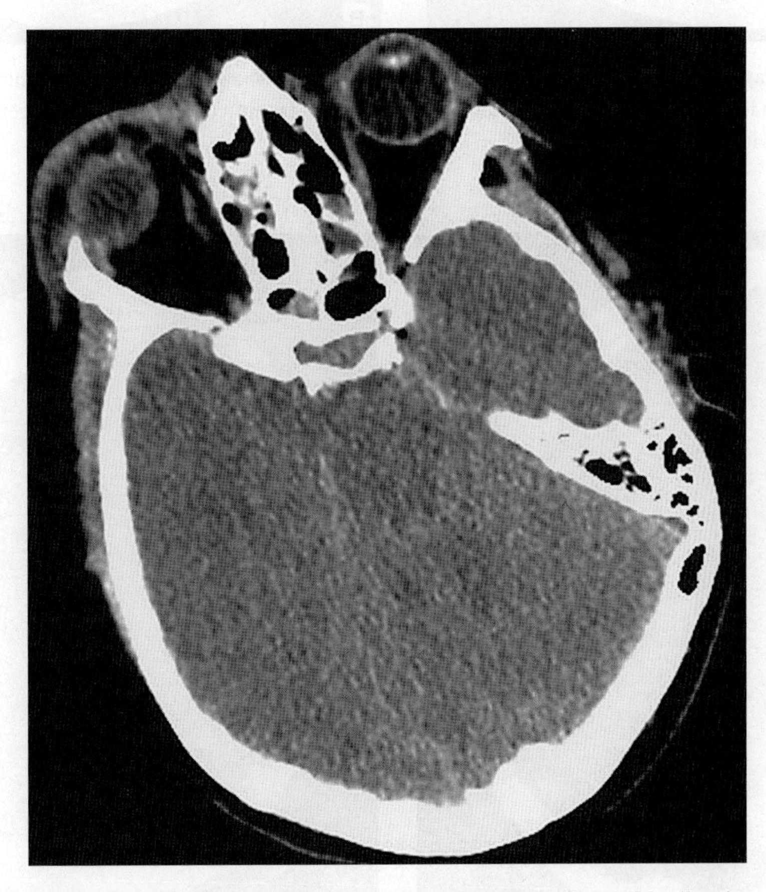

FIGURE 1.29 ■ Cerebral Edema with Uncal Herniation. NECT in trauma shows loss of normal basilar cisterns due to uncal/transtentorial herniation. Note diffuse loss of gray-white differentiation indicating diffuse edema. The cerebellum is slightly denser than cerebrum due to edema in cerebrum.

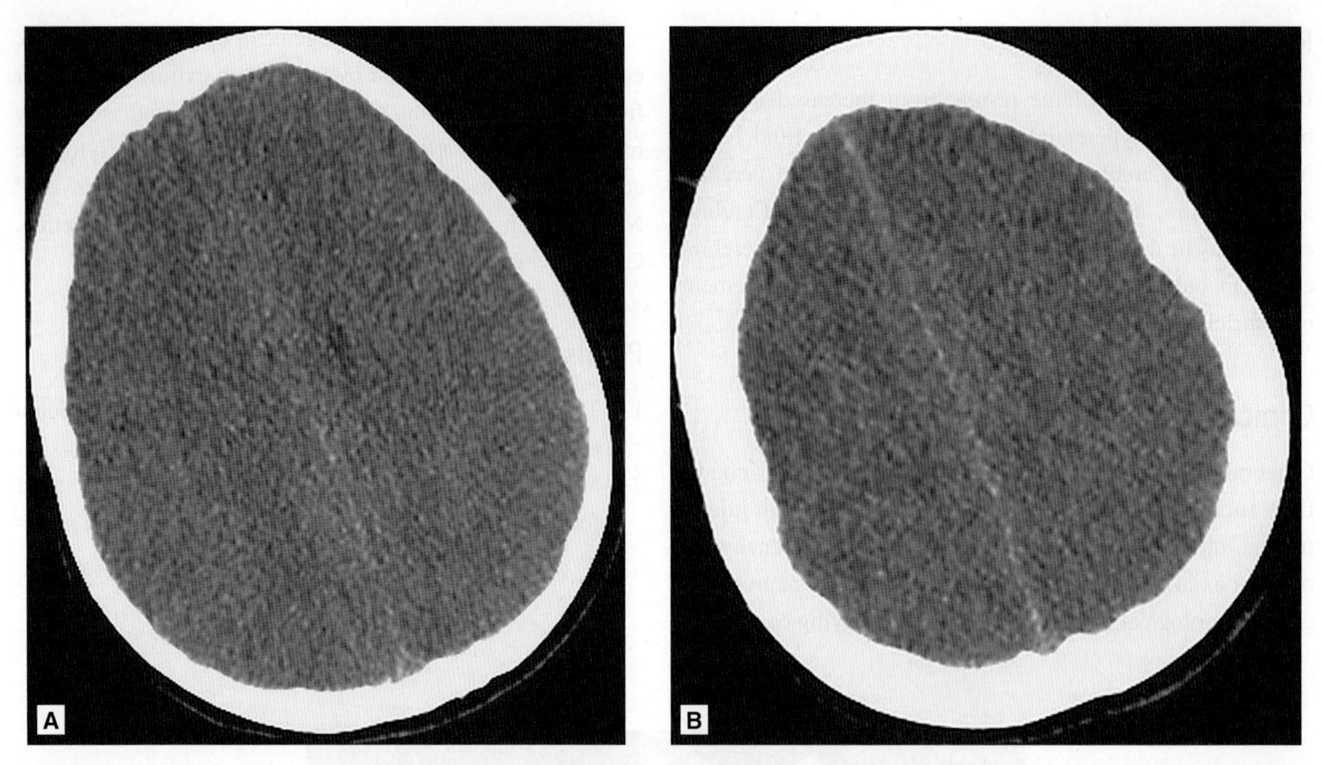

FIGURE 1.30 ■ Loss of Gray-White Differentiation. **A, B:** NECT at the vertex shows loss of the gray-white differentiation and diffuse cerebral edema. There is also loss of the normally seen sulci (although this can be difficult to detect in younger patients who have less CSF within their sulci compared with elderly patients).

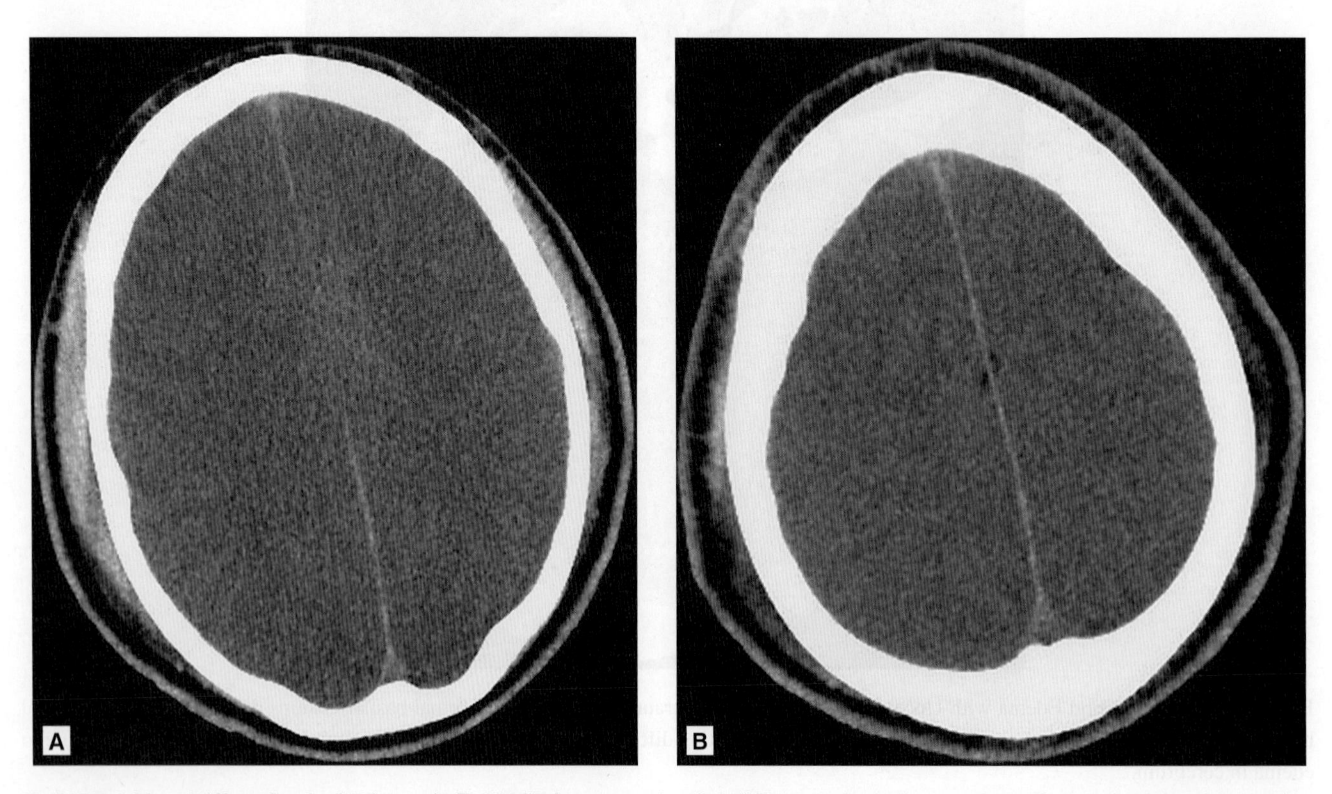

FIGURE 1.31 ■ Diffuse Cerebral Edema. **A, B:** NECT in trauma showing diffuse cerebral edema as loss of normal sulci and gray-white differentiation.

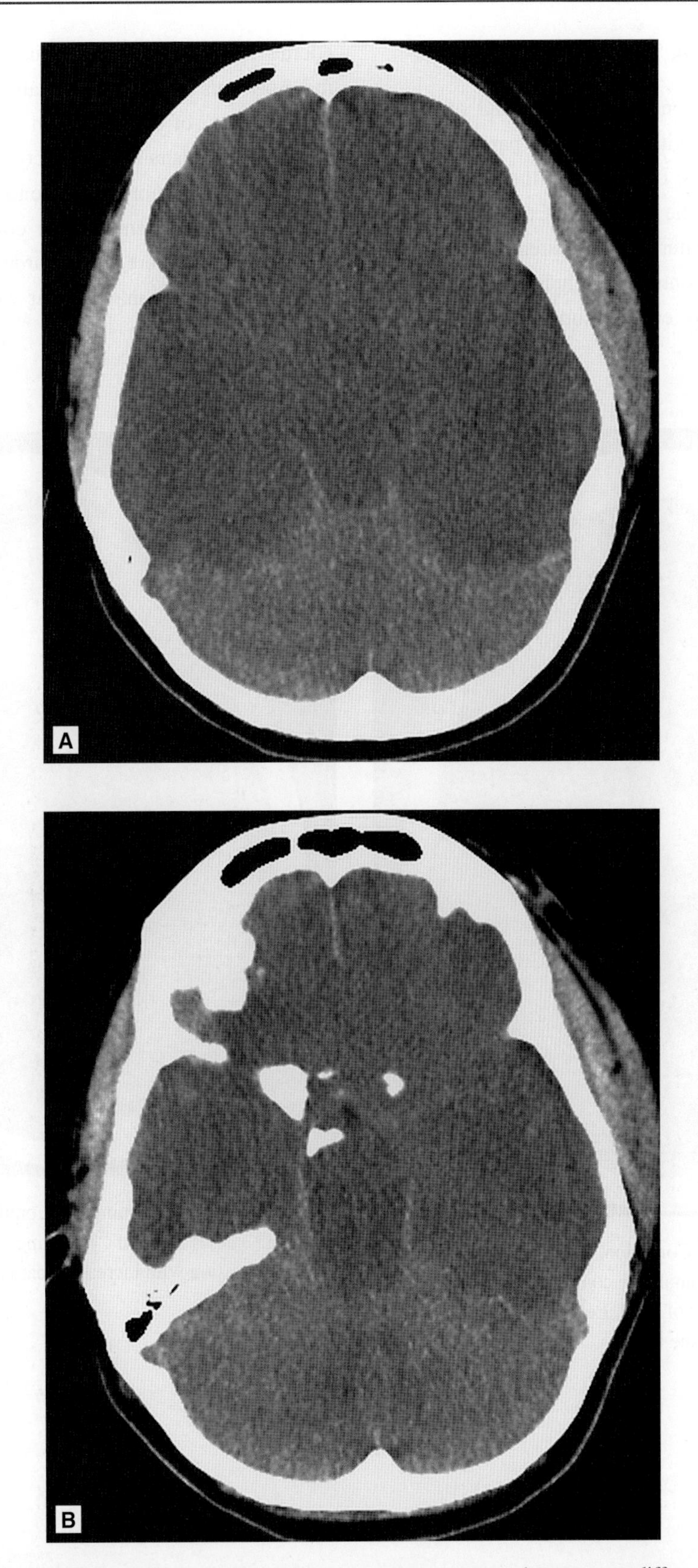

FIGURE 1.32 ■ White Cerebellum Sign. **A, B:** Axial CT without intravenous contrast demonstrates diffuse supratentorial cerebral edema with resulting hypodensity of parenchyma, loss of gray-white matter differentiation, and effacement of sulci and basilar cisterns. Cerebellum looks "whiter" because it is not as edematous as cerebrum. This is a very poor prognostic sign as it indicates severe brain edema.

Radiographic Features

Acute hemorrhagic contusion appears as round or irregularly shaped hyperdensity within the brain parenchyma on noncontrast CT (NCCT) and occurs when the brain impacts the irregular inner table of the calvarium. Contusions always involve the cortical gray matter and may extend into the white matter. Common areas of contusion include frontal and temporal lobes. As contusions evolve, surrounding vasogenic edema becomes more pronounced, making the contusion more obvious on CT. Additionally, there may occasionally be "blossoming" of contusions on follow-up imaging as further hemorrhage occurs inside the contusion.

MRI is much more sensitive than CT to detect acute hemorrhagic and nonhemorrhagic contusions, especially along the convexity, where beam-hardening artifact limits CT. A chronic contusion may appear as a wedge-shaped area of enchephalomalacia.

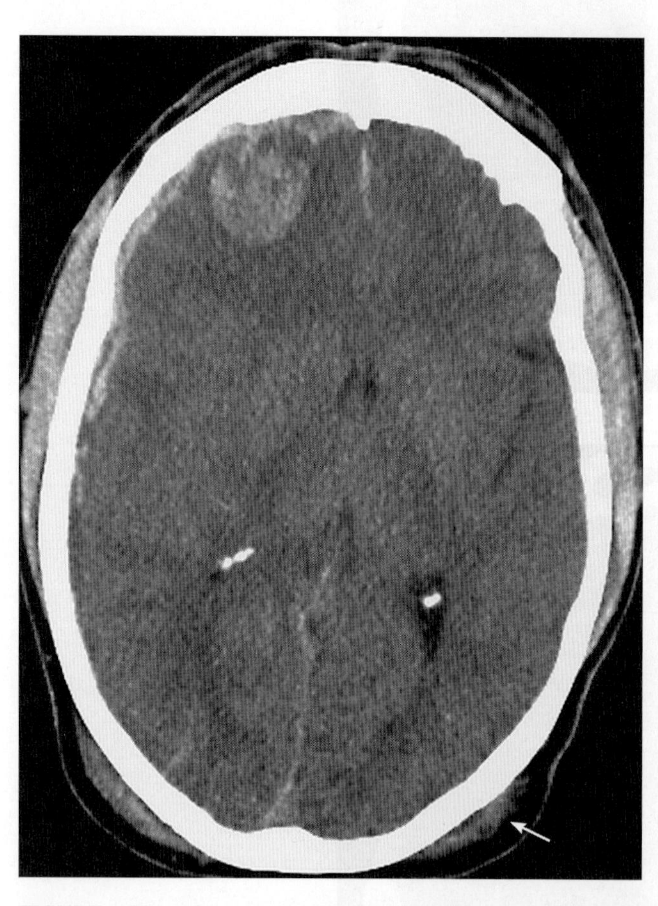

FIGURE 1.33 ■ Contrecoup Contusion. NECT following trauma shows a round-shaped right frontal lobe contrecoup contusion, overlying SDH, and a small amount of SAH. Left posterior parietal scalp swelling indicates the "coup" site (arrow).

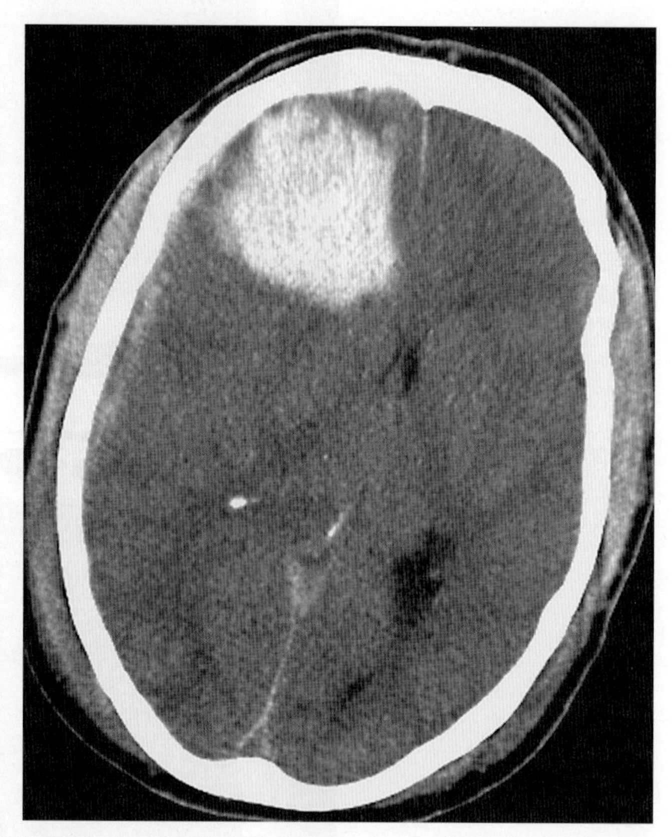

FIGURE 1.34 ■ Blooming of Contusion. NECT 24 hours after Fig. 1.33 shows marked "blooming" or enlargement of the right frontal contusion with increased mass effect and edema.

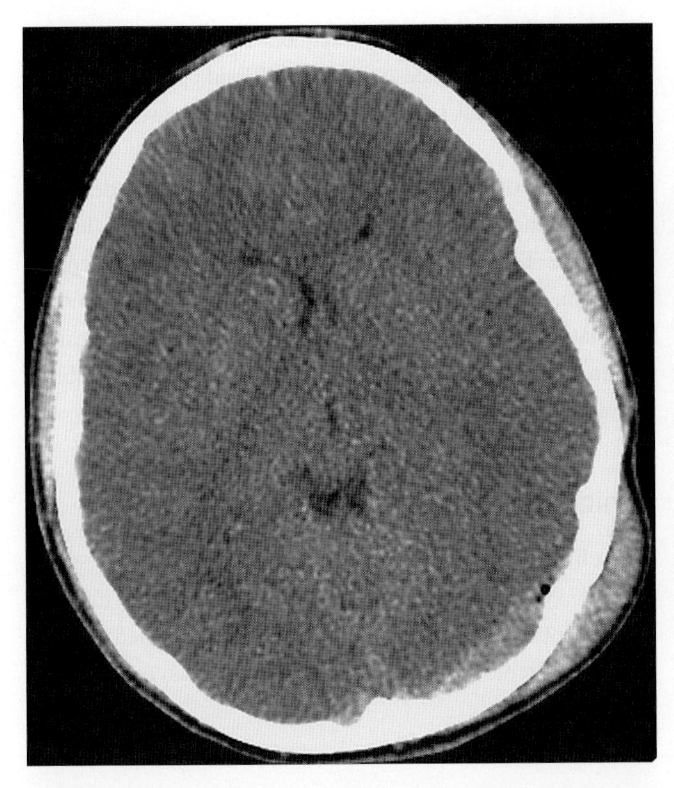

FIGURE 1.35 ■ Coup Lesion. NECT shows left parietal scalp swelling and underlying intracranial subdural hematoma and pneumocephalus (indicating fracture). This is the "coup" site.

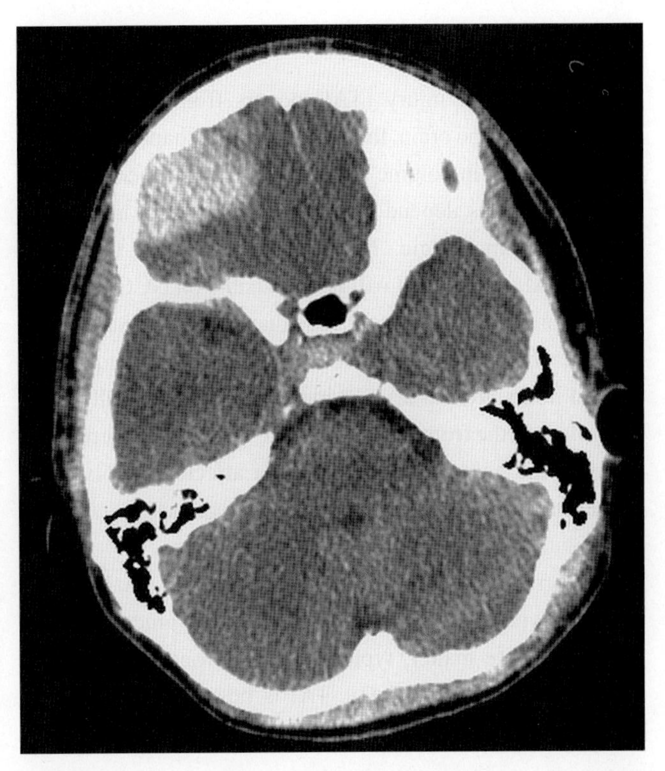

FIGURE 1.36 ■ Contrecoup Contusion. NECT shows a "contrecoup" contusion along the inferior right frontal lobe. This is a common location for traumatic contusions due to the irregular surface of the skull base.

Clinical Implications

All patients with hemorrhagic contusion require neurosurgical consultation. Hemorrhagic contusions in the temporal lobe are of particular concern because of the potential for uncal herniation if the contusion blossoms. Thus, patients with temporal lobe contusions are usually admitted.

Pearls

1. Hemorrhagic contusions occur in up to 43% of moderate and severe head injury patients.
2. Contusions may be coup or contrecoup injuries, and may underlie depressed skull fractures.

Radiographic Features

Traumatic axonal injury (TAI) occurs from a shear-strain deformation of the brain, that is, a change in shape of the brain without change in volume that causes severe injury to axons. Imaging features depend on whether the TAI is nonhemorrhagic or hemorrhagic. Nonhemorrhagic shear comprises 80% of TAI injuries and will not be visible on NCCT. MRI is much more sensitive to nonhemorrhagic TAI, which will be visible in the acute phase on both FLAIR and DWI sequences. Several hours after injury, T2 hyperintensity is usually seen, most often in the frontal/parietal white matter. The corpus callosum is the next most common area affected. Involvement of the brainstem and cerebellar hemispheres suggests severe injury.

Hemorrhagic TAI may on NCCT appear as small collections of hyperdense fluid collections at the junction of the gray and white matter, typically in the frontal or temporal lobes. However, hemorrhagic TAI is best seen on susceptibility-weighted MR sequences, which are sensitive to blood breakdown products. These sequences include GRE/SWI/T2* (pronounced "tee-two-star"). Blood products create a "dropout" signal (dark black signal) in the areas of acute hemorrhage.

Location of the TAI determines the grade. Grade I TAI occurs at the gray-white matter junction. Grade II lesions (moderate TAI) involve lobar white matter and the corpus callosum, which is susceptible to shear due to its immobility relative to adjacent brain parenchyma. Grade III lesions (severe TAI) additionally involve the dorsolateral midbrain and upper pons.

Clinical Implications

The clinical manifestations of TAI range from postconcussive syndrome (headaches, light-headedness, inability to concentrate) to coma. MRI should be obtained in head trauma patients where CT is normal but symptoms are persistent.

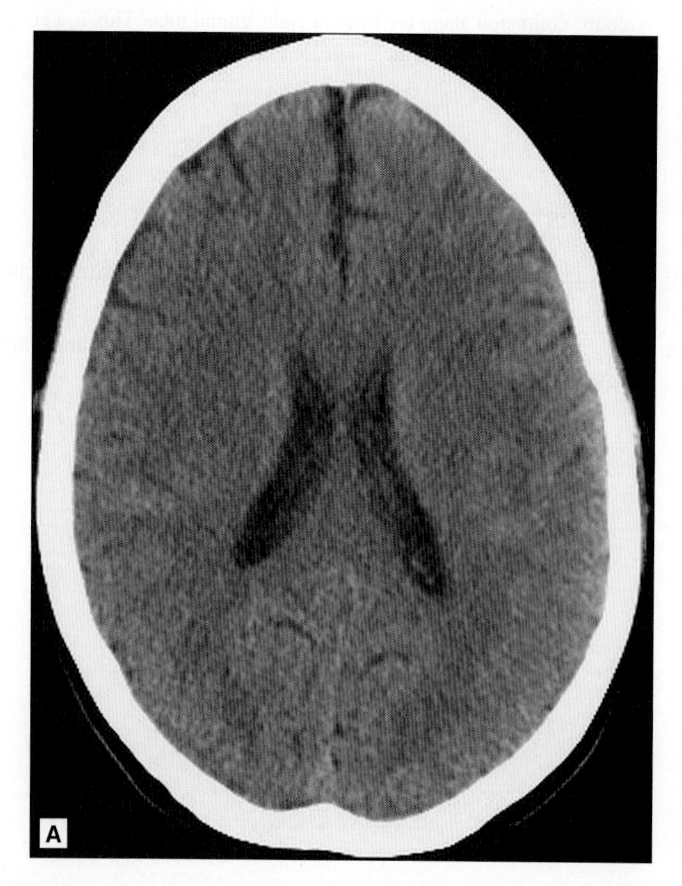

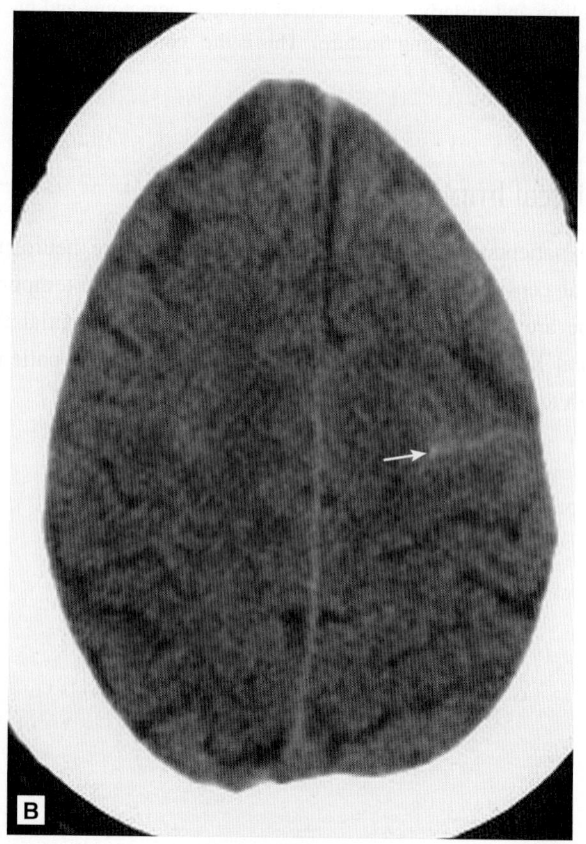

FIGURE 1.37 ■ tSAH. **A, B:** NECT following car accident is nearly normal, with subtle SAH in the posterior left frontal lobe (arrow). The exam did not fit the CT findings, so an MRI was ordered.

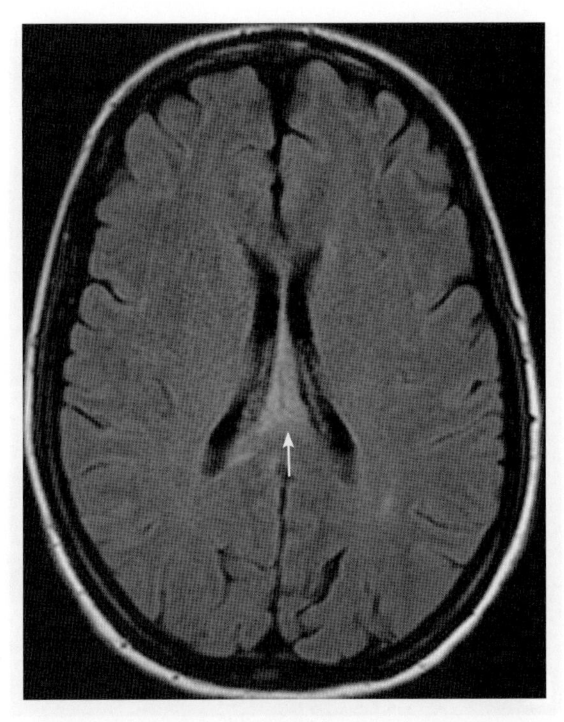

FIGURE 1.38 ■ Hemorrhagic TAI. FLAIR MR image shows abnormal intensity in the body and splenium of the corpus callosum (arrow). The corpus callosum white matter is densely packed, and in the traumatic setting, this injury strongly suggests axonal injury.

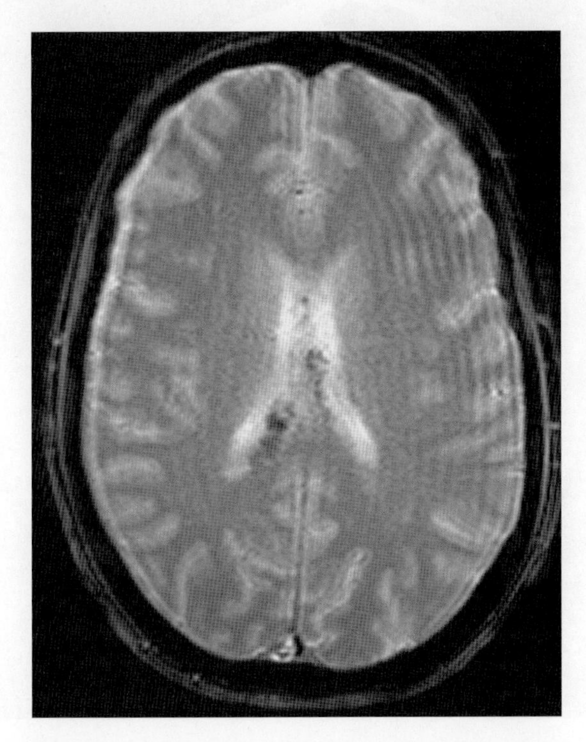

FIGURE 1.39 ■ Hemorrhagic TAI. T2*/GRE MR image shows hemorrhagic foci (dark signal) in the corpus callosum. This is the best sequence to detect hemorrhage due to the dark signal artifact caused by blood products.

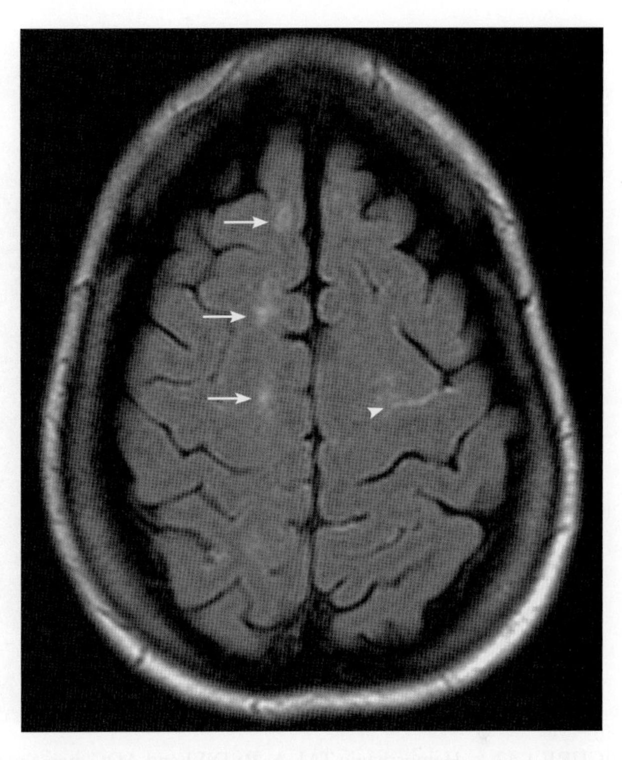

FIGURE 1.40 ■ Hemorrhagic TAI. FLAIR MR image near the vertex shows several foci of white matter hyperintensity in the right frontal lobe (arrows) representing lobar axonal injury in this clinical setting. Note small amount of bright SAH near the left frontal precentral gyrus (arrowhead) (corresponding to CT in Fig. 1.37).

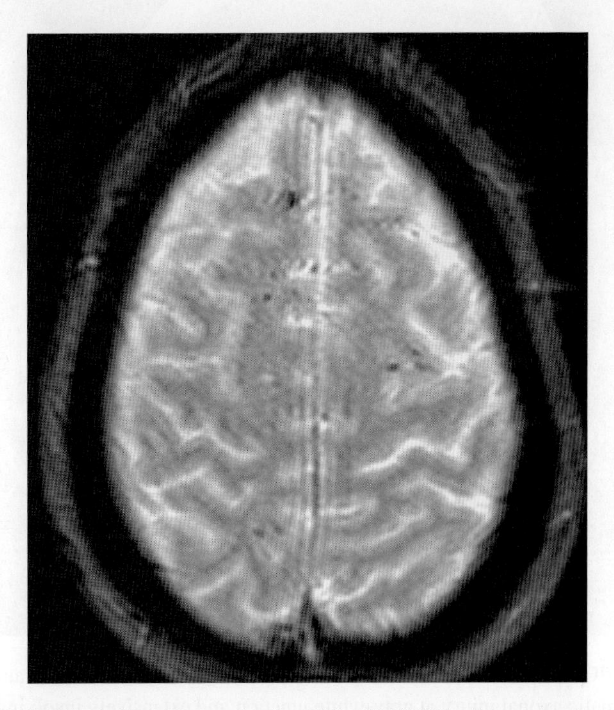

FIGURE 1.41 ■ Hemorrhagic TAI. T2*/GRE shows scattered hemorrhagic foci in the bilateral hemispheres (not appreciated on other sequences).

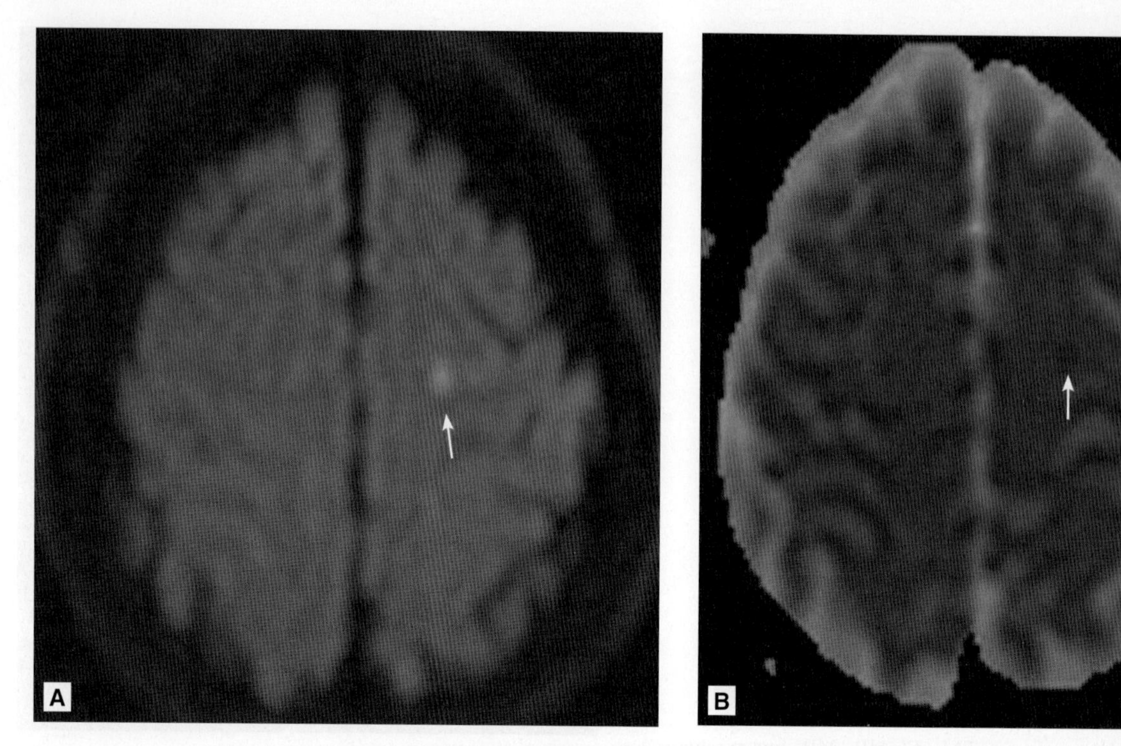

FIGURE 1.42 ■ Hemorrhagic TAI. **A, B:** DWI and ADC map show a small focus of restricted diffusion (infarct) in the high left fontal lobe (arrows). Axonal injury can occasionally demonstrate this finding.

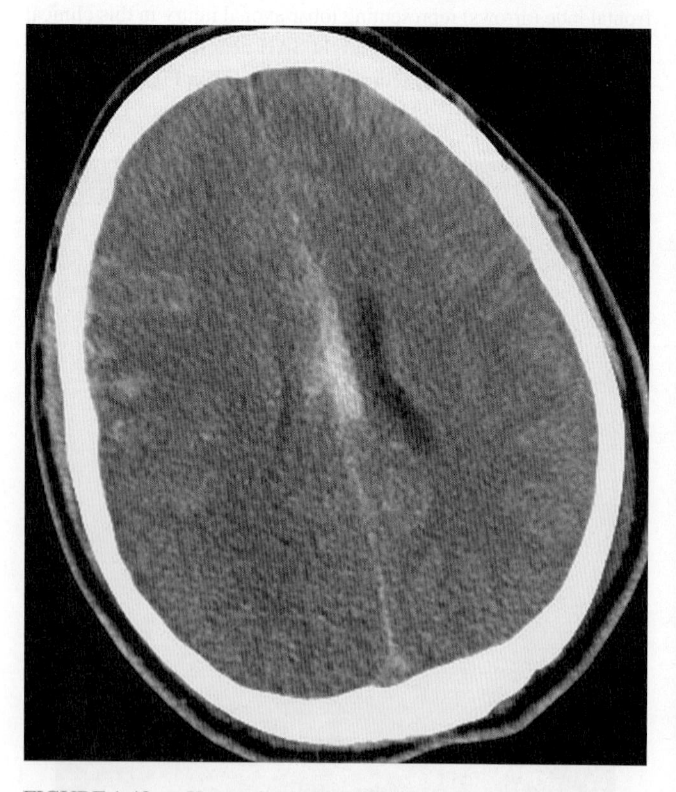

FIGURE 1.43 ■ Hemorrhagic TAI. NECT shows hemorrhagic traumatic axonal injury at gray-white junction and extensively involving the corpus callosum.

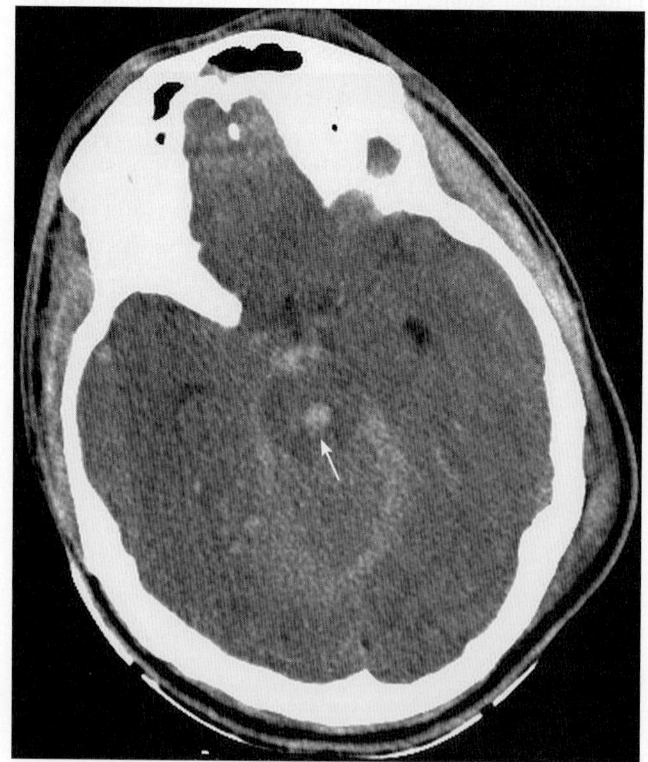

FIGURE 1.44 ■ Hemorrhagic TAI of the Pons. NECT shows punctate focus of blood in the dorsal pons of the brainstem (arrow). SAH is present in the basilar cisterns. Punctate hemorrhagic foci are seen in the temporal lobes.

TABLE 1.3 ■ MRI SEQUENCE UTILITY

Sequence	Utility
T1	Anatomy CSF is dark Subacute blood is bright (due to methemoglobin)
T2	CSF is bright Subacute blood is bright Pathology is bright
FLuid Attenuation Inversion Recovery (FLAIR)	CSF is dark Pathology is bright Much better than conventional T2 for cortical contusions, SAH, and nonhemorrhagic TAI
Diffusion-weighted imaging (DWI)	Sensitive for TAI and infarct
T2*/GRE/SWI (GRadient Echo) susceptibility-weighted imaging	Identification of acute or chronic blood breakdown products, particularly hemorrhagic TAI
T1 postcontrast	Conditions that breach BBB such as tumor, subacute infarctions, abscess, and cerebritis

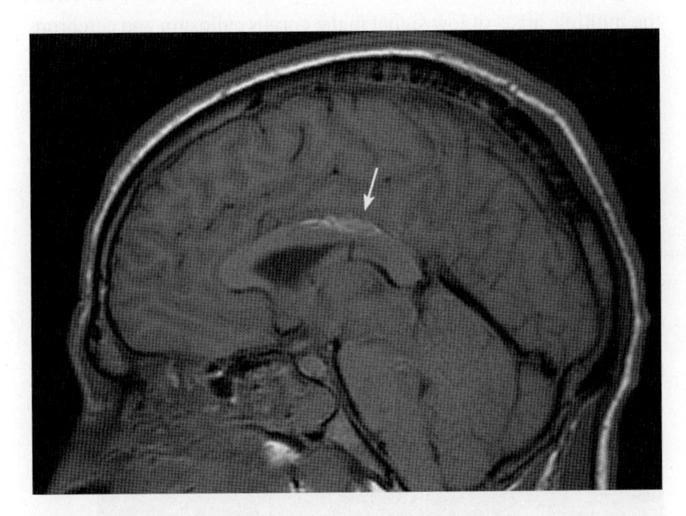

FIGURE 1.45 ■ Hemorrhagic TAI of the Pons. Same patient as in Figs. 1.43 and 1.44 but MRI 3 days later. Sagittal T1 MRI shows bright signal along the superior aspect of the corpus callosum (arrow) representing subacute blood. This is a common site of injury in TAI.

Pearls

1. The "shear injury triad" includes the lobar gray-white junction, corpus callosum, and the dorsolateral midbrain. These are the most common locations of TAI.
2. FLAIR, GRE/T2*/SWI, and DWI are the most useful MRI sequences in the evaluation of TAI. See Table 1.3 for the utility of the MRI sequences.
3. Eighty percent of TAIs are nonhemorrhagic and not visible on CT.
4. Susceptibility-weighted imaging sequences are extremely sensitive for the identification of microhemorrhagic TAI.
5. Older names for TAI include shear injury and diffuse axonal injury (DAI).

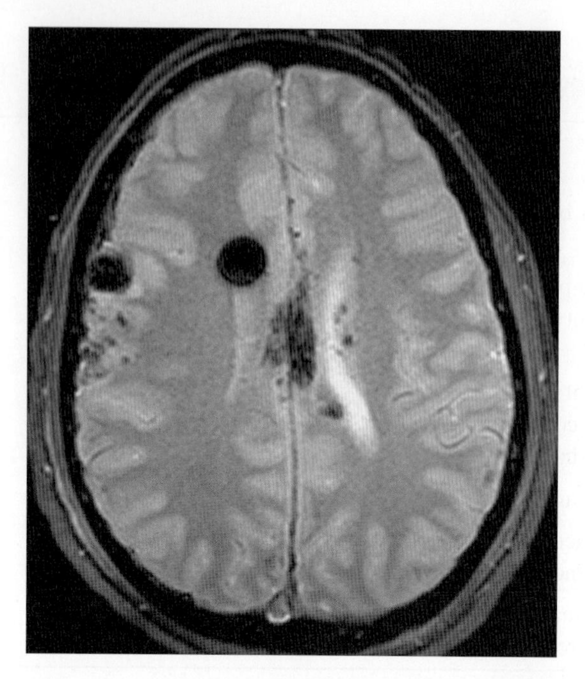

FIGURE 1.46 ■ Hemorrhagic TAI on T2*/GRE. T2*/GRE shows low signal along the corpus callosum and right convexity indicating hemorrhagic foci and/or contusions. This is the best conventional MR sequence for detecting prior blood products. The large round black signal void in the right frontal lobe is an artifact related to extraventricular drain placed between the CT and MRI exams.

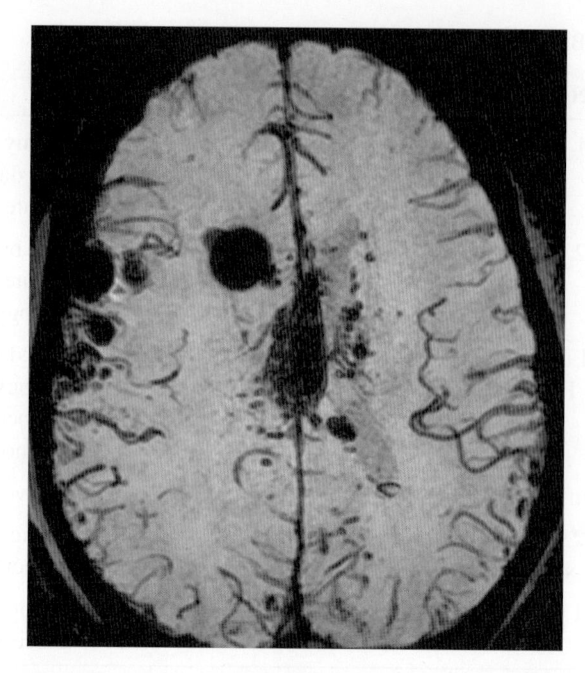

FIGURE 1.47 ■ Hemorrhagic TAI on SWI. Susceptibility-weighted image (SWI) at the same level as in Fig. 1.46 shows to better effect the multiple areas of low signal in the corpus callosum and cerebrum of hemorrhagic TAI. SWI is 3 to 6 times more sensitive to blood products than conventional T2*/GRE and is included in all trauma MRI exams at our institution. The serpiginous dark structures are the cerebral vessels (the deoxyhemoglobin contributes to the low signal).

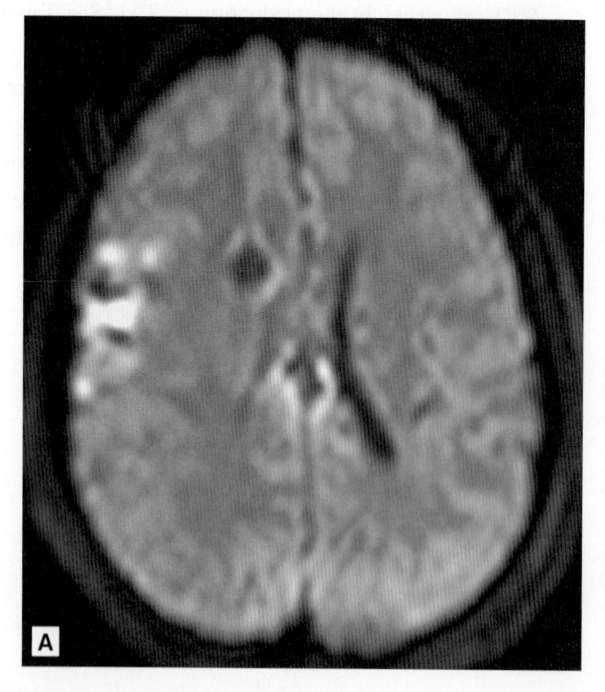

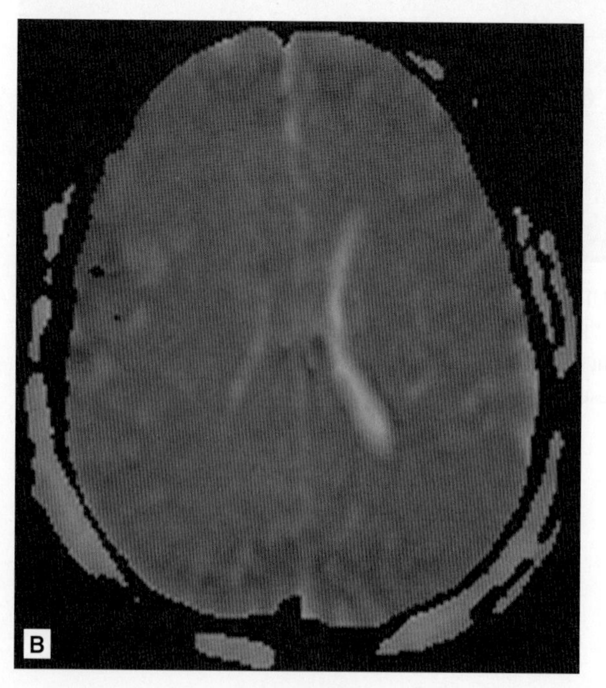

FIGURE 1.48 ■ Hemorrhagic TAI on DWI/ADC. **A, B:** DWI and ADC map show areas of restricted diffusion at the sites of TAI. This can be seen with TAI as well as at sites of contusion. Differentiating this from ischemic infarcts is normally straightforward based on the clinical history.

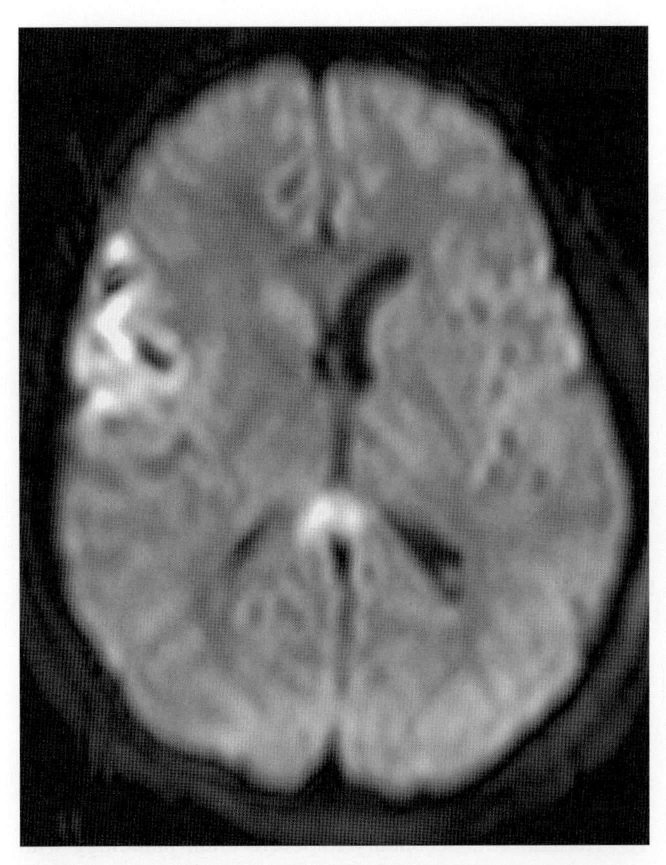

FIGURE 1.49 ■ Hemorrhagic TAI on DWI. DWI at slightly lower level better shows the restricted diffusion in the splenium of the corpus callosum as well as along the site of right frontal lobe contusion.

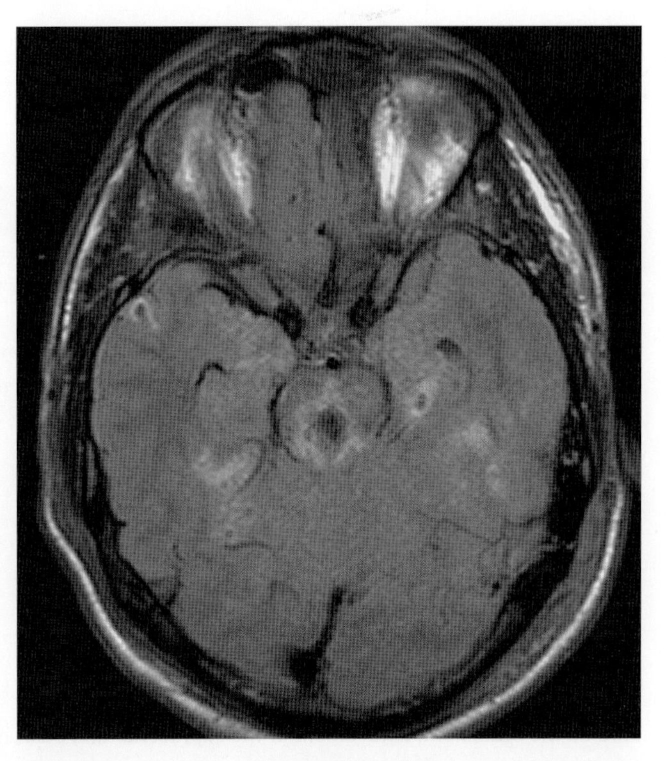

FIGURE 1.50 ■ Pontine TAI. FLAIR at the level of the pons shows abnormal high signal in the brainstem consistent with edema, as well as round area of low signal that represents pontine hemorrhage related to TAI. TAI that involves the brainstem carries the worst prognosis.

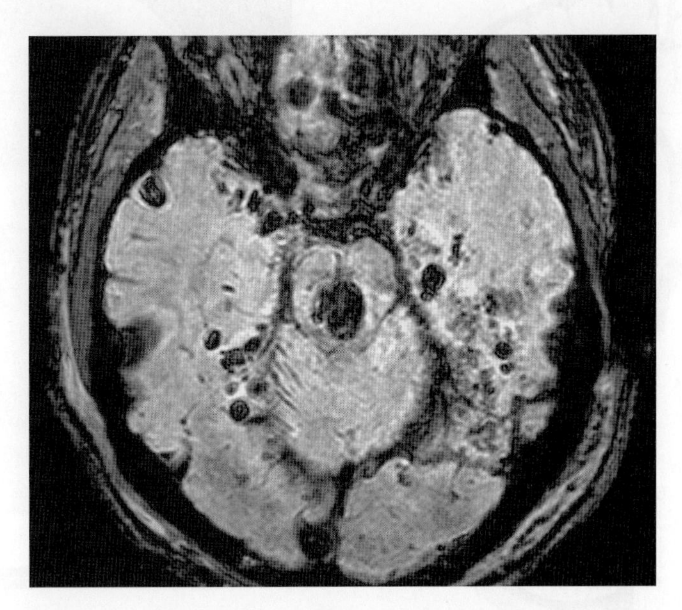

FIGURE 1.51 ■ Pontine TAI. SWI sequence at the same level exploits the susceptibility effect caused by blood to showcase the multiple areas of hemorrhagic TAI and contusion, the largest involving the pons.

Radiographic Features

Six distinct herniation syndromes have been described and findings on NCCT scan may be subtle. *Subfalcine herniation* occurs when the cingulate gyrus of the frontal lobe is displaced underneath the falx. Hemispheric edema with falcine shift from midline suggests subfalcine herniation. Branches of the anterior cerebral arteries may be compressed, causing ischemia or infarction of the ACA territories in the frontal lobes.

Uncal herniation occurs when the medial portion of the temporal lobe is displaced inferiorly through the tentorium. Effacement or asymmetry of the suprasellar cistern is a frequent finding. The posterior cerebral artery and cranial nerve III may be compressed between the herniating brain and tentorium. PCA territory infarcts may occur. Patients with CN III compression present with the characteristic "blown pupil" of herniation.

Central or downward herniation is caused by mass effect of the supratentorial compartment placing downward pressure on the brainstem. Effacement of the supracellar and basilar cisterns occurs. Progression of this syndrome can cause brainstem infarction.

When mass effect occurs in the posterior fossa, portions of the cerebellum may decompress through the foramen magnum or through the superior cerebellar cisterns. In *cerebellar tonsillar herniation*, the cerebellar tonsils herniated through the foramen magnum. Tonsillar herniation may compress the posterior inferior cerebellar artery (PICA). In *upward herniation*, quadrigeminal and superior cerebellar cisterns are effaced by cerebellar tissue.

External herniation occurs when severe edema of the cerebral hemispheres causes external protrusion of the brain. This may occur with a large overlying skull fracture or following craniectomy.

Clinical Implications

Brain herniation is a form of delayed or secondary head injury. Clinical manifestations may include depressed levels of consciousness, decorticate or decerebrate posturing, seizures, or unequal pupils. Clinical or CT evidence of brain herniation should prompt the clinician to consider treatment aimed at reducing intracranial pressure.

Pearl

1. Herniation is secondary to severe brain pathology with increased intracranial pressure.

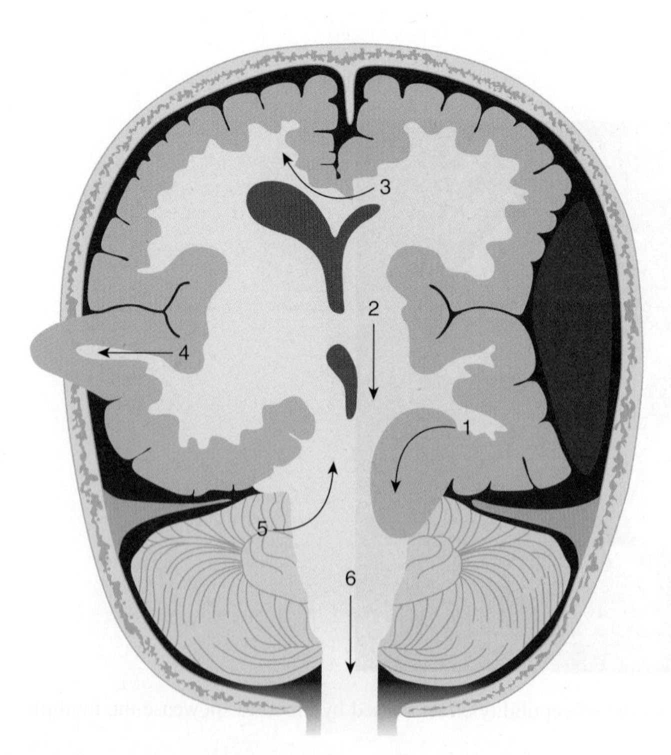

FIGURE 1.52 ■ Herniation Syndromes. (1) Uncal; (2) central transtentorial; (3) subfalcine; (4) external; (5) upward; (6) tonsillar.

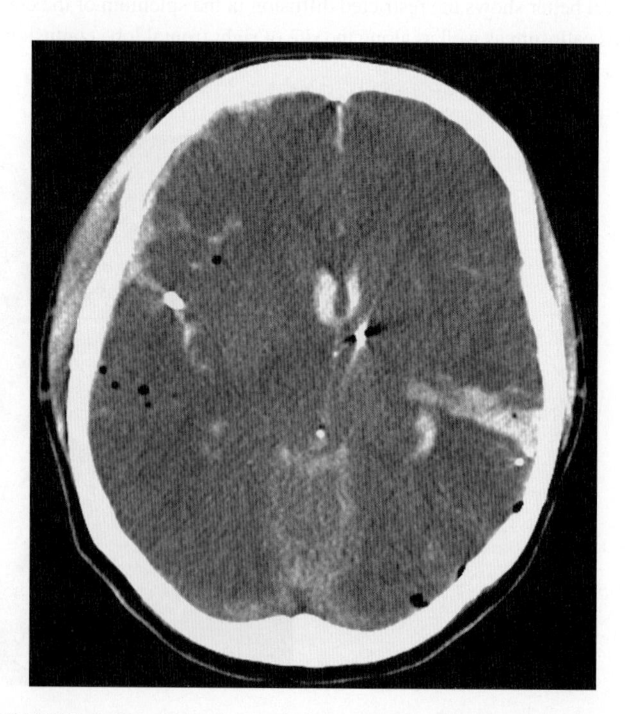

FIGURE 1.53 ■ Uncal Herniation. Ballistic injury to the brain demonstrates a right *uncal herniation* (medial temporal lobe compressed against the midbrain). Other findings include SAH, SDH, IPH, and pneumocephalus.

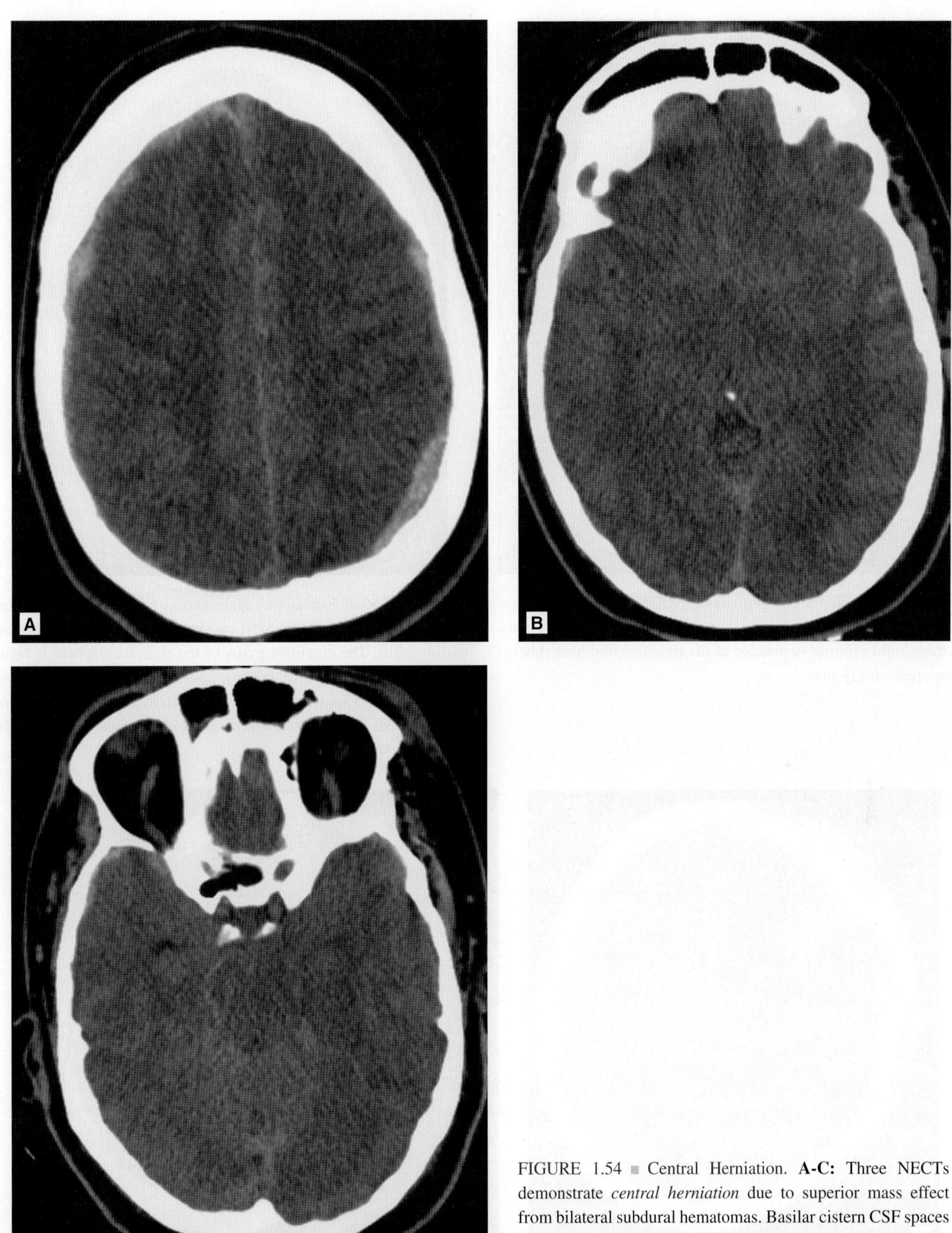

FIGURE 1.54 ■ Central Herniation. **A-C:** Three NECTs demonstrate *central herniation* due to superior mass effect from bilateral subdural hematomas. Basilar cistern CSF spaces have been obliterated. This is a hard diagnosis to make on CT imaging.

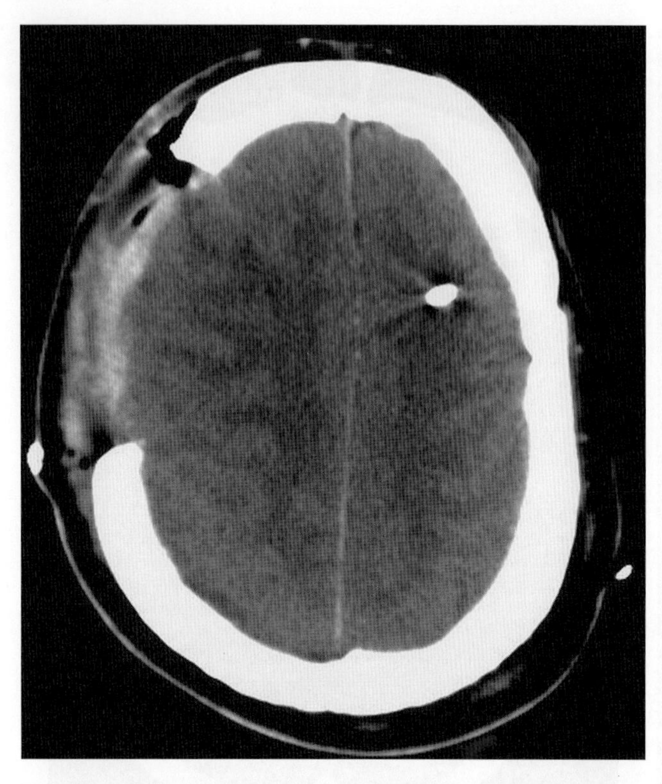

FIGURE 1.55 ■ External Herniation. NECT following craniectomy due to increased intracranial pressure following trauma demonstrates mild *external herniation* of the right cerebral hemispheres at the craniectomy site.

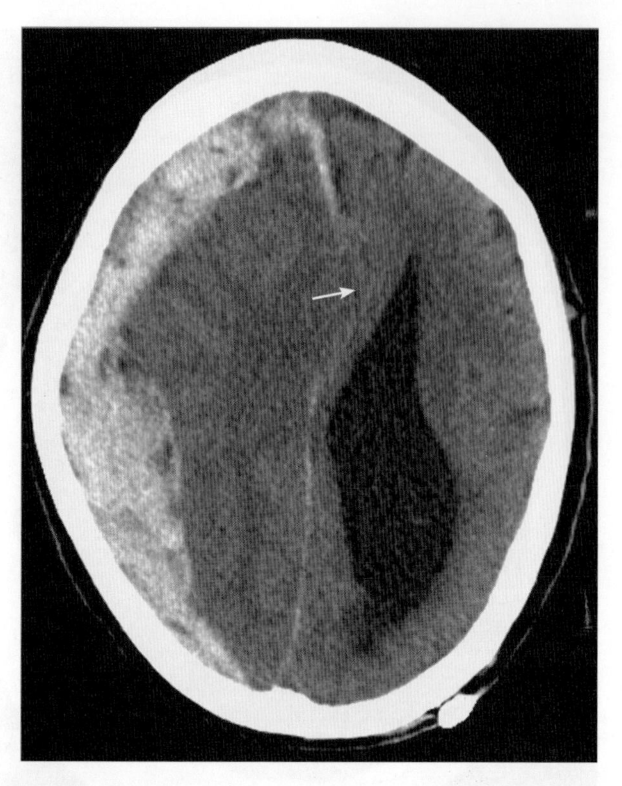

FIGURE 1.56 ■ Subfalcine Herniation. NECT shows a large hyperdense right convexity SDH causing significant mass effect and midline shift. The cingulate gyrus of the right hemisphere is being displaced beneath the falx cerebri, constituting a *subfalcine herniation* (arrow). This type of herniation places the anterior cerebral artery at risk for injury as it runs along the medial surface of the cingulate gyrus.

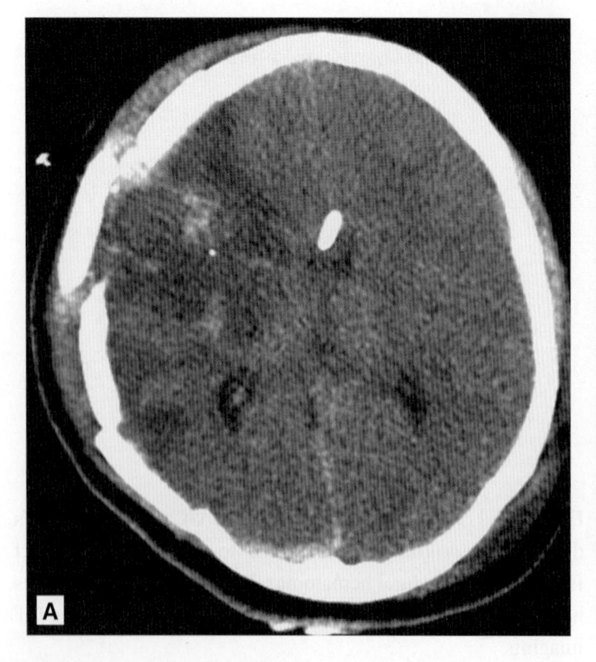

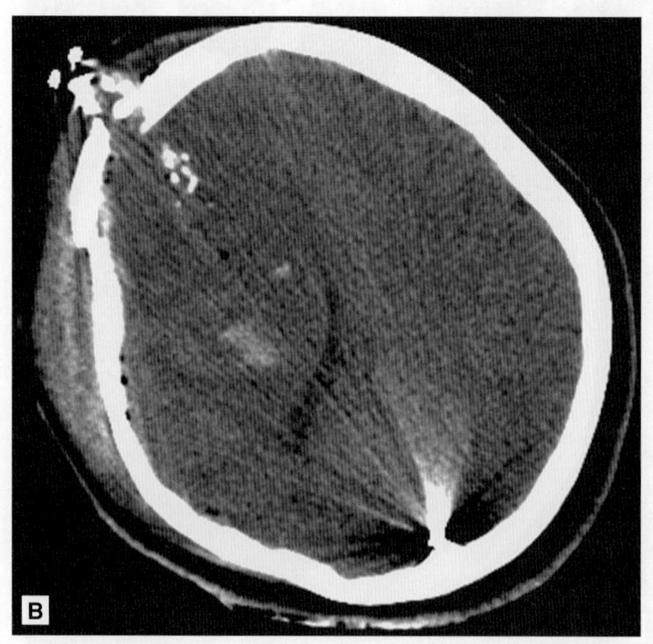

FIGURE 1.57 ■ External Herniation. **A, B:** NECTs demonstrate mild right frontal *external herniation* following ballistic injury. There is also suggestion of subfalcine herniation.

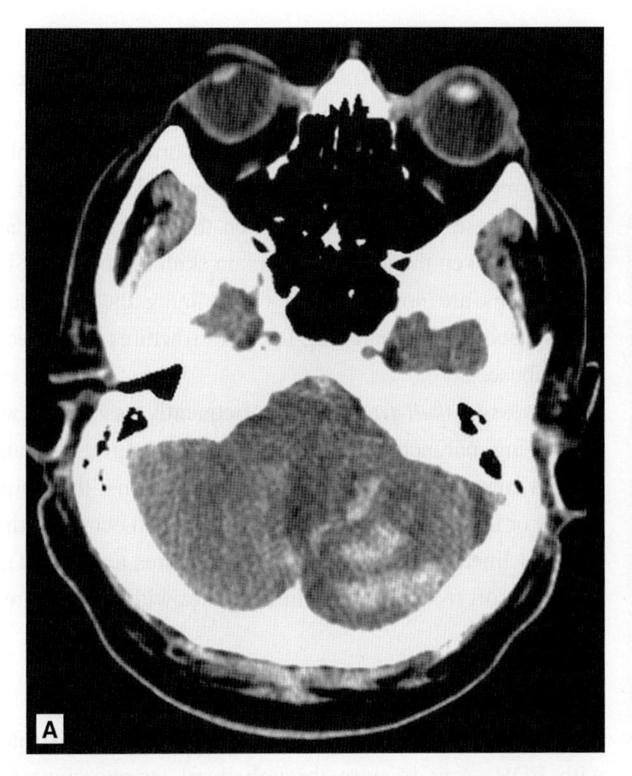

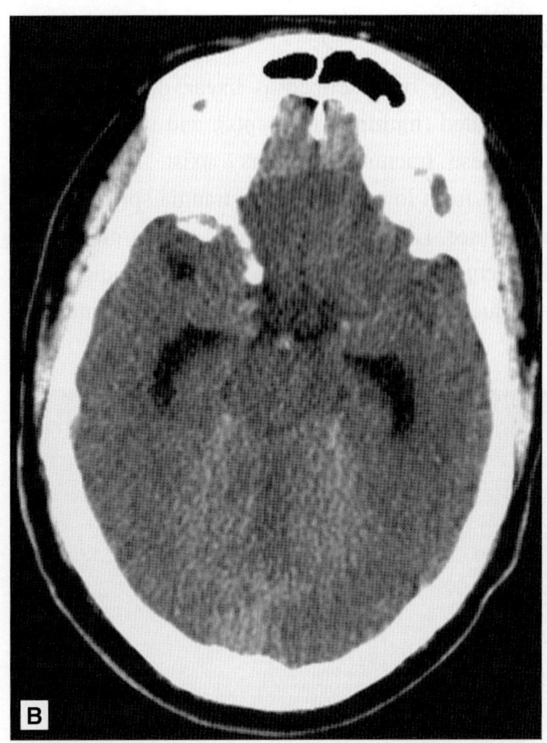

FIGURE 1.58 ■ Upward Herniation. **A, B:** NECTs demonstrate intraparenchymal hemorrhage in the posterior fossa obliterating the fourth ventricle and causing hydrocephalus (note dilation of the temporal horns). There is *upward herniation* of the cerebellum through the incisura of the tentorium cerebelli.

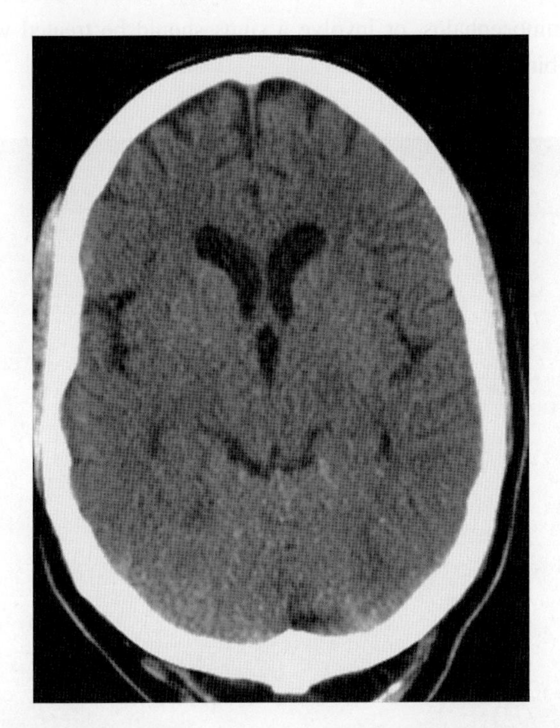

FIGURE 1.59 ■ Resolved Upward Herniation. NECT of the same patient as in Fig. 1.58 demonstrates return to normal basilar cisterns (quadrigeminal) surrounding the midbrain and resolution of the hydrocephalus.

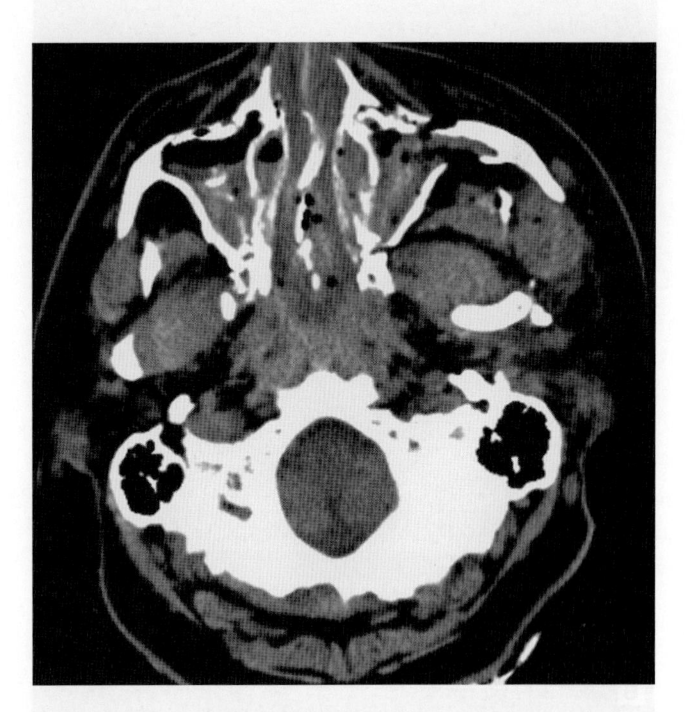

FIGURE 1.60 ■ Tonsillar Herniation. NECT at the level of the foramen magnum demonstrates downward herniation of the cerebellar tonsils, representing *tonsillar herniation*. Also note extensive facial fractures related to patient's traumatic event.

Radiographic Summary

Skull fractures may be described as linear, depressed, diastatic, comminuted (multiple fragments), and open. A combination of these fracture types may exist. *Linear skull fractures* result from low-energy blunt trauma spread over a wide skull surface. Linear skull fractures are the most common skull fracture. They appear on CT or plain radiographs as a straight lucent break in the calvarium. Suture lines and vascular grooves may be mistaken for fractures. Suture lines are distinguished from fracture by irregular margins. Vascular grooves will also be more serpentine than linear fractures, with corticated margins. Linear fractures oriented in the plane of imaging may be missed on conventional axial head CT images. These are more obvious on the CT "scout" image, which has taken the place of the plain skull radiograph. Skull radiographs are now reserved for defining the location of foreign bodies and searching for skull fractures in suspected child abuse.

Depressed skull fractures are frequently associated with underlying parenchymal injury. Fractures through cranial sutures may cause sutural diastasis, widening the normal (2 mm or less) cranial sutures. Diastasis often occurs with an adjacent linear skull fracture. Skull fractures are considered *open* if a soft tissue defect communicates with the fracture.

Clinical Implications

Linear fractures are the most common fracture associated with EDH. Any fracture through dural venous sinus may cause venous sinus thrombosis. Depressed skull fractures are typically explored neurosurgically. Skull fractures that are open, are caused by a ballistic injury, are associated with pneumocephalus, or involve a sinus should be treated with antibiotics.

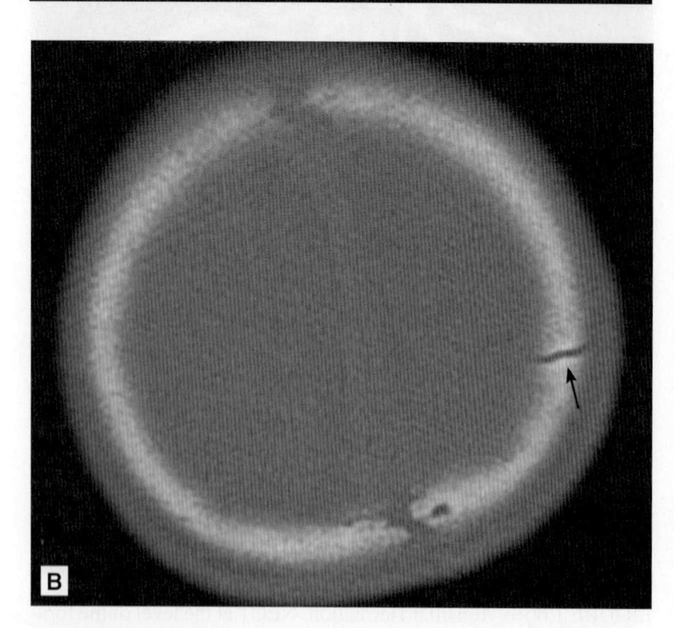

FIGURE 1.61 ■ Linear Skull Fracture. **A, B:** Axial NECT of a young child (note nonfused cranial sutures) shows linear left parietal skull fracture (arrows).

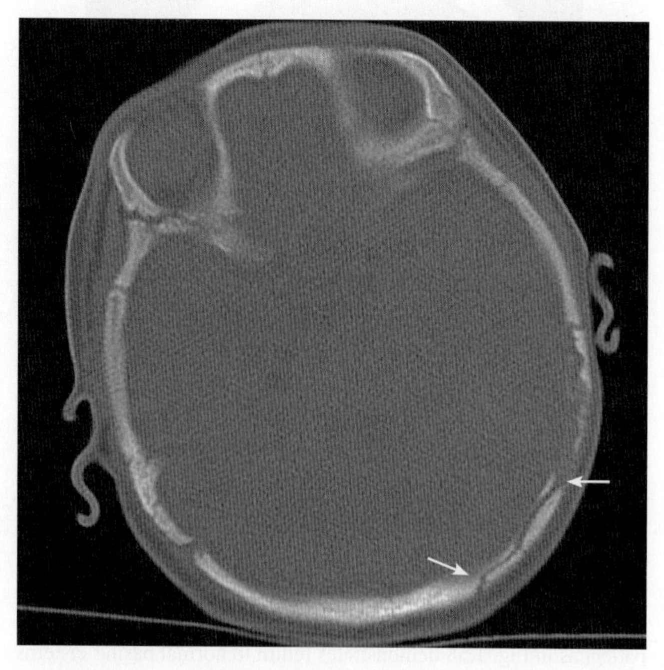

FIGURE 1.62 ■ Occipital Skull Fracture. Axial NECT shows a nondepressed linear left occipital bone fracture (arrows).

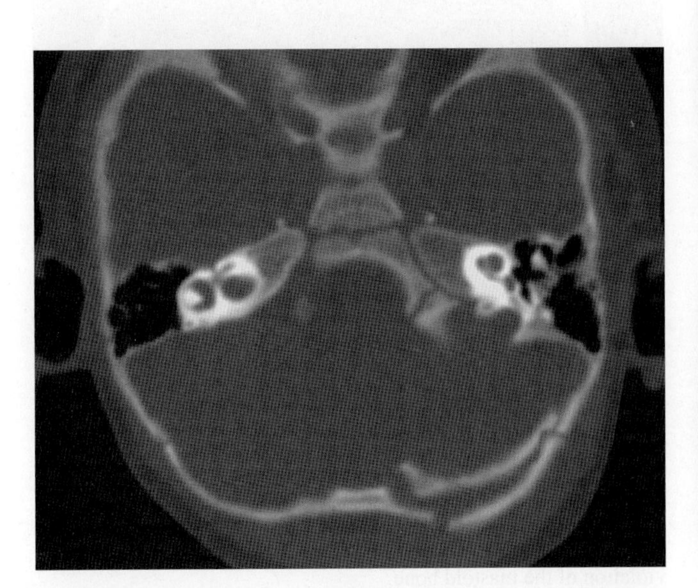

FIGURE 1.63 ▪ Depressed Skull Fracture. NECT of a child shows a depressed left occipital skull fracture with overlying soft tissue swelling.

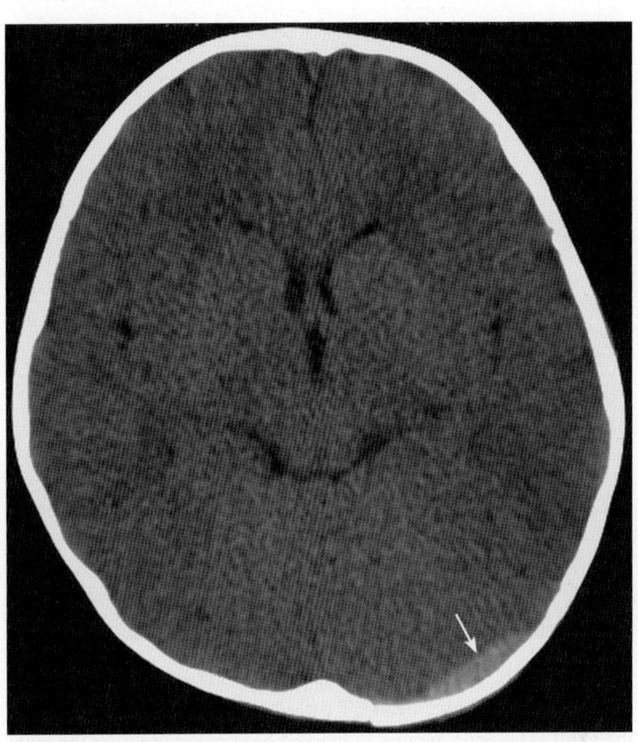

FIGURE 1.64 ▪ Depressed Skull Fracture and SDH. CT of the same child as in Fig. 1.63 shows a small epidural hematoma over the left occipital lobe under the fracture (arrow).

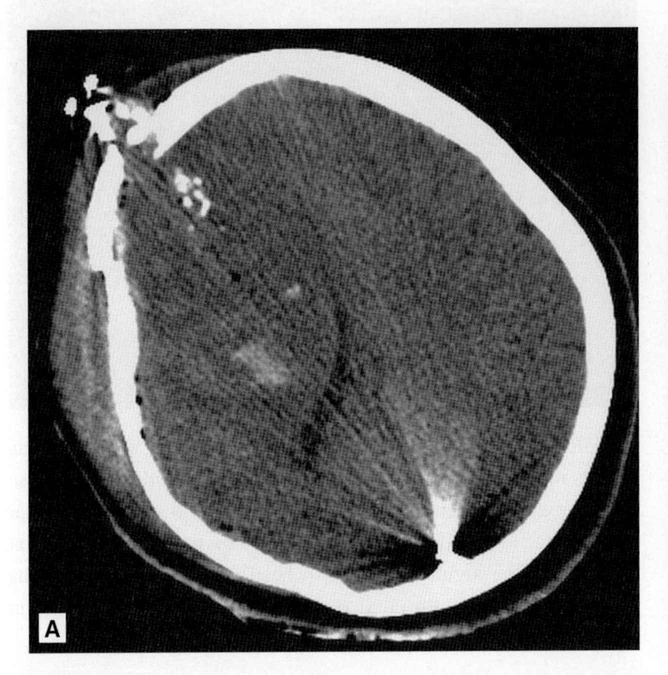

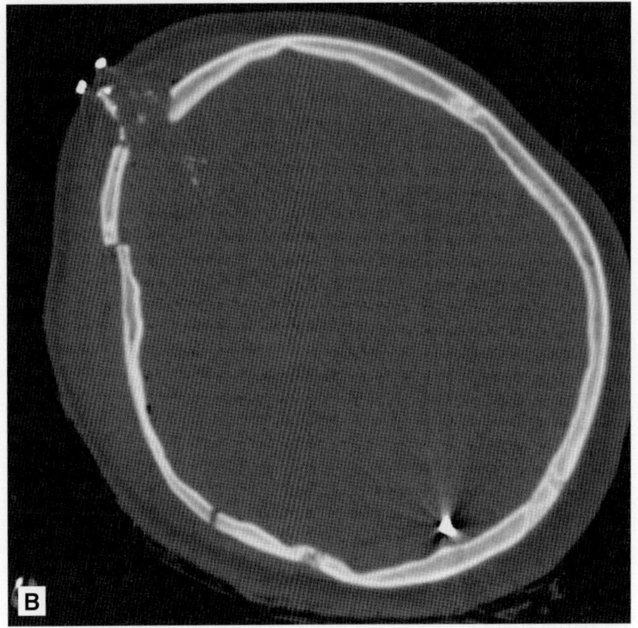

FIGURE 1.65 ▪ Ballistic Skull Fracture. **A, B:** Gunshot wound with entrance at the right frontal bone. Blood and bone fragments line the tract with a small metallic fragment in the posterior cranial vault. SAH and edema are present (note the leftward midline shift on the image "A" and likely early subfalcine herniation).

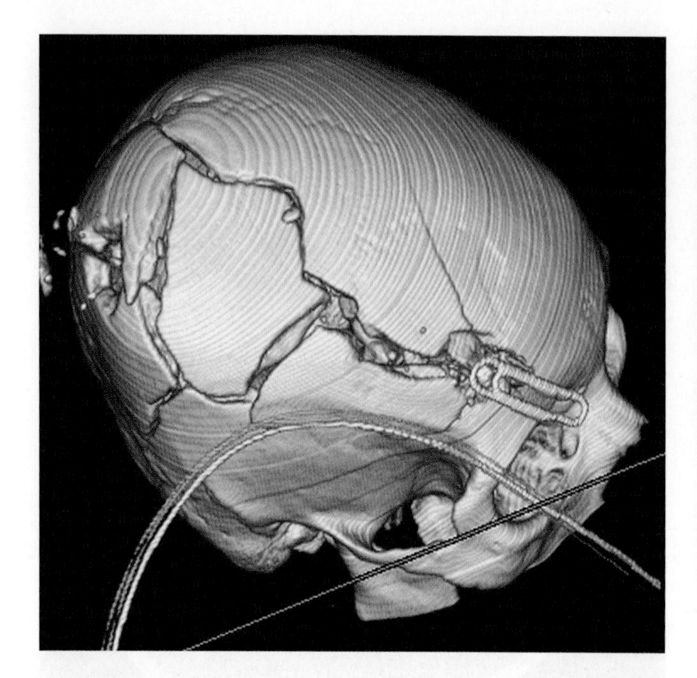

FIGURE 1.66 ■ Ballistic Skull Fracture. 3D surface reformatted image from the source head CT data shows comminuted fracture of the skull. The entry wound is marked by a paperclip over the right frontal skull; the exit wound is in the right parietal skull.

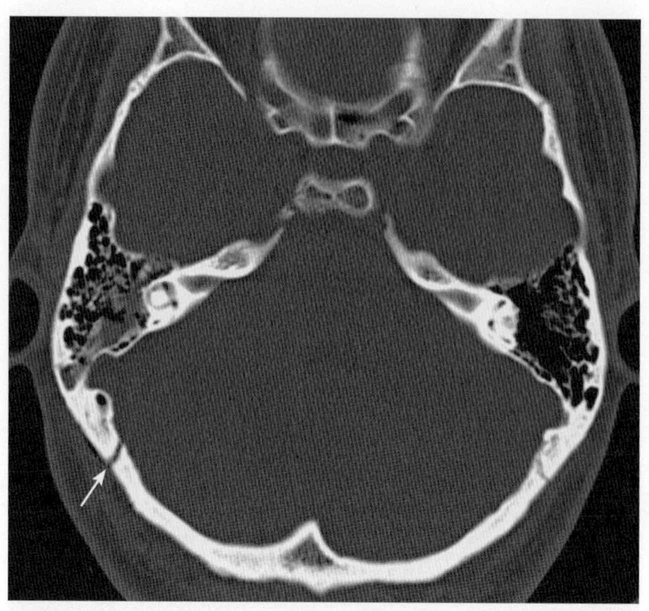

FIGURE 1.67 ■ Diastatic Skull Fracture. CT shows diastasis of the right occipitomastoid suture on the right (arrow) (note the normal left side). Some fluid is seen in the right mastoid air cells suggesting violation of the mastoid bone.

Pearls

1. Coup injuries, especially those with overlying fracture, should prompt careful inspection for cortical contusions, SDH or EDH, and foreign bodies.
2. Use bone window settings (window 1500, level 450) on CT to evaluate for pneumocephalus.
3. Table 1.4 summarizes comparative finding of cranial sutures and fractures on CT scan.

TABLE 1.4 ■ SKULL FRACTURE VERSUS SKULL SUTURES ON CT

Skull Fracture	Skull Suture
>3 mm	<2 mm
Widest at center, narrow at ends	Same width throughout
Appears darker	Appears lighter
Usually over temporal–parietal area	Located at known anatomical sites
Straight	Irregular
Angular turns	Serpentine turns

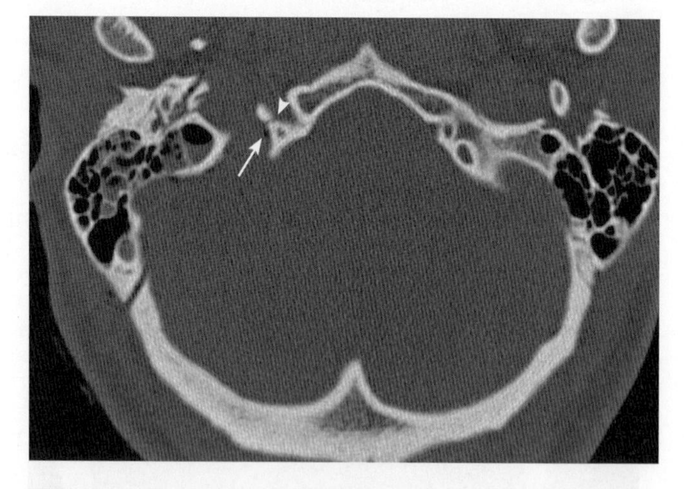

FIGURE 1.68 ■ Diastatic Skull Fracture. Coned view of same area as in Fig. 1.67 shows diastasis of the skull suture. There is also pneumocephalus seen in the region of the sigmoid sinus and jugular foramen (arrow). A faint fracture is seen crossing the skull base at the level of the jugular fossa (arrowhead). CT venogram could be considered to assess for dural venous sinus injury or thrombosis in this case since the fracture crosses the sinuses.

Radiographic Features

The dental alveoli are sockets in which roots of teeth are housed. The alveolar ridge is the bony ridge of the mandible or maxilla that holds the alveoli. Alveolar ridge fractures are identified by disruptions of the normal bony contours of the alveolar ridge as seen on axial and coronal reconstructions of the maxillofacial NCCT.

Clinical Implications

The maxillary alveolar ridge is more prone to injury than the mandibular alveolar ridge because of the thinner bone in the maxilla. Cosmetic deformity, tooth loss, and malocclusion may result from alveolar ridge fractures if improperly managed. Consult facial surgeons for management.

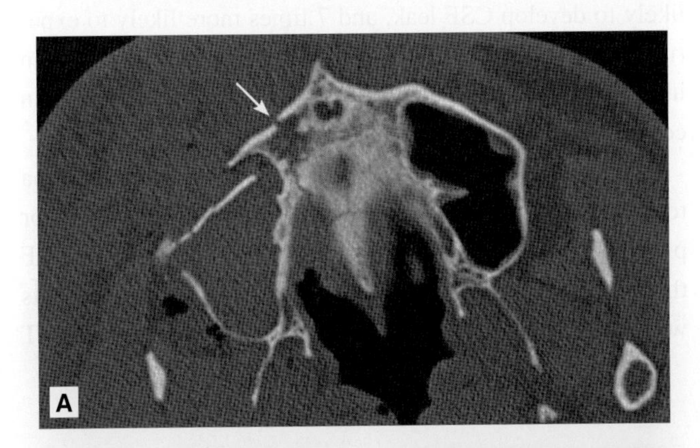

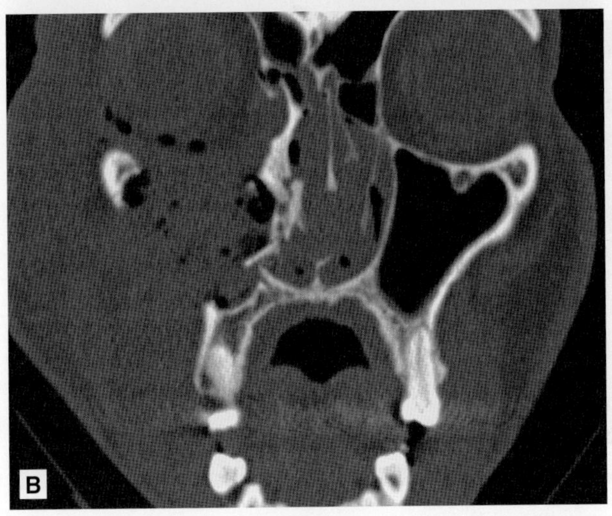

FIGURE 1.69 ■ Alveolar Ridge Fracture. **A, B:** Axial and coronal CT images show a fracture through the most anterior aspect of the maxilla (alveolar ridge arrow). Also noted are maxillary sinus wall fractures, medial orbital wall fracture, and air in the masticator space along the right mandible due to the fractures. With alveolar ridge fracture, evaluate mouth for dental avulsion injuries.

Pearls

1. The maxillary alveolar ridge is used in correct enunciation of specific sounds [t], [d], [z], [n], and [l] produced when the tongue touches the alveolar ridge.
2. Panorex views of the mouth are often used to evaluate dental infections, but facial CT is preferred for trauma.
3. There are 32 adult teeth, which are conventionally numbered begining with the right upper third maxillary molar. Tooth 32 is the right mandibular third molar.

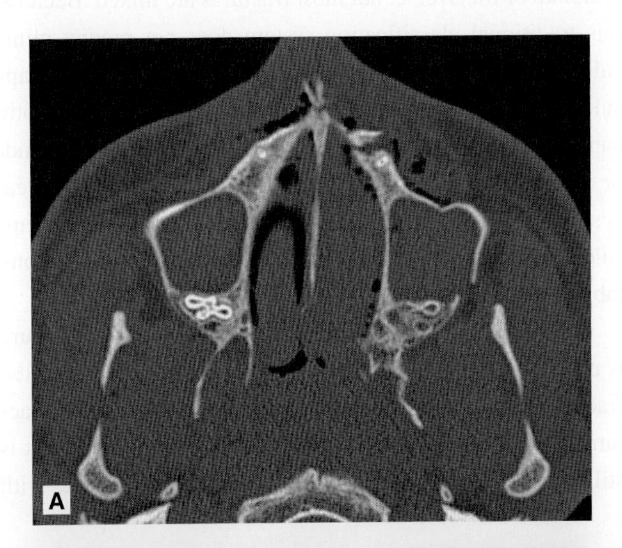

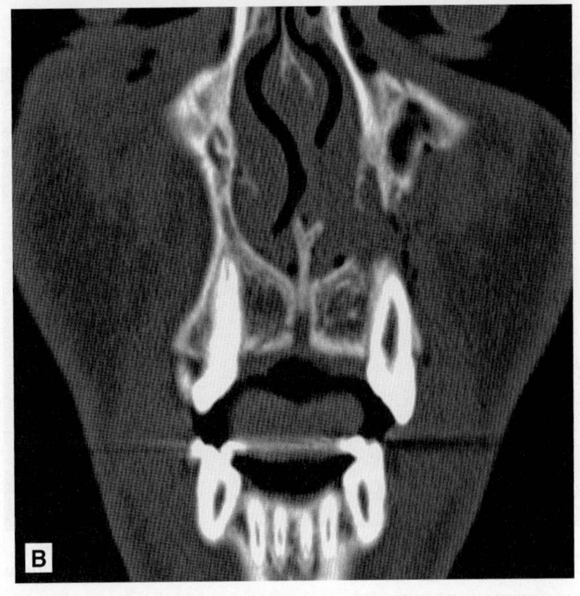

FIGURE 1.70 ■ Alveolar Ridge Fracture. **A, B:** Axial and coronal CT images show a fracture through the anterior tip of the alveolar ridge and a fracture along the left maxillary process. The left lateral pterygoid process is fractured as is the left posterolateral maxillary wall.

Radiographic Features

The skull "base" is made up the frontal bone, occiput, occipital condyles, clivus, posterior sphenoid wall, carotid canals, and the petrous portions of the temporal bones. A basilar skull fracture is essentially a linear skull fracture at the base of the skull. It is typically associated with a dural injury. Indirect radiographic signs of basilar skull fracture include pneumocephalus and air–fluid levels in the sphenoid sinus.

Temporal bone fractures (TBF) comprise 75% of basilar skull fractures. Traditionally TBF have been classified as longitudinal or transverse, but most fractures are mixed. Because this traditional classification system does not predict clinical outcomes, more recent nomenclature defines "otic capsule sparing" and "otic capsule involving" fractures. In otic capsule violating fractures, the fracture line courses into and/or through the bony labyrinth, which includes the cochlea, vestibule, and semicircular canals of the inner ear. In otic capsule sparing fractures, the fracture does not involve the bony labyrinth.

Occipital condyle fractures include 3 types. Type I fracture is due to an axial compression injury causing a comminuted fracture of the occipital condyles and is typically a stable fracture. Type II is a more extensive basioccipital fracture, but is still considered stable. Type III is an avulsion fracture, with displacement of the avulsed condyle. Type III fractures are potentially unstable.

Clival fractures can be described as longitudinal, transverse, or oblique, with the longitudinal fracture carrying the worse prognosis due to involvement of the vertebrobasilar system. Cranial nerve VI and VII deficits may also occur.

Clinical Implications

Basilar skull fractures are associated with significant injury that may involve the internal carotid and vertebral arteries, the sigmoid and transverse sinuses, and cranial nerves, and to the middle or inner ear.

Patients with otic capsule violating TBF fractures are 2 times more likely to develop facial paralysis, 4 times more likely to develop CSF leak, and 7 times more likely to experience profound hearing loss, and more likely to sustain intracranial complications including EDH and tSAH when compared with otic capsule sparing fractures.

Vascular injuries are common in patients with trauma to the skull base. An internal carotid artery dissection or pseudoaneurysm occurs in 35% of patients with TBF through the carotid canal. Additionally, 40% of patients with dissections do not have an associated fracture. CT

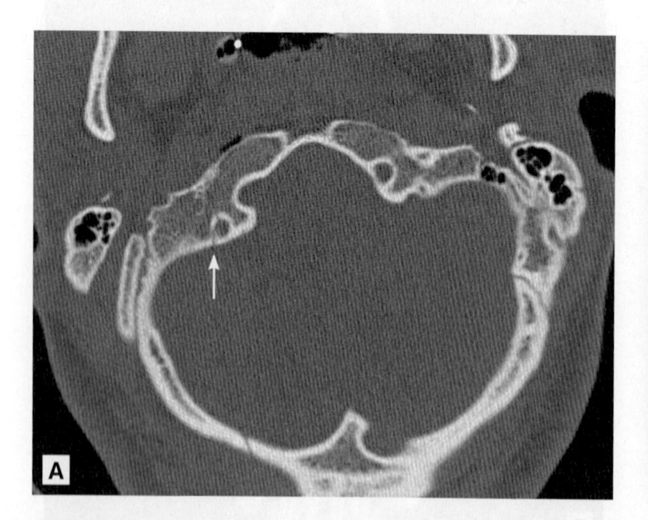

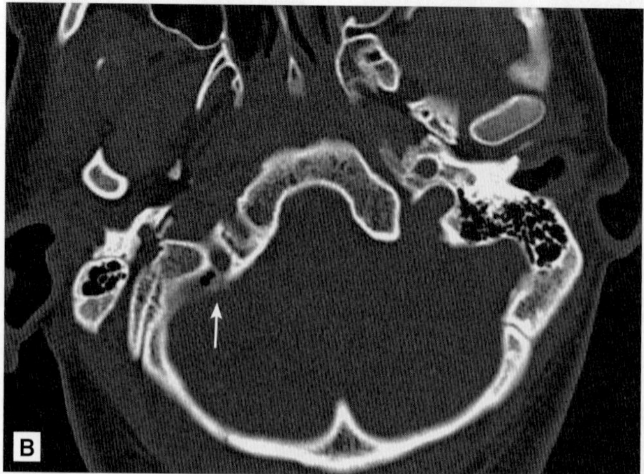

FIGURE 1.71 ■ Basilar Skull Fracture. **A, B:** NECT with bone windows shows fracture crossing the inferior right occipital bone (both posterior squamous portion and more anterior condylar portion) and involving the right jugular foramen. Image "A" shows fracture line extending across the hypoglossal canal on the right (arrows) that transmits the hypoglossal cranial nerve.

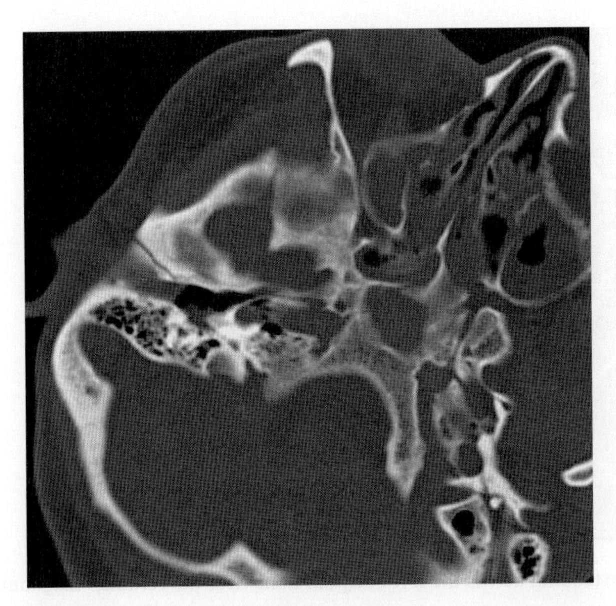

FIGURE 1.72 ■ Temporal Bone Fracture. A fracture extends through the right petrous carotid canal into the sphenoid sinus. Patients with basilar skull fractures often have arterial injury, which typically occurs in the cervical region (despite the higher level of the skull fracture). CTA of the head and neck is indicated.

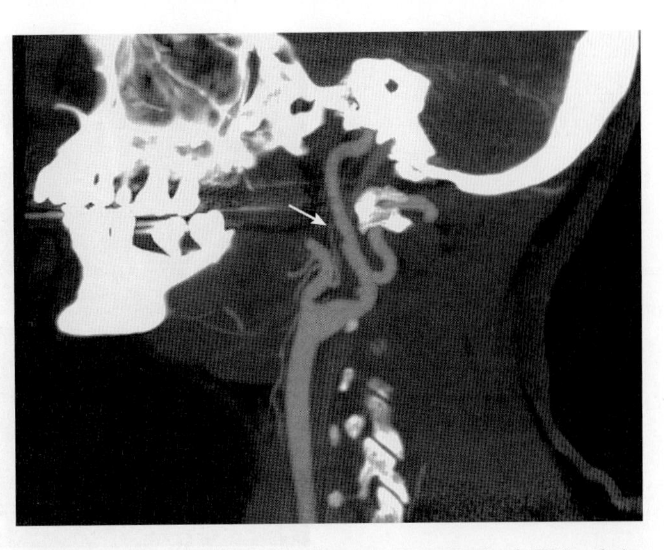

FIGURE 1.73 ■ Carotid Artery Dissection. Sagittal CTA of the neck demonstrates luminal irregularity of the midportion of the left ICA representing a carotid dissection with pseudoaneurysm (arrow). CTA is preferred over MRA for traumatic vessel injury as it has higher spatial resolution to detect subtle intimal injuries.

angiography (CTA) has become the initial screening study of choice to evaluate for vascular injury, although the diagnosis can be made with conventional angiography and MR angiography.

Pearls

1. Occipital condyle fractures are rarely seen on plain radiographs but are easily identified on cervical spine CT.
2. Fluid in the mastoid air cells is not specific for basilar skull fracture.

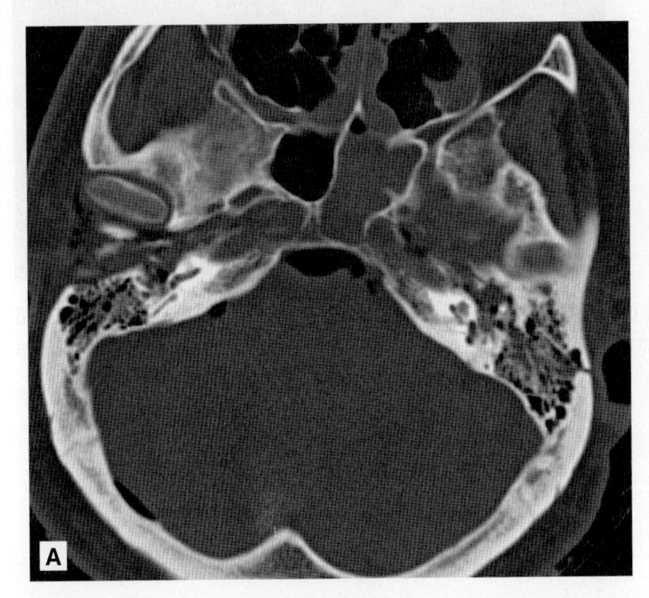

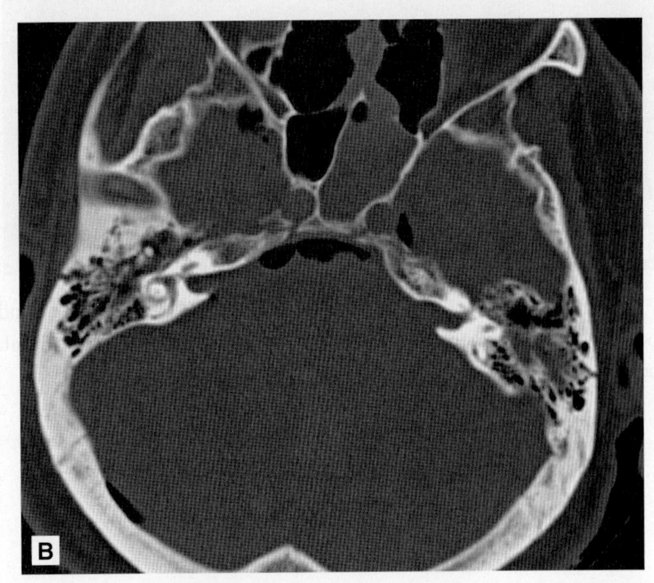

FIGURE 1.74 ■ Temporal Bone Fracture. **A, B:** Axial NECT shows bilateral temporal bone/petrous pyramid fractures. Fractures extend across both carotid canals. Pneumocephalus is seen anterior to the brainstem indicating a breach of the dura. CTA of the head and neck would be recommended.

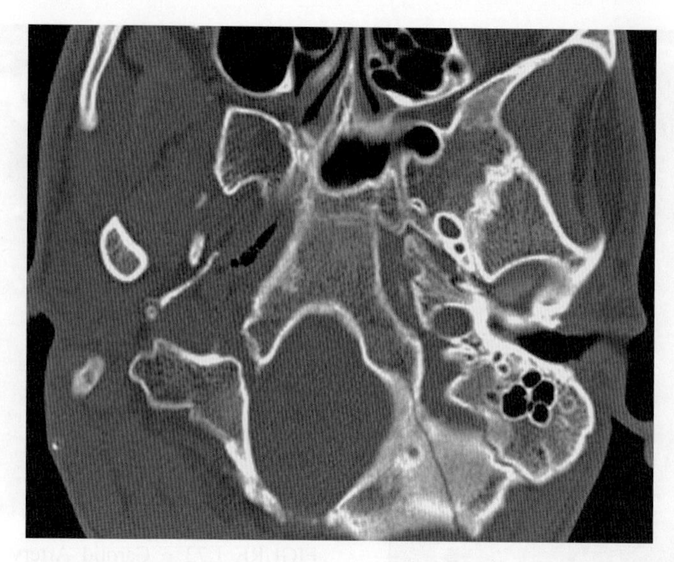

FIGURE 1.75 ■ Occipital Bone Fracture. Axial NECT shows fracture extending across the left occipital bone near the foramen magnum. Significant force must have occurred to sustain a fracture in this site.

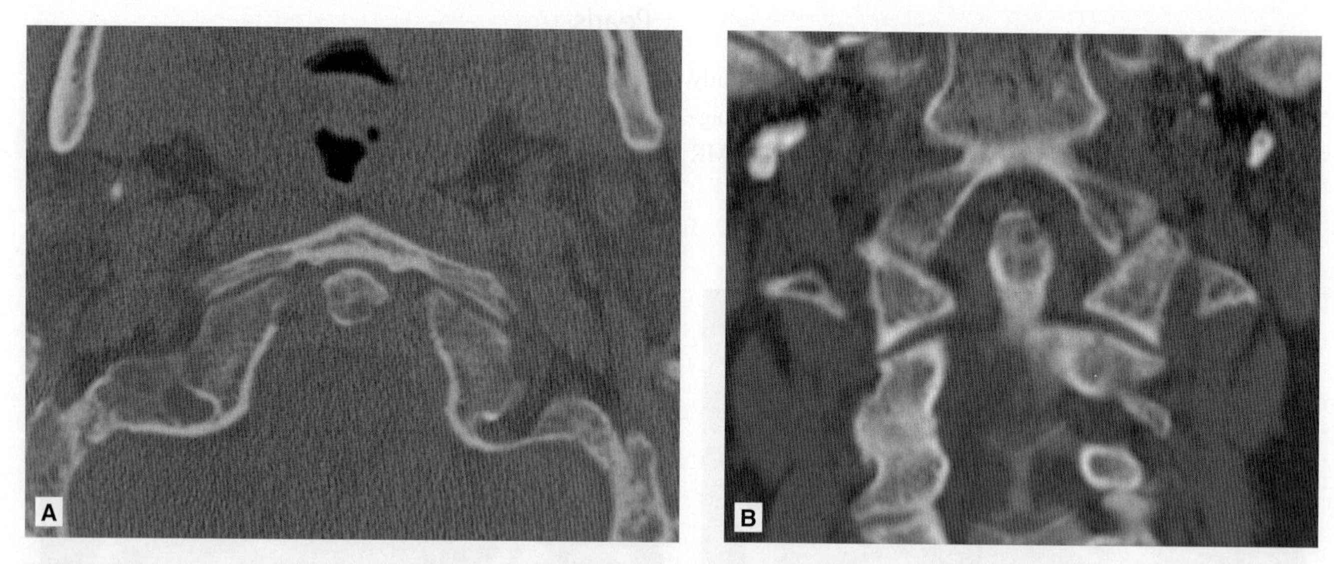

FIGURE 1.76 ■ Occipital Condyle Fracture Type I. **A, B:** Axial and coronal NECTs of the cervical spine show bilateral nondisplaced occipital condyle fractures (type I) due to axial loading injury. When bilateral, this can be unstable as the dens loses its anchor to the occipital condyles.

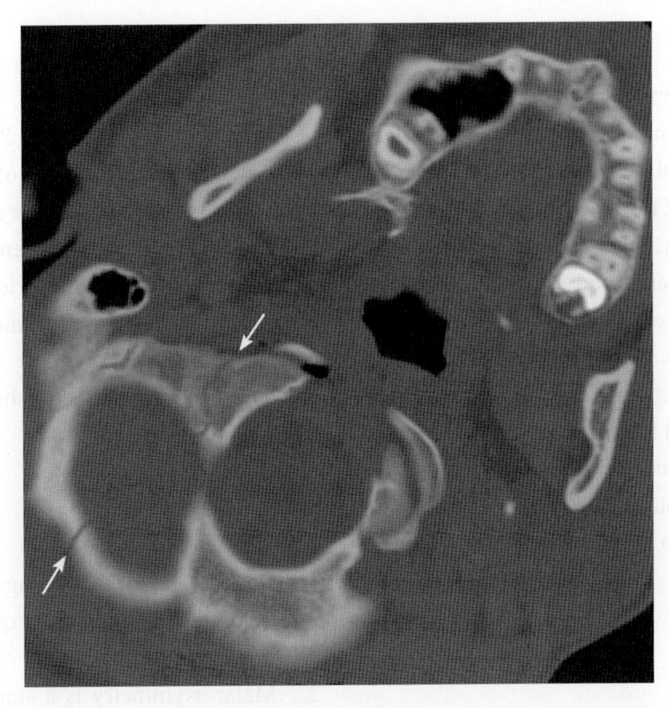

FIGURE 1.77 ■ Occipital Condyle Fracture Type II. Axial NECT shows a right occipital condyle fracture (type II) with occipital skull fracture (arrows).

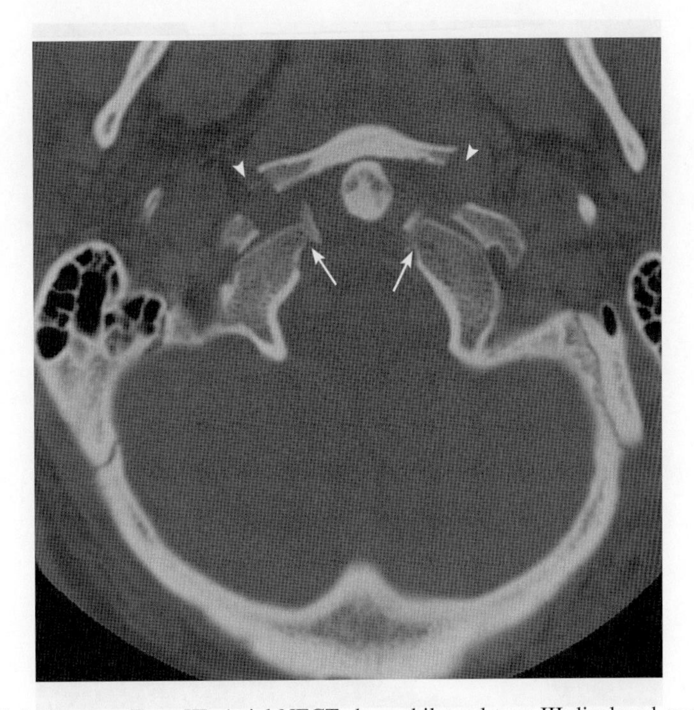

FIGURE 1.78 ■ Occipital Condyle Fracture Type III. Axial NECT shows bilateral type III displaced occipital condyle fractures (arrows) with anterior ring fractures of C1 (arrowheads).

Radiographic Features

The zygomaticomaxillary complex (ZMC) has articulations with the frontal, maxillary, temporal, and sphenoid bones, creating the zygomaticofrontal (ZF), zygomaticomaxillary (ZM), zygomaticotemporal (ZT), and zygomaticosphenoid (ZS) articulations, respectively. The ZF articulation is disrupted by fractures of the lateral orbital rim. The ZM articulation is disrupted by inferior orbital rim, orbital floor, and maxillary sinus wall fractures. The ZT articulation is disrupted by zygomatic arch fractures. The ZS articulation is disrupted by lateral orbital wall fractures.

ZMC fractures represent a spectrum of injuries; thus, all 4 articulations may not be disrupted. The ZF articulation is the strongest and is often the last to break.

Clinical Implications

ZMC fractures are common, second only to nasal fractures in frequency. Nondisplaced ZMC fractures do not require surgery. Depressed fractures of the zygomatic arch can cause trismus from masseter muscle spasm or from impingement of the coronoid process on the temporalis muscle. Other complications of a ZMC fracture include enophthalmos, entrapment, orbital compartment syndrome (OCS), sinusitis, and cheek hypesthesias.

Facial trauma surgeons should be consulted to manage ZMC fractures.

Pearls

1. ZMC fractures involving all 4 articulations are more accurately described as "quadripod" rather than "tripod" fractures.
2. Malar asymmetry is a significant complication of ZMC fractures.

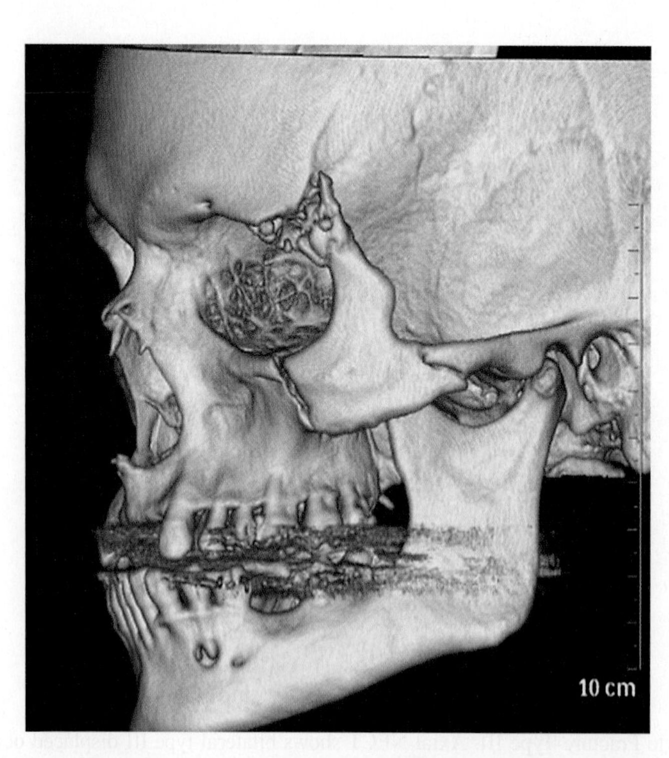

FIGURE 1.79 ■ ZMC Articulations. A 3D surface reformatted image of the patient in Fig. 1.80 demonstrating the articulations of the zygoma with the skull and maxilla.

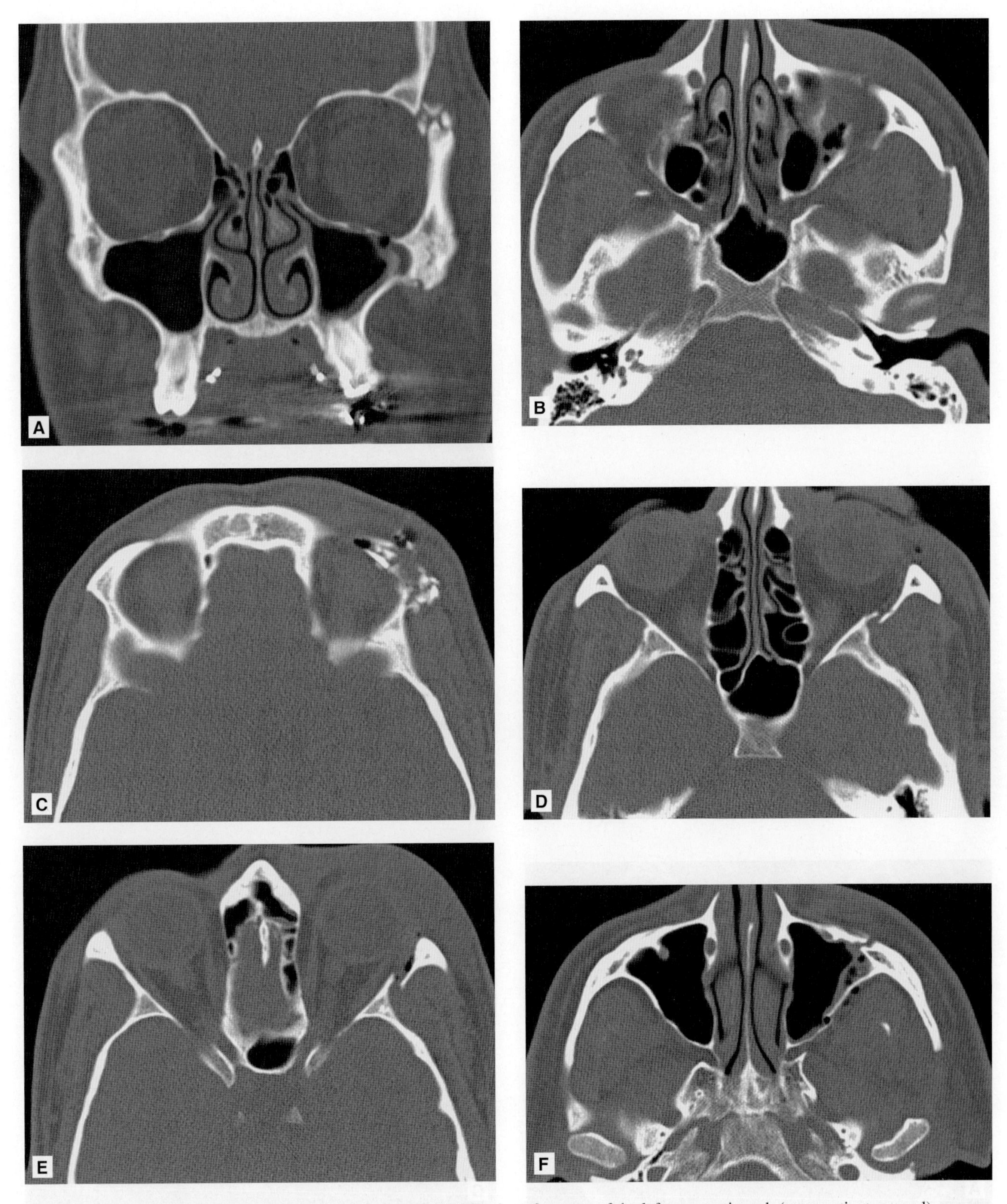

FIGURE 1.80 ■ ZMC Fractures. **A-F:** Axial and coronal NECTs show fractures of the left zygomatic arch (zygomaticotemporal), superolateral orbital buttress (zygomaticofrontal), greater sphenoid wing at the zygomaticosphenoid articulation, and zygomaticomaxillary articulation. These are the 4 articulations the zygoma makes with the face. All are fractured.

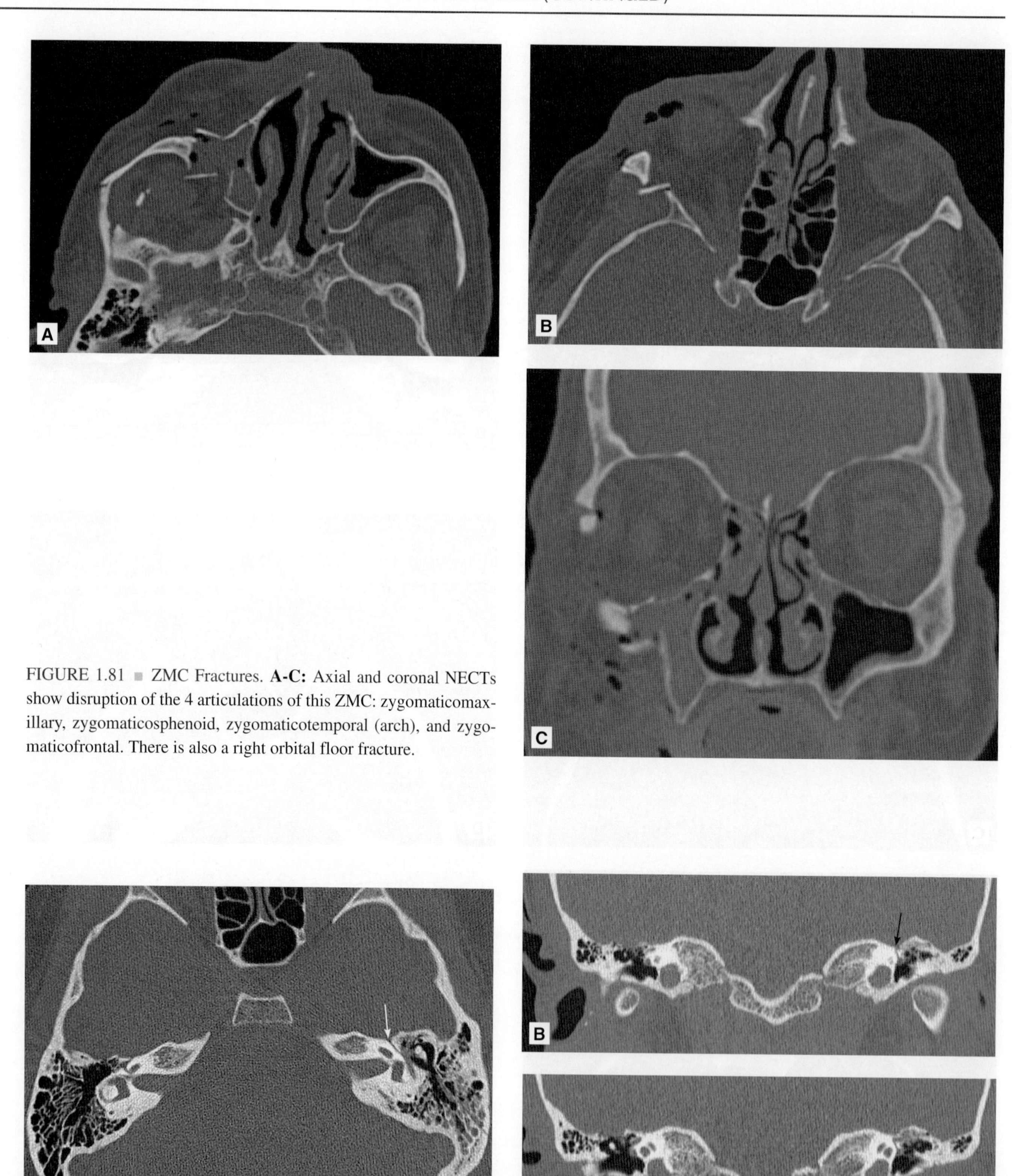

FIGURE 1.81 ■ ZMC Fractures. **A-C:** Axial and coronal NECTs show disruption of the 4 articulations of this ZMC: zygomaticomaxillary, zygomaticosphenoid, zygomaticotemporal (arch), and zygomaticofrontal. There is also a right orbital floor fracture.

FIGURE 1.82 ■ Otic Sparing Temporal Bone Fracture. **A-C:** Axial and coronal NECTs show otic sparing temporal bone fracture that crosses the genu and tympanic section of the facial nerve canal (arrows).

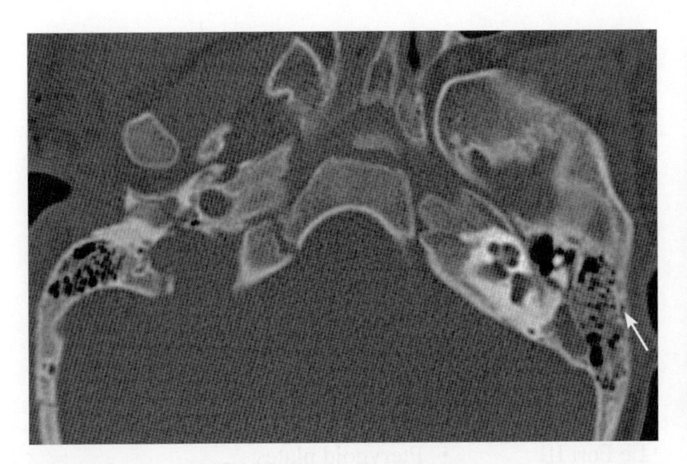

FIGURE 1.83 ■ Otic Violating Temporal Bone Fracture. Longitudinal fracture extends along the axis of the left temporal bone (arrow). It crosses the left otic capsule but the visualized malleus and incus remain in appropriate locations.

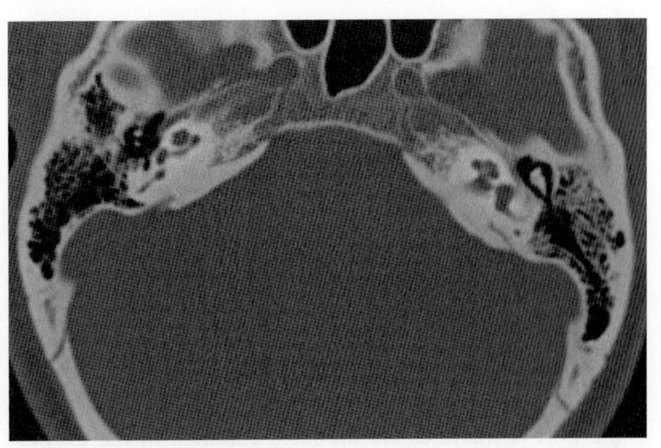

FIGURE 1.84 ■ Normal Ossicles. Axial CT in a different patient demonstrates the normal appearance of the malleus and incus bones. The middle ear should also normally be air filled.

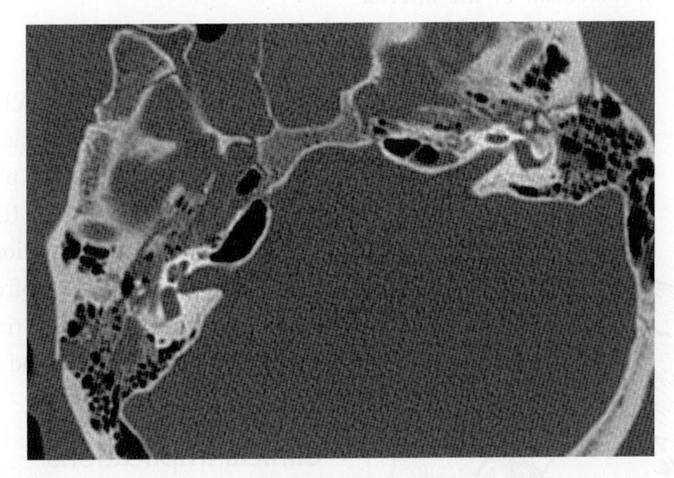

FIGURE 1.85 ■ Ossicular Disruption. Axial CT shows ossicular disruption in the left middle ear. The normal "ice cream cone" configuration of the malleus and incus is disrupted in this 19-year-old male following trauma.

Radiographic Features

All Le Fort fractures involve fractures through bilateral medial and lateral pterygoid plates. Pure Le Fort fracture patterns are infrequent and the most frequent fracture patterns are mixed.

Le Fort I fracture is a horizontal fracture across the maxilla separating the maxilla from the rest of the facial bones. This injury is best seen on coronal images that demonstrate bilateral disruption of the medial and lateral pterygoid plates with fractures of all walls of the maxillary sinus (the distinguishing feature of a Le Fort I fracture), and the nasal septum.

Le Fort II fractures are the most common of the Le Fort fractures. The fracture extends in a triangular configuration to involve the pterygoid plates, medial orbital wall, orbital floor, inferior orbital rim, and the maxillary antra. Le Fort II fractures spare the medial wall of the maxillary sinus. The distinguishing feature of a Le Fort II fracture, compared with the other Le Fort fractures, is involvement of the inferior orbital rim.

TABLE 1.5 ■ LE FORT FRACTURE CLASSIFICATION AND INJURIES

Fracture	Injuries
Le Fort I	• Pterygoid plates • All maxillary sinus walls*
Le Fort II	• Pterygoid plates • Anterior and posterolateral maxillary sinus wall • Nasofrontal articulation • Orbital floor* • Orbital medial wall
Le Fort III	• Pterygoid plates • Lateral orbital rim • Lateral orbital wall • Medial orbital wall • Nasofrontal articulation • Zygomatic arch*

*Distinguishing feature.

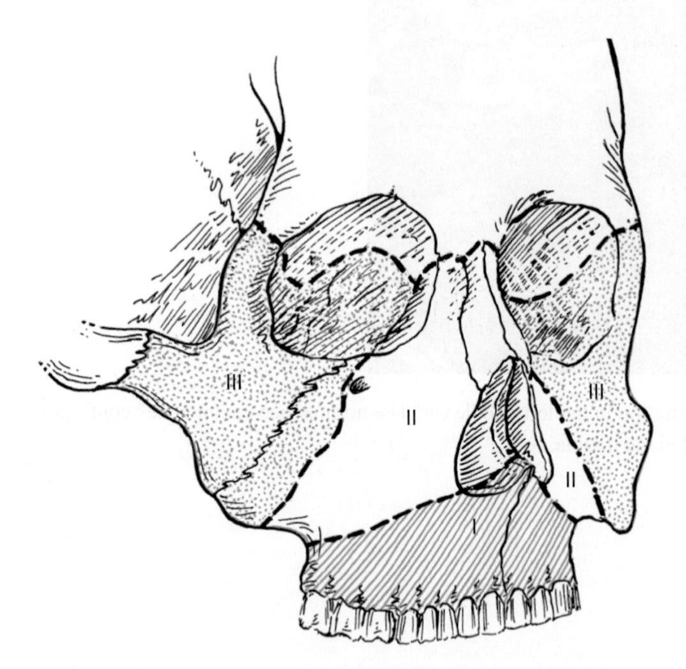

FIGURE 1.86 ■ Le Fort Facial Fracture Classification. (Reproduced with permission from Knoop KJ, Stack LB, Storrow AB, Thurman RJ, eds. *The Atlas of Emergency Medicine*. 3rd ed. New York: McGraw-Hill; 2010:11. © 2010 McGraw-Hill.)

Le Fort III fractures dissociate the midface from the more posterior cranium (cranial–facial separation). Injured structures include the pterygoid plates, zygomatic arch (distinguishing feature of Le Fort III fracture from other Le Fort fractures), and medial, posterior, and lateral orbital walls. The medial orbital rim and nasofrontal articulation is disrupted instead of the inferior orbital rim. A summary of Le Fort classification and injuries is found in Table 1.5.

Clinical Implications

The utility of the Le Fort classification is limited because pure Le Fort fractures are infrequent; however, it is still used to describe midface injuries. The most serious complication of a Le Fort fracture is airway obstruction due to posterior displacement of the midface. Le Fort I injures are associated with dentoalveolar trauma. Le Fort II and III fractures have a higher association with cerebrovascular injury, such as internal carotid artery dissection or pseudoaneurysm. Other complications include nasolacrimal duct injury. Orbital floor fractures may impinge on the exiting infraorbital nerve or cause extraocular muscle entrapment. Cerebral spinal fluid leak occurs most often with Le Fort III fractures.

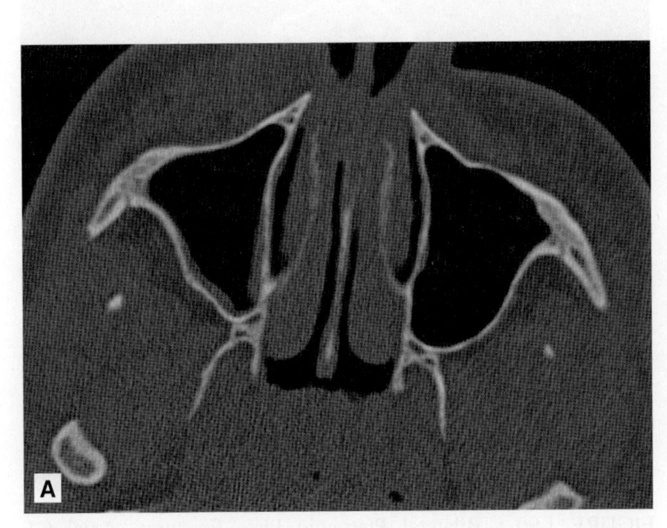

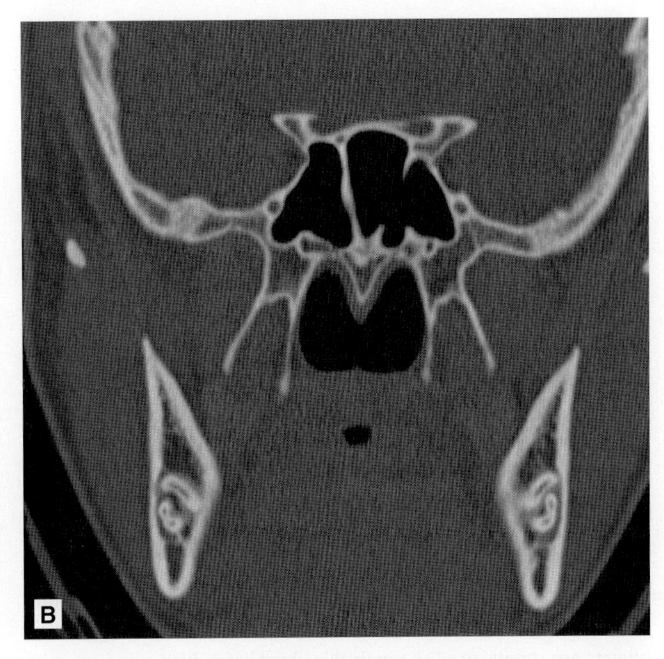

FIGURE 1.87 ■ Pterygoid Plate Fractures. **A, B:** Axial and coronal CT images demonstrate normal medial and lateral pterygoid plates. These are always fractured in a Le Fort injury.

Pearls

1. Midface fractures account for 75% of all facial fractures.
2. All Le Fort fractures include bilateral pterygoid plate fractures.
3. A pure Le Fort fracture is infrequent and most are mixed fractures.
4. René Le Fort, a French army surgeon, developed his facial fracture classification system by delivering blunt forces to skulls of cadavers. The force he generated is much less than that experienced by trauma patients today.

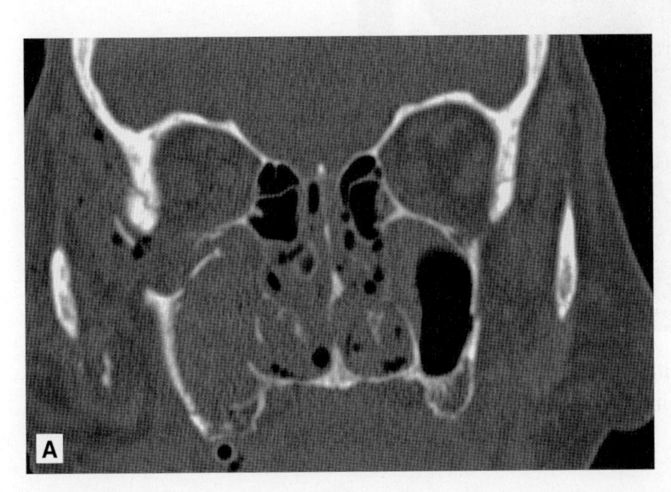

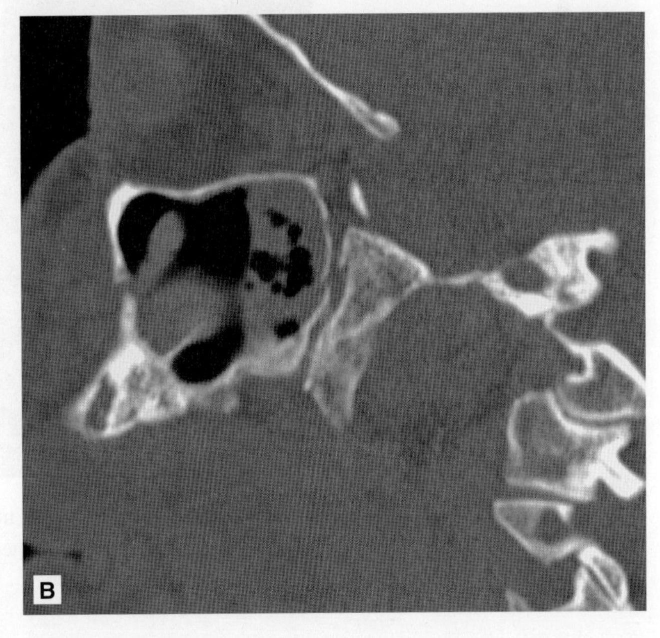

FIGURE 1.88 ■ Le Fort I and II Fractures. **A, B:** Coronal and sagittal NECTs show horizontal fracture plane through the walls of the left maxillary sinus, constituting a Le Fort I on the left side. The inferior orbital rim is involved on the right side, making this a Le Fort II fracture.

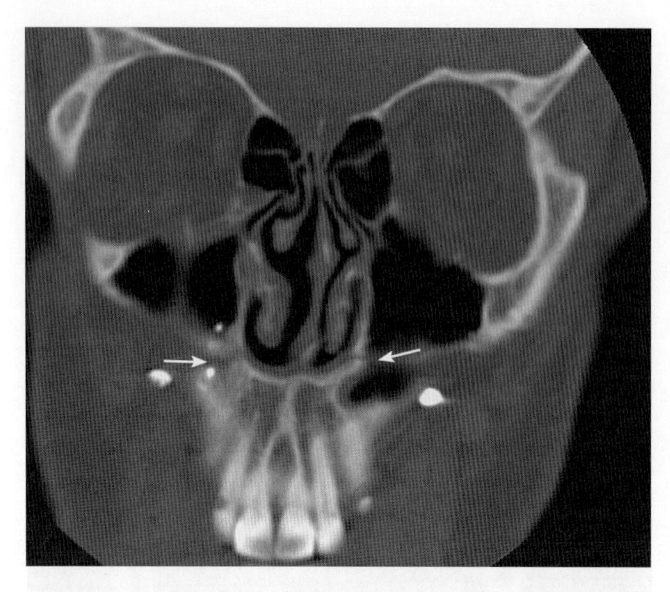

FIGURE 1.89 ■ Le Fort I Fracture. Coronal NECT shows fracture line crossing beneath nose across maxilla (arrows). The metallic objects are screws used to repair this chronic fracture.

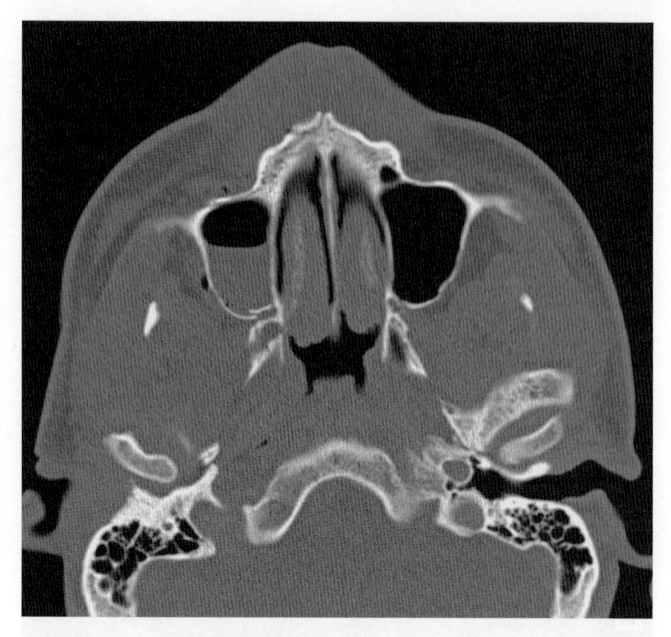

FIGURE 1.90 ■ Bilateral Pterygoid Plate Fractures. Axial CT shows bilateral pterygoid plate fractures (not fully shown on this 1 image), fractures of the right maxillary walls inferiorly, and a fracture plane crossing the maxillary alveolar ridge.

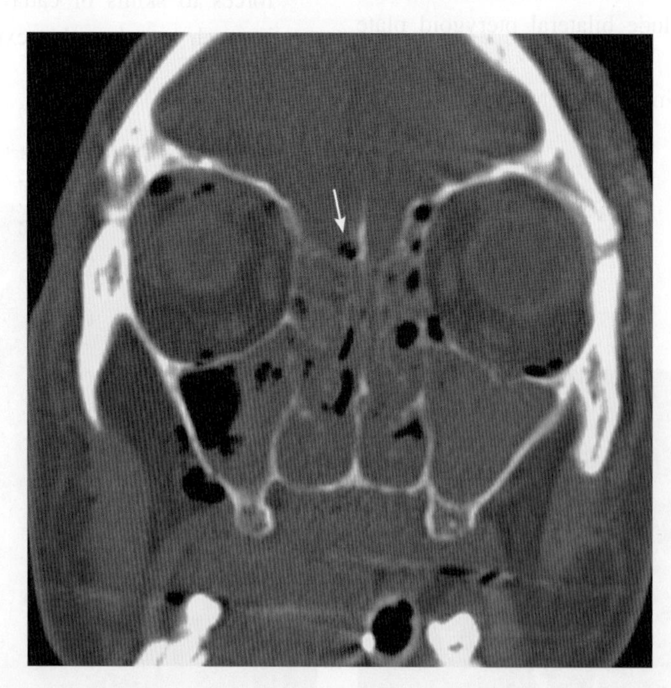

FIGURE 1.91 ■ Le Fort II Fracture. Coronal reformatted CT shows multiple facial fractures extending through both maxillary sinuses to the ethmoid sinuses. Abnormal air is seen above the cribiform plate in the intracranial vault (arrow). There is also orbital emphysema.

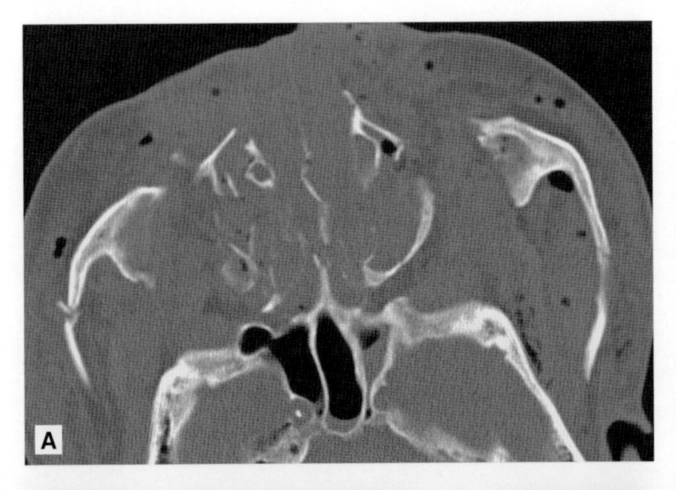

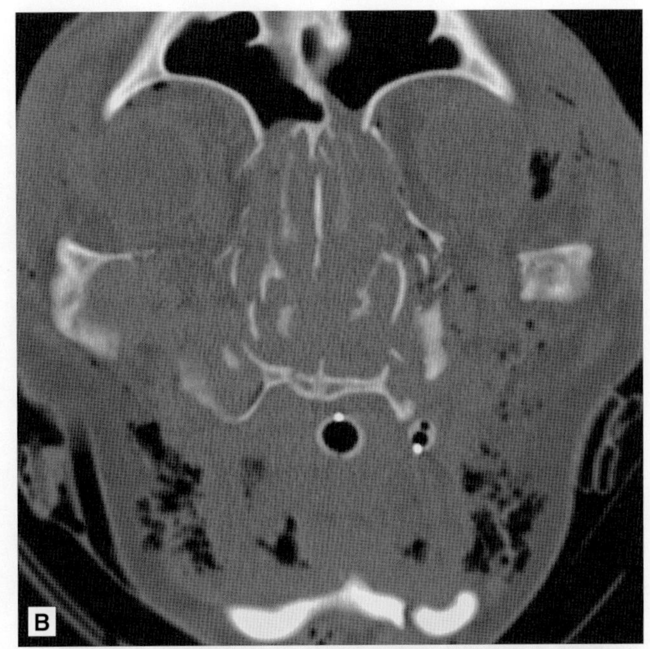

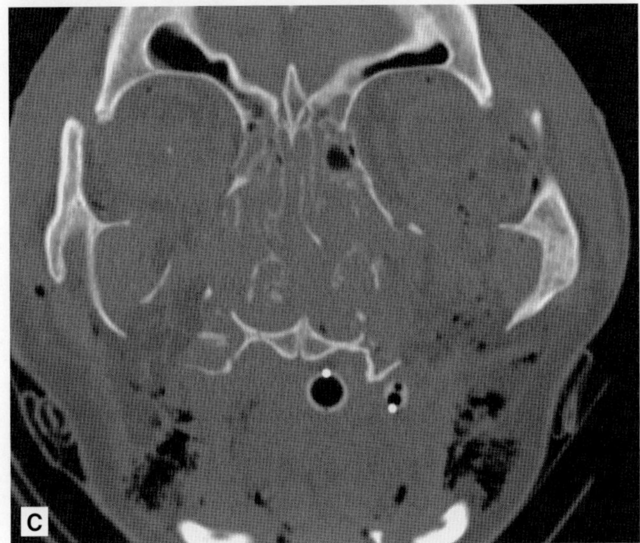

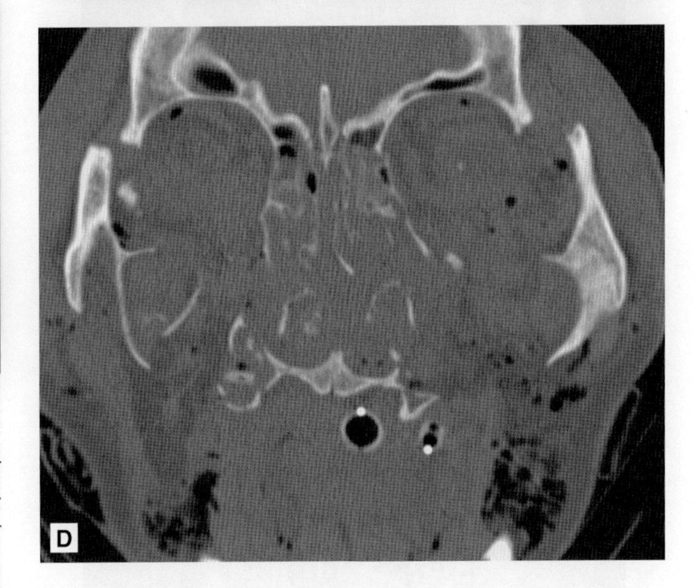

FIGURE 1.92 ■ Le Fort III Fracture. **A-D:** Axial and coronal NECTs show extensive facial fractures and subcutaneous air. Fractures through both zygomatic arches cause complete dissociation of the midface.

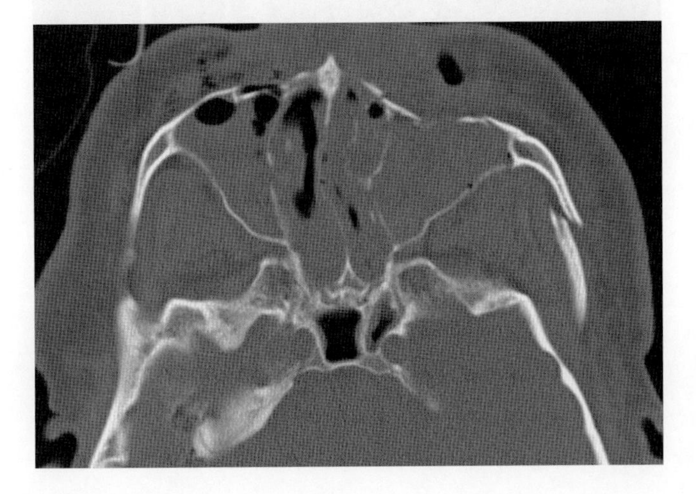

FIGURE 1.93 ■ Left Le Fort III Fracture. Axial image shows a depressed fracture of the left zygomatic arch. In some cases with this fracture, trismus can be a presenting sign following trauma. The zygomatic arch involvement makes this a Le Fort III fracture on the left.

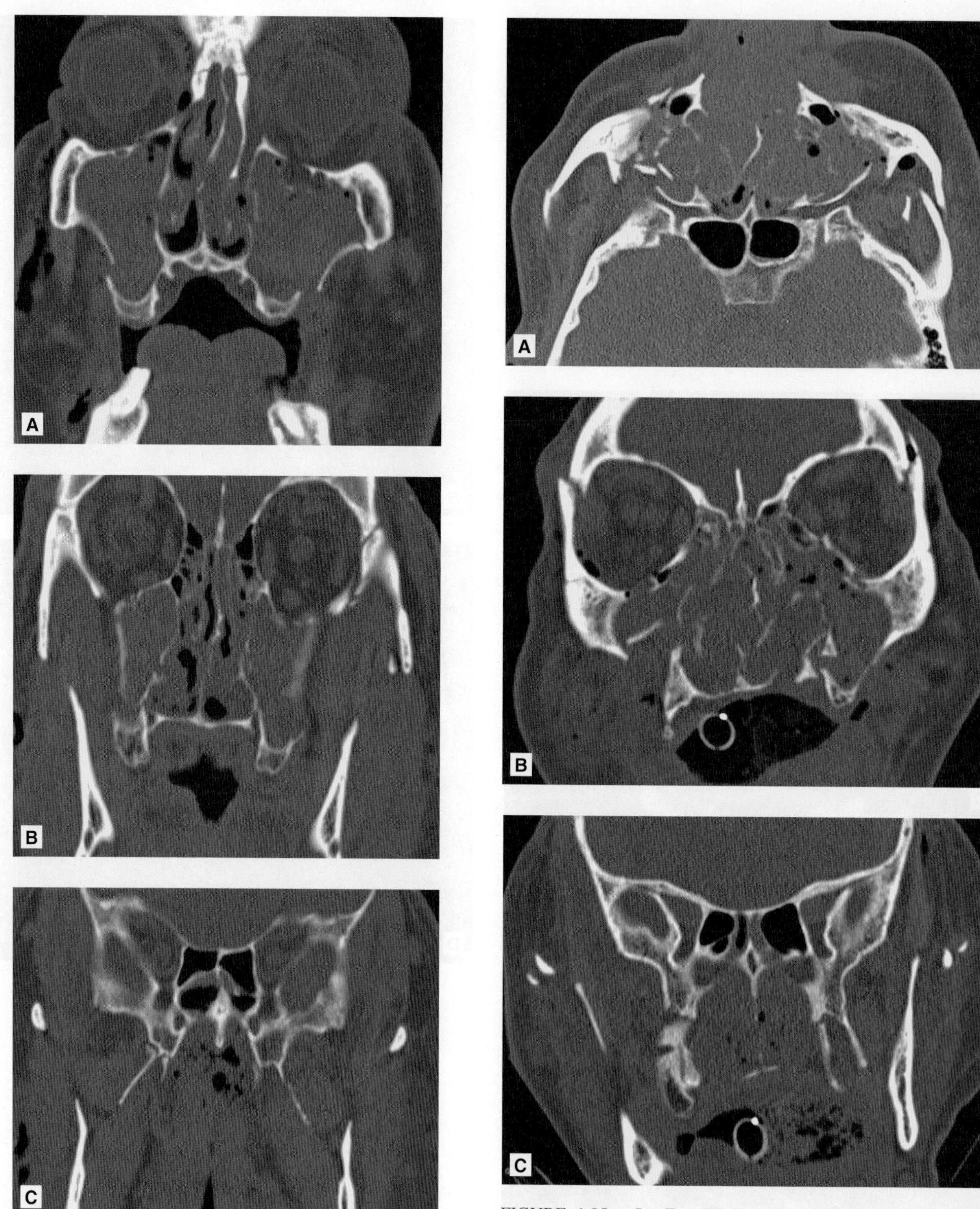

FIGURE 1.94 ■ Left Le Fort III Fracture. **A-C:** Coronal NECT shows a left Le Fort III fracture. Zygomatic arch involvement makes this a Le Fort III fracture. This is distinguished from a ZMC fracture by involvement of the pterygoid plates (see Figs. 1.12 to 1.14) and medial orbital wall.

FIGURE 1.95 ■ Le Fort III Fracture. **A-C:** Axial and coronal NECTs show fractures of all maxillary sinus walls, both pterygoid processes, medial, inferior, and lateral orbital rims, and both zygomatic arches. This pattern constitutes a Le Fort III injury.

Radiographic Features

The nasal bones are rectangular-shaped bones that articulate with the frontal bone superiorly, the frontal processes of the maxilla laterally, and the end plate of the ethmoid bone forming a tent-like configuration. Nasal fractures are frequently comminuted.

Occipitomental (Waters) and lateral views of the nose are used to evaluate suspected nasal bone fractures. Deviation, displacement with sharp angulation, and soft tissue swelling when inspecting the nasal septum and arch are signs suggesting fracture. On the lateral view, short lucent line that extends to the anterior cortex suggests fracture, rather than suture.

Clinical Implications

Complications of nasal bone fractures that require acute intervention include epistaxis, septal hematoma, and severely displaced fracture fragments. Open nasal bone fractures should be treated with antibiotics.

Pearls

1. Isolated nondisplaced nasal bone fractures typically do not require imaging.
2. Nasal bone fractures on the lateral view are more lucent than sutures or nasociliary groove.

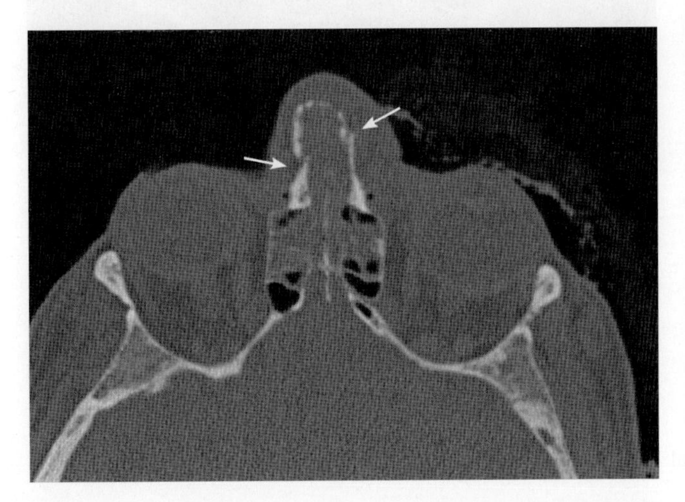

FIGURE 1.96 ■ Nasal Bone Fracture. Axial NECT shows displaced fractures of the nasal bones (arrows) in this 55-year-old female.

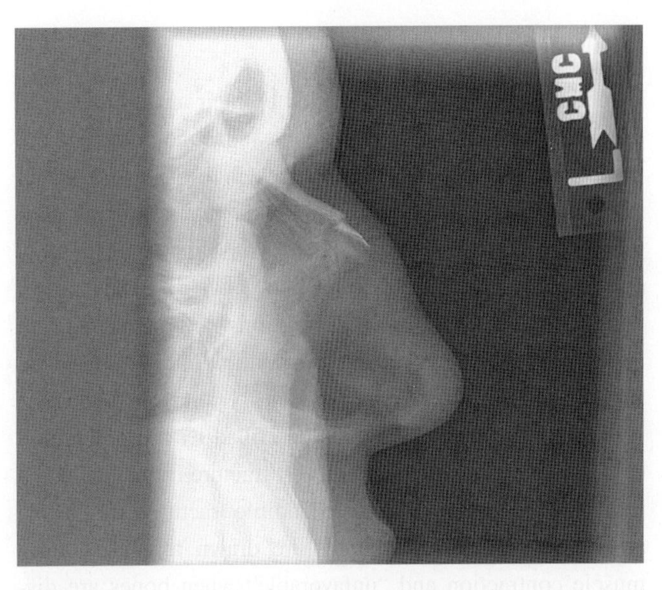

FIGURE 1.97 ■ Nasal Bone Fracture. A lateral view of the nasal bones shows a minimally depressed fracture.

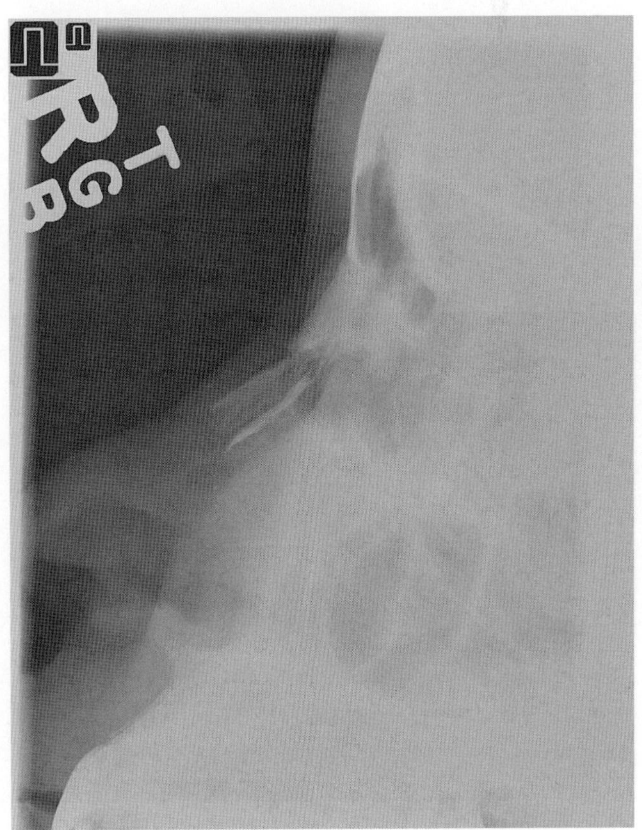

FIGURE 1.98 ■ Nasal Bone Fracture. A lateral view of the nasal bones in a different patient shows comminuted and significantly depressed fractures of the nasal bones.

Radiographic Features

Mandibular fractures are classified by their anatomical location and most commonly involve the angle and body. Greater than 50% of mandibular fractures have multiple breaks due to the ring structure of the bone. Panorex is the best plain radiograph to identify injury if isolated to the mandible. If panorex is unavailable, PA, oblique, and Towne (AP axial) plain radiograph are used. Cortical disruptions are typically easy to identify. NECT is best utilized if multiple facial injures are suspected and is often needed to identify condylar fractures.

Mandibular fractures can be described by the orientation of the fracture line and the effect on fracture fragments when mastication muscles contract. Mandible fractures are "favorable" when fracture fragments are drawn together during muscle contraction and "unfavorable" when bones are displaced during muscle contraction. Fractures of the angle and body of the mandible tend to be unfavorable.

Clinical Implications

Mandibular fractures are second to the nose as the most common facial fracture, mainly due to their prominence on the face. Bilateral parasymphyseal fractures may cause airway obstruction in the supine patient. Open fractures, displaced fractures, and those associated with dental trauma require immediate consultation. Open fractures require admission for IV antibiotics.

Pearls

1. Parasymphysis and symphysis fractures are inherently unfavorable, meaning mastication muscle contraction results in distraction of bony fragments from each other.
2. The condyles are the most common location of mandibular fracture in children less than 10 years of age.

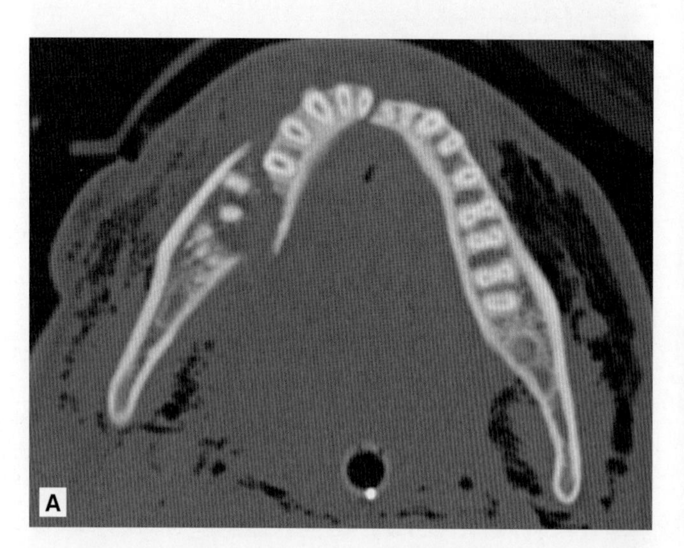

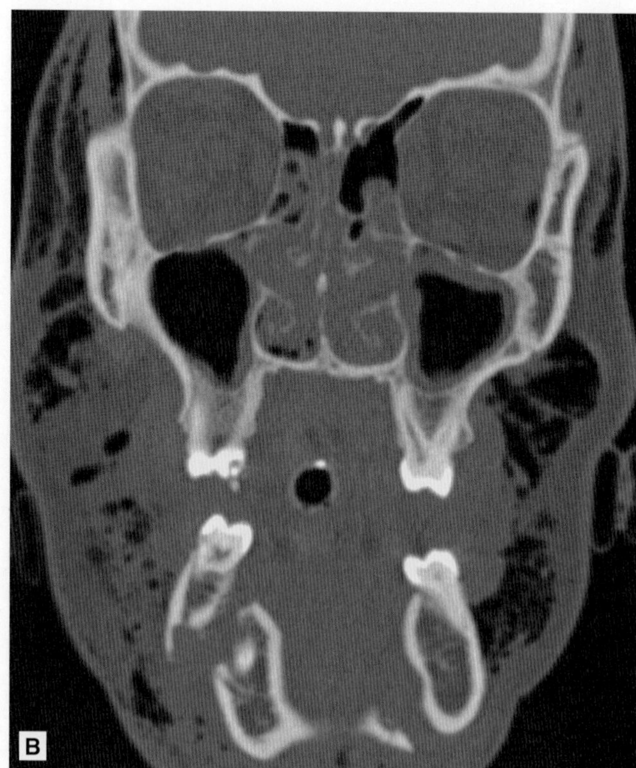

FIGURE 1.99 ■ Mandibular Body Fracture. **A, B:** Axial and coronal NECTs show displaced parasymphyseal and right mandibular body fractures. The molar roots are involved on the right.

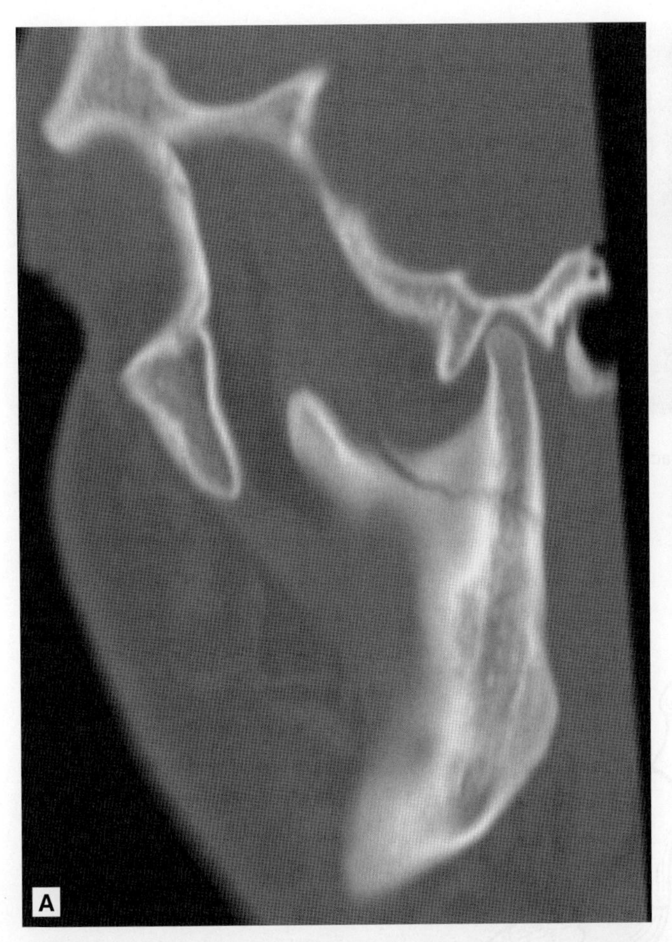

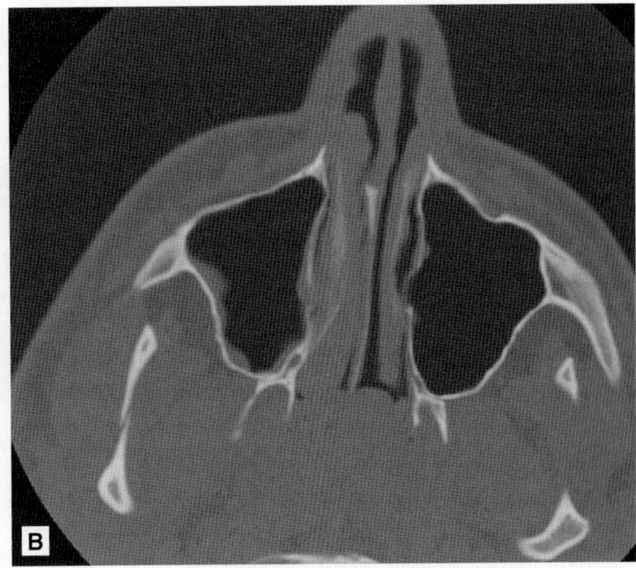

FIGURE 1.100 ■ Subcondylar Mandibular Fracture. **A, B:** Axial and sagittal NECTs show nondisplaced right subcondylar mandibular fracture (seen best on sagittal view).

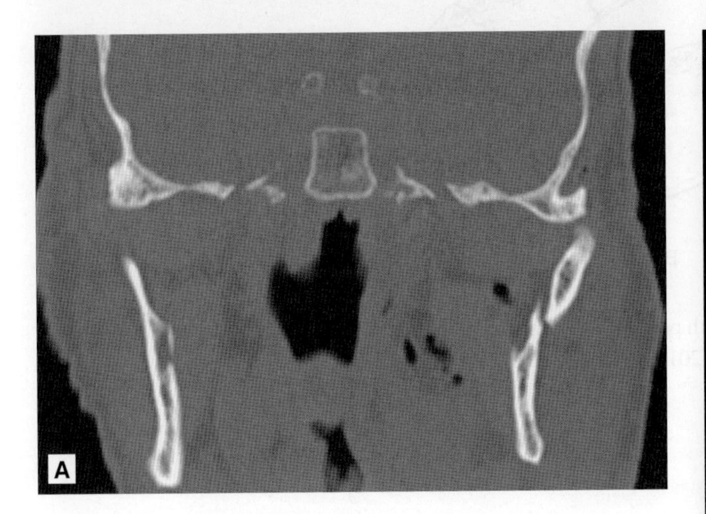

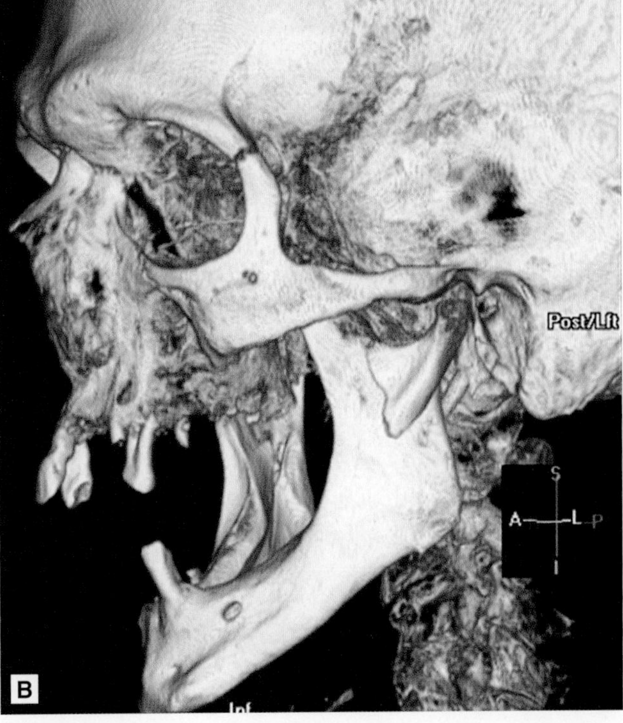

FIGURE 1.101 ■ Condylar Neck Fracture. **A, B:** Coronal and 3D NECTs show displaced left condylar neck fracture.

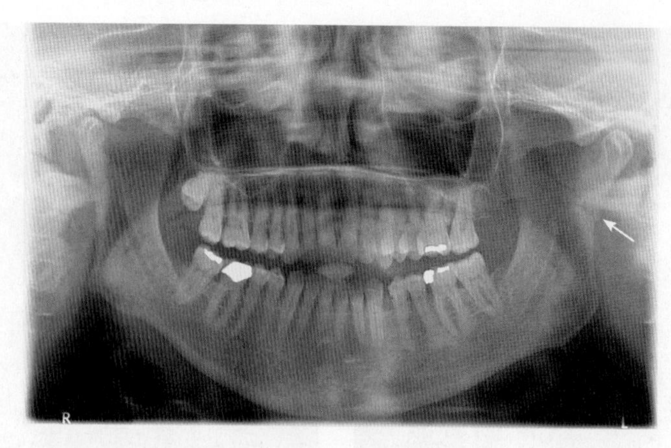

FIGURE 1.102 ■ Mandibular Condylar Fracture. Panorex shows a fracture through the left mandibular condyle (arrow) with some displacement of the condyle.

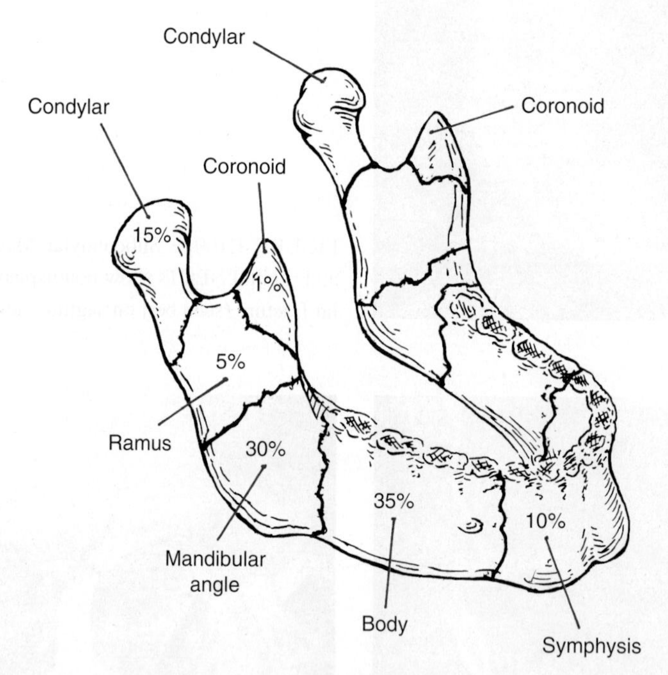

FIGURE 1.103 ■ Mandibular Fracture Frequency. (Reproduced with permission from Knoop KJ, Stack LB, Storrow AB, Thurman RJ, eds. *The Atlas of Emergency Medicine*. 3rd ed. New York: McGraw-Hill; 2010:15. © 2010 McGraw-Hill.)

Radiographic Features

Fractures of the conical orbit may involve the floor, medial wall, roof, or lateral wall. Orbital wall fractures may be part of a ZMC fracture or Le Fort II or III fractures. Fractures of the *orbital floor* are best evaluated in the coronal plane with NC maxillofacial CT. With depressed orbital floor fractures, bone and orbital contents may herniate into the maxillary sinus. An indirect sign of an orbital floor fracture is blood products in the maxillary sinus.

Fractures of the *medial wall of the orbit* (lamina papyracea) can be seen on both coronal and axial CT images. The force required to fracture the orbital floor or medial wall is small because these walls are thin (papyracea is Greek for "like paper-like"). Buckling of the cortex with blood in the ethmoid air cells suggests a fracture. Normally the medial wall is straight and smooth. Bony fragments may be depressed into the ethmoid sinuses. Air within the orbit (orbital emphysema) strongly suggests fracture.

Fractures of the orbital roof are best seen on coronal images, and may extend into the frontal sinus. Pneumocephalus deep to the frontal sinus suggests a fracture of the posterior cortex of the frontal sinus.

Clinical Implications

Traumatic optic neuritis, orbital compartment syndrome, and globe injury are the most important injuries associated with orbital fractures. Enophthalmos is a significant cosmetic concern. Generally, surgery is recommended if greater than 50% of the orbital floor is depressed. A longitudinal medially based fracture may cause a trapdoor effect with entrapment of orbital soft tissue. This occurs when an orbital floor fracture allows herniation of orbital soft tissue but then the bony fragment returns to its normal position. CT findings may be minimal.

Pearls

1. Any orbital emphysema requires a search for subtle fractures.
2. Extraocular muscle entrapment is a clinical diagnosis but can be suggested on CT scan by displacement or stretching of the inferior rectus muscle.
3. Gingival and cheek numbness suggests infraorbital nerve (V2) impingement. The infraorbital foramen is located within the orbital floor.
4. Soft tissue windows on facial CT allow viewing of the extraocular muscles and extraocular hematomas.
5. Hematomas within the orbit may require evacuation if increased intraocular pressure causes proptosis.

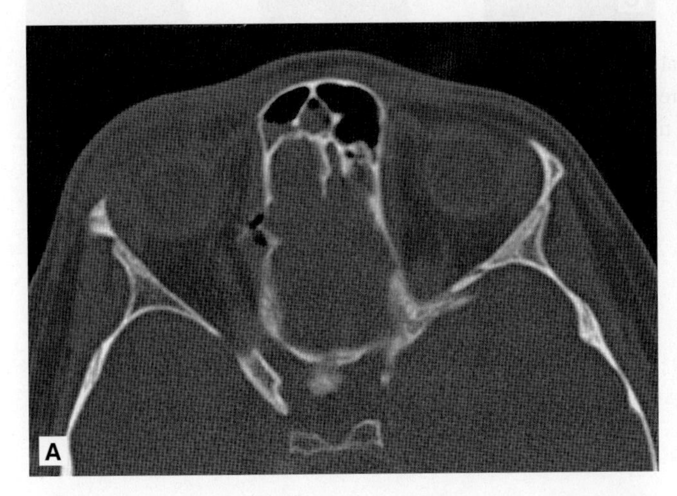

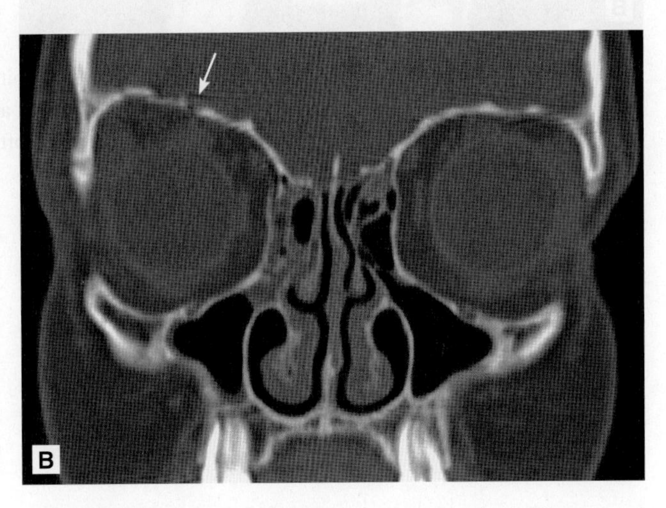

FIGURE 1.104 ■ Minimally Depressed Right Medial Orbital Wall Fracture with Extraconal Air Marking the Fracture. **A, B:** The coronal view shows an associated orbital roof fracture (arrow). Both the orbital roof and floor are best seen in the coronal plane.

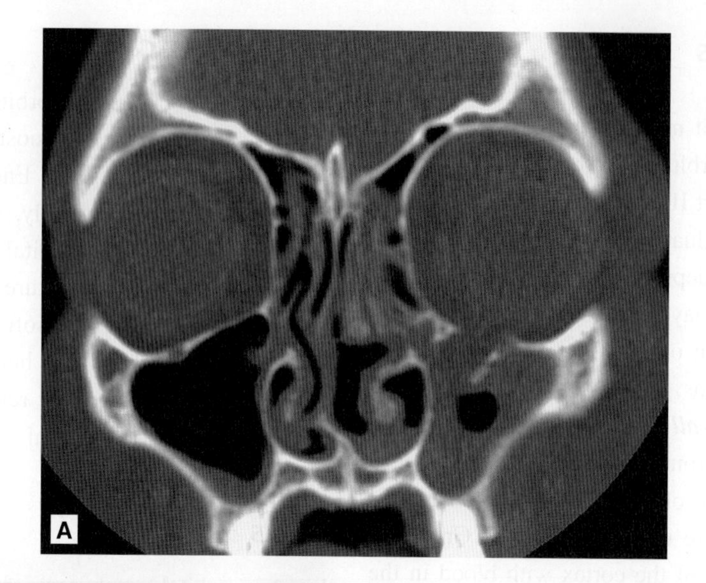

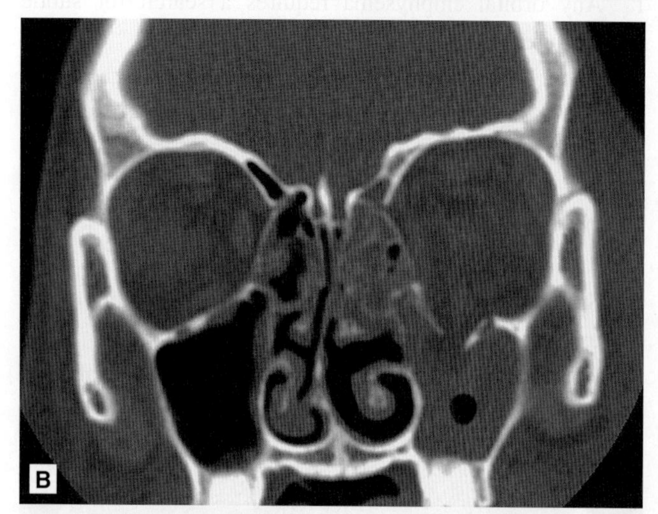

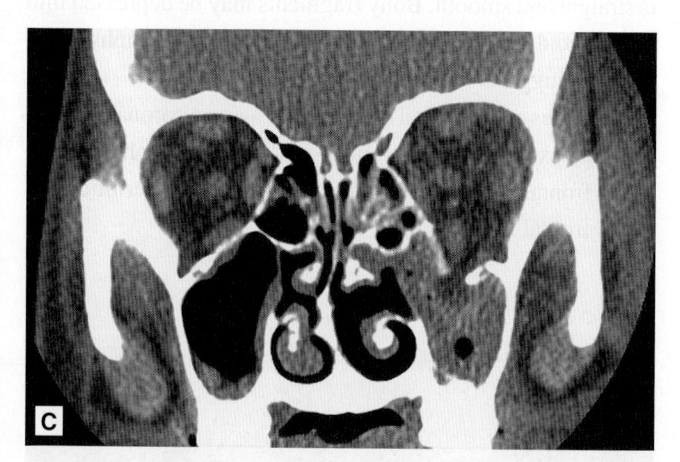

FIGURE 1.105 ■ Orbital Floor Fracture. **A-C:** A depressed left orbital floor fracture through the inferior orbital foramen allows extraconal fat to herniate into the maxillary sinus. The inferior rectus muscles are also displaced downward. Blood fills the maxillary sinus (note the high attenuation of acute blood). Image "C" is same CT but with soft tissue windows that allow for better visualization of soft tissues such as fat and muscle.

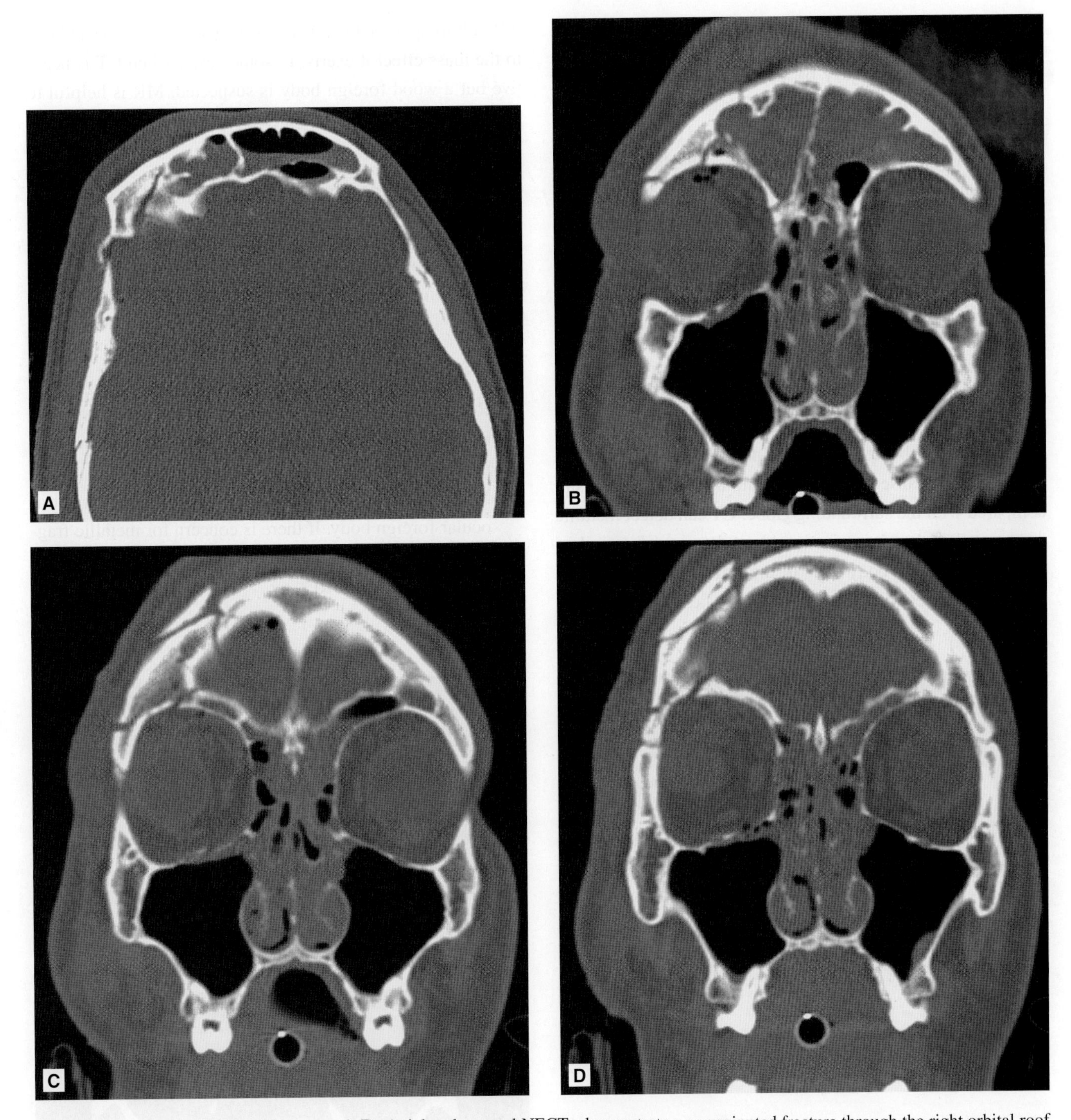

FIGURE 1.106 ■ Orbital Roof Fracture. **A-D:** Axial and coronal NECTs demonstrate a comminuted fracture through the right orbital roof that also involves the right frontal sinus. Note air within the orbit (orbital emphysema) and fluid in the frontal sinuses. The superolateral orbital rim (zygomaticofrontal process) is also involved.

Radiographic Summary

Evaluation of globe injury by CT may detect lens dislocation, globe hemorrhage, open globe, intraocular foreign body, and retinal detachment. Ocular lenses should be located in the anterior portion of the eye and symmetric. Displacement from their normal location should raise suspicion for lens dislocation. Hyperdense fluid within the globe suggests acute retinal, choroidal, or vitreous hemorrhage.

CT findings suggestive of an open globe injury include loss of spherical shape ("flat tire" sign), loss of volume, scleral discontinuity, intraocular air, and intraocular foreign body. Decreased volume of the anterior chamber due to corneal perforation appears as a diminished anterior to posterior distance of the lens compared with the normal globe.

Most foreign bodies are easily identified on CT. Metallic foreign bodies cause streak artifact and have a higher density compared with the surrounding globe. CT can detect metallic fragments less than 1 mm in size. It can detect a 1.5 mm glass intraocular foreign body 96% of the time and is superior to MRI in the detection of most foreign bodies. Wood is more difficult to appreciate on CT, and may only be suspected due to the mass effect it exerts. In some cases, when CT is negative but a wood foreign body is suspected, MR is helpful to identify inflammation related to the foreign body.

Clinical Implications

Intraocular hemorrhage, open globe, intraocular foreign body, and retinal detachment require immediate ophthalmology consultation.

Pearls

1. Retinal detachment extends to the optic nerve, whereas choroidal hemorrhage is biconcave and does not extend to the optic nerve.
2. MRI is contraindicated in patients with metallic intraocular foreign body. If there is concern for metallic fragments in orbits, a plain radiograph of the sinuses can be obtained prior to MRI.

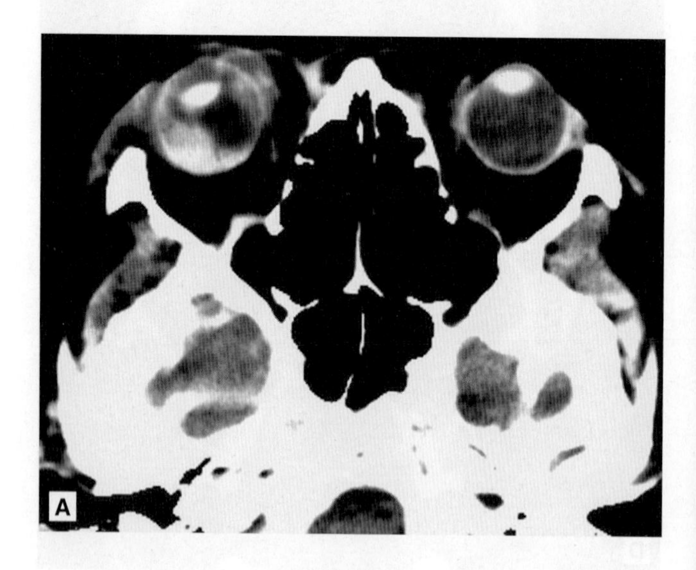

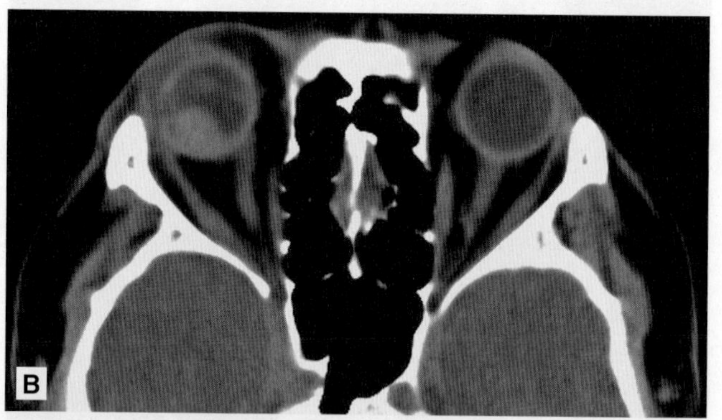

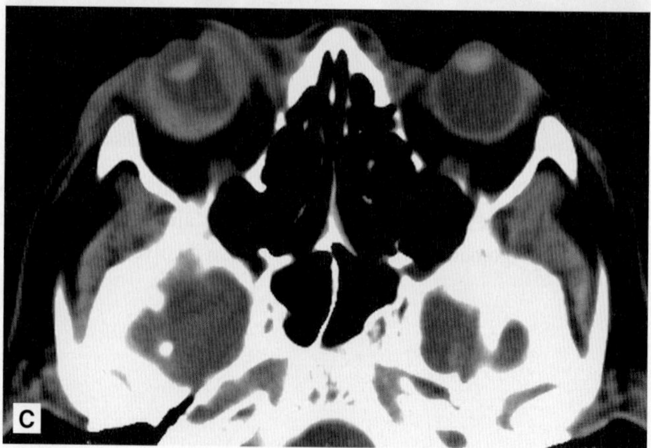

FIGURE 1.107 ■ Globe Hemorrhage. **A-C:** Axial NECT shows hyperdense collection of blood in the posterior chamber of the right eye layering along the retinal surface. In image "A", note how the right lens is more posteriorly located compared with the left, representing lens dislocation.

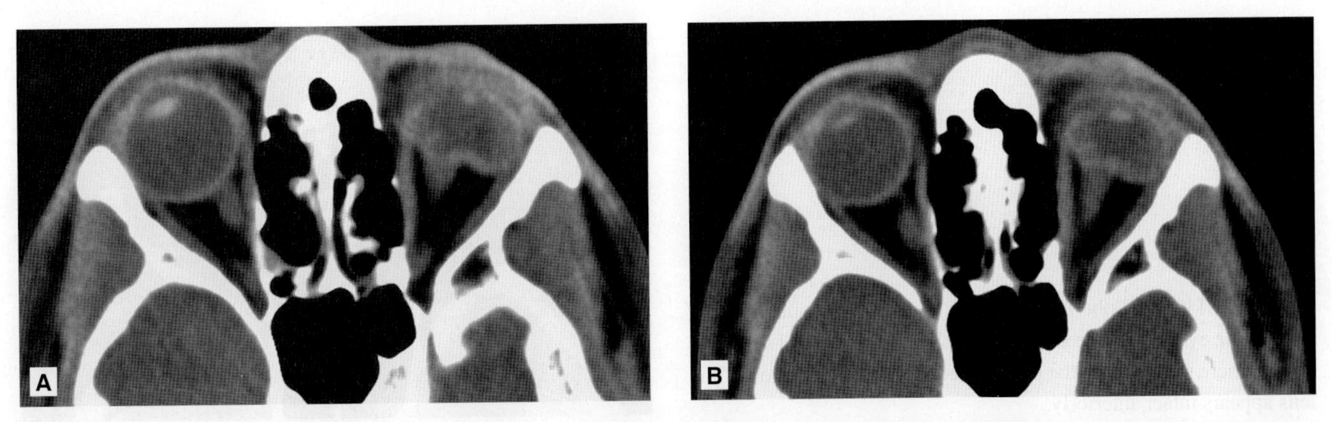

FIGURE 1.108 ■ Open Globe—“Flat Tire” Sign. **A, B:** An 11-year-old male hit in eye with baseball. Axial NECT shows loss of the normal spherical shape of the left globe following trauma. This is called the “flat tire sign.”

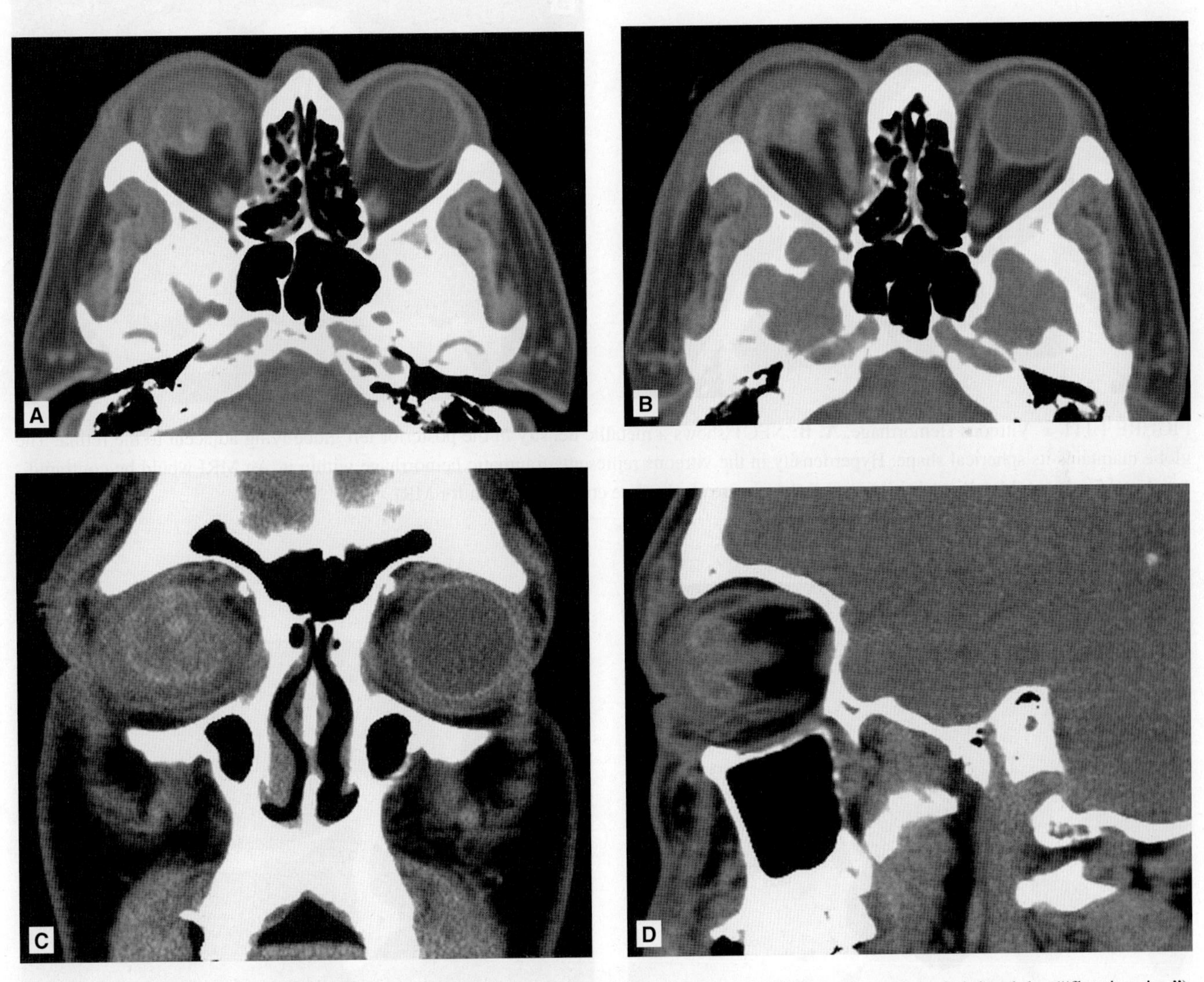

FIGURE 1.109 ■ Open Globe—“Flat Tire” Sign. **A-D:** Axial, coronal, and sagittal NECTs show a ruptured right globe (“flat tire sign”). Note that the right lens is traumatically dislocated and lies adjacent to the retina.

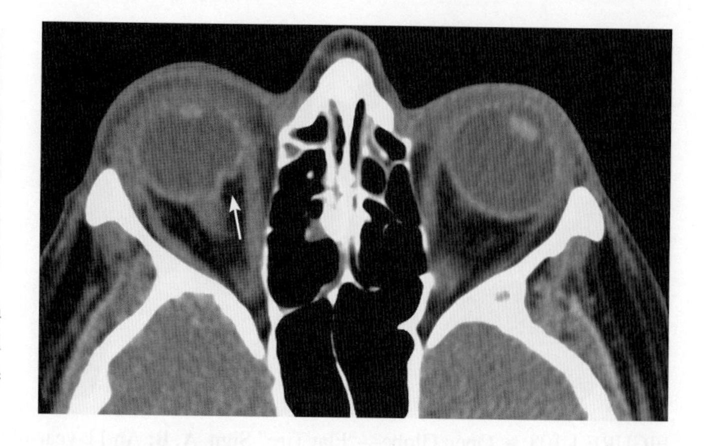

FIGURE 1.110 ■ Globe Foreign Body. Adolescent with a foreign body in the eye. The globe should maintain a nearly perfect spherical shape. There is a defect in the posteromedial right globe (arrow). The lens appears intact anteriorly.

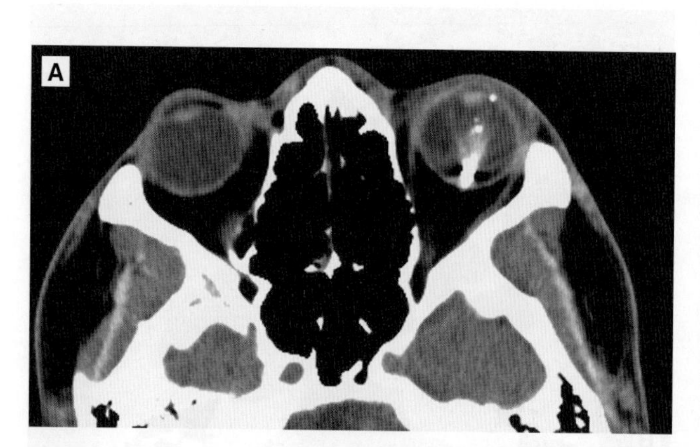

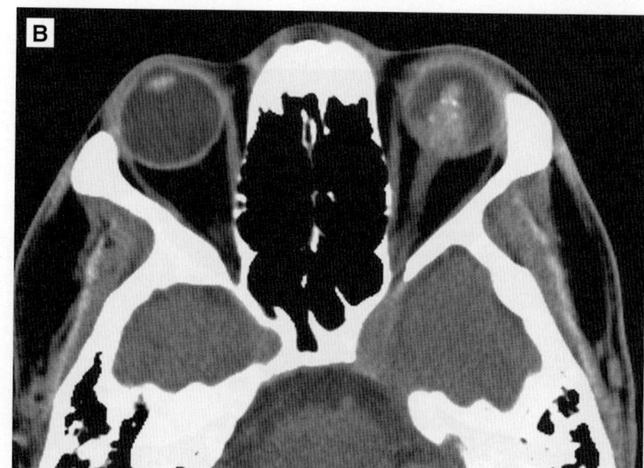

FIGURE 1.111 ■ Vitreous Hemorrhage. **A, B:** NECT shows a metallic density in the posterior left globe lying adjacent to the retina. The globe maintains its spherical shape. Hyperdensity in the vitreous represents traumatic hemorrhage within it. An MRI would be contraindicated in this patient. Metallic debris in or near the eye are an absolute contraindication for MRI.

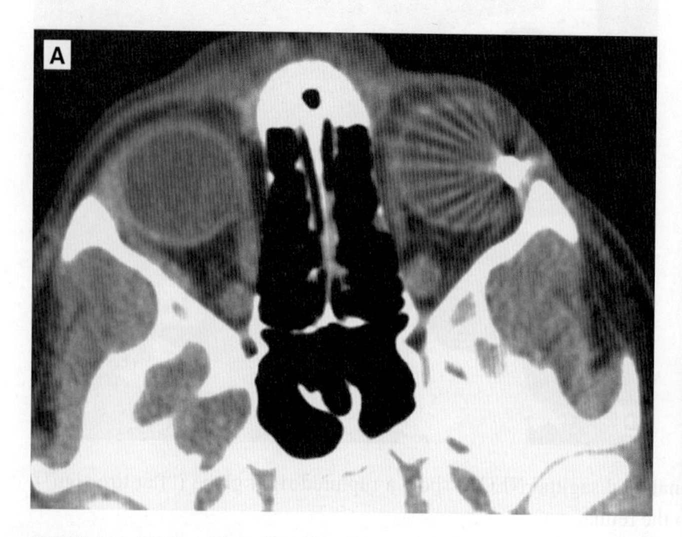

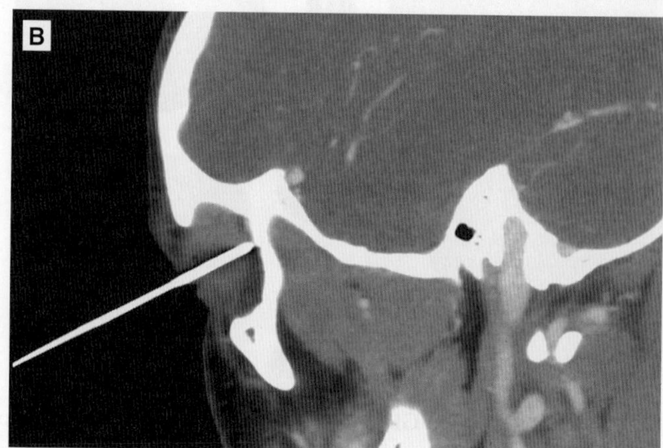

FIGURE 1.112 ■ Globe Foreign Body. **A, B:** Axial and sagittal NECTs show a metallic object near the lateral left eye (blow dart) with rupture of the globe.

Radiographic Features

The ocular muscles and their fasciae form a muscle cone. Outside the muscle cone, but within the orbit, is the "extraconal" space. Traumatic blood on soft tissue windows may have the same density as the extraocular muscles. Hematomas may displace the muscles from their normal position. Proptosis can be secondary to intraorbital pressure from expanding extraconal blood or air. When intraorbital pressure rises, the globe may displace anteriorly due to mass effect, stretching the optic nerve.

Clinical Implications

Ocular compartment syndrome (OCS) results when intraorbital pressure rises. Hematoma, from the injury to the infraorbital artery or one of its branches, is the most common injury resulting in OCS. When intraorbital pressure exceeds the central retinal artery pressure, ischemia may occur. Orbital fractures allow air to enter the orbit through a one-way valve mechanism. The orbital emphysema that results may raise orbital pressure and cause ischemia. OCS is an eyesight-threatening condition that requires immediate decompression with lateral canthotomy.

Pearls

1. Direct traumatic optic neuropathy occurs from impingement, transection, or crush injury to the optic nerve and may cause irreversible visual loss.
2. An afferent pupillary defect and signs of increased intraocular pressure following facial trauma should prompt careful examination for extraconal hematoma or other cause of traumatic optic neuropathy.

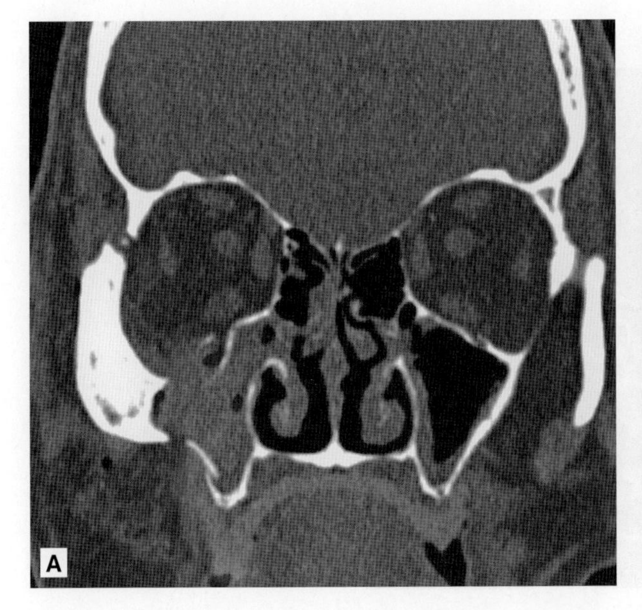

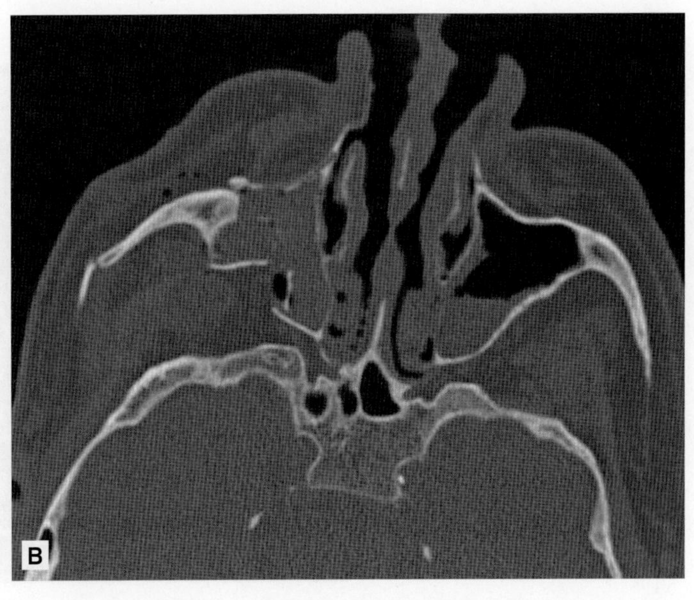

FIGURE 1.113 ■ Extraconal Hematoma. **A, B:** Axial and coronal NECTs of the face show displaced right orbital floor fracture with extraconal hematoma as well as a right ZMC fracture and blood in the maxillary sinus.

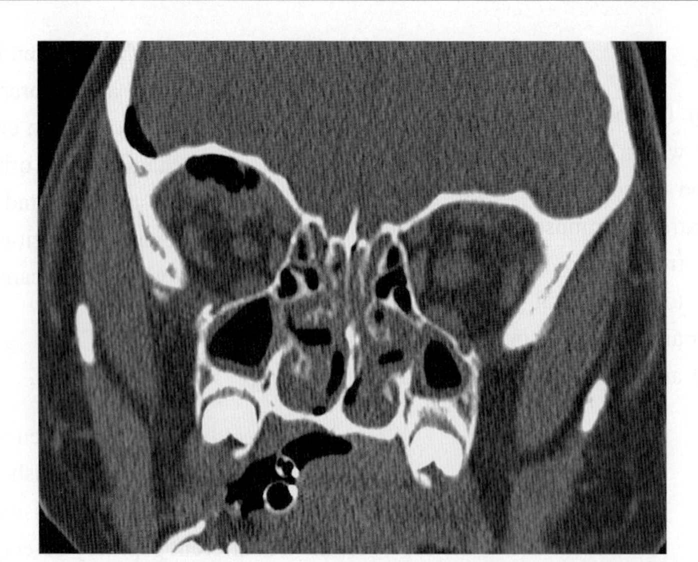

FIGURE 1.114 ■ Extraconal Hematoma. Coronal NECT in a 3-year-old male shows a large right superior extraconal hematoma and orbital emphysema (air in orbit). The superior rectus is displaced inferiorly (compare to the normal left side). Also noted is pneumocephalus related to skull base fractures (not shown on this image).

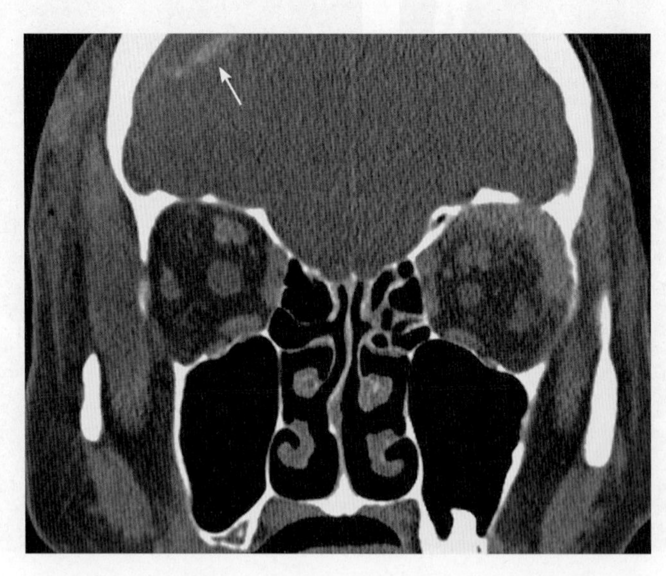

FIGURE 1.115 ■ Extraconal Hematoma. Coronal NECT in a middle-aged female shows extraconal hematoma in the superior and lateral aspect of the left orbit. Also noted is intraparenchymal hemorrhage in the right frontal lobe (arrow).

Chapter 2

ATRAUMATIC CONDITIONS OF THE HEAD AND FACE

Matthew D. Dobbs
Camiron L. Pfennig
Dorris Elise Powell-Tyson
Cari L. Buckingham

Radiographic Summary

Suspected ischemic stroke is one of the most common indications for neurological imaging in the ED. Initial imaging includes NECT and/or MRI. Stroke MRI protocols may be completed in 10 minutes if resources permit, including perfusion imaging. CT findings of acute stroke may include "hyperdense MCA sign" or "dot sign", which is due to thrombus within the proximal MCA or Sylvian MCA branch, "insular ribbon sign" due to obscuration of the insular cortex due to edema, and parenchymal hypodensity. Most commonly however, NECT will be normal in the initial stages of ischemic stroke. Later findings include the development of hypodensity, gyral swelling and sulcal effacement. Hemorrhagic transformation is most common after 1-2 days.

Many centers include CTA or CT Perfusion (CTP) immediately following NECT. CTA allows assessment of stenoses, dissections, vasculitis, or intracranial large vessel thrombus. CTP assesses cerebral blood flow and identifies the core infarct and surrounding tissue-at-risk (penumbra).

DWI is the most sensitive MR sequence for acute ischemia. Findings of "restricted diffusion" are a bright signal on DWI with a corresponding dark signal on ADC. Findings become positive within minutes of ischemia and remain positive for 10 days. MRA can be obtained as an alternative to CTA.

MR perfusion-weighted imaging (PWI) can be obtained with contrast analogous to CTP. In combination with DWI, mismatches between DWI infarct and PWI ischemic tissue can be used to determine if any salvageable penumbra tissue exists.

Clinical Implications

An ischemic stroke results from brain hypoperfusion due to thrombus, emboli, dissection, stenosis, or hypotension. Patients with ischemic stroke may present with the sudden onset of focal neurologic deficits such as motor weakness, sensory deficits, or speech difficulties. Current NINDS guidelines recommend that the ED physician complete the initial assessment and NECT within 25 minutes of patient arrival to maximize potential benefit for reperfusion therapy.

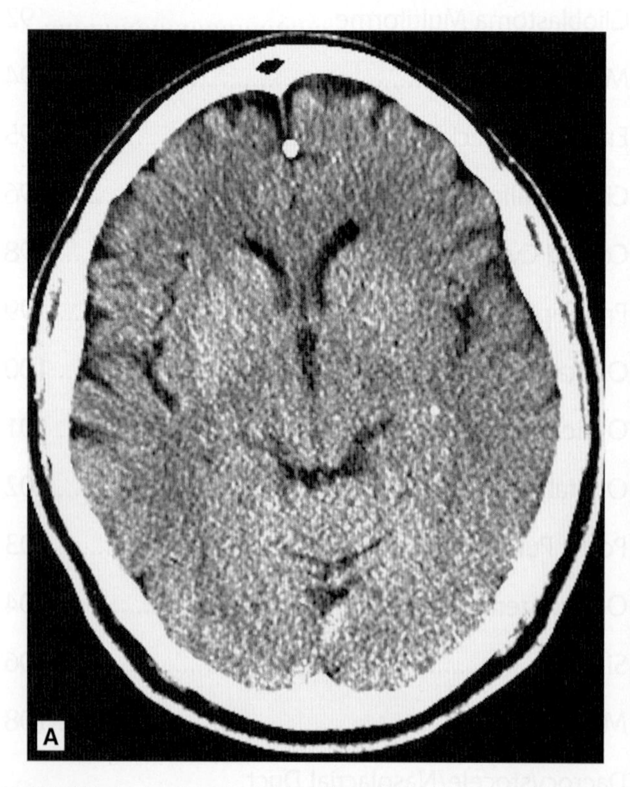

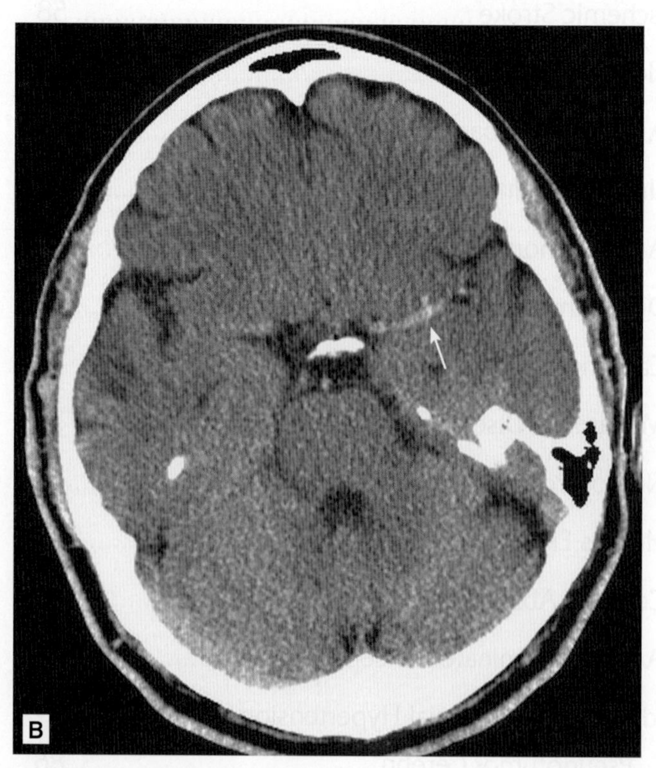

FIGURE 2.1 ■ Ischemic Stroke. **A:** NECT shows subtle loss of the left insular ribbon (region between the lentiform nuclei and Sylvian fissure), sulcal effacement, and mild edema that blurs the gray-white interface. Findings suggest acute MCA infarction. **B:** NECT shows hyperdensity in the region of the left middle cerebral artery ("hyperdense MCA sign") (arrow).

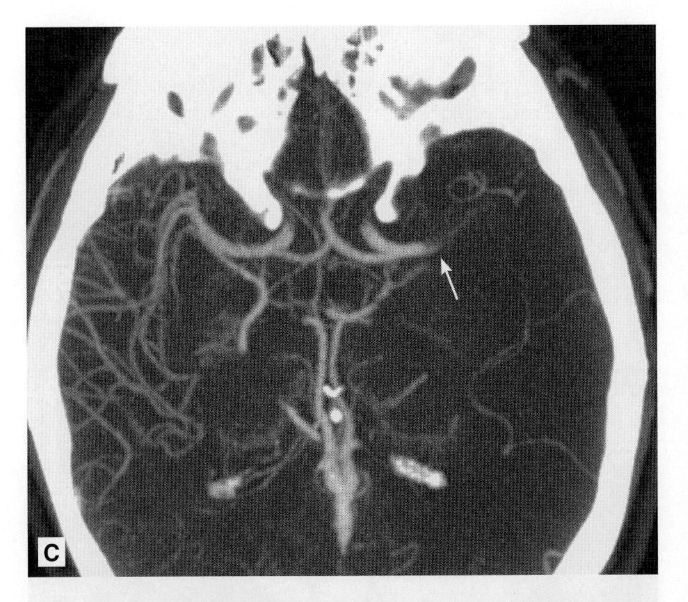

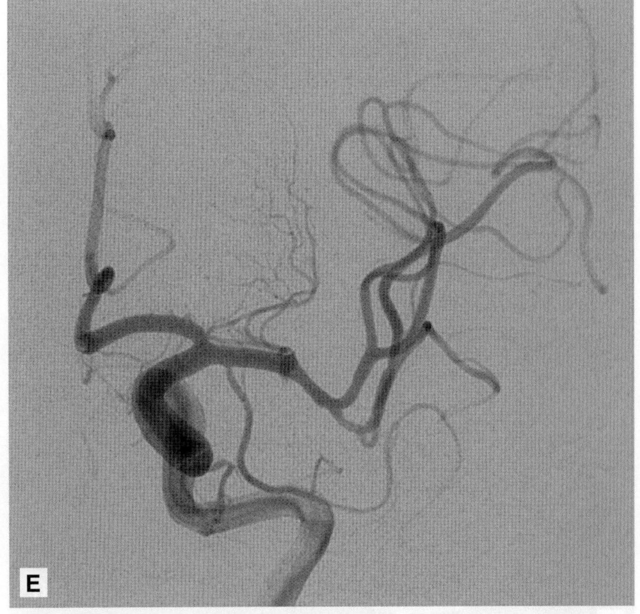

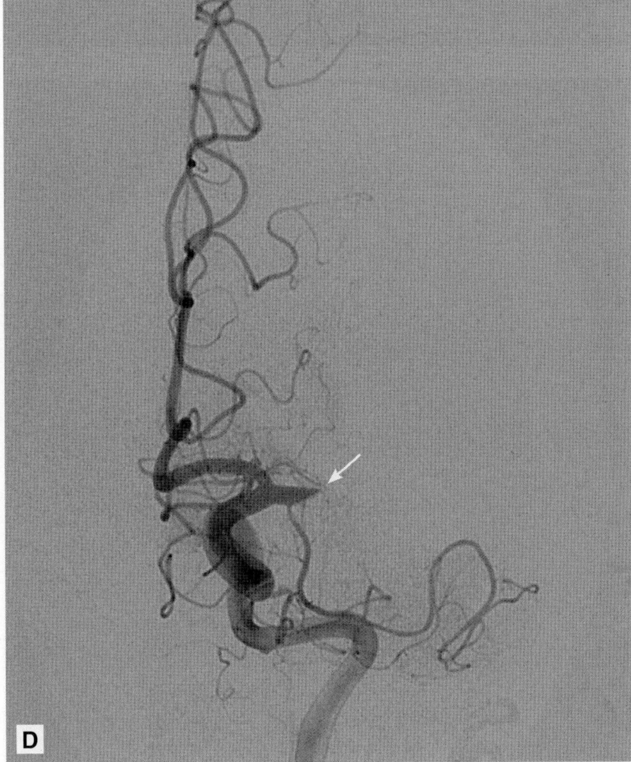

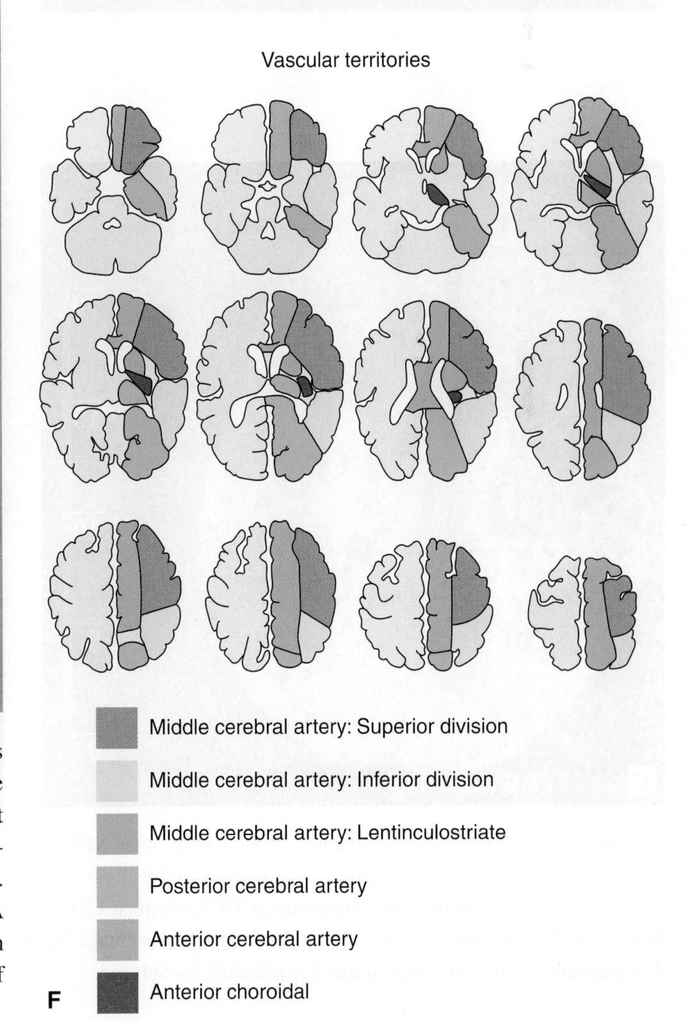

FIGURE 2.1 ■ (*Continued*) **C:** Axial CTA confirms the thrombus occluding the proximal (M1) segment of the left MCA with little collateral flow distally (arrow). **D:** Conventional angiogram of left carotid injection shows cut-off of middle cerebral artery on left corresponding to the CTA (arrow). Normal filling is seen in the ACA. **E:** Angiogram of left carotid injection following intra-arterial tPA and MERCI thrombus removal device intervention shows restoration of blood flow into the left MCA vessels. **F:** Schematic diagram of cerebrovascular territories.

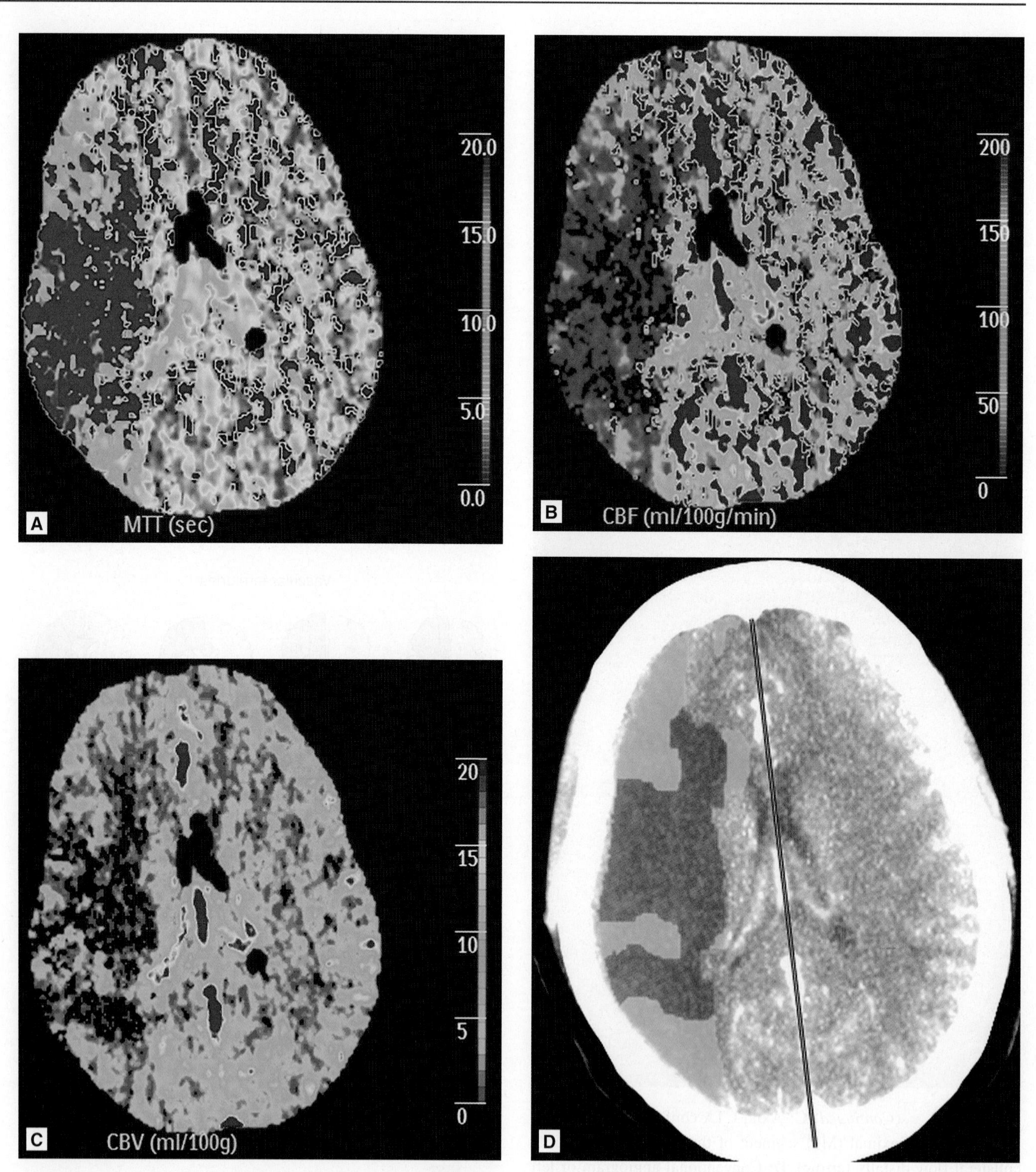

FIGURE 2.2 ■ CT Perfusion Obtained Immediately After NECT. **A:** Mean transit time (MTT) map at level of basal ganglia shows prolonged transit through the right MCA territory indicating sluggish blood flow in this region. **B:** CT Perfusion cerebral blood flow (CBF) map shows decreased blood flow in corresponding MCA territory. **C:** CT Perfusion cerebral blood volume (CBV) map shows markedly decreased delivery of blood volume to this region. **D:** CT Perfusion image based on calculations indicates area of infarct (red) and penumbra (green). The penumbra is the only region that has potential for salvage.

The most recent American Heart Association guidelines recommend that IV tPA may be given up to 4.5 hours after the onset of ischemic stroke. It is crucial to obtain imaging studies prior to the administration of thrombolytics as acute hemorrhage must be ruled out prior to treatment. The more rapidly that studies can be obtained, the sooner treatment decisions can be made, a critical element of emergent stroke care as the earlier the treatment is begun the higher the odds ratio is for positive clinical outcome.

Pearls

1. Edema related to an infarct typically involves gray and white matter. If edema only involves white matter, consider alternative diagnoses such as tumor.
2. Diffusion MRI becomes positive within minutes of acute ischemic stroke, but it usually takes at least 4.5 hours for FLAIR sequences to demonstrate hyperintensity.
3. A dense MCA sign corresponds to a significant acute clot in the proximal cerebral vasculature. Patients with this radiographic finding may benefit from neurointerventional procedures to aid in clot lysis or mechanical clot removal in order to reperfuse ischemic brain tissue.

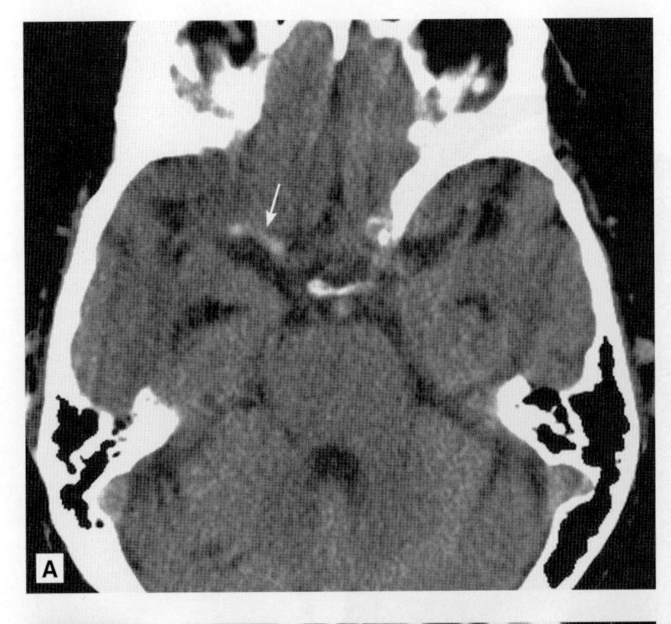

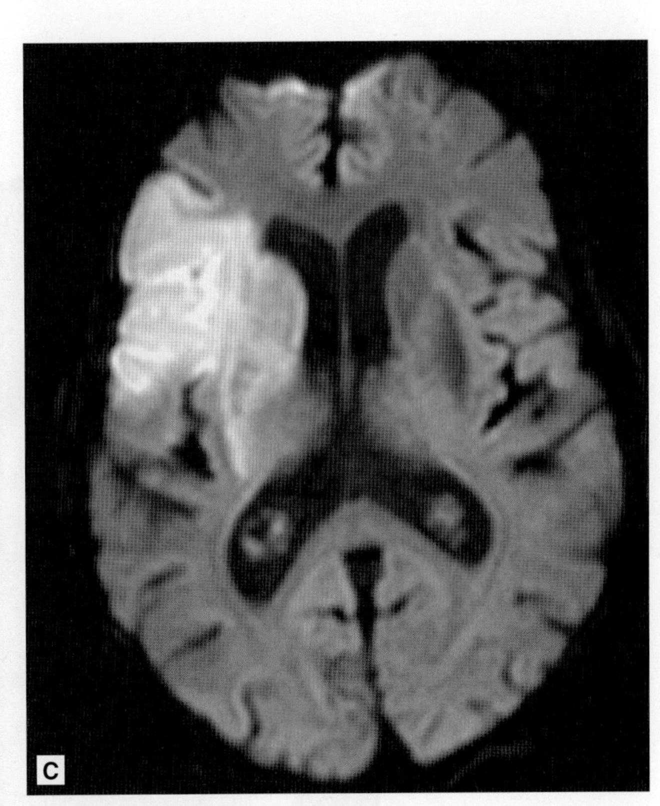

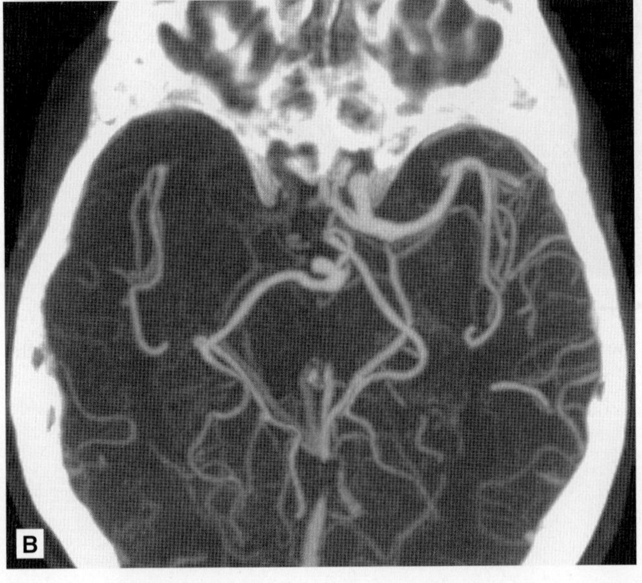

FIGURE 2.3 ■ Ischemic Stroke. **A:** 80-year-old female NECT shows hyperdensity in right MCA (hyperdense MCA sign) (arrow). **B:** Axial CTA MIP shows cutoff of right MCA indicating thrombus. **C:** DWI MRI shows restricted diffusion in the right MCA territory involving the basal ganglia, right frontal, and right temporal lobes indicating acute infarction.

Radiographic Summary

Hemorrhagic strokes are acute bleeding events in the brain and may result in the rapid development of neurological impairment, respiratory failure, and death. In suspected acute stroke, NECT of the brain or MRI is necessary for treatment planning. MRI with gradient-based sequences is superior to CT for detection of hemorrhage, but is less often used in most centers due to its time, expense, and availability.

Acute parenchymal hemorrhage on CT will be hyperdense (bright). MRI of hyperacute (less than 12 hours) blood will be T1 isointense, T2 hyperintense, and hypointense on T2*/GRE. Common locations for hypertensive hemorrhage are the basal ganglia, thalamus, pons, and cerebellum. Occasionally blood can seep into the adjacent ventricular system. Hemorrhages in other locations suggest an alternate etiology, such as vascular malformation (AVM, cavernous malformation), tumor, or amyloid angiopath.

Clinical Implications

Hemorrhagic stroke accounts for about 10-15% of all strokes, with a higher mortality rate when compared to ischemic stroke. It is important to ask about usage of any anti-platelet agents or warfarin when obtaining history. Patients with acute ICH may have additional clinical symptoms that go along with focal neurological deficits such as headache, seizures, persistent nausea and vomiting, altered mental status, and

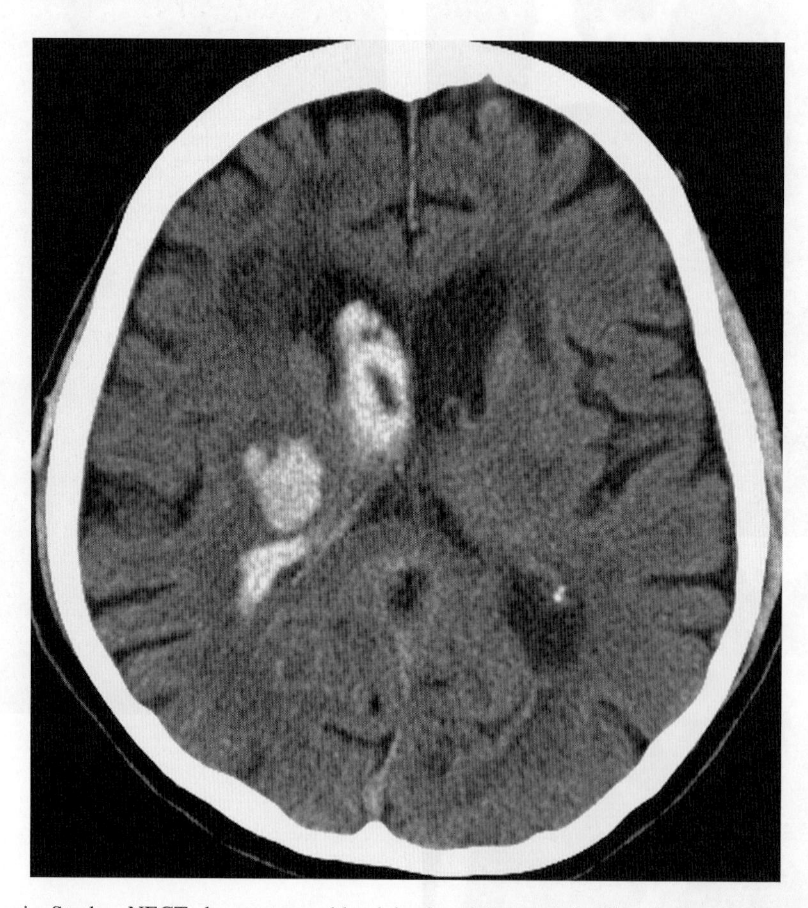

FIGURE 2.4 ■ Hemorrhagic Stroke. NECT demonstrates blood in the right posterior basal ganglia/thalamus as well as within the lateral ventricle.

cardiopulmonary failure. The mechanism of ICH is thought to be leakage from small intracerebral arteries damaged by long-standing high blood pressure. Other causes include cerebral amyloidosis, iatrogenic anticoagulation, bleeding diathesis, and use of cocaine. In addition to the focally injured area, there is additional pressure produced by the mass effect of the hematoma and bleeding that subsequently may lead to rapid increases in intracranial pressure. Decompressive craniotomy may be required in some instances.

Pearls

1. Morbidity and mortality rates are higher for hemorrhagic strokes than ischemic strokes.
2. Acute respiratory failure and need for emergent airway management are much more common with acute hemorrhagic stroke than with ischemic stroke.
3. NECT is the first-line imaging for the detection of acute hemorrhagic stroke.

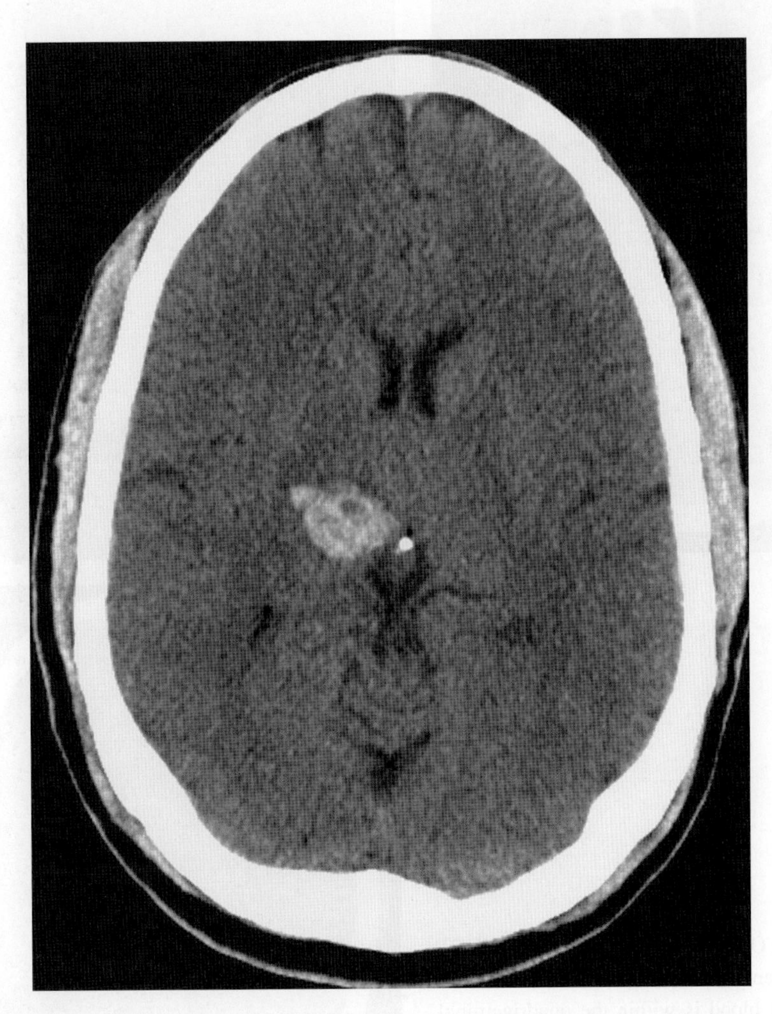

FIGURE 2.5 ■ Hemorrhagic Stroke. NECT in a 41-year-old male with left-sided weakness and systolic blood pressure of 175 mmHg shows acute hemorrhage in the right thalamus.

Radiographic Summary

Atraumatic subarachnoid hemorrhage (SAH) usually results from a ruptured aneurysm, 90% of which arise from the circle of Willis. NECT is the initial choice for imaging patients with suspected SAH. Blood appears as a hyperdensity within the basilar cisterns and sulci but may also be commonly seen along the sylvian fissure and interpenduncular fossa. MRI is nearly as sensitive as CT for hyperacute (less than 12 hours) SAH detection. After 24 hours, MRI is superior to CT for detection of blood products as the sensitivity of CT for SAH detection drops to 93% by 24 hours and 50% at 7 days as the SAH is cleared by the CSF circulation. FLAIR demonstrates SAH as a bright signal along the cerebral sulci or within the basilar cisterns and T2*/GRE sequences show areas of a dark signal within the sulci.

The location of SAH may suggest where the aneurysm is located. Blood in the anterior interhemispheric fissure suggests aneurysm of the ACOM (anterior communicating) artery. Sylvian fissure blood correlates with the middle

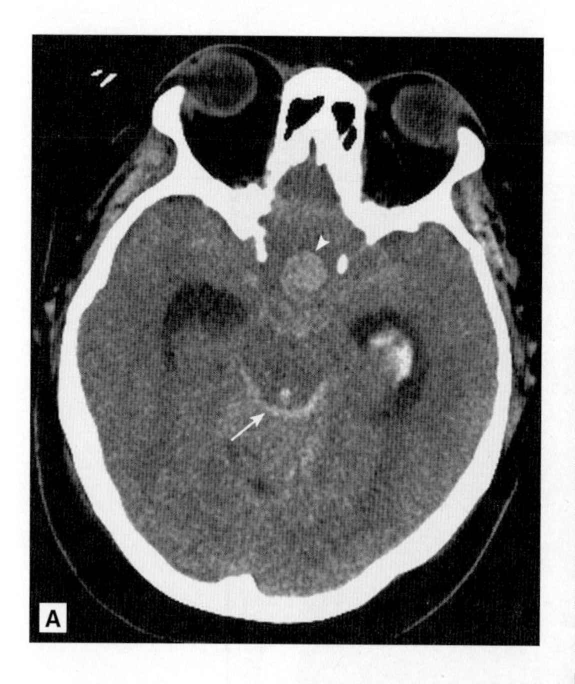

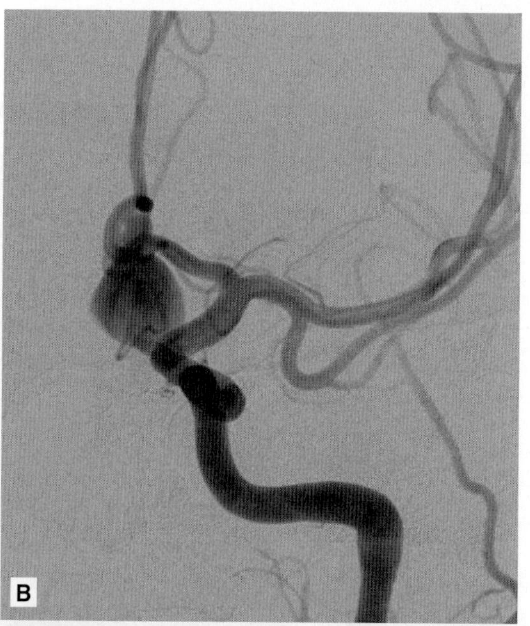

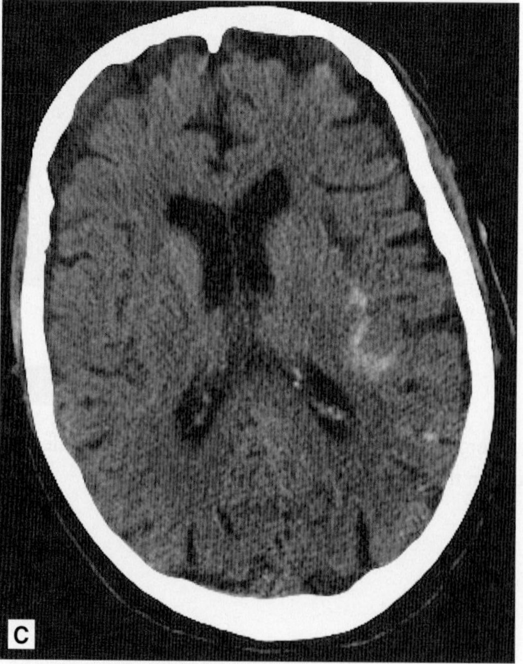

FIGURE 2.6 ■ ACOM Aneurysm with SAH. **A:** NECT shows dilation of temporal horns with blood in the left side. Subarachnoid blood is within the quadrigeminal and ambient cisterns (arrow). A round gray object is seen in the interhemispheric fissure representing a large ACOM aneurysm (arrowhead). **B:** Magnified frontal angiogram of carotid injection shows saccular aneurysm arising from the anterior communicating artery. **C:** (In a different patient): Axial NECT shows small amount of SAH in the left Sylvian fissure.

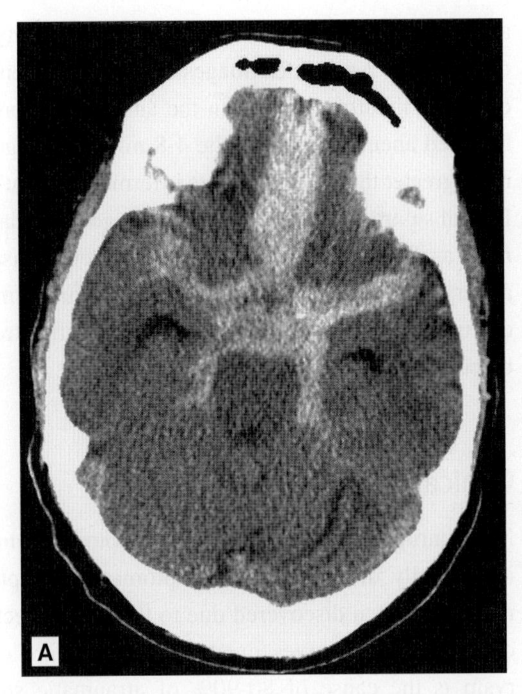

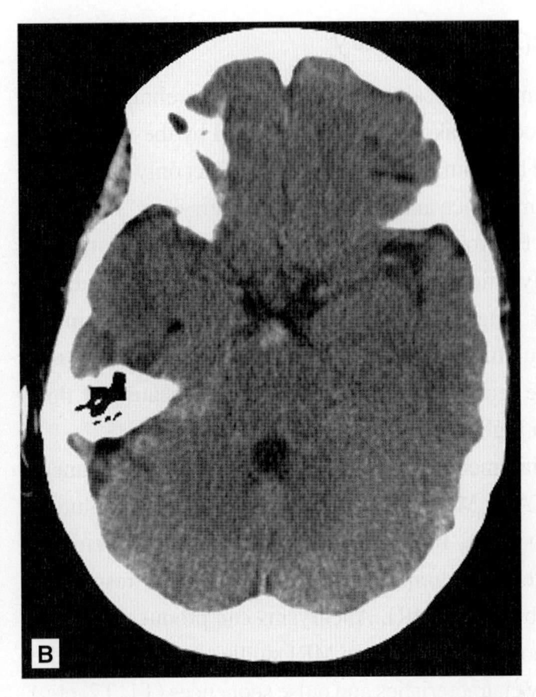

FIGURE 2.7 ■ Atraumatic Subarachnoid Hemorrhage. **A:** NECT (different patient from images 8a-8d) shows extensive SAH throughout the basilar cisterns, prepontine cistern, and anterior interhemispheric fissure. **B:** NECT shows small focus of SAH in the interpeduncular fossa. Angiography was negative. Patient was diagnosed with a perimesencephalic nonaneurysmal SAH.

cerebral artery (MCA), and blood located in the posterior fossa correlates with a posterior circulation aneurysm (basilar artery or PICA).

An entity called perimesencephalic nonaneurysmal SAH exists in which SAH is present in the preponting cistern, interpeduncular fossa, or ambient cisterns; however, angiography will fail to reveal an aneurysm. The source is thought to be venous and the risk of re-bleeding is exceedingly low with a benign clinical course.

Clinical Implications

Patients with SAH often present with sudden onset of severe headache "thunderclap headache" accompanied by possible syncope, nausea, vomiting, photophobia, and focal neurological deficits. Meningeal irritation or neck stiffness may be a sign of a ruptured aneurysm. Grading of SAH depends on the patient's neurological state, with a higher mortality rate associated with more profound disability on presentation. Treatment is based upon the availability of interventional neuroradiology/endovascular neurosurgery. Some studies have shown lower morbidity and mortality with coil embolization versus surgical clipping. SAH can cause hydrocephalus by obstructing the arachnoid villi and interrupting the normal flow of CSF. After several days, SAH can also cause dangerous vasospasm of the cerebral vessels.

If there is high clinical suspicion for SAH in the face of a negative CT scan, a lumbar puncture must be performed to assess for RBC's and xanthrochromia in order to rule out hemorrhage. There is emerging literature to suggest a NECT plus CT angiography may become a suitable approach to rule out SAH, but this method has not been proven to date.

Pearls

1. Emergent NECT is the initial preferred imaging modality for patients with suspected SAH with nearly 100% sensitivity if performed within 12 hours.
2. If NECT reveals SAH, CTA or cerebral angiography is the next step. If this is normal, a repeat CTA in 7-14 days is recommended to re-assess for a bleeding source. If the 2nd CTA is negative, an MRI is recommended to assess for vascular malformations of the brain, brainstem, or spinal cord.
3. If NECT reveals no SAH, lumbar puncture is the next step. If lumbar puncture reveals xanthochromia or elevated red-cell count, CTA or cerebral angiography is indicated.

Radiographic Summary

An aneurysm is a focal outpouching of a cerebral artery at an area of focal weakness that is contained by the media and adventitia. These intracranial aneurysms affect only part of the vessel circumference and are also called "berry" or "saccular" aneurysms. Fusiform aneurysms are long areas of dilation of a vessel. Mycotic aneurysms are an entity due to infection (bacterial or fungal). They are often found in the distal intracranial vasculature near branch-points. They lack a true vessel wall and are technically pseudoaneurysms. Because of this, they are at a high risk of rupture.

The initial method for evaluation of intracranial aneurysms is CTA or MRA. CTA offers greater spatial resolution compared to MRA. If CTA is equivocal and concern remains high, catheter angiography is needed as it offers resolution unmatched by CT or MRI. Aneurysms can produce hyperintense or hypointense signals on MRI studies depending on the specific flow characteristics and pulse sequences (T1, T2, etc.) used. The typical aneurysm lumen with rapid flow is visible as a well-delineated mass that shows high-velocity signal loss on T1- and T2-weighted images. Signal heterogeneity may be observed if turbulent flow in the aneurysm is present. Most ruptured aneurysms are in the 4-8 mm size range. An aneurysm greater than 25 mm in size is termed a "giant" aneurysm. Digital subtraction angiography is the gold standard for diagnosis as this modality affords the most accurate assessment of aneurysm size, configuration (saccular or fusiform), and neck evaluation (narrow or broad). Coil embolization treatment can be performed during the same procedure.

Clinical Implications

Most unruptured aneurysms are asymptomatic and are often incidentally discovered. If symptomatic, unruptured aneurysms are often discovered due to the mass effect they exert on surrounding nerves or structures. Rupture of an aneurysm is the cause of 80-90% of atraumatic subarachnoid hemorrhage.

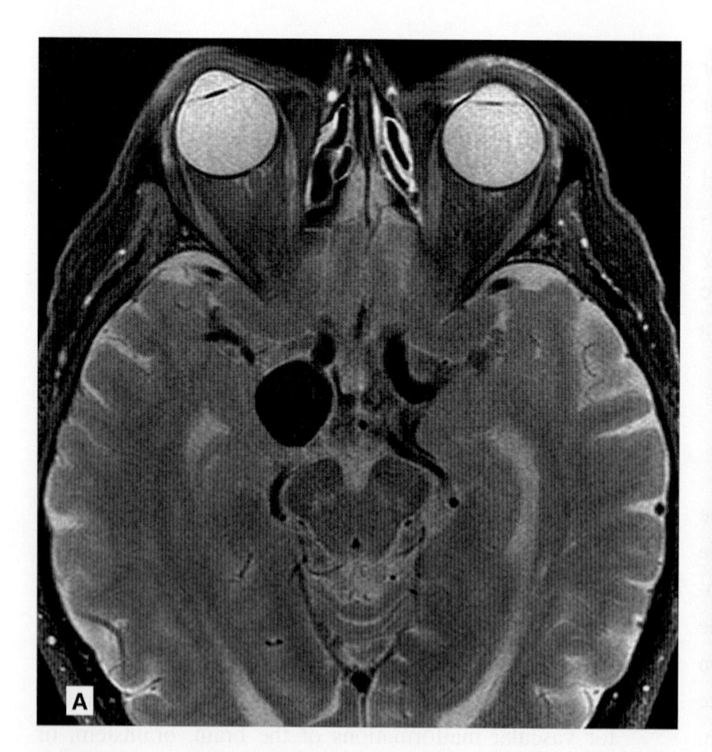

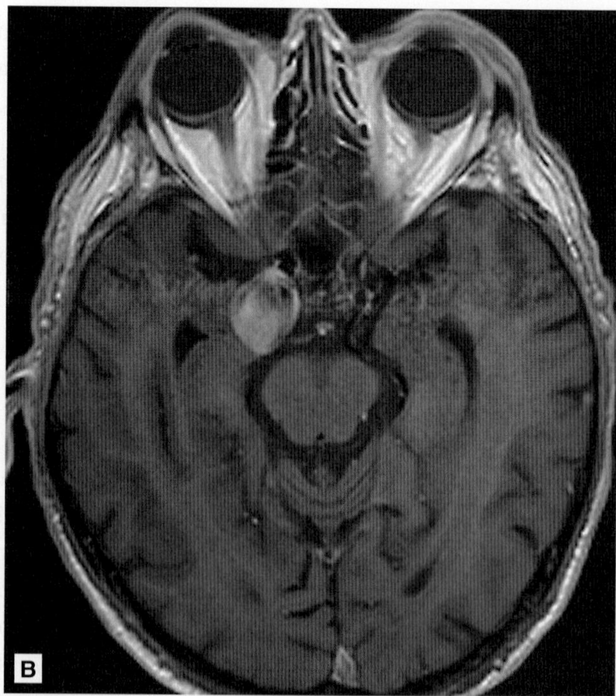

FIGURE 2.8 ■ MCA Aneurysm. **A:** A 77-year-old-male presenting with right CN III palsy. T2 MR shows a large round lesion in the right parasellar region. **B:** T1+C MR, shows pulsation artifact and enhancement within the lesion, confirming an aneurysm. The pulsation artifact is due to the movement of blood.

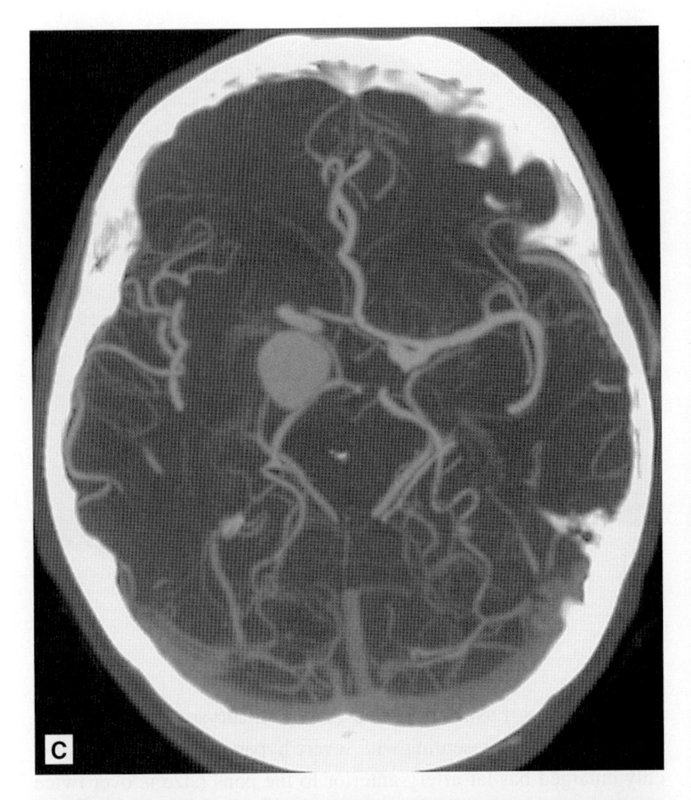

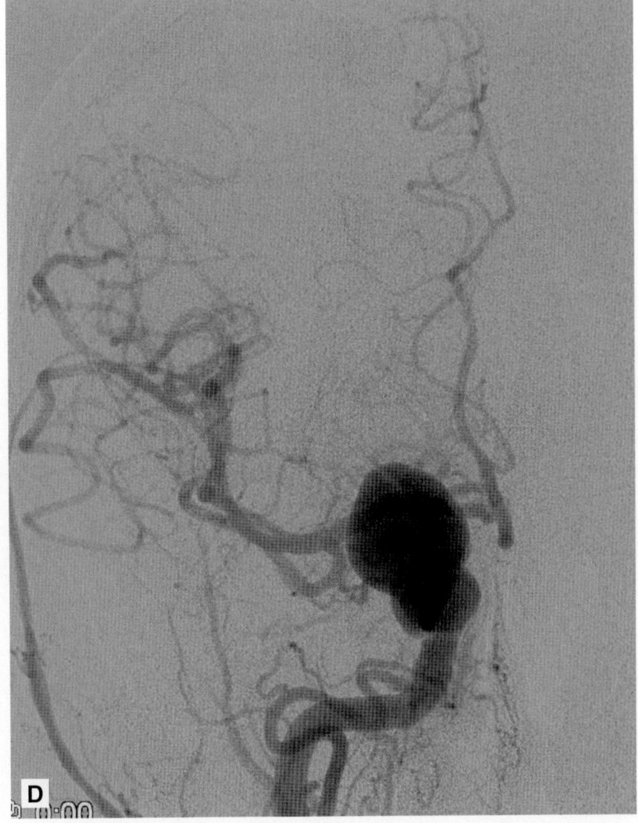

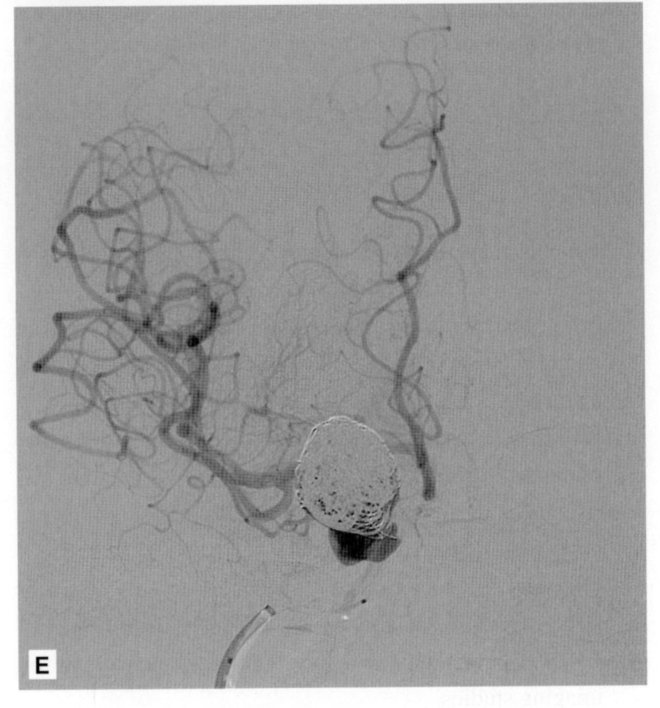

FIGURE 2.8 ■ (*Continued*) **C:** Axial CTA shows the large aneurysm that is actually arising from the ICA terminus. On this image, the aneurysm is seen displacing the PCOM artery. The 3rd cranial nerve runs adjacent to the PCOM, and is being impinged upon by the aneurysm causing a 3rd nerve palsy. **D:** Frontal angiogram from right carotid artery injection demonstrates a large aneurysm sac filling with contrast confirming the findings seen on CT/MRI. **E:** Frontal angiogram following endovascular coil embolization of the large aneurysm with minimal residual filling of the neck of the aneurysm.

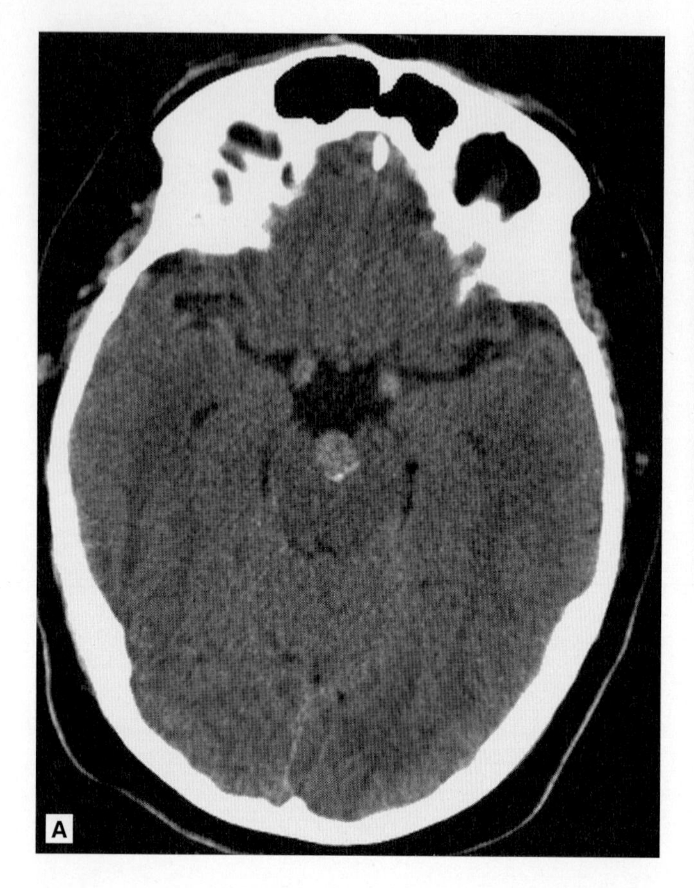

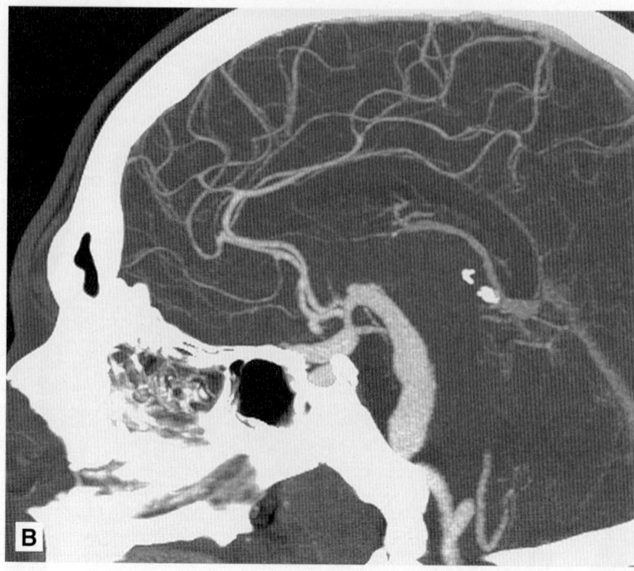

FIGURE 2.9 ■ Fusiform Basilar Artery Aneurysm. **A:** NECT in a 39-year-old male presenting with severe hypertension shows a markedly enlarged basilar artery anterior to the pons (size is over twice that of internal carotid arteries). **B:** Sagittal CTA shows long segment fusiform aneurysm of the basilar artery without rupture.

A classic symptom of an unruptured aneurysm is a PCOM aneurysm causing painful third nerve palsy with a "blown pupil." The oculomotor nerve (CN III) passes directly lateral to the PCOM and may be compressed by an enlarging aneurysm. The PCOM branches off the ICA as it enters the brain. The junction of the PCOM and the ICA is the most common site for a PCOM aneurysm. Coil embolization or surgical clipping are the treatments of unruptured aneurysms.

Unruptured aneurysms vary in their risk of rupture based on their size and location. The larger the aneurysm, the higher the risk of rupture, with anterior circulation aneurysms having a lower 5-year risk of rupture than posterior circulation aneurysms.

Pearls

1. Patients may report headache on the same side as the aneurysm. Painful compression of the third nerve resulting in ipsilateral 3rd nerve palsy is a common symptom and may be the only deficit in patients harboring a PCOM aneurysm.
2. CTA or MRA is the preferred initial imaging. Angiography remains the gold standard. Due to the invasive nature and risks of conventional angiography, noninvasive imaging is pursued first.
3. CTA and MRA can reliably detect aneurysms 3 mm or larger with 90% sensitivity.
4. 15-20% of patients will have multiple aneursysms on imaging studies.

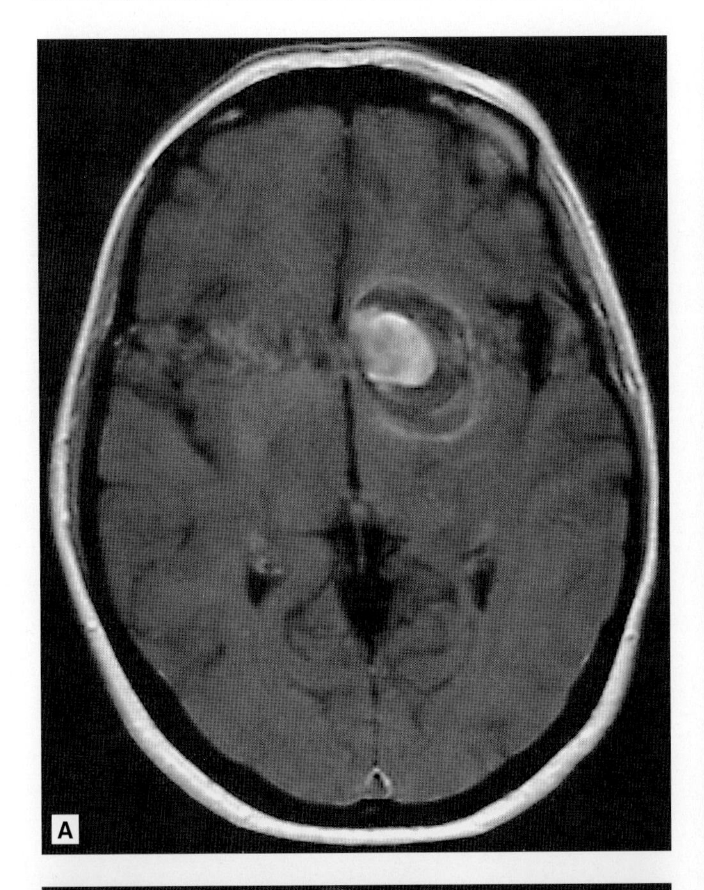

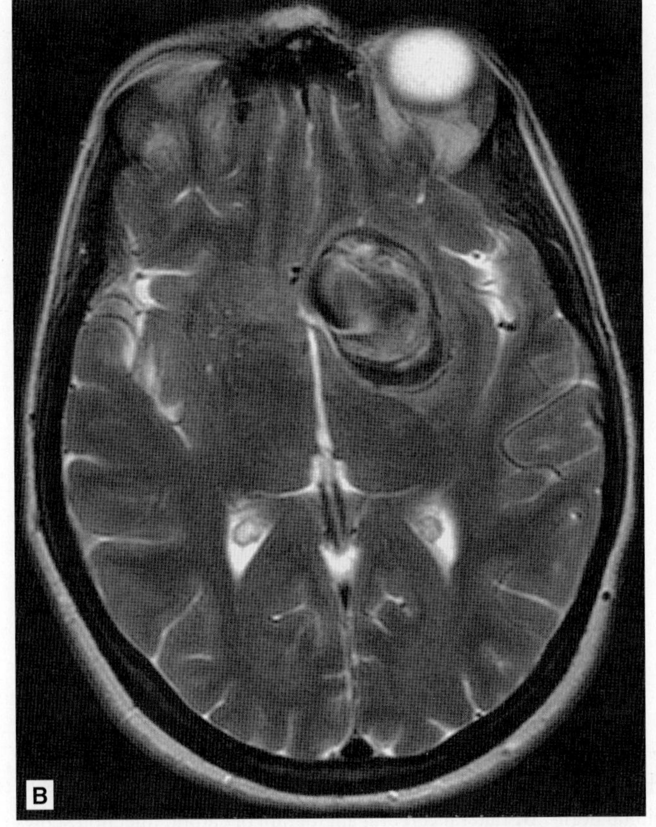

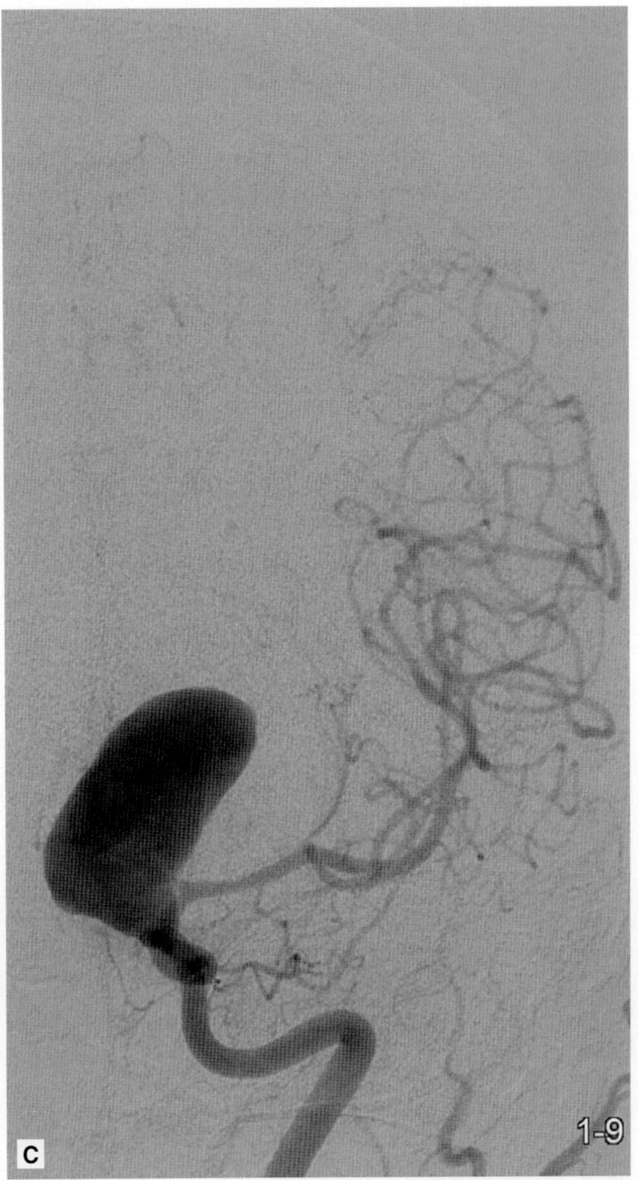

FIGURE 2.10 ■ MCA Aneurysm. **A:** Axial T1 MRI without contrast demonstrates a large mass near the inferior left basal ganglia containing areas of bright signal (thrombus or slow-moving blood). The horizontal pulsation artifact indicates that this is an aneurysm as a tumor would not cause a MRI pulsation artifact. **B:** Axial T2 image shows mixed bright and dark T2 signal within this large aneurysm representing areas of flowing blood (dark signal) and slow-moving blood or thrombus (brighter signal). **C:** Frontal angiogram demonstrates a giant aneurysm arising from the ICA terminus/MCA.

Radiographic Summary

Arteriovenous malformations (AVM) are masses of abnormal blood vessels characterized by direct connection of arteries to veins without the normal intervening capillary network. If an AVM has not hemorrhaged, the appearance on CT is that of enlarged vessels with a density that may be only slightly higher than the adjacent brain tissue. The vessels may have the appearance of a high-density mass, with calcification present 15-20% of the time. When associated with hemorrhage, an AVM will present as a high-density mass within the brain on NECT, and acute hyperdense blood may obscure other diagnostic features. On MRI, dilated arteries and enlarged draining veins from an AVM are dark in signal on T2WI. These will enhance with contrast (CTA or MRA). The nidus may have the appearance of a "bag of worms" due to the cluster of serpentine vessels. Digital subtraction angiography remains the gold standard of diagnosis and pre-treatment planning as it allows exquisite detail of the location and number of feeding vessels, flow dynamics, and the drainage pattern.

Clinical Implications

AVMs may present with headache, acute neurologic dysfunction, and signs and symptoms as a consequence of acute intracranial hemorrhage. Slowly progressive neurological deficits may also occur and are thought to relate to siphoning of blood flow away from the adjacent brain tissue ("steal phenomenon"). Neurological deficits may be explained alternatively by the mass effect of an enlarging AVM or venous hypertension in the draining veins. Neurologic findings are rare in the absence of seizure or hemorrhage in patients with cerebral AVMs, but are more common in brainstem and deeply situated AVMs. If parenchymal hemorrhage is present, physical findings are indistinguishable from those due to intracranial hemorrhage of other causes.

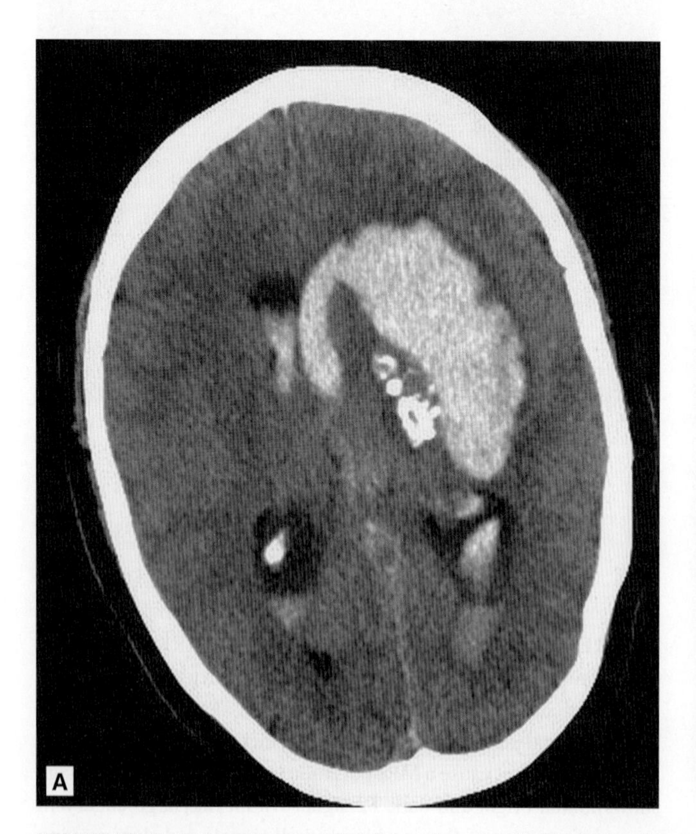

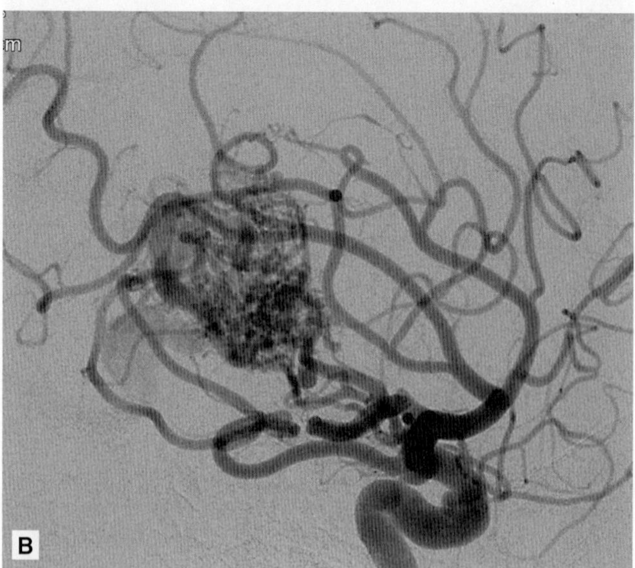

FIGURE 2.11 ■ Arteriovenous Malformation. **A:** NECT shows a large parenchymal hemorrhage in the lateral left basal ganglia. A coarsely calcified mass is present in the left basal ganglia medial to the hemorrhage. The mass represents thrombosed chronically calcified vessels. Blood is present within the ventricles (notice hematocrit level in the occipital horns. **B:** Lateral cerebral angiogram of carotid injection shows a tangle of vessels arising from the middle cerebral artery territory representing the AVM.

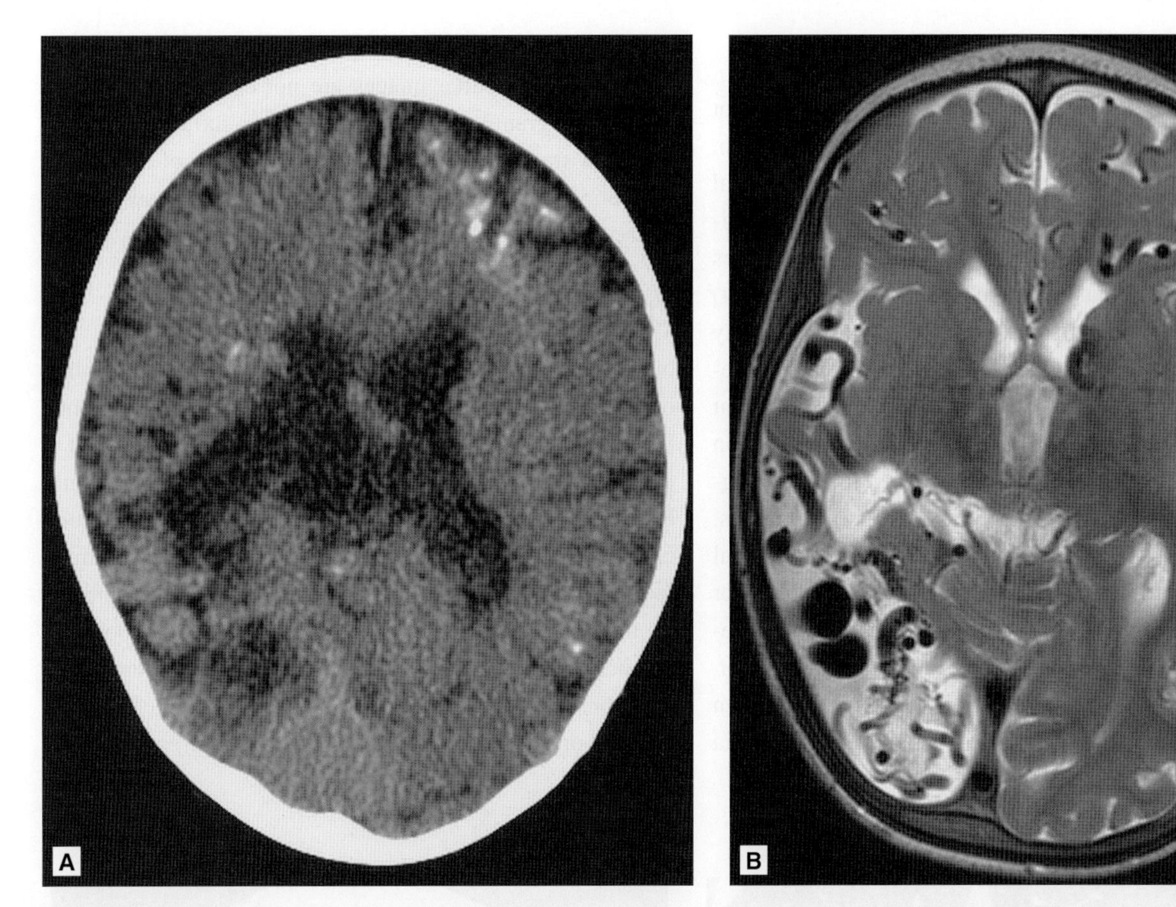

FIGURE 2.12 ■ Arteriovenous Malformation. **A:** NECT in a 3-year-old male shows dystrophic calcification in the left frontal lobe from prior hemorrhage or infection. There is a poorly characterized lesion in the right parietal lobe consisting of tubular structures better seen on subsequent MRI. **B:** T2WI shows enlarged and tortuous abnormal vessels predominantly in and around the right parietal lobe, but also in each frontal lobe.

Pearls

1. MRI with MRA will provide a more detailed evaluation of the brain and vasculature than CTA alone. In cases of hemorrhage, repeat imaging several weeks after the acute bleeding has subsided provides the best imaging evaluation.
2. Young adults with spontaneous intracranial hemorrhage should trigger a search for an AVM. Treatment can entail embolization, surgical resection, or radiation.
3. Peak presentation is in 3rd and 4th decades of life.

Radiographic Summary

Cerebral venous sinus thrombosis results from a blood clot of the dural venous sinuses that drain blood from the brain. NECT may demonstrate hyperdensity within the dural sinuses or cortical veins, termed the "cord sign." MRI initially demonstrates T1 isointense signal within the sinuses but in the subacute phase of illness (2-3 days after onset) T1 hyperintense signal is present. CECT or MRI may show the "empty delta sign," which consists of enhancement of the outer venous walls, but no central enhancement due to thrombus. CTV or MRV is the preferred evaluation for sinus thrombosis. If equivocal, conventional angiography provides definitive evaluation. As time progresses, increased venous hypertension can cause intraparenchymal hemorrhage or infarction due to back pressure. Superior sagittal sinus thrombosis maybe associated with involvement of the parasagittal frontal and parietal white matter. Internal cerebral vein or straight sinus involvement can affect the thalami or basal ganglia. Asymmetric hypoplasia of the transverse sinuses is often present and can mimic stenosis if the source images are not examined carefully. Arachnoid granulations and acute extra-axial hematomas near the transverse sinus can mimic areas of thrombus. Patients with elevated hematocrit can also show falsely dense sinuses on NECT.

Clinical Implications

Ninety percent of people with dural sinus thrombosis complain of headache, while about half have stroke-like symptoms. Some patients may have memory loss or aphasia. Unless it is contraindicated, patients with dural sinus thrombosis should be anticoagulated in order to prevent extension of the blood clot and formation of new thrombus. If symptoms continue to progress despite anticoagulation, endovascular thrombolysis may be considered. The use of D-Dimer as a laboratory adjunct may be helpful in the diagnosis of acute dural sinus thrombosis. Signs of increased ICP such as papilledema and elevated opening pressure on LP may also be present.

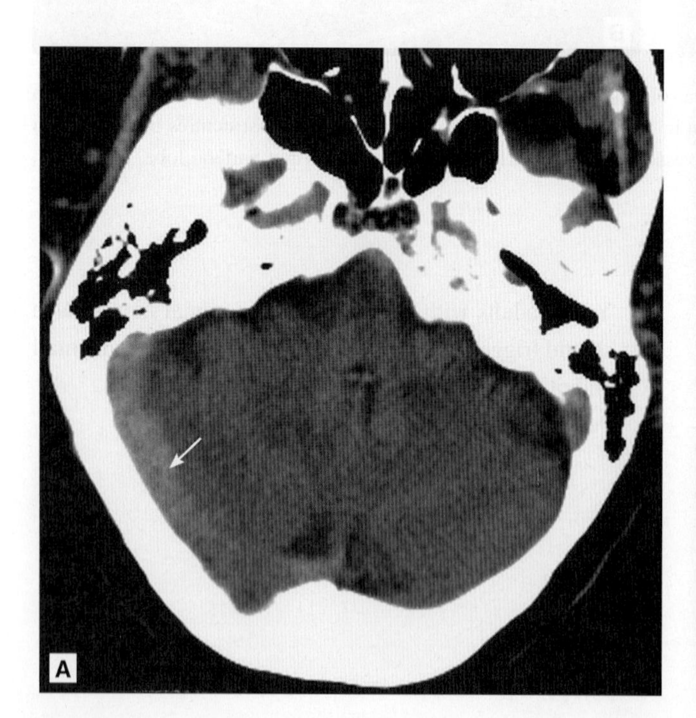

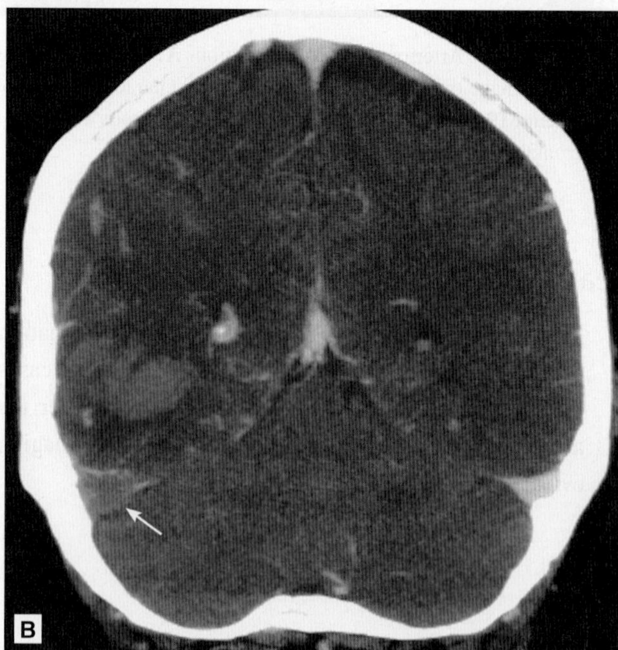

FIGURE 2.13 ■ Transverse Sinus Thrombosis. **A:** NECT shows hyperdense structure in the region of the right transverse sinus ("cord sign") (arrow). **B:** Coronal CTA in the venous phase shows filling of the superior sagittal and left transverse sinuses but only enhancement of the outer wall of the right transverse sinus ("empty delta sign") (arrow).

Pearls

1. Dural sinus thrombosis presents in a clinical manner similar to idiopathic intracranial hypertension, making radiographic imaging important.
2. CTV or MRV is the imaging modality most likely to definitively identify the thrombus.
3. One percent of strokes are due to dural sinus thrombosis. They are often misdiagnosed or missed because they can be hard to diagnose with imaging and are often not considered clinically.
4. Imaging pitfalls include congenital asymmetric size of venous sinuses, arachnoid granulations, and elevated hematocrit levels mimicking thrombus.

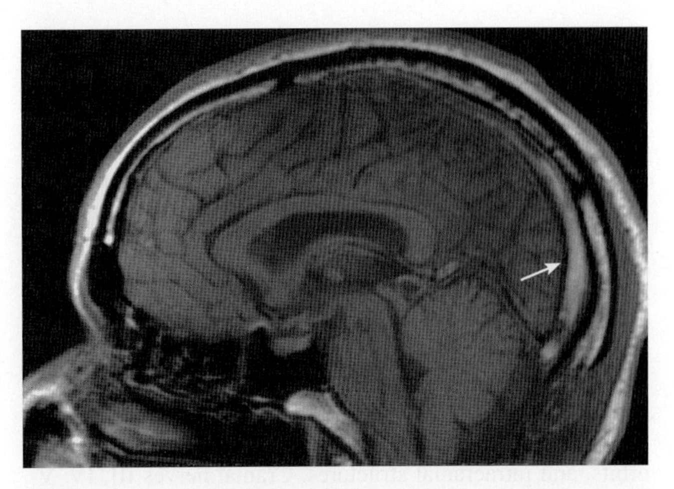

FIGURE 2.14 ■ Sagittal Sinus Thrombosis. Sagittal T1 MRI shows abnormal hyperintense signal within the superior sagittal sinus indicating subacute thrombus. Normally, this should be a black signal void (arrow).

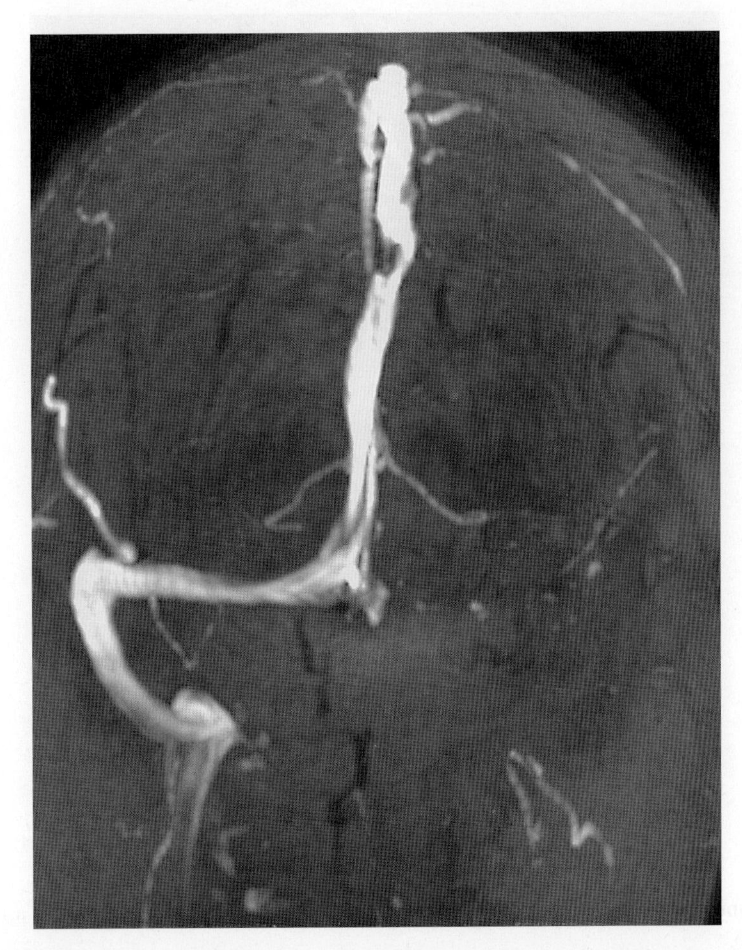

FIGURE 2.15 ■ Transverse Sinus Thrombosis. 3D MIP image of MRV shows no flow in the left transverse sinus. After confirming that this is not an anatomically hypoplastic sinus in the source images, these findings support venous thrombosis.

Radiographic Summary

Cavernous sinus thrombosis is a rare complication of orbital, sinus, or facial infection. CTA or CECT of the brain may demonstrate an abnormally convex margin to the cavernous sinus that should normally be flat or concave. Engorgement or dilation of the superior ophthalmic vein is often seen as the pressure extends back into the draining veins. There may be narrowing of the internal carotid artery as it passes through the cavernous sinus. Orbital MRI with fat-saturation best demonstrates the anatomy of this region. MR also provides important information about the adjacent soft tissues, sinuses, orbits, and intracranial structures. Cranial nerves III, IV, V_1, and V_2, and VI run through the cavernous sinus. Catheter angiography may be required for final diagnosis.

Clinical Implications

Patients with cavernous sinus thrombosis often have fever, severe headache or facial pain, usually unilateral and localized to retro-orbital and frontal regions. Later developments may include ophthalmoplegia, proptosis, and diminished or absent facial sensation. Decreased level of consciousness, confusion, seizures, and focal neurologic deficits are signs of spread to the CNS. Patients may also have anisocoria or mydriasis, papilledema, and vision loss. Complications include meningoencephalitis, brain abscess, stroke, blindness, and pituitary insufficiency. Imaging is important to assess for other diagnoses that can present in a similar manner such as idiopathic orbital inflammatory syndrome/orbital pseudotumor, Wegener's, neurosarcoidosis, sinusitis with orbital extension,

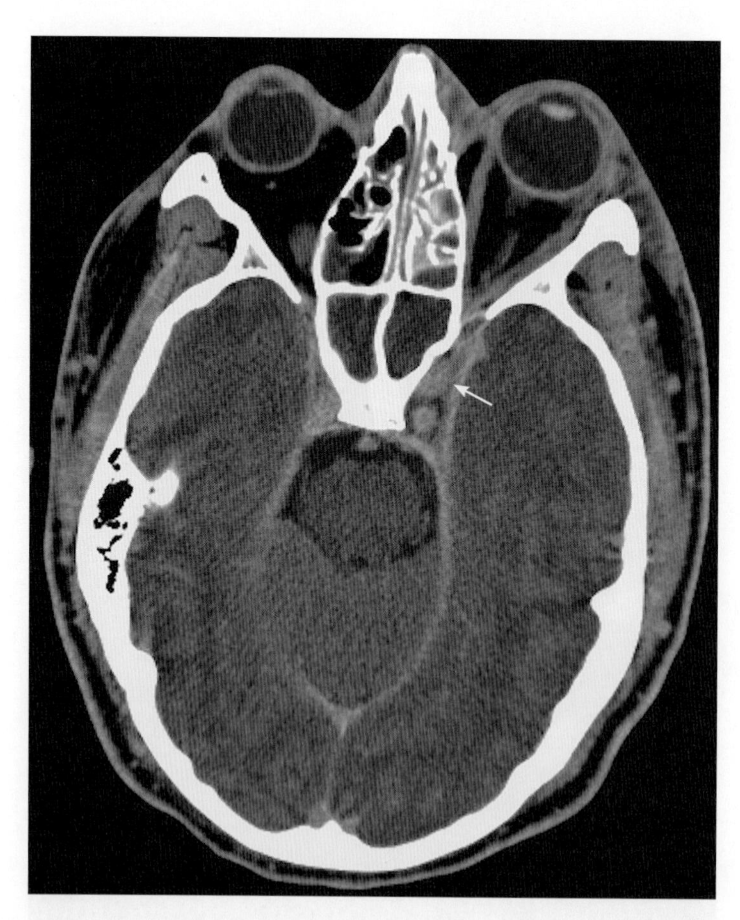

FIGURE 2.16 ■ Cavernous Sinus Thrombosis. Axial CTA shows enlargement of the left cavernous sinus in a 19-year-old male who initially presented with sinusitis (arrow).

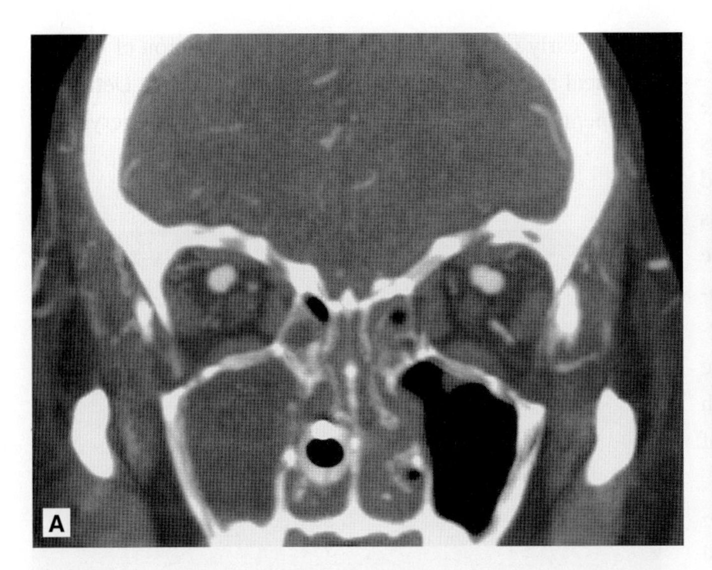

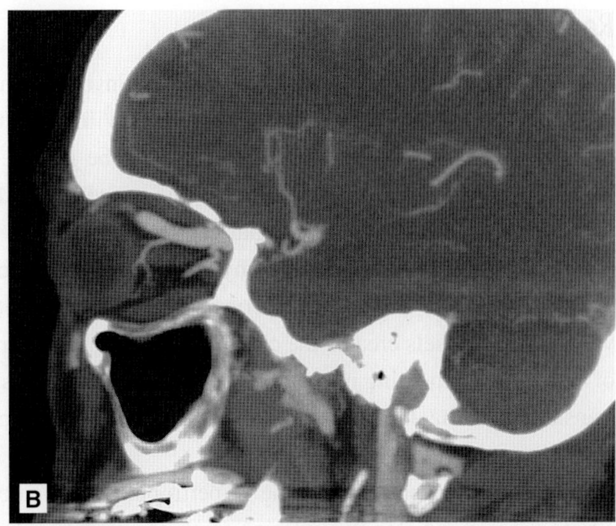

FIGURE 2.17 ■ Cavernous Sinus Thrombosis. **A:** Coronal CTA in a 70-year-old female with proptosis and bruit over the eye shows marked enlargement of both superior ophthalmic veins (these are commonly enlarged in both cavernous sinus thrombosis and carotid-cavernous fistula). **B:** Sagittal CTA shows the engorged superior ophthalmic vein.

tumors, or masses. Treatment includes IV antibiotics with possible surgical intervention. Secondary treatment may include corticosteroids for cranial nerve dysfunction; anticoagulation is controversial because most patients respond to antibiotics, and adverse effects of anticoagulation may exceed benefits of the therapy.

Pearls

1. Look for asymmetric engorgement of the cavernous sinus on the ipsilateral side of involvement on contrast-enhanced images as a sign of cavernous sinus thrombosis.
2. Proptosis, ptosis, chemosis, and cranial nerve palsy beginning in one eye and progressing to the other eye suggests the diagnosis.
3. Dilation of the superior ophthalmic veins is often seen ipsilateral to the thrombosed sinus.
4. CT and MR venography are not preferred over CTA or CECT for the diagnosis of cavernous sinus thrombosis even though the involved structures are part of the venous vasculature.

Radiographic Summary

Moyamoya disease is a vaso-occlusive disease involving the distal internal carotid arteries and the circle of Willis and its branches. The term moyamoya disease should be reserved for an idiopathic, sometimes familial condition, which leads to characteristic intracranial vascular changes. An extensive collateral network develops from hypertrophied lenticulostriate, dural, and meningeal arteries. This collateral network of tiny vessels creates the classic angiographic picture of contrast disappearing into a cloud of tiny vessels (English translation of the Japanese word "moyamoya" is "puff of smoke").

CTA or MRA may show the hypertrophied lenticulostriate vessels and stenotic anterior cerebral circulation but traditional catheter angiography is needed for ultimate diagnosis and pre-operative planning. Axial MRI images may show small flow voids insinuating around the basal ganglia and midbrain due to the collateral vessels. Contrasted imaging and FLAIR may show the "ivy sign" (diffuse leptomeningeal enhancement representing engorgement of the pial vasculature) due to slow flow in meningeal collaterals. Diffusion-weighted imaging (DWI) is helpful to determine acute versus chronic infarcts as these patients have often had prior insults.

Clinical Implications

Moyamoya disease, although initially described in the Japanese population, can be seen in any ethnicity. However, this condition is the most common cause of stroke in Asian children. It is believed to be due to a genetic defect in chromosomes 3p, 17q, and possibly others. Other causes of acquired moyamoya pattern are sickle cell disease, Down syndrome, brain irradiation, neurofibromatosis, tuberous sclerosis, vasculitis (inflammatory or infectious), and connective tissue disorders. If the patient is non-Asian, non-genetic etiologies should be considered. Children often present with TIA or ischemic stroke, while adults more commonly present with subarachnoid or parenchymal hemorrhage. Recognition of disease early in the course with prompt institution of therapy is critical to achieve the best outcomes in patients. Definitive treatment may include revascularization bypass surgery.

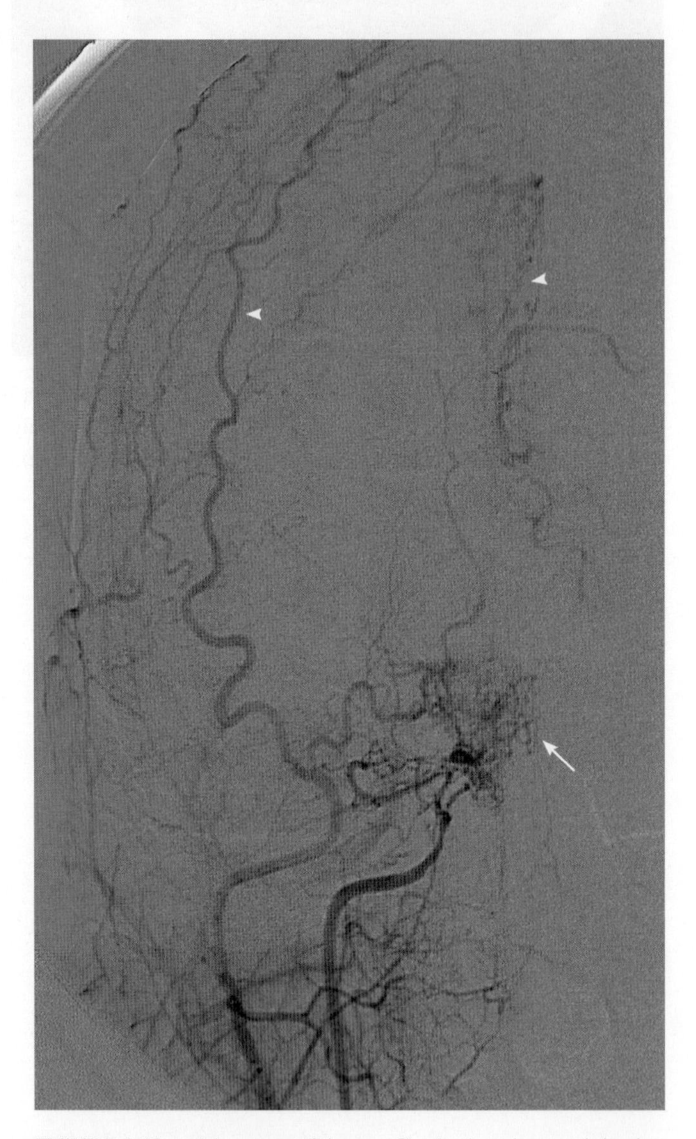

FIGURE 2.18 ■ Moyamoya Disease. Cerebral angiogram injection of carotid artery in a 27-year-old female shows terminal occlusion of the ICA with a "puff of smoke" appearance of the contrast as it dissipates into small lenticulostriate vessels (arrow). Note the enlarged meningeal and pial collaterals supplying the anterior and middle cerebral vessels peripherally (arrowheads).

Pearls

1. MRI is more sensitive than CT in demonstration of cerebral ischemia and infarcted regions. CTA and MRA can both demonstrate the abnormal vessels.
2. On catheter angiography, small collateral lenticulostriate arteries produce the characteristic "puff of smoke" appearance.
3. Moyamoya is the leading cause of stroke in Asian children.

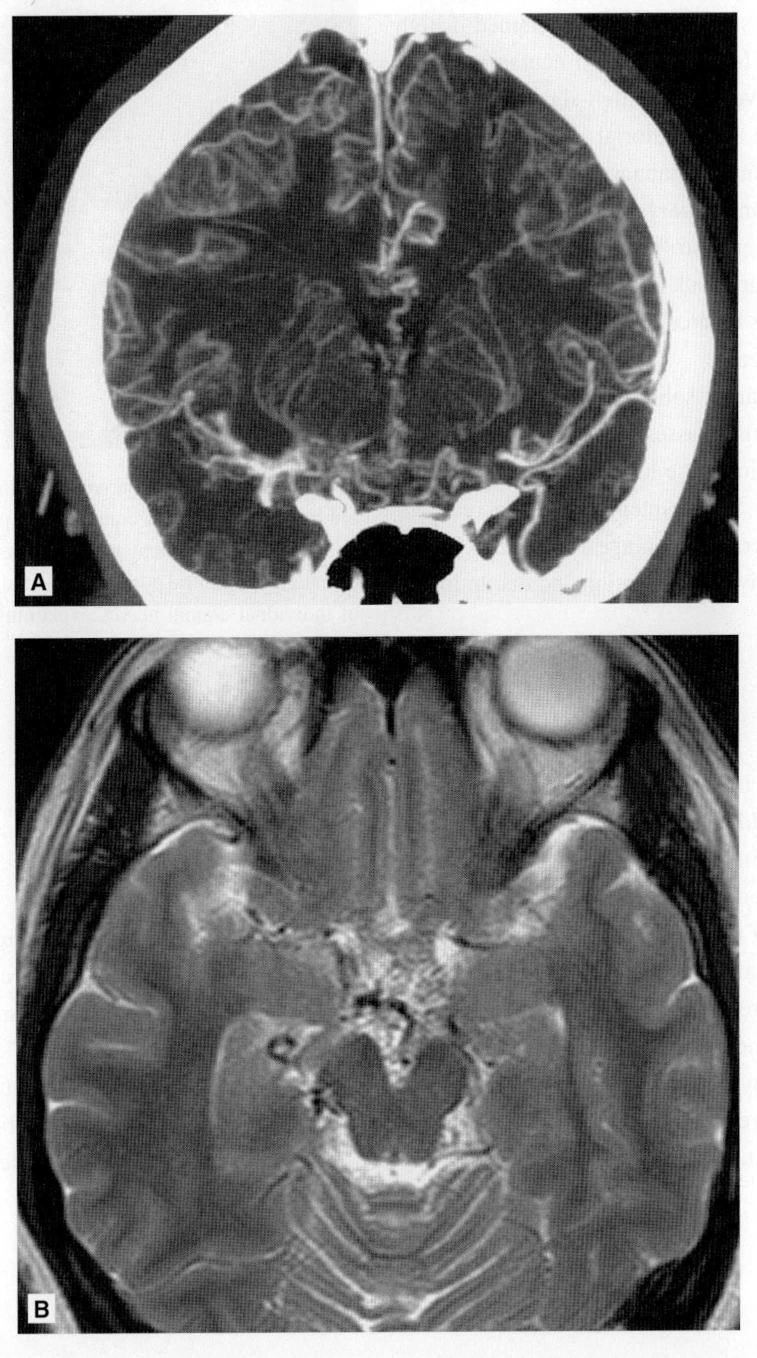

FIGURE 2.19 ■ Moyamoya Disease. **A:** Coronal CTA in a 20-year-old Asian female shows severe narrowing of bilateral middle cerebral arteries. There is marked hypertrophy of the lenticulostriate vessels that supply the basal ganglia. **B:** T2 shows numerous serpentine flow voids surrounding the midbrain representing tiny collateral vessels.

Radiographic Summary

Neurosarcoidosis is a complication of sarcoidosis in which inflammation occurs in the brain, spinal cord, and other areas of the nervous system. CECT is neither sensitive nor specific but may show leptomeningeal involvement seen as linear and nodular meningeal enhancement. Concomitant hydrocephalus may also be seen. CE MRI is superior in identifying neurosarcoidosis and should be obtained if high clinical suspicion exists. In a patient with neursarcoidosis, CE MRI may show periventricular high-signal lesions on FLAIR images, multiple supratentorial and infratentorial brain lesions, leptomeningeal enhancement, optic nerve enhancement, and intramedullary spinal cord lesions. Enhancing lesions are often distributed near the basilar cisterns and along the pituitary stalk and cranial nerves, which can mimic entities such as tuberculosis, leptomeningeal carcinomatosis, or Lyme disease.

Neurosarcoid lesions can be solitary or multiple and typically present as hyperintense masses on MR FLAIR images. After contrast administration these lesions typically enhance when biologically active. Signal intensity will decrease in response to effective therapy. Meningeal or parenchymal enhancement suggests active inflammation and disruption of the blood–brain barrier.

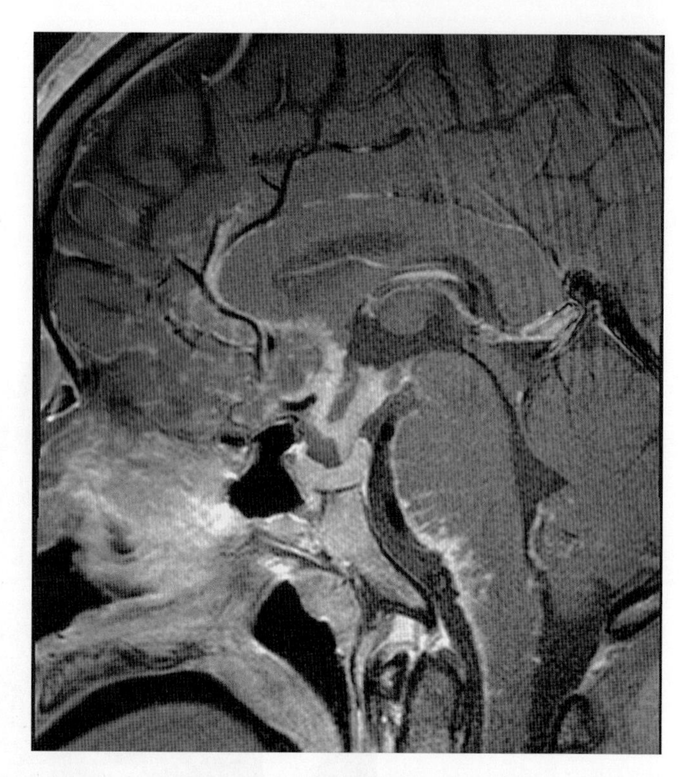

FIGURE 2.20 ■ Neurosarcoidosis. Sagittal T1+C MR in a 31-year-old male with multiple cranial nerve palsies shows extensive leptomeningeal enhancement in the suprasellar region, basilar cisterns, and along the ventral pons. Parasagittal images showed enhancement of individual cranial nerves explaining the patient's clinical symptoms caused by neurosarcoidosis.

Clnical Implications

Neurosarcoidosis occurs in approximately 5% of patients with sarcoidosis and should be considered in sarcoid patients who develop neurologic findings without any other underlying etiology. African-Americans have a higher incidence due to increased prevalence of underlying sarcoidosis. Common presentations include cranial mononeuropathy, neuroendocrine dysfunction, seizures, encephalopathy, myelopathy, hydrocephalus, aseptic meningitis, peripheral neuropathy, or myopathy. Patients may present with dysfunction of the facial nerve followed by reduction in visual perception due to optic nerve involvement. Corticosteroids are the mainstay of treatment, with methotrexate sometimes used as a second-line agent.

Pearls

1. The facial nerve is the most frequently symptomatic cranial nerve but is often radiographically normal on MRI.
2. Up to 60% of patients with subsequently proven neurosarcoidosis have negative CT scans.
3. The MRI findings seen in neurosarcoidosis can be nonspecific and may mimic tuberculosis, leptomeningeal carcinomatosis, and Lyme disease.

Radiographic Summary

Herpes (HSV) encephalitis is a viral infection of the central nervous system caused by retrograde transmission of the reactivated HSV-1 virus from a peripheral site on the face, along a nerve axon, to the brain. Classic radiographic findings of HSV encephalitis are seen best with MRI demonstrating T2/FLAIR hyperintensity of the medial temporal lobes, insular cortex, and inferior frontal lobes (cingulate gyrus). The basal ganglia are typically spared, helping to distinguish HSV encephalitis from a middle cerebral artery infarct. NECT may reveal hypodensity in the temporal lobes either unilaterally or bilaterally, with or without frontal lobe involvement. CT will often be normal in these patients making it important to consider MRI if HSV encephalitis is in the differential diagnosis. Bright DWI can be one of the first findings seen in this life-threatening process. Hemorrhage can be seen as well as patchy or gyriform contrast enhancement.

Clinical Implications

HSV encephalitis is typically caused by reactivation of the HSV-1 virus that had been dormant in the trigeminal ganglion. This explains the typical location of infection in the limbic system that is adjacent to the trigeminal ganglion.

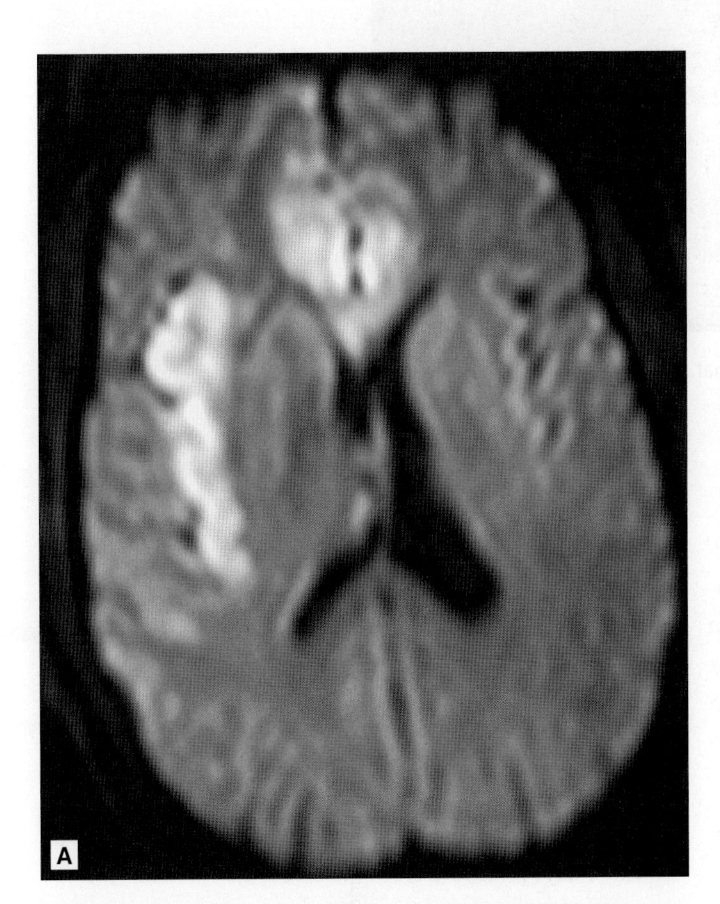

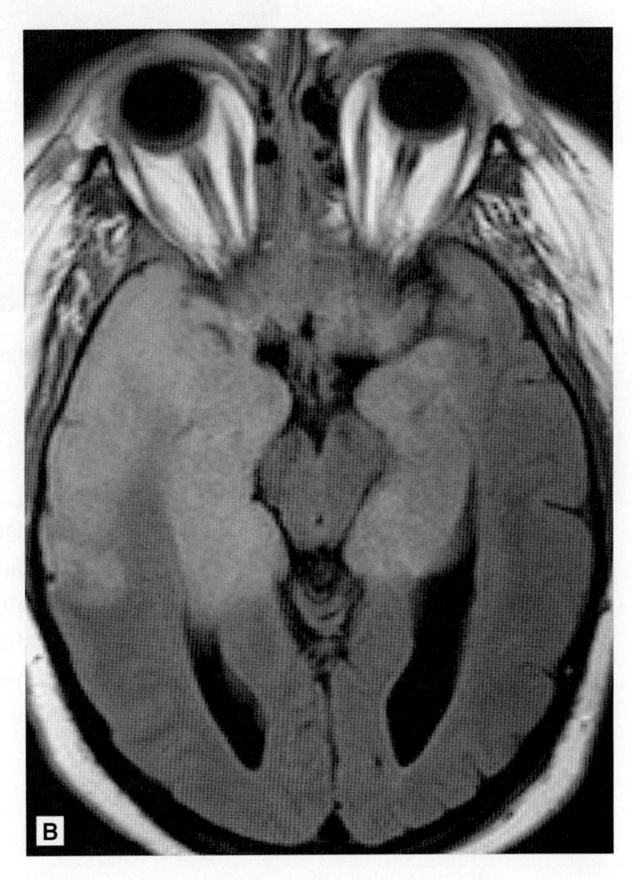

FIGURE 2.21 ■ Herpes Encephalitis. **A:** A 42-year-old-female with renal transplant presents with headache and subsequent mental status decline. DWI MRI shows restricted diffusion in the right insula and cingulate gyri. **B:** FLAIR shows abnormal high signal in both medial temporal lobes and the lateral right temporal lobe.

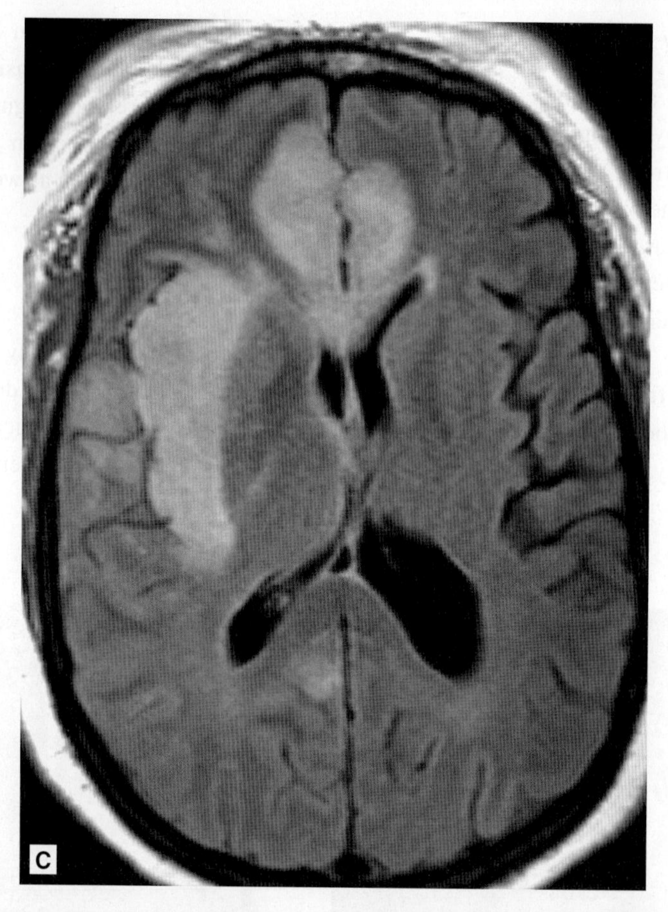

FIGURE 2.21 ■ (*Continued*) **C:** FLAIR shows hyperintense signal abnormality in the cingulate gyri and right insula. There is sparing of the basal ganglia commonly seen in HSV-1 encephalitis.

HSV-1 causes 95% of herpes encephalitis and occurs primarily in older children and adults over 50 in both immune competent and compromised individuals. HSV-2 is often seen in neonates. Patients may present with confusion, personality changes, fever, or seizures. It is crucial to make the diagnosis early as there is a 60-70% mortality rate when the disease process is left untreated.

Pearls

1. MRI is the preferred modality for the radiographic diagnosis of HSV encephalitis. However, a negative MRI does not exclude HSV encephalitis.
2. When findings typical of HSV encephalitis are observed on CT scan, they often are associated with brain damage and a poor prognosis.
3. MRI in HSV encephalitis may show positive findings up to 2 days prior to CT.

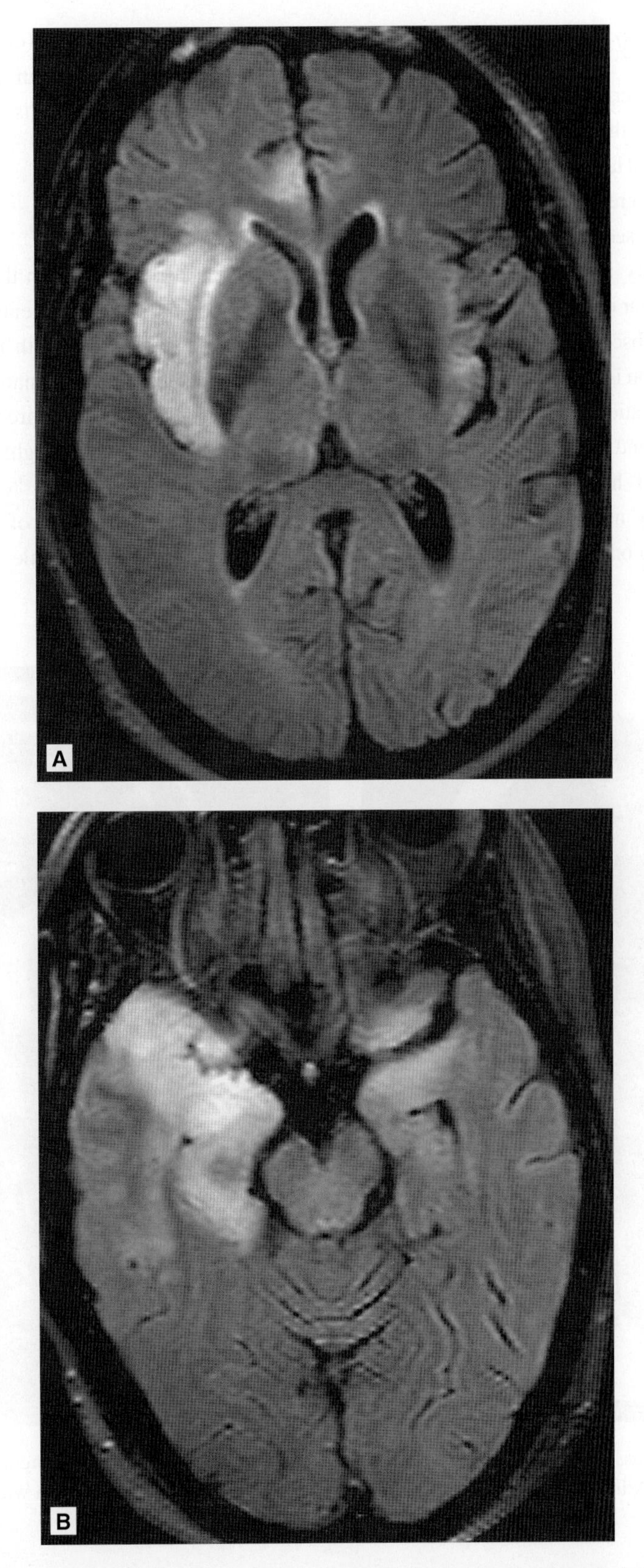

FIGURE 2.22 ■ Herpes Encephalitis. **A, B:** FLAIR images in a 57-year-old female show abnormal signal in the medial right temporal lobe, right insular cortex, and cingulate gyrus with sparing of the basal ganglia. There is early involvement of the medial left temporal lobe. Findings are classic for HSV-1 encephalitis.

Radiographic Summary

Cerebral abscesses are characterized by inflammation and collections of infected material in the brain. Brain abscesses progress through 4 stages: early and late cerebritis followed by early and late capsule formation. Cerebritis evolves into a localized abscess in a series of stages seen with imaging. NECT may show nonspecific hypodensity in the region of cerebritis or abscess. CECT shows irregular enhancement of late cerebritis and rim enhancement of an abscess. However, MRI is the preferred modality when infection is suspected as it affords higher specificity and allows evaluation of adjacent complications such as subdural empyemas and subdural effusions.

On MRI, abscesses will have a thin rim of contrast enhancement and a centrally necrotic center with restricted diffusion (very bright signal) on DWI. Other helpful features include a T2 hypointense (dark) rim. Surrounding T2 hyperintense vasogenic edema in the adjacent brain is commonly seen. Associated meningitis may be seen as leptomeningeal enhancement.

Clinical Implications

Brain abscesses are rare in the general population; however, immunocompromised patients have an increasing incidence of brain abscess, often with fungal or protozoan organisms. Common sources are hematogenous spread, post-operative brain or skull base procedures, sinus, teeth, or temporal bone infections, trauma, or right-to-left cardiovascular shunts. Inflammation during the "early cerebritis" stage evolves into a necrotic collection of pus, eventually surrounded by a well-vascularized capsule after approximately 2 weeks.

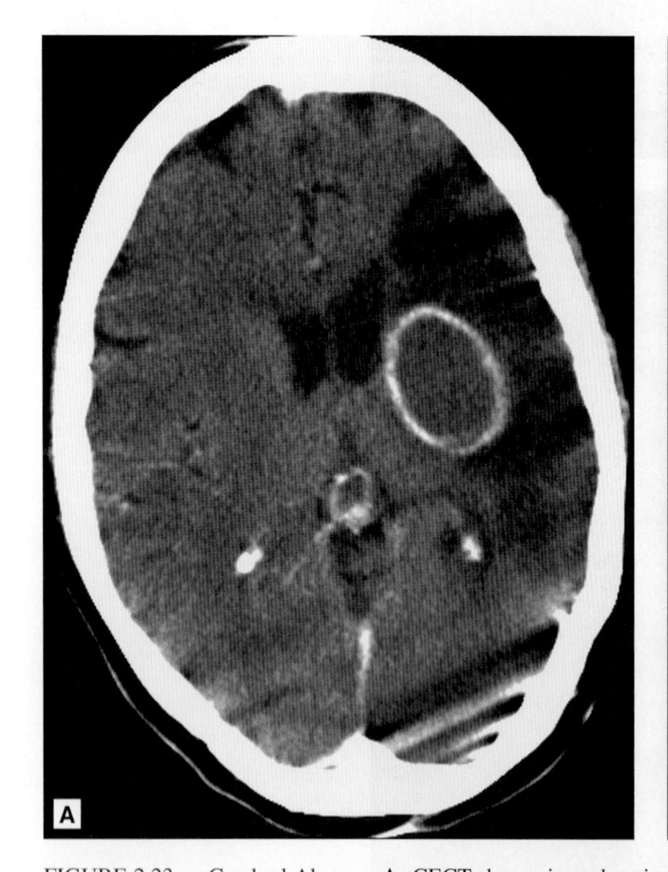

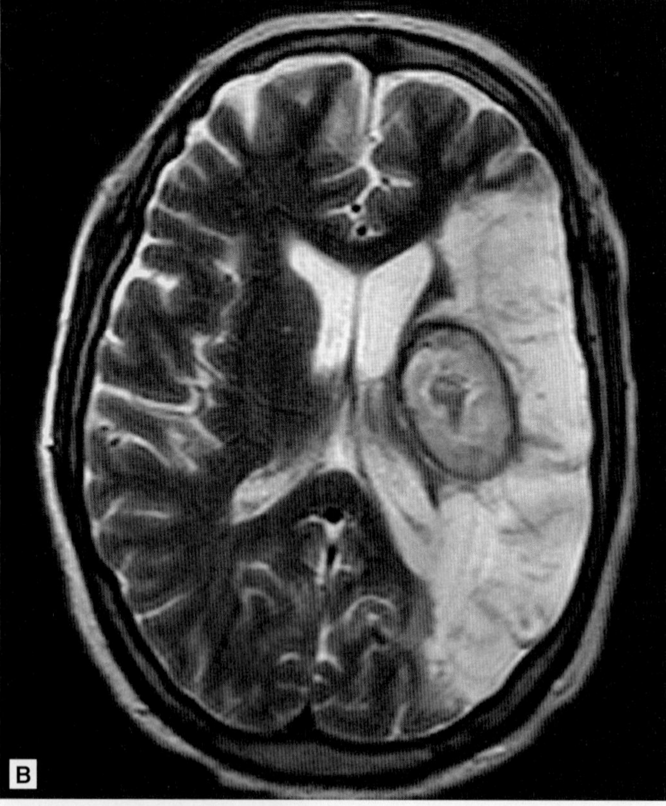

FIGURE 2.23 ■ Cerebral Abscess. **A:** CECT shows rim-enhancing round lesion in the left basal ganglia within a background of encephalomalacia from a prior left MCA infarct. **B:** Axial T2WI shows ovoid lesion in the left basal ganglia with a characteristic hypointense rim surrounding it.

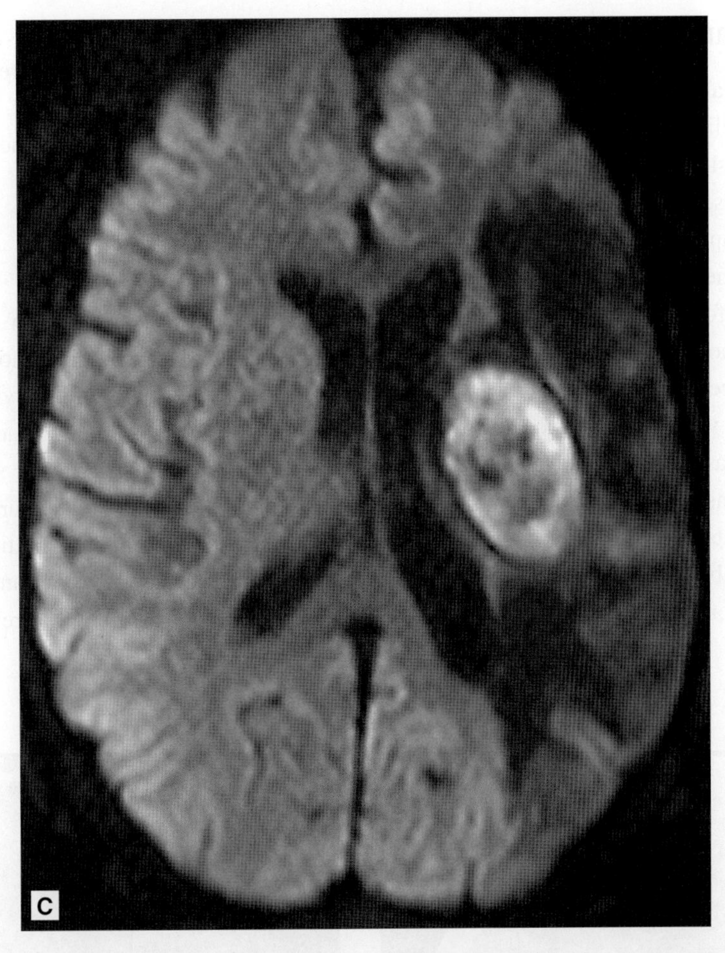

FIGURE 2.23 ■ (*Continued*) **C:** Axial DWI shows restricted diffusion within the ovoid lesion, a characteristic finding in pyogenic abscess.

Near drowning, foreign body aspiration, application of dental braces, tongue piercing, and upper endoscopic procedures have also been associated with brain abscess. Selection of appropriate antimicrobials with adequate CNS penetration and coverage of typical anaerobic and aerobic organisms is critical. In almost all cases, definitive treatment of brain abscess requires surgical drainage.

Pearls

1. MR diffusion-weighted-imaging is helpful to differentiate abscess from other ring-enhancing brain lesions.
2. If initial NECT raises concern for infection, MRI with contrast is the best imaging modality for a more definitive evaluation and confirmation of an intracranial abscess.

Radiographic Summary

Acute disseminated encephalomyelitis (ADEM) is a monophasic inflammatory demyelinating disease of the CNS with findings progressing over a short period of time (in contradistinction to multiple sclerosis, which has similar demyelinating lesions, but with a multiphasic course). This can occur at any age, but the average patient age is 5-8 years. This condition often occurs 1-2 weeks following a viral infection or vaccination. ADEM is best demonstrated on T2 and FLAIR MRI sequences. Contrast enhancement is seen at times in acute lesions. MRI abnormalities vary in appearance and location but are typically bilateral, asymmetric, and poorly marginated. T2 hyperintense lesions range from punctuate to large confluent areas. Most patients have multiple lesions of demyelination in the deep and subcortical white matter. The periventricular white matter is often spared. Gray matter lesions sometimes accompany the white matter abnormalities, especially in children. CT scans are often normal, particularly early in the course of the disease. ADEM can affect the spinal cord, and if symptoms refer to the cord, MRI of the spine may also be helpful.

Clinical Implications

ADEM should be suspected in a child who develops systemic signs and neurologic abnormalities, including altered level of consciousness, after a viral infection. Patients may present with fever, vomiting, headache, irritability, and a stiff neck. Progression of neurologic signs to the maximum deficit occurs typically over the course of a week. Patients with ADEM usually present with multifocal signs of motor deficits and impaired consciousness. Cranial nerve abnormalities may occur as well. Rarely, ADEM presents as an acute psychosis.

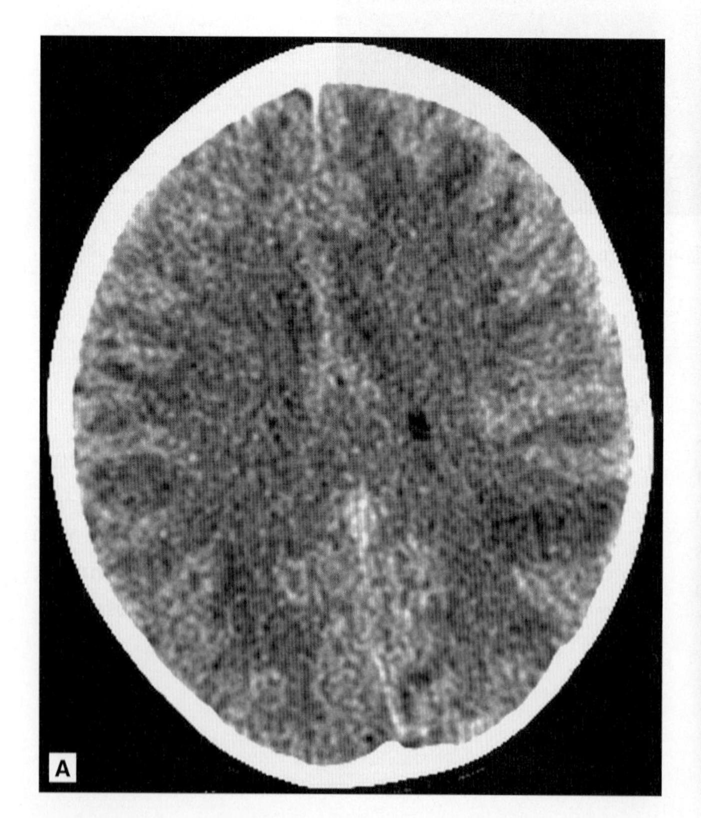

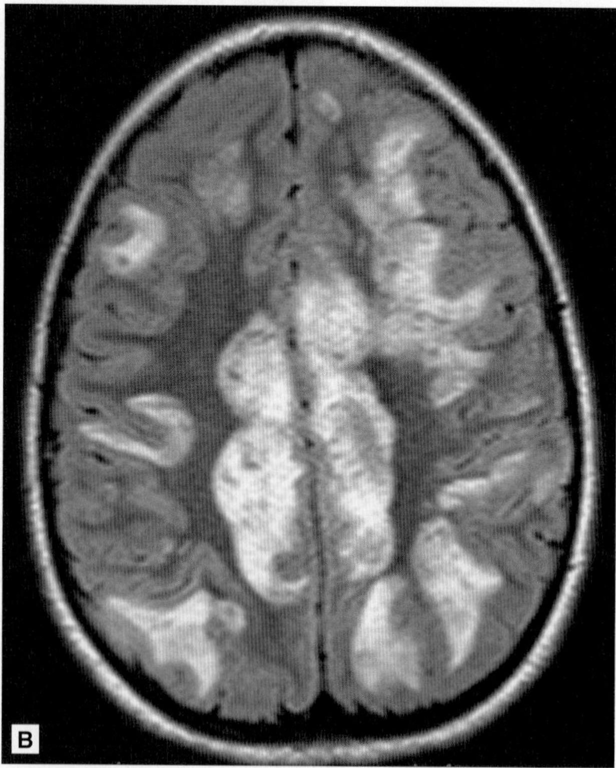

FIGURE 2.24 ■ Acute Disseminated Encephalomyelitis. **A:** NECT in a 9-year-old female shows subtle low attenuation in the subcortical white matter. **B:** FLAIR MRI sequence shows corresponding extensive edema bilaterally within the deep and subcortical white matter.

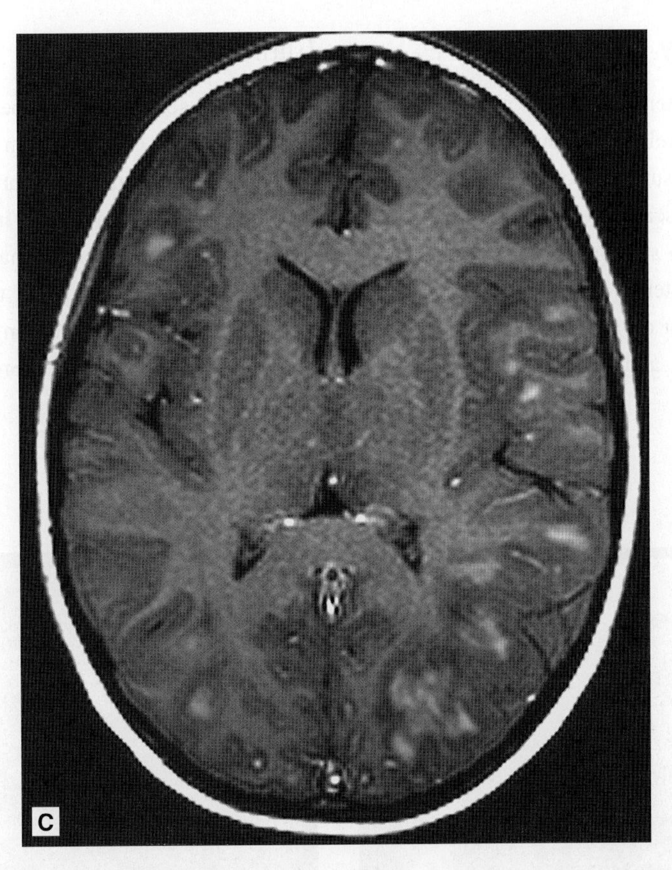

FIGURE 2.24 ■ (*Continued*) **C:** T1+C MR shows patchy areas of enhancement in the subcortical white matter. Findings represent acute disseminated encephalomyelitis (ADEM). The FLAIR signal abnormalities are characteristic. Patchy enhancement is not seen with all cases.

Evidence of inflammation is common in CSF, with pleocytosis and increased protein concentration in the majority of patients.

As these patients present with meningeal signs, empiric treatment protocols typically include broad-spectrum antibiotics and acyclovir until CSF analysis excludes infection. The mainstay of treatment is IV glucocorticoids. Intravenous immunoglobulin and plasmapheresis can also be considered.

Most patients recover slowly over 4-6 weeks, with up to 90% having no residual long-term neurologic deficits. Present day mortality is close to 0% unless the patient develops the hemorrhagic variant of ADEM (acute hemorrhagic leukoencephalitis), which carries a much worse prognosis.

Pearls

1. ADEM mandates close clinical and MRI follow-up as the initial imaging can mimic multiple sclerosis or other demyelinating disorders. ADEM is monophasic and additional lesions should not appear on follow-up studies in comparison to a multiphasic disease such as MS. The diagnosis of multiple sclerosis requires lesions to be "disseminated in time and space."
2. Lesions of ADEM are commonly larger than those of MS. They also tend to involve the deep gray matter and basal ganglia more often than MS.
3. Studies have shown that the location and severity of lesions on MRI do not predict the clinical course.

Radiographic Summary

Idiopathic intracranial hypertension (IIH), also known as pseudotumor cerebri, is a constellation of signs and symptoms of increased intracranial pressure without a causative mass or hydrocephalus. On NECT scan, slit-like ventricles and an enlarged partially empty sella support the diagnosis of IIH. MRI may show flattened posterior sclera in many patients, enhancement of the prelaminar optic nerve, distension of the perioptic subarachnoid space, and vertical tortuosity of the orbital optic nerve.

Clinical Implications

IIH is often seen in young obese females. However, the diagnosis should be considered in any patient with chronic daily headaches, transient visual problems, pulsatile tinnitus, and papilledema. With moderate increased CSF pressures, imaging of the brain may be normal. However, CT and MRI findings will often help support the final diagnosis. There is a strong correlation between an "empty sella," caused by herniation of subarachnoid cerebrospinal fluid through an absent

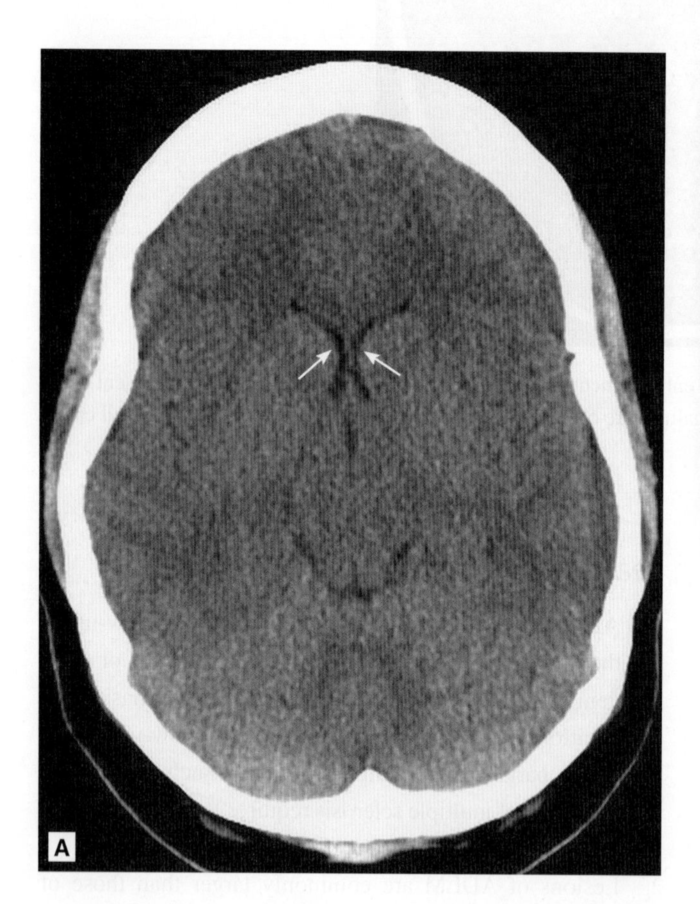

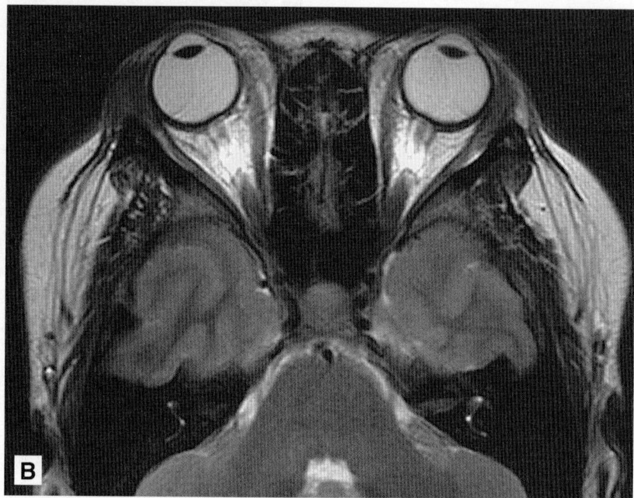

FIGURE 2.25 ■ Pseudotumor Cerebri. **A:** NECT shows slit-like ventricles in this patient with pseudotumor cerebri (idiopathic intracranial hypertension) (arrows). **B:** Axial T2WI in a 15-year-old male with papilledema shows increased CSF fluid within the optic nerve sheaths.

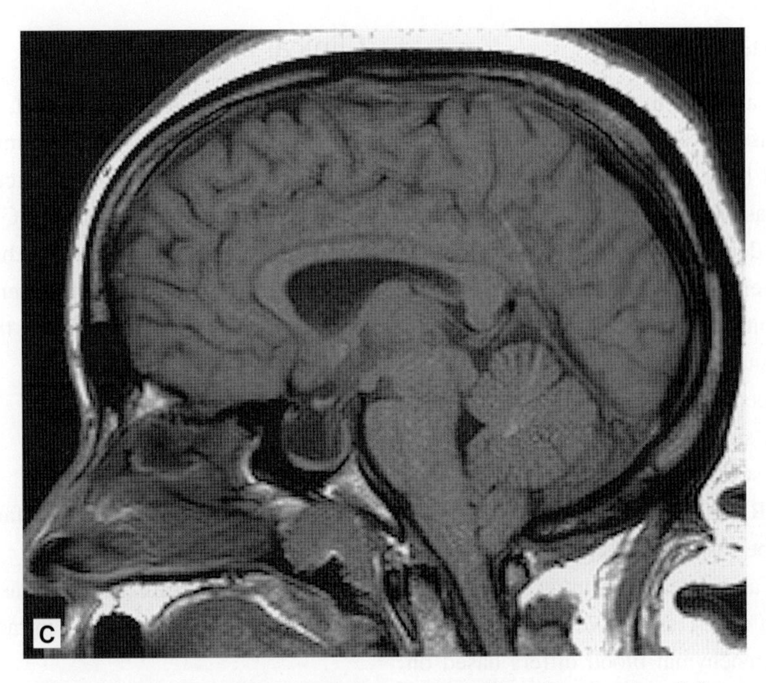

FIGURE 2.25 ■ (*Continued*) **C:** Sagittal T1WI in a 25-year-old shows a markedly enlarged and partially empty sella turcica. The pituitary gland is pressed against the bottom of the sella.

or patulous diaphragm, with IIH. The diagnostic test of choice for IIH is lumbar puncture with measurement of opening pressure, as CSF pressure can still be elevated with normal imaging. Opening pressure varies in patients, but normal CSF should range from 6-20 cm H_2O in adults. IIH is treated mainly through the reduction of CSF pressure utilizing agents such as acetazolamide, repeat lumbar punctures, weight loss, or surgical shunting.

Pearls

1. Radiographic signs suggestive of IIH include flattening of the posterior orbit at the optic nerve, distended subarachnoid spaces of the optic nerve, and slit-like ventricles.
2. Brain imaging is important to exclude intracranial masses or venous obstructions.
3. Lumbar puncture is both diagnostic and therapeutic in patients with IIH. Accurate opening pressure measurements in the lateral decubitus position are needed as the diagnostic criteria for pressures are based on this body position.

Radiographic Summary

NECT most often shows areas of hypodensity surrounding metastatic lesions due to associated vasogenic edema. CECT will show enhancement of large metastatic lesions, but many small subcentimeter metastases may be missed with CT. Calvarial metastases will demonstrate lytic/lucent lesions in the skull. CE MRI is the preferred imaging modality for metastatic evaluation unless contraindicated. Edema (bright signal on T2/FLAIR and low signal on T2) is often seen surrounding metastatic lesions, especially in the white matter. Small cortical lesions often lack surrounding edema and will only be seen on the post-contrast images. Metastases can be identified in the skull with MRI, as the normal bright T1 signal of bone marrow fat will be lost due to tumor infiltration of the marrow. Hemorrhage associated with intracranial metastatic lesions may be seen on CT as hyperdensity. On MRI, the appearance of intraparenchymal blood differs based on the age of the blood. Acute blood will be isointense to brain on T1 and subacute blood will be bright on T1.

Clinical Implications

If a solitary brain lesion is present, there is a 50% chance that it is a metastasis from a remote primary source. Evaluation for a primary neoplastic lesion is indicated to help exclude metastatic disease, often including a CT of the chest, abdomen, or pelvis. Symptoms may include headache, meningeal irritation, or seizure due to cerebral edema and increased intracranial pressure. Dexamethasone is the treatment of choice to reduce cerebral edema.

Pearls

1. Metastatic brain tumors are far more common than primary brain neoplasms.
2. MRI of the brain with contrast is superior to CT in its sensitivity for identifying intracranial metastatic lesions.

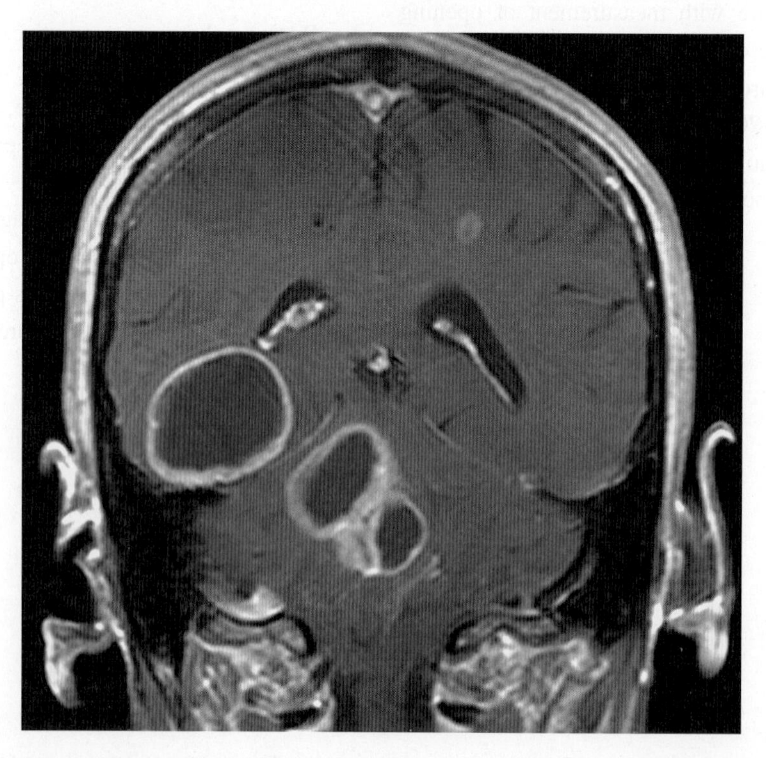

FIGURE 2.26 ■ Intracranial Metastatic Lesions. Coronal T1+C image shows rim-enhancing lesions throughout the brain. Pathology showed neuroendocrine cell lung cancer with metastases to the brain.

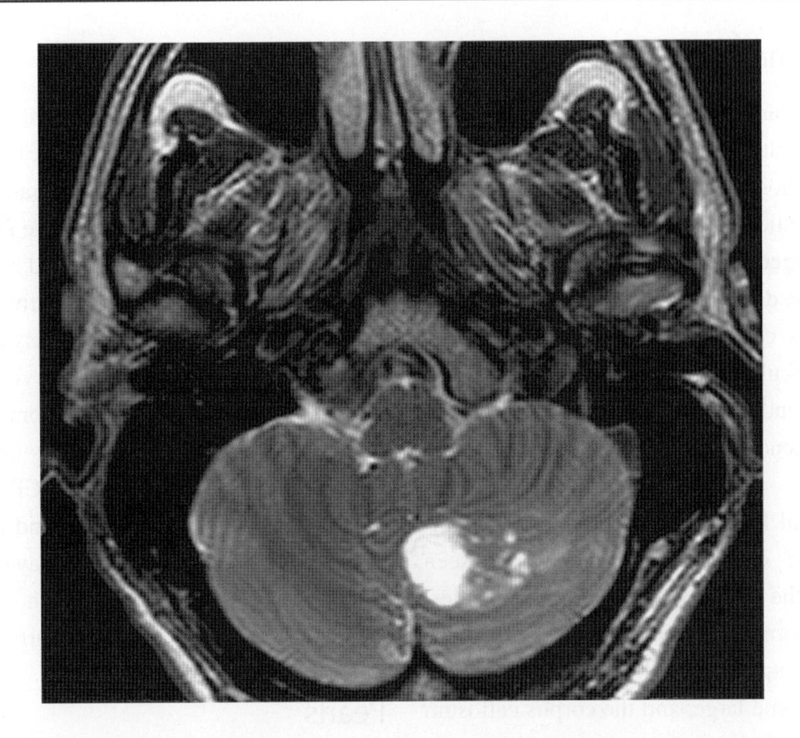

FIGURE 2.27 ■ Intracranial Metastatic Lesions. T2WI shows a cystic and solid lesion in the left cerebellar hemisphere. The solid portion enhanced on contrast sequences. The primary source was identified as bronchogenic carcinoma.

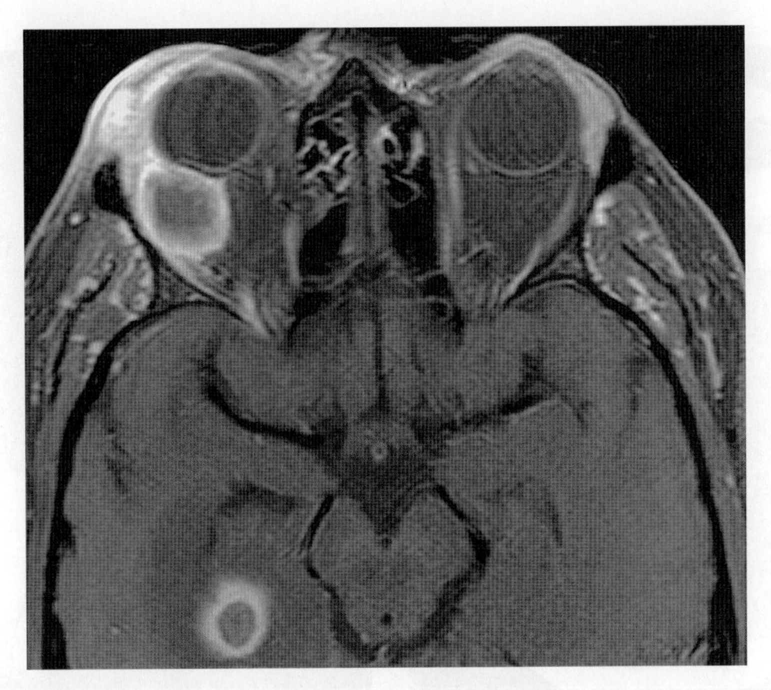

FIGURE 2.28 ■ Intracranial Metastatic Lesions. Fat-saturated T1+C MR of the orbits in a patient with a past history of nephrectomy years ago for RCC, presenting with proptosis. Enhancing biopsy-proven RCC metastases are seen in the right hippocampus and the lateral right orbit leading to proptosis.

Radiographic Summary

Hydrocephalus is the enlargement of the ventricles due to accumulation of CSF resulting from inhibition of its normal flow pathway. Imaging choices are based on the clinical situation and the age of the patient. NECT is usually obtained initially and will show enlarged ventricles. In cases of congenital malformations, MRI best delineates the extent of associated brain anomalies such as corpus callosum agenesis, Chiari malformations, and vascular malformations. T2-weighted images can show transependymal flow of CSF in acute hydrocephalus. On CT, transependymal flow manifests are periventricular low attenuation.

Dilatation of temporal horns may be the earliest manifestation of ventricular obstruction and may be seen before enlargement of the bodies of the lateral ventricles. Ballooning of frontal horns of lateral ventricles and third ventricle may indicate aqueductal obstruction. In severe cases, the ventricles become large, and the corpus callosum becomes thinned and bowed forming an arch. In chronic hydrocephalus, the third ventricle may herniate into the sellaturcica.

Clinical Implications

Acute hydrocephalus occurs over days, subacute hydrocephalus occurs over weeks, and chronic hydrocephalus occurs over months or years. Infants demonstrate poor feeding, vomiting, and irritability. Children may have slowing of mental capacity, headaches, vomiting, blurred vision, or ataxia. Adults have symptoms that show cognitive deterioration, morning headaches (as CSF is resorbed less efficiently in the recumbent position), vomiting, blurred vision, horizontal diplopia, ataxia, and urinary and fecal incontinence. Normal pressure hydrocephalus (NPH) presents as an enlargement of ventricles with little or no increase in ICP with the clinical triad of gait instability, mild dementia, and urinary incontinence. In untreated hydrocephalus, death may occur by tonsillar herniation secondary to raised ICP with compression of the brain stem and subsequent respiratory arrest.

Pearls

1. NECT is the preferred initial imaging in suspected hydrocephalus. Some centers have begun performing limited fast T2-weighted MRI sequences in children to avoid the risk of CT ionizing radiation.

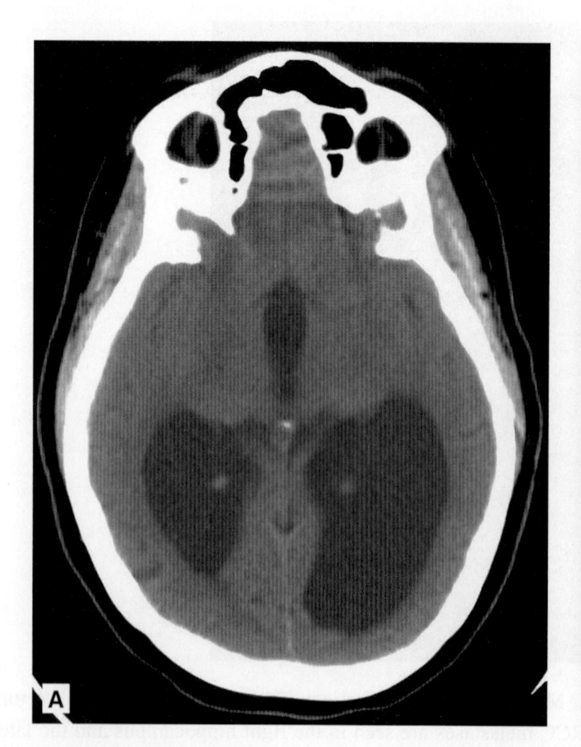

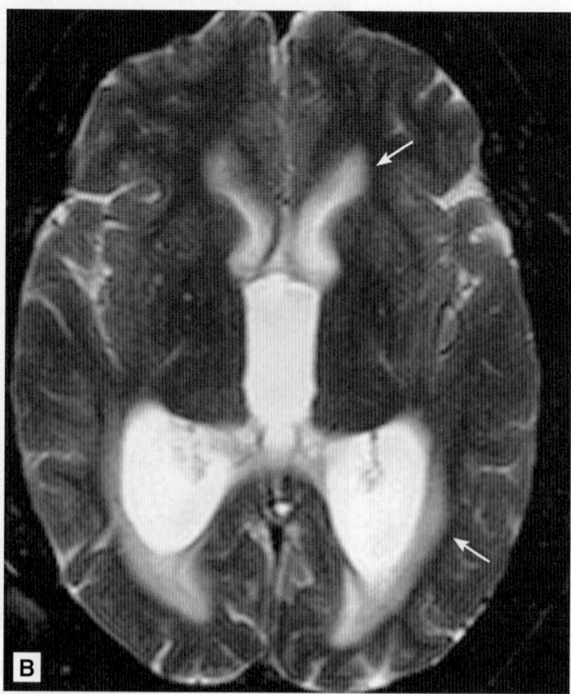

FIGURE 2.29 ■ Acute Hydrocephalus. **A:** Non-contrasted CT in a 15-year-old female who presented with acute progressive headache. Note the massively dilated lateral ventricles as well as the dilated 3rd ventricle. **B:** T2WI shows dilated lateral and 3rd ventricles. The bright signal that extends into the adjacent white matter indicates acute onset of obstruction with transependymal CSF flow (arrows).

2. It is important to differentiate hydrocephalus from brain atrophy. With atrophy the cerebral sulci will be enlarged, whereas in hydrocephalus, the sulci will be normal or small.

3. Patients with shunt-dependent hydrocephalus should have a shunt series x-ray obtained to evaluate the shunt for kinking or discontinuity.

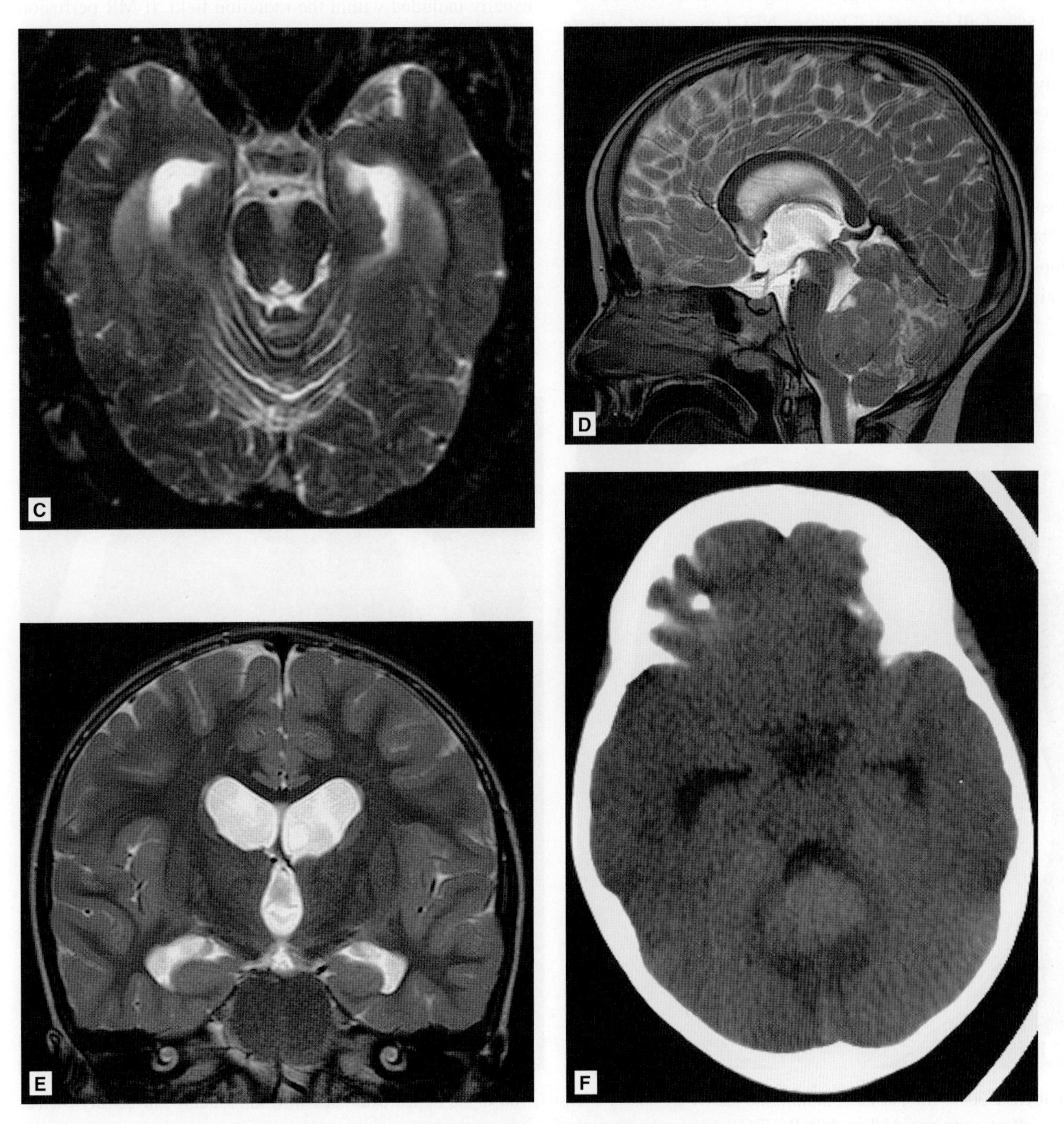

FIGURE 2.29 ■ (*Continued*) **C:** T2WI shows dilation of the temporal horns. **D:** Sagital T2WI shows a large mass in the 4th ventricle causing hydrocephalus with upward bowing of the corpus callosum and distention of the 3rd ventricle. Significant brainstem compression is also present due to the mass (medulloblastoma). **E:** Coronal T2 shows dilated lateral and 3rd ventricles. **F:** Axial NECT shows dilated temporal horns of the lateral ventricles due to the mass present within the 4th ventricle on this image (medulloblastoma).

Radiographic Summary

Glioblastoma Multiforme (GBM) is the most common and most aggressive malignant primary brain tumor. These tumors are typically large at diagnosis and account for 12-15% of all intracranial tumors. NECT may show a mass with a large area of surrounding vasogenic edema and possibly an area of central low attenuation if necrosis is present. CECT demonstrates irregular solid enhancement and thick rim enhancement with central necrosis. GBM is one of the few brain tumors (along with CNS lymphoma), which can cross the thick white matter of the corpus callosum (termed a "butterfly glioma"). MRI typically demonstrates a large amount of surrounding T2 hyperintensity representing vasogenic edema and tumor infiltration, which normally extends well beyond the borders of the contrast enhancement. GBM does not stop at the edge of the contrast enhancement, as tumor cells infiltrate diffusely beyond the tumor margin. For treatment, the entire region of T2/FLAIR hyperintensity is usually included within the radiation field. If MR perfusion is performed, there will be increased relative cerebral blood flow (rCBV) reflecting the increased neo-angiogenesis of the tumor.

Clinical Implications

A GBM may occur at any age, but is most common in patients over age 40-50. Typically patients present with neurological deficits, increased ICP, and possibly seizures. Despite multimodality treatment consisting of gross tumor surgical

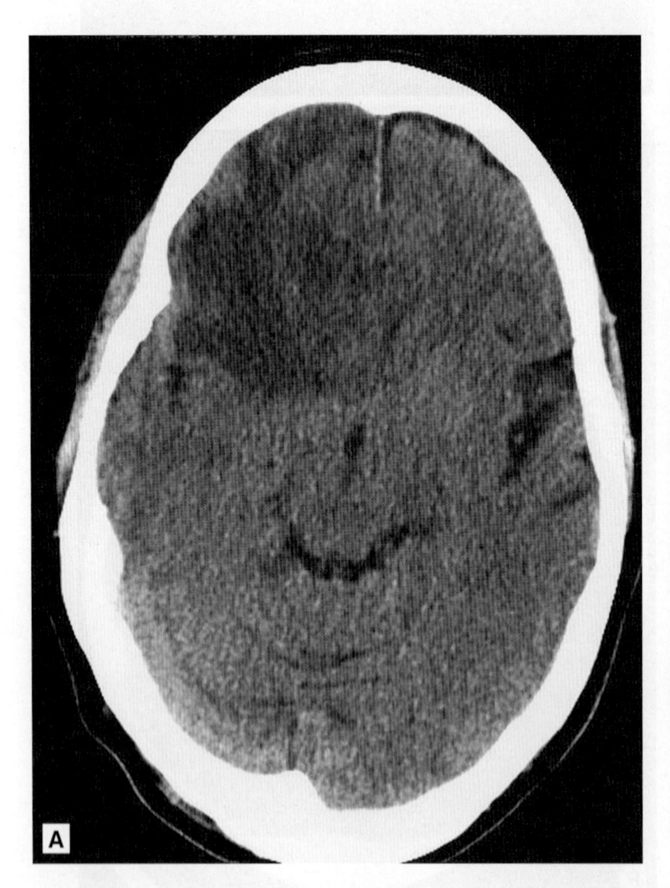

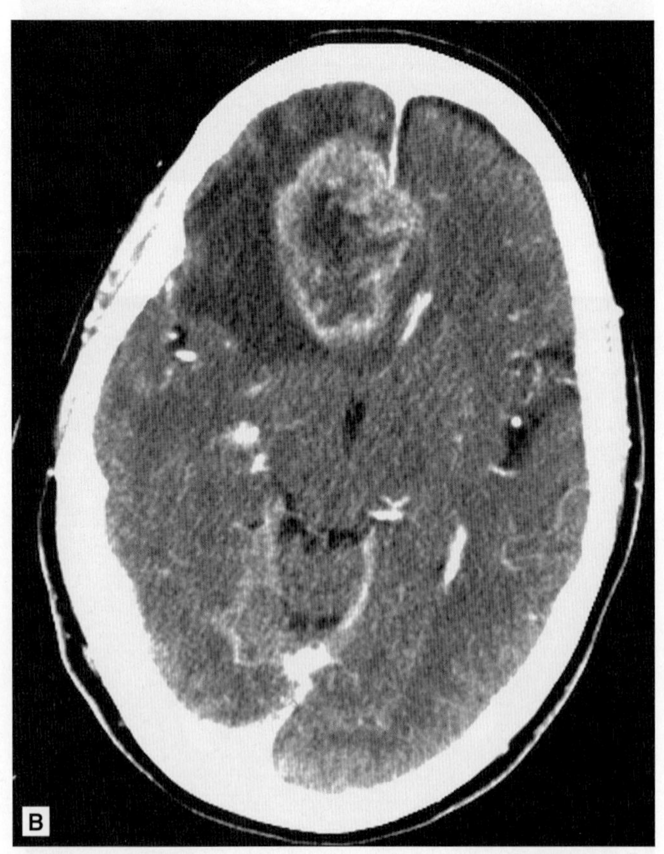

FIGURE 2.30 ■ Glioblastoma Multiforme. **A:** NECT shows a mass lesion in the right frontal lobe with surrounding low-density edema, mass effect, and some midline shift. **B:** CECT shows enhancement of the rim of the tumor with central necrosis.

resection followed by chemotherapy (temozolide), radiation, and anti-angiogenic therapy (bevacizumab), median survival is still only 14 months. Patients that do survive may have cognitive problems, persistent neurologic deficits, communicating hydrocephalus, and cranial neuropathies and polyradiculopathies from leptomeningeal spread. After the initial successful therapy, patient should have frequent neurologic exams and repeat MRI scans every 2 months with chemotherapy cycles.

Pearls

1. GBM is one of the few tumors that may invade the corpus callosum.
2. MRI is the preferred imaging for brain tumor evaluation unless contraindicated.
3. Often, patients have very advanced disease by the time any imaging is obtained.

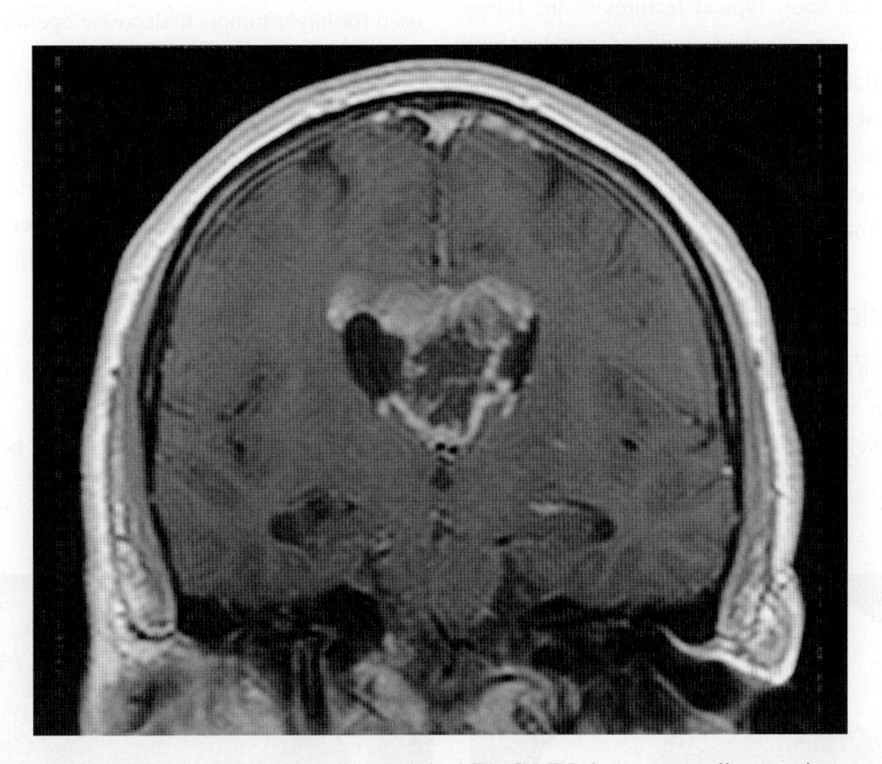

FIGURE 2.31 ■ Glioblastoma Multiforme. Axial, coronal, and sagittal T1+C MRI shows a centrally necrotic mass centered in the corpus callosum that extends down the septum pellucidum. A classic differential for corpus callosum tumors is GBM versus lymphoma.

Radiographic Summary

Meningiomas are typically benign and are the second most common primary neoplasm of the central nervous system. They arise from the arachnoid cap cells of the arachnoid villi in the meninges and are frequently attached to the dura. Common locations include the parasagittal surface of frontal and parietal lobes, the sphenoid ridge, the olfactory grooves, the sylvian region, the superior cerebellum, along the falxcerebri, cerebellopontine angle, and the spinal canal. Meningiomas are usually dome-shaped, with the base lying on the dura. CECT can show typical features of the tumor including a sharply circumscribed, unilobular mass with broad-based dural attachment. Hyperostosis of the adjacent skull and intratumoral calcification may be present. On MR, the classic features are isointensity to gray matter on T1 and T2 and avid contrast enhancement. Meningiomas are hypervascular masses and may be associated with flow voids.

Clinical Implications

Meningiomas are often asymptomatic and are commonly found incidentally on brain imaging. Tumors located near critical structures are more likely to be symptomatic. Meningiomas can irritate the underlying cortex, compress the brain or the cranial nerves, or induce vascular injuries to the brain. Compression of the brain can give rise to focal or generalized cerebral dysfunction presenting as weakness, dysphasia, apathy, and somnolence. By irritating the underlying cortex, meningiomas can also lead to seizure activity. Meningiomas in the vicinity of the sellaturcica may produce panhypopituitarism while meningiomas that compress the visual pathways produce various visual-field defects. Treatment is usually with surgical excision. If only incomplete resection is possible, then external-beam radiation therapy can be used. Pre-operative embolization can be used for larger tumors to decrease operative bleeding.

Pearls

1. CT and MRI showing the dural attachment site, location of edema, and displacement of neurovascular structures are helpful in predicting the likelihood of being able to remove the meningioma.
2. Plain radiographs of the skull may show calcification in meningiomas but in most patients these images will be normal.
3. Posterior fossa meningiomas may be missed by NECT.

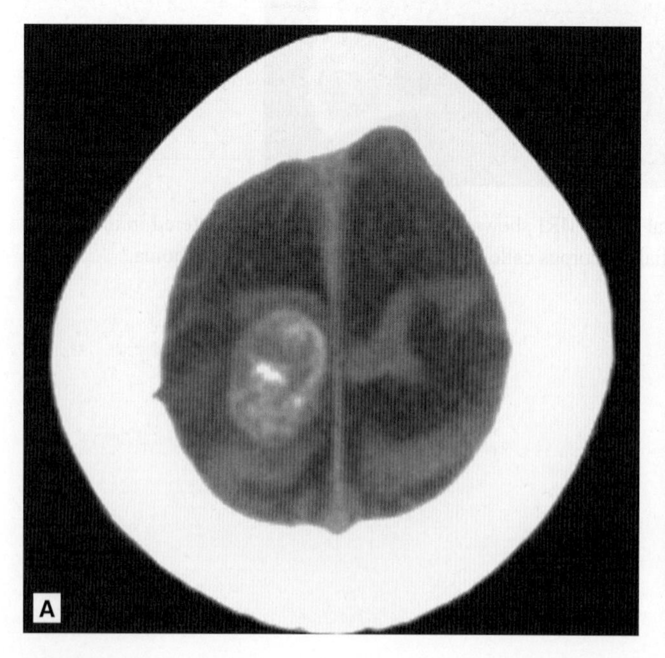

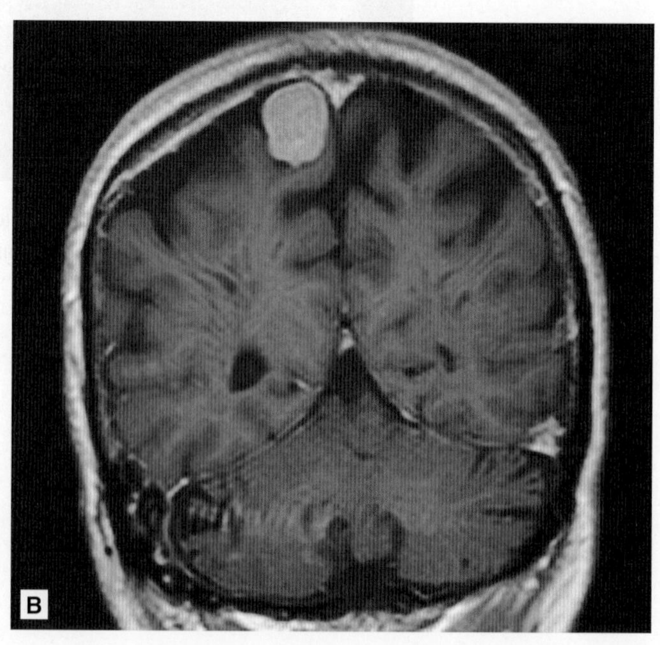

FIGURE 2.32 ■ Meningioma. **A:** Axial NECT at the skull vertex shows a partially calcified smooth extra-axial mass. **B:** Coronal T1+C MR shows the extra-axial nature of the homogenously enhancing mass.

Radiographic Summary

Encephalomacia is softening of the brain tissue usually caused by vascular insufficiency or degenerative changes. The underlying white matter may demonstrate CT hypodensity, T1 hypointensity, and T2 hyperintensity. Encephalomalacia appears with associated volume loss and the cortex may appear thin with heterogeneous signal reflecting varying degrees of gliosis, vacuolation, and residual gray matter integrity. T1W MRI can demonstrate ribbon-like cortical hyperintensity ("laminar necrosis") at sites of prior infarction. Decreased size of white matter tracts is due to wallerian degeneration and parenchymal loss can allow ex-vacuo ventricular enlargement. Areas of encephalomalacia associated with a prior ischemic insult correspond to the corresponding affected vascular territory. Newborns and infants can have periventricular cystic encephalomalacia as a result of perinatal or prenatal hypoxia.

Clinical Implications

Encephalomalacia refers to any loss of brain matter in response to infections, inflammation, ischemia, or hemorrhage. Disturbances in cognition that persist over time may be a source of psychosocial, intellectual, and vocational impairment, often leading to depression and a sense of futility. Intellectual and memory impairment may be accompanied by development of post-traumatic epilepsy.

Pearls

1. Encephalomalacia is very common and should not be confused with acute infarcts or neoplastic processes.
2. Areas of encephalomalacia hinder imaging evaluation of new infarctions on CT. MRI with diffusion imaging is most helpful for finding new areas of infarction as DWI will only be "bright" for approximately 10 days following an acute stroke.

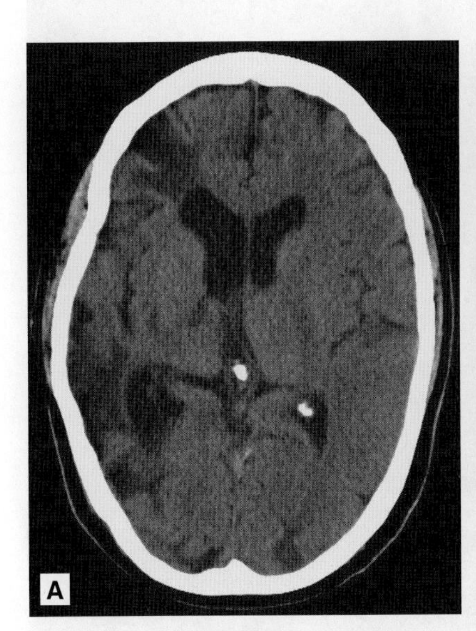

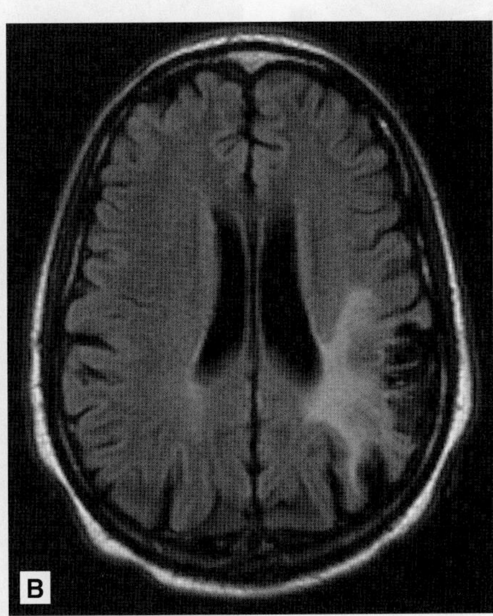

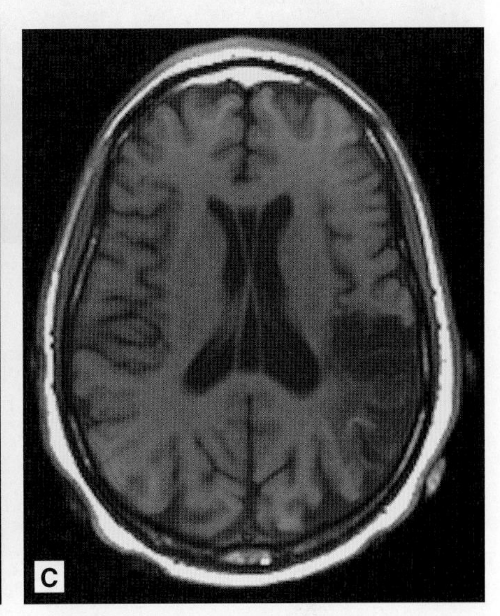

FIGURE 2.33 ■ Encephalomacia. **A:** NECT shows low attenuation from prior right MCA infarction. Note the enlargement of the right frontal horn ventricle due to volume loss in the adjacent white matter (ex-vacuo enlargement). **B:** Axial FLAIR image in a different patient (55-year-old male) shows increased T2 signal, volume loss, and encephalomalacia in the left parietal lobe due to a prior infarction. **C:** T1WI in the same patient shows volume loss. Subtle ribbon-like hyperintensity along the left parietal cortex represents laminar necrosis from prior infarction.

Radiographic Summary

The underlying problem in Chiari malformations is a congenitally small posterior fossa. Arnold-Chiari 1 malformation is caudal protrusion of "peg-shaped" cerebellar tonsils more than 5 mm below the foramen magnum. CT shows a "crowded" foramen magnum but MRI is the test of choice, with measurements made on the midline sagittal images. Phase contrast MR sequences can be used when considering surgery to evaluate the CSF flow at the foramen magnum. A syrinx in the cervical spine is present in up to 75% of patients. Chiari 2 malformation is usually identified at birth, if not during prenatal ultrasound. Prenatal ultrasound can show ventriculomegaly, "lemon sign" of calvarium, and "banana sign" of the posterior fossa. MRI findings include a small posterior fossa, protrusion of cerebellar tissue through foramen magnum, tectal beaking, callosal dysgenesis, an elongated 4th ventricle, and interdigitation of sulci.

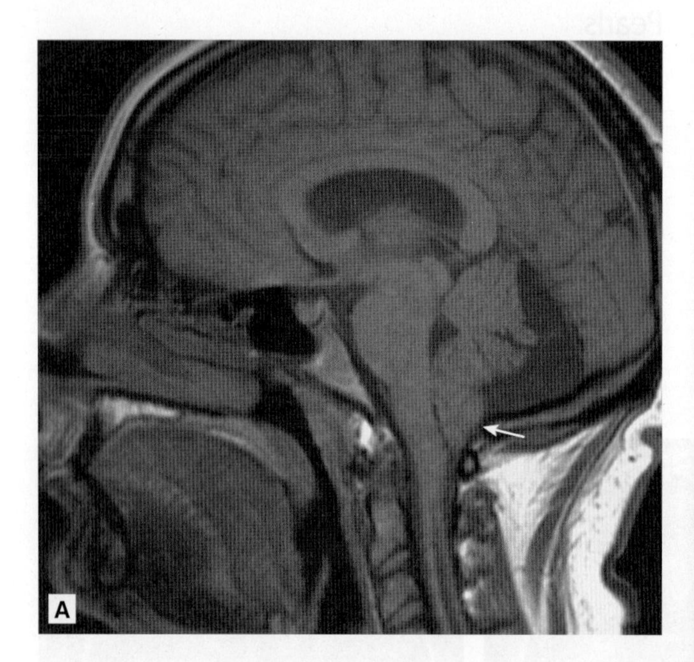

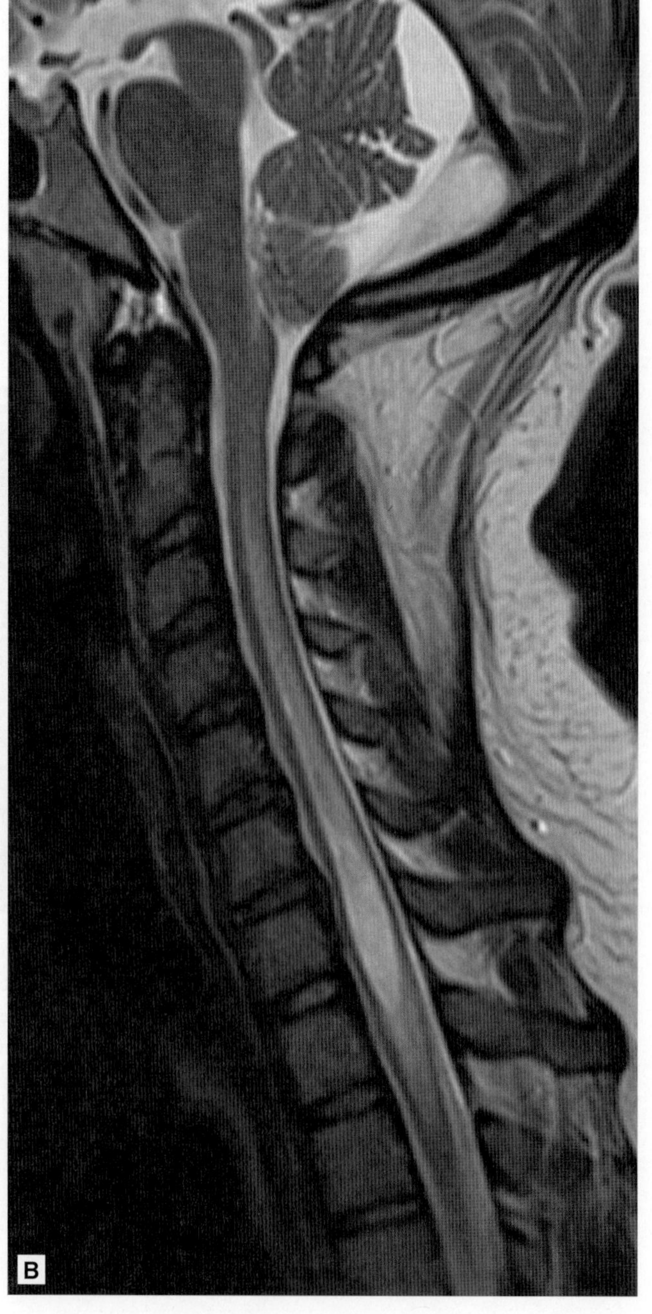

FIGURE 2.34 ■ Chiari I Malformation. **A:** Sagittal T1 MR shows descent of the cerebellar tonsils >5 mm through the foramen magnum (arrow). Low signal in cervical spinal cord represents a syrinx. **B:** Sagittal T2 shows a large syrinx within the cervical and upper thoracic spinal cord. These findings are commonly associated with Chiari I.

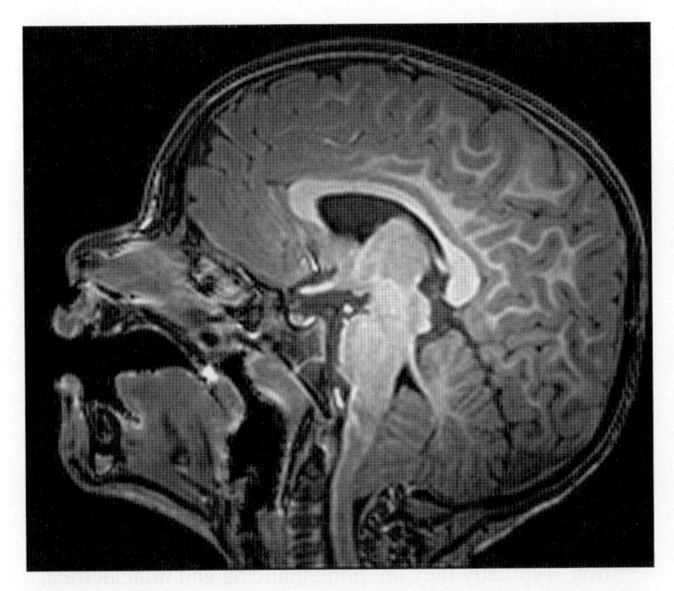

FIGURE 2.35 ■ Chiari I Malformation. Sagittal T1WI shows descent of peg-shaped cerebellar tonsils through the "crowded" foramen magnum in this child.

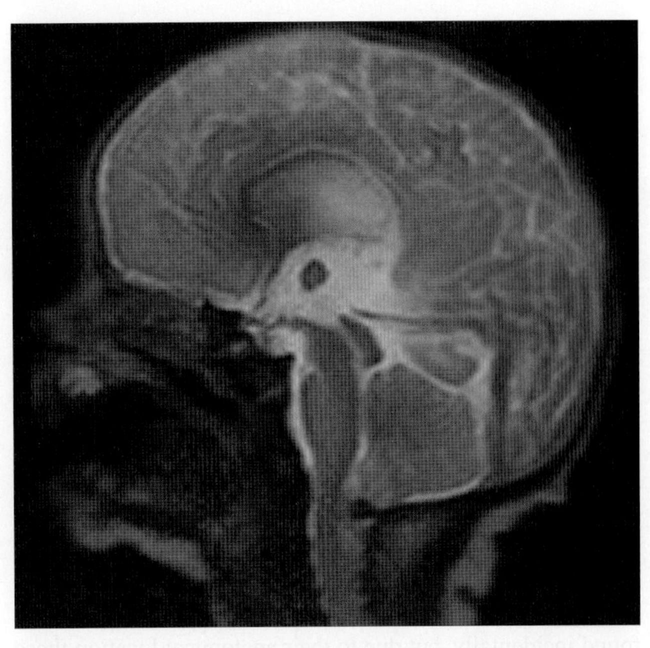

FIGURE 2.37 ■ Chiari I Malformation. Sagittal T2WI in a 1-month-old male with myelomeningocele shows a small posterior fossa, tectal beaking, dysgenetic corpus callosum, and an elongated 4th ventricle.

Clinical Implications

Despite the fact that Chiari 1 malformation is usually present at birth, the symptoms of the malformation are usually not experienced until the patient is in the 3rd to 4th decade of life. Complaints may include neck pain, ataxia, muscle weakness, numbness in the extremities, dizziness, vision problems, tinnitus, vomiting, or headache worsened by coughing or straining ("Chiari spells"). Infants may have difficulty swallowing, irritability, excessive drooling, a weak cry, vomiting, arm weakness, and failure to thrive. Up to 50% of Chiari 1 malformations are asymptomatic and are discovered incidentally. If symptomatic or accompanied by syrinx, neurosurgical treatment often entails a suboccipital decompression to create space in the posterior fossa to allow unimpeded CSF flow.

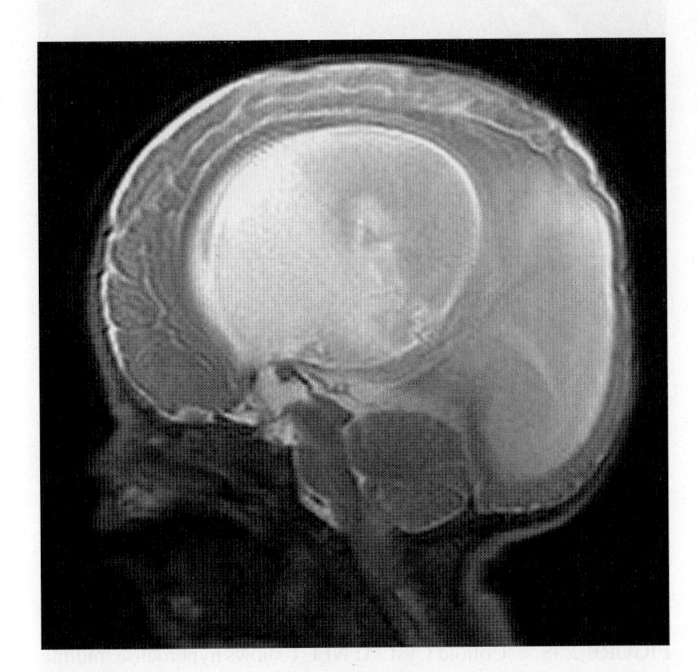

FIGURE 2.36 ■ Chiari II Malformation. Sagittal T2WI in a 2-month-old male with Chiari II malformation and myelomeningocele. There is massive dilation of the lateral ventricle, small posterior fossa, and tectal beaking.

Pearls

1. Chiari 1 is often discovered incidentally as many patients are asymptomatic. If symptomatic, neurosurgical evaluation and additional advanced imaging is recommended.
2. Chiari 2 has a nearly 100% association with myelomeningocele, and is obvious on prenatal ultrasound or at the time of birth.
3. The underlying problem with most Chiari malformations is congenital underdevelopment of the posterior fossa, which leads to crowding at the foramen magnum and abnormal CSF flow.

Radiographic Summary

On NECT, most colloid cysts are hyperdense oval or rounded masses that arise from the anterior third ventricle just posterior to foramen of Monro. Hydrocephalus may occur due to the "ball-valve" effect of the mass plugging the foramen of Monro preventing normal CSF flow. The appearance of colloid cysts on MRI is variable, but their location is nearly pathognomonic. Due to the proteinaceous nature of the contents of a colloid cyst, the most common appearance on MRI demonstrates hyperintensity on T1, hypointensity on T2, and thin rim enhancement usually representing enhancement of the adjacent and stretched septal veins.

Clinical Implications

Colloid cysts are benign congenital lesions that are often found incidentally, but due to their anatomical location these cysts can cause serious morbidity and mortality when they lead to obstructive hydrocephalus and increased intracranial pressure. Both CT and MR can be used in the diagnosis of colloid cysts. CT scans are important preoperatively as the viscosity of cystic contents correlates to the radiodensity of the fluid seen on CT. Although colloid cysts do not have malignant potential, they are often managed surgically because of the potential to cause hydrocephalus by obstructing cerebrospinal fluid flow at the third ventricle. All patients with findings concerning colloid cysts should be referred for neurosurgical evaluation.

Pearls

1. On both CT and MRI, colloid cysts occasionally have a thin rim of peripheral enhancement after contrast injection. Typically they are nonenhancing and noncalcified.
2. Even though colloid cysts are benign masses, they can cause intermittent hydrocephalus, reflecting the importance of obtaining CT or MRI.
3. MRI is superior to CT in fully characterizing the lesion.

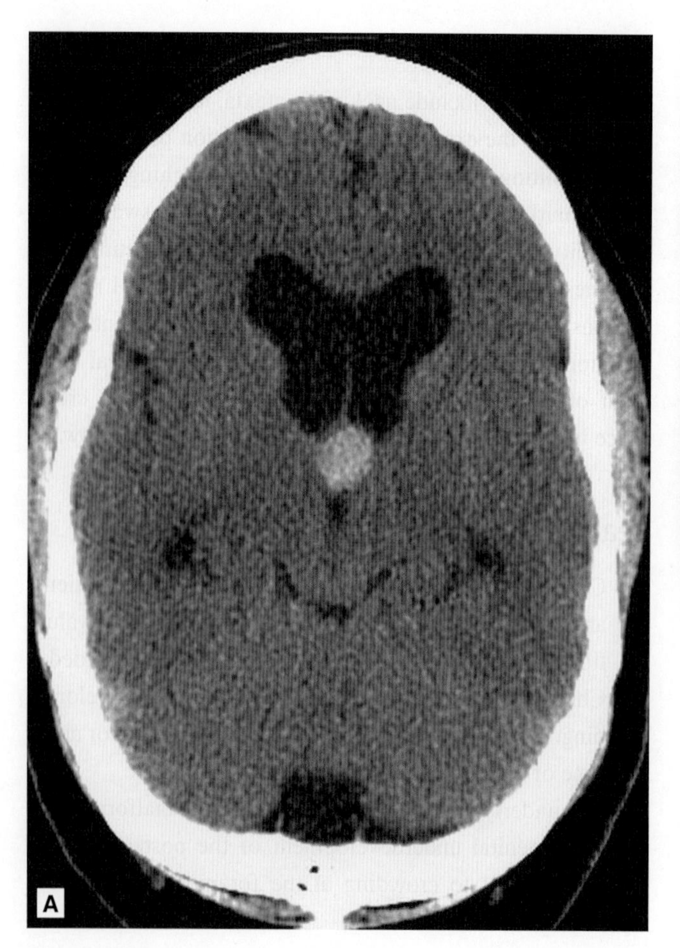

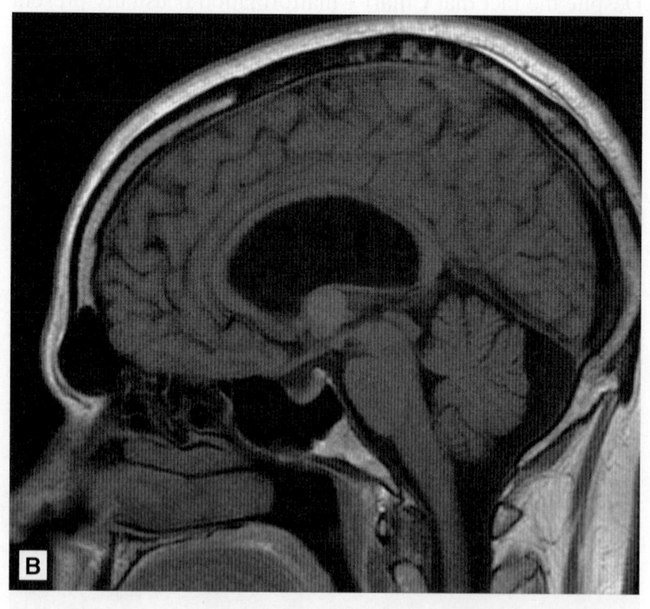

FIGURE 2.38 ■ Colloid Cyst. **A:** NECT shows hyperdense midline mass near the foramen of Monro with hydrocephalus. **B:** Sagittal T1WI shows a mildly hyperintense midline mass near the foramen of Monro with dilation of the lateral ventricles. There is no enhancement on contrasted scans. Findings are typical for a colloid cyst.

Radiographic Summary

Preseptal cellulitis is infection of tissues anterior to the orbital septum. CECT findings include swelling of the eyelid and adjacent preseptal soft tissues. Fat stranding and edema are noted, but there is no extension of infectious changes posterior to the orbital septum. Orbital MRI with contrast is an imaging option, but CECT is superior as it allows better evaluation of adjacent ethmoid sinuses.

Clinical Implications

Preseptal cellulitis is an infection of the eyelid and periorbital soft tissues characterized by eyelid erythema and edema. The orbital septum serves as a barrier to the spread of infection into the orbit. Patients will present with a painful, swollen eyelid and they may not be able to open the affected eye. There is typically no disturbance in visual acuity or ocular motility. Bacterial infection usually results from the local spread of adjacent upper respiratory tract infections such as sinusitis, external ocular infection (stye), or following trauma to the eyelids.

Pearls

1. A CECT scan of the head is also indicated for any neurological findings on examination in patients with preseptal cellulitis.
2. The orbital septum is the dividing line between preseptal and orbital cellulitis.
3. Outpatient management of preseptal cellulitis may be considered in appropriate patients, while true orbital cellulitis represents a surgical emergency.

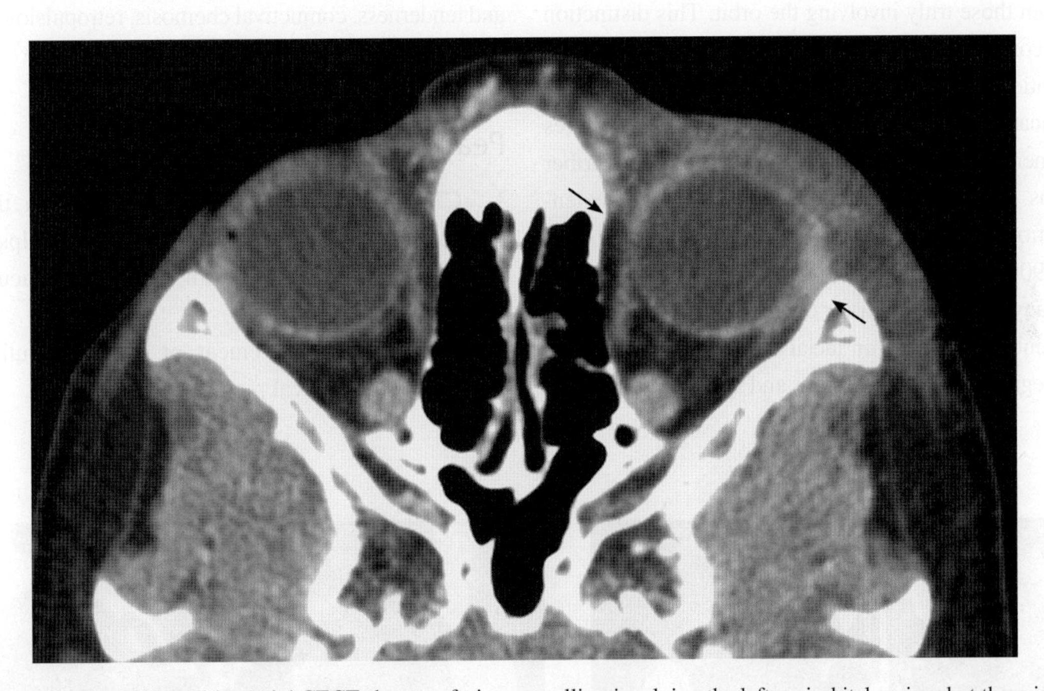

FIGURE 2.39 ■ Pre-Septal Cellulitis. Axial CECT shows soft tissue swelling involving the left periorbital region, but there is no extension of infection posterior to the orbital septum confirming the diagnosis of preseptal cellulitis. The location of the orbital septum is demonstrated by the arrows.

Radiographic Summary

Orbital cellulitis is inflammation of the soft tissues posterior to the orbital septum, a thin tissue that divides the eyelid from the eye socket. Orbital CECT can confirm extension of inflammation into the orbit, detect coexisting sinus disease, and identify an orbital or subperiosteal abscess. CECT will show fat stranding and enhancement and often edema of the eyelid. CT scan can also detect detachment of the periorbita seen with subperiosteal abscess or true orbital abscess. MRI or CECT of the orbits can be helpful in assessing intracranial extension of the infection into the cavernous sinus or adjacent structures. CT or MR venography provides no additional help in assessing cavernous sinus involvement.

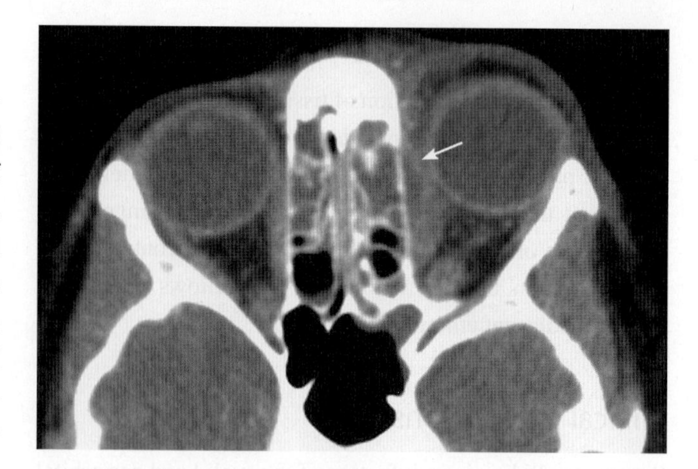

FIGURE 2.40 ■ Subperiosteal Orbital Abscess. Axial CECT shows fluid-filled ethmoid sinuses with extension of inflammation into the medial left orbit. There is a small low-attenuation region with enhancing rim representing a subperiosteal orbital abscess (arrow).

Clinical Implications

Diagnostic imaging can help distinguish primary inflammatory processes occurring in front of the orbital septum (preseptal cellulitis) from those truly involving the orbit. This distinction is crucial secondary to the potential need for surgical intervention in patients with orbital cellulitis as well as to identify acute complications of the condition. Orbital cellulitis requires urgent treatment to preserve visual acuity and prevent further complications. Orbital cellulitis is most often caused by extension of infection from adjacent sinuses, especially the ethmoid sinus (75 to 90%); it is less commonly caused by direct infection accompanying local trauma or contiguous spread of infection from dental infections or facial surgery. Proptosis and ophthalmoplegia are the cardinal signs and symptoms of orbital cellulitis, but pain with extraocular eye movement, orbital pain and tenderness, conjuctival chemosis, retropulsion of the globe, and even nasal drainage may be seen.

Pearls

1. CECT of the orbits is used to confirm the cause in patients with periorbital swelling and helps distinguish true orbital cellulitis from more benign acute preseptal cellulitis.
2. Radiologic improvement of orbital cellulitis will lag behind the clinical picture by several days.

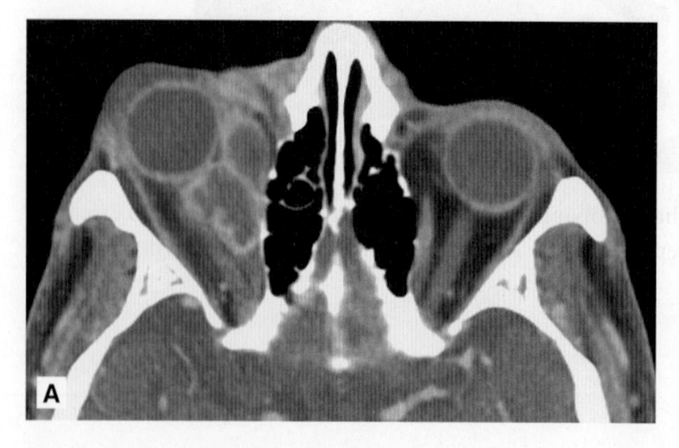

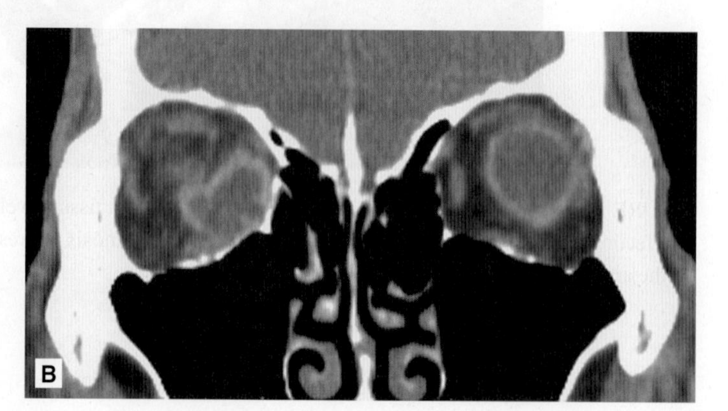

FIGURE 2.41 ■ Orbital Abscess. **A, B:** Axial and coronal orbit CECT show rim-enhancing abscess near the right medial rectus muscle with concomitant orbital proptosis. This patient was surgically managed with favorable outcome.

Radiographic Summary

Optic neuritis is the inflammation of the optic nerve that may cause a complete or partial loss of vision. In patients with optic neuritis, MRI of the brain and orbits with contrast and fat-suppression may show abnormal enhancement of the affected optic nerve. Thin-slice T2-weighted images through the optic nerves may show characteristic high-signal intensity in the minimally expanded nerve. In those patients with optic neuritis presenting as a complication of MS, the MRI may show characteristic periventricular white matter lesions that are seen best on FLAIR sequences.

Clinical Implications

Optic neuritis is an inflammatory demyelinating condition of the optic nerve causing acute monocular vision loss. Many cases of optic neuritis are associated with multiple sclerosis or neuromyelitis optica (Devic's disease), but optic neuritis can occur in isolation. In patients with multiple sclerosis, optic neuritis is commonly the first manifestation of the disease. Over a 15-year period, 50% of patients with optic neuritis will eventually be diagnosed with MS.

Acute optic neuritis presents with vision loss developing over hours to days and may be associated with an afferent pupillary defect and acute eye pain. Treatment for patients with optic neuritis focuses on vision improvement and treatment of underlying MS. Patients with optic neuritis with two or more brain lesions on brain MRI may have a significantly decreased risk in developing chronic sequelae of MS if given intravenous methylprednisolone. For patients with optic neuritis whose brain lesions on MRI indicate a high risk of developing MS, treatment may also include immunomodulator therapy.

Pearls

1. CT scanning has a very limited role in the setting of optic neuritis. Size differences in the optic nerve can be appreciated, but this is neither sensitive nor specific.
2. Contrasted orbital MRI is the best imaging for suspected optic neuritis.

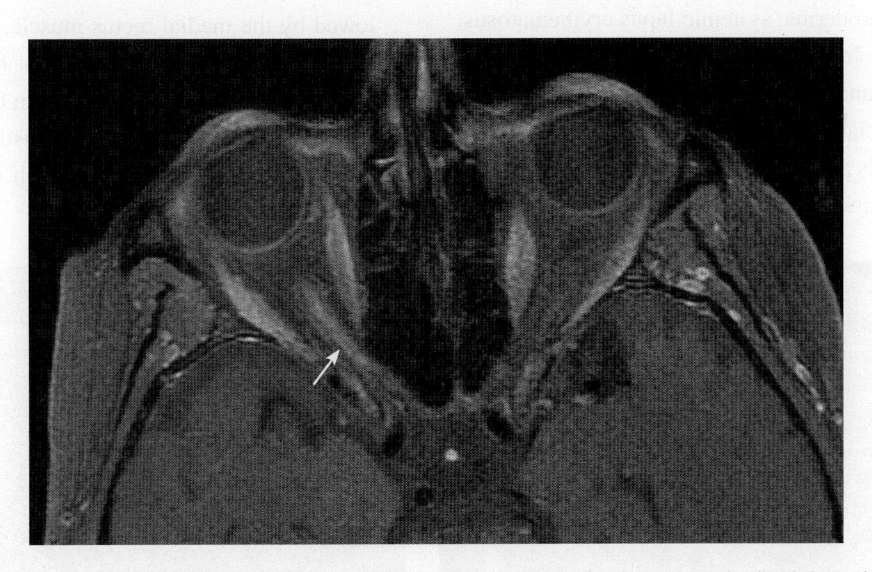

FIGURE 2.42 ■ Optic Neuritis. Axial fat-saturated T1+C orbit MRI shows abnormal enhancement in the right optic nerve consistent with optic neuritis (arrow).

Radiographic Summary

Orbital pseudotumor is a benign idiopathic inflammation that may encompass the entire orbit or be present in a localized fashion involving the anterior orbit, posterior orbit, lacrimal gland, or extraocular muscles. CECT of the orbit in orbital pseudotumor typically reveals marked swelling and enhancement in the lacrimal glands or in one or more of the extraocular muscles (EOM). Stranding is often seen in the orbital fat. When orbital pseudotumor affects the EOM, swelling typically involves the belly of the muscle(s) as well as the insertion (myotendinous junction) adjacent to the globe. Imaging can be performed with either CT or MRI of the orbits with contrast. When orbital pseudotumor extends posteriorly into the superior orbital fissure or cavernous sinus, it is then termed Tolosa–Hunt Syndrome.

Clinical Implications

Differentiating between orbital infections and orbital pseudotumor can be challenging. Although often idiopathic in origin, orbital pseudotumor has been associated with several noninfectious diseases including thyroid-related eye disease, psoriatic arthropathy, scleroderma, systemic lupus erythematosus, and Crohn's disease. Infectious etiologies such as Lyme disease, herpes zoster, and various upper respiratory infections have also been associated with this entity. Prompt treatment with corticosteroids is associated with improvement in symptoms and a reduced risk of muscle fibrosis and recurrence.

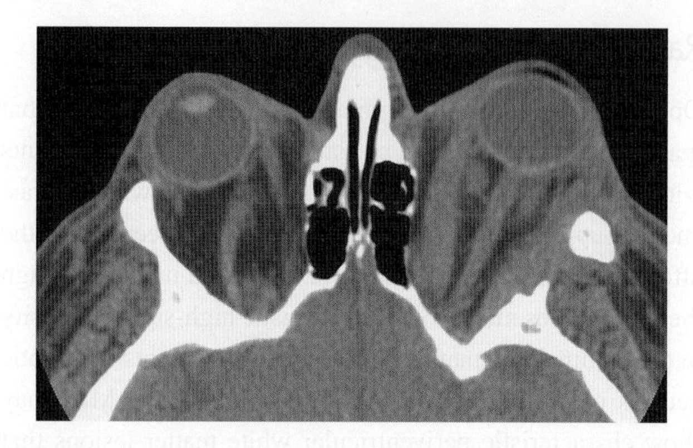

FIGURE 2.43 ■ Orbital Pseudotumor. NECT of the orbits in a 40-year-old male shows inflammation within the left orbital fat. There is marked enlargement of the extraocular muscles that involves the myotendinous junction (an important distinction from thyroid orbitopathy).

Pearls

1. Most cases of orbital pseudotumor tend to be unilateral. This helps differentiate it from thyroid orbitopathy, which is usually bilateral.
2. Any muscle can be affected, including isolated lateral rectus involvement, while in thyroid-related eye disease there is predilection for the inferior rectus muscle followed by the medial rectus muscle. An important imaging distinction is the involvement of the myotendinous junction in pseudotumor, but not in thyroid orbitopathy.
3. Pain on presentation helps to distinguish from orbital lymphoma and sarcoidosis, which can appear identical on imaging.

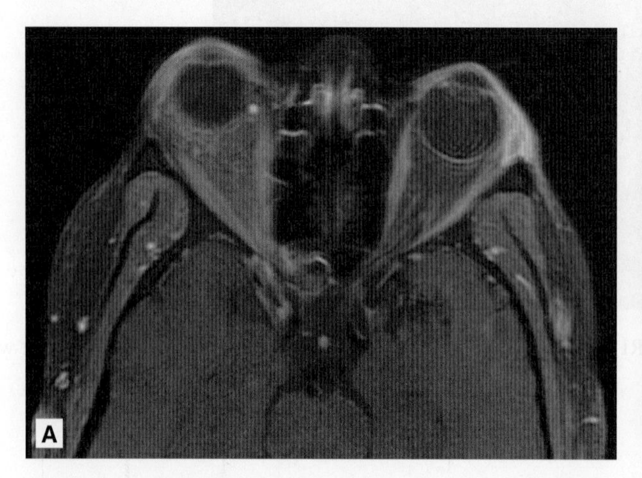

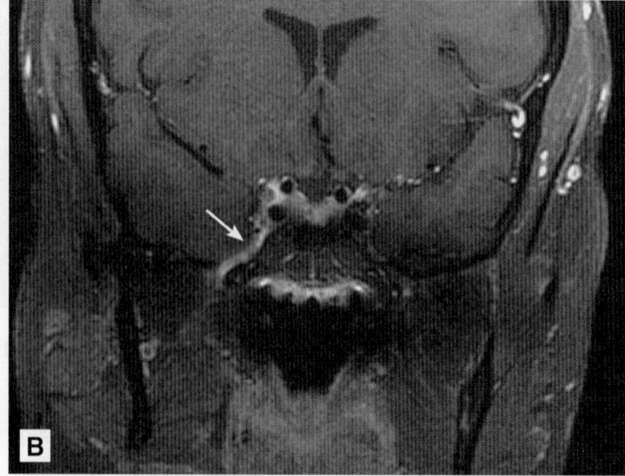

FIGURE 2.44 ■ Orbital Pseudotumor. **A:** Axial fat-saturated T1+C orbit MRI demonstrates proptosis and inflammation within the right orbit that extends through the orbital apex to the cavernous sinus (Tolosa–Hunt Syndrome). **B:** Coronal T1+C fat-saturated MRI shows enhancement that extends inferiorly from the right cavernous sinus along cranial nerve V_3 via foramen ovale at the skull base (arrow). The patient had a history of breast and thyroid cancer as well as lupus, so orbital biopsy was obtained to exclude metastases. Ultimately the pathology revealed inflammation consistent with Tolosa–Hunt Syndrome.

Radiographic Summary

Pott's puffy tumor is an anterior extension of a frontal sinus infection that results in frontal bone osteomyelitis and subperiosteal abscess. CT is utilized to evaluate Pott's Puffy Tumor as it depicts optimal detail of bony structures, soft tissue, and air in the setting of sinus disease. IV contrast helps assess soft tissue infection or abscess as well as any intracranial subdural or parenchymal infection. On CT scan, fluid in the frontal sinuses is seen with adjacent destruction of the anterior sinus wall and infection spreading out into forehead soft tissues causing a subgaleal abscess. MRI is the preferred imaging modality if there is concern for concomitant intracranial involvement.

Clinical Implications

Pott's puffy tumor is typically seen in children and adolescents as a complication of frontal sinusitis or trauma. Patients may present with swelling of the forehead, headache, photophobia, fever, rhinorrhea, vomiting, and lethargy. Although a decrease has been seen in the incidence of disease of the frontal sinuses since the development of broad-spectrum antibiotics, Pott's puffy tumor can cause significant complications if the diagnosis is not made quickly. There is potential for intracranial spread of thrombophlebitis from the frontal sinus through the diploic veins leading to empyema over the frontal lobe, meningitis, venous sinus thrombosis, or cerebral abscess. The mainstay of treatment includes broad-spectrum antibiotics combined with surgical drainage.

Pearls

1. Pott's puffy tumor is often misdiagnosed as a neoplasm, infected hematoma, or other soft tissue infection. The diagnosis should be included on the differential for any patient with swelling on the forehead and frontal sinus disease.
2. Concomitant intracranial involvement should be considered and ruled out in patients with Pott's puffy tumor.

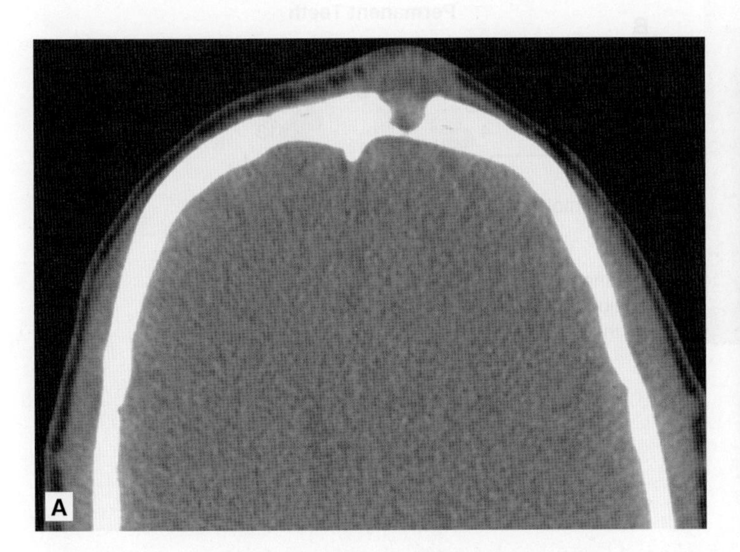

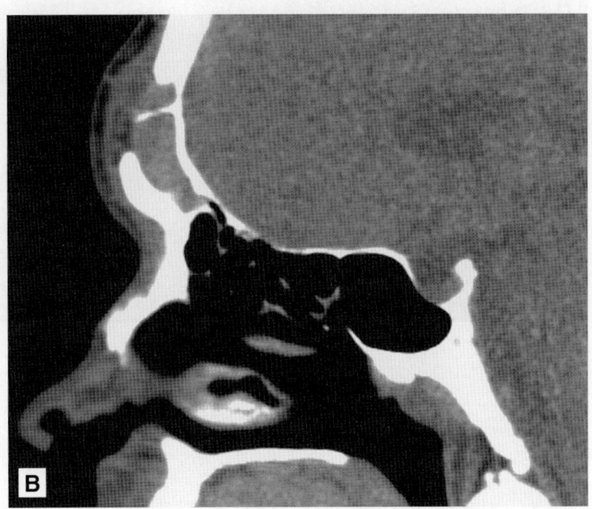

FIGURE 2.45 ■ Pott's Puffy Tumor. **A, B:** Axial and sagittal NECT of sinuses show opacification of the normally air-filled frontal sinuses with cortical destruction of the anterior wall. Extension of inflammation into the soft tissues overlying the anterior skull is evident (subgaleal tissue).

Radiographic Summary

A periapical abscess is a collection of pus surrounding the tooth apex, usually from an infection that has spread from a tooth to the surrounding tissues. When a periapical abscess is suspected, panoramic radiography is the most helpful emergency imaging because it provides the most information for all the teeth and surrounding bone. A periapical abscess will appear as a radiolucency around the apex (root) of the tooth. Dental caries may also be seen on the radiograph as areas of lucency within the crown of the tooth. As the decay process proceeds, the mineral content of the enamel and dentin decreases with a resultant decrease in attenuation of the x-ray beam as it passes through the teeth.

If there is concern for infectious spread into the adjacent buccal or lingual soft tissues, a CECT of the face may help identify abscess collections in potential spaces such as the buccal or canine space. CT lacks the spatial resolution of a Panorex radiograph, but still nicely demonstrates periapicallucencies and caries, with the added benefit of soft tissue evaluation.

Clinical Implications

A periapical abscess usually occurs secondary to dental caries. Dental caries erode the enamel and dentin and allow bacteria to invade the pulp leading to necrosis, invasion of the alveolar bulb, and ultimately the development of an abscess. Patients often present with severe localized tooth pain, thermal sensitivity, pain with chewing, halitosis, and may have a fever. Treatment of a periapical abscess requires incision and drainage and endodontic therapy or extraction of the diseased tooth. Antibiotics are often added as an adjunct therapy. The acute abscess should be treated aggressively to alleviate the patient's pain and to prevent worsening sequelae such as cellulitis or soft tissue abscess. When associated abscesses extend into the potential spaces of the face, oral surgery consultation may be appropriate for emergent incision and drainage. Ludwig angina, extension of abscess into the submandibular and sublingual spaces, has the potential for acute airway compromise and is a surgical emergency.

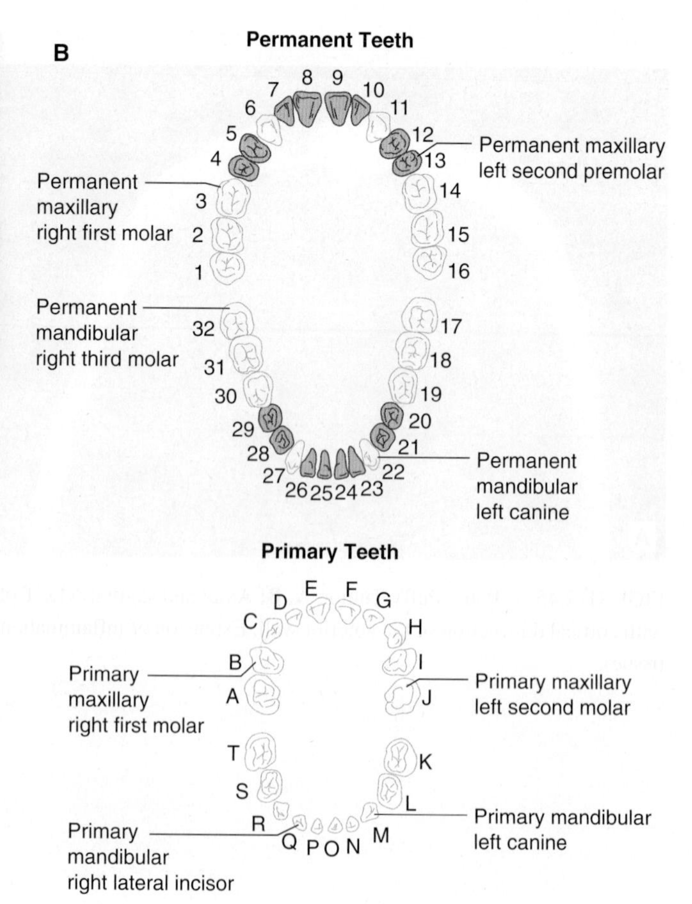

FIGURE 2.46 ■ Odontogenic Abscess. **A:** Mandibular panorex radiograph shows a small periapical lucency surrounding the roots of tooth #18 (arrow). Multiple dental caries are present throughout the remainder of the teeth. **B:** Identification of teeth. (Reproduced with permission from Tintinalli JE, Stapczynksi JS, Ma OJ, Cline DM, Cydulka RK, Meckler GD, eds. *Tintinalli's Emergency Medicine: A Comprehensive Study Guide.* 7th Edition. New York: McGraw-Hill; 2011:1573.)

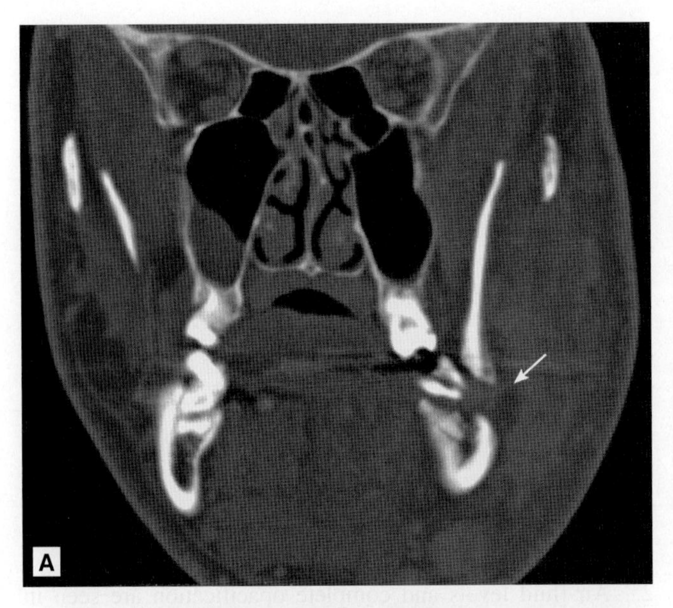

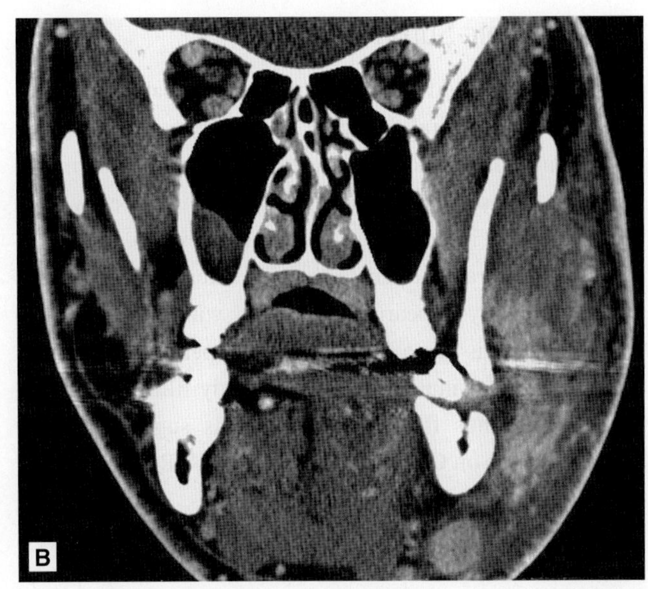

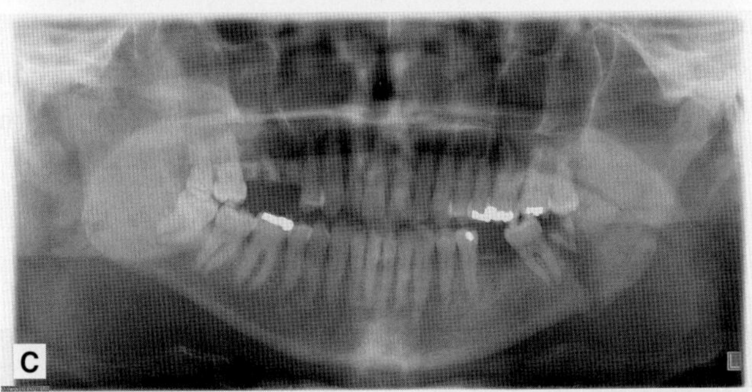

FIGURE 2.47 ■ Odontogenic Abscess. **A, B:** Coronal CECT in bone and soft tissue windows shows a large left mandibular molar periapical abscess with adjacent buccal space abscess (arrow). **C:** Mandibular panorex of the same patient shows the large left mandibular abscess with destruction of the cortical bone creating a sinus tract to the buccal space.

Pearls

1. Understanding of the American Dental Association Universal Numbering system helps in management and description of patients with dental pain.
2. If there is concern for extension of the periapical abscess into the soft tissues, CECT of the face is helpful to determine the location, size, extent, and relationship of the inflammatory process and extension of infection into the surrounding structures.

Radiographic Summary

Sinusitis refers to inflammation of the sinus that occurs with infection from a viral, bacterial, or fungal source. If indicated, sinus CT without contrast is the first line of imaging. MRI is reserved for cases of sinus tumors or invasive sinusitis when intracranial or orbital extension is a concern. CT appearance of acute sinusitis often shows air-fluid levels or bubbly appearing secretions within the sinuses. Chronic sinusitis has a more variable appearance with soft tissue lining the sinus walls or completely filling the sinus. Hyperdense sinus fluid or calcifications suggest chronic fungal sinusitis on CT. Fungal sinusitis on MRI can demonstrate low signal on T2WI.

Clinical Implications

Sinusitis can be acute (<4 weeks), subacute (4-8 weeks), or chronic (>8 weeks). All three types have similar symptoms and are often difficult to distinguish by exam alone. CT scans are recommended for acute sinusitis only if there is a severe infection or a high risk for complications. Patients with poorly controlled diabetes and patients that are immunocompromised are at increased risk for invasive fungal sinusitis and may benefit from imaging studies. CT is superior to MRI for visualization of the paranasal anatomy but MRI should be utilized when there is concern for complications of local sinus infections, particularly intracranial extension.

Pearls

1. Uncomplicated sinusitis does not require radiologic imaging. However, when symptoms are recurrent or refractory despite treatment, further diagnostic evaluations may be indicated.
2. Air-fluid levels and complete opacification are seen in only 60% of sinusitis cases.
3. Sinus CT findings should be interpreted in conjunction with the patient's clinical findings because of the high rate of false-positive studies.

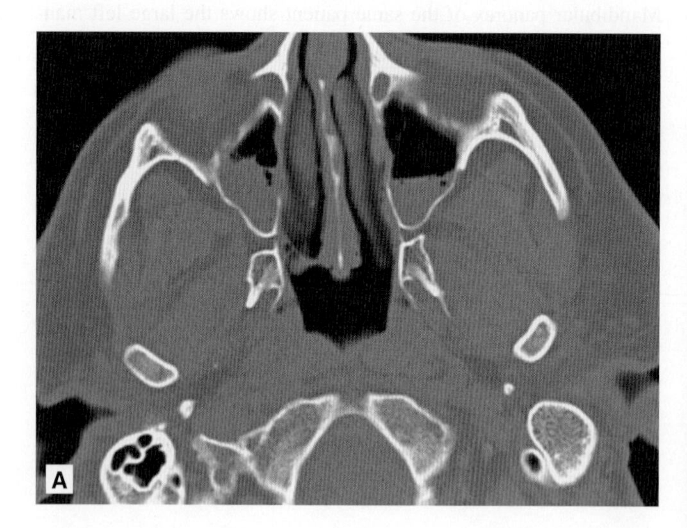

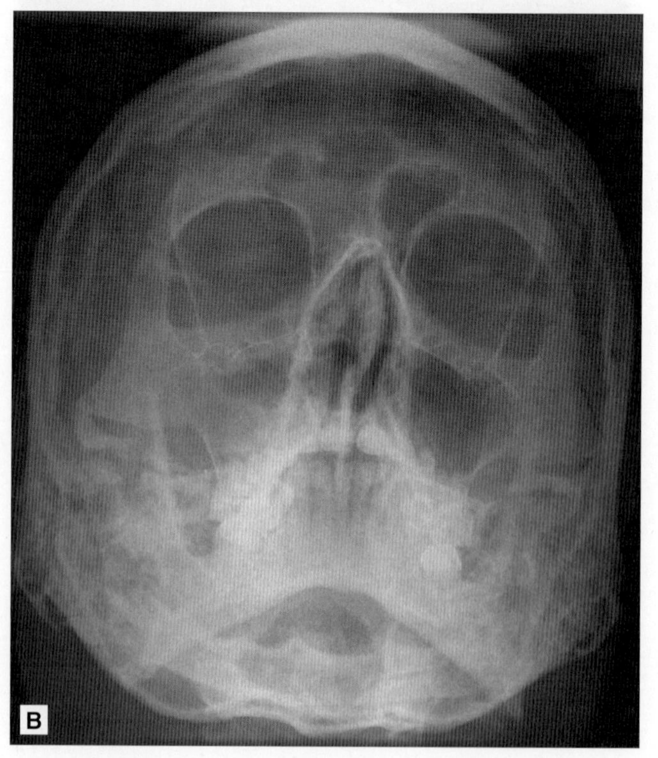

FIGURE 2.48 ■ Acute Sinusitis. **A:** NECT shows air-fluid levels in both maxillary sinuses with locules of air trapped within the fluid suggestive of acute sinusitis. **B:** Waters view of skull shows air-fluid levels with bubbly secretions in the right frontal and maxillary sinuses suggesting acute sinusitis.

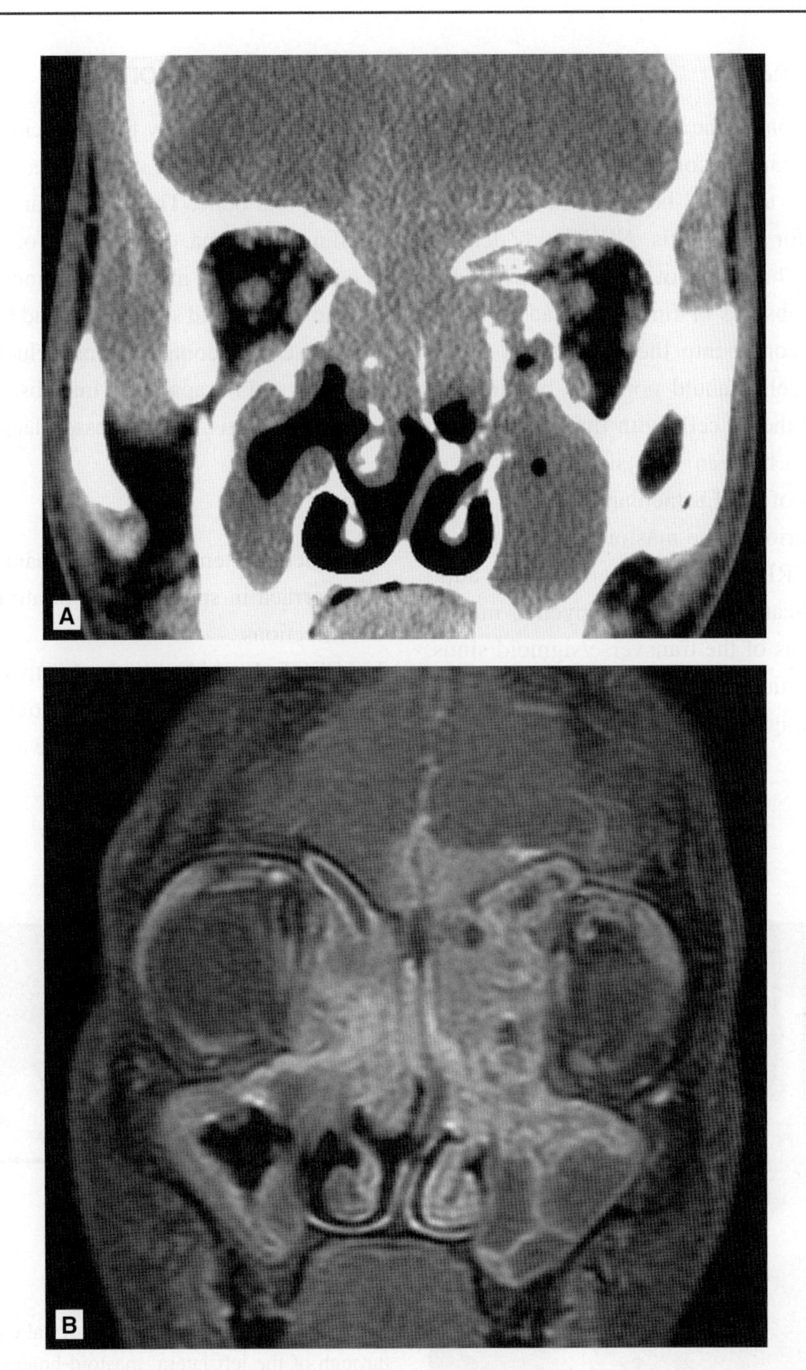

FIGURE 2.49 ■ Invasive Fungal Sinusitis. **A:** Coronal NECT shows opacification of the ethmoid sinus that has eroded through the cribiform plate into the intracranial cavity. **B:** Coronal T1 MR with contrast shows enhancement within the ethmoid sinuses that extends through the cribiform plate into the frontal lobes. Patient was a 20-year-old male with invasive fungal sinusitis.

Radiographic Summary

Mastoiditis is an infection of the portion of the temporal bone located behind the ear that contains open, air-containing spaces. CECT of the temporal bones is the diagnostic imaging test of choice for mastoiditis. NECT may demonstrate acute mastoiditis, but will not help to determine if there is accompanying abscess or further spread of infection through the bony cortex into the soft tissues of the neck. The mastoid air cells should normally be air-filled on CT. Opacification of the air cells with fluid is seen with mastoiditis, but can also be seen with simple effusion or obstruction/dysfunction of the Eustachian tube. A soft tissue abscess located inferior to the mastoid bone is termed a "Bezold's abscess." MRI is reserved for evaluating adjacent intracranial complications such as empyema, meningitis, or septic thrombosis of the transverse/sigmoid sinus. On T2-weighted MRI, fluid signal in the mastoid can be an incidental finding limiting its usefulness in screening for mastoiditis.

Clinical Implications

Mastoiditis is typically found in children, with the diagnosis being based on history and physical combined with CECT of the temporal bone. The findings are based on retro-auricular swelling, erythema, or protrusion of the auricle plus evidence of coexistent otitis media. Extension of the infectious process beyond the mastoid system can lead to a variety of intracranial and extracranial complications including meningitis, epidural, subdural, and intraparenchymal abscesses, vascular thrombosis, osteomyelitis, and abscesses deep within the neck.

Pearls

1. Patients often present with pain or fever and persisting otorrhea in spite of appropriate treatment of middle-ear infections.
2. CECT should be obtained if there is clinical concern for mastoiditis due to the potential for extension of infection into the soft tissues of the neck or development of an intracranial abscess.

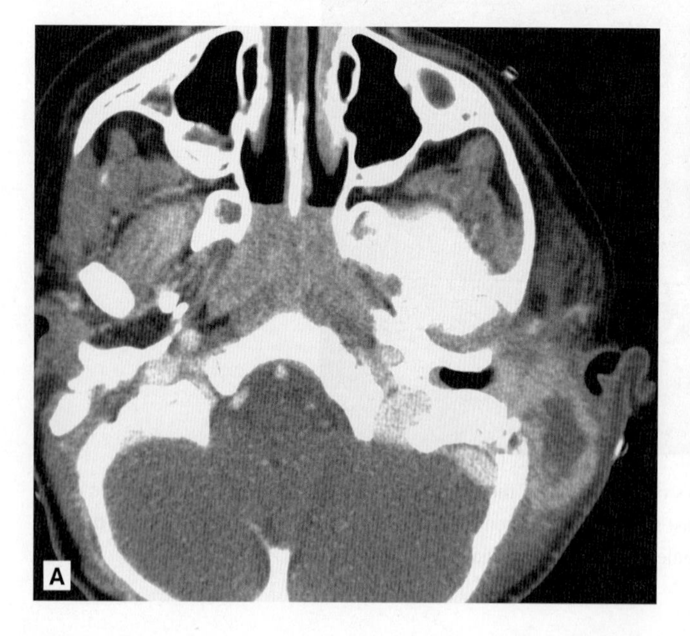

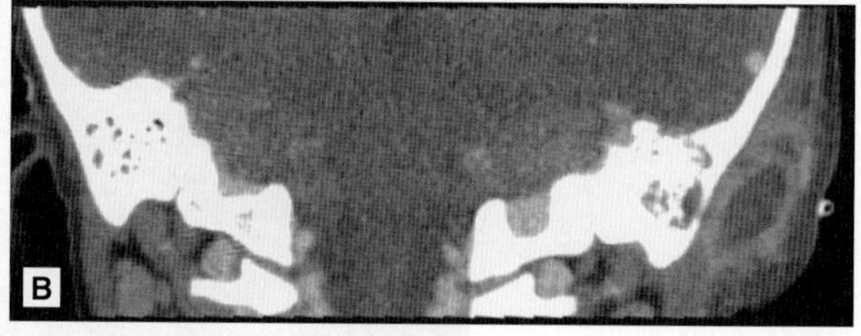

FIGURE 2.50 ■ Mastoiditis. **A:** Axial CECT shows cortical breakthrough of the left lateral mastoid bone with a large abscess in the adjacent soft tissues. **B:** Coronal CECT of temporal bones shows fluid-filled left mastoid air cells with extension of infection into adjacent soft tissues forming a rim-enhancing abscess (Bezold's abscess).

Radiographic Summary

Dacrocystocele is an obstruction of the nasolacrimal sac. On both CT and MRI, dacrocystoceles have a characteristic appearance of a fluid collection with minimal rim enhancement along the course of the affected nasolacrimal duct, with no adjacent solid components. If there is thick rim enhancement and adjacent fat stranding, this suggests superinfection of the dacrocystocele (dacrocystitis). Occasionally, the edema and/or infection can spread to the adjacent periorbital tissues.

This entity is to be distinguished from the similarly named dacryoadenitis, which is an acute or chronic inflammation of the lacrimal glands. Acutely, it could present with swelling of the eyelids with erythema and excess tearing due to a viral or bacterial infection of the superolateral lacrimal gland. Chronic causes include Sjogren's syndrome and sarcoidosis.

Clinical Implications

Dacrocystoceles appear as a blue-gray mass in the inferomedial canthus that forms as a result of a narrowing or obstruction of the nasolacrimal duct, usually during prenatal development. In infants, it is important to consider dacrocystocele when there is a mass that causes an upward slanting of the palpebral fissure nasally or cystic expansion into the nose. A dacrocystocele forms when tears accumulate within the lacrimal sac as a result of distal obstruction. The dacrocystocele may extend intra-nasally forming an endonasal cyst located in the inferior meatus. As obligate nasal breathers, neonates can have respiratory distress during feeding and sleeping due to obstruction by these cysts. First-line therapy is massage of the nasolacrimal region ("Crigler" massage). If this fails to work, ophthalmologists can gently probe the nasolacrimal duct in hopes of opening the obstruction (often an imperforate valve of Hasner).

Pearls

1. If conservative treatment measures fail and imaging is required, CECT of the orbits is recommended to assess for infectious complications and assess the nasolacrimal duct anatomy.
2. As dacrocystocele is the 3rd leading cause of neonatal nasal obstruction (behind mucosal edema and choanal atresia), CT is preferred over MRI as it allows evaluation for all 3 possibilities at the same time (MRI poorly evaluates nasal bone anatomy). CT has the added benefit of being quickly performed without sedation in a neonate.
3. Dacrocystoceles most commonly present in infants between 0 and 10 weeks old.

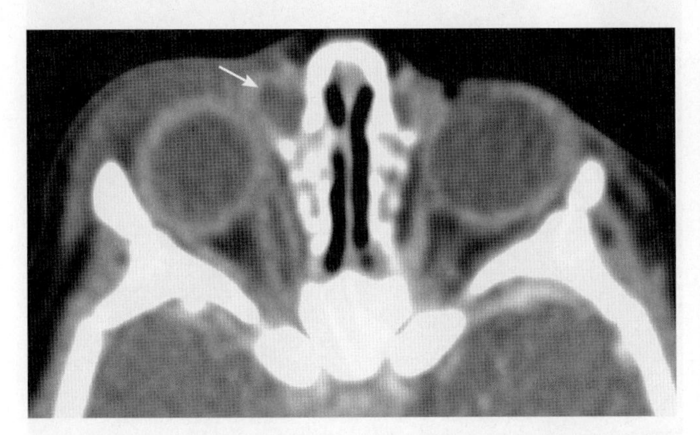

FIGURE 2.51 ■ Dacryocystitis. Axial orbit CECT shows rim enhancement and adjacent fat stranding of a fluid collection centered over the right nasolacrimal duct near the medial canthus in this infant consistent with inflammation of a dacryocystocele (dacryocystitis) (arrow).

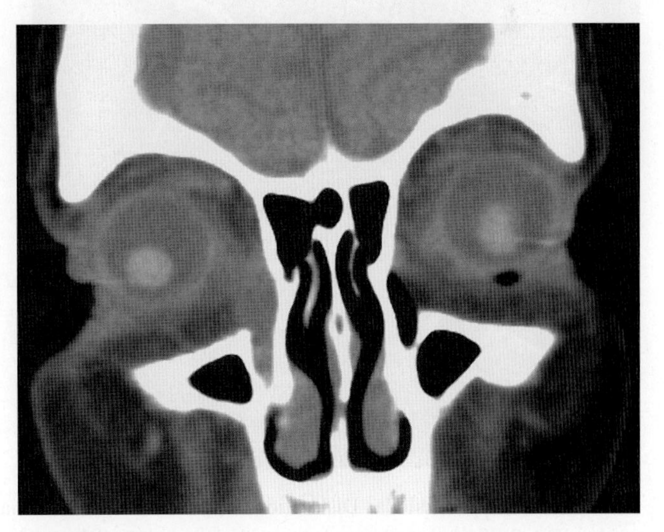

FIGURE 2.52 ■ Dacryocystitis. Coronal orbit NECT shows soft tissue/fluid filling the right nasolacrimal duct (note air-filled left duct) representing obstruction of the nasolacrimal duct outflow with drainage into the inferior nasal meatus.

Radiographic Summary

Mandible dislocation is the displacement of the mandibular condyle from the articular groove in the temporal bone. In noncomplicated cases, a panorex view of the mandible is accurate in detecting and characterizing mandibular fractures and reliably detects dislocations. However, mandibular dislocations are best visualized on NECT scan of the facial bones with multiplanar reformats. Normally, the mandibular condyle lies in the mandibular fossa of the temporal bone when the mouth is closed and moves slightly forward when the mouth is open. When dislocated, the mandibular condyle typically moves forward and lies anterior to the articular eminence, which prevents its return to the mandibular fossa of temporal bone.

Clinical Implications

Most patients with mandibular dislocations present with jaw pain, inability to close the jaw with normal occlusion, and drooling after mouth opening (commonly yawning), dental procedures, seizure activity, or after a traumatic blow to the jaw. People prone to dislocation may have natural laxity of the TMJ ligaments. Symmetric dislocation is most common, but unilateral dislocation with jaw deviating to the opposite side can also occur. Palpation of the TMJ will reveal one or more condyles trapped in front of the articular eminence and spasm of the muscles of mastication. Radiographs of TMJ are not always necessary but should be obtained if there is any suspicion of an associated fracture. If a history, physical exam, and NECT reveal an isolated mandibular dislocation, a closed reduction in the ED can be safely completed. However, oral maxillofacial surgery consultation should be considered for patients with dislocations associated with fractures or in patients with recurrent dislocations.

Pearls

1. After reduction, the patient should be able to move the mandible freely. However, if there is local bony tenderness, a post-reduction image should be obtained to evaluate for reduction-associated mandibular condyle fracture.
2. MRI is useful in visualizing structural abnormalities of the TMJ in cases of chronic jaw pain associated with TMJ syndrome.

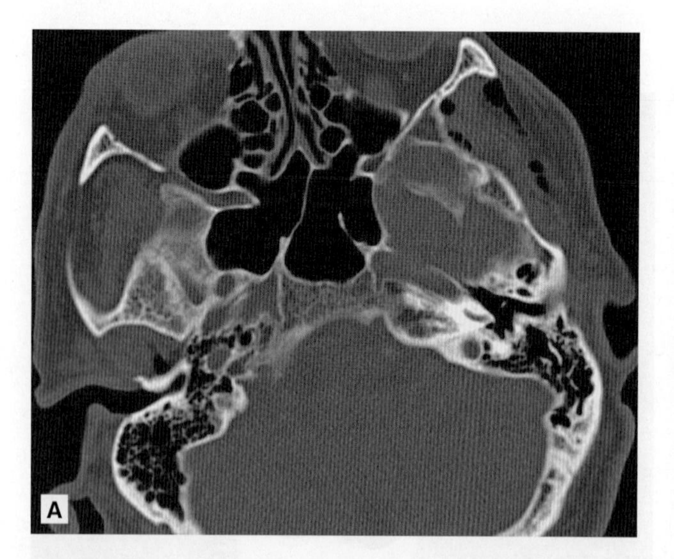

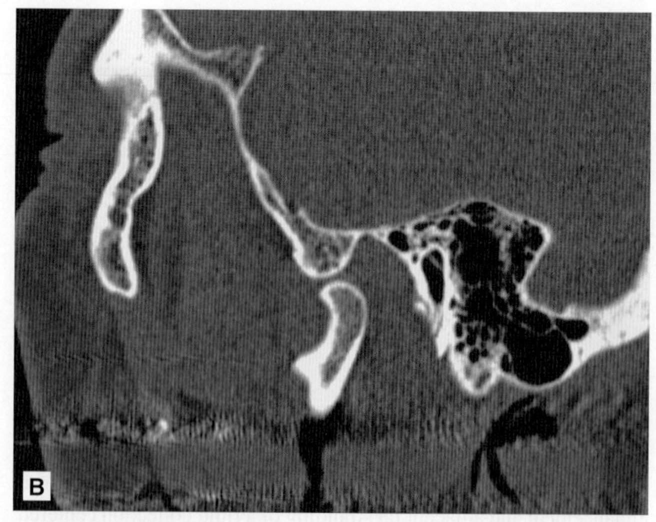

FIGURE 2.53 ■ Mandibular Dislocation. **A, B:** NECT of the facial bones after trauma shows an empty TMJ fossa on the axial image on the right. Sagittal view shows the mandibular condyle dislocated anterior to the TMJ joint. The jaw was reduced under anesthesia.

Chapter 3

SOFT TISSUE CONDITIONS OF THE NECK

Matthew D. Dobbs
Marc Mickiewicz
Cari L. Buckingham

Radiographic Summary

A laryngeal fracture is an injury to one of the components of the laryngeal apparatus. These include injuries to the hyoid bone, thyroid cartilage, or cricoid cartilage. These injuries are best evaluated with a CT of the neck. Although contrast is not necessary to evaluate laryngeal injury, CECT and/or CTA is preferred for penetrating trauma. Cartilage fracture may appear as a step-off of the normally smooth contour of the cartilage. Signs of cartilage dislocation include abnormal rotation of the arytenoids cartilage and widening at the articulations. Indirect signs include submucosal edema, hematoma, and airway narrowing. Presence of extra-luminal air suggests injury to the larynx and/or esophagus.

Clinical Implications

Laryngeal fracture is more commonly caused by blunt than penetrating trauma. Assess the patient's ability to phonate, listen for the presence of stridor, and palpate for tenderness in the anterior neck. If the patient is stable, flexible laryngoscopy is performed (along with CT) to determine the extent of the injury. Patients in need of emergent airway management may be difficult or impossible to intubate via the oral route, and cricothyrotomy may be impossible depending on the level of injury. In severe cases, emergent tracheotomy may be the only way to secure the patient's airway.

Pearls

1. Blunt trauma force sufficient to cause a laryngeal fracture often results in other injuries to the vasculature, spine, and/or esophagus. Consider CT angiography (CTA) of the neck to exclude arterial injury in patients with laryngeal fracture.
2. Findings of laryngeal injury may be subtle. Always review the cervical spine CT in bone and soft tissue windows when looking for these injuries as the amount of calcification within the cartilage may vary.

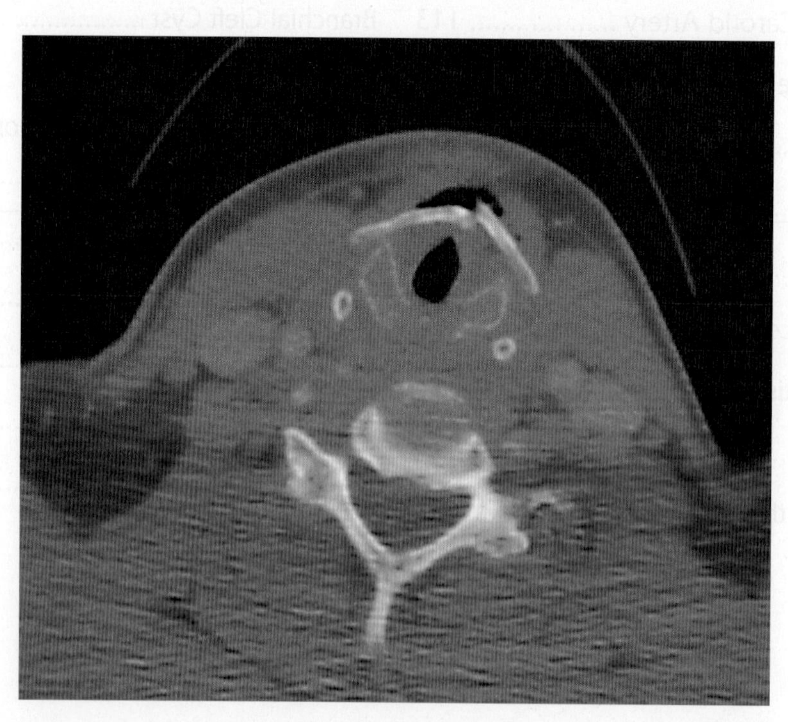

FIGURE 3.1 ■ Thyroid Cartilage Fracture. Axial CT image at the level of the larynx demonstrates a fracture of the normally V-shaped thyroid cartilage. Note air located anterior to the cartilage within the soft tissues.

Radiographic Summary

Penetrating arterial injury is the disruption of the vessel wall by a foreign body entering the neck such as with a gunshot wound or knife injury. CTA has largely replaced conventional angiography and/or surgical neck exploration in excluding injury to the major arteries and veins of the neck. CTA findings include neck hematoma, extravasation of contrast, dissection, and pseudoaneurysm formation. A pseudoaneurysm is a saccular defect of the arterial wall where an indwelling hematoma is contained only by the adventitia of the arterial wall as opposed to a true aneurysm, where an intact arterial wall is maintained. Pseudoaneurysms are significantly more likely to rupture due to their weak architecture.

Clinical Implications

Expanding hematoma, change in phonation, and stridor after penetrating neck injury should prompt definitive airway management, and typically occur prior to the radiographic identification of a carotid artery injury. Absence of these clinical findings may allow the angiographic evaluation prior to definitive airway management.

Pearls

1. CTA of the neck has replaced surgical exploration of penetrating neck injuries.
2. The most common vascular injuries are dissection, hematoma, and pseudoaneurysm.

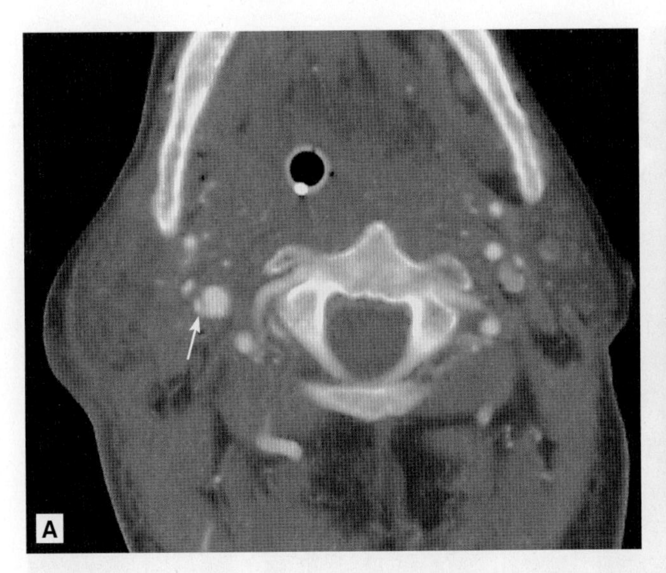

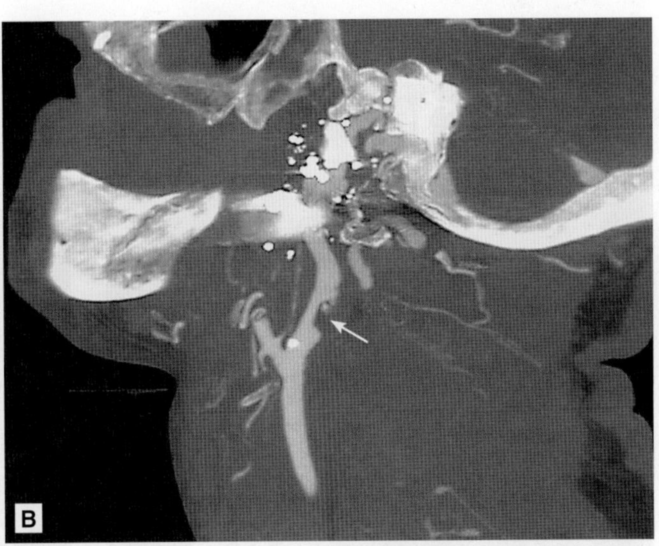

FIGURE 3.2 ■ Penetrating Vascular Injury. **A:** Axial CTA shows intimal dissection flap in the right internal carotid artery (arrow) of a 95-year-old male with a gunshot wound. **B: Dissection and Pseudoaneurysm.** Sagittal CTA shows the dissection and pseudoaneurysm of the ICA (arrow). Metallic debris from a gunshot wound project over the skull base.

Radiographic Summary

Dissection is the disruption of the intima of the vessel wall with blood tracking between the intima and media of the wall, creating an "intimal flap." CTA is the test of choice to evaluate for carotid artery dissection. CT angiographic findings of traumatic carotid artery dissection include an intimal flap separating the true and false lumens, a narrowed and irregular vessel lumen, thickened vessel wall due to intramural hematoma, and cone-like tapering of the vessel lumen.

A fat-suppressed axial T1-weighted sequence does an excellent job in demonstrating subacute blood products within the vessel wall. Subacute blood products are hyperintense (bright) on T1-weighted images due to the presence of methemoglobin. MR angiography findings are similar to CTA. Conventional angiography remains the gold standard if CTA or MRI/MRA is equivocal.

Clinical Implications

Carotid artery dissection may be spontaneous or occur in the setting of blunt trauma. Missed carotid artery dissection will likely progress to stroke. Clinical features that should prompt evaluation for carotid artery dissection include neck hematoma, ipsilateral seat-belt ecchymosis, head, neck, or face pain, partial Horner's syndrome, TIA, and stroke-like symptoms. Minor trauma such as overhead painting or chiropractic manipulation may precipitate a carotid artery dissection.

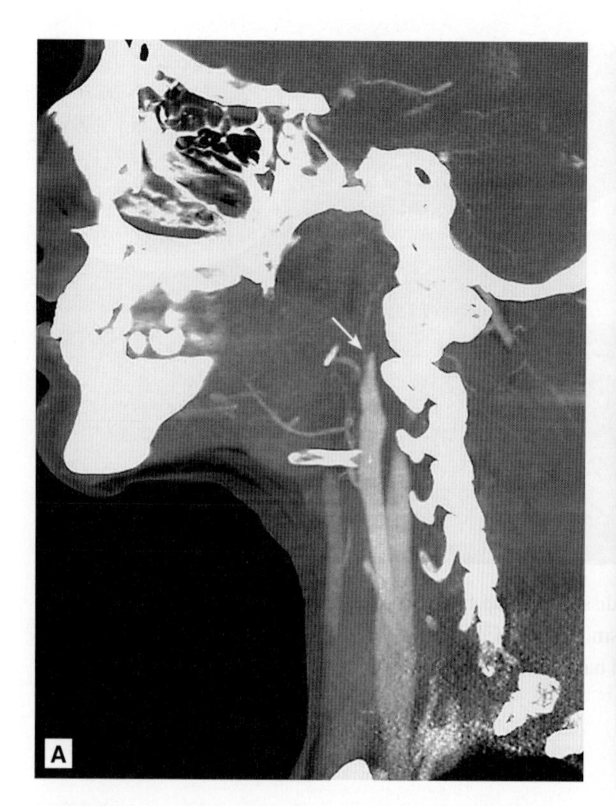

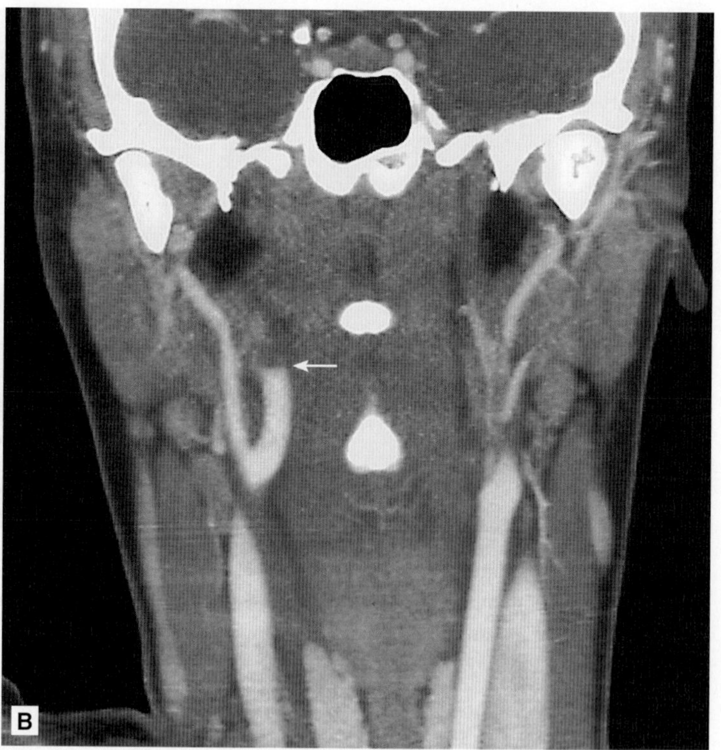

FIGURE 3.3 ■ Traumatic Carotid Artery Dissection. **A:** Sagittal CTA shows abrupt occlusion of the right ICA (arrow) following a car accident in a 19-year-old female. **B:** Coronal CTA shows abrupt occlusion of the right ICA (arrow).

Pearls

1. Cervical spine fractures should raise the clinical suspicion for carotid artery dissection after major trauma.
2. An axial fat-saturated T1-weighted sequence is routinely used to evaluate for carotid dissection.
3. CTA of the neck is nearly 100% sensitive and specific for the evaluation of carotid artery dissection when compared to arterial angiography.

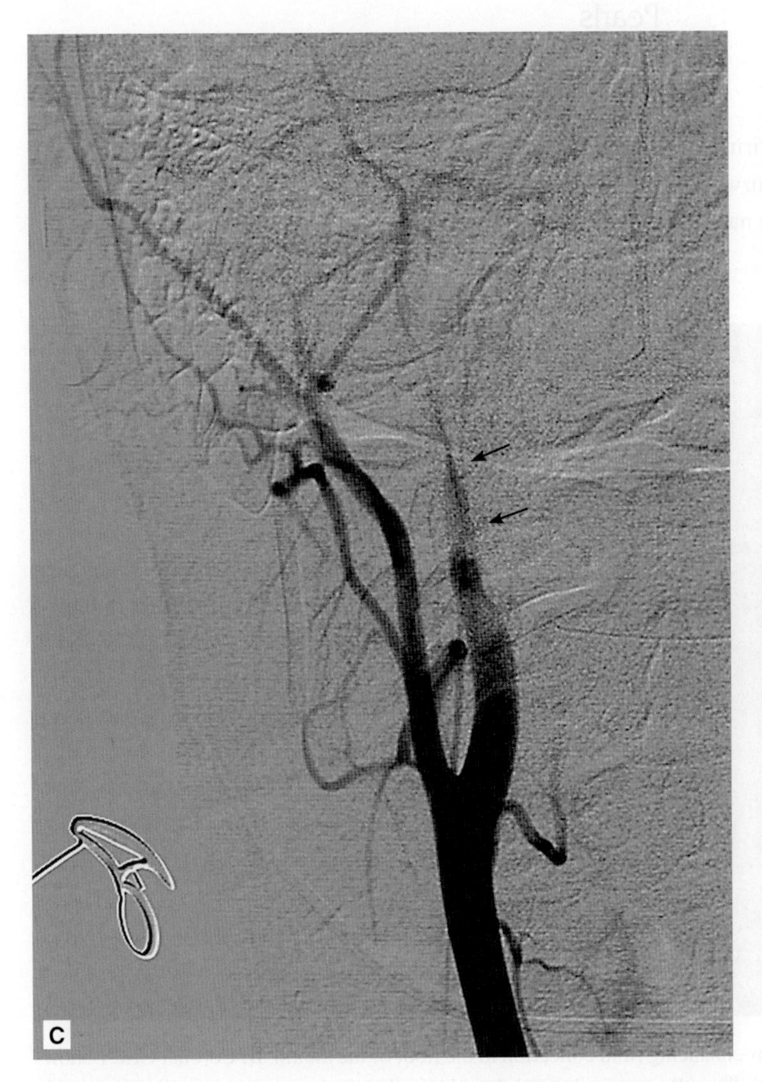

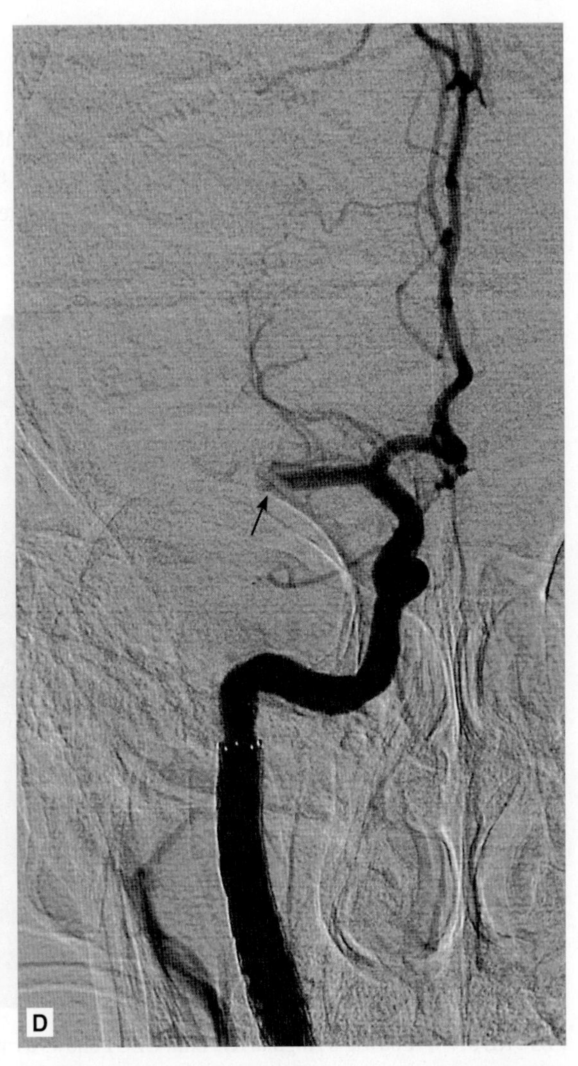

FIGURE 3.3 ■ (*Continued*) **C:** AP view of common carotid artery injection angiogram shows severe narrowing of the proximal ICA (arrows). **D:** AP view of common carotid angiogram following placement of stent in ICA shows thrombus in M1 segment of middle cerebral artery (arrow) subsequently treated with intra-arterial tPA and MERCI retrieval device (thrombus present initially due to dissection).

Radiographic Summary

Ludwig's angina is a severe infection involving the sublingual, submandibular, and submental spaces causing induration and elevation of the tongue. Most cases are odontogenic in origin. Contrast-enhanced neck CT demonstrates a phlegmon with inflammation beneath the tongue, and may also show the presence of an abscess (fluid collection with contrast enhancing rim) or spread of the infection to the mediastinum.

Clinical Implications

Ludwig's angina is diagnosed clinically, and confirmed with CECT. The greatest immediate threat to life is airway obstruction. Preparation should be made for immediate nasal fiberoptic intubation in case of decompensation. Oral intubation or cricothyrotomy may be impossible due to swelling and landmark distortion. Clues that a patient needs a secure airway prior to imaging include respiratory distress, air hunger, and an inability to tolerate laying flat. Many cases require operative drainage, though improvement with medical management alone is also possible.

Pearls

1. Mandibular panorex radiographs or CT scan may demonstrate an ododentogenic cause of the infection.
2. Severe submental lymphadenopathy may be clinically confused with Ludwig's angina obviating the need for diagnostic imaging.

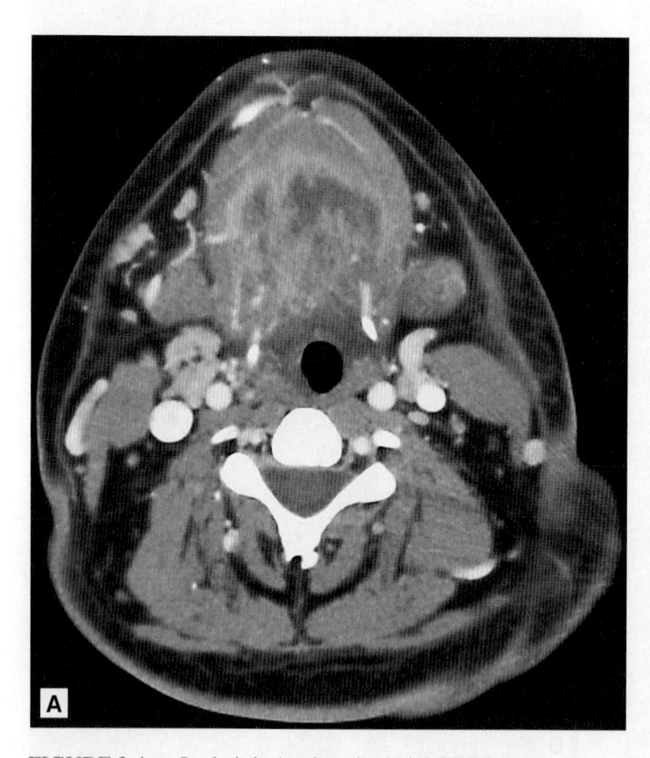

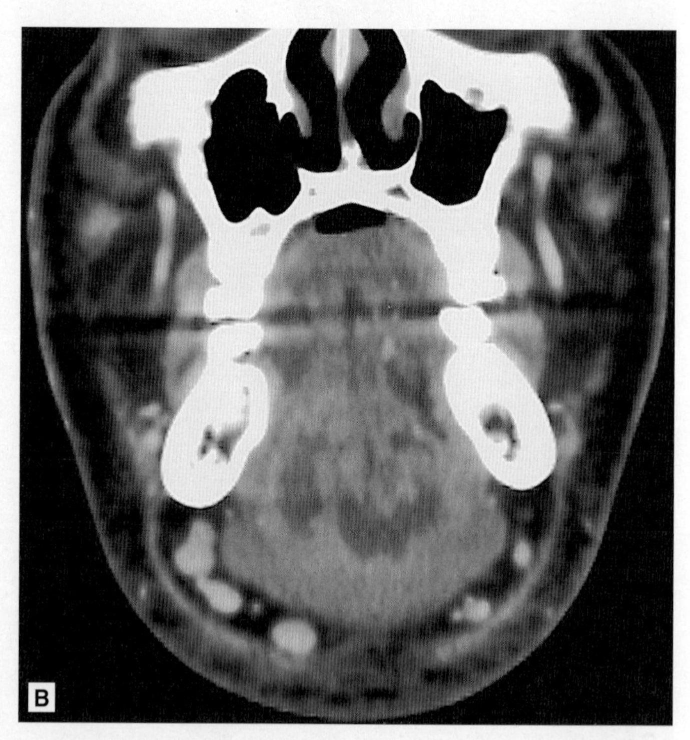

FIGURE 3.4 ■ Ludwig's Angina. **A:** Axial CECT shows a rim-enhancing fluid collection in the floor of the mouth. **B:** Coronal CECT shows a rim-enhancing fluid collection in the floor of mouth. Beneath the collection is the mylohyoid muscle which contains the collection within the sublingual space.

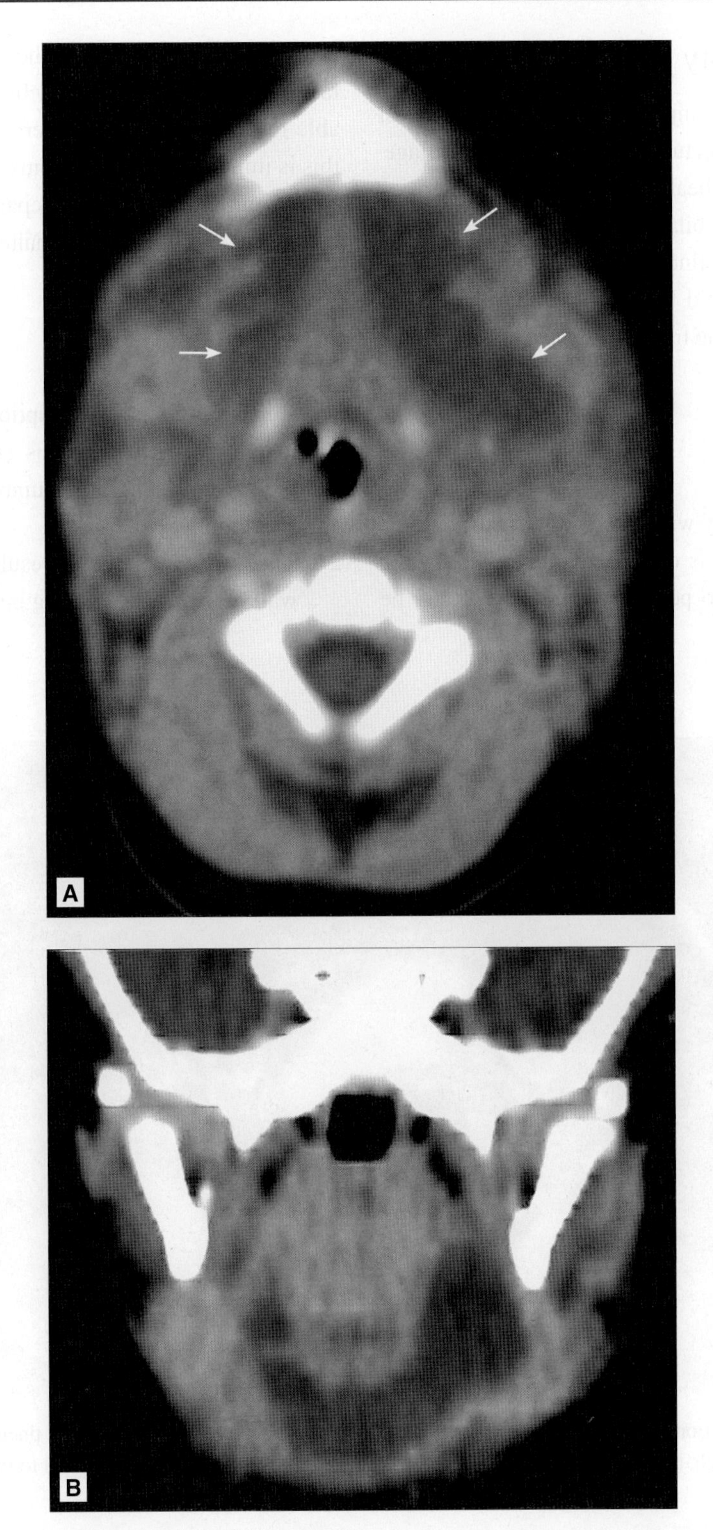

FIGURE 3.5 ■ Ludwig's Angina. **A:** Axial CT in a young child shows a large fluid collection in the sublingual space (arrows). **B:** Coronal CT shows a U-shaped configuration of the fluid in the sublingual space, bounded inferiorly by the mylohyoid muscle.

Radiographic Summary

Tracheal disruption is a rare injury, which includes tears of the connective tissue and fractures of the tracheal cartilage. CXR and CT findings of tracheal disruption include extensive subcutaneous emphysema, bilateral pneumothoraces, and pneumomediastinum. Other findings include an abnormally superior position of the hyoid bone (above the 3rd cervical vertebra) or penetration of the trachea by the distal end of an endotracheal tube.

Clinical Implications

Most patients with this injury will die in the pre-hospital setting as airway management is often extremely challenging. In cases of disruption due to penetrating trauma, it may be possible to intubate the trachea distal to the injury through laceration. In cases caused by blunt trauma, the injury may be able to be bridged using fiberoptic intubation techniques. If this is impossible, tracheostomy will be required. These injuries often require operative repair; however, if the defect can be bridged and the air leak halted, expectant management is possible.

Pearls

1. Consider tracheal disruption in a patient with large amounts of subcutaneous emphysema, pneumomediastinum, and bilateral pneumothoraces after blunt or penetrating neck trauma.
2. This injury can be the result of trauma to the posterior wall of the trachea during intubation.

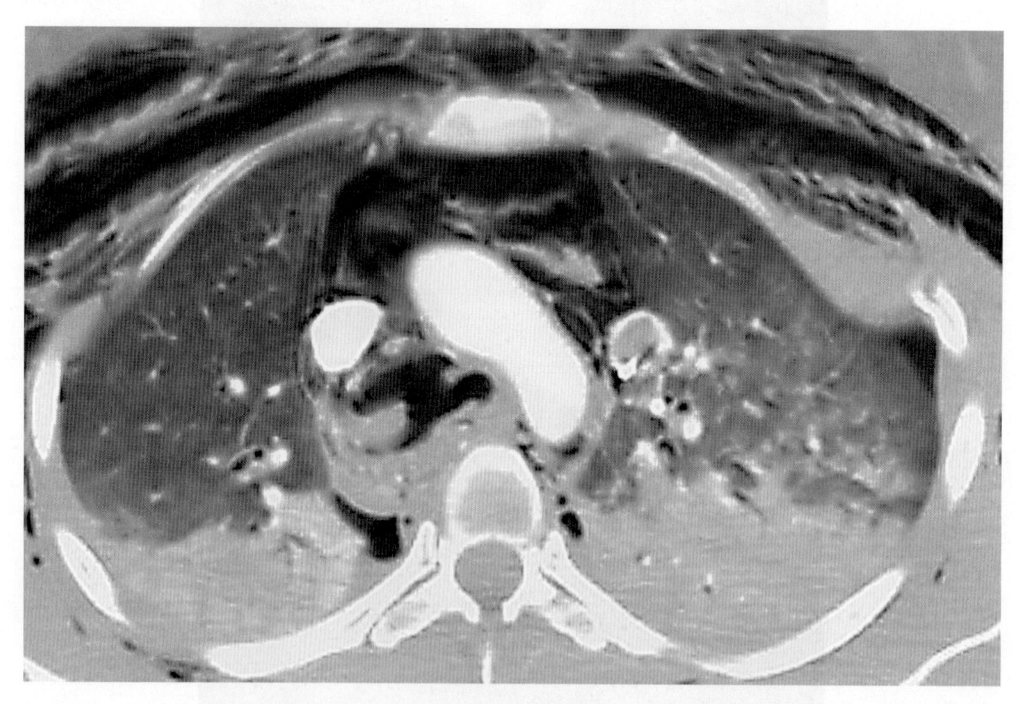

FIGURE 3.6 ■ Tracheal Disruption. Axial CT image demonstrates extensive subcutaneous emphysema, pneumomediastinum, and pneumothorax. Posterior to the aortic arch, there is a large collection of air. The trachea is ruptured just proximal to the carina.

Radiographic Summary

A peritonsillar abscess (PTA) is a collection of pus located between the palatine tonsillar capsule and the pharyngeal muscles. CECT of the neck is the preferred method for imaging PTA. PTA appears as a fluid collection with a rim of contrast enhancement in the tonsillar fossa. Narrowing and contralateral displacement of the airway is seen to varying degrees. Peritonsillar cellulitis or phlegmon may have a similar clinical appearance, but will lack a well defined abscess collection (though sometimes an early abscess can be difficult to distinguish from a phlegmon). Other CT findings include obscuration of the adjacent parapharyngeal fat. Bedside ultrasound can rapidly confirm the presence of PTA. An endocavitary transducer is placed gently within the mouth and the symptomatic side scanned in both the sagittal and tranverse planes. The abscess will appear as a hypoechoic structure. This technique allows for the precise localization of the abscess and the internal carotid artery.

Clinical Implications

The diagnosis of a PTA is primarily clinical. Confirmation with imaging is not necessary in most cases. Clinical findings include unilateral sore throat, trismus, swelling of the

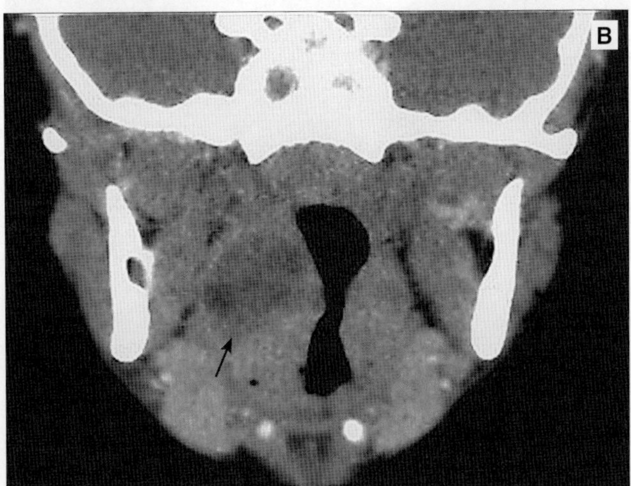

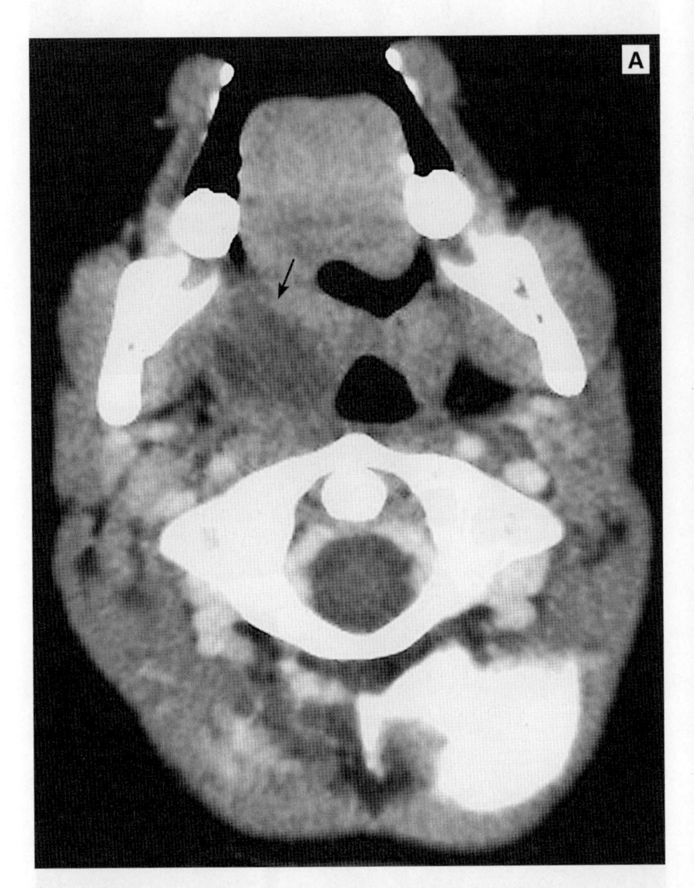

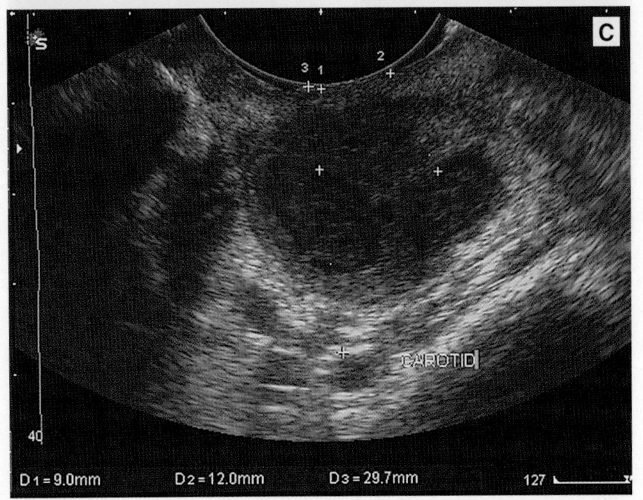

FIGURE 3.7 ■ Tonsillar Abscess. **A:** Axial CECT shows a rim-enhancing fluid collection in the right tonsillar fossa (arrow). There is some inflammation in the right parapharyngeal fat. **B:** Coronal CECT shows a rim-enhancing fluid collection in the right tonsillar fossa (arrow). **C:** Intraoral ultrasound performed at the bedside demonstrates two hypoechoic regions within a swollen tonsil representing a tonsillar abscess. Depth measurements can be made for needle entry. The distance to the ipsilateral carotid artery can be determined as well.

tonsillar pillar, and deviation of the uvula. Definitive treatment of a PTA is ED drainage (often needle aspiration is sufficient) combined with antibiotics. A CT or ultrasound can confirm the presence or abscence of fluid and avoid an unnecessary procedure. Obtain a CT in cases where the patient is immunosuppressed, appears extremely toxic, or if there is concern for spread of the infection to the deep neck spaces and/or mediastinum.

Pearls

1. Pre-drainage CT or US can help establish the presence of an abscess versus phlegmon and delineate the regional anatomy.
2. CT should be preformed if bilateral PTA is suspected as there may be a higher chance of the trans-spatial spread of infection in these patients.

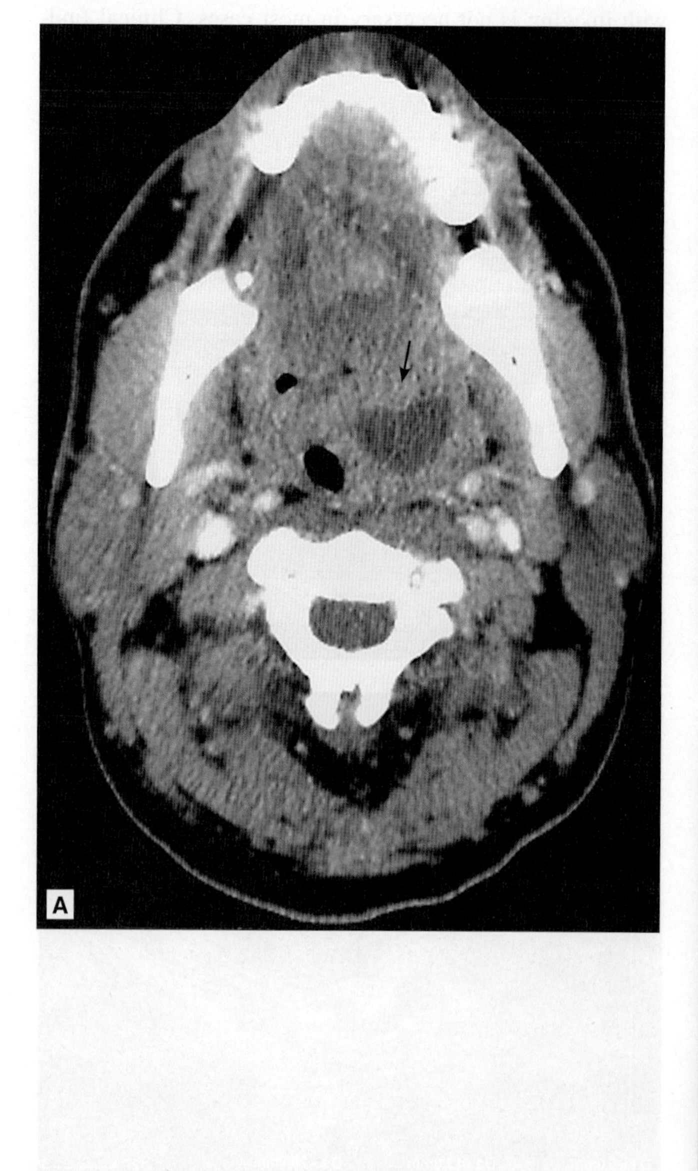

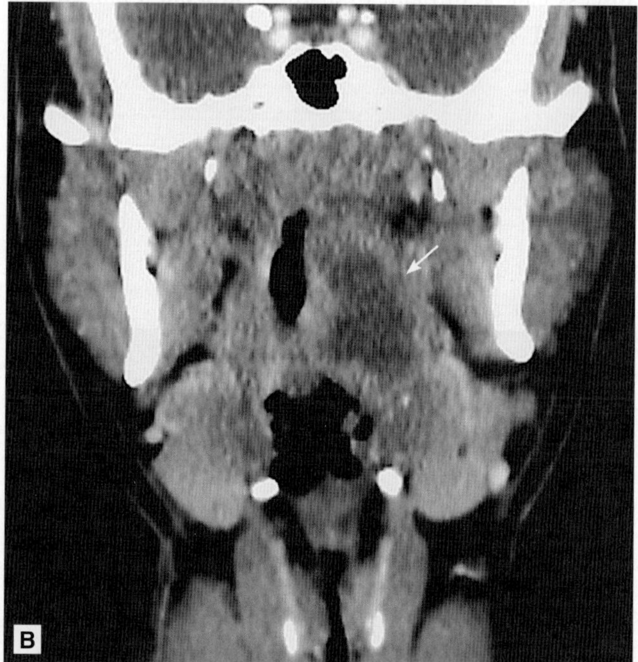

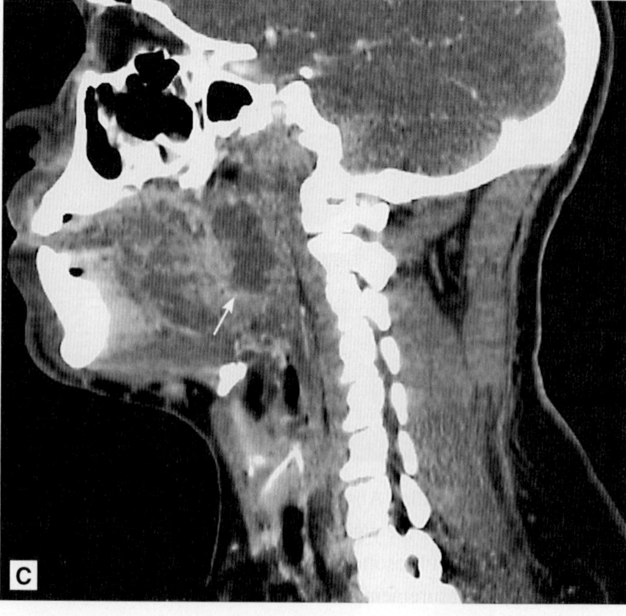

FIGURE 3.8 ■ Tonsillar Abscess. **A-C:** Axial, coronal, and sagittal CECT images show a low attenuation focus in the left tonsillar fossa with rim enhancement (arrows). Edema extends into the left parapharyngeal space and causes some oral airway narrowing.

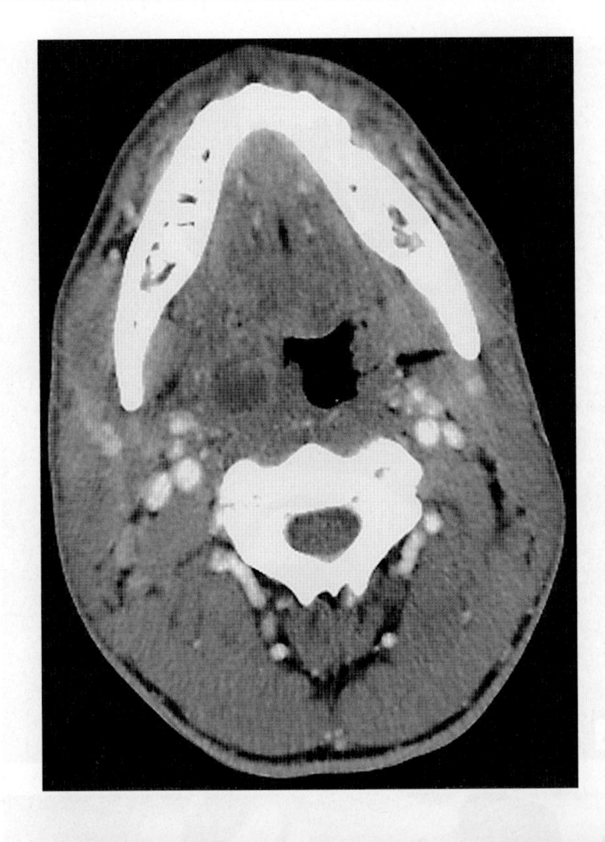

FIGURE 3.9 ■ Tonsillar Abscess. Axial CECT shows low attenuation in the right palatine tonsil with rim enhancement. Minimal edematous narrowing of the airway is present.

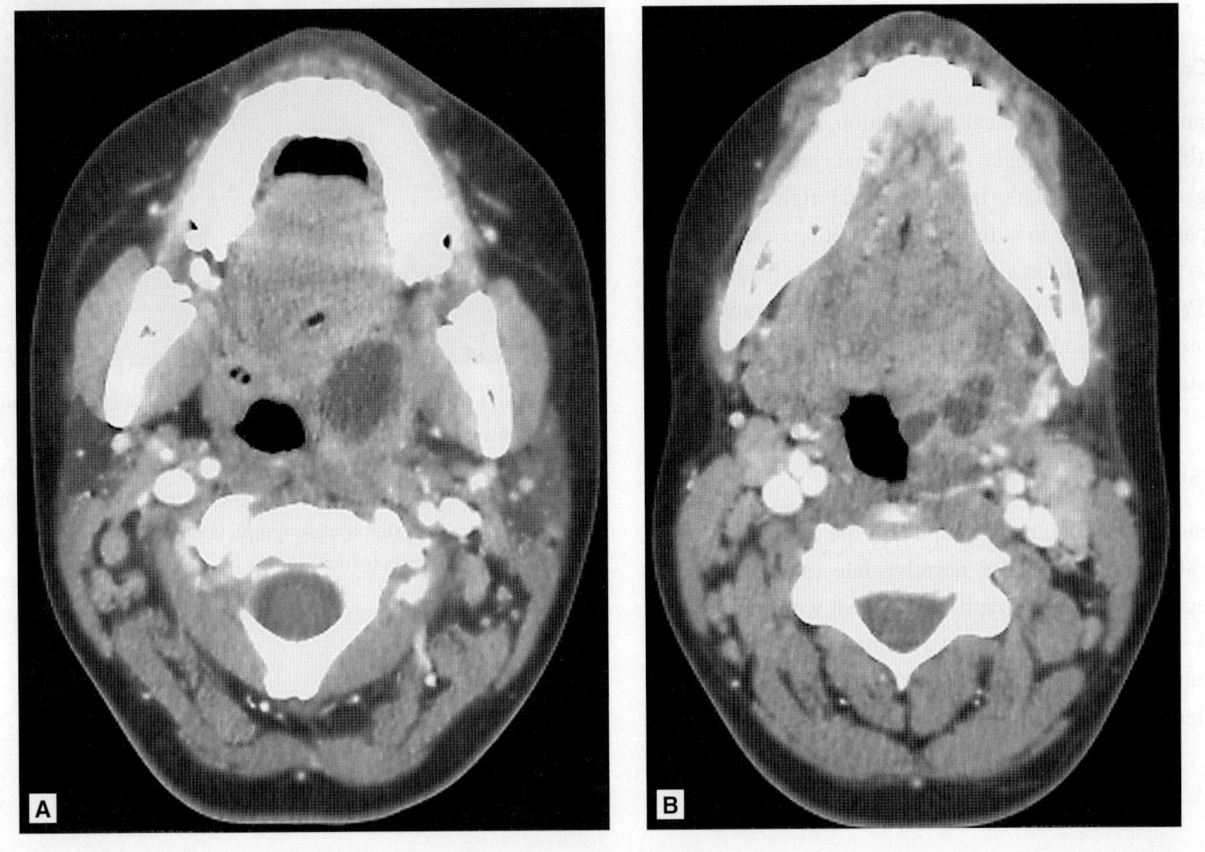

FIGURE 3.10 ■ Tonsillar Abscess. **A, B:** Axial CECT show a rim-enhancing low-attenuation region in the left tonsillar fossa that extends out of the tonsillar fossa into the surrounding parapharyngeal region and submandibular space.

Radiographic Summary

A retropharyngeal abscess (RPA) is a collection of pus in the retropharyngeal space due to trauma or extension of a parapharyngeal infection. Contrast-enhanced neck CT of an RPA typically demonstrates a dark fluid collection distending the retropharyngeal space posterior to the oropharynx with or without a contrast-enhancing rim. Differentiation from suppurative retropharyngeal lymphadenitis can be difficult, but lymph nodes tend to be located off-midline. An early abscess or retropharyngeal phlegmon may not demonstrate rim enhancement. CT is very sensitive for RPA and alternative diagnoses. Traditionally, soft tissue lateral neck radiographs have been used to evaluate for abnormal swelling in the prevertebral/retropharyngeal tissues (>7 mm at C2 and >14 mm at C6 in children and > 22 mm at C6 in adults). Detection of gas within the prevertebral soft tissues is highly suggestive, but rarely seen. As expiration and neck flexion can both spuriously thicken the prevertebral soft tissues, the specificity is low. Optimal technique is crucial, including true lateral positioning, and obtaining the radiograph during inspiration and neck extension.

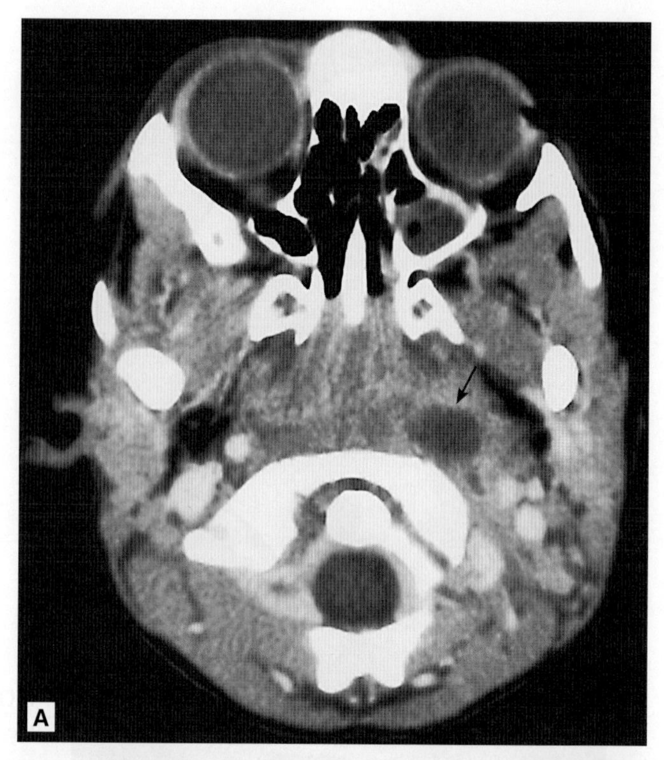

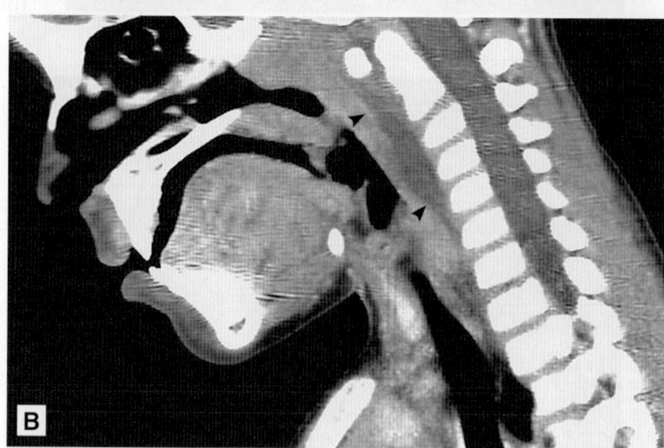

FIGURE 3.11 ■ Retropharyngeal Abscess. **A, B:** Axial and sagittal CECT shows a faintly rim-enhancing fluid collection in the left retropharyngeal space (arrow). The sagittally-reformatted image shows the pre-vertebral fluid collection tracking inferiorly (arrowheads). This could either be a suppurative lymph node with effusion or early retropharyngeal abscess formation.

Clinical Implications

RPA can have a subtle clinical presentation. Fever, sore throat, neck stiffness, odynophagia, and dysphagia are common presenting symptoms. Signs include nuchal rigidity, cervical adenopathy, lethargy in children, and drooling. Inability of a child to look upward is another valuable clue. Identification of a RPA should prompt ENT evaluation for operative management. Stridor and respiratory distress should prompt one to consider advanced airway management.

Pearls

1. Sensitivity of plain radiographs for the detection of RPA is 80% but has a false negative rate as high as 33%. Negative plain radiographs in a patient with a high clinical suspicion should prompt a contrasted neck CT.
2. Contrasted neck CT is nearly 100% sensitive for the detection of RPA.

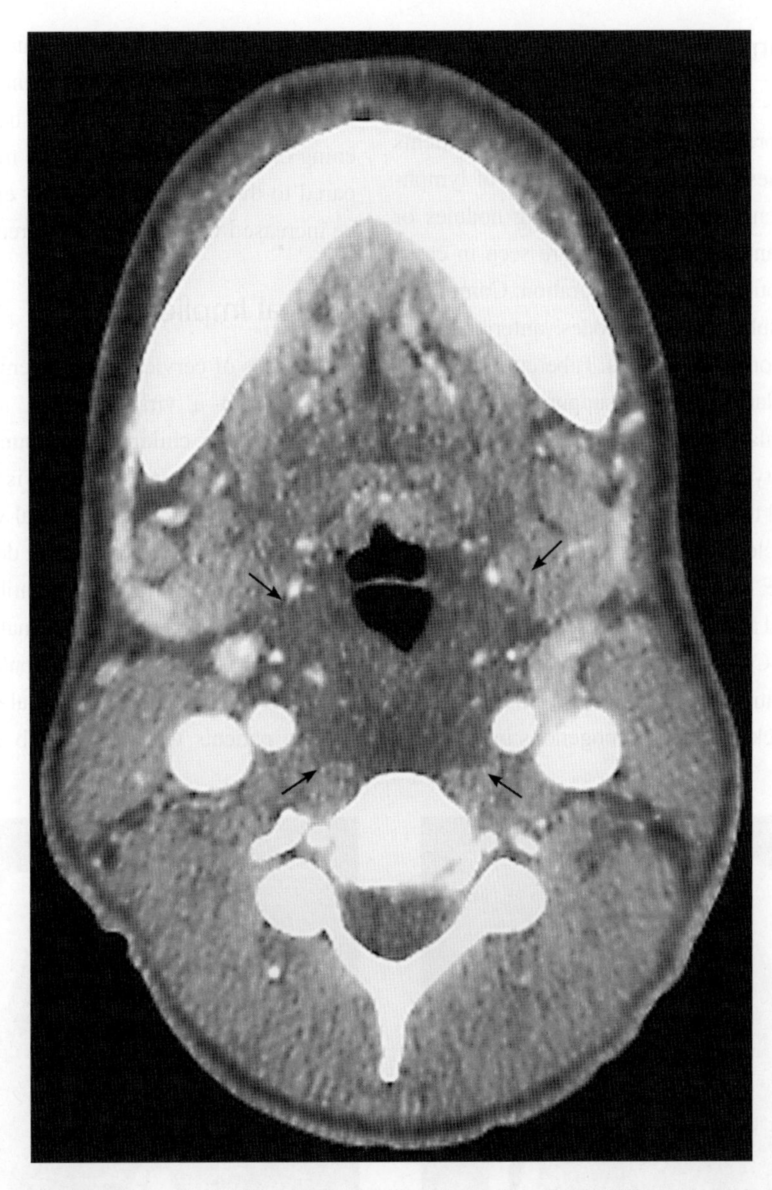

FIGURE 3.12 ■ Retropharyngeal Abscess. Axial CECT in a patient with neck swelling shows diffuse edema throughout the retropharyngeal space (arrows). There is no rim-enhancement or well-defined fluid collection. This represents retropharyngeal edema/effusion.

Radiographic Summary

Cervical lymphadenitis is enlargement of lymph nodes due to infection. CECT is the preferred method to evaluate patients with palpable neck masses. Lymph nodes in cases of lymphadenitis will appear as enlarged, hyperenhancing nodules or masses. Central nonenhancing (dark) areas are seen in cases of necrosis or super-infection causing suppuration. Commonly involved areas are the submandibular nodes, anterior chain, jugular chain, and posterior triangle nodes. Tuberculous lymphadenitis can appear similar to bacterial suppurative lymphadenitis. TB often causes enlarged nodes with central low density or necrosis. In children, atypical mycobacterial lymphadenopathy is sometimes referred to as "scrofula."

Neck ultrasound can clearly demonstrate lymph nodes and their internal architecture. Normal nodes are reniform in shape with an echogenic central hilum (the increased echogenicity is due to fat in the hilum). Color Doppler US will show vessels emanating from the central hilum. The surrounding cortex should be uniform in thickness, and homogenous in texture.

Reactive lymph nodes have thickened cortices, but maintain their normal fatty hilum. Malignant lymph nodes have their fatty hilum replaced by tumor. They also have irregular thickening of the cortex, and become more globular in shape compared to the normal reniform or elongated shape. There may be increased vascularity in both reactive and malignant nodes.

Clinical Implications

Most cases of cervical lymphadenitis are the result of inflammation from a viral infection and resolve spontaneously (particularly in children and young adults). Antibiotics may be used if a bacterial etiology is suspected. Close observation and follow-up within several weeks is essential. Imaging should be reserved for cases that do not resolve spontaneously or are resistant to a course of antibiotics. Concern for a neck abscess or a high suspicion for malignancy (age > 40, tobacco history, chronic alcohol use) should also prompt the provider to obtain a CECT. Mycobacterial infection (scrofula) can be seen in patients with HIV or Tb exposure. Non-tuberculosis

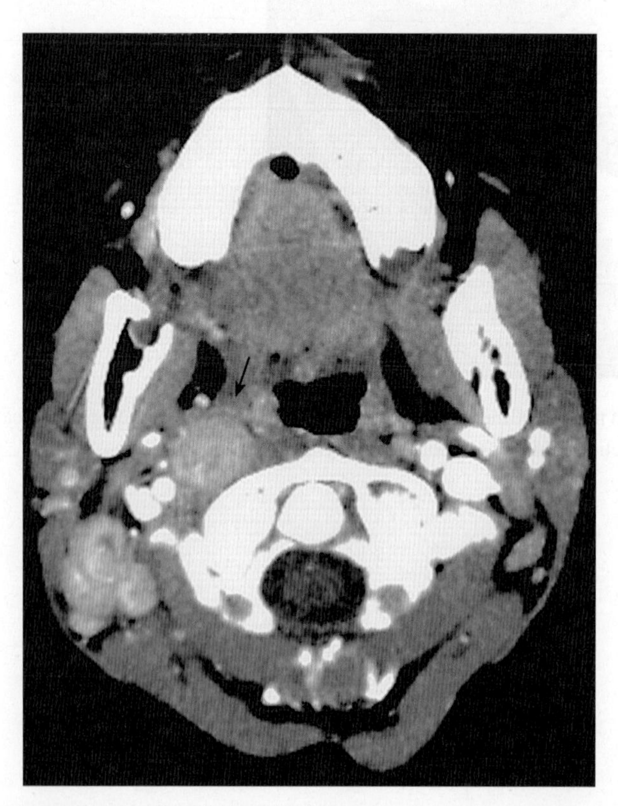

FIGURE 3.13 ■ Lymphadenitis. Axial CECT shows hyperenhancing right-sided nodes in levels IIA and IIB (jugulodigastric chain). The largest node is located medial to the carotid space (arrow) and displaces the black parapharyngeal fat anteriorly. Small areas of low attenuation represent early suppurative change.

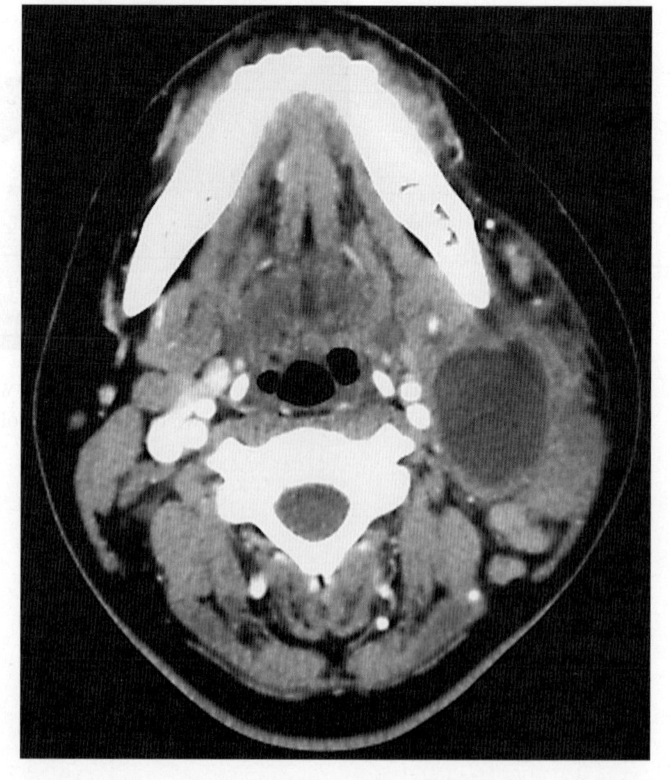

FIGURE 3.14 ■ Lymphadenitis. Axial CECT shows a large area of low attenuation in the left-level IIA lymph node region. Surgical drainage confirmed an infected, suppurative lymph node. The differential diagnosis would include a branchial cleft cyst in a child, or a necrotic metastasis in an adult.

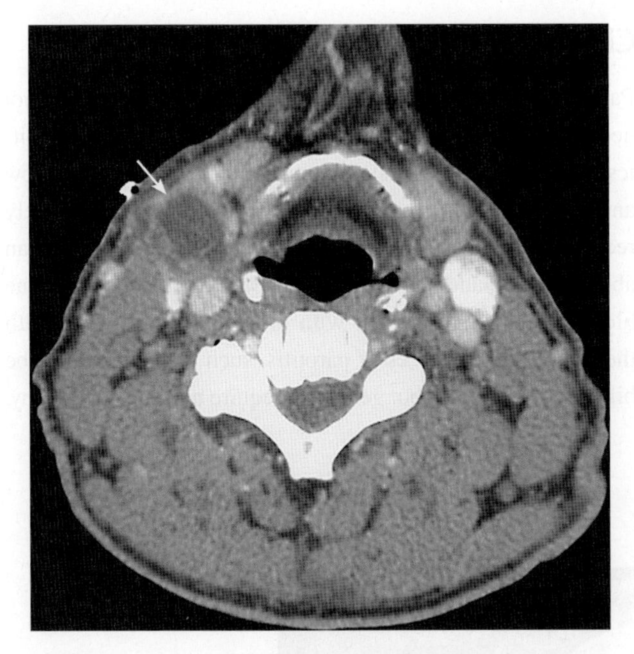

FIGURE 3.15 ■ Lymph Node Metastases. Axial CECT in a 61-year-old male shows a rim-enhancing low-attenuation region in the right (arrow) neck. This is a level IIA lymph node at the level of the hyoid bone. This was originally called a branchial cleft cyst. Biopsy revealed metastases from squamous cell carcinoma (the primary was a right base of the tongue lesion).

mycobacterial lymphadenitis is caused by *Mycobacterium avium-intracellulare* and presents as a "cold abscess," (fluctuant but lacking warmth). For both mycobacterial infection and malignancy a fine needle biopsy or aspirate allows for definitive diagnosis.

Pearls

1. Many cases of lymphadenitis will resolve spontaneously. Proper follow-up, is essential.
2. Consider imaging patients who are older than 40, have risk factors for head and neck cancer, are from TB endemic areas, or have HIV.
3. Benign lymph nodes have a reniform shape, a fatty hilum, and are typically smaller than 1 cm in short axis. This normal morphology can be appreciated on CT and ultrasonography alike. The fatty hilum is hyperechoic on US and hypodense on CT.
4. Malignant lymph nodes lose their fatty hila and become round in shape. Malignant lymph nodes are typically larger than 1 cm in short axis.
5. Reactive nodes can enlarge significantly but maintain their hilar fat and reniform shape.

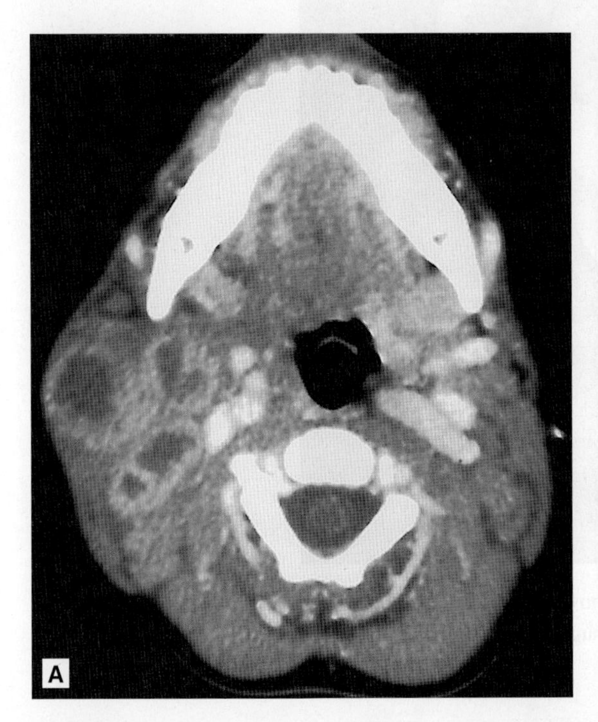

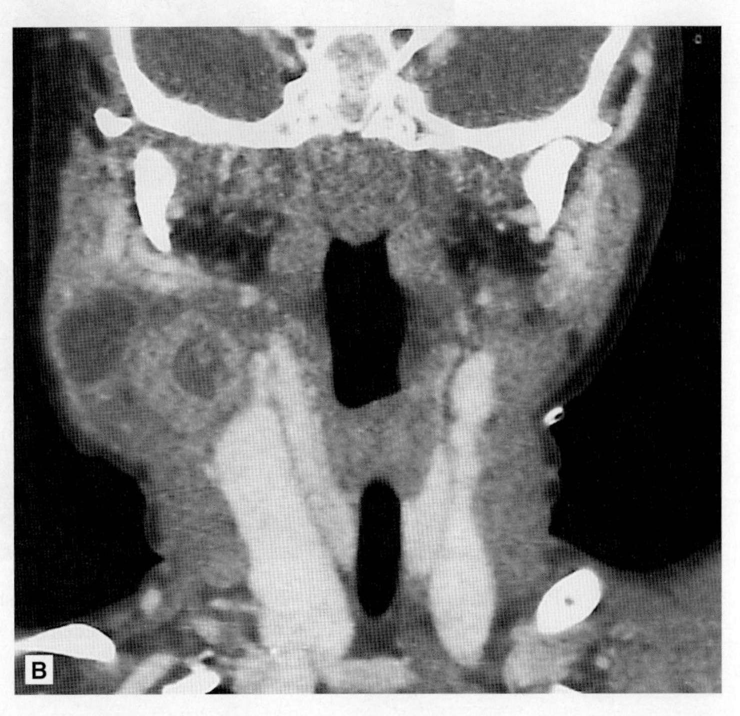

FIGURE 3.16 ■ Lymphadenitis. **A, B:** Axial and coronal CECT in a 2-year-old child with neck mass unresponsive to 2 weeks of antibiotics shows a conglomerate mass of necrotic neck lymph nodes with thick enhancing rims and low-attenuation centrally. Cultures grew *Mycobacterium avium.* Diagnosis is nontuberculous mycobacterial adenitis ("scrofula").

Radiographic Summary

Parotitis is the infection of the parotid gland. Contrast-enhanced CT findings in acute parotitis include gland edema and fat stranding. The parotid gland will be enlarged and may enhance more than the normal gland. A dark collection with a contrast-enhancing rim will be seen if an abscess is present. A stone within Stenson's duct may cause obstruction and subsequent infection of the parotid. A stone appears as a round, small, and bright object in the duct as it courses to the oral cavity adjacent to the 2nd maxillary molar tooth.

Clinical Implications

Parotitis is a clinical diagnosis and routine CT imaging is not necessary in most cases. Treatment may include antibioitics and frequent use of sialogogues to promote salivary flow and resolution of duct blockage. Surgical drainage is rarely required. Bedside ultrasound may be used to identify an abscess. Submandibular glands are even more prone to stone blockage and may present with unilateral swelling beneath the tongue. Viral causes of parotitis, such as mumps, may be bilateral and painful but generally require no specific therapy.

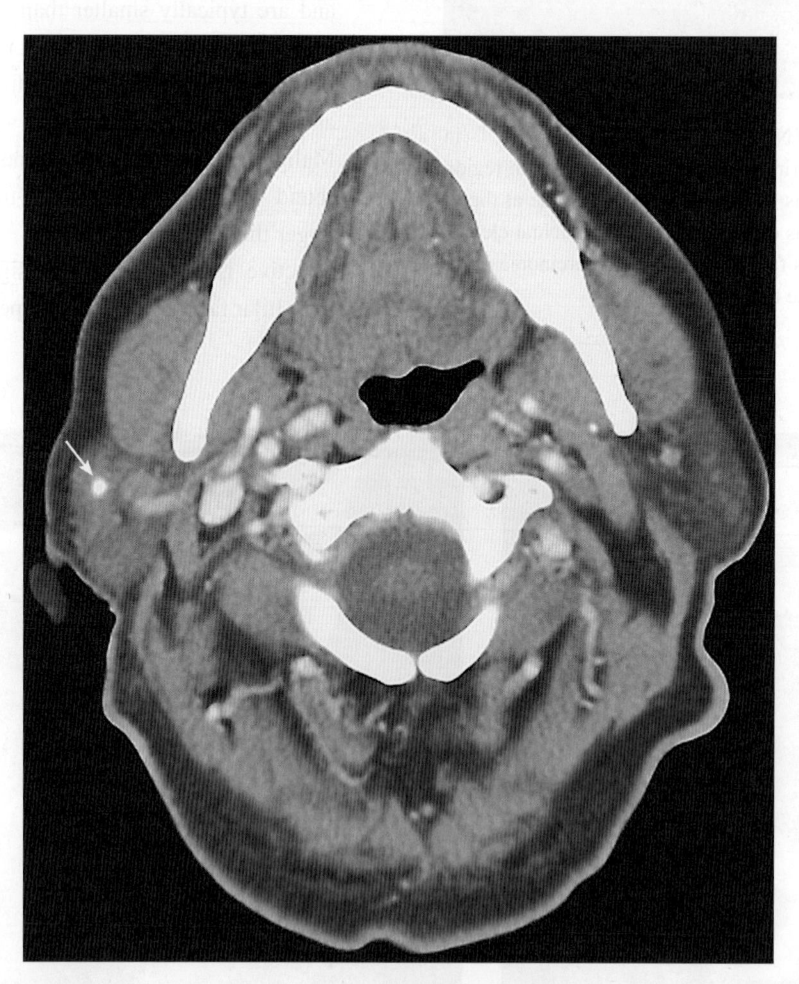

FIGURE 3.17 ■ Parotid Sialolithiasis. Axial CECT in a 75-year-old patient shows increased density in the right parotid gland with a small stone (sialolith) within it (arrow). There is no overlying stranding or edema to suggest acute inflammation.

Pearls

1. Reserve imaging for cases of parotitis that do not respond to antibiotics or sialogogues.
2. Concern for malignancy is an indication for a CT scan.
3. Always evaluate the entire parotid duct, which courses anteriorly and medially. A stone can be easily overlooked when it is small and similar in density to the adjacent bone and teeth.
4. CT can detect a salivary duct stone as small as 1-2 mm.

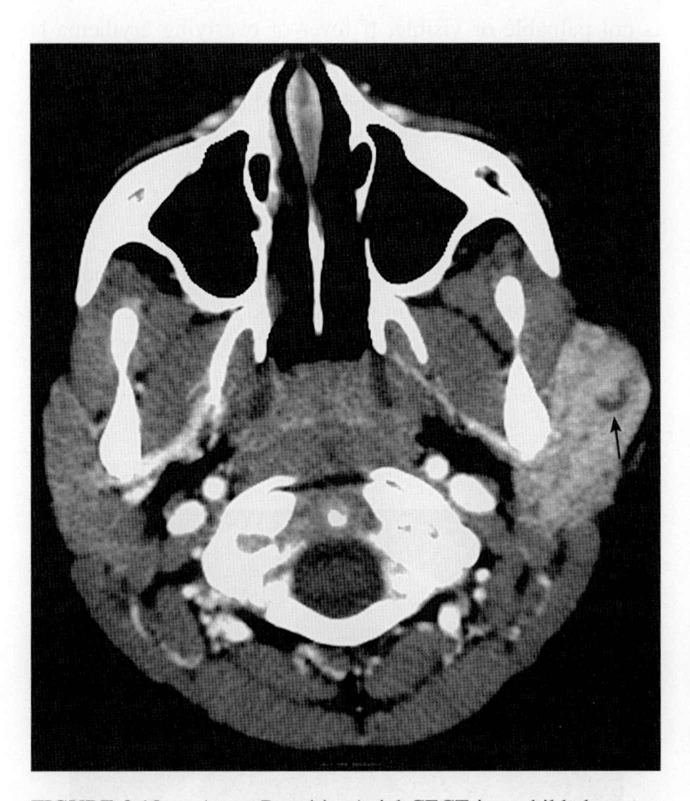

FIGURE 3.18 ■ Acute Parotitis. Axial CECT in a child shows an enlarged and hyperenhancing left parotid gland. A small area of low density within it may represent a microabscess or suppurative intraparotid lymph node (arrow).

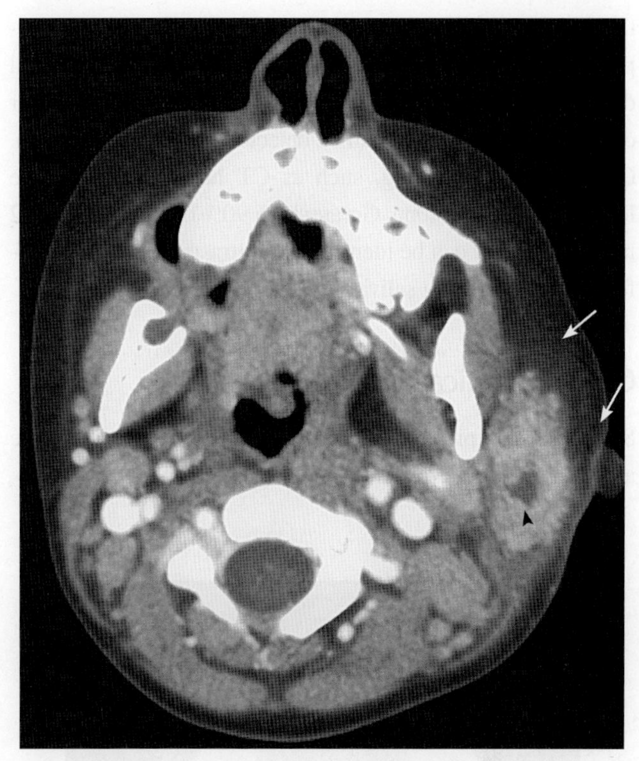

FIGURE 3.19 ■ Acute Parotitis with Microabscess. Axial CECT shows an enlarged and hyperenhancing left parotid gland with overlying infiltration of the fat indicating inflammation (arrows). There is a microabscess within the gland (arrowhead).

Radiographic Summary

Sialolithiasis is the presence of a calculus in the salivary gland or duct. More than 80% of stones originate from the submandibular gland. Twenty percent arise from the parotid gland. Noncontrast neck CT is the preferred imaging method for submandibular sialolithiasis and can demonstrate stones as small as 1-2 mm within the gland or along the course of the 5 cm Wharton's duct. Use contrast when infection is suspected or if alternative diagnoses are suspected. The proximal duct is typically dilated. Ninety percent of submandibular calculi are calcified and can be detected on plain radiograph. Cross-sectional imaging, such as CT helps in the precise localization of the stone. Greater than 90% of stones at least 2 mm in diameter can be identified by ultrasound. MRI is ineffective in identifying salivary-duct stones.

Clinical Implications

Sialolithiasis typically presents with pain and swelling of the affected gland and is exacerbated by eating. Symptoms wax and wane with gustatory anticipation and activity. Saliva can normally be seen flowing from a duct by compressing the corresponding gland. Lack of flow suggests duct obstruction. Stones may be visible at the duct orifice and may be coaxed into view by compressing the floor of the mouth or the salivary gland. Imaging is most often used to identify the cause of pain and swelling of a salivary gland or facial pain if a stone is not palpable or visible. If fever or overlying erythema is present, contrast-enhanced CT will provide the most information to make the diagnosis and will not obscure the presence of a stone.

Pearl

1. Imaging modalities for sialolithiasis include enhanced or unenhanced CT, plain radiographs, ultrasound, and sialography. The best initial test is an unenhanced CT of the neck.

FIGURE 3.20 ■ Submandibular Sialolithiasis. Axial CECT shows a large stone in the left submandibular duct of Wharton (arrow).

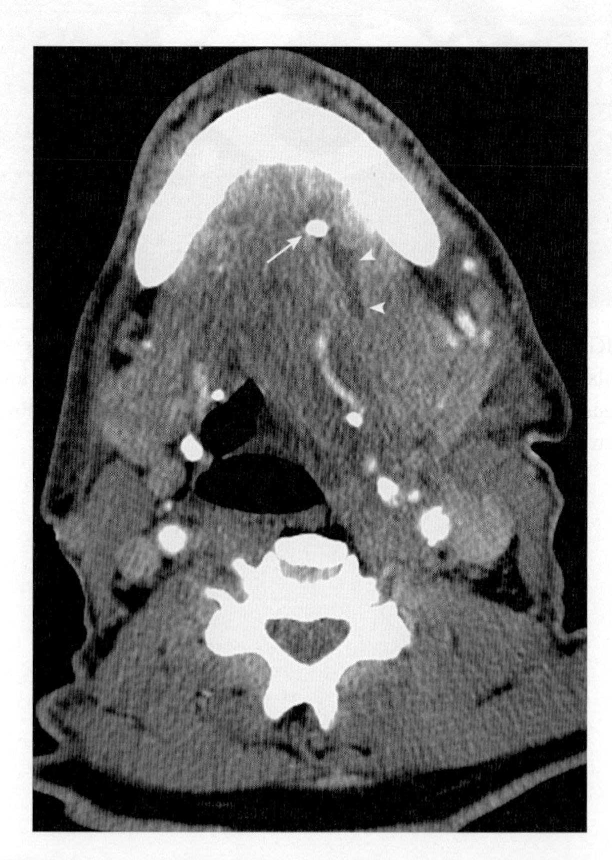

FIGURE 3.21 ■ Submandibular Sialolithiasis. Axial CECT in soft tissue windows shows a small stone in the distal left submandibular duct (Wharton's duct arrow). Note the proximal dilation of the duct (arrowheads). Note that stones can be easily seen with a contrasted study, and pre- and post-contrast CT scans need not be performed.

Radiographic Summary

Thyroglossal duct cyst (TDC) is a cystic lesion in the anterior mid-neck that is a remnant of the thyroglossal duct. It is the most common congenital neck mass. Ultrasound is an effective imaging modality and allows for evaluation without ionizing radiation in children. Findings can be variable, but a thin walled, anechoic structure that enhances posteriorly is most common. TDCs commonly occur near the level of the hyoid bone. Contrast-enhanced CT allows for excellent visualization of the cyst and its relationship to nearby neck structures.

Clinical Implications

A TDC usually presents as a painless neck mass early in life, but may become infected. Cysts may become large enough that swallowing or respiration is impaired. Treatment is with surgical excision of the cyst, thyroglossal duct remnant, and the middle of the hyoid bone. If it is not removed, there is a rare risk of malignant transformation, most commonly to papillary thyroid carcinoma.

Pearls

1. TDC is the most common congenital neck mass. Both US and CT can demonstrate the cyst, but CT provides better visualization of the anatomy of the surrounding structures for presurgical planning.
2. Patients may present with recurrent appearance of a mass or recurrent abscess.
3. Though most commonly presenting before age 20, TDC may go undetected until later in life.

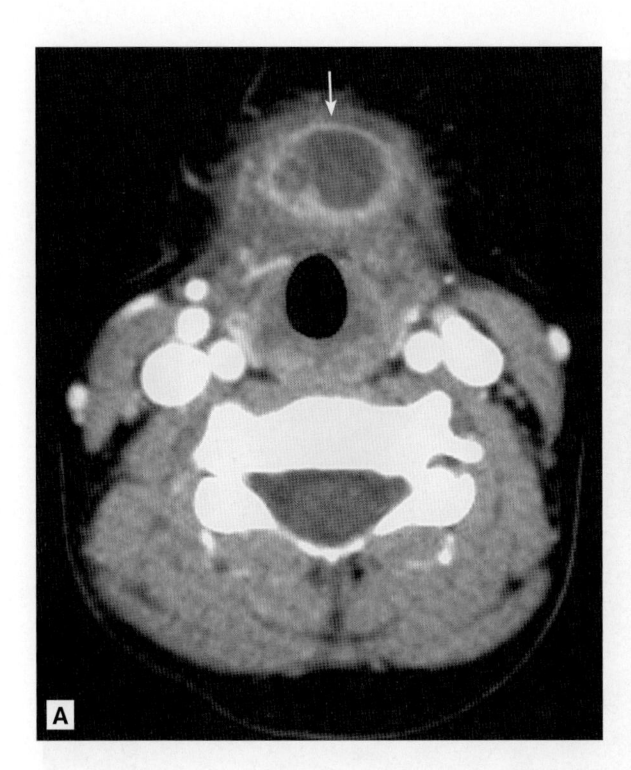

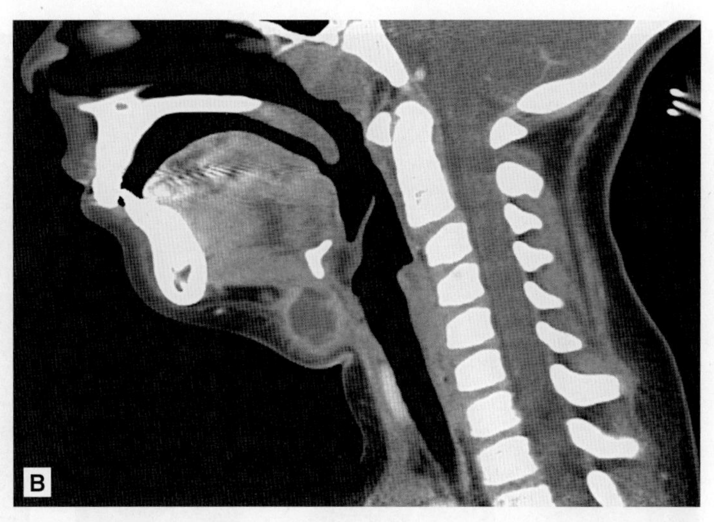

FIGURE 3.22 ■ Thyroglossal Duct Cyst. **A, B:** Axial and sagittal CECT in a child shows an inflamed cystic structure in the midline just below the hyoid bone and contained within the strap muscles (arrow). The findings are consistent with a thyroglossal duct cyst.

Radiographic Summary

Branchial cleft cysts (BCC) are congenital lesions that arise when a portion of the branchial apparatus fails to involute during development. The location can range from the ear to the mediastinum, depending on which cleft remains. Second BCC are the most common type so far and are typically found adjacent to the upper third of the sternocleidomastoid muscle. CT and MRI are the preferred imaging modalities. A BCC will appear as a nonenhancing fluid-filled mass. If infected, a BCC may have a thick enhancing wall, septations, and surrounding inflammatory stranding.

Clinical Implications

Typically, a BCC presents as a neck mass in a child or young adult. Usually they are painless and relatively asymptomatic, though if infected they can cause painful and local compressive effects. It is very rare for BCC to present in adulthood, and a mass adjacent to the muscle in the characteristic region is far more likely to be malignant (necrotic metastatic squamous cell carcinoma of the head and neck). Treatment of BCC is surgical excision.

Pearls

1. Second BCC are a common cause of lateral neck mass in children and young adults. Neck CT or MRI is the best imaging examination.
2. The diagnosis cannot be made in an older adult until malignancy is excluded.

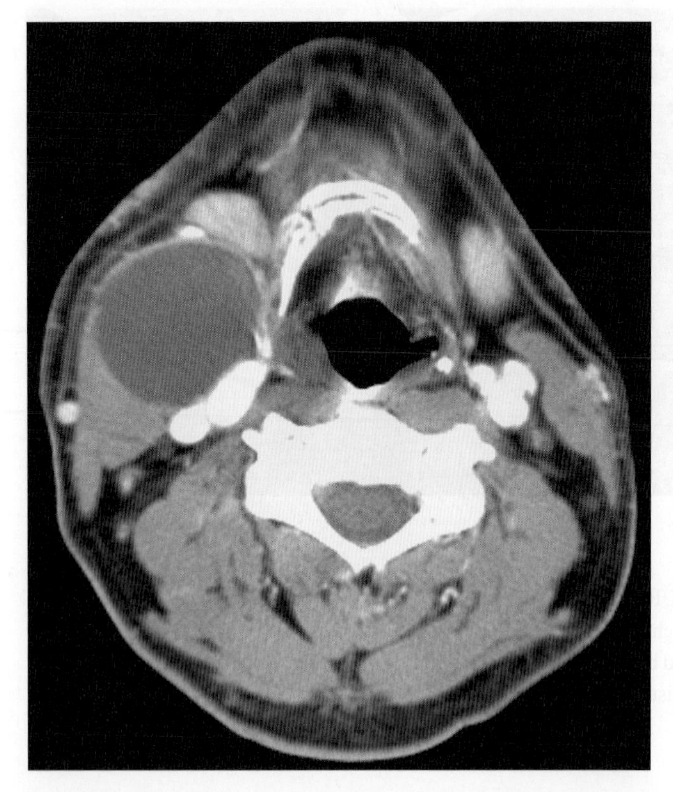

FIGURE 3.23 ■ Branchial Cleft Cyst. Axial CECT image in a teenager shows a noninflammed cystic mass in the right neck posterior to the submandibular gland, anteromedial to the sternocleidomastoid muscle, and lateral to the carotid. This is the classic location of a 2nd branchial cleft cyst.

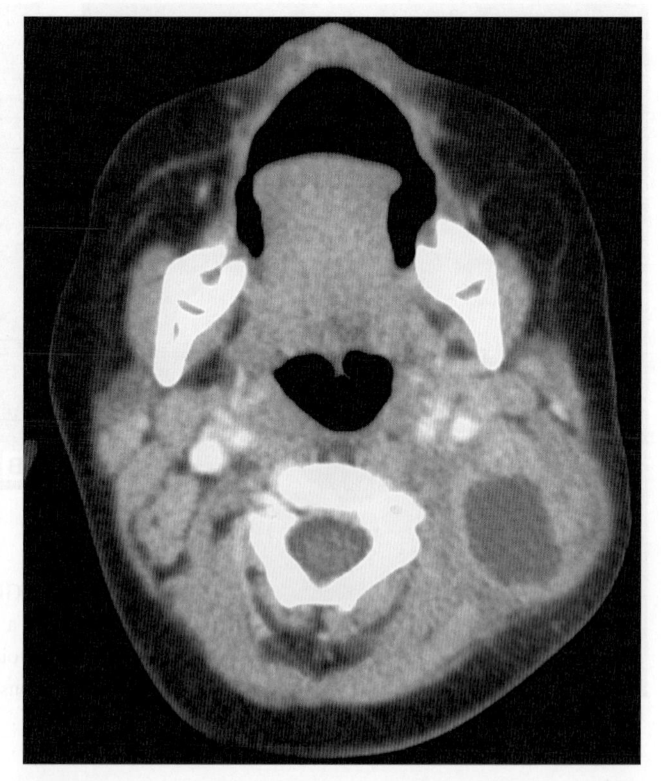

FIGURE 3.24 ■ Branchial Cleft Cyst. Axial CECT in a child shows a low-attenuation cystic mass in the left neck with surrounding inflammation within the fat and soft tissues. This was an inflamed 2nd branchial cleft cyst, but a necrotic lymph node would be another leading differential diagnosis in a child.

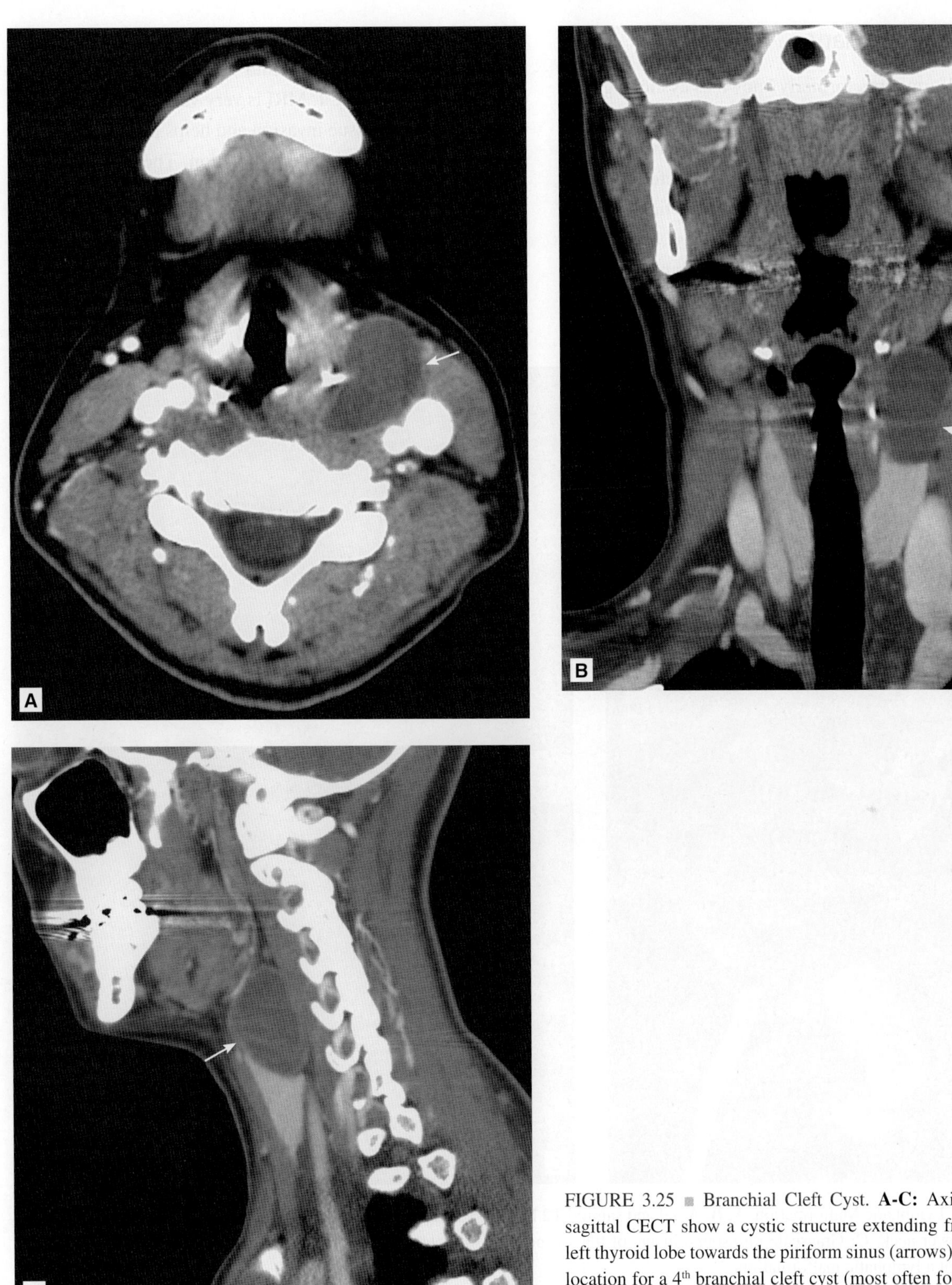

FIGURE 3.25 ■ Branchial Cleft Cyst. **A-C:** Axial, coronal, and sagittal CECT show a cystic structure extending from the superior left thyroid lobe towards the piriform sinus (arrows). This is a classic location for a 4th branchial cleft cyst (most often found arising from the left, closely associated with the thyroid).

LYMPHATIC MALFORMATION (ALSO KNOWN AS LYMPHANGIOMA OR CYSTIC HYGROMA)

Radiographic Summary

Lymphatic malformation, formerly known as cystic hygroma or lymphangioma, is a congenital dilation of lymphatic channels typically detected early in life as a mass in the neck, axilla, or groin. Ultrasound and MRI are the preferred imaging modalities. Ultrasound is useful for superficial lesions and will reveal a septated, hypoechoic mass, sometimes with internal debris. CT is faster than MRI but carries the risk of radiation exposure. Lymphatic malformations appear isodense to cerebral spinal fluid and are best demonstrated on contrast enhanced CT. MRI is very valuable if there is any concern for deep-tissue invasion and helps plan the operative approach and avoids ionizing radiation. The cystic contents will appear bright on T2-weighted images and somewhat dark on T1-weighted images. Lymphatic malformations should not enhance.

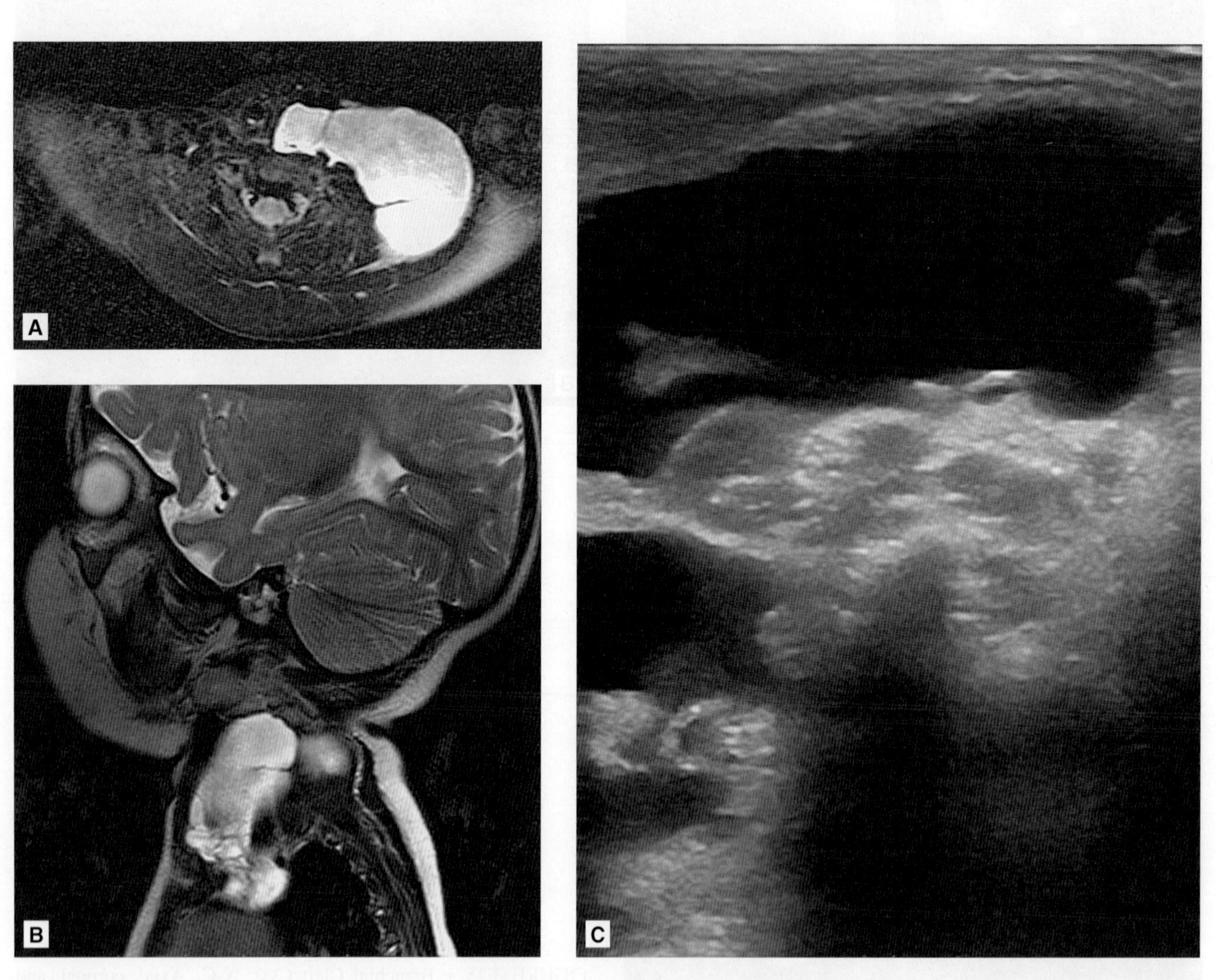

FIGURE 3.26 ■ Lymphatic Malformation. **A, B:** Axial and sagittal T2 MRI in a 10-month-old male show a large multiseptated cystic structure in the left lower neck. **C:** Grayscale ultrasound image of the left neck shows a large anechoic fluid collection and areas of septations. Findings represent a lymphatic malformation.

Clinical Implications

These masses typically present as large, soft, compressible lesions that readily transluminate. They may compress the trachea and cause stridor or extend to the oral tract and affect swallowing. Rapid growth due to infection or bleeding from minor trauma may result in respiratory distress. Oral intubation may be impossible and the patient will require emergent tracheotomy. Definitive therapy is surgical resection, though some lymphatic malformations are treated with injections of a sclerosing agent.

Pearls

1. Lymphatic malformations of the neck or tongue are a rare cause of pediatric difficult airway. Oral intubation may be impossible, mandating co-management with a specialist skilled in pediatric surgical airway placement.
2. Most lymphatic malformations will present in the neck, but they may occur anywhere. US, CT, and MRI have complementary roles in diagnosing these lesions and presurgical planning.

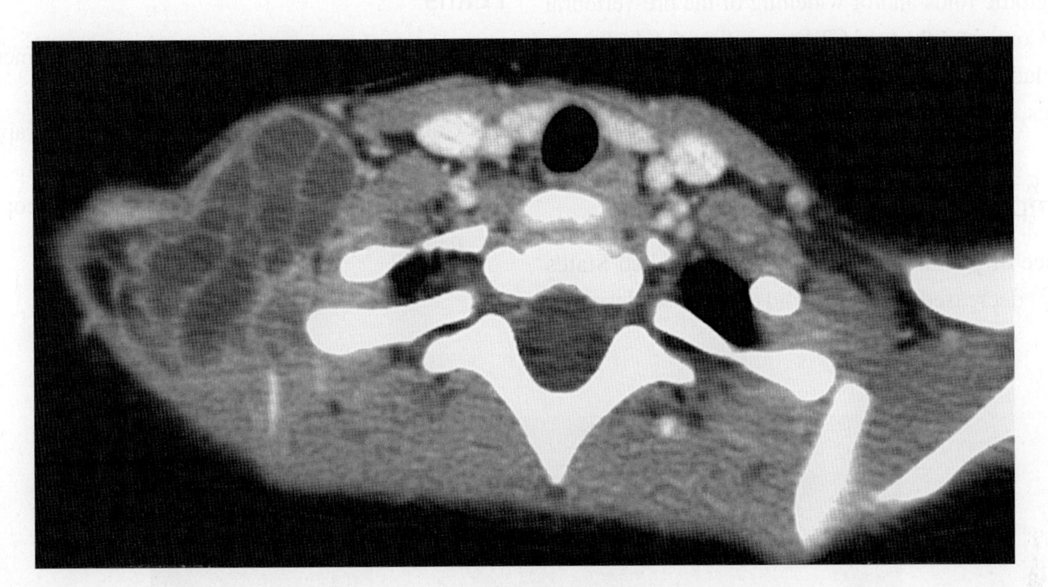

FIGURE 3.27 ■ Lymphatic Malformation. Axial CECT shows a multiseptated fluid collection in the right lower neck. There were no signs of infection clinically. A cystic neoplasm is a consideration and should be excluded. This is an example of a lymphatic malformation.

Radiographic Summary

Epiglottitis is a rapidly progressive, life-threatening inflammation of the supraglottic larynx. A portable soft tissue lateral neck radiograph is highly sensitive and specific in diagnosing epiglottitis. Ideally, the radiographs are taken with the neck held in extension and the mouth closed. Normally, the epiglottis will appear as a thin, curved structure. There should be a column of air seen above it, representing the vallecula. If the epiglottis is infected or inflamed it will appear swollen, and can at times obliterate the vallecular space. This is the so-called "thumbprint sign." Other findings include abnormally thick aryepiglottic folds and/or widening of the pre-vertebral soft tissues. Contrast-enhanced CT can confirm the diagnosis. Findings include enlarged epiglottis, edema with loss of normal fat planes, regional abscess, and gas.

Clinical Implications

The incidence of pediatric epiglottitis in the United States dramatically decreased after the advent of widespread immunization against *Haempholis influenzae B* (HIB). Cases still occur, however, and children who are not fully immunized remain at risk. The classic clinical presentation is a drooling child with fever, stridor, and respiratory distress. Due to the small caliber of the pediatric airway, it is vital to keep small children as calm as possible. Children should be kept in a position of comfort, usually in the mother's lap. Medical measures to decrease epiglottic inflammation should be initiated while emergent otolaryngology care is coordinated.

Pearls

1. Suspected pediatric epiglottitis requires emergent otolaryngology and anesthesia consultation.
2. Consider obtaining conventional radiographs on adult patients with a sore throat but no pharyngitis. Direct visualization with a fiberoptic nasopharyngoscope is an alternative method to evaluate the epiglottis.

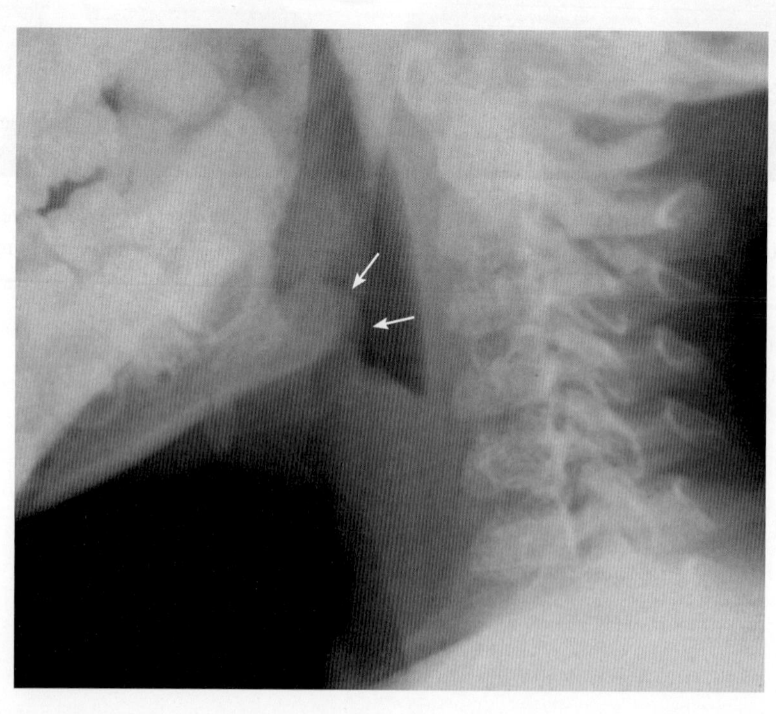

FIGURE 3.28 ■ Epiglottis. Coned down lateral view of a child's neck soft tissues shows a markedly thickened epiglottis ("thumbprint sign") arrows.

Radiographic Summary

Croup, also called laryngotracheobronchitis, is a viral illness that causes inflammation and narrowing of the subglottic larynx and trachea. An antero-posterior radiograph of the neck or chest demonstrates subglottic narrowing described as a "steeple sign" due to the tapered narrowing of the subglottic tracheal air column. Soft tissue lateral neck radiographs typically demonstrate hyperexpansion of the hypopharynx.

Clinical Implications

Plain radiographs of the chest and neck should be obtained in the acutely stridulous patient when the etiology is unclear. Patients with croup most often present with a sudden onset of stridor, barking cough, and respiratory distress, preceded by a viral illness of several days duration. Symptoms quickly improve during the drive to the ED or with nebulized racemic epinephrine. Patients with a typical history for croup do not require imaging to confirm the diagnosis. Consider plain radiographs in unimmunized patients with acute onset of stridor or when other causes of stridor are considered likely.

Pearls

1. Imaging is not required in acutely stridulous patients where the diagnosis of croup is certain.
2. The "steeple sign" may also be seen in patients with bacterial tracheitis, thermal injury, and allergic reaction.

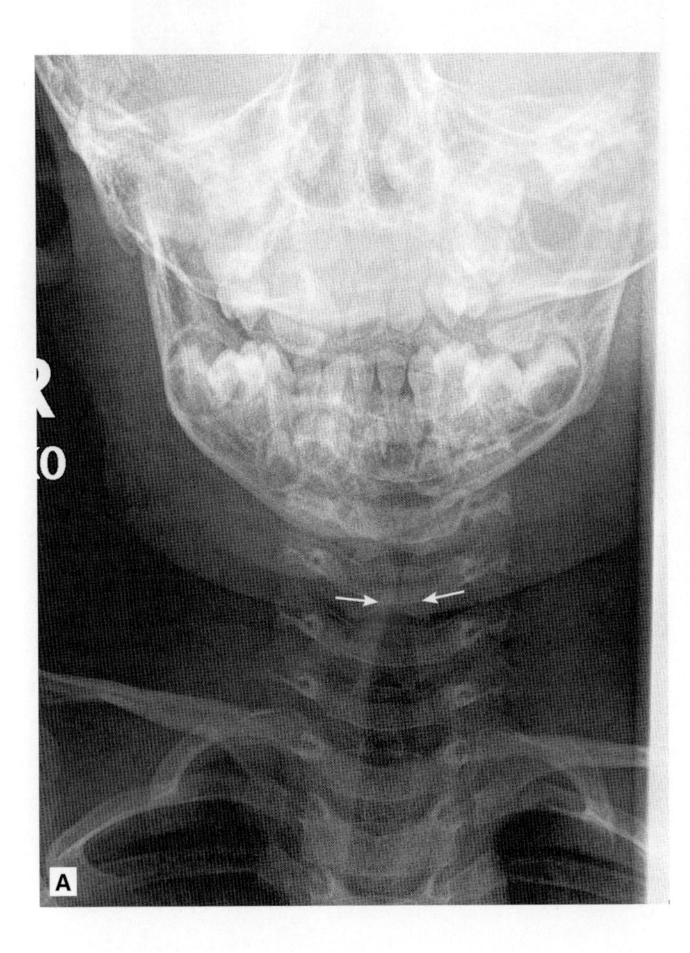

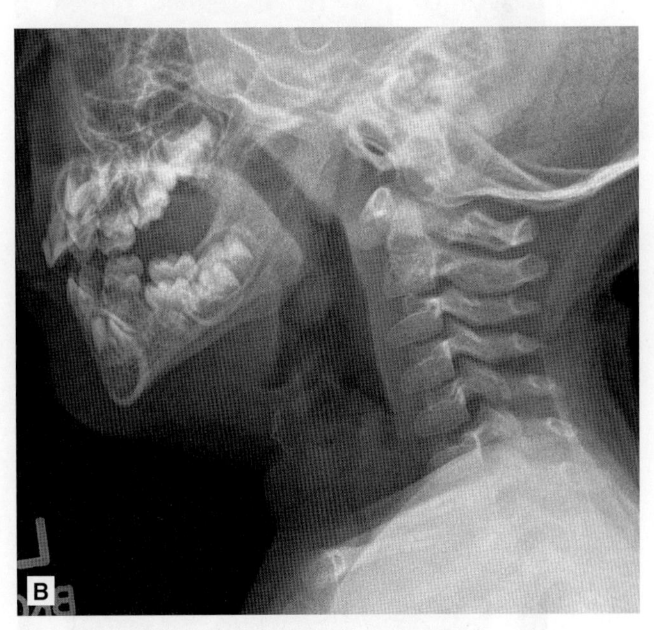

FIGURE 3.29 ■ Croup. **A:** Frontal view of neck soft tissues shows subglottic edema ("steeple sign" arrows). **B:** Lateral radiograph of the neck shows hyperexpansion of the hypopharynx. Findings are consistent with croup.

Radiographic Summary

Lymphoma describes a group of malignancies that are generally either Hodgkin disease or non-Hodgkin lymphoma. Lymphoma may present in the ED as painless cervical lymphadenopathy or as enlarged mediastinal lymph nodes as an unexpected finding on CXR. Contrast-enhanced CT of the neck and chest best evaluates lymphoma. Lymph nodes may appear enlarged and confluent, with enhancing rims

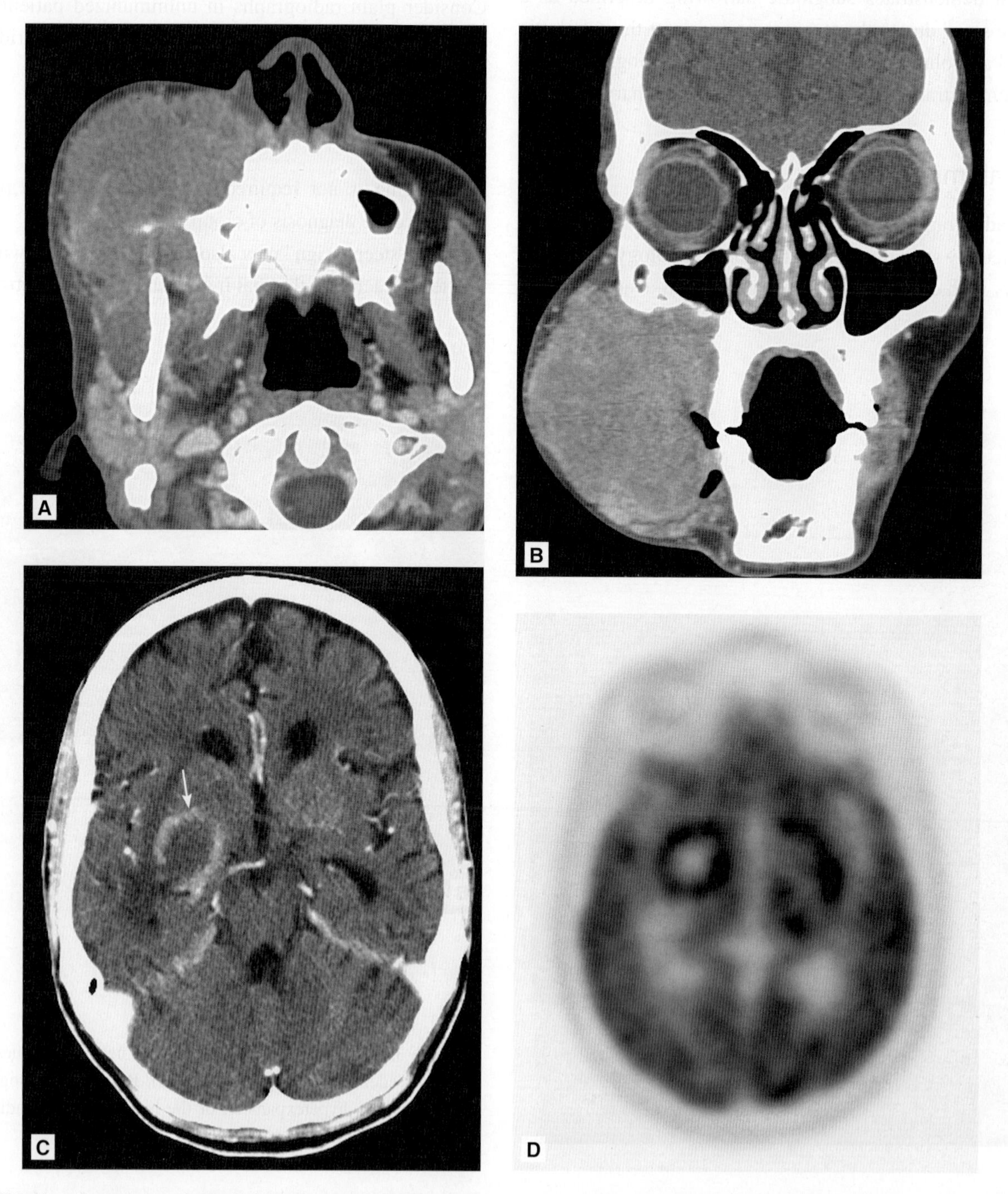

FIGURE 3.30 ■ Lymphoma. **A, B:** Axial and coronal CECT images of the face show a very large irregular mass arising from the right cheek. Biopsy found aggressive diffuse large B-cell lymphoma. **C:** Axial CECT image of the brain shows a rim-enhancing lesion in the right basal ganglia (arrow). HIV testing was recommended based on the unusual presentation of lesions in both the brain and face, and the patient was unknowingly HIV positive. **D:** Axial 18-F FDG PET image of the brain shows hypermetabolic activity corresponding to the area of enhancement in the right basal ganglia. This confirms lymphoma in an HIV patient (toxoplasmosis would not have increased activity on PET imaging).

and/or central necrosis. Lymphoma found outside the nodes will appear to have uneven margins and findings of necrosis are less common.

Clinical Implications

Lymphoma most commonly presents as painless adenopathy (typically of the head or neck, axilla, or groin) but associated systemic symptoms can include fever, night sweats, weight loss, and fatigue. Diagnosis is made by biopsy; the diagnostic yield of core biopsy and surgical biopsy is better than fine-needle aspiration.

Pearls

1. Lymphoma often presents as a bland appearing bulky adenopathy of the neck, axillary, or mediastinal lymph node groups.
2. Contrast-enhanced neck CT or US is the best initial test for the evaluation of a neck or mediastinal mass.
3. Lymphadenopathy that persists after antibiotic treatment should be considered for CT- or ultrasound-guided biopsy depending on the location of the targeted lesion.

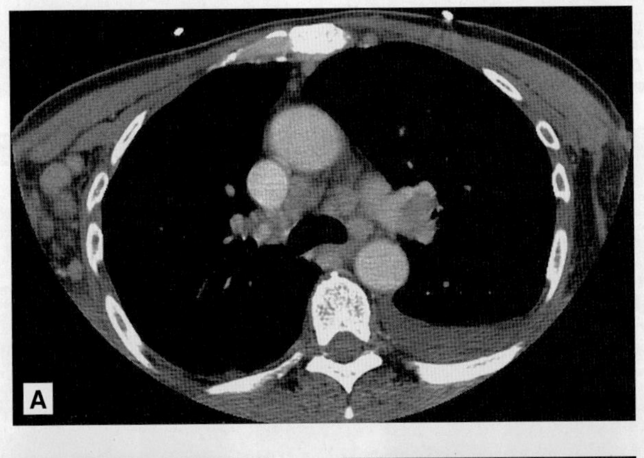

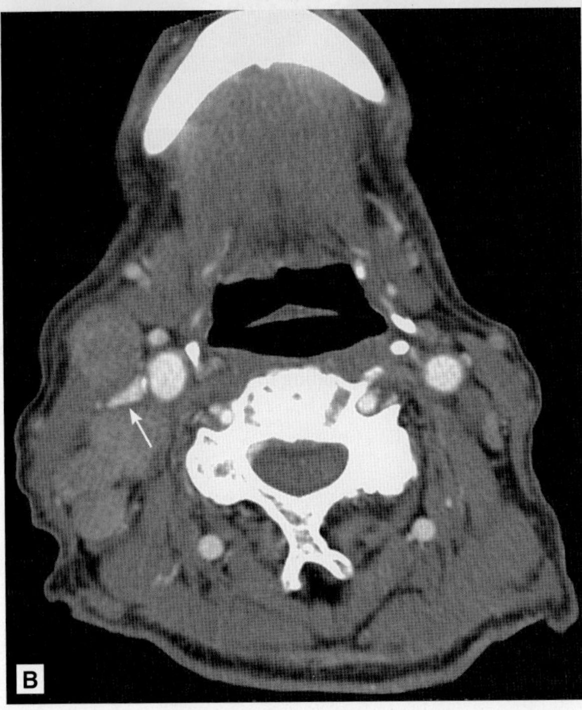

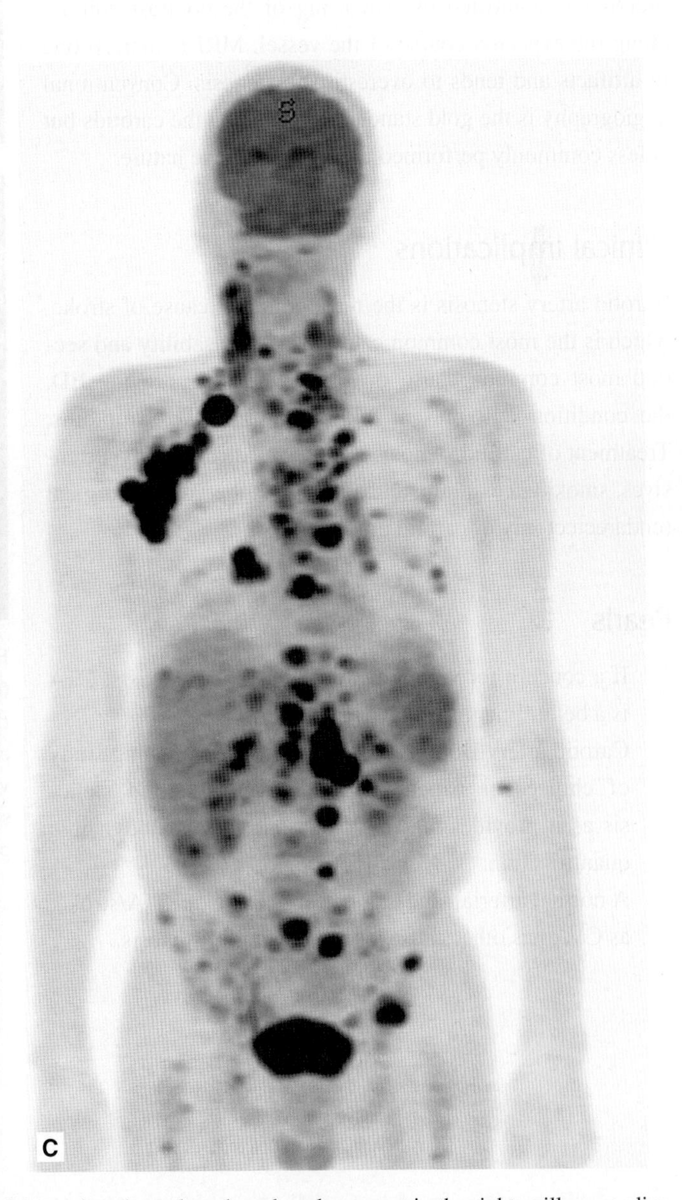

FIGURE 3.31 ■ Lymphoma. **A:** Axial CECT image at the level of the carina shows lymph-node enlargement in the right axillary, mediastinal, and hilar regions. A small left pleural effusion is present. **B:** Axial CECT of the neck shows large right cervical lymph nodes which cause compression upon the internal jugular vein (arrow). Biopsy revealed Hodgkin lymphoma in this 63-year-old male. **C:** MIP image from a whole-bed PET shows numerous areas of abnormal metabolic activity in lymph nodes of the neck, chest, axilla, abdomen, and pelvis.

Radiographic Summary

Carotid artery athersosclerotic occlusive disease may contribute to ischemic stroke by embolism or low blood flow states. Multiple imaging modalities may be utilized to evaluate carotid artery blood flow. Duplex ultrasound is a screening tool to identify patients at risk for stroke. Velocity measurements accurately estimate luminal stenosis. CTA and magnetic resonance angiography (MRA) provide detailed, non-invasive images of the carotid arteries and their branches. These studies are sensitive for the presence of stenosis or aneurysm. Stenosis is identified by narrowing of the contrast column along the expected course of the vessel. MRI is more prone to artifacts and tends to overestimate stenosis. Conventional angiography is the gold standard for imaging the carotids but is less commonly performed due to its invasive nature.

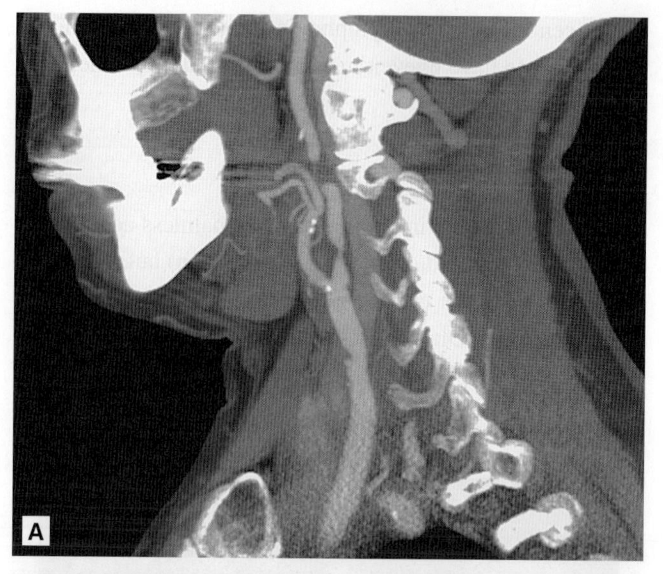

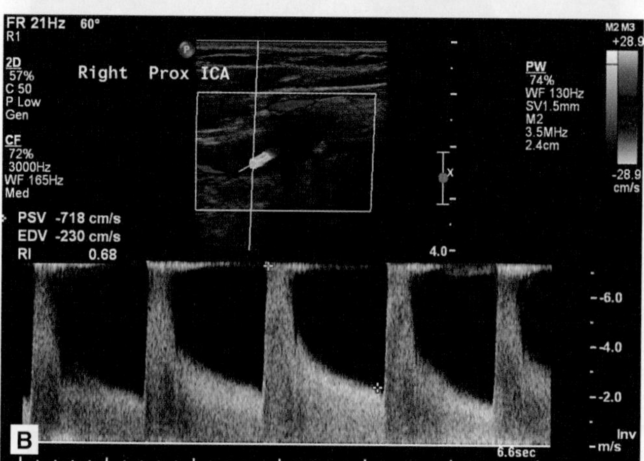

FIGURE 3.32 ■ Carotid Artery Stenosis. **A:** Sagittal CTA in a 66-year-old female shows severe focal narrowing of the proximal right ICA just beyond the carotid bifurcation. **B:** Spectral Doppler carotid ultrasound of the proximal right ICA shows markedly elevated systolic velocities (718 cm/second, normal is <125 cm/s) and spectral broadening. Grayscale images confirm diffuse atheromatous plaque in this region corresponding to severe (80-99%) stenosis.

Clinical Implications

Carotid artery stenosis is the most common cause of stroke, which is the most common cause of adult disability and second most common cause of death worldwide. In the ED, the condition will present with TIA or stroke symptoms. Treatment of carotid stenosis is either medical (antihypertensives, smoking cessation, and antiplatelet therapy) or surgical (endarectectomy or carotid artery stenting).

Pearls

1. If a concern for vertebral artery disease also exists, CTA is a better imaging choice than MRA.
2. Carotid artery Doppler US should be the screening study of choice for patients with suspected carotid stenosis as it provides not only anatomic, but hemodynamic quantification.
3. A normal arterial study alone cannot rule out TIA/stroke, as CVA has other causes than just arterial stenosis.

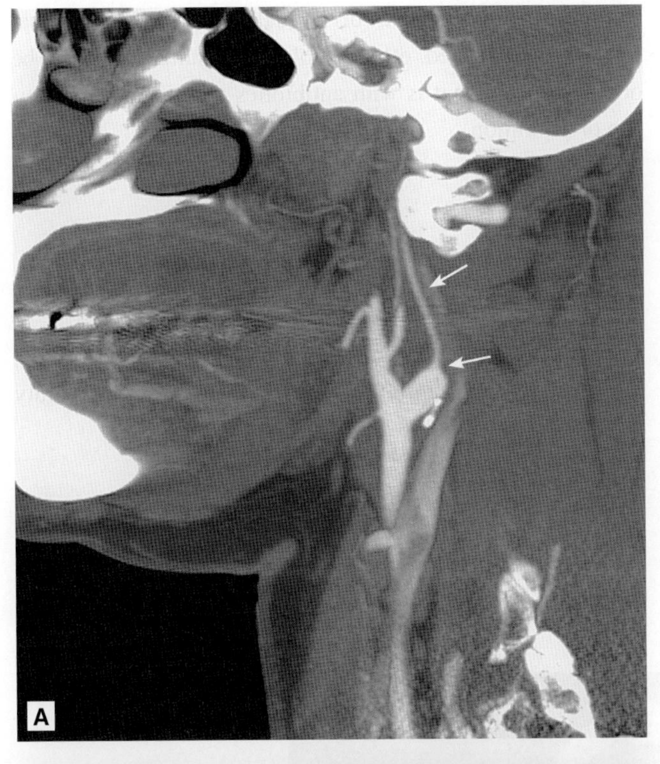

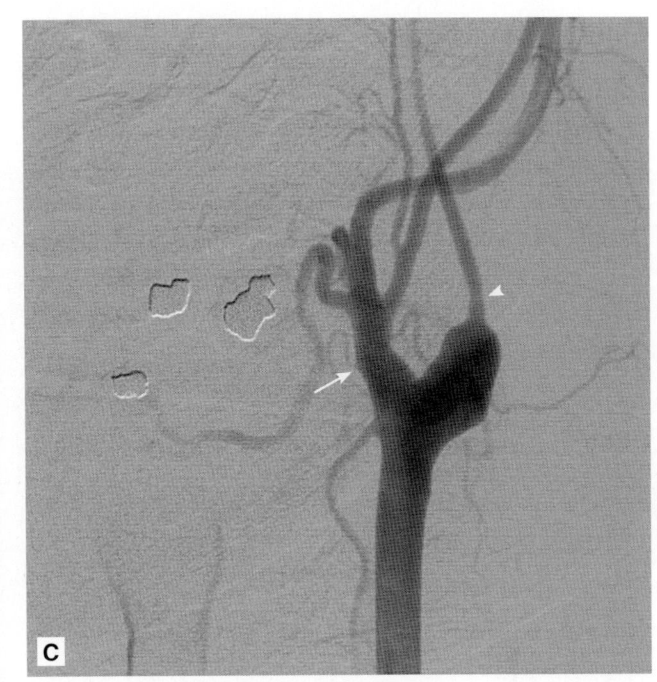

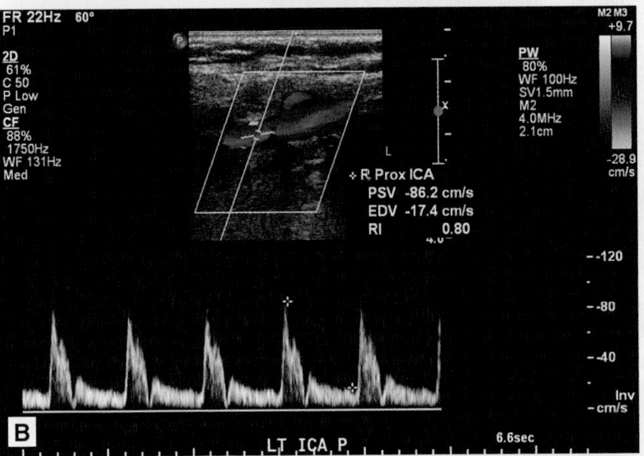

FIGURE 3.33 ■ Carotid Artery Stenosis. **A:** Sagittal CTA shows severe smooth, long segment narrowing of the left internal carotid artery (arrows) in this 42-year-old female with right upper extremity parasthesias. **B:** Spectral Doppler carotid ultrasound shows narrowed lumen of the ICA, but no atherosclerotic changes to explain the narrowing. The velocities and vessel waveforms were all within normal range leading to the conclusion that this stenosis was congenital in origin. **C:** Lateral angiogram image shows the long smooth stenotic appearance of the internal carotid artery (note how the external carotid artery (arrow) has a much larger diameter than the internal carotid arrowhead).

Clinical Summary

Lingual abscess is a rare soft tissue bacterial infection of the head and neck caused by *Staphylococcal* and *Streptococcal species,* and anaerobes. Contrast-enhanced neck CT demonstrates a rim-enhancing lesion with central hypodense fluid located within the tongue. CT will differentiate lingual abscess from other causes of tongue swelling and pain which include angioedema, hemorrhage, tumor, lingual artery aneurysm, and cellulitis.

Clinical Implications

Swelling, redness and pain of the tongue, drooling, and odynophagia should prompt a contrast-enhanced neck CT to confirm the diagnosis of lingual abscess. Once lingual abscess is confirmed, otolaryngology consultation should be obtained. Treatment is with antibiotics and incisional drainage or aspiration.

Pearls

1. The imaging modality of choice for lingual abscess is a contrast-enhanced neck CT.
2. MRI is capable of identifying lingual abscesses. However, there may be significant limitations in the image quality due to motion artifact.

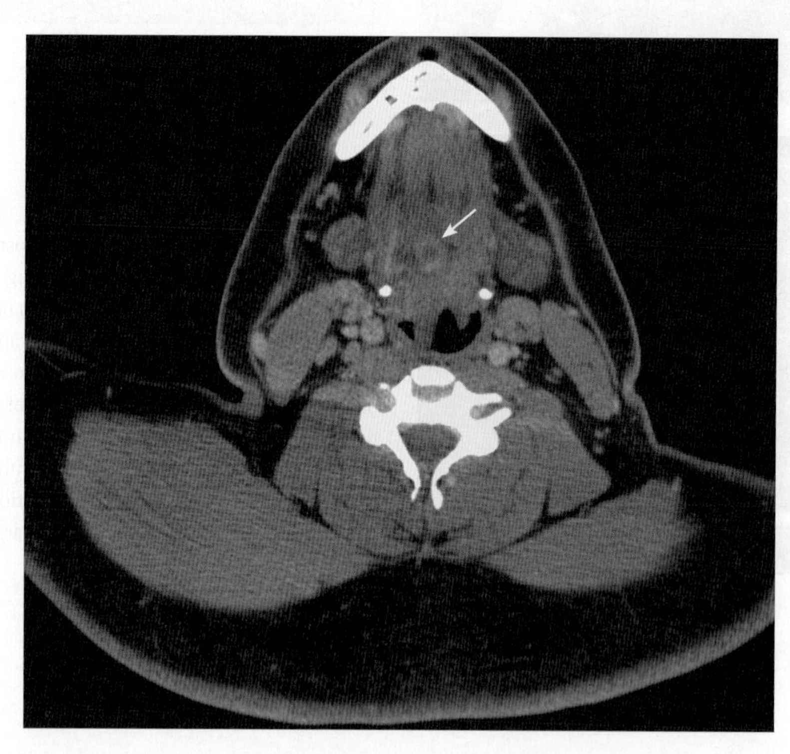

FIGURE 3.34 ■ Lingual Abscess. Axial and sagittal CECT in a 21-year-old male with muffled voice and dysphagia show a small rim-enhancing abscess at the base of the tongue (arrow) just superior to the hyoid bone (the hyoid bone is not shown on this image). The findings represent a lingual abscess.

Chapter 4

TRAUMATIC CONDITIONS OF THE CHEST

Joseph Blake
Charles Seamens
R. Jason Thurman

Radiographic Features

A majority of sternal fractures occur transversely across the midbody, but may also be seen at the manubrium. In general, the sternum is initially imaged with PA and lateral chest radiographs, but more sensitive dedicated sternal views are also available when clinical suspicion is high. The lateral chest x-ray provides more value in identifying sternal fractures and their degree of displacement than the PA view. With the advent of later generation CT scanners and their expanded use in trauma patients, CT often identifies sternal fractures and is greater in sensitivity and specificity than plain radiographs. CT is also useful to identify associated thoracic or cardiopulmonary injuries, which are of greater clinical importance than the fracture itself.

Clinical Implications

Sternal fractures are usually associated with direct blunt traumatic injury to the chest sustained in a motor vehicle crash, but stress fractures may also be encountered. Sternal fractures are painful injuries resulting in decreased respiratory excursion and pulmonary atelectasis, so outpatient management

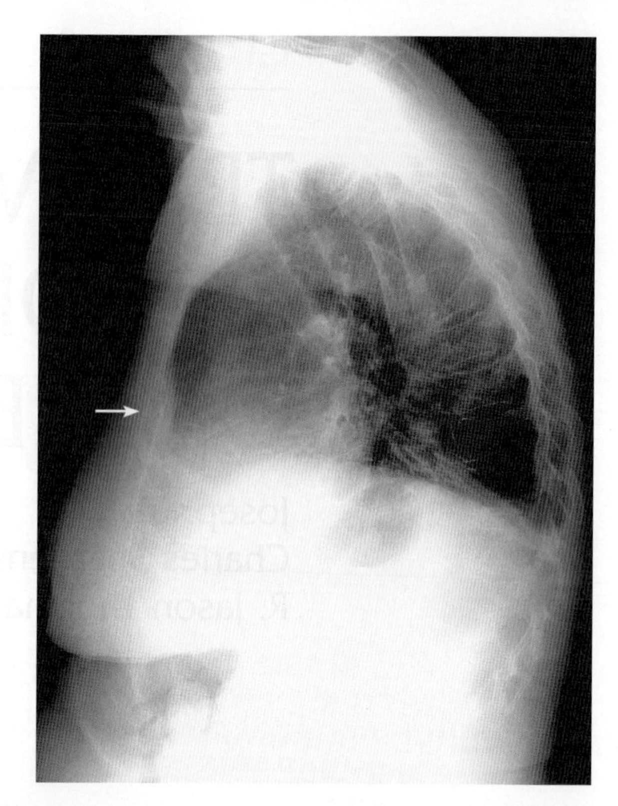

FIGURE 4.1 ■ Sternal Fracture. The lateral chest radiograph adequately shows the mildly posteriorly displaced fracture of the sternal body (arrow).

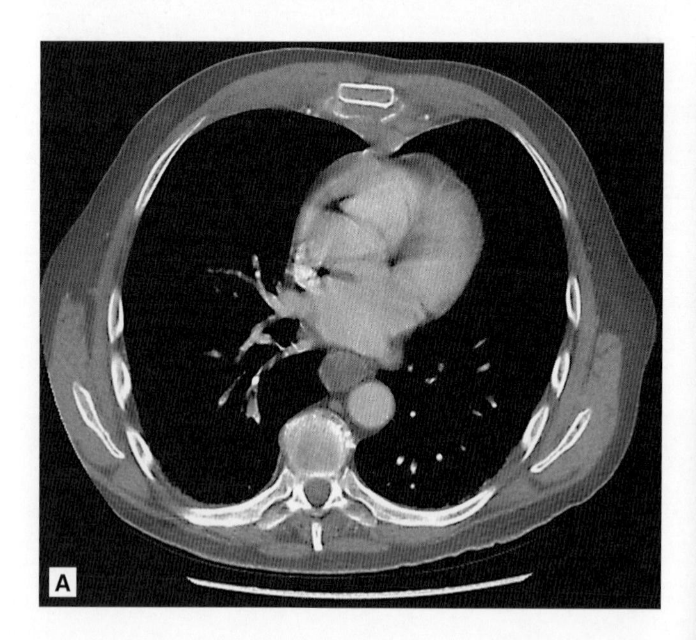

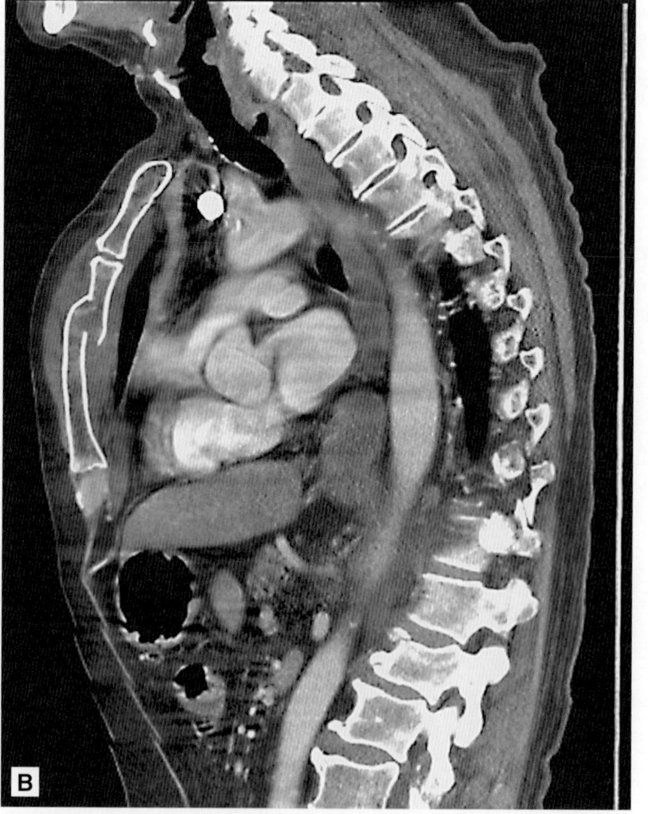

FIGURE 4.2 ■ Sternum Fracture. **A, B:** An axial and a sagittal CT image of the chest in another patient show a mildly displaced sternal fracture with hematoma formation about the fracture site. Anteriorly displaced sternal fractures, such as this, have a high association with flexion injury of the thoracic spine.

should consist of adequate analgesia and incentive spirometry. Sternal fractures may be associated with acute life-threatening intrathoracic injuries such as cardiac contusion, mediastinal injury and bleeding, aortic injury, flail chest, pneumothorax or hemothorax, pulmonary contusions and lacerations, and compression fractures of the ribs and thoracic spine. Because of the high morbidity and mortality of concomitant injuries, a high index of suspicion should be held for associated injuries when sternal fracture is diagnosed.

Pearls

1. Identification of associated injuries carrying high morbidity and mortality is of paramount importance when considering the diagnosis of sternal fracture.
2. Dedicated sternal views are more sensitive than PA and lateral chest radiographs in identifying sternal fractures by changing the viewing angle and exposure of the radiograph. These should be considered when clinical suspicion is high and chest radiographs are negative, unless a CT is to be performed.
3. A clue to look for a subtle sternal fracture on CT is retrosternal hematoma formation.
4. Anteriorly displaced sternal body fractures are commonly associated with flexion injuries of the thoracic spine.

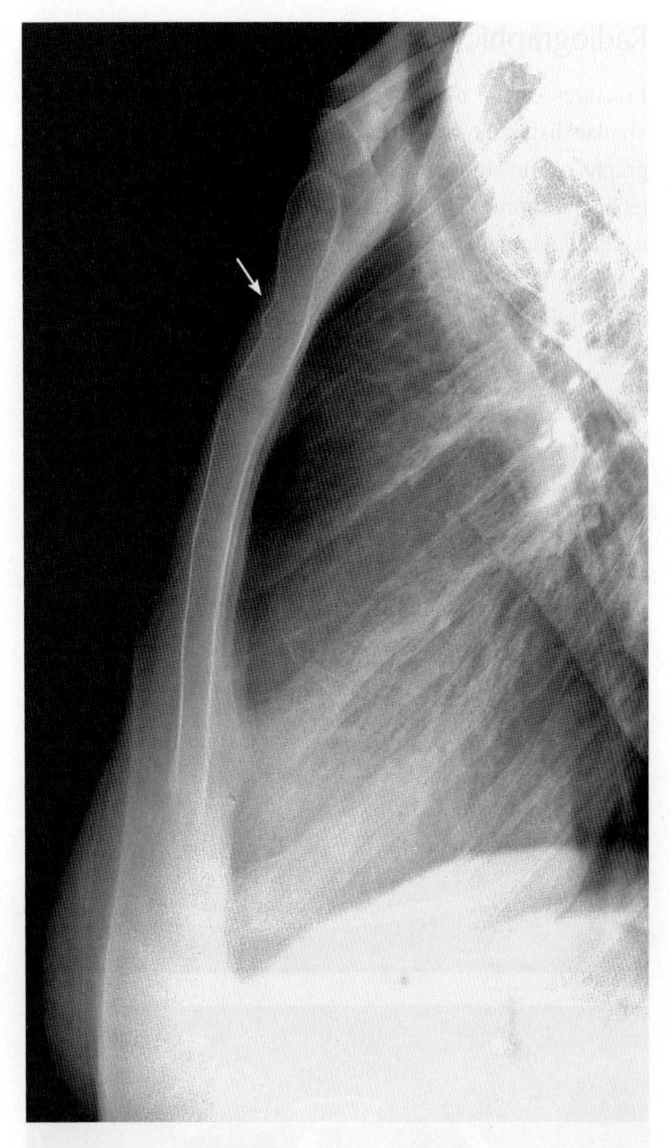

FIGURE 4.3 ■ Manubrium Fracture. A lateral view of the sternum nicely demonstrates buckling of the manubrium in this nondisplaced fracture (arrow).

Radiographic Summary

Fractures of the medial third of the clavicle and sternoclavicular dislocations are difficult to visualize on plain radiographs of the shoulder or the chest. Because of radiographic technique, some subtle injuries will be better detected on dedicated clavicular views. If one suspects a displaced sternoclavicular injury, a contrasted CT scan should be obtained. CT is important not only in determining if underlying structures are being compressed by the medial clavicle but also perhaps in elucidating associated intrathoracic injuries. Findings may include demonstration of sternoclavicular disruption, fractures of the sternum and clavicle, mediastinal hematoma, and vascular injury to aorta and its branches or the superior vena cava. These injuries usually occur in the setting of high-energy trauma and concomitant intrathoracic injuries such as pneumothoraces, pulmonary contusions, and head and neck injuries are commonly present.

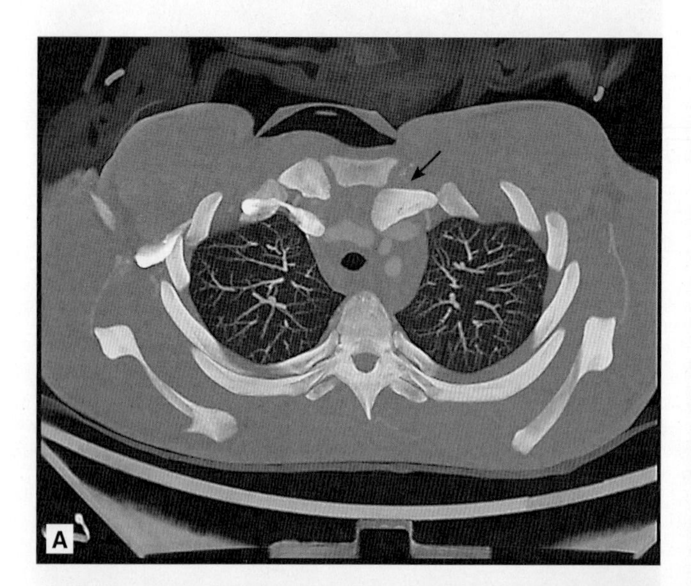

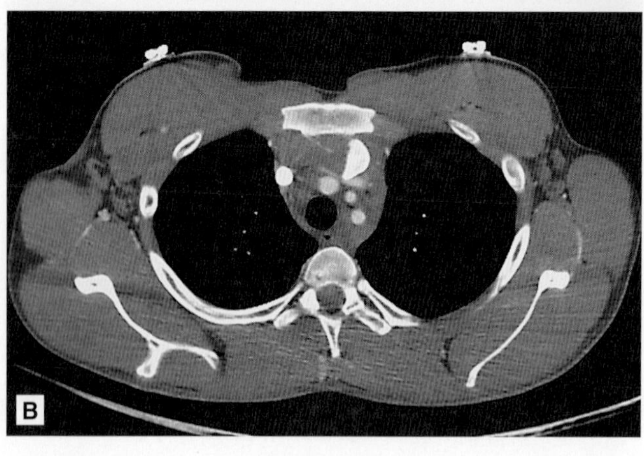

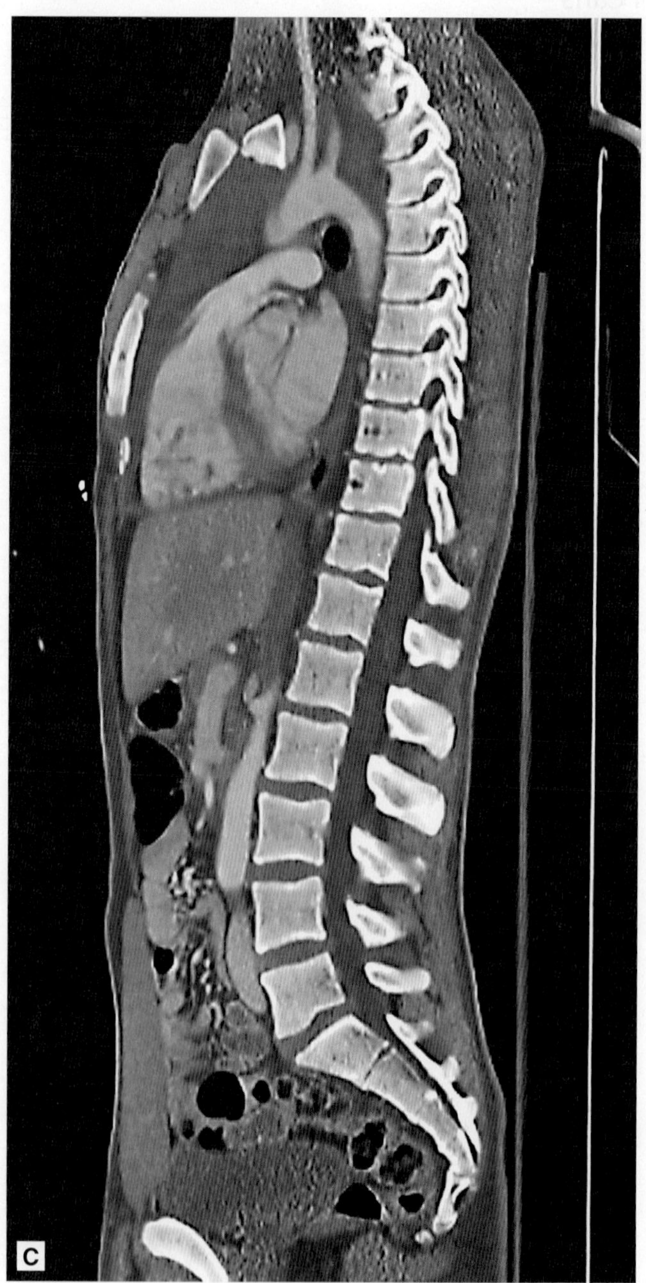

FIGURE 4.4 ■ Sternoclavicular Dislocation. **A-C:** The left clavicular head is dislocated posteriorly (arrow) (normal right side for comparison). The head of the dislocated clavicle narrows the lumen of the left brachiocephalic vein. There is mediastinal hematoma present.

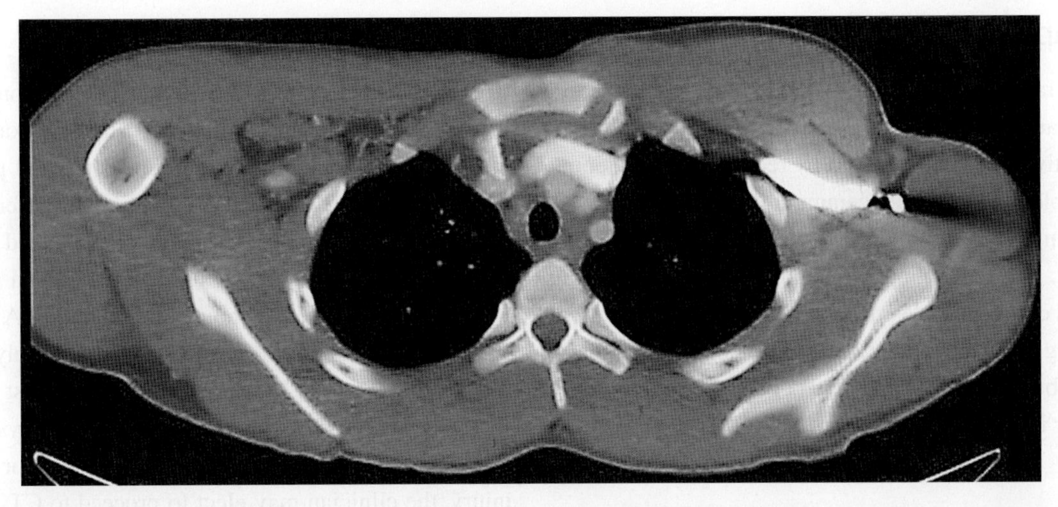

FIGURE 4.5 ■ Sternoclavicular Dislocation. Axial CT image at the level of the sternoclavicular joints demonstrates posterior dislocation of the right clavicular head. Note the normal alignment of the left sternoclavicular joint.

Clinical Implications

Injuries to the sternoclavicular joint are potentially life-threatening by causing injury to underlying vital mediastinal structures. Dislocations at the sternoclavicular joint may be either anterior or posterior, with posterior dislocations potentially resulting in injury to adjacent structures through direct anatomical compression. Anterior dislocations can occur as the arm is forcefully abducted above the head. Patients with anterior dislocations tend to have much less pain than patients with retrosternal dislocations. Posterior dislocations may be accompanied by other symptoms depending on the structure being compressed such as hoarseness, stridor, or venous congestion of the head and neck. Both dislocations have pain exacerbated by movement of the upper extremity.

Anterior dislocations can be treated with conscious sedation and closed reduction. Once reduced, the clavicle should be immobilized for 4 to 6 weeks. If recurrent dislocations occur, surgical fixation may be required. Posterior dislocations may require urgent reduction if significant compression of underlying structures is present.

Pearls

1. The medial aspect of the clavicle may not be adequately visualized on plain radiographs. If the clinical setting suggests a sternoclavicular dislocation, contrasted CT scan of the chest provides more information on not only the extent of the clavicular injury but also the status of the underlying vascular structures, trachea, and lung.
2. Many sternoclavicular dislocations in patients younger than 25 years old are actually fractures through the physeal plate and represent Salter–Harris type I or II fractures.

Radiographic Summary

Plain chest radiography is generally the initial study used to detect rib fractures, although the overall sensitivity of CXR is poor. Sensitivity can be increased by recognizing thickening of the extrapleural soft tissues commonly accompanying these injuries. If higher sensitivity is desired, oblique rib views can be obtained. Plain radiography may miss fractures occurring in the costal cartilages unless the cartilage is heavily calcified. CT scanning is far more sensitive than plain radiographs in detecting rib fractures, but the test is generally unnecessary unless other injuries are of concern.

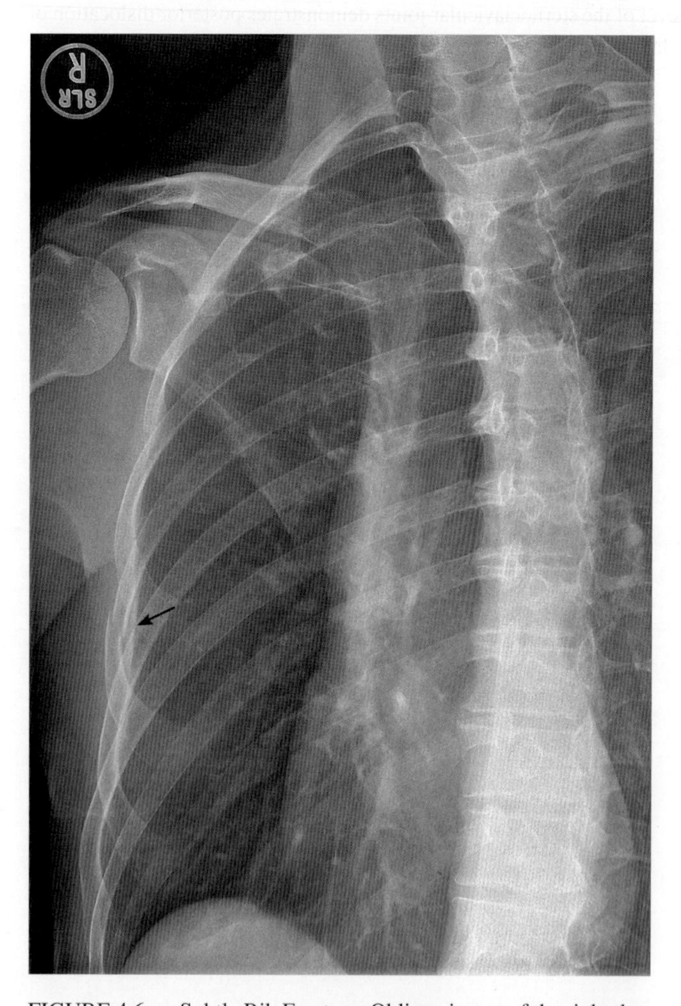

FIGURE 4.6 ■ Subtle Rib Fracture. Oblique image of the right thorax demonstrates a minimally displaced fifth anterolateral rib fracture. Note the slight amount of extrapleural soft tissue thickening accompanying this acute injury (arrow). See the section "Diagnosis: Flail Chest" for additional examples of rib fracture.

Clinical Implications

Rib fractures are clinically suspected based on history of direct trauma to the area of the chest and pain exacerbated by movement, inspiration, cough or sneezing, and palpation of the injured area. Depending on the amount of energy transferred, rib fractures may be isolated or associated with underlying injuries. For patients with isolated trauma to the chest without major force, the choice of an upright PA chest x-ray is a reasonable option. Rib radiographs are rarely necessary, as the results do not change management in most cases.

Patients whose mechanism of injury, physical exam, or symptoms suggest underlying pulmonary or abdominal injury, the clinician may elect to proceed to CT scan. CT is more sensitive for detecting injury to underlying lung and pneumothorax. A contrasted CT is used to diagnose injury to pulmonary vasculature and detection of intra-abdominal and retroperitoneal injuries. Isolated rib fractures are not life-threatening in and of themselves, but are extremely painful and may cause life-threatening complications, especially in elderly patients with borderline pulmonary reserve. Due to splinting of the chest wall, there is limitation of deep breathing and subsequent atelectasis and resultant pneumonia. For this reason, pain control, incentive spirometry, and pulmonary toilet are the mainstays for the treatment of rib fractures.

Pearls

1. Conventional upright PA view is far more sensitive for detection of rib fracture than a supine portable AP ("trauma") view; CT may show fractures not otherwise visible on plain radiographs.
2. For patients with normal CXR in whom it is important to determine the presence of isolated rib fracture, ultrasound at the site of maximal tenderness may be of benefit. The fracture and subperiosteal hematomas can be detected in the osseous and cartilaginous portions of the rib. However, ultrasound is less helpful in detecting upper rib and subscapular fractures.
3. PA and lateral views of the chest serve to evaluate for complications of rib injury, such as pneumothorax, pulmonary contusion, or hemothorax. Dedicated rib views for localization of nondisplaced fractures are generally unnecessary.

Radiographic Features

With scapulothoracic dissociation, chest x-ray may show significant lateral displacement of the scapula, indicating severe injury to the upper extremity and what amounts to a closed amputation of the extremity. Patients often have associated fractures of the clavicle, scapula, and humerus that may be evident on plain radiographs as well as intrathoracic injuries best demonstrated on CT scan. Selective angiography is needed to diagnose injuries to the subclavian and axillary arteries. MRI is the imaging modality of choice for associated brachial plexus injuries and may also demonstrate muscular and ligamentous injuries in detail.

Clinical Implications

Scapulothoracic dissociation is a rare injury most often resulting from motor vehicle collisions, especially in motorcyclists. The injury is associated with complete or partial injuries to muscles of the shoulder girdle, brachial plexus, and arteries supplying the upper extremity. Patients may complain of motor weakness and decreased sensation of the arm along with severe pain. Neurovascular injuries may be difficult to detect in intubated patients, underscoring the importance of adequate imaging in the multisystem trauma patient. On physical examination the shoulder area may be massively edematous or the upper extremity may be mottled, making vascular injury more apparent. Complete injuries to the brachial plexus may result in the need for amputation because the limb is rendered functionless.

Pearls

1. Test strength and sensation of the upper extremity in all distributions of the brachial plexus and assess vascular integrity in all patients with fractures of the scapula and clavicle.
2. Compare the distance from the medial border of the scapula to midline on both sides of the thorax with the arms in similar position. A widening of this space may indicate scapulothoracic dissociation.
3. If patient's condition allows, obtain MRI to further delineate injuries to the brachial plexus.
4. Complete disruption of the brachial plexus (even more so than vascular injury due to collaterals) portends dismal prognosis for limb salvage.

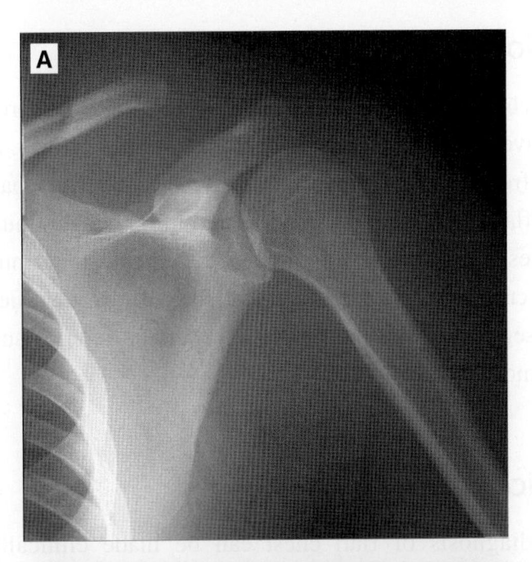

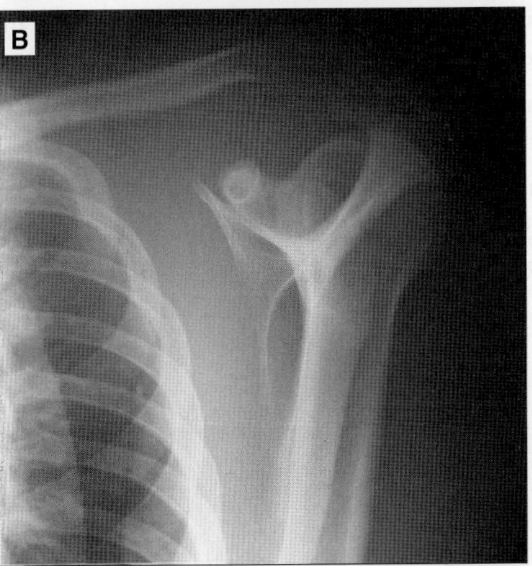

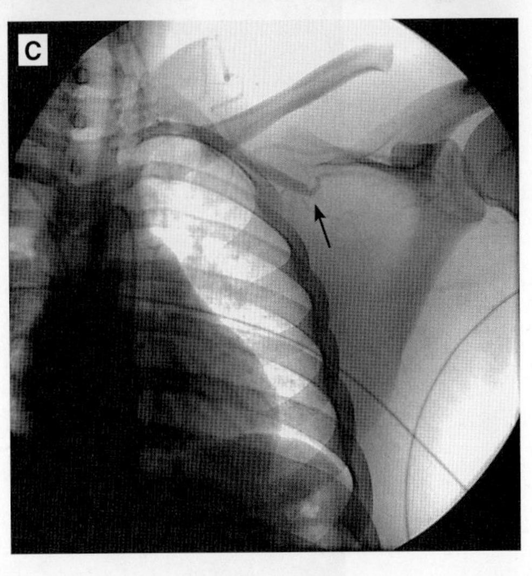

FIGURE 4.7 ■ Scapulothoracic Dissociation. **A, B:** Very wide separation and displacement at the acriomioclavicular joint with separation of the scapula from the chest wall. **C:** An arteriogram in the same patient with abrupt cutoff or occlusion of the left subclavian artery (arrow). (Image used with permission from David A. Taber, MD.)

Radiographic Summary

Flail chest occurs when there are fractures of 3 or more consecutive ribs with at least 2 fracture sites of each rib, creating a free-floating segment of the thoracic wall. Most patients with flail chest have other associated intrathoracic traumatic injuries. Plain chest radiographs may demonstrate multiple consecutive rib fractures, but CT scan better identifies the flail segment and other associated thoracic injuries such as pneumothorax and pulmonary contusion.

Clinical Implications

The diagnosis of flail chest can be made clinically by observing a paradoxical motion of the chest wall in a spontaneously breathing patient. With inspiration, the uninjured chest moves up and out while the flail segment is pulled inward due to the movement of the flail segment in response to negative intrathoracic pressure. This flail segment causes focal chest wall instability and atelectasis, pneumonia, and ARDS. Flail chest may not be obvious clinically in an intubated patient and the diagnosis may have to be made radiographically. The force that fractures the segment of ribs is usually enough to cause significant underlying pulmonary contusion. Depending on the patient's underlying pulmonary reserve, the extent of the lung injury, and the size of the flail segment, patients may require mechanical ventilation. If the flail chest is an isolated injury, the patient will need aggressive pulmonary toilet and pain control for the multiple rib fractures. If the size of the flail segment is large enough, a traumatic pulmonary herniation can occur through this defect. This is a rare injury and usually occurs through the anterior chest wall where there is little soft tissue support.

Pearls

1. On chest x-ray, segmental rib fracturing may not be obvious, as often only 1 of the 2 fracture planes is visible.
2. CT scan may detect lung herniation through the flail window that mandates urgent surgical repair if large or causing ventilatory compromise.

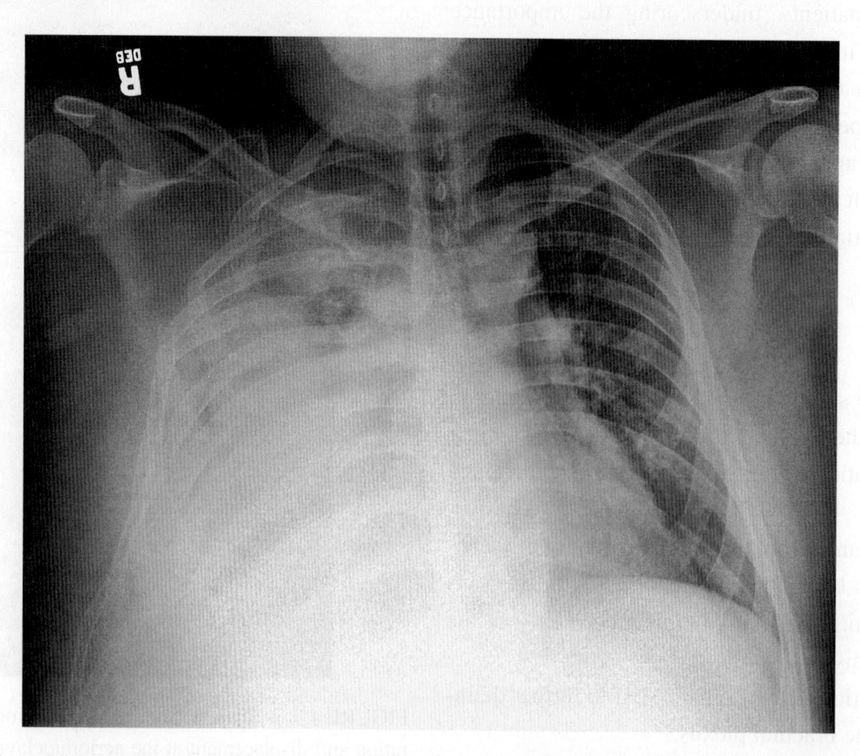

FIGURE 4.8 ■ Flail Chest. Multiple right rib fractures at contiguous levels. Many of the rib fractures are segmental. Large right hemothorax and lung opacity compatible with contusion and atelectasis are also present.

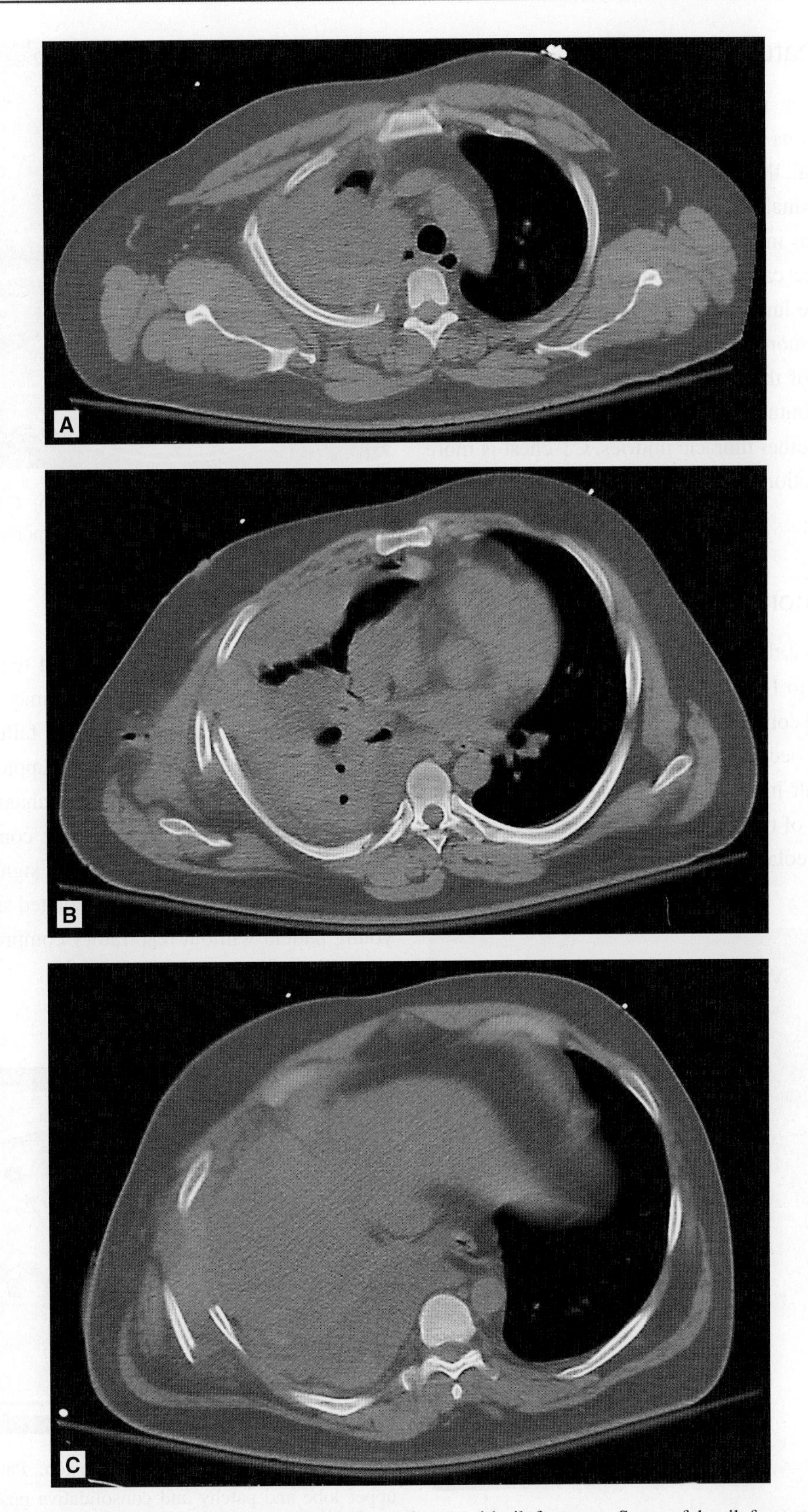

FIGURE 4.9 ■ Flail Chest. **A-C:** CT image shows a large right hemothorax with rib fractures. Some of the rib fractures are widely displaced. Most are segmental fractures.

Radiographic Features

Pulmonary contusions resulting from blunt chest trauma appear as opacifications of varying size and density on chest radiograph. In general, there are no air bronchograms present due to the fact that small airways may be filled with blood. Pulmonary contusions may appear as scattered patchy opacifications or, in severe cases, as extensive confluent opacification throughout the lung fields. Associated pneumothorax, hemothorax, and pulmonary lacerations may be identified on contrasted CT scan of the chest. Rapid radiographic resolution of pulmonary contusions over a period of days is common. As with many other thoracic injuries, CT chest is more sensitive for the detection of pulmonary contusions than chest radiograph.

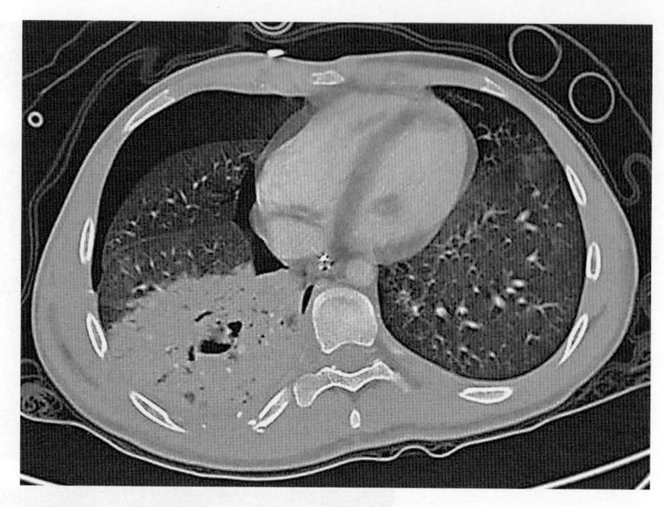

FIGURE 4.11 ■ Pulmonary Contusion. CT image in the same patient as in Fig. 4.10 demonstrates pulmonary contusion, pneumatocele, and pneumothorax.

Clinical Implications

Pulmonary contusion is detectable within 6 hours of injury and usually resolves in 3 to 14 days depending on size of the contusion and associated comorbidities. Some contusions worsen over a few days and become more symptomatic. Pulmonary contusions may result in hypoxia and hypoventilation from splinting due to pain of traumatic injury as well as decreased ventilation due to alveolar hemorrhage. Clinical findings vary based on the severity of injury and the respiratory reserve of the injured patient, but patients may exhibit pain, tachypnea, hypoxia, and even respiratory failure. Aggressive pulmonary toilet, pain control, and supplemental oxygen are the mainstays of therapy, while mechanical ventilation may be required with severe pulmonary contusions. Pulmonary contusions may be complicated by significant hemorrhage, respiratory failure, and ARDS. Isolated small contusions in a young patient without respiratory compromise do not necessitate hospitalization.

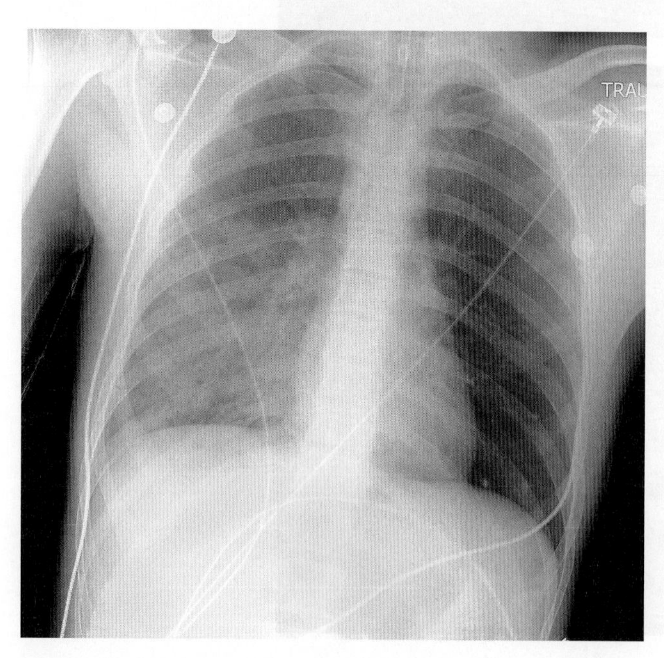

FIGURE 4.10 ■ Pulmonary Contusion. AP chest x-ray demonstrates extensive right-sided pulmonary contusion. Note multiple adjacent rib fractures.

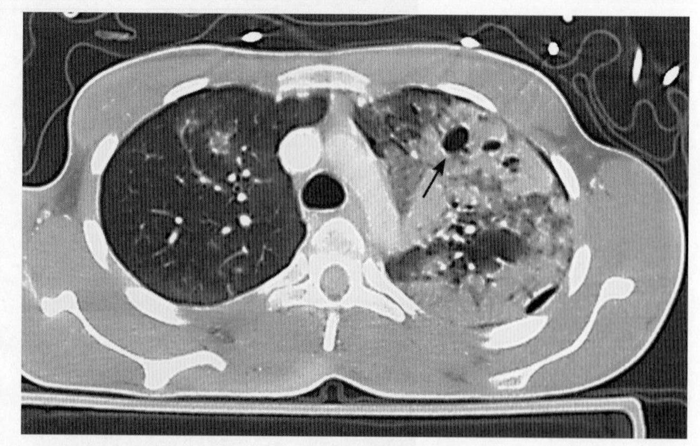

FIGURE 4.12 ■ Pulmonary Contusion. Patchy opacity in right upper lobe and patchy and consolidative opacity in the left upper lobe are compatible with contusions, worse on the left. Round lucencies in the midst of the left lung contusion represent traumatic pneumatocele formation (arrow).

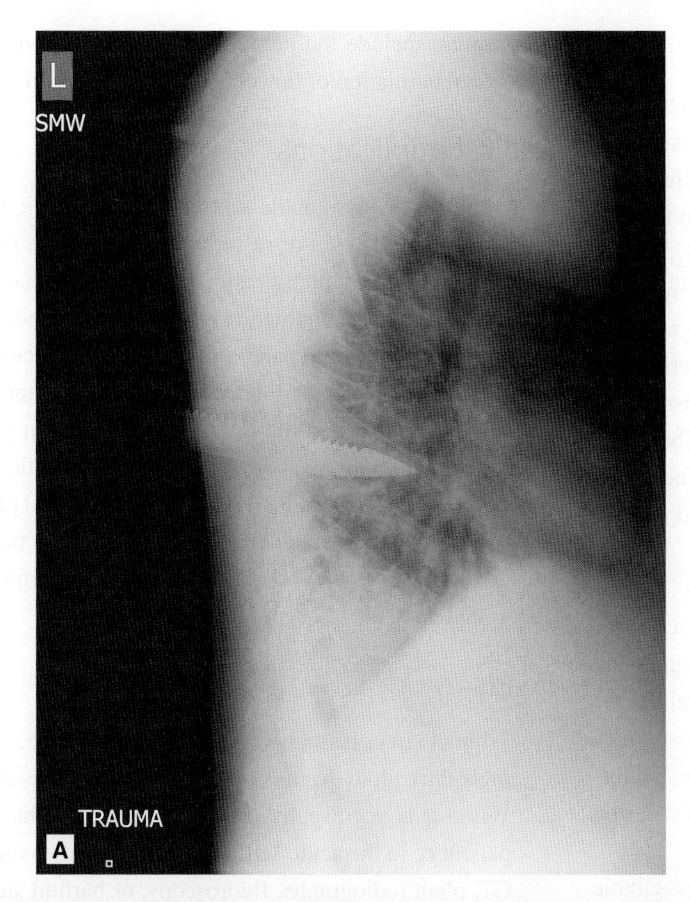

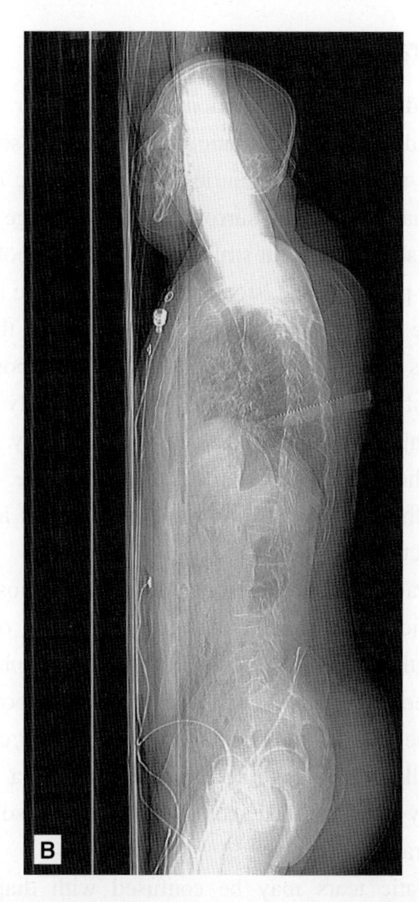

FIGURE 4.13 ■ Penetrating Injury with Resultant Pulmonary Contusion. **A, B:** A lateral chest radiograph and a lateral scout CT image show a serrated knife in the inferior and posterior thorax.

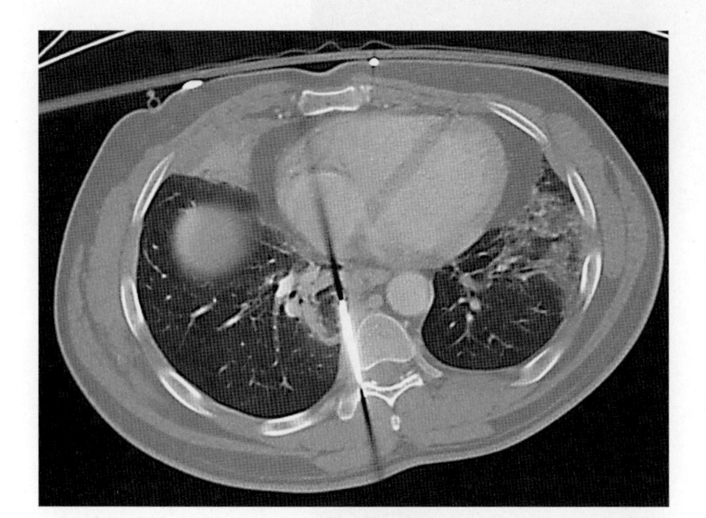

FIGURE 4.14 ■ Penetrating Injury Causing Pulmonary Contusion. A CT image details the relationship of the knife with the adjacent structures. Note the focal region of pulmonary contusion surrounding the tip of the knife. Fortunately for this patient, there was no significant injury to the vessels or the heart.

Pearls

1. Children are much more susceptible to pulmonary contusions due to the elasticity of their rib cages, leading to greater compressive forces transmitted to the lung parenchyma.
2. Pulmonary contusions are associated with significant compressive forces to the thorax and therefore associated injuries are common. The most common associated injuries are hemothorax, pneumothorax, and rib fractures.
3. Pulmonary contusions are often indistinguishable radiographically from lung opacities of various other causes.

Radiographic Summary

Contrasted CT scan of the abdomen is the most practical diagnostic study for diaphragmatic rupture and is also useful for diagnosis of coexisting injuries. Diaphragmatic defects are often visualized without surrounding hemorrhage to the diaphragm itself or adjacent structures. Most commonly, visualization of peritoneal fat, stomach, or bowel in the hemithorax makes the injury obvious. Injury to the lung in the adjacent area helps detect diaphragmatic rupture. The posterolateral portions of both hemidiaphragms are most readily visualized, making injuries to these areas easier to identify. The dome is often the most difficult area to detect rupture. The sensitivity of the CT scan is improved with coronal and sagittal reconstructions.

Two radiographic signs may aid in diagnosis of diaphragmatic rupture: the "collar sign" (pinching of a hollow viscus with a waist-like constriction at the diaphragm) and the "dependent viscera" sign (the stomach or bowel on the left, or the liver on the right abuts the posterior chest wall). Abnormally thick diaphragm indicating edema or hemorrhage may be present but should not be used as sole criterion for diaphragmatic rupture.

Traumatic tears may be confused with diaphragmatic defects that may develop in elderly patients. Clues to suggest true rupture include the presence of air bubbles posterior to the defect, herniation of bowel, and the "collar sign."

Clinical Implications

Symptoms of diaphragmatic rupture are nonspecific but may include abdominal pain or respiratory compromise from visceral herniation. Diaphragmatic rupture is associated with other severe injuries and can occur in blunt and penetrating trauma. Splenic and hepatic injuries are most commonly associated with this injury. The left side of the diaphragm is injured more often than the right due to protection provided by the liver. Operative repair of acute diaphragmatic injuries is generally the standard. Patients may have delayed presentation for months or years after the initial trauma as the defect in the diaphragm becomes large enough for herniation of abdominal contents to occur.

Pearls

1. Without viscus herniation, diaphragmatic rupture is exceedingly difficult to diagnose with plain radiographs alone.
2. While it is not usually practical in the unstable trauma patient or in the acute setting, MRI is more sensitive than CT, plain radiographs, fluoroscopy, or barium studies in detecting diaphragm rupture.

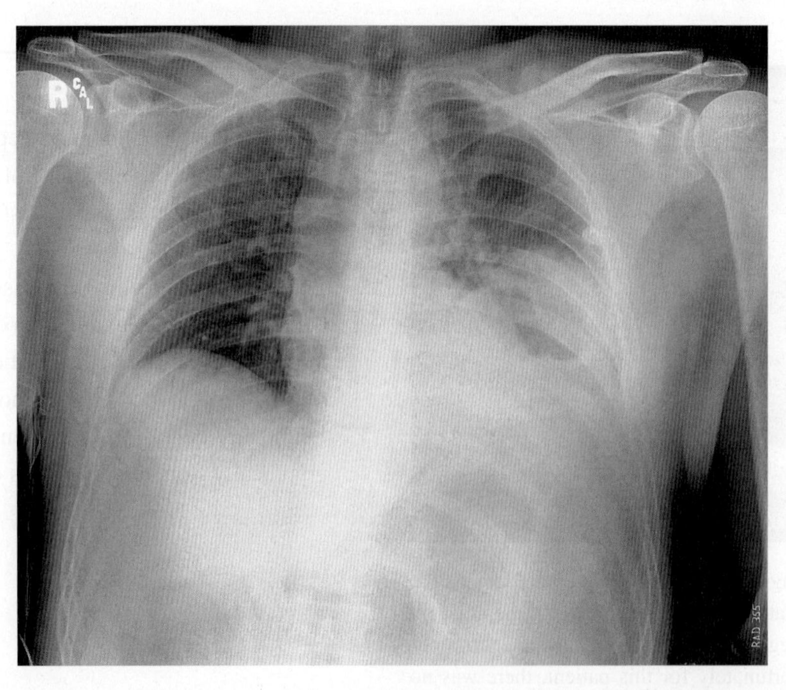

FIGURE 4.15 ■ Diaphragm Rupture. An indistinct and elevated diaphragm contour on the left along with gas collection in the left chest. In the setting of trauma, these findings should be considered as evidence of diaphragmatic rupture until otherwise proven with CT.

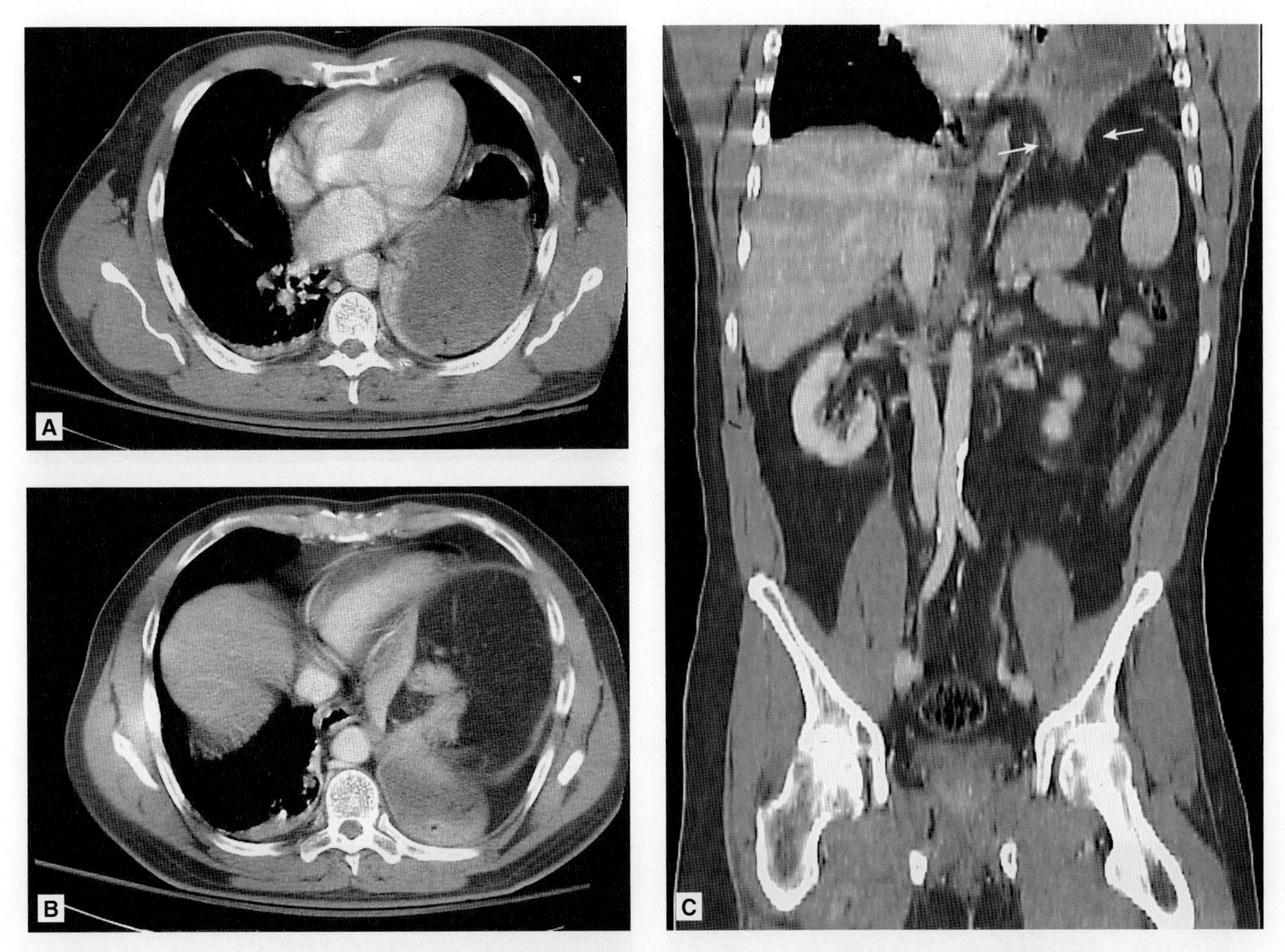

FIGURE 4.16 ■ Diaphragm Rupture. **A-C:** The stomach is herniated into the left hemithorax through a visible defect in the left hemidiaphragm. A "waist" or "collar" sign is often produced when stomach contour is narrowed as it extends through the diaphragmatic defect, as shown on the coronal reformatted image (arrows).

Radiographic Features

Pneumothorax is the presence of air within the pleural space. The diagnosis is made on plain chest radiograph by the visualization of the outer visceral pleural border (pleural line) outlined by gas in the pleural space. This gaseous space features the absence of the vascular markings seen within normally aerated lung. Small pneumothoraces may be difficult to detect on plain radiograph, and soft tissue folds as well as scapular borders may mimic pleural lines. Pleural lines are also often difficult to detect on supine radiographs, and the presence of air in the subpulmonic region (deep sulcus sign) may be the only radiographic clue to the presence of pneumothorax. Expiratory radiographs or lateral decubitus radiographs may accentuate the findings of pneumothorax on chest x-ray. The presence of mediastinal shift or compression of thoracic structures implies the presence of tension pneumothorax, but this diagnosis should be based on clinical presentation ideally. CT of the chest is far more sensitive for detecting pneumothorax than plain radiographs and should be considered when the diagnosis of pneumothorax is suspected but chest radiographs are indeterminate.

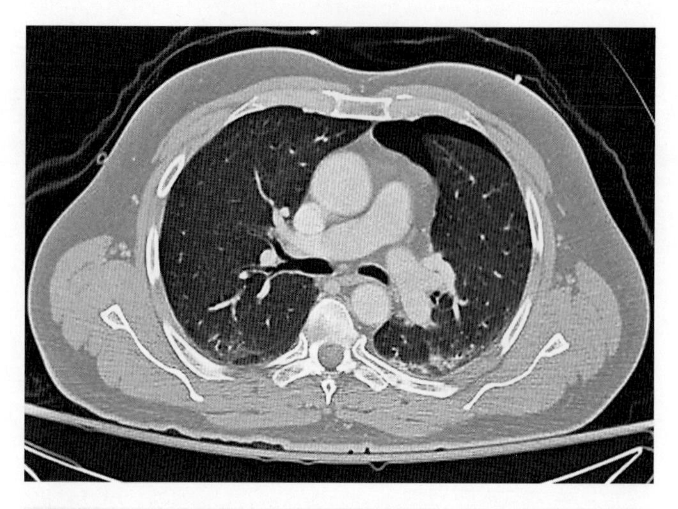

FIGURE 4.18 ■ Pneumothorax. CT image in a different patient demonstrating a small anteromedial left-sided pneumothorax.

Clinical Implications

Pneumothorax is most commonly caused by traumatic injury, but spontaneous pneumothorax is also frequently encountered in the emergency department and may arise from a number of predisposing conditions. Patients with pneumothorax may

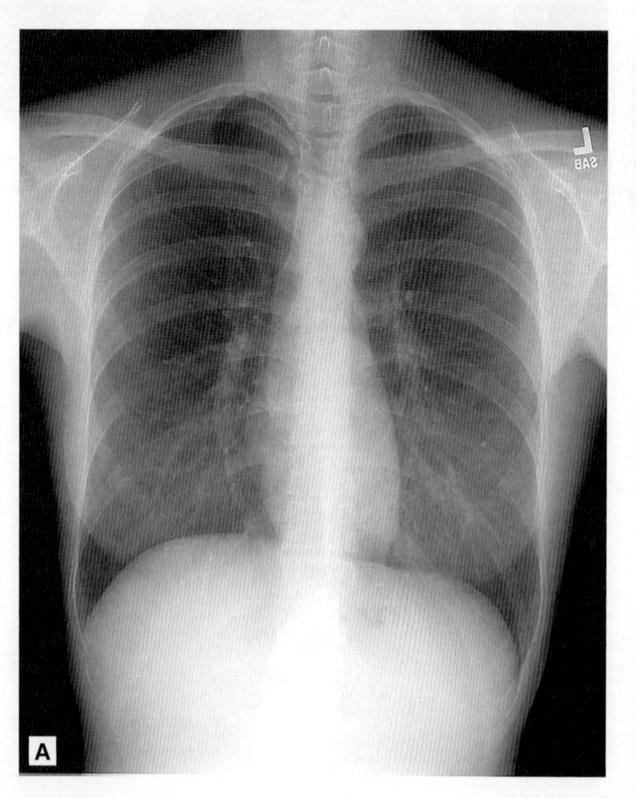

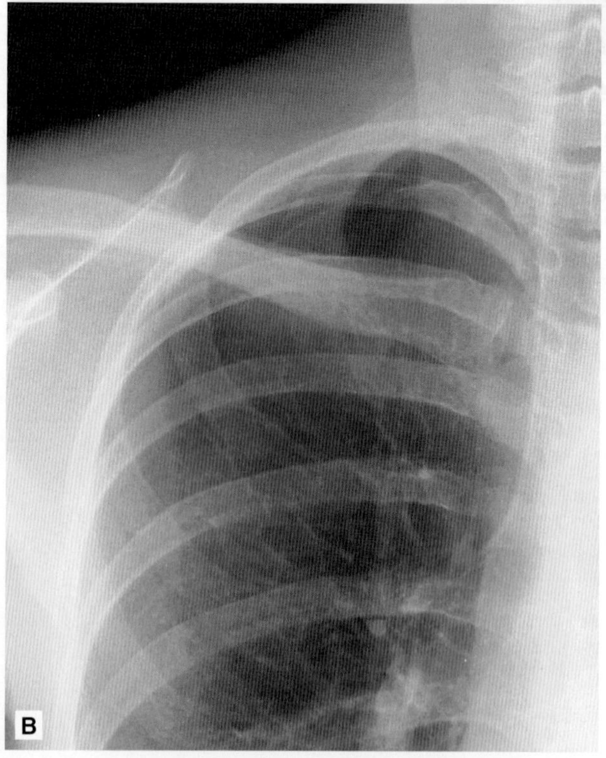

FIGURE 4.17 ■ Pneumothorax. **A, B:** This PA view of the chest demonstrates a subtle pneumothorax, distinguished by a crisp white line, outlined by adjacent air in the pleural space and lung. The magnified image clearly demonstrates the lack of pulmonary markings peripheral to the pleural edge.

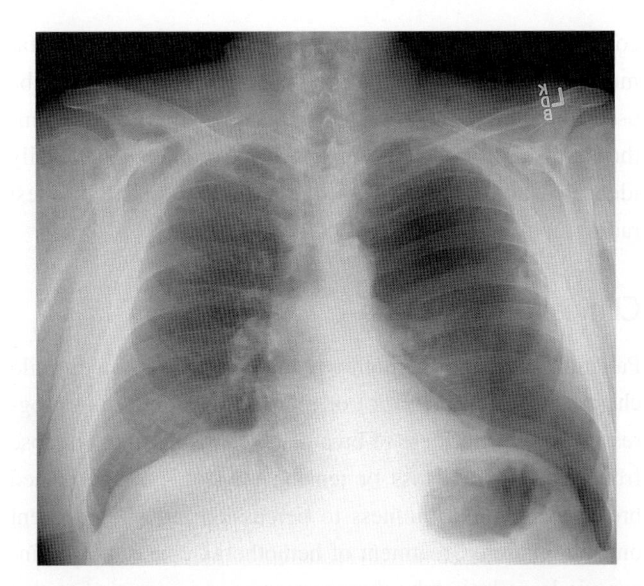

FIGURE 4.19 ■ Pneumothorax. A large left pneumothorax without shift of mediastinum. A left fifth rib fracture is also visible.

present only with mild chest pain (often pleuritic) or mild dyspnea, but may progress to severe shortness of breath and, in the case of tension pneumothorax, cardiovascular collapse. Treatment of pneumothorax ranges from observation and supplemental oxygen to simple aspiration or tube thoracostomy. Needle thoracostomy should be considered for immediate decompression of a tension pneumothorax.

Pearls

1. In cases of suspected tension pneumothorax, treatment should not be delayed in favor of confirmatory imaging.

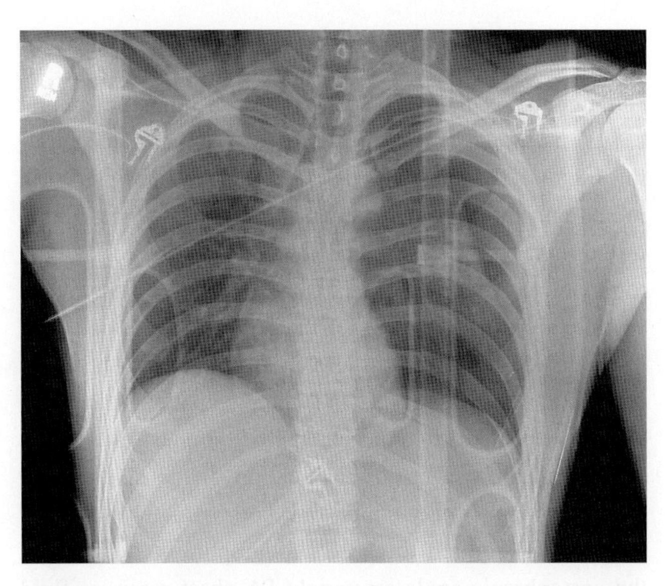

FIGURE 4.21 ■ Pneumothorax. A large left pneumothorax with shift of mediastinal structures (eg, trachea and heart) to the right. This is compatible with a tension pneumothorax.

2. Skin folds and scapular borders may mimic pneumothorax, leading to unnecessary invasive procedures. A pneumothorax typically results in a "white" line, while skin folds have been described as "black" edges. In stable patients, consider CT scanning as a superior test when pneumothorax is strongly suspected, but not confirmed on radiographs.
3. In cases of pneumothorax caused by procedures, sensitivity of testing is not improved with the use of expiratory chest radiographs.

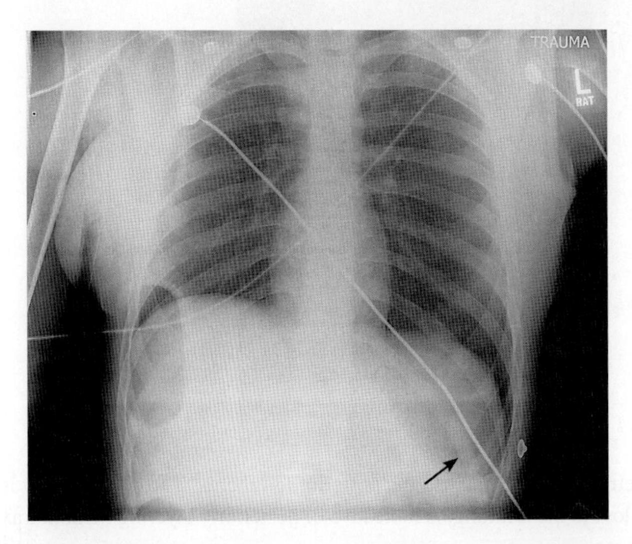

FIGURE 4.20 ■ Pneumothorax. A moderate-sized pneumothorax on the left results in a "deep sulcus sign" on the left with a deepened and lucent left costophrenic angle (arrow).

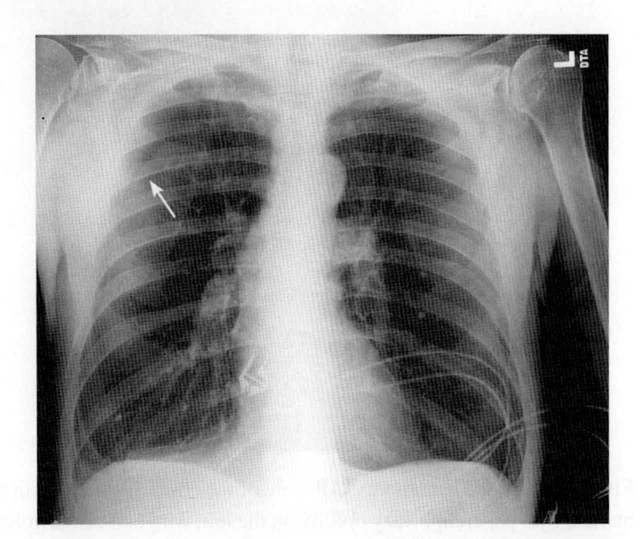

FIGURE 4.22 ■ Skin Fold. A curvilinear black edge parallels the right chest wall, compatible with a skin fold (arrow). This is a common mimicker of pneumothorax.

Radiographic Features

Hemothorax is the presence of blood within the pleural cavity and is most frequently caused by blunt or penetrating trauma. The diagnosis is made on plain upright chest radiograph by the visualization of fluid (blood) collecting in the right or left hemithorax causing blunting of the costophrenic angle and in larger hemothoraces, layering out of blood occupying a portion of the hemithorax. Blood may also be seen tracking up the pleural margins of the chest wall on upright radiograph. In the supine patient, the blood will layer posteriorly and may appear on chest radiograph as a subtle diffuse hazy opacification of the hemithorax, mimicking pulmonary contusion. Approximately 400 cm^3 of blood is required to cause radiographic obliteration of the costophrenic angle on upright PA chest x-ray, as fluid typically accumulates in the subpulmonic location prior to extending into the costophrenic sulcus. Lateral decubitus views are much more sensitive. Associated injuries such as rib fractures, pulmonary contusion, and pneumothorax are common in the presence of hemothorax. Chest CT is far more sensitive for hemothorax than chest x-ray and may be used to quantify the amount of blood occupying the hemithorax. In addition, posteriorly layering blood is more easily identified and quantified on chest CT than on plain chest radiography.

Clinical Implications

Patients with minor hemothorax may present only with mild chest pain (often pleuritic) or mild dyspnea, but may progress to severe shortness of breath and cardiovascular collapse from severe blood loss or tension physiology. Diminished breath sounds and dullness to percussion are often present on examination. Treatment of hemothorax consists of drainage via large-bore tube thoracostomy and in cases of severe bleeding (greater than 1000-1500 cm^3 of blood evacuated immediately after tube thoracostomy or continued bleeding of 150-250 cm^3/h for 2-4 hours) emergent surgical thoracotomy is warranted.

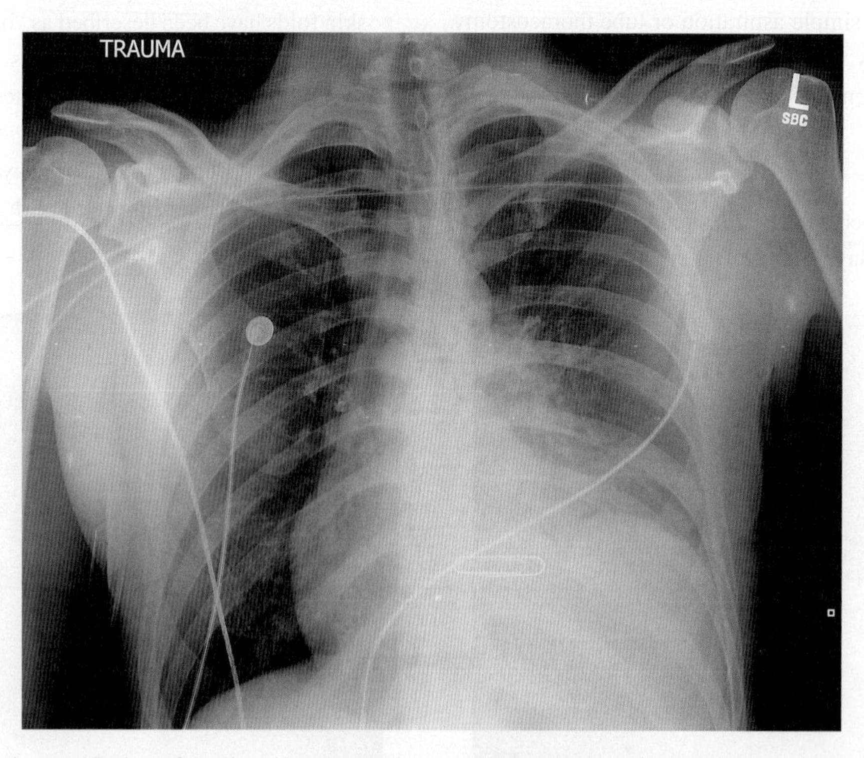

FIGURE 4.23 ■ Hemothorax. AP view of the chest in patient with penetrating knife injury to the posterior left thorax. The site of injury is marked by a paperclip. Hazy opacity on the left, with associated volume loss in the left lung, is indicative of posteriorly layering hemothorax and atelectatic change.

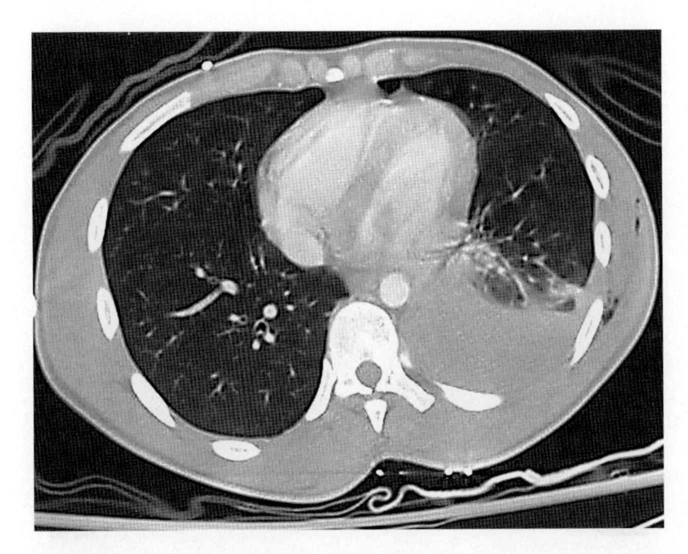

FIGURE 4.24 ■ Hemothorax. CT image in the same patient as in Fig. 4.23 showing large hemothorax layering dependently in the supine patient.

Pearls

1. Care must be taken in the interpretation of supine chest radiographs in the traumatized patient. The presence of a large hemothorax on supine radiographs may appear only as a vague diffuse haziness in the hemithorax as the blood layers posteriorly along the chest wall.
2. Chest tubes should be inserted and secured in a dependent area to insure adequate drainage of hemothorax.
3. A hemothorax can be differentiated from a simple pleural effusion on CT by measuring attenuation of the collection to a value similar to soft tissue (>40 HU).

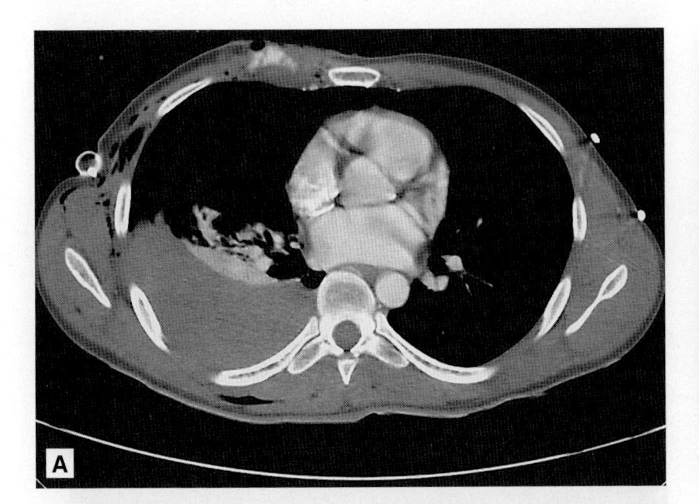

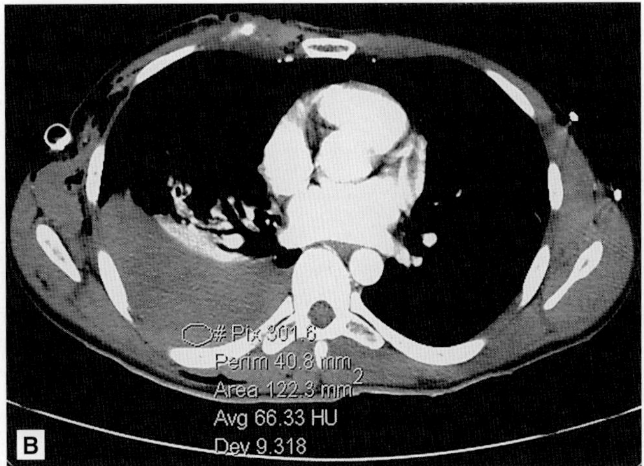

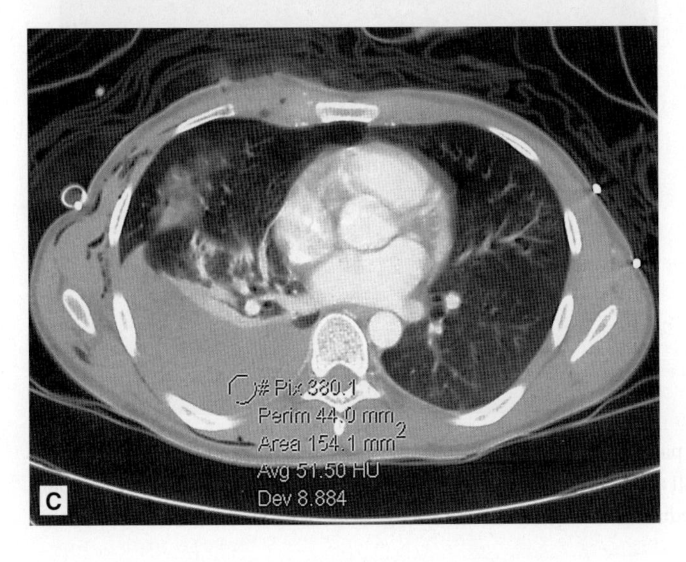

FIGURE 4.25 ■ Hemothorax. **A-C:** A large right pleural fluid collection with rib fractures. The attenuation measures greater than 50 HU or more, indicating a hemothorax. Additionally, there is active contrast extravasation in the right anterior chest wall, indicating active bleeding and vessel injury. Right lung contusion is also evident.

Radiographic Summary

Air in the mediastinum is seen as a thin lucency where there is usually a solid confluence of shadows of the heart, great vessels, and esophagus. It may appear most conspicuously along the left heart border. CT imaging is more sensitive than plain radiography for detection of pneumomediastinum. Air can localize anywhere in the mediastinum but commonly collects adjacent to the aorta and pulmonary veins. The amount of air is not usually very large given the small space available for collection but can be confused with pneumothoraces in some instances. Other studies may need to be performed if the source is not discernable on CT. These studies include esophagoscopy or contrast barium study and bronchoscopy and should wait until the patient has been stabilized.

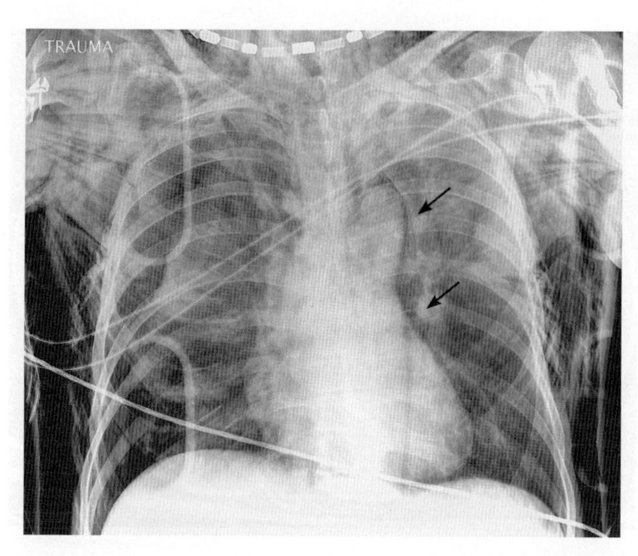

FIGURE 4.26 ■ Pneumomediastinum. In addition to a large right pneumothorax, there is lucency along the heart border and aortic arch (arrows) as well as extensive subcutaneous emphysema with lucency throughout extrathoracic soft tissues.

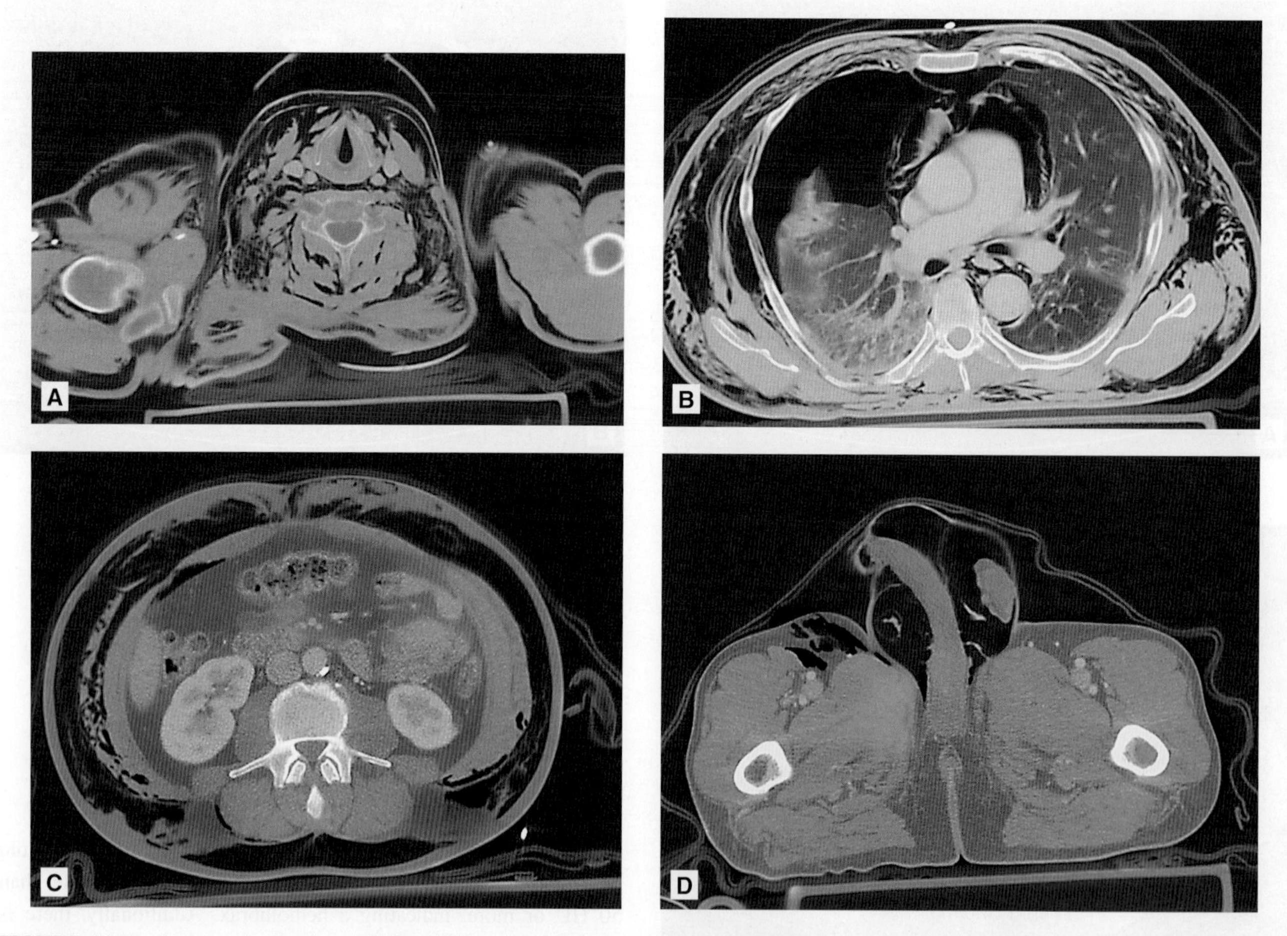

FIGURE 4.27 ■ Pneumomediastinum. **A-D:** CT images of the same patient as in Fig. 4.26 show extensive subcuatenous emphysema along the neck, axillae, and shoulders, extending along the anterior chest wall and abdominal wall. Gas dissects into the scrotum. The large amount of gas outlines the mediastinal structures, compatible with pneumomediastinum. Again, there is a large pneumothorax as well.

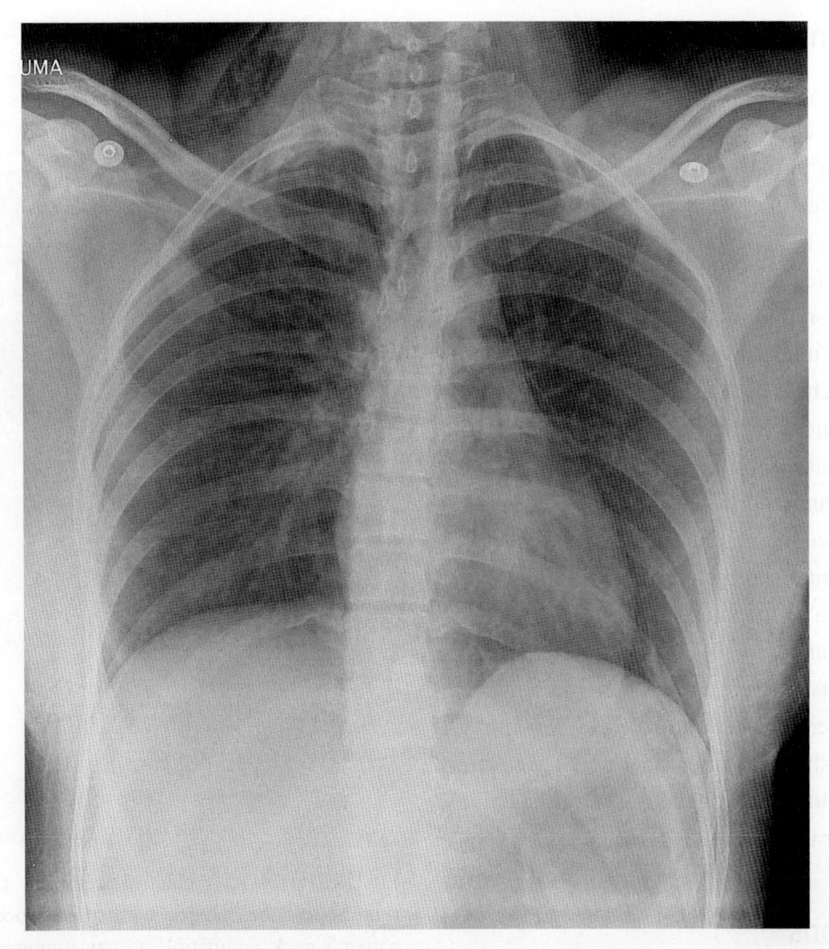

FIGURE 4.28 ■ Pneumomediastinum. A more subtle case of pneumomediastinum with lucency along left heart border, giving it an "extra crisp" appearance. Also, gas is present in the soft tissues of the neck.

Clinical Implications

While air may enter the mediastinum from several sources such as esophagus, the neck, or retroperitoneal injuries, most commonly traumatic pneumomediastinum results from air tracking back to the mediastinum from a bronchial injury along the bronchial tree. Even in the absence of trauma, pneumomediastinum may develop after coughing, forceful inhalation/exhalation, or esophageal rupture. Mediastinal air rarely causes a problem itself but signifies potentially more serious injuries of the tracheobronchial tree or the esophagus. Penetrating injuries of the mediastinum, especially high-energy gunshot wounds, will often leave a "track" of metallic fragments, bone, blood, and air making injured structures easier to identify. Compared with low-energy knife wounds, GSWs create a larger track of hemorrhage. The termination of the wound may be the presence of the bullet or the exit site from the body but the extent of a knife wound may not be so obvious. For this reason, delayed complications from chest stab wounds are well recognized.

Pearls

1. The presence of mediastinal air in a patient involved in blunt trauma should prompt one to search for the source, beginning with the tracheobronchial tree.
2. CXR can be used to screen for peripheral lung injuries caused by a knife or bullet, but injuries to the mediastinum are best diagnosed by CT.
3. A predominately medially positioned pneumothorax can mimic pneumomediastinum. While not always present, a key discriminator is the presence of subcutaneous emphysema in the neck, frequently seen in patients with pneumomediastinum.

Radiographic Summary

Ten percent of patients with tracheobronchial injury may not show any radiographic abnormality initially and up to 30% of cases are missed on initial evaluation. Plain radiographs of the chest may manifest nonspecific findings such as subcutaneous emphysema, a pneumothorax, or pneumomediastinum (most sensitive feature for airway rupture on CXR), but tracheobronchial disruption is more often detected by CT. Approximately 85% of tracheal lacerations occur 2 cm above the carina. Smaller tracheal injuries may present with pneumomediastinum incidentally noted on CT scan. Another clue for the presence of an air leak from a tracheobronchial injury is the presence of a pneumothorax. Pneumothoraces are more common with right-sided injuries because the right mainstem bronchus enters the pleura shortly after its origin in contrast to the left that enters the pleura more distally.

If a tracheobronchial injury is not recognized after the initial evaluation, persistent subcutaneous emphysema may give a clue to its presence. Once intubated, a patient's CT scan of the chest may show deviation of the ETT, deformity of the endotracheal balloon cuff, or protrusion of the balloon through a tracheal laceration.

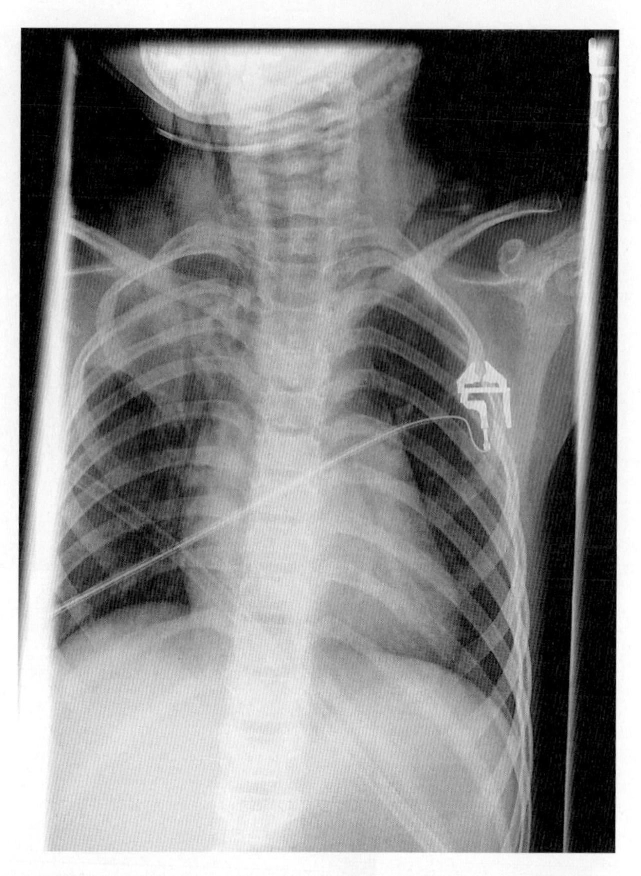

FIGURE 4.29 ■ Tracheal Laceration. Chest radiograph shows right upper lobe collapse with streaky lucencies extending into the patient's neck, compatible with pneumomediastinum.

Clinical Implications

The intrathoracic trachea bifurcates into the right and left bronchi at the tracheal carina that is about at the level of T4. Tracheobronchial injuries are relatively uncommon and occur in less than 5% of blunt trauma patients and less than 10% of penetrating trauma patients. The mediastinal structures are protected by the sternum and thoracic spine as well as more vital structures such as the esophagus and great vessels. Because of their central location, the forces needed to cause disruption of the trachea and bronchi are associated with closed head injury and injuries to the aorta, lungs, chest wall, abdomen, and spinal cord. In blunt trauma, the right mainstem bronchus is injured more commonly than the left because there is less protection from other mediastinal structures. The trachea is most commonly ruptured transversely rather than longitudinally.

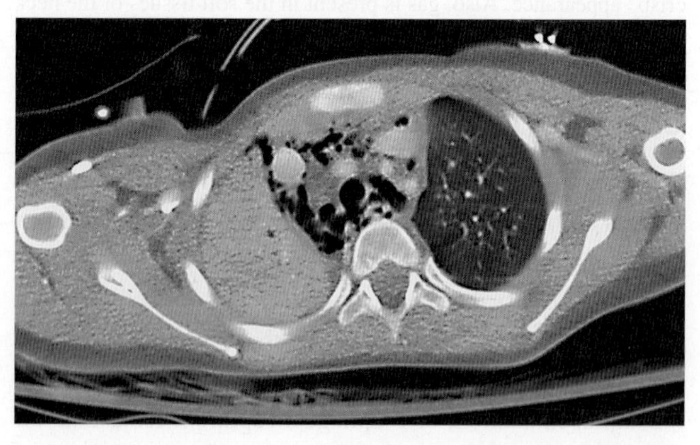

FIGURE 4.30 ■ Tracheal Laceration. CT of the same patient as in Fig. 4.29 shows disruption of the posterior wall of the trachea, the location of the laceration. Pneumomediastinum and right upper lobe collapse are as seen on the radiograph.

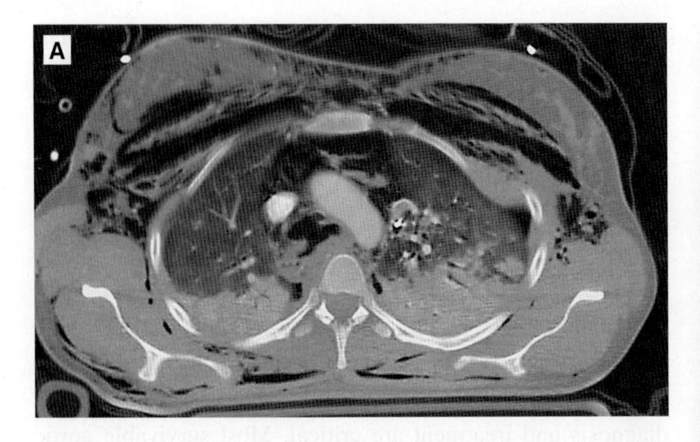

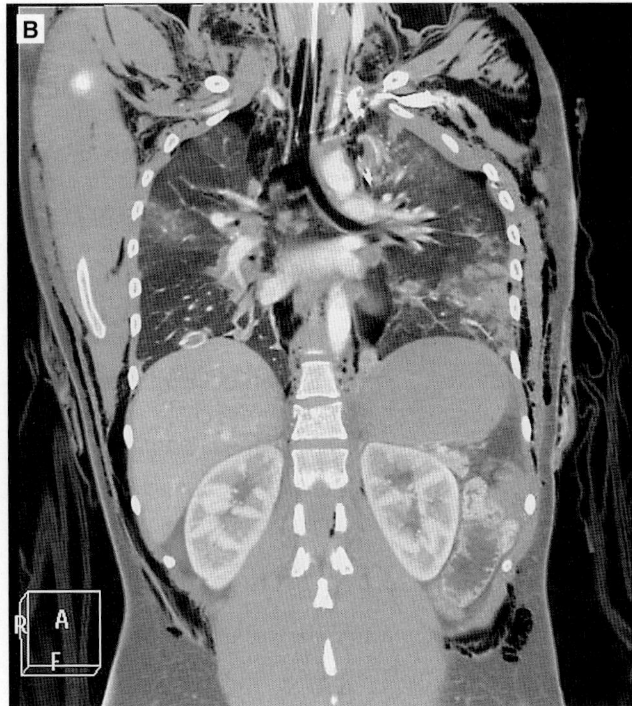

FIGURE 4.31 ■ Bronchial Tree Disruption. **A, B:** Axial and coronal CT images demonstrating disruption of the tracheobronchial tree at the junction of the right mainstem bronchus. Note extensive pneumothorax, pneumomediastinum, and subcutaneous gas.

Once the possibility is recognized, establishing a definitive airway should be undertaken being careful to not convert a partial tear to a complete tear. Bronchoscopy should be obtained in patients with suspicion of tracheobronchial injuries for definitive diagnosis and treatment.

Pearls

1. Isolated trachea injuries generally do not cause pneumothoraces but can cause deep cervical emphysema (air beneath the deep cervical fascia seen as lucency anterior to the spine on lateral neck x-rays).
2. If complete disruption of a bronchus occurs, the affected lung becomes atelectatic and will “fall” to the most dependent portion of the pleural space. This appears as a “fallen lung sign” on imaging studies.

Radiographic Summary

Supine AP chest x-ray is often the initial study done in resuscitation of trauma patients. CXR is not able to definitively diagnose aortic injury but can provide some clues. Findings suggesting aortic injury include widened mediastinum (>8 cm at the arch), apical pleural cap, abnormal contour of the aortic knob, and rightward deviation of the trachea or nasogastric tube. If clinical suspicion for aortic injury exists, contrasted helical CT of the thorax should be obtained. Findings suggestive of traumatic aortic injury include abnormal aortic contour, pseudoaneurysm, intimal flap, periaortic hemorrhage, and displacement of the trachea to the right by associated hematoma. Less common findings include luminal clots, active extravasation of contrast, or abrupt tapering of the descending aorta relative to the ascending aorta. Mediastinal hematoma is not specific for aortic injury and can occur with sternal fractures or thoracic spine fractures. Pseudoaneurysm is an aortic rupture contained by the adventitia or periaortic tissues and is characteristically seen as an outpouching of the aorta on CT. Intimal disruptions or flaps are seen as a small intimal irregularity, typically at the level of the ligamentum arteriosum that tethers the aorta. Aortic rupture is most commonly seen distal to the left subclavian artery. The accuracy of helical CT has markedly decreased the need for aortography but this additional study may be necessary with equivocal findings on CT scan.

Clinical Implications

Traumatic injury to the aorta has potentially rapid fatal results. In fact, 90% of patients with traumatic aortic injuries die before they receive emergency care. Therefore, prompt diagnosis and treatment are critical. Most survivable aortic injuries occur at the aortic isthmus just distal to the left subclavian artery. The descending thoracic aorta is an uncommon site of injury. The lethality of injury and the need to diagnose associated trauma is one of the reasons CT has supplanted catheter angiography in evaluation of traumatic aortic injuries. Aortography as a diagnostic study is less available, is more expensive and invasive, has more of a dye load, and has a higher stroke risk, so it is now used only for uncertain CT results and to guide stent/graft placement. Transesophageal echocardiogram (TEE) can be performed at bedside but has limited availability and is operator dependent.

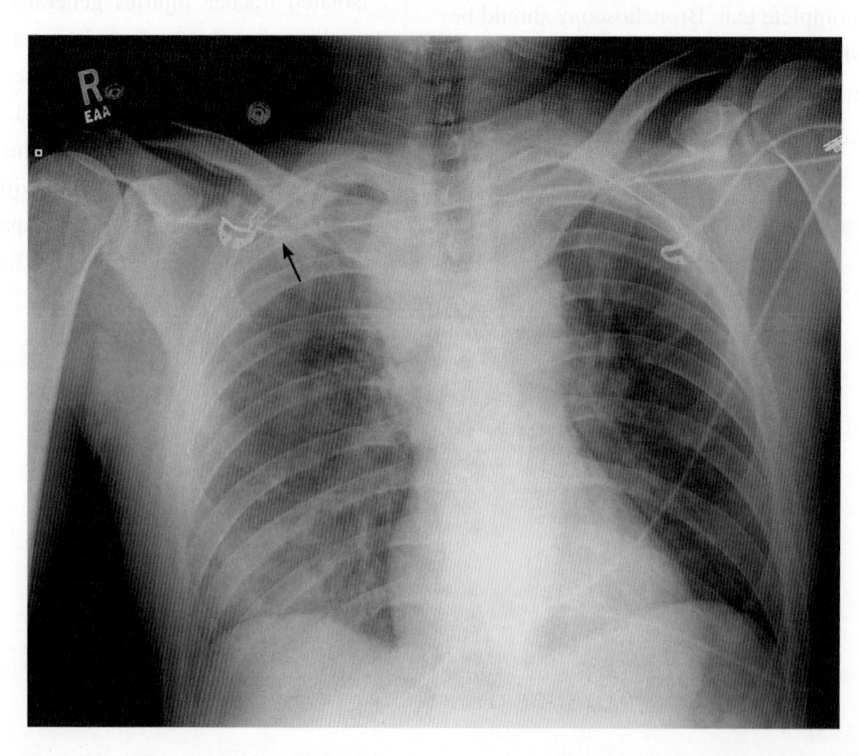

FIGURE 4.32 ■ Aortic Disruption. AP portable view of the chest demonstrates a widened upper mediastinum, with thickened paratracheal stripes. Note the presence of a right apical "cap (arrow)."

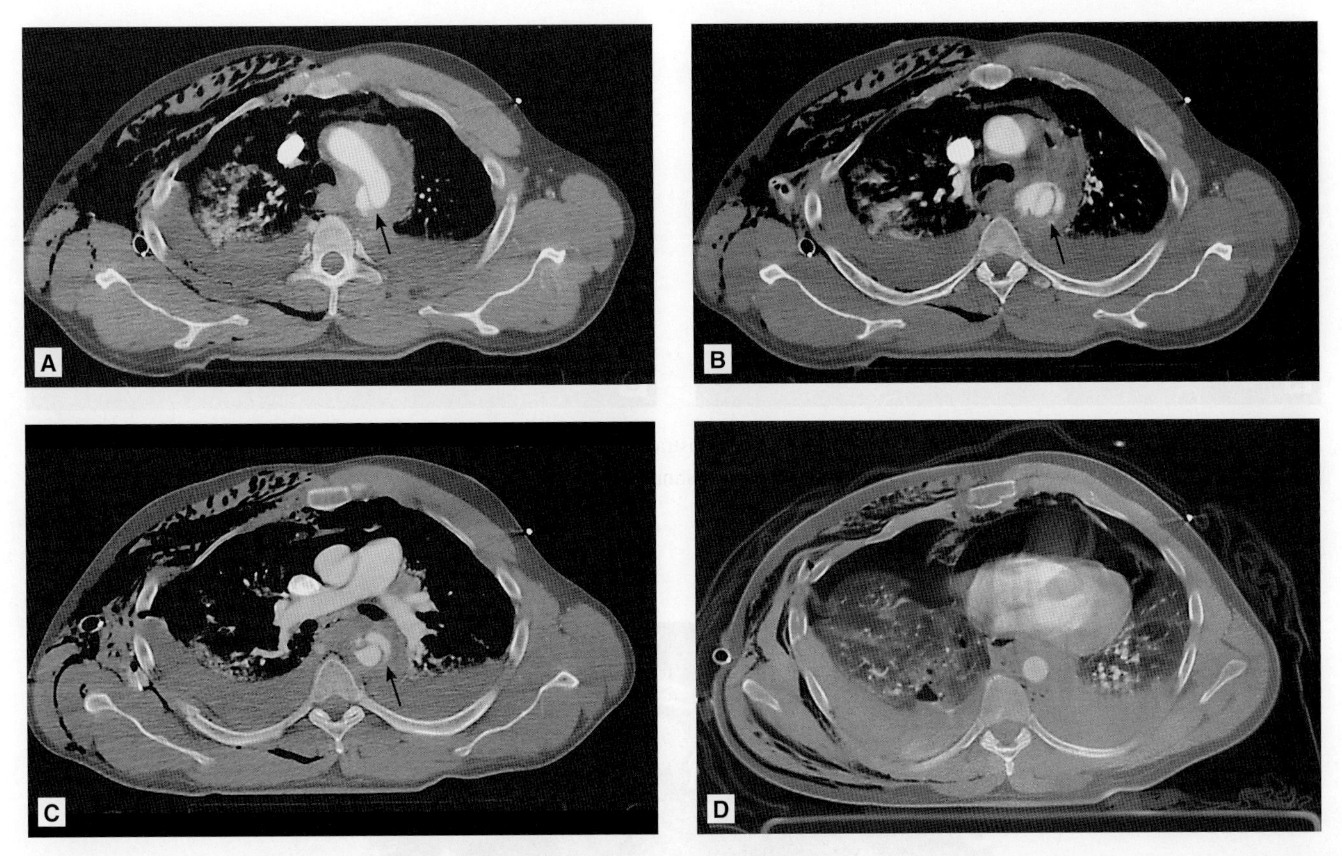

FIGURE 4.33 ■ Aortic Disruption. **A-D:** CT images with soft tissue windowing show the injury with intimal disruption and flap (arrows) beginning proximally just beyond the left subclavian takeoff, a common location. Also a large mediastinal hematoma is present along with bilateral effusions. CT image with lung window in the same patient shows bilateral pneumothoraces and very large pneumopericardium with mass effect on the heart.

Pearls

1. In the stable patient, there are few physical clues to the presence of aortic injury and diagnosis is made radiographically.
2. Patients with no mediastinal widening and normal mediastinal/cardiac width ratios can have traumatic aortic injury. However, it is unusual to have blood in the mediastinal tissues and have a normal mediastinal width and contour.
3. Mediastinal hemorrhage identified on CT is not specific for injury of the great vessels. A majority of mediastinal hemorrhage results from thoracic spinal or sternal fracture.
4. Recognize there are variations of normal aortic anatomy at the aortic isthmus (such as the ductus "bump") that can cause confusion, especially when mediastinal hemorrhage is present.

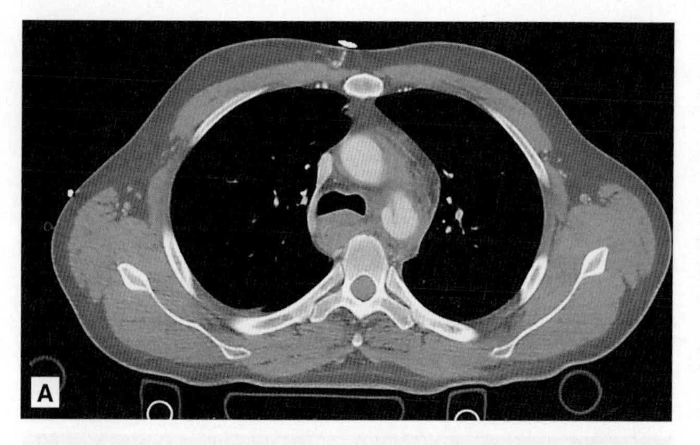

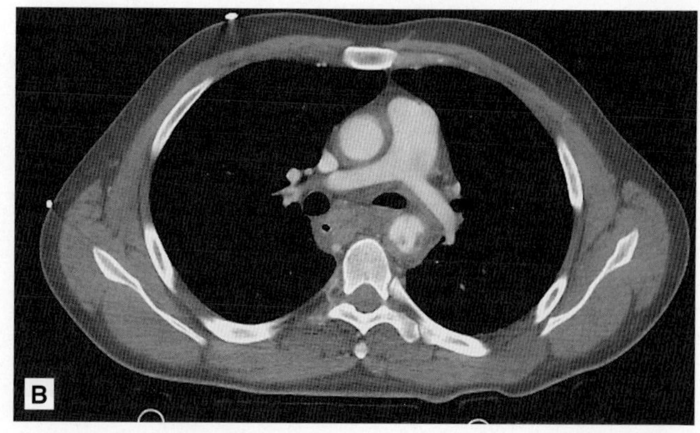

FIGURE 4.34 ■ Acute Traumatic Aortic Injury. **A, B:** A CT demonstrates the aortic injury with intimal disruption and flap in the proximal descending thoracic aorta. There is hematoma throughout the mediastinum as seen on the radiograph.

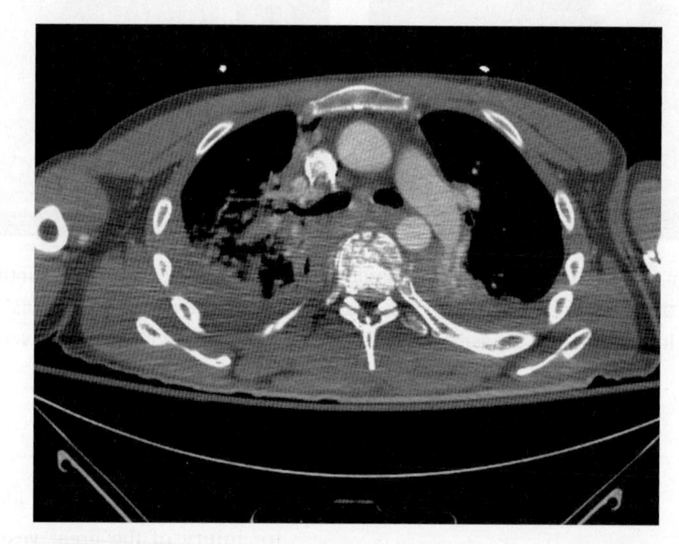

FIGURE 4.35 ■ Mediastinal Hematoma Without Aortic Rupture. CT scan of the thorax demonstrates extensive mediastinal hematoma. Note that in this patient the aortic contour is normal. The hematoma formation is caused by the underlying thoracic vertebral burst fracture.

Chapter 5

ATRAUMATIC CONDITIONS OF THE CHEST

Christopher Kuzniewski
Christie Sullivan
Kurt A. Smith

Radiographic Summary

A hiatal hernia is a herniation of elements of the abdominal cavity through the esophageal hiatus of the diaphragm. On an upright chest radiograph, a gastric bubble containing an air fluid level can be seen above the diaphragm, usually in the mid-chest in the retrocardiac region. There are four types of hiatal hernia (I–IV). Type I, or sliding hiatal hernia, accounts for >95% of cases. This is caused by laxity of the phreno-esophageal membrane, allowing a portion of the gastric cardia to herniate upward. Most of these are asymptomatic. Types II–IV hiatal hernias are varieties of paraesophageal hernias where the GE junction remains fixed while a portion of the stomach herniates through the esophageal hiatus and lies beside the esophagus.

Clinical Implications

The majority of patients with hiatal hernia are asymptomatic. When symptoms do occur, the most common symptoms are intermittent epigastric or substernal pain, postprandial fullness, nausea, and vomiting. Shortness of breath can occur due to diaphragmatic irritation and palpitations can occur due to vagus nerve irritation. If a hiatal hernia is noted on plain radiographs and further characterization of the defect is needed, the best radiographic modality is a barium swallow.

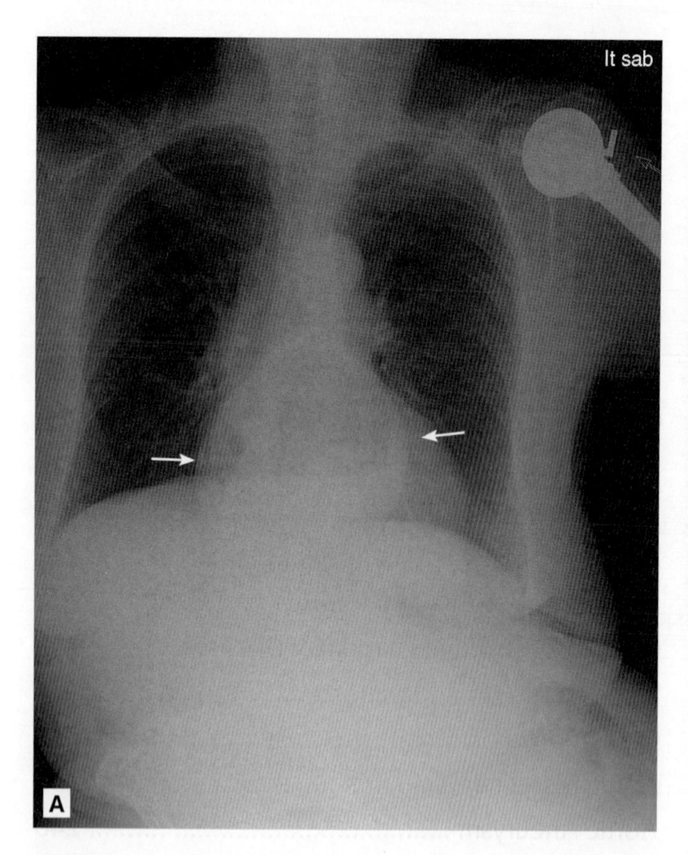

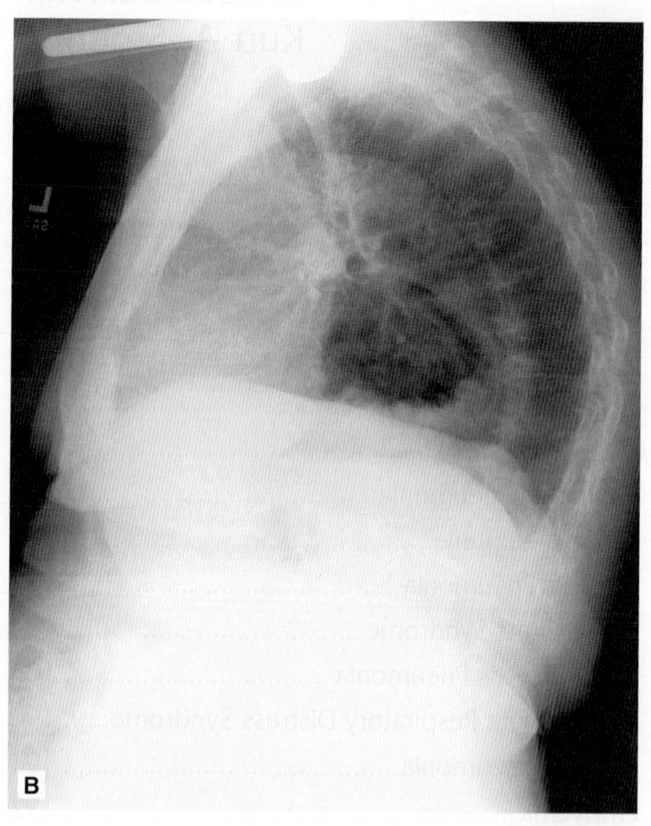

FIGURE 5.1 ■ Hiatal Hernia. **A, B:** Frontal radiograph demonstrates a midline retrocardiac rounded mass with an air fluid level (arrows). The lateral view confirms a rounded and air-filled middle mediastinal mass. This is the typical appearance for a hiatal hernia. The patient has had shoulder replacement surgery.

The natural progression of a type II, III, or IV hernia is progressive enlargement. They never regress spontaneously. For this reason, these are referred for surgical treatment, even in the absence of symptoms. Complications of an enlarging hernia include gastric volvulus, torsion, bleeding, incarcerated hernia pouch, and respiratory complications from mechanical lung compression. Type I hernias rarely require any intervention.

Pearls

1. Most hiatal hernias are asymptomatic. If patients present with GERD symptoms, optimize PPI and H2 blocker therapy prior to referral for surgical management.
2. Barium swallow is the follow-up study of choice, if required.

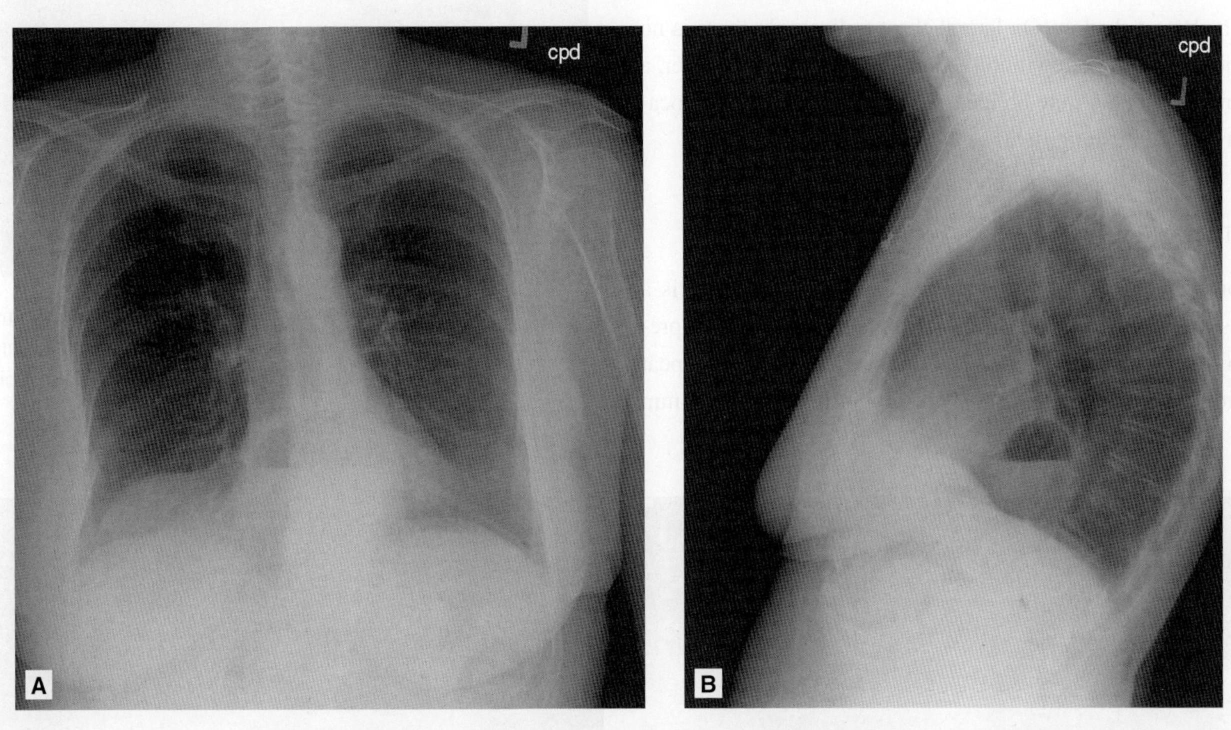

FIGURE 5.2 ■ Hiatal Hernia. **A, B:** Frontal radiograph demonstrates a midline retrocardiac rounded mass with an air fluid level. The lateral view confirms a rounded and air-filled middle mediastinal mass. This is the typical appearance for a hiatal hernia.

Radiographic Summary

Nipple shadows appear as hyperdense opacities in the lower lung fields on the PA view of the chest. The nipple of the male or female breast projects into the air and can create a radiographic shadow that resembles an intraparenchymal pulmonary nodule. Nipples tend to have fuzzy margins and are bordered by a radiolucent halo created by the projection of air from around the nipple. They are typically located at the level of the fifth or sixth anterior ribs or near the bottom of the breast shadow. On lateral chest radiograph, there is no orthogonal correlate within the lung parenchyma; however, a prominent nipple may be identified in a corresponding location outside the lung field.

Clinical Implications

If only an AP view of the chest is available, and there is a question whether the hyperdensity in the inferior chest represents a nipple shadow versus a pulmonary nodule, then repeat radiographs should be taken with nipple markers—1.5 mm

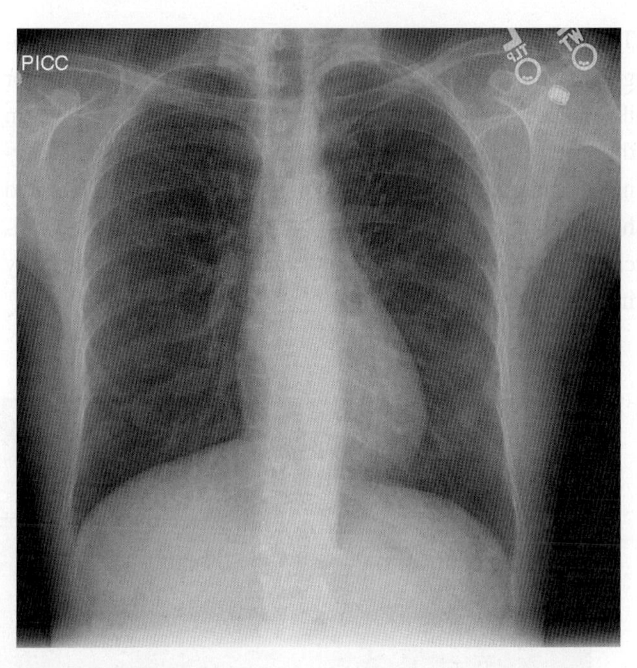

FIGURE 5.3 ■ Nipple Shadows. There are bilateral and symmetric nodular densities in the lower lungs, slightly more prominent on the left. Incidental note is made of a right PICC. This is the typical appearance and location of nipple shadows.

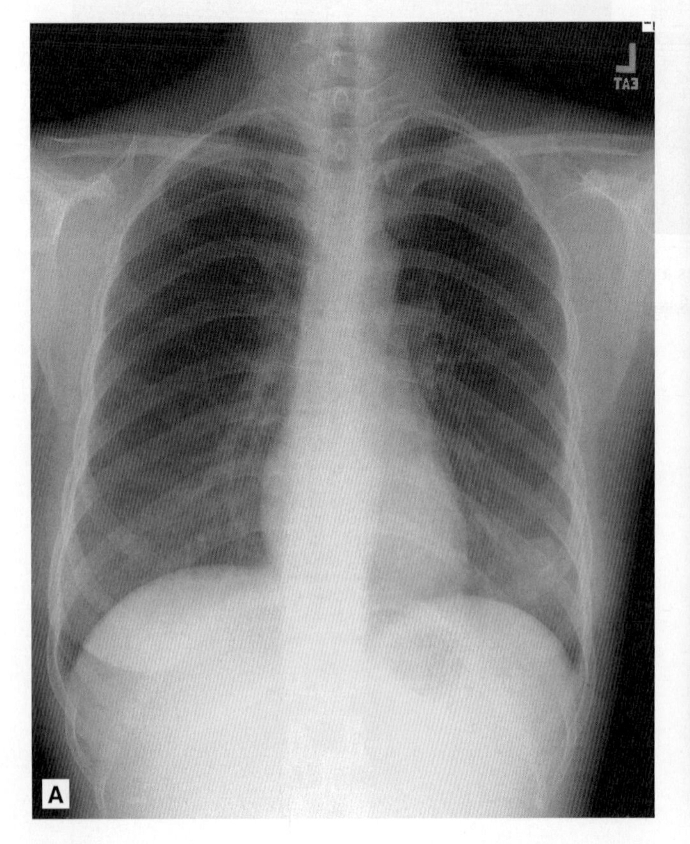

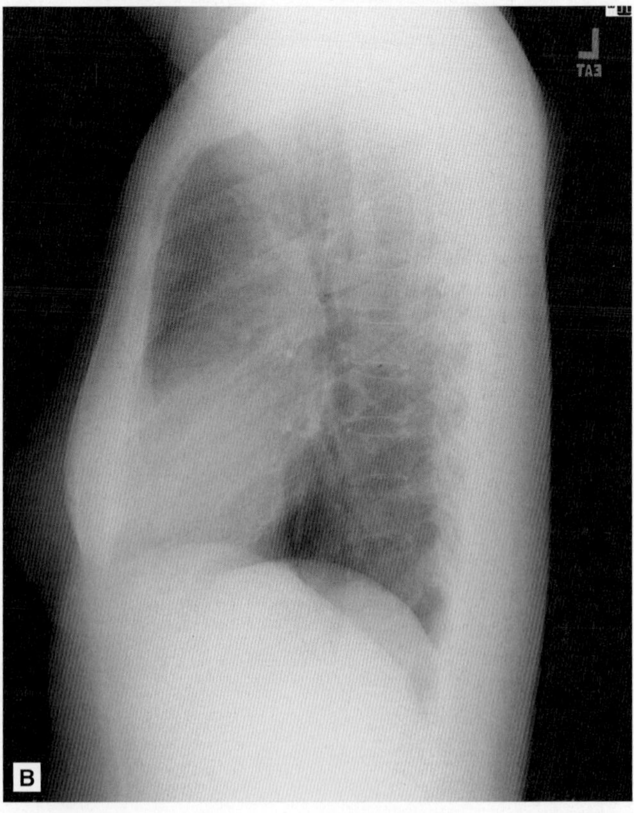

FIGURE 5.4 ■ Nipple Shadows. **A, B:** There are bilateral and symmetric lower lung densities. No orthogonal correlate is seen on the lateral view.

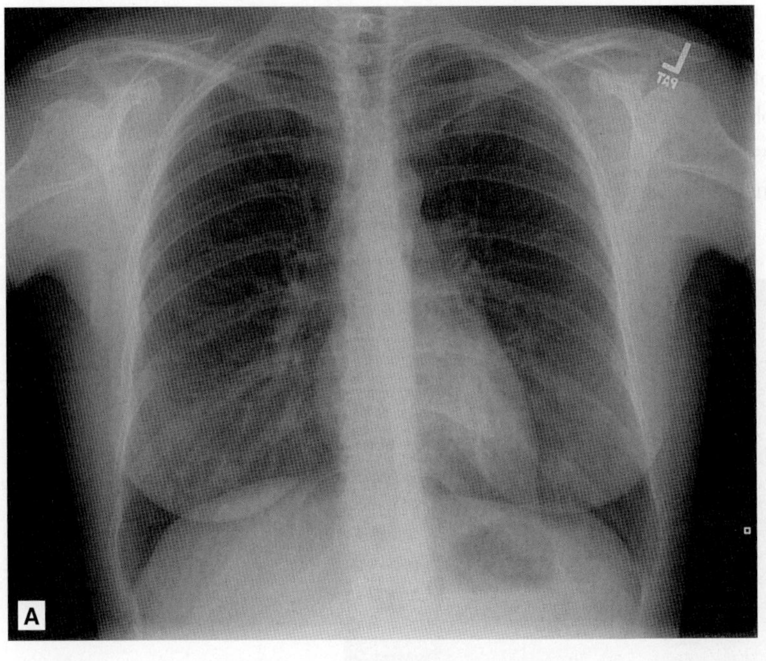

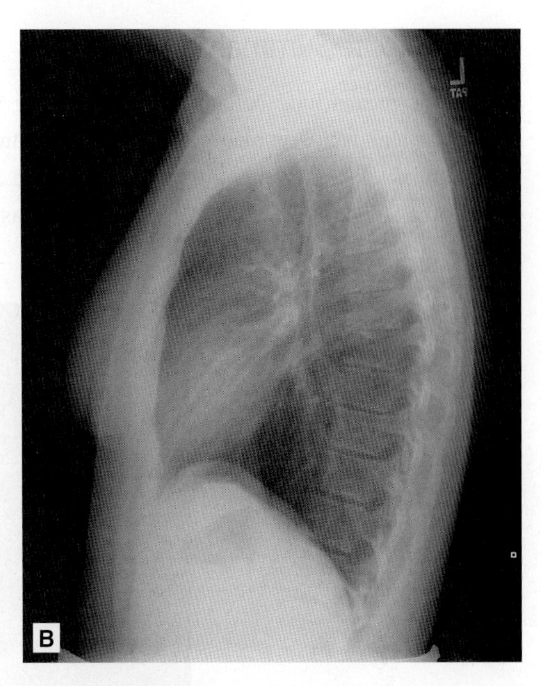

FIGURE 5.5 ■ Nipple Shadows. **A, B:** There are bilateral and symmetric lower lung densities. No orthogonal correlate is seen on the lateral view.

lead objects that overlie the nipple—in order to determine if the opacity on imaging correlates with the location of the physiologic nipple.

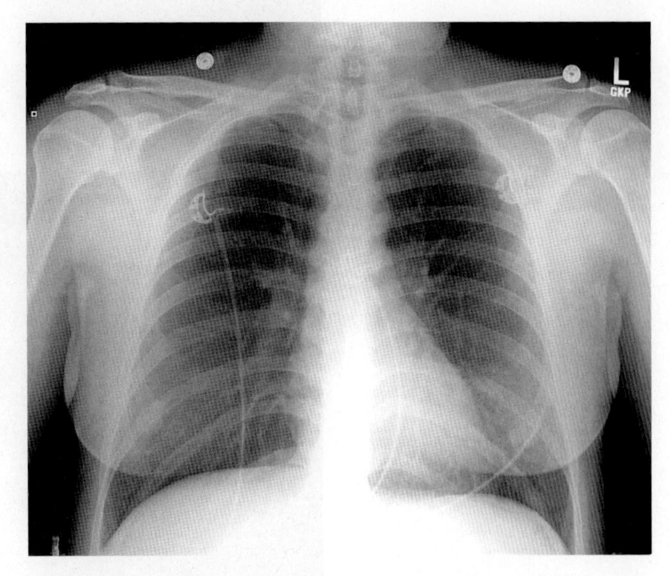

FIGURE 5.6 ■ Nipple Shadows. There are bilateral and symmetric lower lung densities.

Pearls

1. If there is question about whether a lower lung field opacity represents a nipple shadow or a pulmonary nodule, obtain an additional AP view with nipple markers.
2. Nipple shadows are seen in approximately 10% of chest radiographs.

Radiographic Summary

Atelectasis means lung collapse or loss of lung volume. It appears as an opacity on plain radiographs that can obscure a lobe, part of a lobe, or an entire lung field. In the absence of any appreciable volume loss or fissural or mediastinal shift, atelectasis can be difficult to distinguish from a consolidation as both may appear as lung opacities. Pneumonia may result in signs of volume expansion due to mass effect. Atelectasis, however, is typically associated with signs of volume loss because alveoli have collapsed and lung volume has been lost. Signs of volume loss include elevation of the ipsilateral

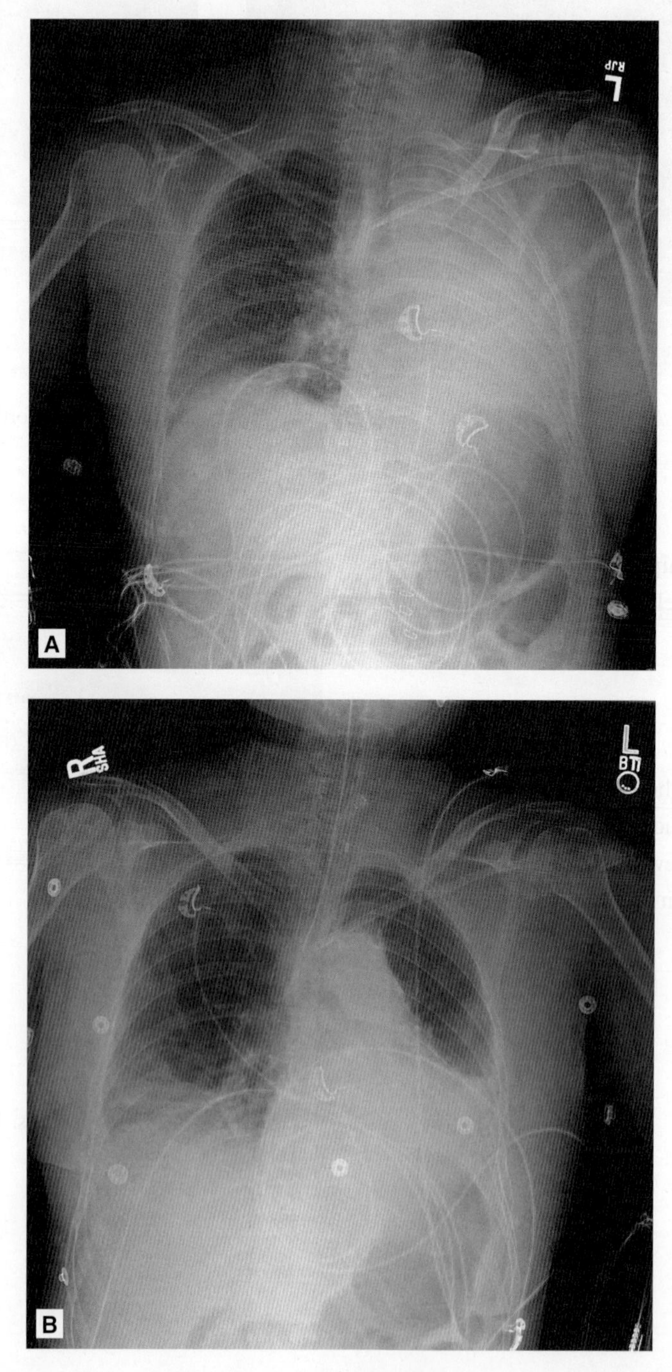

FIGURE 5.7 ■ Complete Left Lung Atelectasis. **A-B:** There is complete opacification of the left lung with shift of the trachea and heart to the left, consistent with volume loss from complete left lung atelectasis. This patient underwent emergent bronchoscopy where a mucous plug was discovered. The left lung is significantly better aerated on the post bronchoscopy images.

hemidiaphragm, graying of the ipsilateral lung base, migration of a fissure toward the atelectatic lung, and deviation of the trachea and mediastinum toward the affected side.

Clinical Implications

Treatment of atelectasis should be directed at the underlying cause of collapse. The most common cause of atelectasis is post-surgical collapse secondary to splinting and pain, which is treated with appropriate pain control, chest physiotherapy, positive pressure ventilation, and early ambulation. Other causes of atelectasis include bronchus or bronchiole obstruction from a mucus plug or aspirated foreign body. The bronchial cut-off sign, in which a bronchus suddenly disappears without visible tapering into smaller bronchioles, is usually due to large mucus plugging.

Pearls

1. Atelectasis and consolidation may be difficult or impossible to distinguish radiographically, especially on portable AP radiographs.
2. Signs of volume loss (midline shift, fissure migration) favor atelectasis over consolidation.

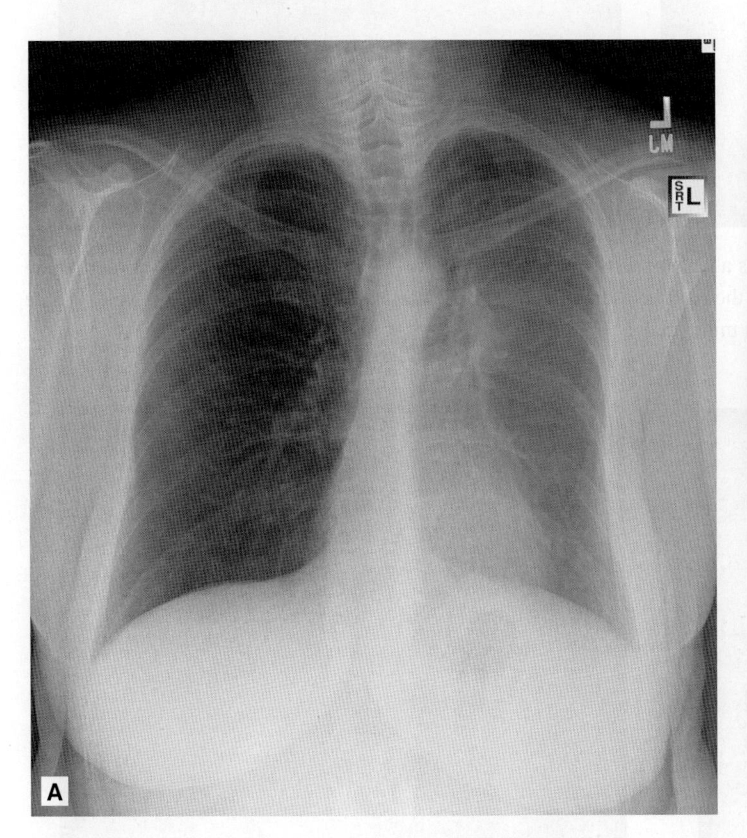

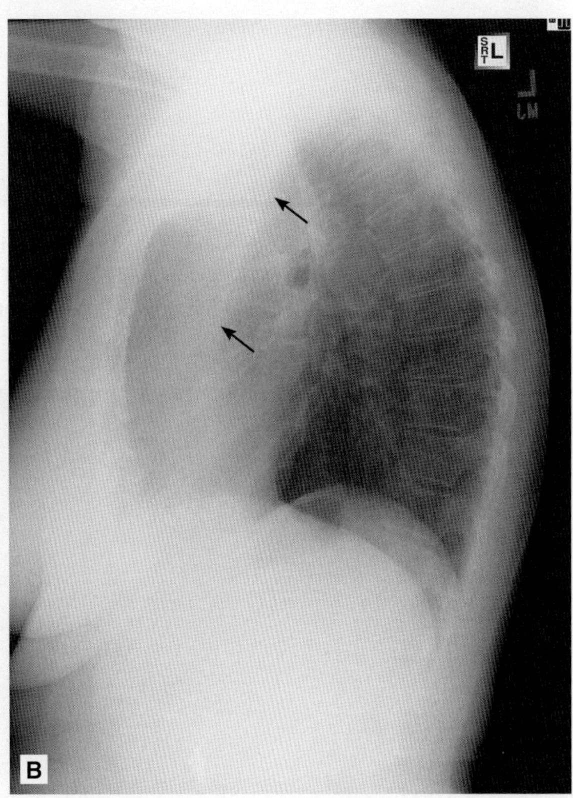

FIGURE 5.8 ■ Left Upper Lobe Atelectasis. **A, B:** There is hazy opacification of the left lung compared to the right with a subtle crescent-shaped lucency adjacent to the aortic arch. On the lateral view, the left major fissure is displaced anteriorly (arrows) and the left lower lobe demonstrates compensatory hyperinflation.

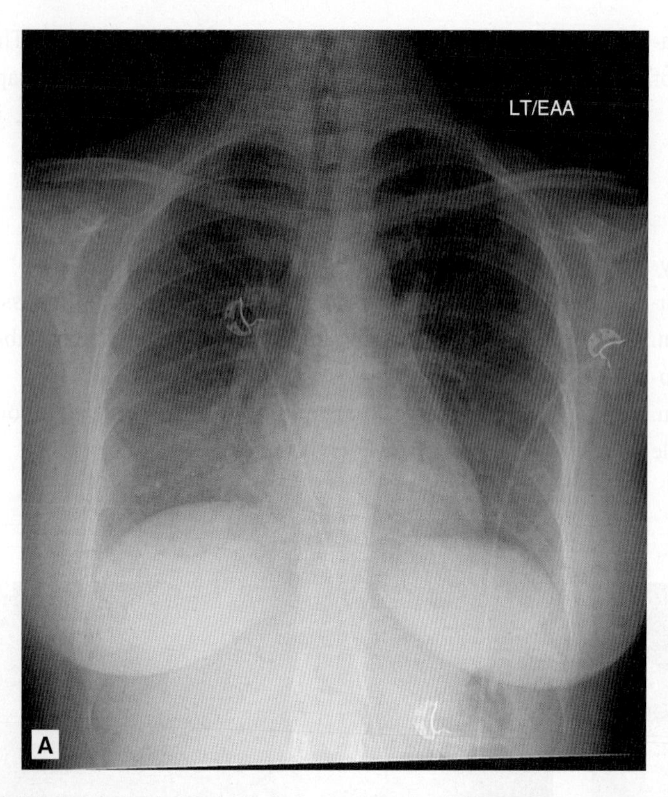

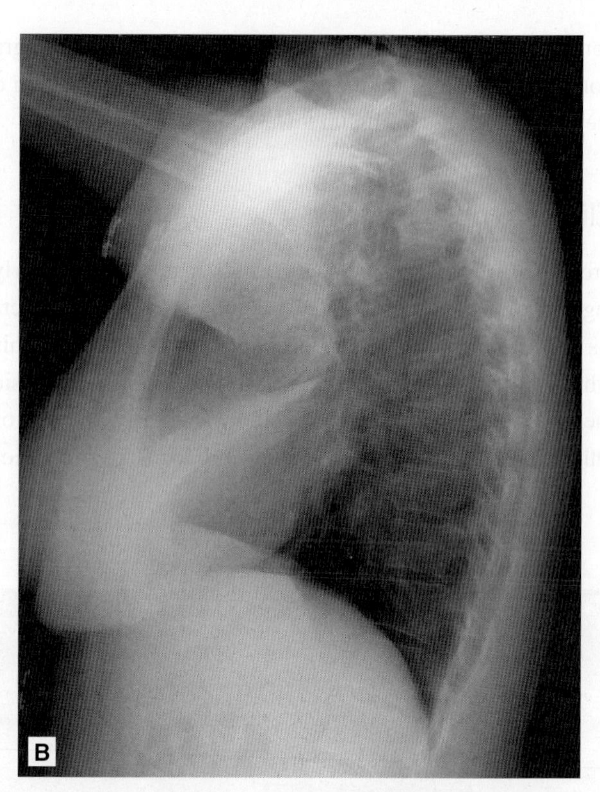

FIGURE 5.9 ■ Right Middle Lobe Atelectasis. **A, B:** There is a hazy opacity in the right lung base obscuring the right heart border. There is only minimal associated volume loss with mild elevation of the right hemidiaphragm. On the lateral view, a wedge-shaped opacity can be seen projecting anteriorly, which represents the collapsed right middle lobe.

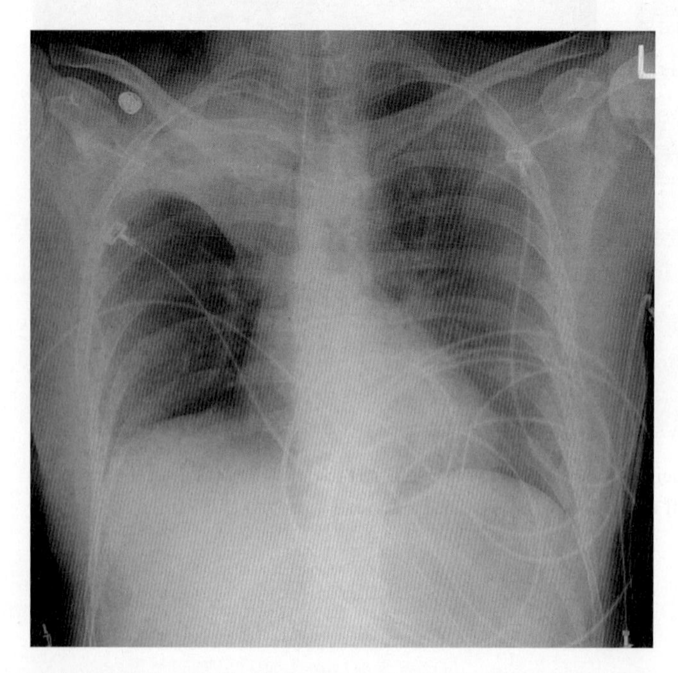

FIGURE 5.10 ■ Right Upper Lobe Atelectasis. There is an opacity in the right upper lung with elevation of the minor fissure and some deviation of the esophagus to the right indicating volume loss—the "S sign of Golden" —and underlying malignancy should be excluded. This patient had adenocarcinoma.

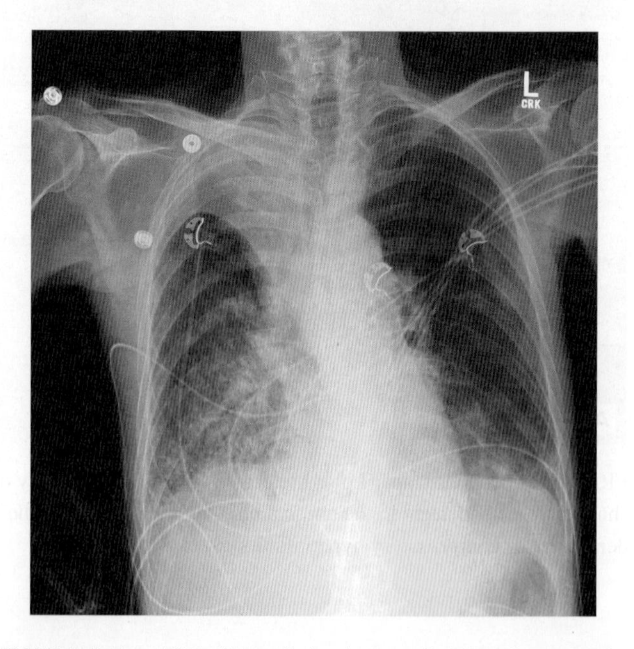

FIGURE 5.11 ■ Right Upper Lobe Atelectasis. There is an opacity in the right upper lung with elevation of the minor fissure and mild deviation of the trachea to the right, indicating volume loss. This appearance of the RUL and minor fissure is often referred to as the "S sign of Golden" and underlying malignancy should be excluded. This patient had adenocarcinoma.

Radiographic Summary

Dextrocardia refers to the position of the heart within the right hemithorax. Dextrocardia may take several forms: *dextroposition*, in which a normally configured heart points more to the right chest than normal; *dextrocardia with situs inversus* in which the heart is completely on the right side; and *situs inversustotalis,* in which all visceral organs are mirrored on the opposite side of their typical position.

When dextrocardia is suspected, first check that the radiograph is appropriately labeled. The apex of the normal heart sits in the left mid-clavicular line. In dextrocardia, the cardiac apex sits in the right mid-clavicular line. If the stomach bubble is located in the right upper quadrant under the cardiac apex, this suggests situs inversustotalis.

Clinical Implications

The majority of adult patients who have dextrocardia on chest radiograph are already aware of the diagnosis. Isolated dextrocardia without situs inversus is more likely to be associated with severe cardiac defects. One in twenty-five of these are associated with primary ciliary dyskinesia or Kartagener syndrome. These patients tend to present with recurrent sinus and bronchial infections secondary to poorly functioning ciliary clearance.

In patients with dextrocardia *with* situs inversus, there are typically no other associated abnormalities.

EKG changes in dextrocardia reflect the fact that the apex of the heart is in the right hemithorax instead of the left. There is a negative P wave and QRS complex in lead 1 since atrial and ventricular depolarization start on the left and spread toward the right. There is reverse R-wave progression across the precordium with the R wave tallest in V1 and getting progressively smaller through V6.

Pearls

1. Location of the stomach bubble helps determine isolated dextrocardia from dextrocardia with situs inversus totalis.
2. When defibrillating a patient with dextrocardia, the pads should be placed in reverse positions (place pads on the upper left and lower right chest).

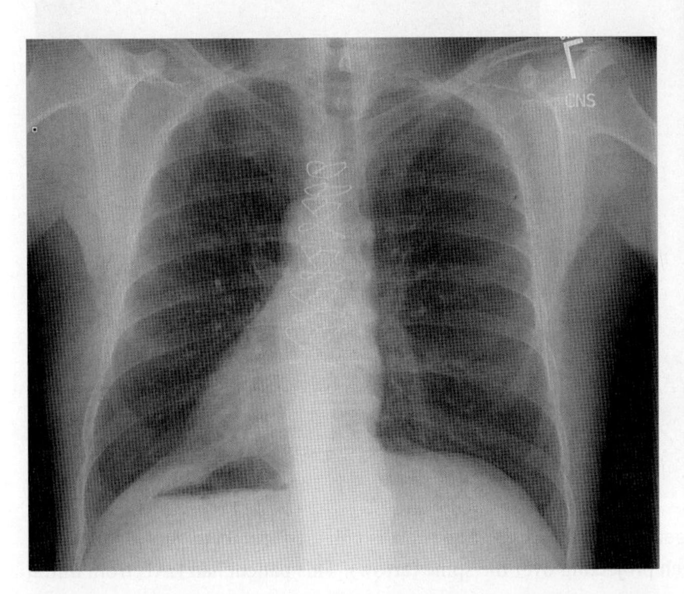

FIGURE 5.12 ■ Dextrocardia. Frontal chest radiograph shows the cardiac apex on the right. The patient has a right arch with subtle deviation of the trachea to the left. The patient has had prior sternotomy and vascular coiling.

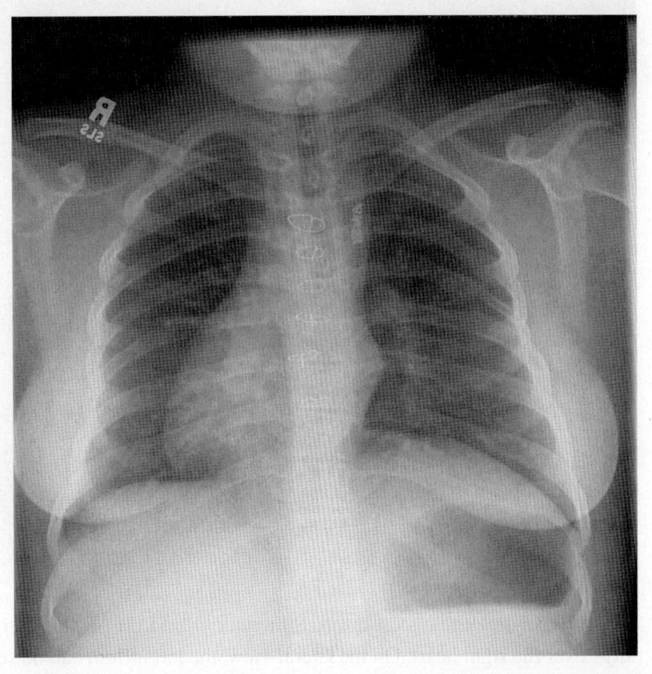

FIGURE 5.13 ■ Dextrocardia. The cardiac apex is on the right. The patient has a right arch with subtle deviation of the trachea to the left. Additionally, the stomach bubble is under the left hemidiaphragm. The patient has had prior sternotomy.

Radiographic Summary

An enlarged cardiac silhouette is defined as a transverse diameter greater than or equal to 50% of the transverse diameter of the chest measured at the lung bases. On a portable AP radiograph, the heart can appear to be artificially enlarged. Since the heart is located within the anterior aspect of the thorax, its size is magnified as the image detector is placed further away from it, behind the patient's back. On plain radiographs alone, it may be difficult to differentiate cardiomegaly from other causes of enlarged cardiac silhouette, including pericardial effusion, mass, left ventricular aneurysm, and pericardial fat pad. If there is cardiomegaly, it is usually possible to determine which cardiac chamber is enlarged. On a PA view, one can visualize the right atrium, left ventricle, and left atrium. The right ventricle can be visualized only on the lateral view.

With right ventricular enlargement, there is increased opacity filling the retrosternal clear space on the lateral view. Right atrial enlargement on the PA view appears as displacement of the right heart border to the right. Left ventricular enlargement appears as displacement of the left heart border laterally and to the left, inferiorly and posteriorly with rounding of the cardiac apex. Signs of left atrial enlargement on the PA view include splaying of the carina with an upward sweep due to the large left atrium. The "double density" sign occurs when the right side of the left atrium pushes into the adjacent lung. On the lateral view, the left atrium can be seen extending posteriorly towards or over the spine.

Clinical Implications

If cardiomegaly is suspected based on a chest radiograph, echocardiography is recommended. An echocardiogram can be used to identify the presence of pericardial effusion, pericardial fat, mass, aneurysm, wall motion abnormalities, chamber dilation, chamber hypertrophy, and valve insufficiency.

Left ventricular hypertrophy is most commonly caused by chronic hypertension, with left ventricular muscle mass increasing in order to compensate for the high resistance that it needs to work against to maintain cardiac output. Common etiologies of chamber dilation include aortic and mitral regurgitation, and the various cardiomyopathies.

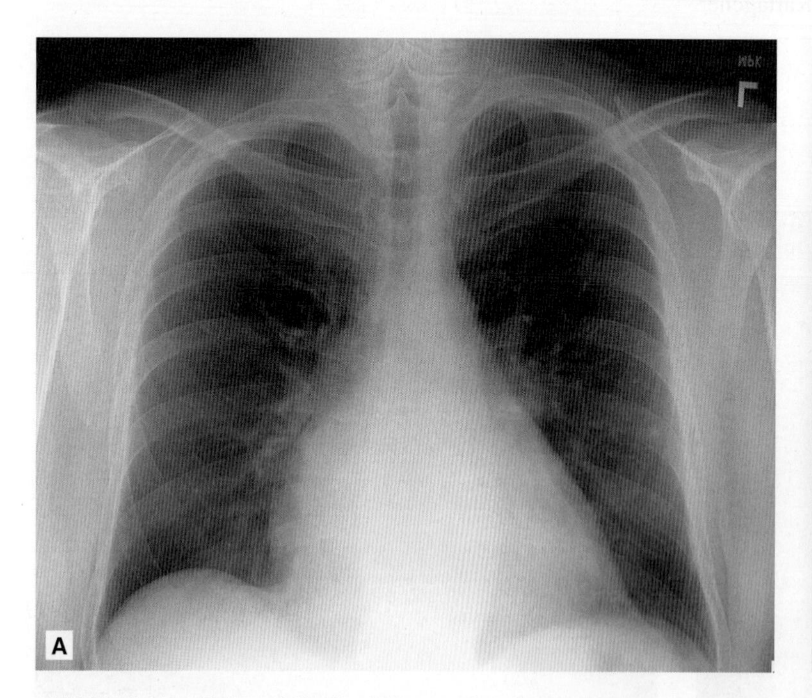

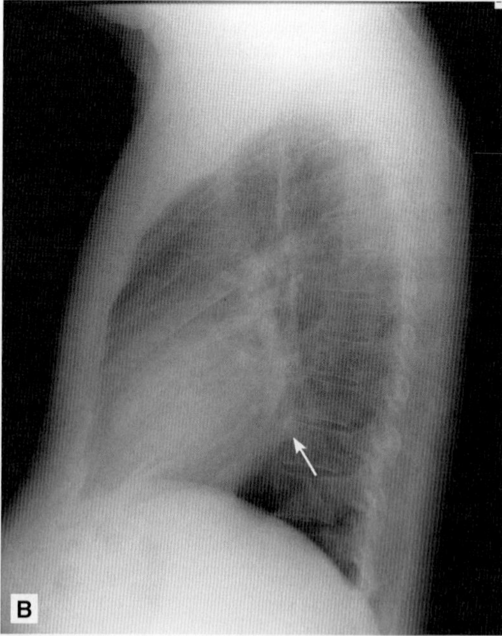

FIGURE 5.14 ■ Enlarged Cardiac Silhouette from Left Atrial Enlargement (LAE). **A, B:** The heart is enlarged and there is a "double density" over the right heart. On the lateral view, the left atrium can be seen projecting over the spine (arrow). This patient had LAE from mitral stenosis.

Pearls

1. An enlarged cardiac silhouette is not synonymous with cardiomegaly. Echocardiography is the modality of choice to differentiate the underlying cause.
2. A lateral view of the chest may be able to diagnose a pericardial effusion: if the effusion is large enough it becomes visible as a radiodense layer sandwiched between the two relatively radiolucent layers of the epicardial and pericardial fat (the "oreo cookie sign").
3. Suspected pathology can be determined based on the chamber/chambers that are enlarged.

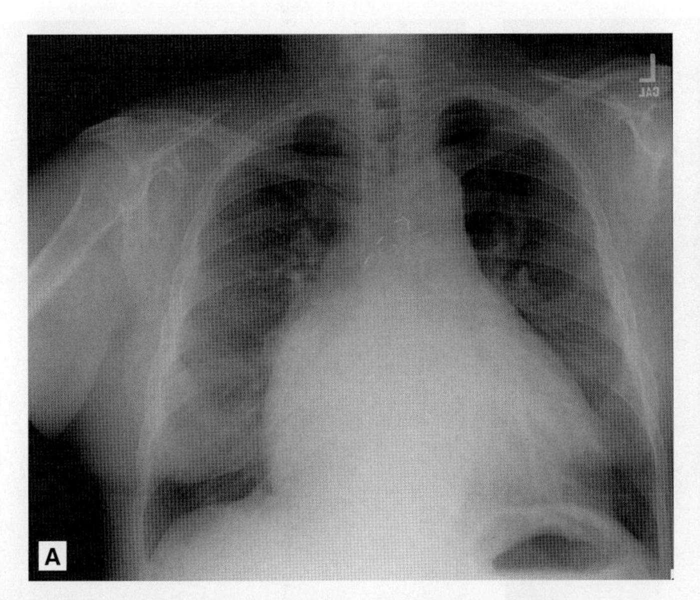

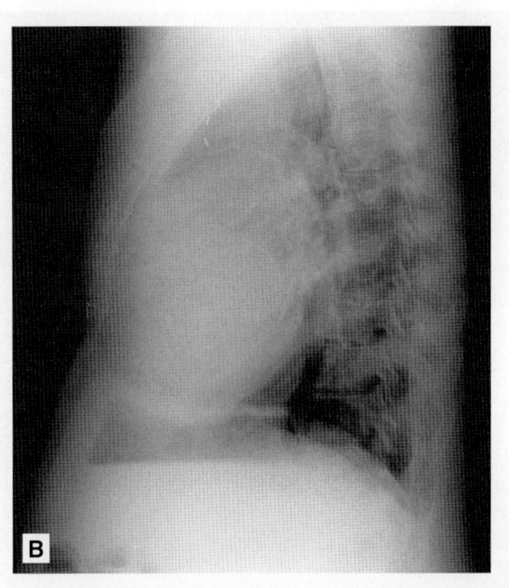

FIGURE 5.15 ■ Enlarged Cardiac Silhouette. **A, B:** On the frontal view, the heart is significantly enlarged with prominence of the right heart border, suggesting right atrial enlargement. On the lateral view, there is filling of the retro-sternal clear space and the left atrium projects over the spine, suggesting right ventricular and left atrial enlargement, respectively. This patient had tricuspid and mitral regurgitation with subsequent valvuloplasty.

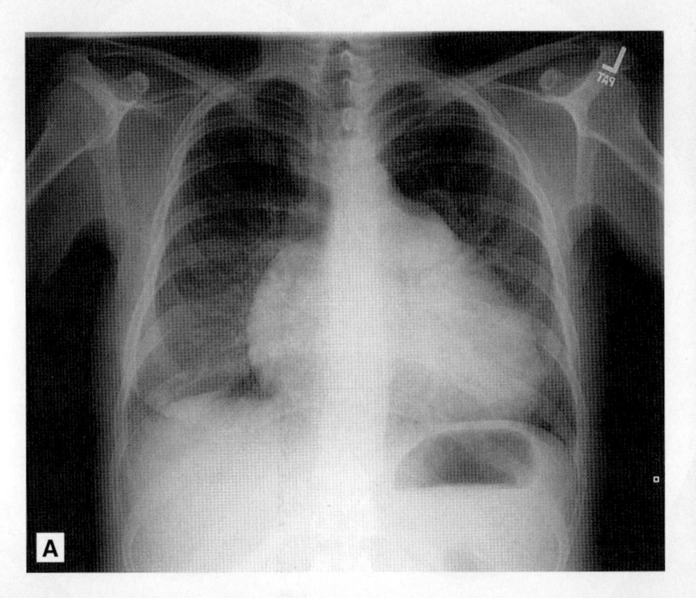

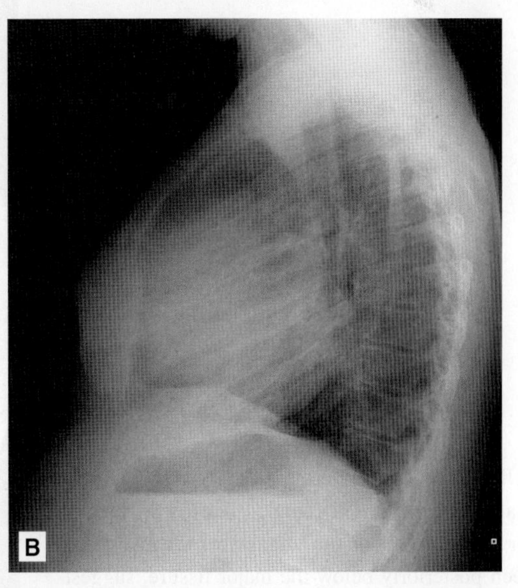

FIGURE 5.16 ■ Enlarged Cardiac Silhouette. **A, B:** On the frontal view, the right heart border is prominent indicating right atrial enlargement. The left atrial appendage is also prominent suggesting left atrial enlargement. On the lateral view, there is filling of the retrosternal clear space, consistent with right ventricular enlargement. This patient had significant right heart enlargement from tricuspid regurgitation and left atrial enlargement from mitral stenosis.

PULMONARY NODULES

Radiographic Summary

Radiographically, a pulmonary nodule is defined as a lesion less than 3 cm in diameter that is both within and surrounded by lung parenchyma. If greater than 3 cm, the lesion is called a mass. Pulmonary nodules are categorized as benign or malignant. The most common causes of a malignant nodule are primary lung cancer, carcinoid tumors, and lung metastases. Malignant nodules, whether primary or metastatic, are rarely calcified. Calcified nodules are usually benign. The most common causes of benign nodules are infectious granulomas (80%) and hamartomas (10%).

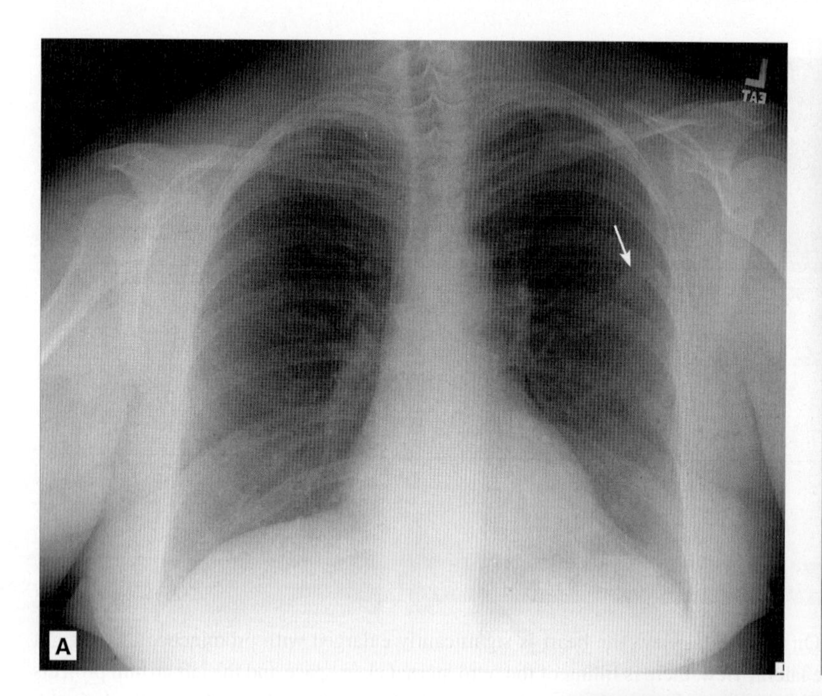

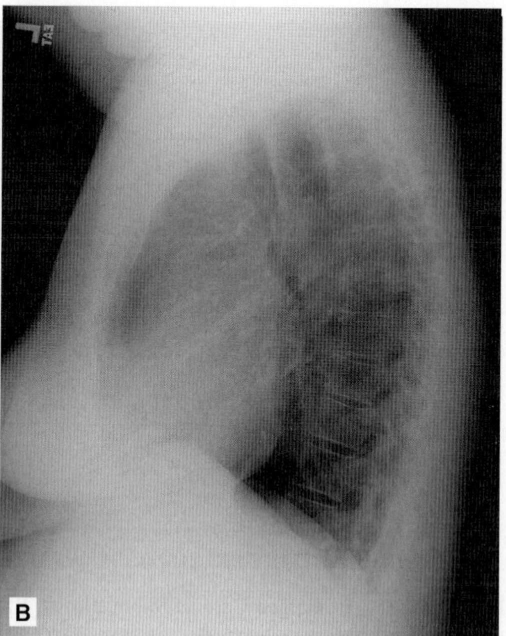

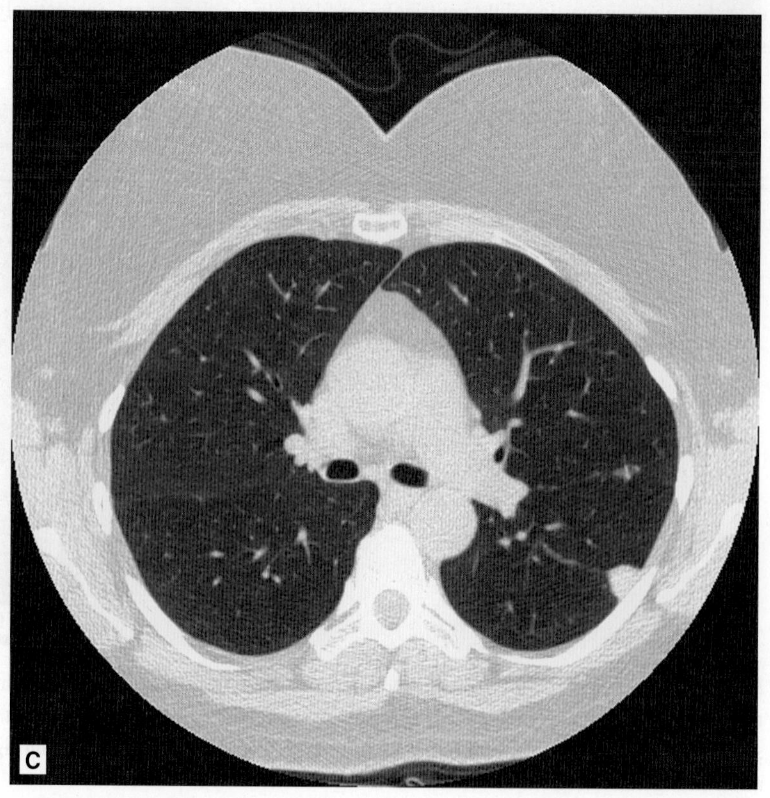

FIGURE 5.17 ■ Pulmonary Nodule. **A-C:** On the frontal view, there is a rounded density in the left upper lung (arrow). On the lateral view, the nodule can be seen posteriorly below the major fissure, suggesting that it is located in the superior segment of the left lower lobe. A CT was ordered, which showed a 1.0 cm pleural-based nodule that remained stable on follow-up and was a presumed granuloma.

When a pulmonary nodule is identified on chest radiograph, every attempt must be made to secure old imaging studies because size comparisons can be used to determine stability versus growth. A nodule that has not grown over 2 years may be considered benign.

Clinical Implications

Clinical features associated with an increased probability of malignancy include advanced age, history of smoking, and prior history of malignancy. Discovery of a new nodule requires that the patient be informed of the nodule, and

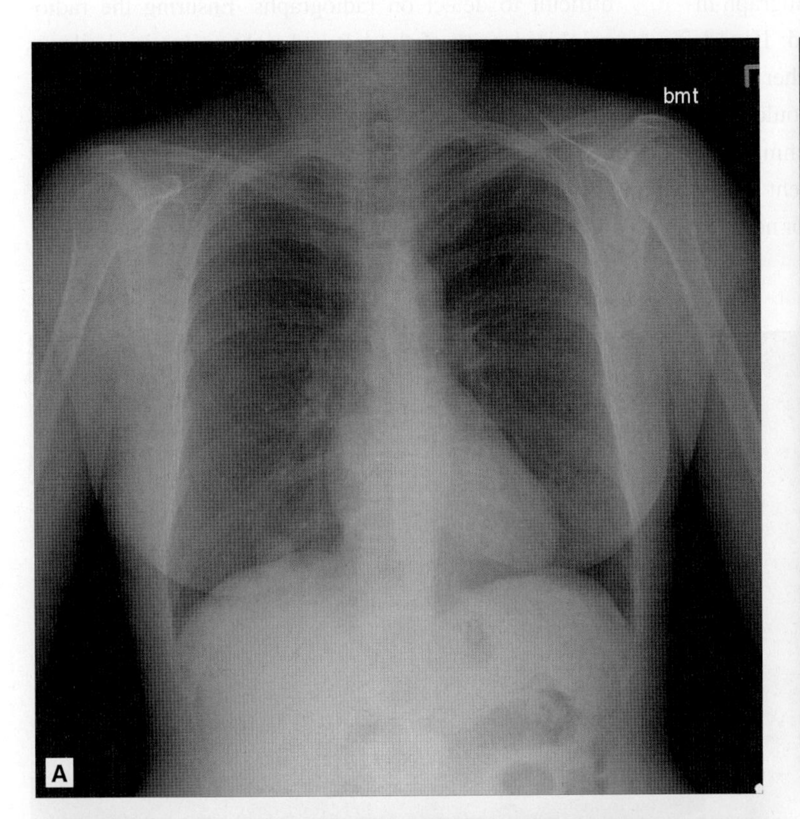

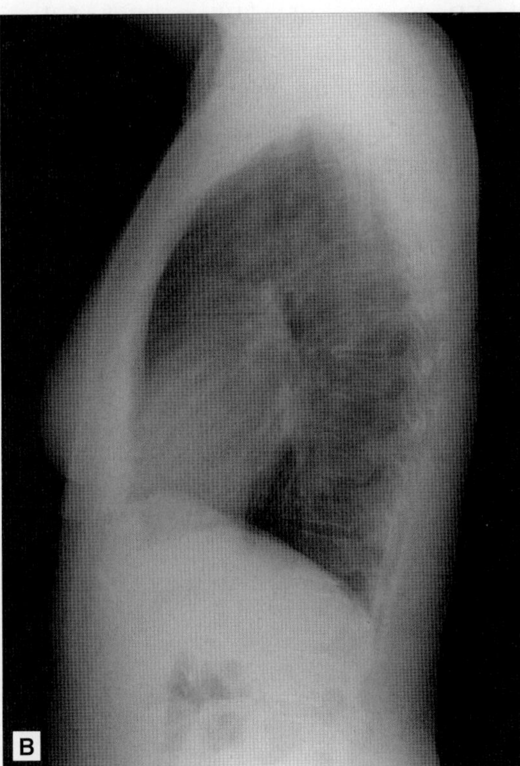

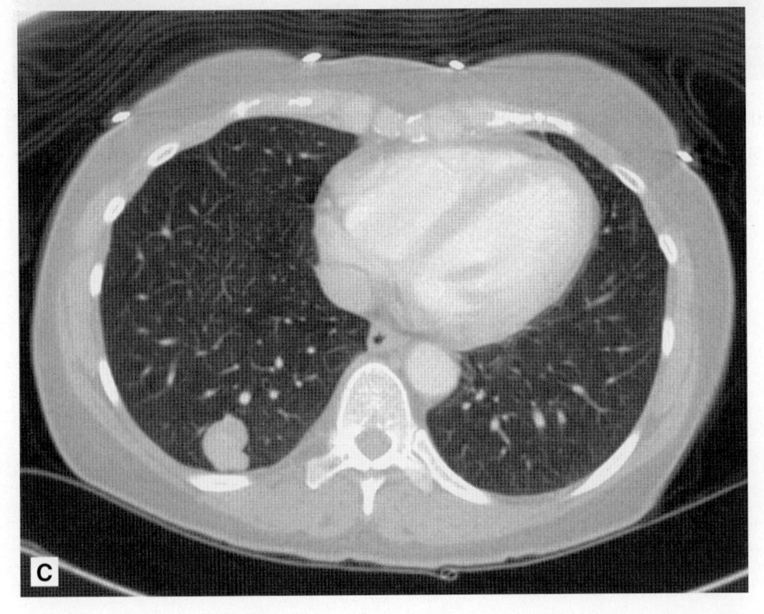

FIGURE 5.18 ■ Pulmonary Nodule. **A-C:** On the frontal view, there is a rounded density in the right lower lung. On the lateral view, the nodule can be seen posteriorly below the major fissure, suggesting that it is located in the right lower lobe. A CT was ordered, which showed a 2.0 cm lobulated nodule with a small central calcification. This remained stable on follow-up and was a presumed hamartoma.

appropriate follow-up arranged. The Fleischner Society guidelines advocate different frequencies of CT scans based upon the size of the nodule and the patient's risk for lung cancer. Patients are considered low risk if they have no history or minimal history of smoking and no other risk factors (such as known carcinogen exposures); otherwise, patients are considered high risk. For a newly diagnosed pulmonary nodule found as an incidental finding on chest radiograph in the ED, these general guidelines may be followed: If nodules are ≤4 mm and the patient is low risk, no further imaging is required. If the patient is high risk, they should have a follow-up CT in 12 months. For nodules 4 to 6 mm, a CT scan should be performed at 12 months if the patient is low risk and at 6-12 months if the patient is high risk. For nodules 6 to 8 mm, a CT scan should be performed at 6-12 months if the patient is low risk, and at 3-6 months if the patient is high risk. For nodules greater than 8 mm, a CT scan should be performed at 3 months whether the patient is low or high risk.

Pearls

1. Nodules occurring in the lung apices may be particularly difficult to detect on radiographs. Ensuring the radiographic density of the left and right apices is similar is reassuring that there is no nodule.
2. Large nodules in the superior sulcus may result in shoulder and arm pain, Horner's syndrome, and weakness and atrophy of the muscles of the hand, a constellation of symptoms referred to as Pancoast's syndrome.

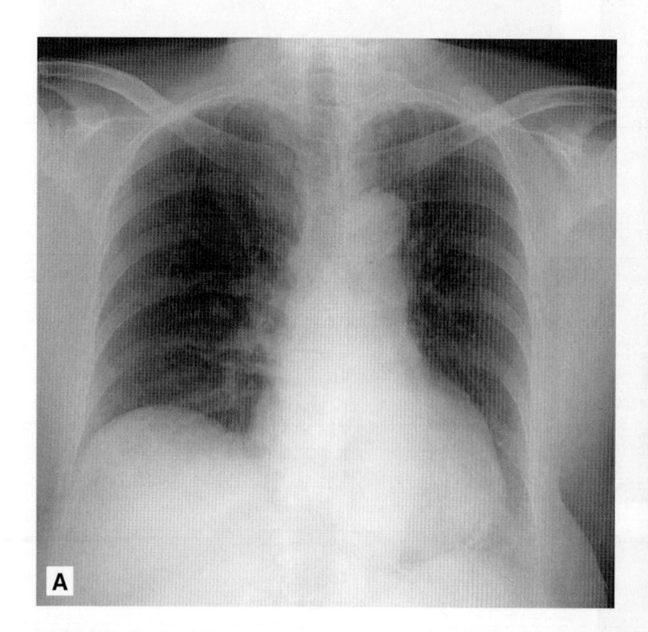

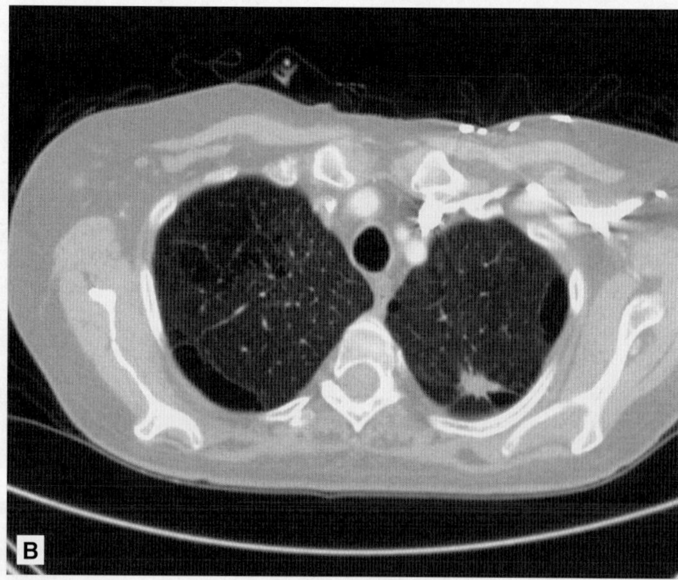

FIGURE 5.19 ■ Pulmonary Nodule. **A, B:** On the frontal radiograph, there is a subtle spiculated density in the left lung apex. A CT scan was ordered, which showed a spiculated nodule with surrounding paraseptal emphysema. This nodule was biopsied and proved to be adenocarcinoma.

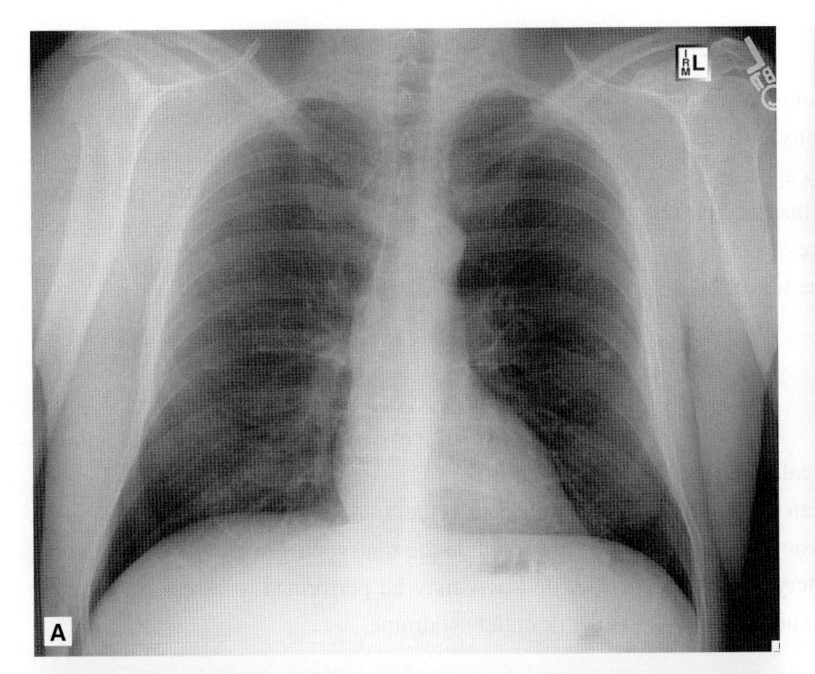

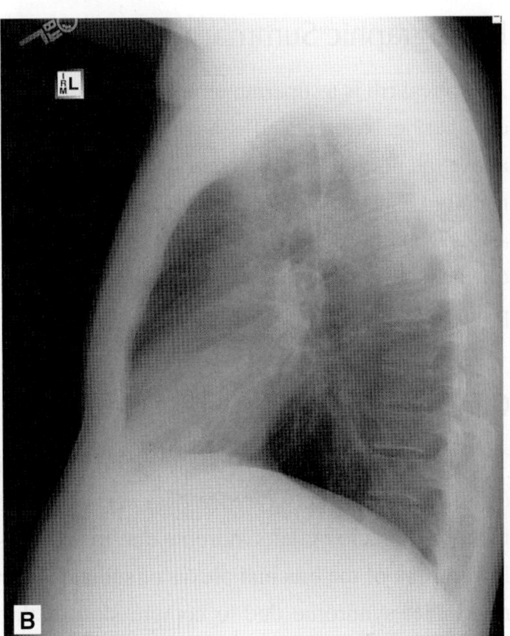

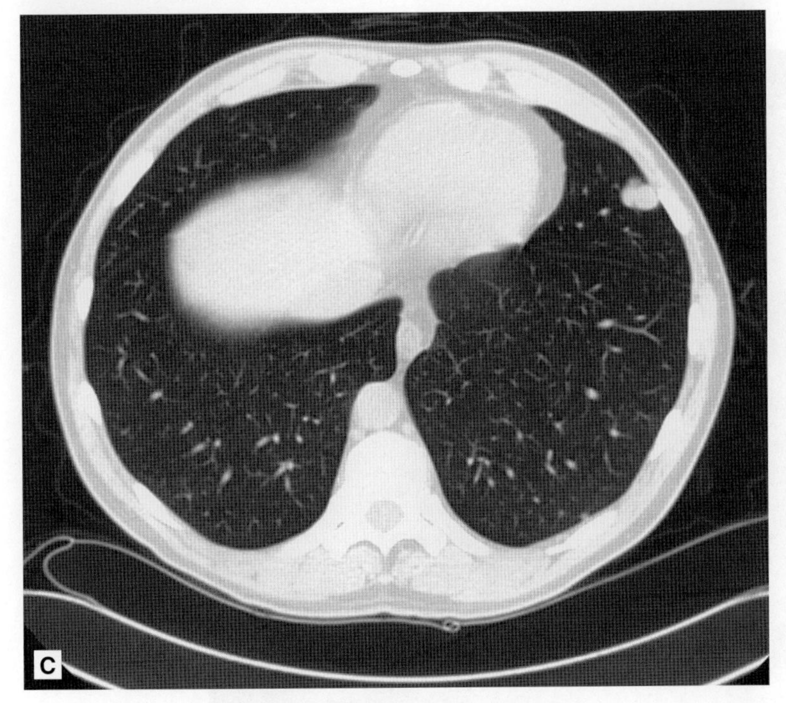

FIGURE 5.20 ■ Pulmonary Nodule. **A-C:** There is a subtle left lower lung density on the frontal view (the smaller more superior density represented a calcified granuloma). This density can be seen over the inferior heart on the lateral view. The CT showed a 1.5 cm nodule in the lingula and was subsequently biopsied. Pathology was consistent with metastatic renal cell carcinoma.

Radiographic Summary

A cervical rib is a supernumerary rib that arises from the seventh cervical vertebra. It is a congenital abnormality located above the normal first rib, overlying the pulmonary apex. It is usually C-shaped and can be identified by noting that the rib arises from a vertebral body whose transverse processes point down, such as C7. In contrast, the transverse processes of T1 point up.

Clinical Implications

The majority of cervical ribs are of limited clinical significance. However, the presence of a cervical rib can cause a form of thoracic outlet syndrome due to compression of the lower trunk of the brachial plexus or subclavian artery or thoracic inlet syndrome due to compression of the subclavian vein. Clinical manifestations of brachial plexus involvement include pain in the neck and shoulder, which radiates into the upper extremities, paresthesias and sensory loss, and weakness of the muscles innervated by the brachial plexus. Subclavian vein compression can present with upper extremity edema and erythema while subclavian artery compression can result in limb ischemia with bluish discoloration and cold hands.

Pearls

1. The majority of cervical ribs are of limited clinical significance.
2. Remember that the transverse processes of C7 point downward while the transverse processes of T1 point up.
3. CTA or MRA may be performed to assess for thoracic inlet or outlet syndrome.

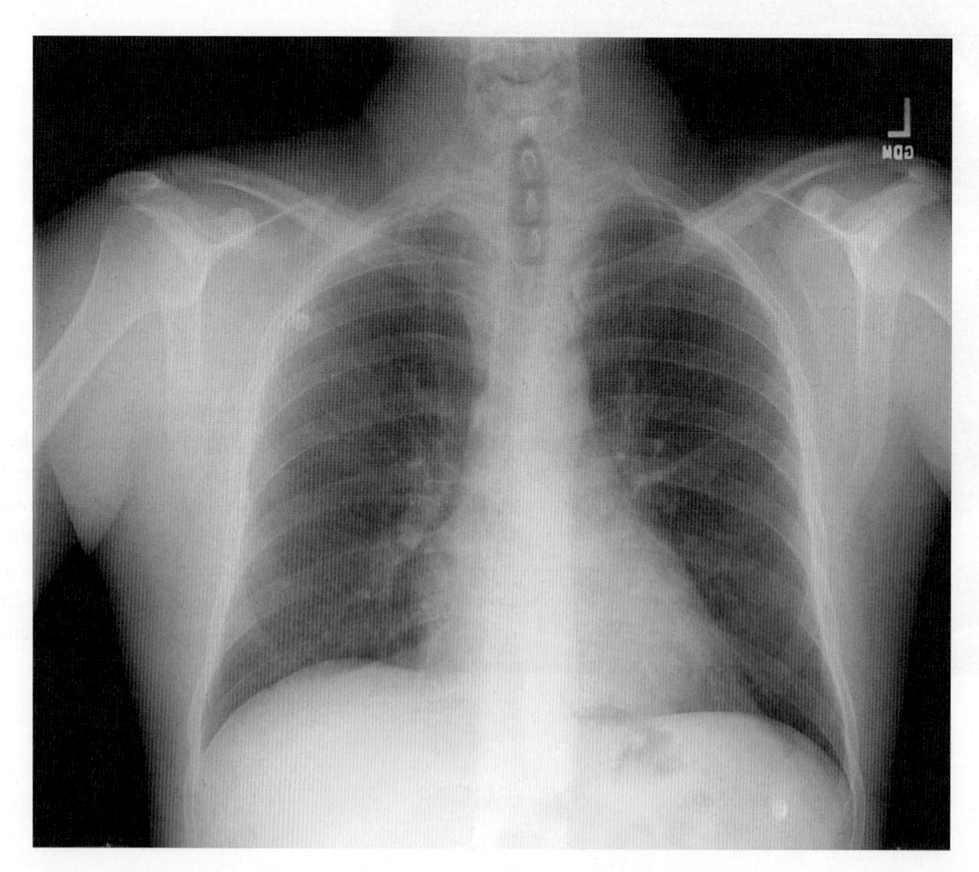

FIGURE 5.21 ■ Cervical Ribs. Rudimentary ribs can be seen projecting bilaterally off the seventh cervical vertebra, consistent with cervical ribs.

Radiographic Summary

Aspiration pneumonia is an inflammation of the lung parenchyma precipitated by the abnormal entry of fluid, particulate exogenous substances, or endogenous secretions into the tracheobronchial tree. Radiographic findings are often delayed, with false-negative radiographs being common early in the disease course. Infiltrates can develop within 6-12 hours and frequently involve the posterior segments of the upper lobes (if aspiration occurred in the supine position) or the superior segments of the lower lobes, most commonly the right lower lobe (if aspiration occurred in the upright position). Later in the disease process, aspiration pneumonia tends to appear as patchy bilateral airspace opacities that are symmetric and somewhat nodular.

CT scanning provides a greater degree of sensitivity and specificity than radiographs alone, however, some of the same diseases that mimic plain radiographic findings of aspiration can also confound the diagnostic interpretation of CT scans. The differential includes: atypical pneumonia, varicella pneumonia, and ARDS.

Clinical Implications

Aspiration is a common event even in healthy individuals and usually resolves without detectable sequelae.

The diagnosis of aspiration pneumonia is usually presumptive based upon the clinical features and course. Treatment of patients with observed or suspected aspiration includes suctioning of the mouth and support of pulmonary function. The use of antibiotics early in the course of aspiration is controversial as damage is mostly due to a chemical pneumonitis. However, antibiotics are commonly given because of the difficulty in excluding bacterial infection as a primary or contributing factor in patients with aspiration.

Pearls

1. False negative findings are common early in the course of the disease, as radiographic findings lag behind clinical findings.
2. Be suspicious for aspiration pneumonitis in a patient who has risk factors such as altered mental status, impaired clearance mechanisms, dysphagia, GERD, and poor oral hygiene.
3. Aspiration pneumonia has a highly variable disease course, with up to 15% mortality.

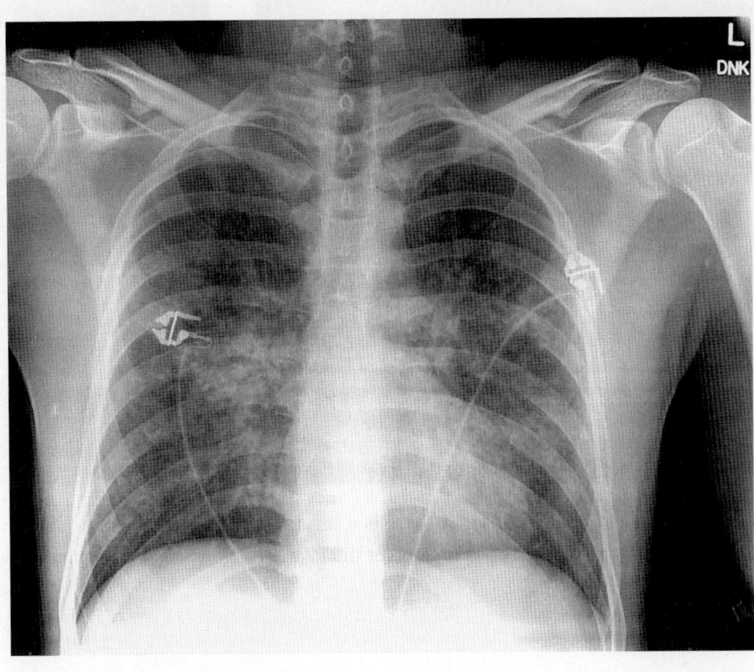

FIGURE 5.22 ■ Aspiration Pneumonia. Bilateral airspace opacities can be diffusely seen in this patient who had a near drowning episode with subsequent aspiration of copious amounts of pool water.

Radiographic Summary

Lobar pneumonia appears radiographically as a focal parenchymal consolidation of a portion or the entire lung lobe. Larger bronchi often remain patent with air, creating characteristic air bronchograms extending into the consolidated parenchyma.

Unlike atelectasis, where the predominant feature is volume loss within the affected segment or lobe of the lung, lobar pneumonia is characterized by mass effect within the involved portion of the lung. Fissures, a hemidiaphragm, or the mediastinal structures may be deviated *away* from the involved lung.

An obscured right heart border on AP view indicates a right middle lobe pneumonia. An obscured right hemidiaphragm on AP view indicates a right lower lobe pneumonia. Similarly, silhouetting of the left heart border on AP view suggests lingular pneumonia and silhouetting of the left hemidiaphragm is consistent with consolidation within the left lower lobe. On the lateral view, as you follow the spine inferiorly, the vertebral bodies get progressively darker on a normal chest radiograph. The "spine sign" is an interruption in the progressive increase in lucency of the vertebral bodies from superior to inferior and is suggestive of left lower lobe pneumonia in the correct clinical setting. Left lower lobe pneumonia can also be seen on AP view as an increased retrocardiac opacity.

Clinical Implications

Pneumonia is classically diagnosed by the presence of an area of consolidation on radiography with a supportive presentation. False negatives can occur early in the disease course. If clinical suspicion is high, it is reasonable to initiate antibiotic therapy based on the clinical picture alone.

The causes, treatment, and prognosis of hospital-acquired pneumonia are different from those of community-acquired pneumonia. Hospital-acquired microorganisms may include resistant bacteria such as MRSA, *Pseudomonas*, and *Enterobacter sp*. Broad-spectrum antibiotic coverage with a multidrug regimen is necessary to cover probable pathogens.

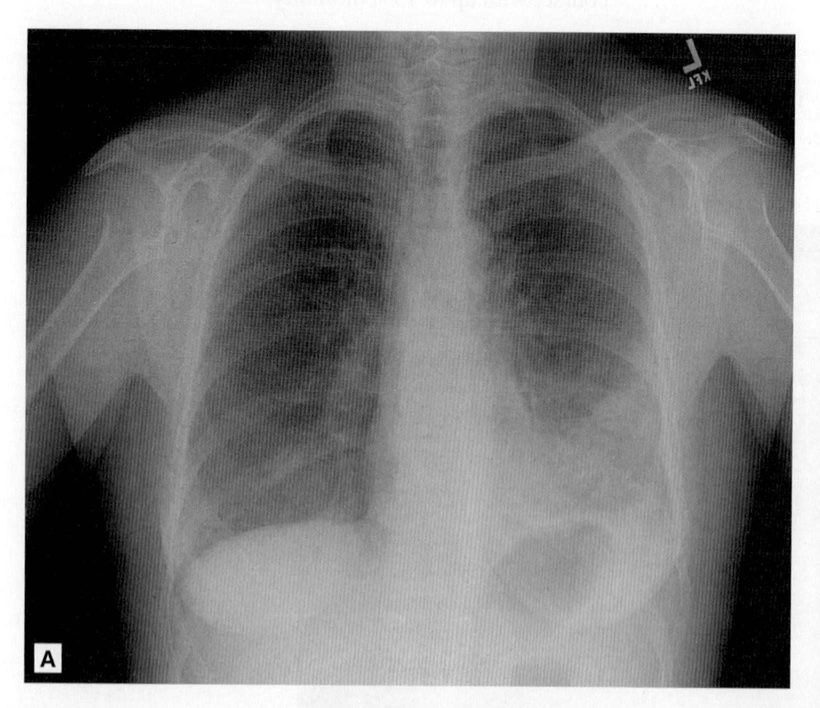

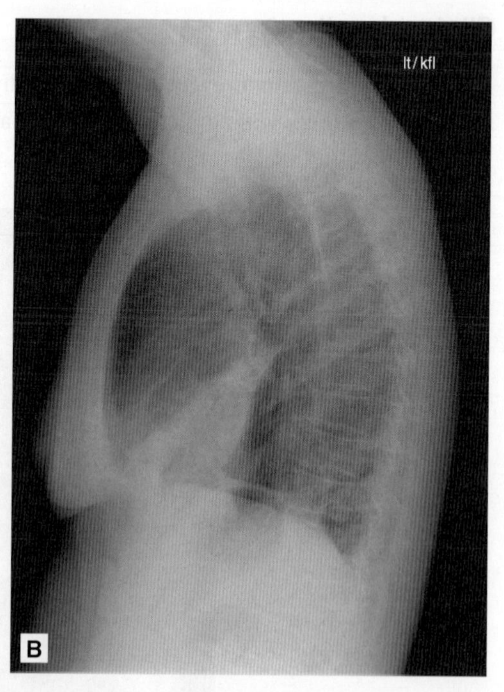

FIGURE 5.23 ■ Lobar Pneumonia. **A, B:** On the frontal view, there is a left lower lung opacity with obscuration of the left heart border. On the lateral view, a wedge shaped opacity can be seen projecting over the heart and anterior to the major fissure. This patient had lingular pneumonia.

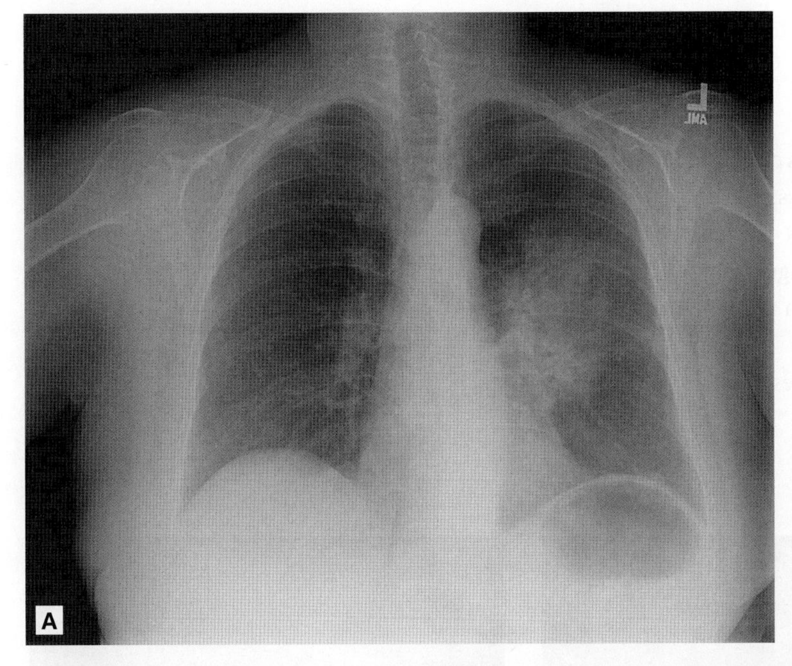

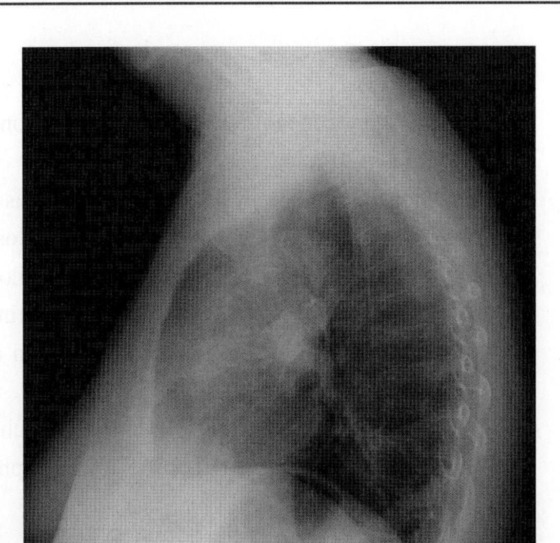

FIGURE 5.24 ■ Lobar Pneumonia. **A, B:** On the frontal view, there is a left mid-lung/peri-hilar opacity with obscuration of the superior left heart border. On the lateral view, an opacity can be seen projecting anterior to the major fissure. This patient had lobar pneumonia within the anterior segment of the left upper lobe with additional early consolidation within the lingula.

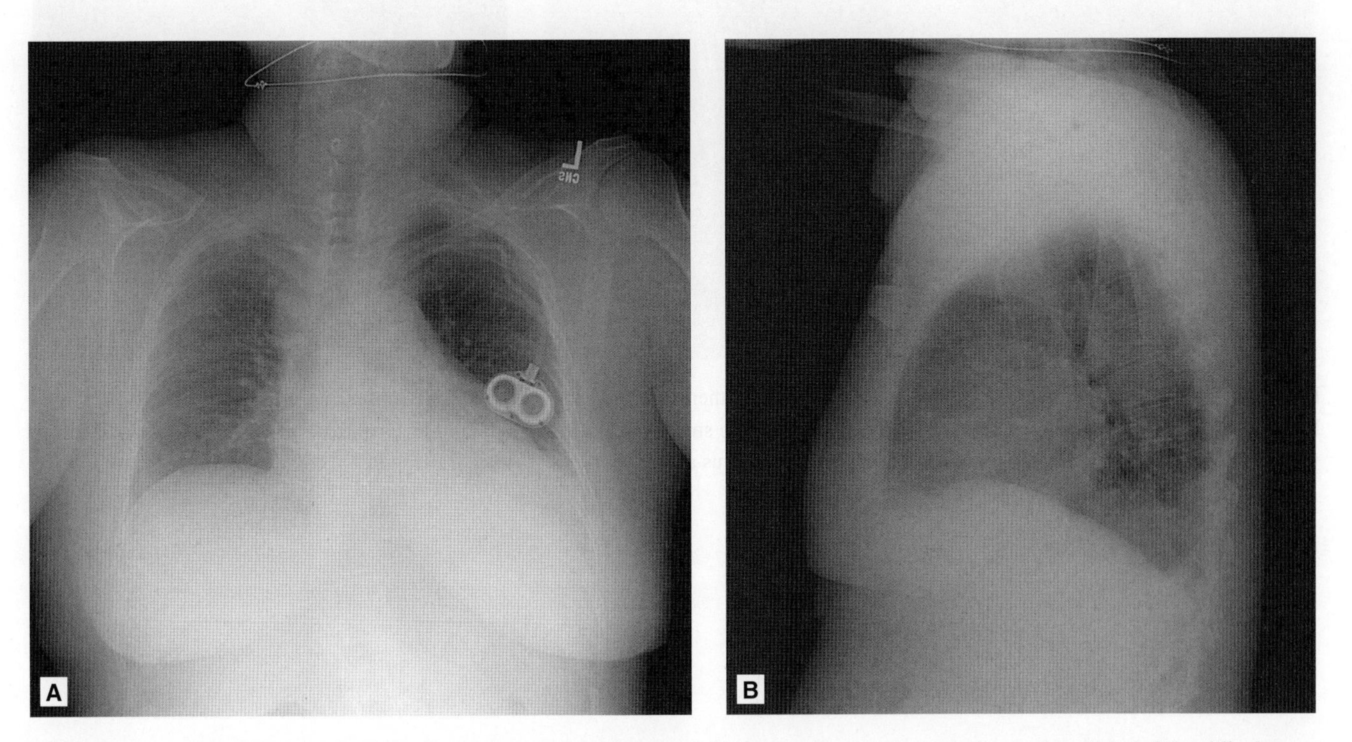

FIGURE 5.25 ■ Lobar Pneumonia. **A, B:** On the frontal view, there is a left retro-cardiac opacity with obscuration of the left hemidiaphragm. On the lateral view, there is obscuration of the lower thoracic spine, the so-called "spine sign." This patient had left lower lobe pneumonia.

Pearls

1. Clinical suspicion with a lobar consolidation on chest radiography is typical for lobar pneumonia.
2. Lobar consolidation may result in regional mass effect, as opposed to atelectasis that results in volume loss.
3. Subtle opacities from early pneumonia do not produce any appreciable mass effect and may be indistinguishable from subsegmental atelectaisis, especially on a portable chest radiograph.
4. Whenever possible, obtain PA and lateral chest radiographs rather than a portable AP radiograph. PA and lateral chest radiographs reveal much more information for half the cost. Portable chest radiographs obtained with the patient supine or recumbent almost always result in some component of atelectasis in the lung bases, which is indistinguishable from early pneumonia. A lateral view allows the evaluation of the retrosternal region, the lower lobes (which hide below the diaphragmatic domes on the AP view), and is much more sensitive for small pleural effusions. The assessment of the heart and mediastinum is also more accurate and complete on a PA and lateral study versus on a portable AP view.

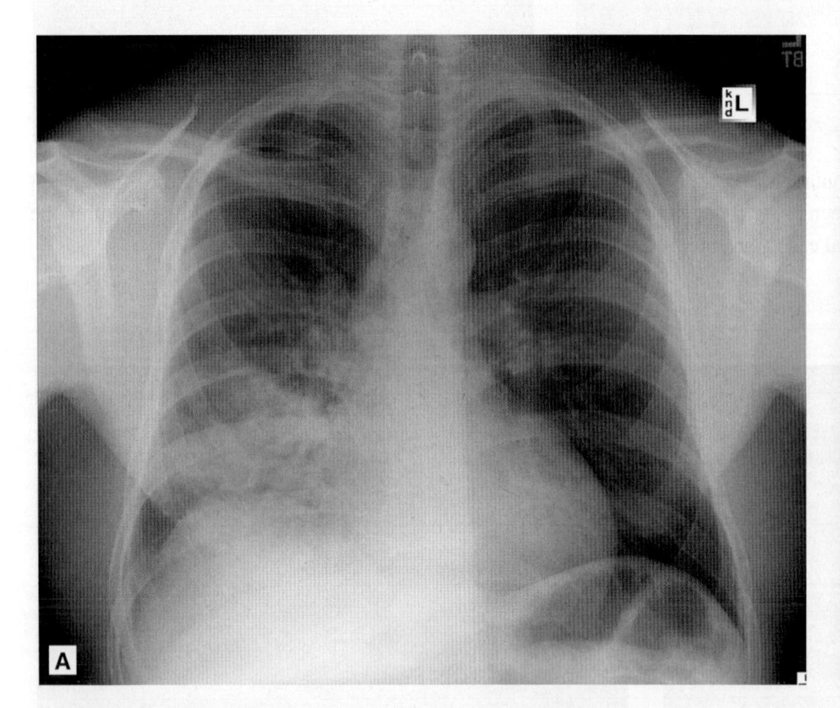

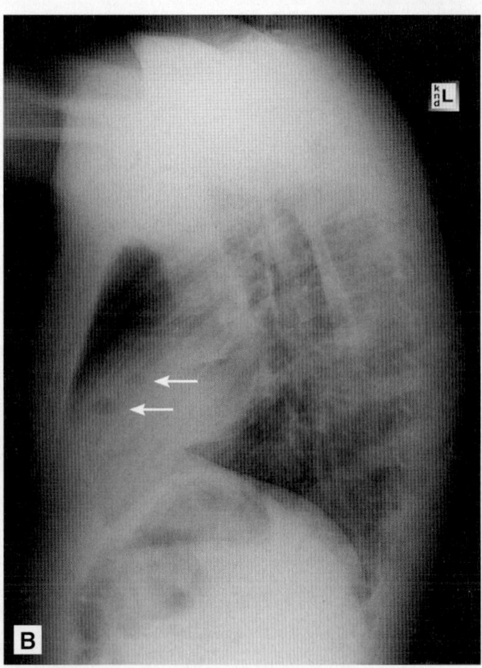

FIGURE 5.26 ■ Lobar Pneumonia. **A, B:** On the frontal view, there is a right lower lung opacity obscuring the right heart border. On the lateral view, the opacity projects anteriorly and contains multiple small abscesses with air-fluid levels (arrows). This patient was diagnosed with necrotizing right middle lobe pneumonia from staphylococcus aureus.

Radiographic Summary

Varicella pneumonia is a rare but rapidly progressive pneumonia with significant mortality. The findings on chest radiography in varicella pneumonia are due to diffuse alveolar damage initially with multiple ill-defined, 5–10 mm nodules that may be confluent and fleeting. These nodules usually resolve within one week after resolution of the skin lesions, but sometimes may persist for months. Sometimes the nodules calcify and persist indefinitely.

The differential diagnosis for amicronodular pattern on plain radiograph includes: alveolar microlithiasis, pulmonary hemosiderosis, miliary tuberculosis, intravenous talc granulomatosis (seen in IV drug users who inject talc), calcified metastases, and early stages of pneumoconioses such as silicosis, talcosis, and coal worker's pneumoconiosis.

Clinical Implications

Varicella pneumonia typically develops slowly within one to six days after the onset of skin lesions. Symptoms are similar to those of other pneumonias, including dry cough, fever, tachypnea, and dyspnea. Varicella pneumonia is the most serious complication of disseminated varicella-zoster virus infection with mortality rates of 10-50%. It is an uncommon complication of varicella in immunocompetent children. In adults, pneumonia accounts for the majority of the morbidity and mortality from varicella infection. More than 90% of cases of adult varicella pneumonia occur in immunocompromised patients and those with lymphoma. If the clinical presentation suggests varicella as the etiology, immediate treatment with IV acyclovir is recommended.

Pearls

1. Immunosuppressed patients who present with varicella skin lesions, respiratory complaints, and suggestive radiography should be immediately treated with IV acyclovir.
2. The calcified nodules that form as sequelae to prior Varicella pneumonia are typically much more numerous and uniform in size and distribution within both lungs than the calcified granulomata resulting from prior granulomatous infection.

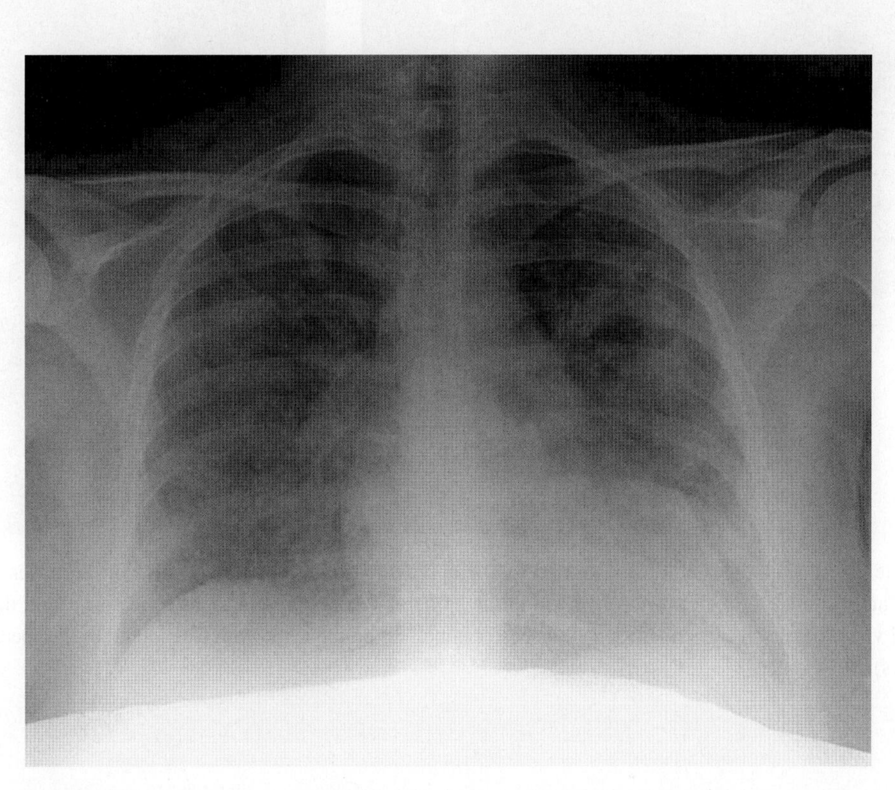

FIGURE 5.27 ■ Varicella Pneumonia. Bilateral interstitial opacities with a somewhat nodular pattern are seen throughout the entire lung bilaterally, but are more pronounced in the lower lungs. This patient was treated for suspected varicella pneumonia.

Radiographic Summary

Acute Chest Syndrome is an acute pulmonary complication of sickle cell disease. Causes include pulmonary infarction, fat embolism, and infection. A chest radiograph typically demonstrates asymmetric opacities with other secondary signs of sickle cell disease, such as sclerosis of the humeral heads (secondary to bony infarcts), cardiomegaly, or Lincoln-log vertebrae.

Without secondary signs of sickle cell disease, it is difficult to diagnose acute chest based on a chest radiograph alone, as it can resemble atypical pneumonia, ARDS, or lobar pneumonia. It is only in conjunction with the clinical history or with secondary signs on the radiograph that the diagnosis of acute chest syndrome can be made.

Clinical Implications

Acute chest syndrome is the second most common cause of hospitalization and most common cause of death in patients with sickle cell disease. Triggers include vaso-occlusive crises and infections such *S. pneumoniae*, *Mycoplasma*, and *Chlamydia*.

The diagnosis of ACS requires a new pulmonary infiltrate on chest radiography that involves at least one complete lung segment. In addition, patients must have one or more of the following: chest pain; temperature >38.5ºC; tachypnea, wheezing, or increased breathing; and hypoxemia relative to the patient's baseline.

Pearls

1. Respiratory complaint with a new opacity on chest radiography in a sickle cell patient is acute chest until proven otherwise. Pneumonia is in the differential.
2. Treatment of acute chest requires volume resuscitation, oxygenation, and pain control.

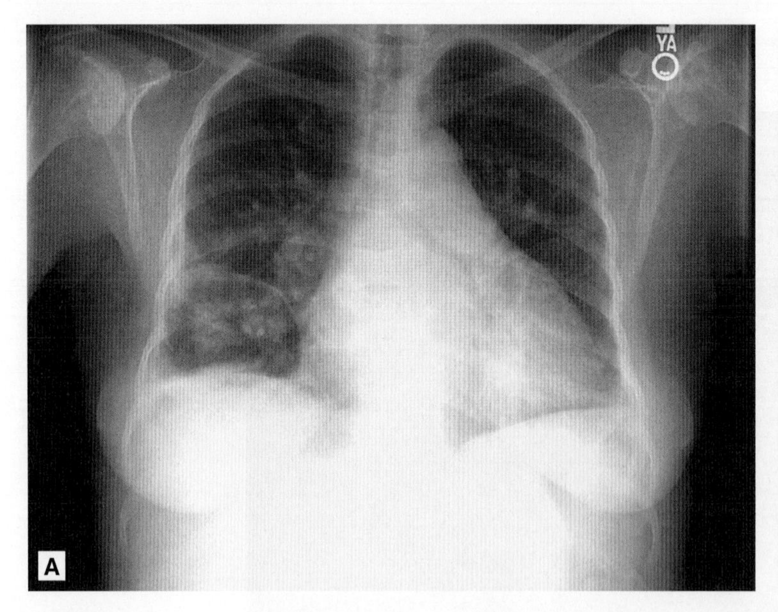

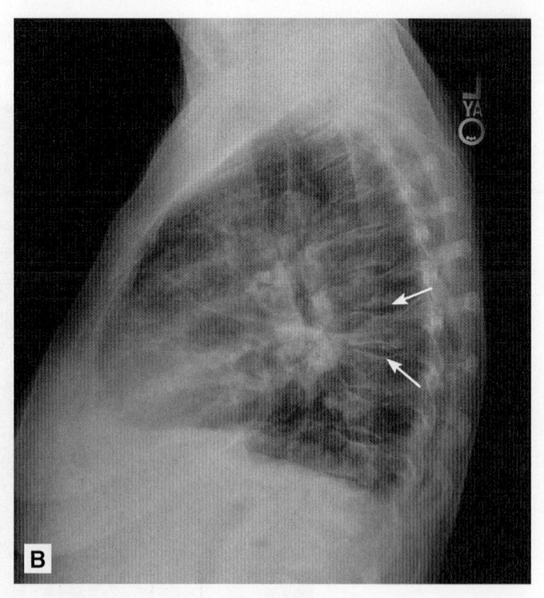

FIGURE 5.28 ■ Acute Chest Syndrome. **A, B:** The frontal radiograph demonstrates patchy opacities in the lower lungs bilaterally with cardiomegaly. Additionally, mild sclerotic changes are noted in the humeral heads representing osteonecrosis from the patient's sickle cell disease. On the lateral view, classic changes of sickle cell disease can be seen in the spine with a "Lincoln log" appearance of the vertebral body endplates (arrows).

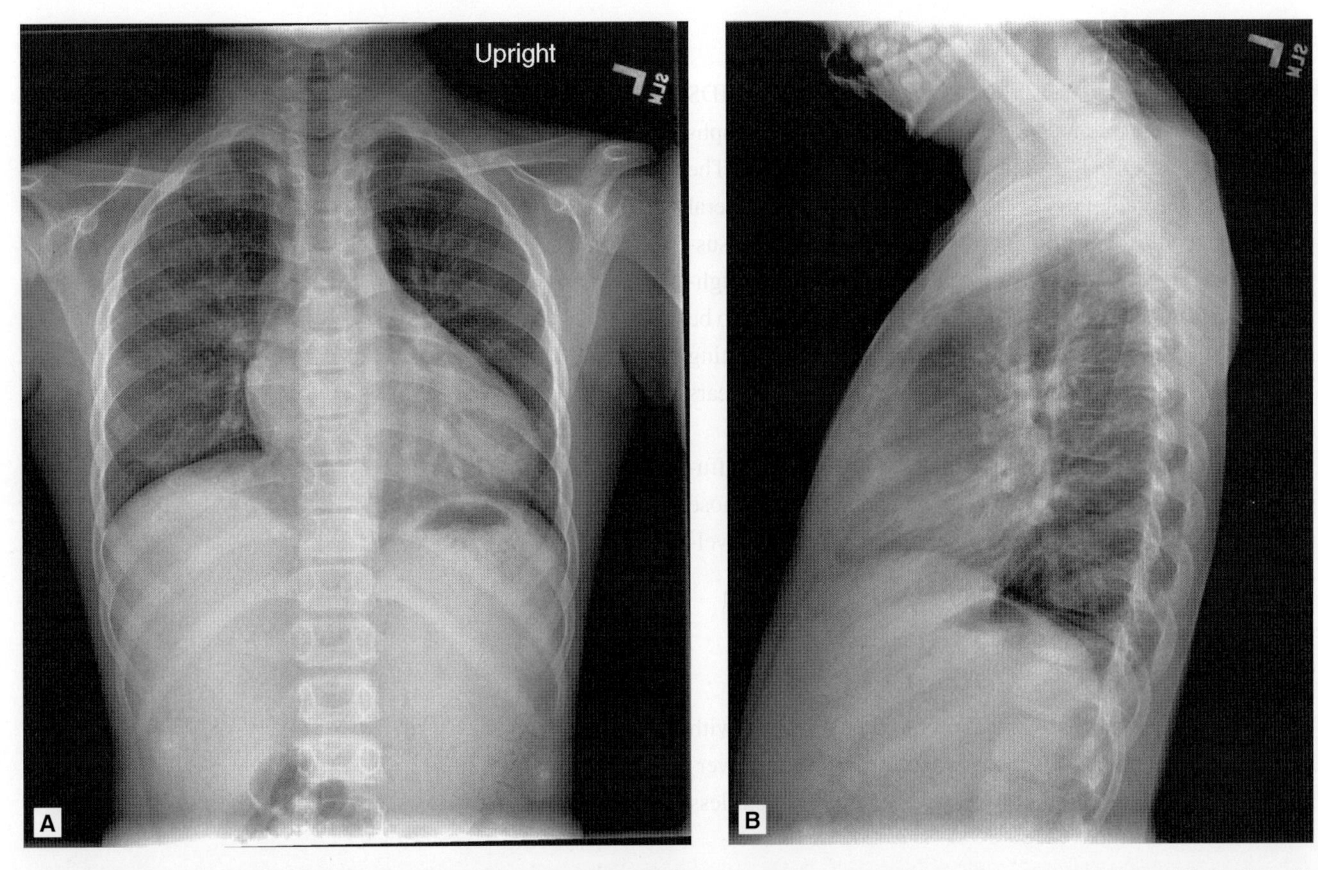

FIGURE 5.29 ■ Acute Chest Syndrome. **A, B:** The frontal radiograph demonstrates patchy opacities in the lower lungs bilaterally with cardiomegaly. On the lateral view, the opacities project in the perihilar region. This child had sickle cell disease and was admitted for management of acute chest syndrome. No osseous changes of sickle cell disease are noted in this patient.

Radiographic Summary

Pneumocystis pneumonia is a common complication of AIDS resulting in severe pulmonary compromise. Chest radiographs may initially be normal in patients with PCP pneumonia. The most common radiographic findings are diffuse bilateral perihilar opacities. For immunosuppressed patients with suspected PCP pneumonia and equivocal chest radiograph, high-resolution CT scan is recommended and has been shown to be nearly 100% sensitive and nearly 90% specific for detecting PCP in HIV-positive patients. PCP pneumonia on CT appears as patchy or nodular ground-glass opacities.

PCP pneumonia can also be associated with pleural effusions, lobar infiltrates, nodules, and pneumothorax. Those receiving pentamidine prophylaxis are more prone to developing predominantly apical infiltrates.

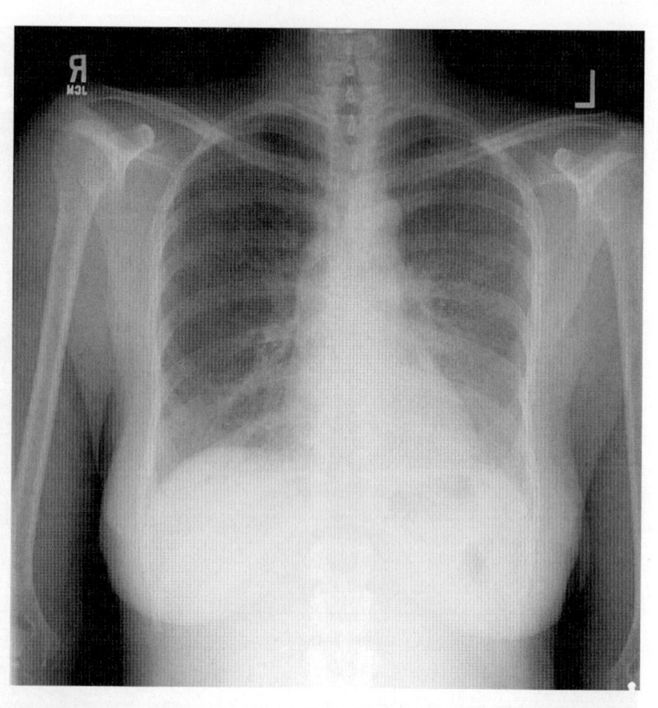

FIGURE 5.30 ■ Pneumonia—PCP. Frontal radiograph shows bilateral perihilar interstitial opacities in this HIV-positive patient. The patient was diagnosed with PCP pneumonia.

Clinical Implications

Diagnosis is made via a combination of clinical picture with radiographic findings. Treatment is based on disease severity. Patients with mild to moderate disease (A-a gradient less

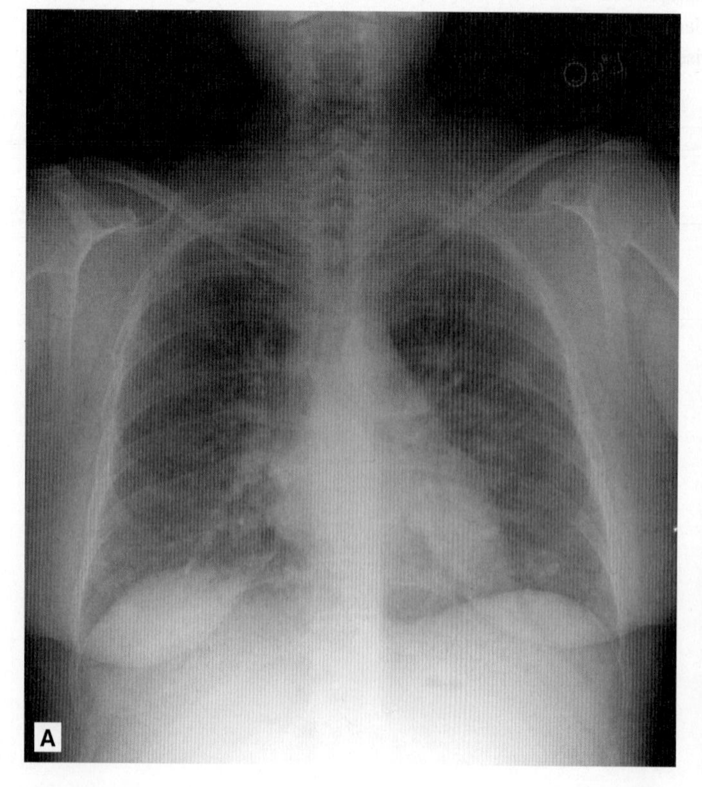

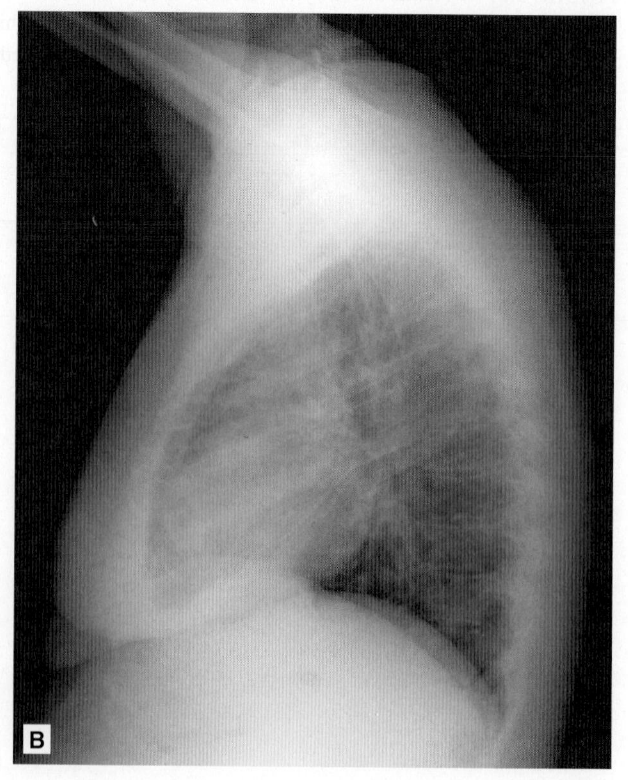

FIGURE 5.31 ■ Pneumonia—PCP. **A, B:** Frontal and lateral radiographs demonstrate bilateral perihilar nodular interstitial opacities in this HIV-positive patient. The patient was diagnosed with PCP pneumonia.

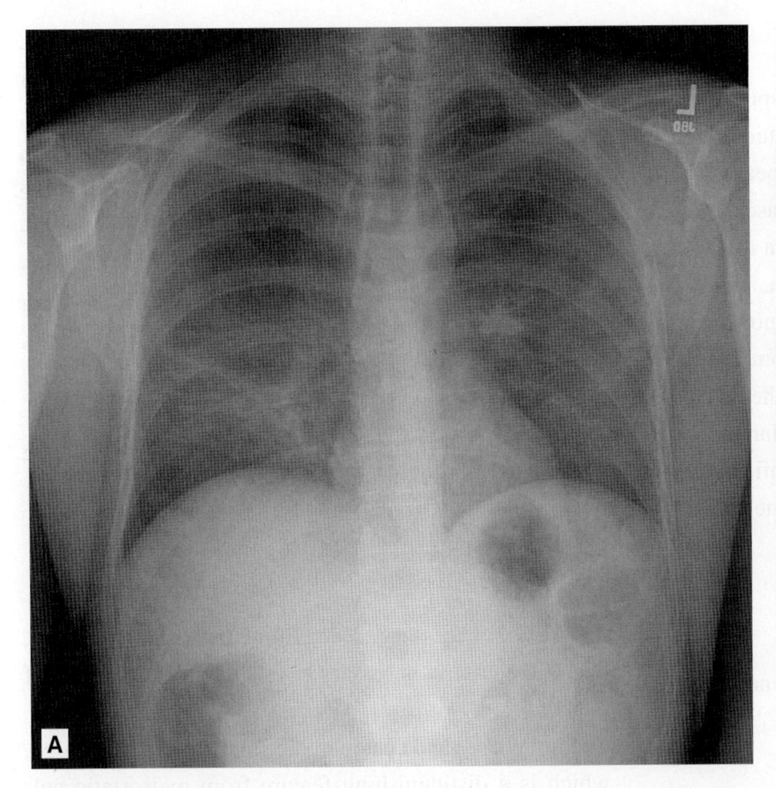

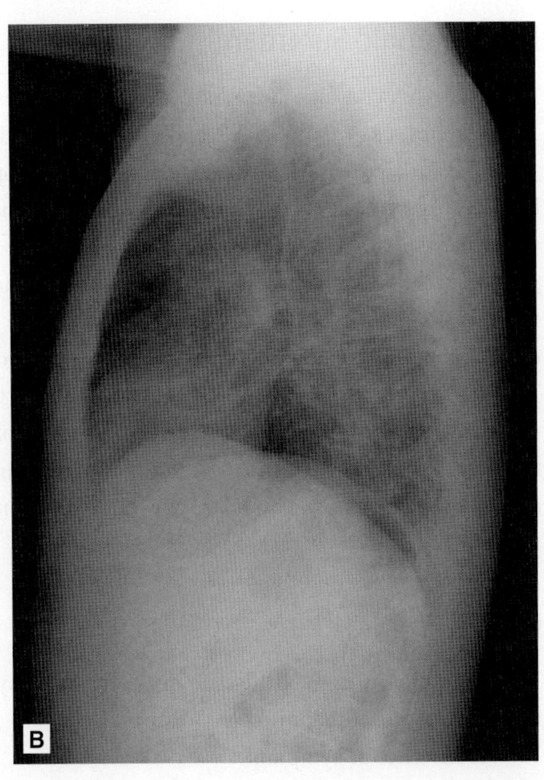

FIGURE 5.32 ▪ Pneumonia—PCP. **A, B:** Bilateral infra-hilar interstitial opacities are seen in this HIV-positive patient. These opacities have a somewhat linear appearance, and the patient was diagnosed with PCP pneumonia.

than 45 mmHg) can receive oral therapy with TMP-SMX, TMP-dapsone, or clindamycin–primaquine, all of which have excellent oral absorption and were found to have no difference in therapeutic failure rate. For patients with severe disease (A-a gradient greater than 45 mmHg), IV therapy combined with corticosteroids is recommended. Patients with PCP typically worsen after two to three days of therapy due to antibiotic-induced death of organisms and subsequent inflammation. Corticosteroids decrease this inflammation and have been shown to decrease the incidence of mortality and respiratory failure when given in patients if room air arterial blood gas reveals a partial pressure of oxygen less than or equal to 70 mmHg or an A-a gradient greater than or equal to 35.

Pearls

1. PCP is still the most common opportunistic infection in HIV-positive patients.
2. Always check an ABG in patients with PCP, as the degree of hypoxemia measured by PaO_2 and the A-a gradient determines the use of adjuvant corticosteroids.
3. Suspected PCP pneumonia warrants admission for observation as the condition can rapidly deteriorate even with appropriate antibiotics.
4. Chest radiographs may be normal or demonstrate perihilar opacities. High-resolution CT shows ground-glass opacities and interstitial prominence.

Radiographic Summary

ARDS is a syndrome of rapidly developing respiratory insufficiency caused by leakage of protein-rich fluid into the alveolar spaces. Radiographically, ARDS appears as bilateral, symmetric air space opacities. The lung bases and costophrenic sulci may be relatively spared. This is a distinguishing feature from hydrostatic pulmonary edema, which is typically most severe in the lung bases. There are no associated pleural effusions or Kerley B lines or cardiomegaly. Typically, there is a 12 hour radiographic delay after the onset of clinical symptoms. After 12 hours, patchy alveolar infiltrates are seen in both lungs. After 24 hours, these infiltrates coalesce to form massive air-space consolidation. Sometimes, air bronchograms are observed.

Clinical Implications

The definition of Acute Respiratory Distress syndrome requires all four of the following features:

1. Acute onset of symptoms
2. Bilateral infiltrates on chest radiographs
3. No evidence of elevated left atrial pressure (pulmonary capillary wedge pressure less than or equal to 18 if measured)
4. A PaO_2/FiO_2 ratio less than or equal to 200 mmHg

Patients with ARDS typically present with tachycardia, tachypnea, dyspnea, hypoxemia, and with diffuse rales. Fever is often lacking or low-grade. Given the severity of lung injury, patients typically worsen rapidly, and mechanical ventilation is almost universally required. The most common causes are sepsis, aspiration, pneumonia, severe trauma, massive transfusion, transfusion-related acute lung injury (TRALI), post-op lung and hematopoietic stem cell transplantation, and drug overdose (salicylates and cocaine are commonly implicated). ARDS is a diagnosis of exclusion. Cardiogenic pulmonary edema and other causes of acute hypoxemic respiratory failure with bilateral infiltrates must be excluded prior to making a diagnosis of ARDS.

Pearls

1. An ABG is necessary to determine the PaO_2/FiO_2 ratio, one of the criteria necessary to establish the definition of ARDS.
2. The lung bases and costophrenic sulci are usually spared, which is a distinguishing feature from hydrostatic pulmonary edema which is typically most severe in the lung bases.
3. The absence of pulmonary venous congestion, Kerley B lines, cardiomegaly, and pleural effusions also help distinguish ALI/ARDS from pulmonary edema.

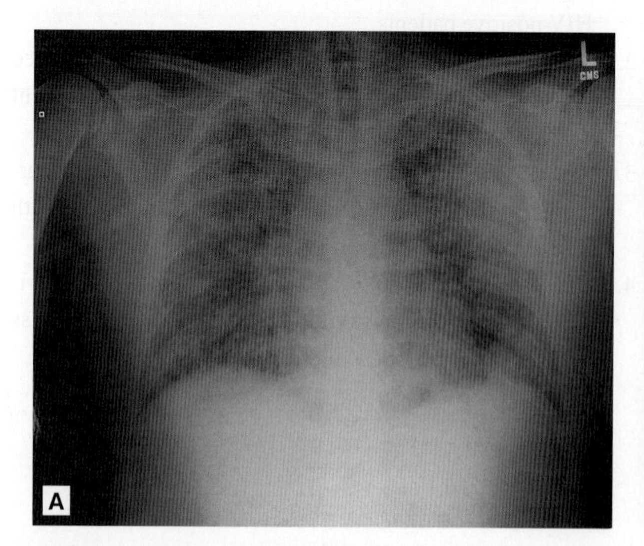

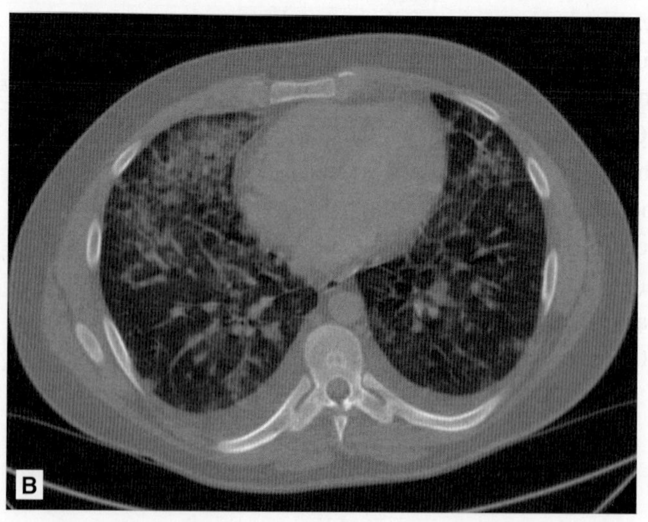

FIGURE 5.33 ■ ARDS. **A, B:** Bilateral patchy airspace opacities are seen throughout both lungs in this patient with acute respiratory failure. The accompanying CT image demonstrates nodular and confluent ground-glass opacities in both lungs. This trauma patient was subsequently diagnosed with ARDS. Notice the relative sparing of the lung bases and costophrenic sulci and the normal heart size and vascular pedicle width; these are distinguishing features from hydrostatic pulmonary edema.

Radiographic Summary

Atypical pneumonia is not caused by traditional pathogens, the most common being *Mycoplasma*, *Chlamydia*, and viruses such as RSV, influenza, parainfluenza, and adenoviruses. Radiographs typically show diffuse, poorly aerated, hazy opacities throughout the lung parenchyma. Opacities tend to be interstitial and linear and less alveolar.

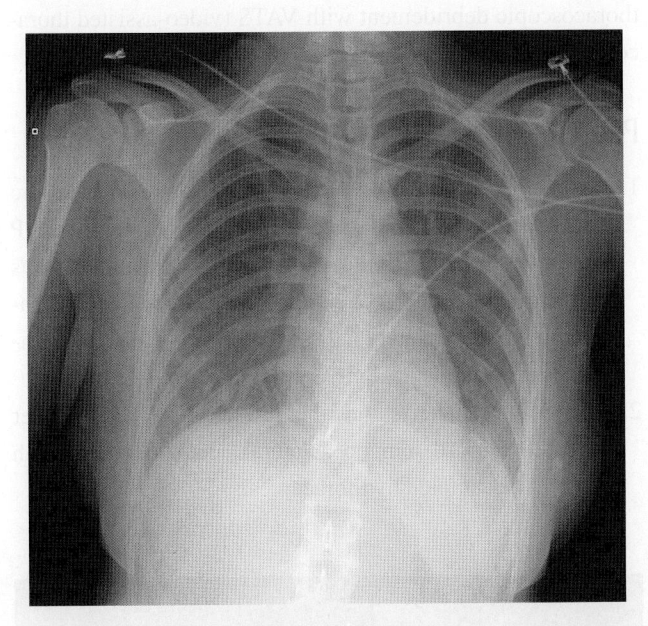

FIGURE 5.34 ■ Atypical Pneumonia. A frontal radiograph demonstrates bilateral interstitial prominence with diffuse bilateral haziness present in this patient with Mycoplasma pneumonia.

Clinical Implications

The diagnosis of atypical pneumonia is based on the clinical presentation in conjunction with radiographic findings. The clinical features include the insidious onset of headache, myalgias, moderate fever, and nonproductive cough. Lab findings include a normal or mildly elevated WBC.

Patients with atypical pneumonias can also appear toxic. Exotic pathogens seen with Q fever (*Coxiella burnetii*), Tularemia (*Francisella tularensis*), and Psittacosis (*Chlamydia psittaci*) can cause a more virulent clinical course.

Pearls

1. *Mycoplasma* and *Chlamydia* are more common causes of atypical pneumonia in younger patients while *Legionella* is more common in older patients.
2. CMV should be considered in transplant recipients and patients with AIDS.
3. Hantavirus should be considered in residents of or recent travelers to the southwestern United States.
4. Q fever pneumonia, due to *Coxiella burnetii*, should be considered in patients who work closely with animals, especially farm livestock. Patients tend to present looking ill, diaphoretic, and febrile.
5. Typical radiographic findings are increased interstitial markings and perihilar linear opacities (rather than focal parenchymal consolidation, as seen in lobar pneumonia).

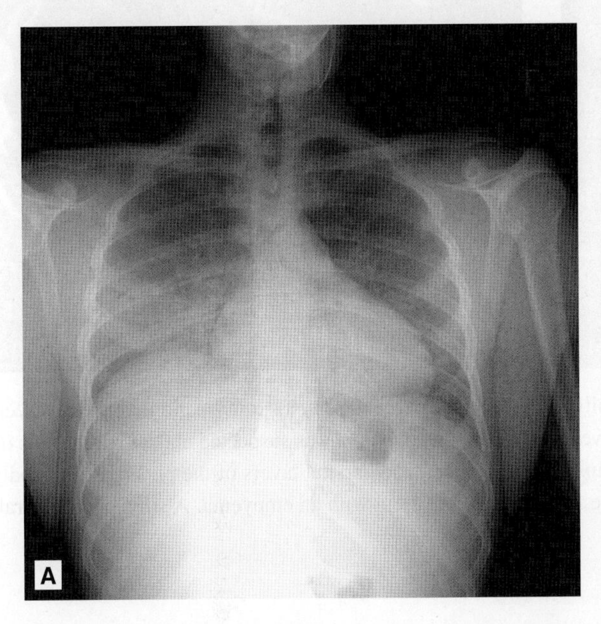

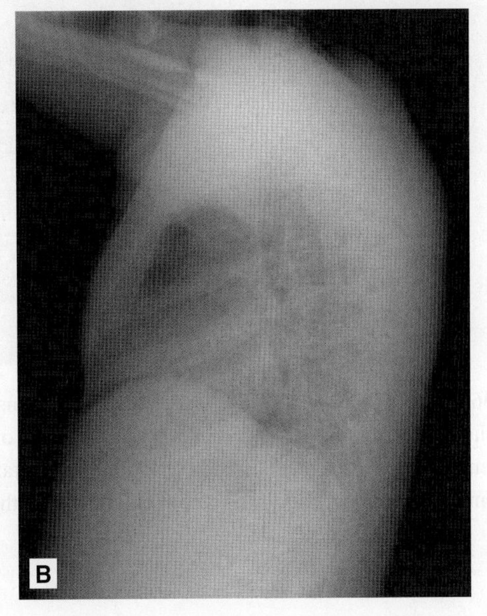

FIGURE 5.35 ■ Atypical Pneumonia. **A, B:** Frontal and lateral views demonstrate bilateral interstitial prominence with diffuse bilateral haziness present in this patient with Mycoplasma pneumonia.

Radiographic Summary

An empyema is a collection of pus in the pleural space or fissures. The initial radiographic study is a standard 2-view chest radiograph, looking for the presence of a pleural effusion.

Thickening of the pleural space on a chest radiograph in the correct clinical setting is suggestive of empyema. Other causes of pleural space thickening include pleural fat, hemothorax, mesothelioma, and benign fibrous tumor of the pleura. Chest CT ideally should be performed with IV contrast because contrast enhances the pleural layers and nonenhancing fluid collection becomes more conspicuous. Ultrasound is superior to CT in differentiating between free or loculated effusions and can guide thoracentesis.

Clinical Implications

An empyema is defined by the presence of bacterial organisms on Gram stain of the pleural fluid or frank pus with pleural fluid aspiration.

Most empyemas are caused by bacterial pneumonia. Indications for thoracentesis in the presence of an effusion include: free-flowing and thicker than 10 mm on decubitus radiograph, presence of loculations, thickened parietal pleura on IV contrast CT scan, or clear delineation by ultrasound. Pleural fluid should be sent for cell count with differential, Gram stain, culture, total protein, lactate dehydrogenase, glucose, and pH. Early intervention decreases the mortality rate associated with empyema. Interventions include tube thoracostomy, intrapleural administration of fibrinolytic agents, thoracoscopic debridement with VATS (video-assisted thoracoscopic surgery), or decortication.

Pearls

1. A lateral radiograph is much more sensitive and specific in detecting small pleural effusions than a portable AP chest radiograph. If the patient can tolerate it, always obtain PA and lateral views of the chest (more information for approximately half the cost). The additional radiation exposure is negligible.
2. Parapneumonic effusions that are free flowing and layer greater than 10 mm on a lateral decubitus radiograph should be sampled by thoracentesis.

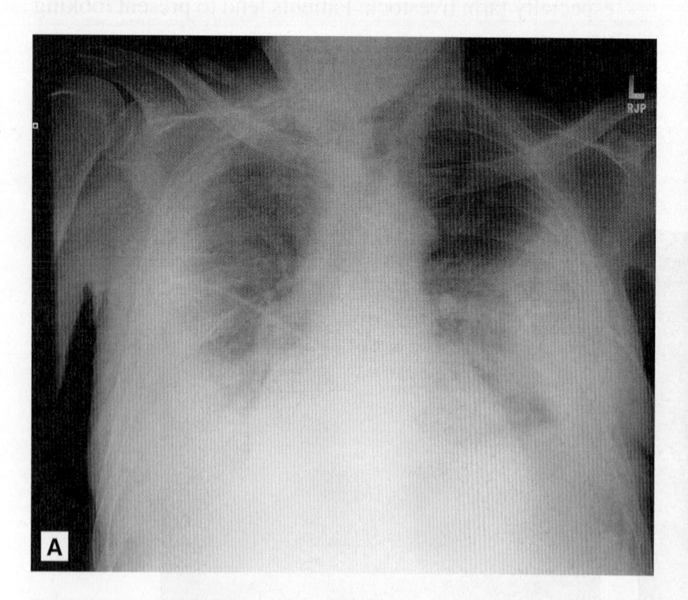

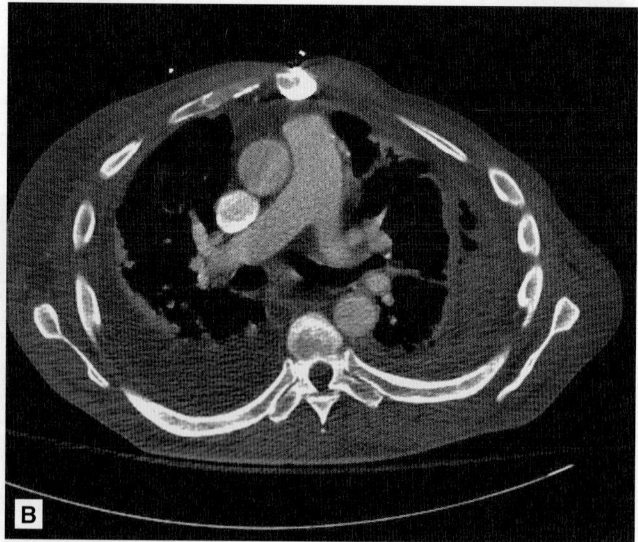

FIGURE 5.36 ■ Empyema. **A, B:** There is a pleural-based density in the left lower lung. Upon closer inspection, a subtle crescent of air can be seen medially within the opacity (partially obscured by the overlying lead). An empyema was suspected and a CT scan was ordered. The CT image demonstrates a left pleural fluid collection that contains air. The visceral and parietal layers of the pleura are markedly thickened and show some enhancement. Notice the "split pleural sign;" the findings are consistent with an empyema. A simple left pleural effusion is also seen.

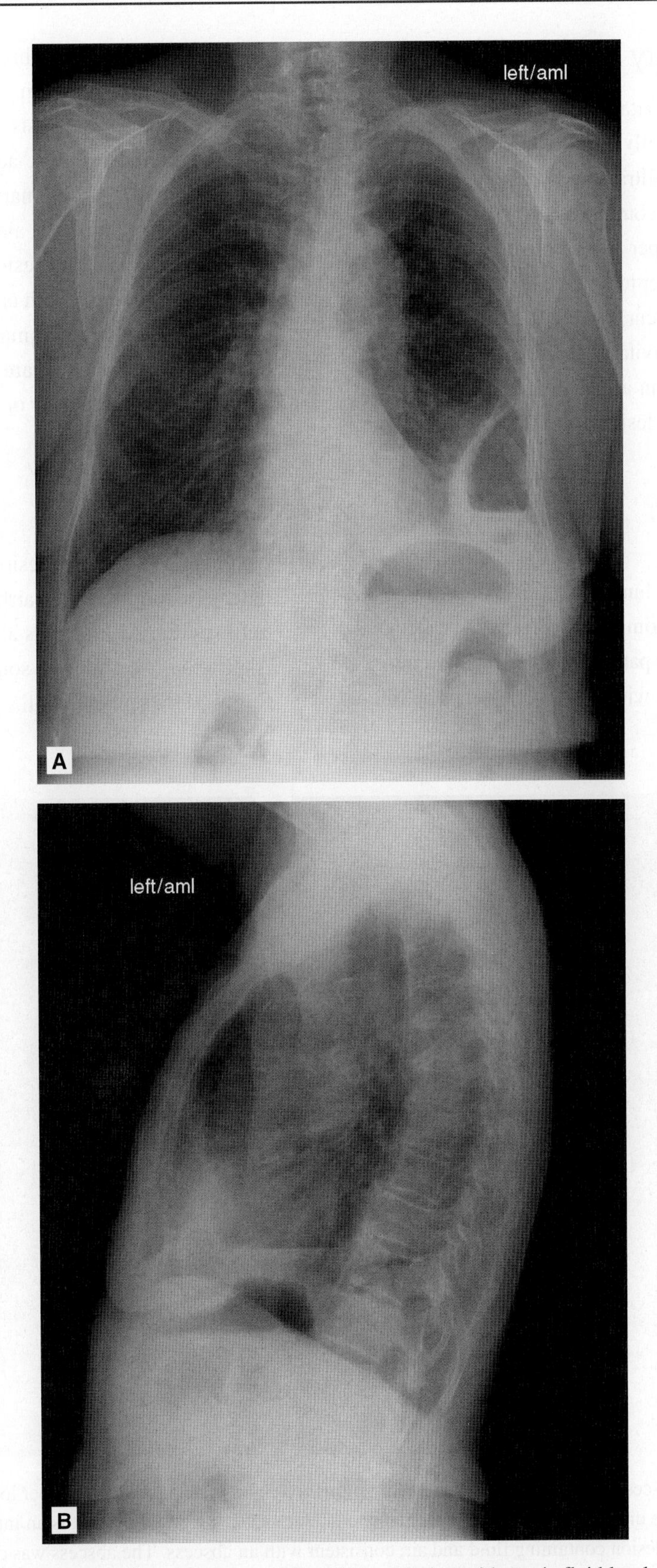

FIGURE 5.37 ■ Empyema. **A, B:** Frontal radiograph shows a pleural-based lesion with an air-fluid level, which projects over the heart on the lateral view, consistent with an empyema. Note that the lesion has different dimensions on the PA view when compared to the lateral view. These findings (flat and oblong) suggest a pleural-based lesion instead of an intra-parenchymal lesion.

Radiographic Summary

A pulmonary abscess is a cavitation of the lung parenchyma resulting from necrosis usually due to microbial infection. Radiographs will show an infiltrate with a cavity, usually with an air-fluid level. The most commonly affected sites are the posterior segment of the upper lobes (mostly right) and the superior segments of the lower lobes (the dependent segments where aspiration tends to occur). A chest radiograph is usually sufficient to identify a cavitary lesion. However, CT scan can be helpful to assess for an associated mass lesion and to differentiate a parenchymal lesion (abscess) from a pleural lesion (empyema).

Clinical Implications

The majority of patients with lung abscesses will present with an insidious course of symptoms that worsens over weeks to months. Necrosis of the lung parenchyma results in a pulmonary abscess, while necrosis within the pleural space, either through direct extension or through a bronchopleural fistula, results in empyema formation.

The differential diagnosis of a cavitary lung lesion includes: anaerobic bacteria, aerobic bacteria, fungi, mycobacteria, neoplasm, pulmonary sequestration, bronchiectasis, cysts and bullae with air-fluid levels, and empyema. Identification of a cavitary lesion prompts immediate initiation of antibiotic therapy with anaerobic coverage. Almost all pulmonary abscesses can be managed with antibiotics alone. Indications for intervention are life-threatening hemoptysis, bronchopleural fistula, tumor or empyema and a residual cavity after treatment.

Pearls

1. An upper lobe cavitary lesion is tuberculosis until proven otherwise, and requires airborne respiratory precautions until sputum AFB smears are negative.
2. Aspiration is a common source of pulmonary abscesses, followed by septic emboli.

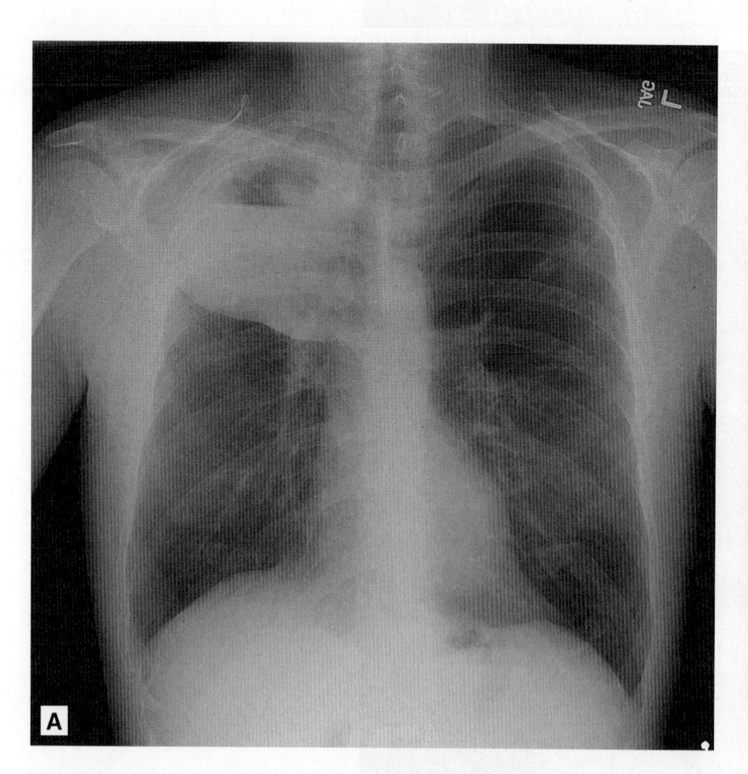

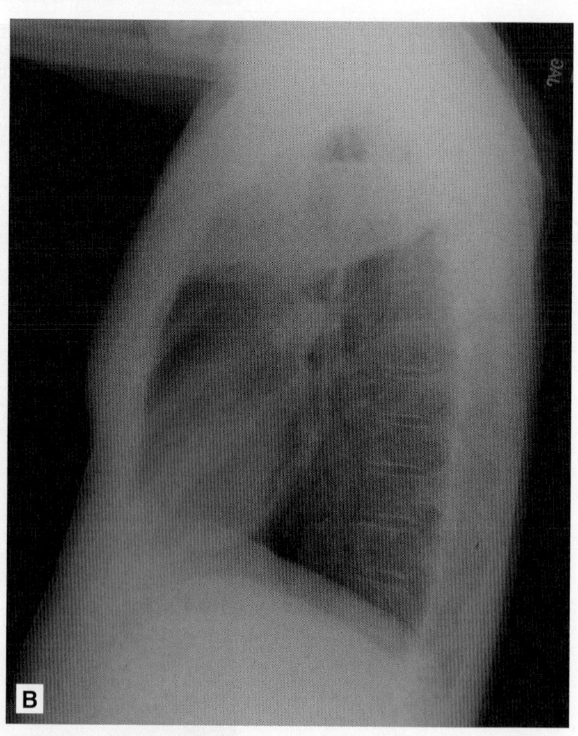

FIGURE 5.38 ■ Pulmonary Abscess. **A-D:** Frontal and lateral radiographs demonstrate a large right upper lobe lesion with an air-fluid level. The lesion is roughly of the same dimensions on both the frontal and lateral views, suggesting that it is an intraparenchymal lesion. CT scan shows a large intraparenchymal lesion containing fluid and air, consistent with an abscess. The abscess was due to *M. kansaii*.

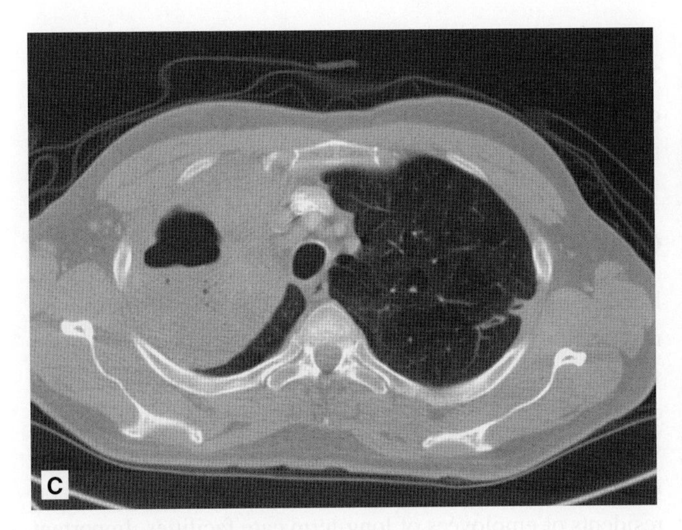

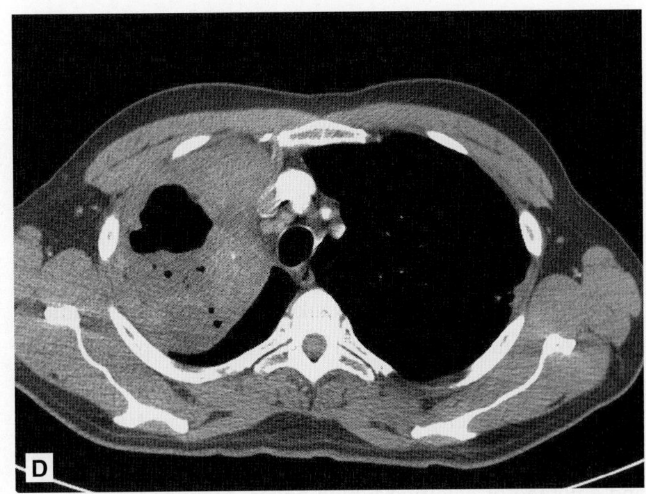

FIGURE 5.38 ■ *(Continued)*

3. To differentiate empyema from a parenchymal abscess, pay attention to the relationship of the visceral pleural to the fluid collection. An empyema is characterized by the "split pleura sign." The two layers of the pleura split around the fluid collection because the collection resides within the pleural space, between the two layers of pleura. A peripherally-located parenchymal abscess does not exhibit this sign. Often, one can appreciate a wedge-shaped remnant of normal lung parenchyma between the abscess and adjacent visceral pleura, indicating that the fluid collection resides within the lung and is invested by the visceral pleura.

Radiographic Summary

Tuberculosis (TB) is an infectious disease caused by *Mycobaterium tuberculosis*, which is transmitted through inhalation of organism from aerosolized saliva or sputum from a patient with active disease. Primary pulmonary TB is asymptomatic in over 90% of patients and can only be identified by the development of a positive TB skin test or the presence of a Ghon focus or Ranke complex on chest radiography. A Ghon focus refers to the initial site of parenchymal involvement at the time of first infection. It appears as a small parenchymal opacity anywhere in the lung, and is nonspecific. A Ranke complex is the combination of a Ghon focus and enlarged or calcified lymph nodes. Lymphadenopathy is the radiologic hallmark of primary pulmonary TB, but this also is very nonspecific.

Postprimary TB, or reactivation TB, is the most common clinical form of TB, triggered by endogenous reactivation of dormant foci. The radiographic hallmark of postprimary TB is parenchymal opacities located in the apical and posterior segments of the upper lobes (84%) and the superior segment of the lower lobes (12%), often associated with cavitation.

Miliary, or disseminated, TB consists of innumerable, 1-3 mm noncalcified nodules distributed uniformly throughout the lung parenchyma. This is called a micronodular pattern, and it has a basilar predominance with miliary TB.

Clinical Implications

Most primary pulmonary TB is asymptomatic. Patients with reactivation TB may present with low-grade fever, night sweats, malaise, weight loss, productive cough. Over time, cough is often associated with hemoptysis. TB should be considered in patients of high-risk groups such as immigrants from endemic regions, IV drug users, patients with AIDS, and residents or employees of long-term care facilities. Important diagnostic testing in high-risk patients who present with respiratory complaints includes TB skin test, chest radiography, and smears for acid-fast bacilli.

All patients with suspected TB should wear a mask and be placed on airborne precautions. Initial therapy is with a four drug regimen until susceptibility tests are available.

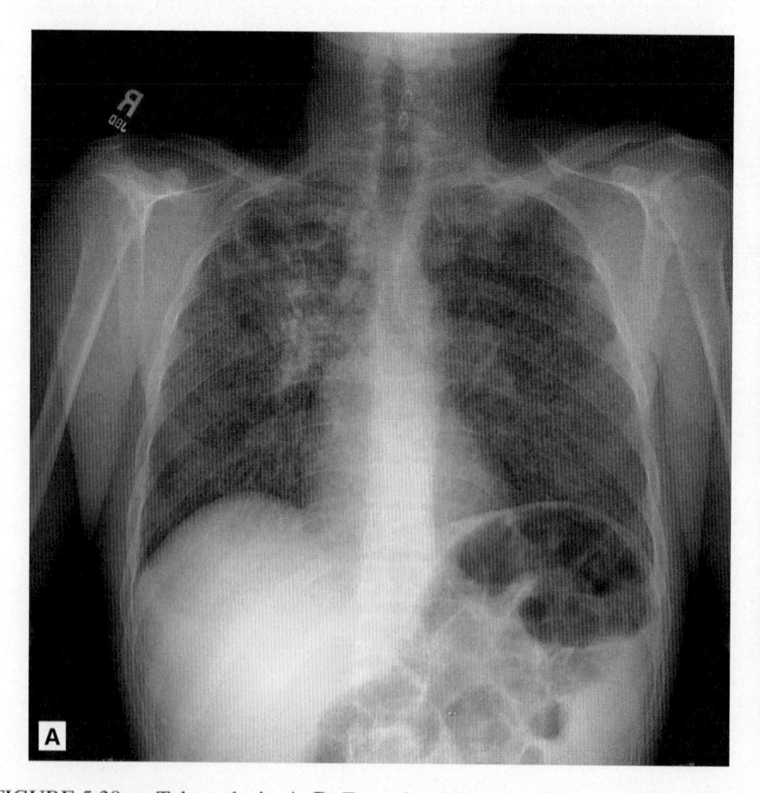

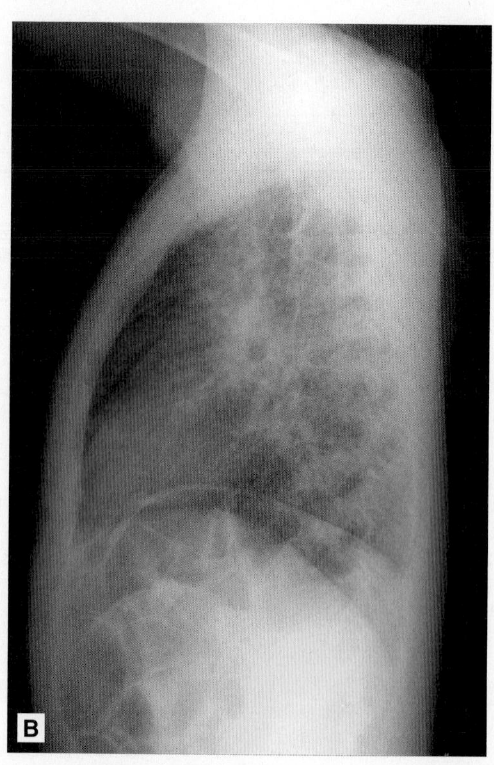

FIGURE 5.39 ■ Tuberculosis. **A, B:** Frontal and lateral radiographs demonstrate a miliary nodular pattern bilaterally. Also, there is a large cavitary lesion in the right upper lobe and a more subtle opacity in the left upper lobe behind the left clavicle. These findings are classic for reactivation tuberculosis.

Pearls

1. Normal chest radiographs are common early in the course of the disease, and occur in 25% to 40% of patients at first presentation.
2. Hilar lymphadenopathy may be the only initial finding.
3. Primary TB may present as a non-specific opacity located anywhere in the lungs. Secondary TB has a predilection for the upper lobes and is typically cavitary.
4. TB is an AIDS-defining illness and should prompt testing.

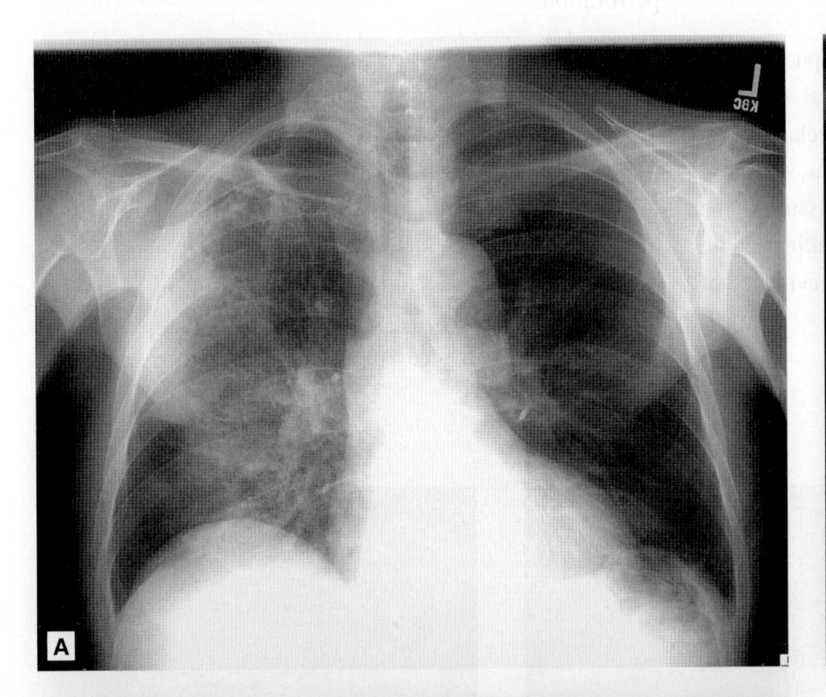

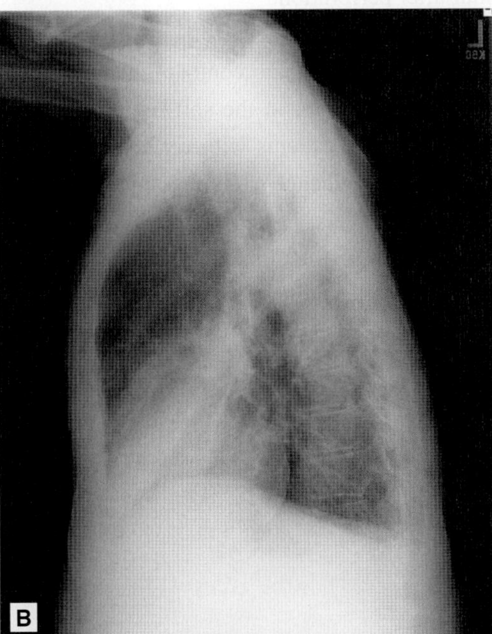

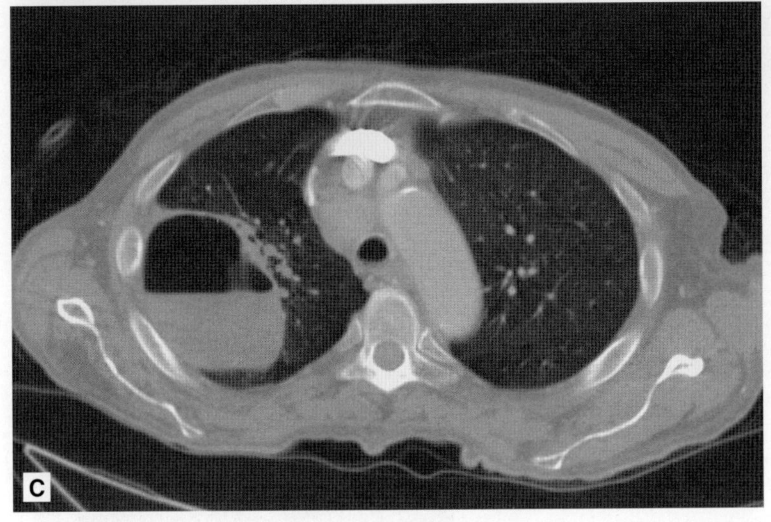

FIGURE 5.40 ■ Tuberculosis. **A-C:** Frontal and lateral radiographs show opacities in the right lower, mid, and upper lung. The lesion in the right upper lung demonstrates cavitation, which is confirmed on the CT scan. This patient was diagnosed with tuberculosis.

Radiographic Summary

Esophageal rupture is a full thickness tear of the esophageal wall with leakage of air and orogastric contents into the mediastinum. Plain radiography has a sensitivity of approximately 80-90% in diagnosing esophageal rupture. Abnormalities may not be evident on chest radiograph until as long as one hour after perforation.

Findings of esophageal rupture may include pneumomediastinum, mediastinal contour changes, pleural effusion, or subcutaneous air in the soft tissues of the neck. Ninety-five percent of patients with cervical perforations will have radiographic evidence of emphysema in the soft tissues of the prevertebral space in the neck, while 40% of patients with intrathoracic perforations will have radiographic evidence of air in the mediastinum.

The diagnosis of esophageal perforation can be confirmed with either CT scan or with water-soluble contrast esophagram. Barium is superior in demonstrating small perforations, but causes an inflammatory response in the surrounding tissue if contrast leak does occur. Endoscopy should not be performed in the evaluation of esophageal perforation.

Clinical Implications

The most common cause of esophageal perforation is iatrogenic, due to medical instrumentation or paraesophageal surgery. A sudden increase in intraesophageal pressure combined with negative intrathoracic pressure, as occurs with intense straining or vomiting, can also result in esophageal rupture known as Boerhaave's syndrome. Patients classically

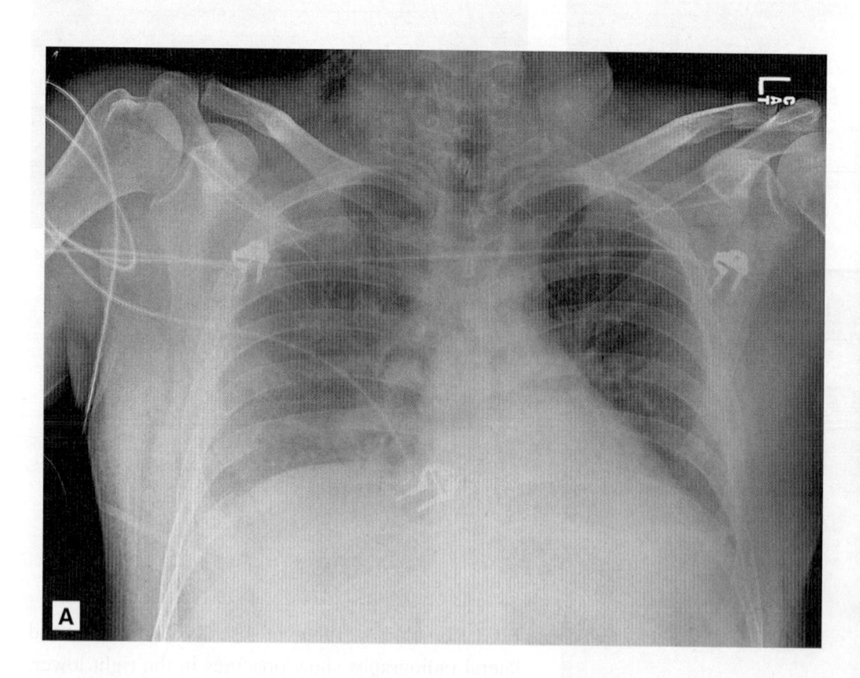

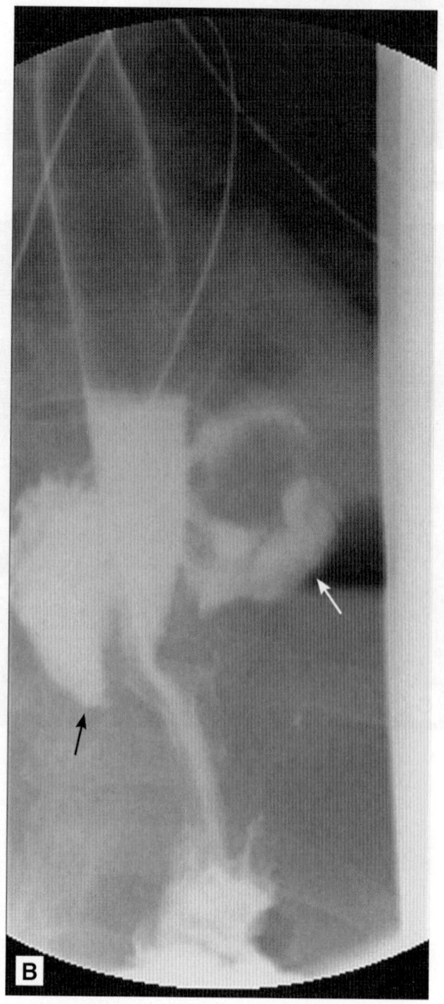

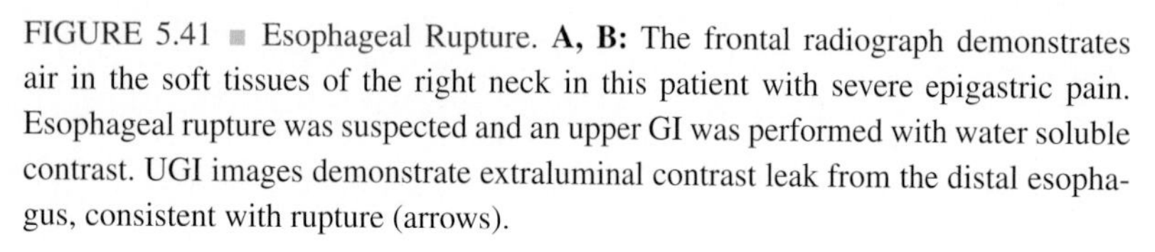
FIGURE 5.41 ■ Esophageal Rupture. **A, B:** The frontal radiograph demonstrates air in the soft tissues of the right neck in this patient with severe epigastric pain. Esophageal rupture was suspected and an upper GI was performed with water soluble contrast. UGI images demonstrate extraluminal contrast leak from the distal esophagus, consistent with rupture (arrows).

present with a history of severe retching and vomiting followed by excruciating retrosternal chest and upper abdominal pain. Caustic ingestions, trauma, Barrett's esophagus, infectious ulcers, and pill esophagitis have also been associated with spontaneous perforation.

Patients may present with a myriad of symptoms including chest, back, or epigastric pain, dysphonia, hoarseness, dysphagia, odynophagia, dyspnea, or hematemesis. Clinical findings may include subcutaneous cervical air, neck hematoma, blood in the NG aspirate, or Hamman's sign, a crunching noise heard when auscultating the chest that corresponds to mediastinal emphysema. If confirmed, surgery is generally required for thoracic perforations, and medical management is often appropriate for cervical perforations.

Pearls

1. Most episodes of esophageal perforation are evident on plain-radiograph radiography.
2. The most common site of rupture in Boerhaave's syndrome is the left posterolateral aspect of the distal esophagus.

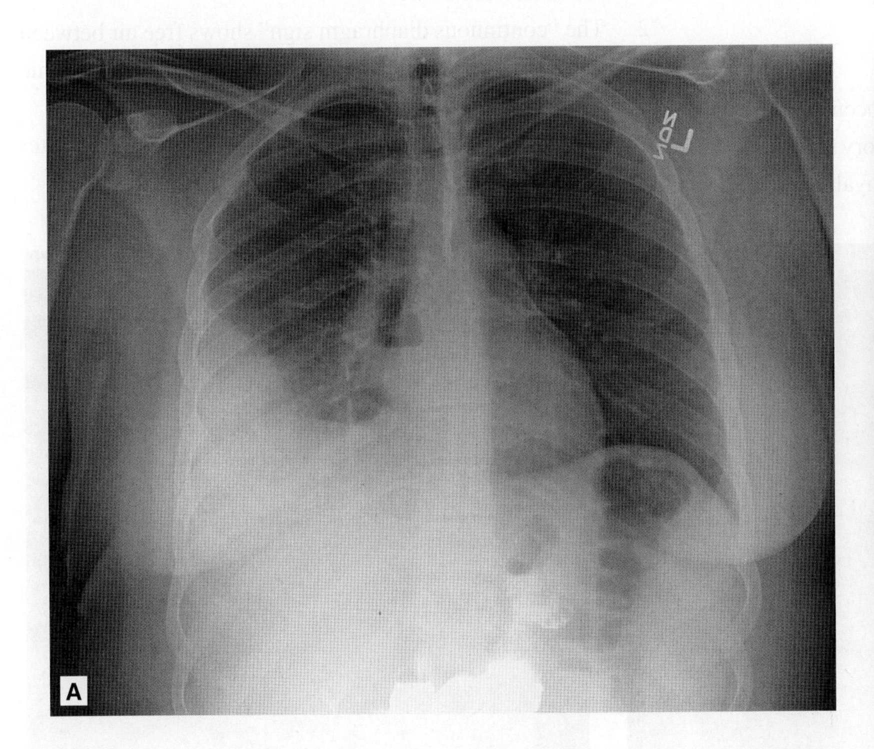

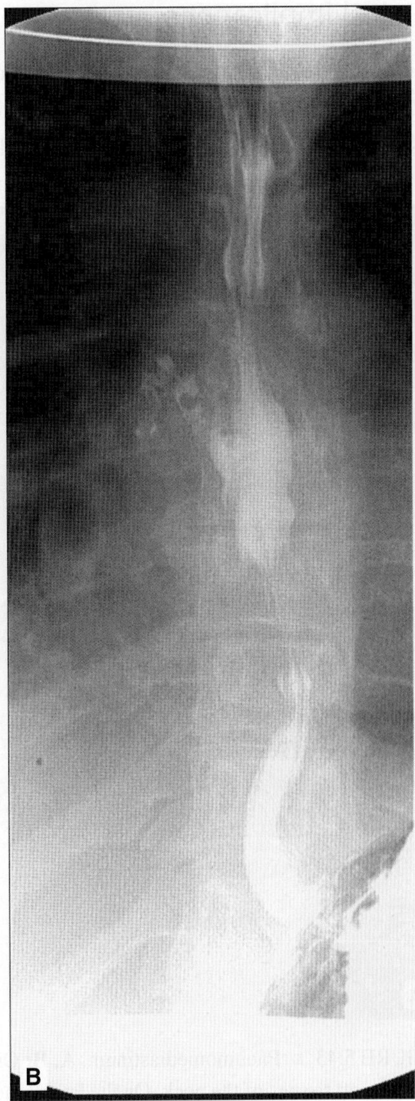

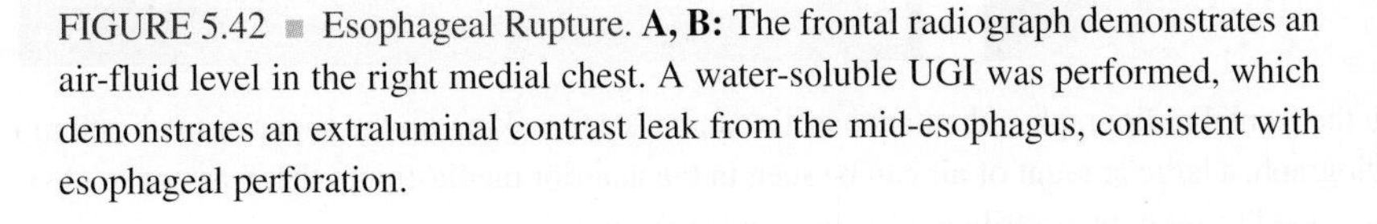
FIGURE 5.42 ■ Esophageal Rupture. **A, B:** The frontal radiograph demonstrates an air-fluid level in the right medial chest. A water-soluble UGI was performed, which demonstrates an extraluminal contrast leak from the mid-esophagus, consistent with esophageal perforation.

Radiographic Summary

Pneumopericardium refers to air in the pericardial space surrounding the heart. It can be seen on conventional chest radiograph as a black stripe of air outlining the normal contour of the heart, with the thin pericardium sharply outlined by air density on either side. This stripe of air can often be seen between the heart and the diaphragm, making the diaphragm visible in the midline where it is normally obscured by the heart. This is known as the "continuous diaphragm sign." Pneumopericardium is differentiated from pneumomediastinum by the degree of superior extension of the air. In pneumopericardium, the air is superiorly confined to the level of the pulmonary artery and ascending aorta. In pneumomediastinum, it can extend up to the superior mediastinum and neck.

Clinical Implications

Pneumopericardium is a rare entity, but occurs most commonly in settings where augmented ventilatory support is necessary, such as in ARDS or in infants with hyaline membrane disease requiring mechanical ventilation. Other causes of pneumopericardium include thoracic surgery, infectious pericarditis with gas-producing organisms, trauma, and fistula between the pericardium and an adjacent air-containing organ.

Prognosis is dependent upon the etiology. Most cases of pneumopericardium will spontaneously resolve with bed rest and close monitoring. If there are any signs of tamponade or infection, immediate drainage is necessary.

Pearls

1. Pneumopericardium extends to the level of the pulmonary artery, whereas pneumomediastinum extends beyond to the neck and above.
2. The "continuous diaphragm sign" shows free air between the mediastinum and diaphragm, and is pathognomonic for pneumomediastinum.
3. Cases of pneumopericardium have been reported after administration of the Heimlich maneuver.

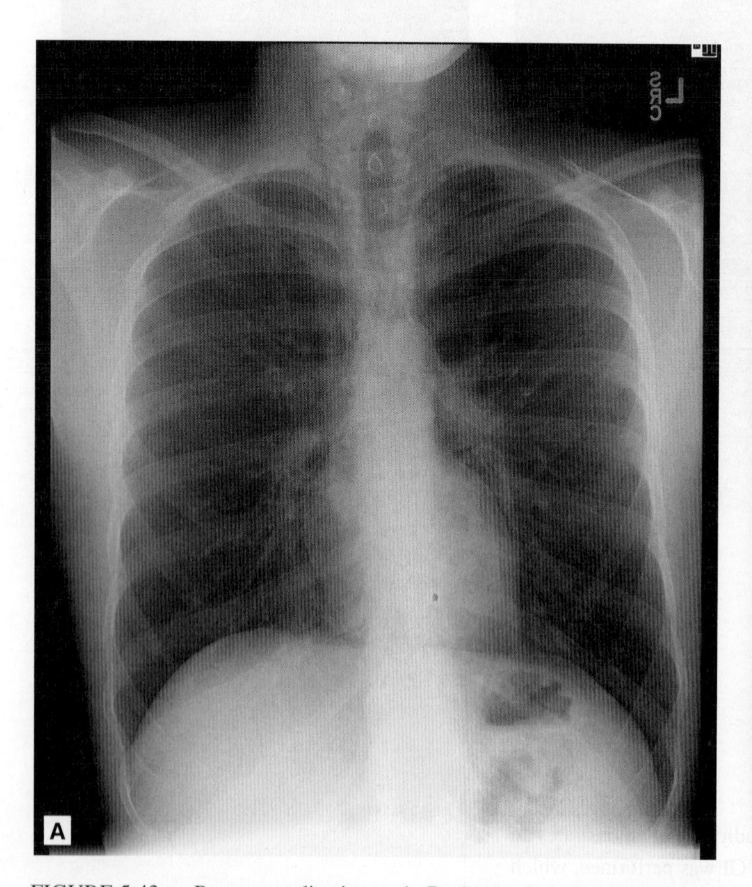

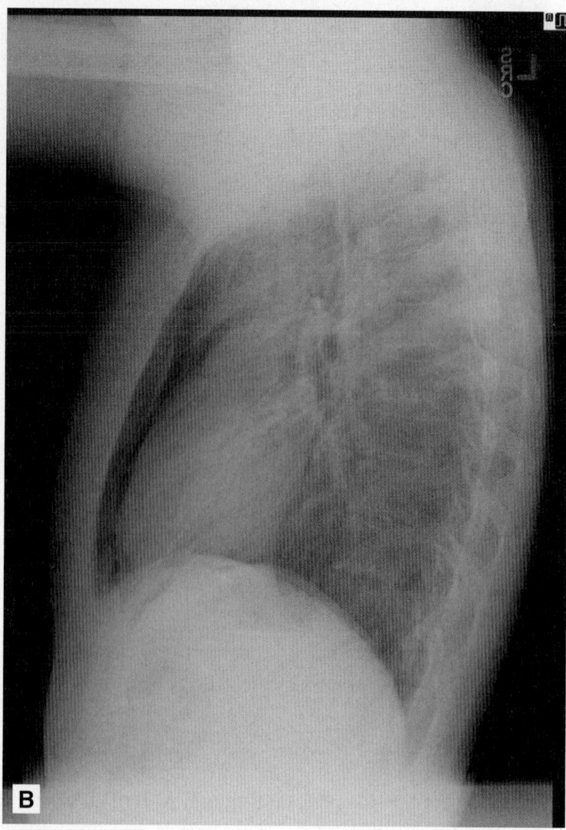

FIGURE 5.43 ■ Pneumomediastinum. **A, B:** On the frontal radiograph, subcutaneous air can be seen tracking up the superior mediastinum into the soft tissues of the neck. On the lateral radiograph, a large amount of air can be seen in the anterior mediastinum that was not so obvious on the frontal radiograph. This patient's pneumomediastinum was attributed to air-trapping from asthma.

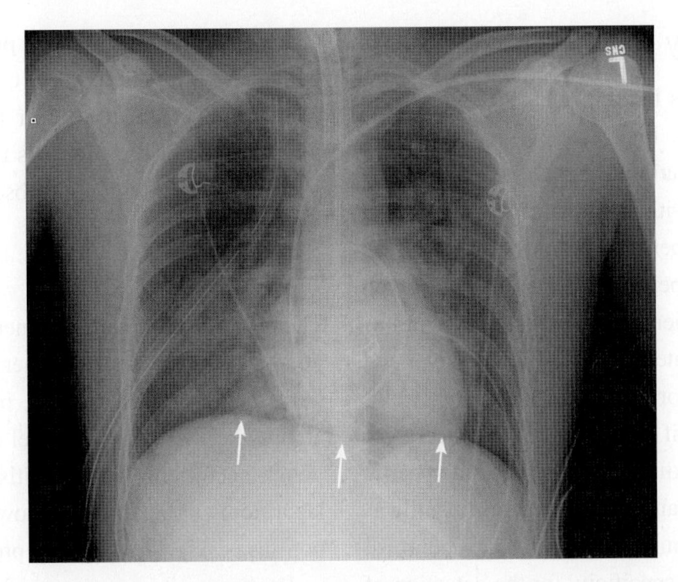

FIGURE 5.44 ■ Pneumomediastinum. This frontal radiograph demonstrates the so-called "continuous diaphragm sign," pathognomonic for pneumomediastinum (arrows). Additionally, a thin crescent of air can be seen adjacent to the right heart border.

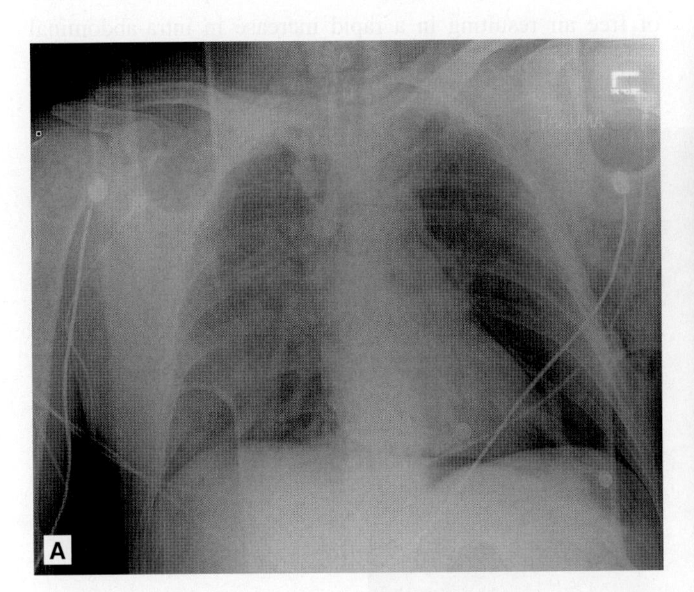

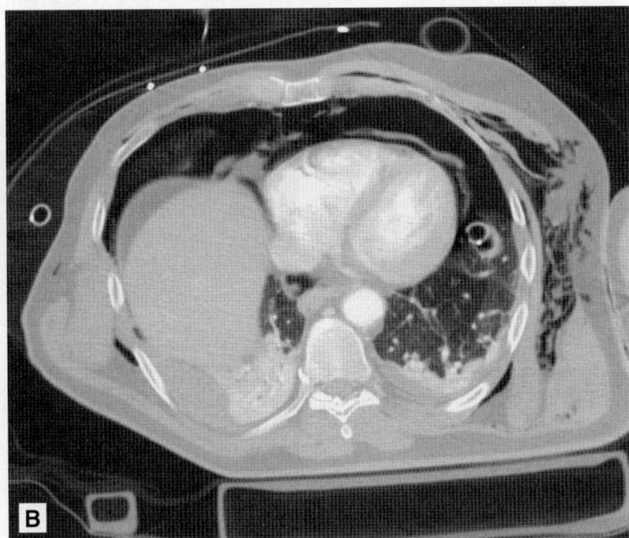

FIGURE 5.45 ■ Pneumopericardium. **A, B:** The frontal radiograph demonstrates multiple findings in this trauma patient. In addition to the left pneumothorax (note the deep sulcus sign), there is also pneumomediastinum and pneumopericardium. Note the sliver of air between the epicardium and the pericardium. The accompanying CT image clearly demonstrates the pneumopericardium as well as bilateral pneumothoraces (the right PTX is not well seen on the frontal radiograph).

Radiographic Summary

Pneumoperitoneum appears as free air under the diaphragm on upright chest radiography. Free air appears as a black stripe under the diaphragm, outlining both edges of the thin diaphragm muscle, with air within the lung parenchyma on one side, and air within the peritoneum on the other. If an upright radiograph cannot be performed, then the radiograph can be performed with the patient in the left lateral decubitus position, and air can be seen interposed between the liver and the abdominal wall. Upright or left lateral decubitus views of the abdomen are essential if there is clinical concern for pneumoperitoneum and are extremely sensitive and specific for the detection of very small amounts of free gas (as little as a few mL of gas). Supine abdominal radiographs, by contrast, have very poor sensitivity and specificity for the detection of pneumoperitoneum.

Abdominal CT also has a high sensitivity and specificity for detecting free air, and should be performed if radiographs are negative and clinical suspicion remains high. A CT can also identify the source of the pneumoperitoneum. The gastric bubble on the patient's left can mimic pneumoperitoneum. Other mimics include linear atelectasis at the base of the lungs, a loop of bowel that is interposed between diaphragm and liver, and a subphrenic abscess.

Clinical Implications

The most common cause of pneumoperitoneum is a perforated duodenal or gastric ulcer. Other causes include ruptured diverticulum, penetrating trauma, perforated megacolon (associated with inflammatory bowel disease or with post-operative ileus), necrotizing enterocolitis, ischemic bowel, status post laparotomy or laparoscopy, bowel injury after endoscopy, and non-invasive positive airway pressure.

Pneumoperitoneum secondary to a perforated viscus requires prompt administration of IV antibiotics to cover intra-abdominal flora, fluids, pain control, and surgical consultation. Tension pneumoperitoneum (TP) is the rapid accumulation of free air resulting in a rapid increase in intra-abdominal

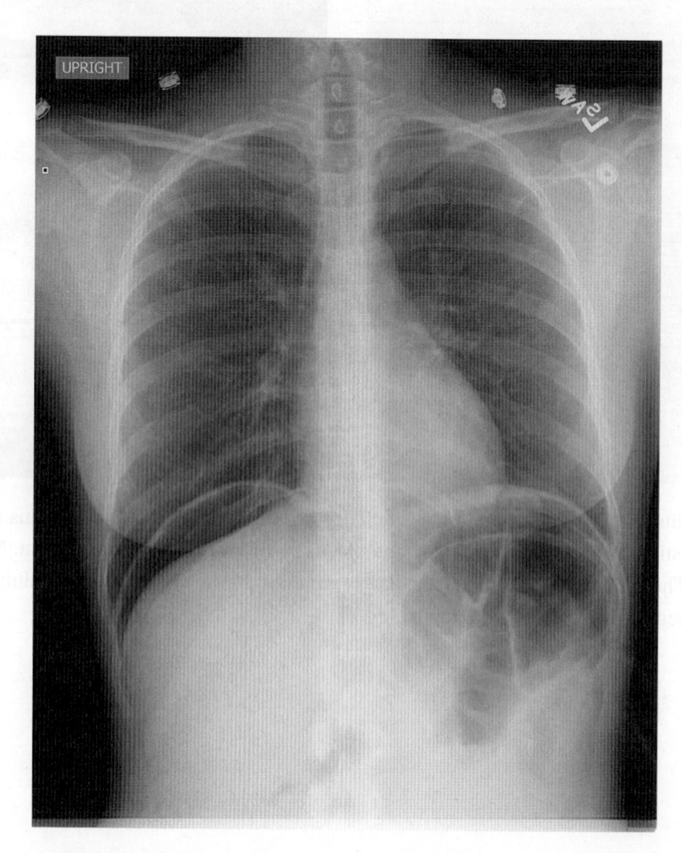

FIGURE 5.46 ■ Free Air under the Diaphragm. This frontal radiograph demonstrates free intraperitoneal air under both hemi–diaphragms. Also, note that air can be seen on both sides of the colon wall, consistent with "Rigler's sign." The source of this patient's free air was from recent abdominal surgery.

pressure. The increased pressure can compress the IVC, leading to decreased venous return to the heart, and subsequent hemodynamic instability. The increased pressure elevates the diaphragm, decreasing lung volume and ventilation, and leading to respiratory failure.

Pearls

1. A pneumoperitoneum is deliberately created when patients undergo laparoscopic surgery. A small amount of free air after laparoscopy is normal in the immediate post-operative period but should gradually resolve within 1 week. Persistent massive pneumoperitoneum or increasing pneumoeritoneum are warning signs and should prompt further evaluation with a CT scan of the abdomen and pelvis.
2. Always obtain upright or left lateral decubitus views of the abdomen when assessing for pneumoperitoneum. Supine radiographs of the abdomen have very poor sensitivity and specificity.
3. On a supine abdominal radiograph, look for Rigler's sign: free intraperitoneal gas outlining the bowel serosa. Another sign is the "football sign": free gas outlining the falciform ligament of the liver. Massive amounts of pneumoperitoneum are needed to produce this appearance.
4. TP should be considered in any decompensating patient with massive abdominal distension.

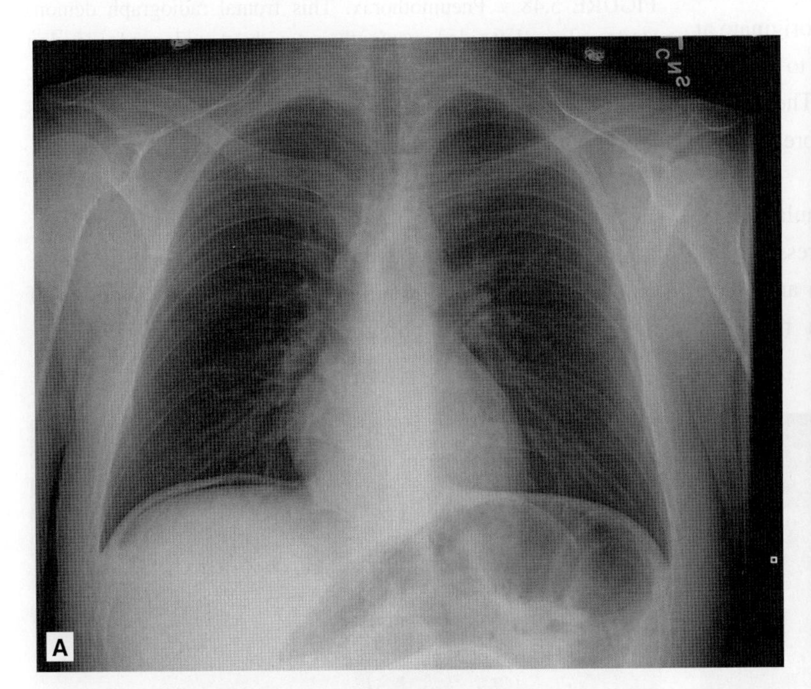

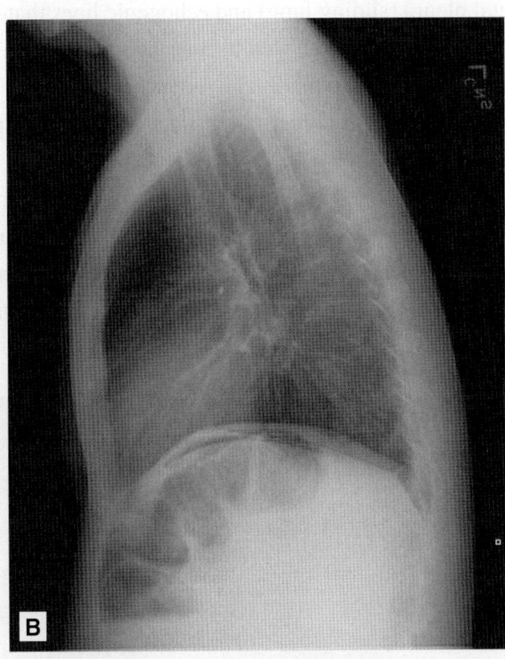

FIGURE 5.47 ■ Free Air under the Diaphragm. **A, B:** Frontal and lateral radiographs demonstrate a thin crescent of air under the right hemidiaphragm consistent with free intraperitoneal air. The source of this patient's free air was from recent abdominal surgery.

Radiographic Summary

A pneumothorax is a collection of air in the pleural space. The main radiographic finding on chest radiography is the presence of a white, curvilinear visceral pleural line that runs parallel to the chest wall with the absence of lung markings in the lung periphery in the space beyond this line. A pneumothorax may be identified on an upright, supine, or lateral decubitus chest radiograph. On the upright view, the pleural air accumulates in an apicolateral location. On a supine AP view, pleural air will accumulate along the costophrenic sulcus, creating a "deep sulcus sign."

The first-line modality in imaging a pneumothorax has traditionally been with chest radiography. Pneumothorax may be detected by bedside ultrasonography. Pneumothorax is assessed by looking for sliding of the visceral pleura on parietal pleura (sliding lung) and echogenic lines that originate at the visceral–parietal pleural interface and extend to the bottom of the ultrasound image (comet tail artifact). The lack of sliding lung and comet tail artifact indicates the presence of air in the pleural space.

Tension pneumothorax refers to the accumulation of air under pressure in the pleural space compressing the ipsilateral lung, and displacing the mediastinum and other structures toward the opposite side. This can result in cardiopulmonary collapse and is a medical emergency. Radiographs may show a shift of the trachea and mediastinum to the contralateral side and flattening or inversion of the ipsilateral hemidiaphragm.

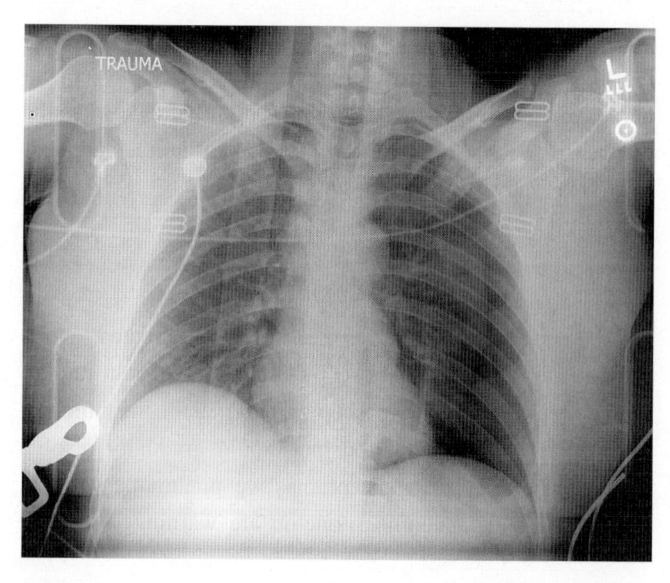

FIGURE 5.48 ■ Pneumothorax. This frontal radiograph demonstrates a large left sided pneumothorax without evidence for tension as there is no significant shift of the mediastinal contents to the right. The etiology of the patient's pneumothorax was from blunt chest trauma.

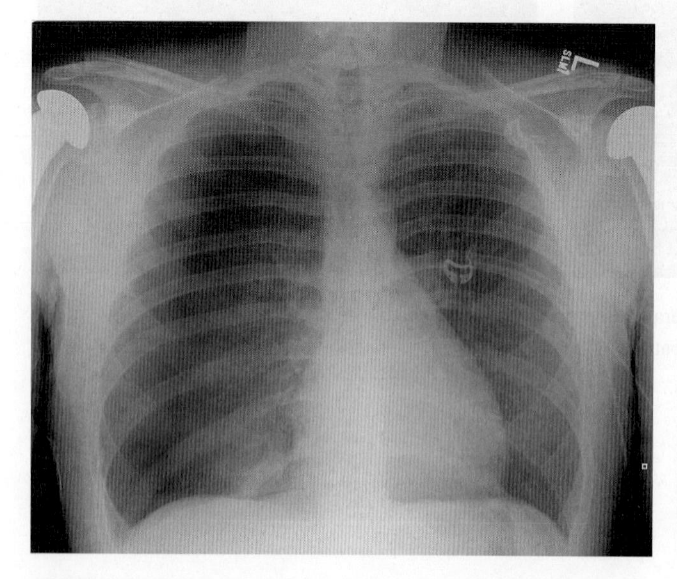

FIGURE 5.49 ■ Pneumothorax. This frontal radiograph demonstrates a large right sided pneumothorax without evidence for tension as there is no significant shift of the mediastinal contents to the left. The etiology of this pneumothorax was never established. Bilateral shoulder hemiarthroplasties are noted.

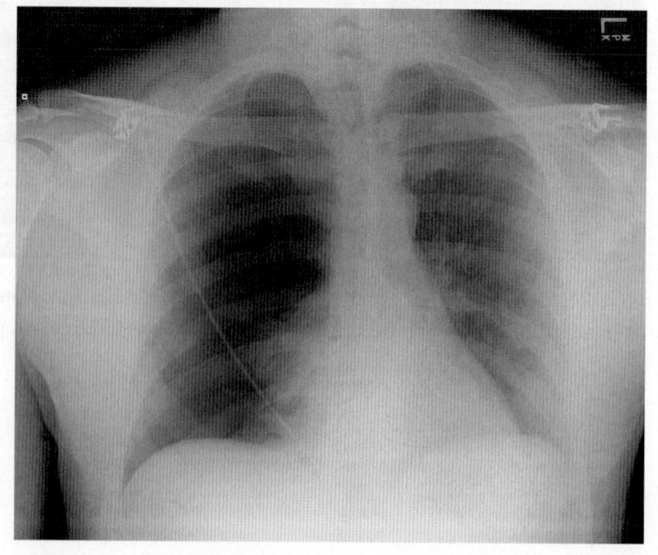

FIGURE 5.50 ■ Tension Pneumothorax. There is a very large right sided pneumothorax with deviation of the mediastinal contents to the left.

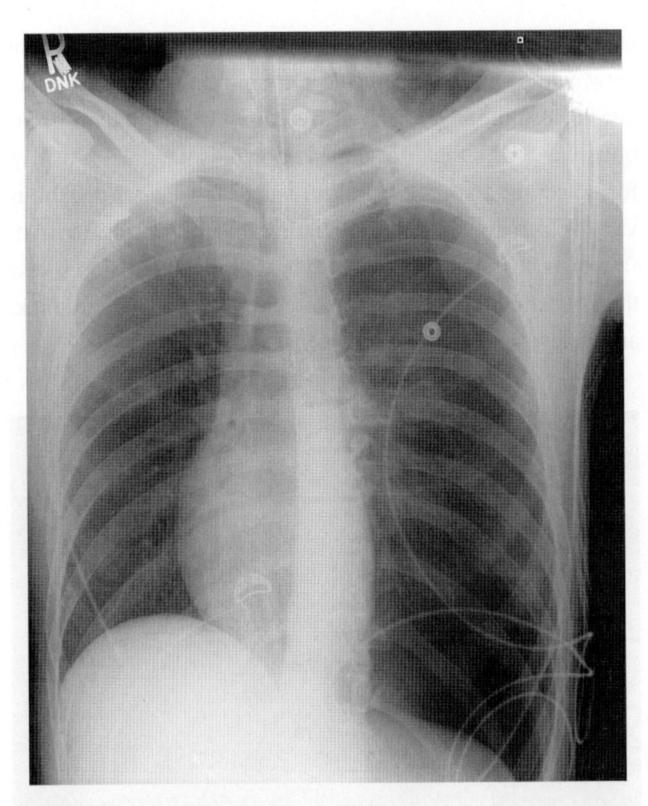

FIGURE 5.51 ■ Tension Pneumothorax. There is a very large left sided pneumothorax with deviation of the mediastinal contents to the right (note the tracheal and cardiac deviation).

Clinical Implications

A spontaneous pneumothorax may present with tachypnea, hypoxia, and unilateral diminished or absent breath sounds.

Treatment of pneumothorax ranges from observation to tube thoracostomy. All patients should be placed on supplemental oxygen as this may increase the rate of pneumothorax resorption. Any hemodynamic compromise necessitates decompression with a needle or chest tube.

Pearls

1. A pneumothorax is easiest to identify on an upright AP or a lateral decubitus view of the chest. Look for the white line of the visceral pleura, which has collapsed away from the chest wall.
2. In the presence of hemodynamic compromise and suspected pneumothorax, decompression should be performed prior to radiographic imaging.
3. A tension pneumothorax is a clinical entity and radiographically, produces a contralateral shift of the mediastinum.
4. It is important to distinguish severe bullous emphysema from a pneumothorax.

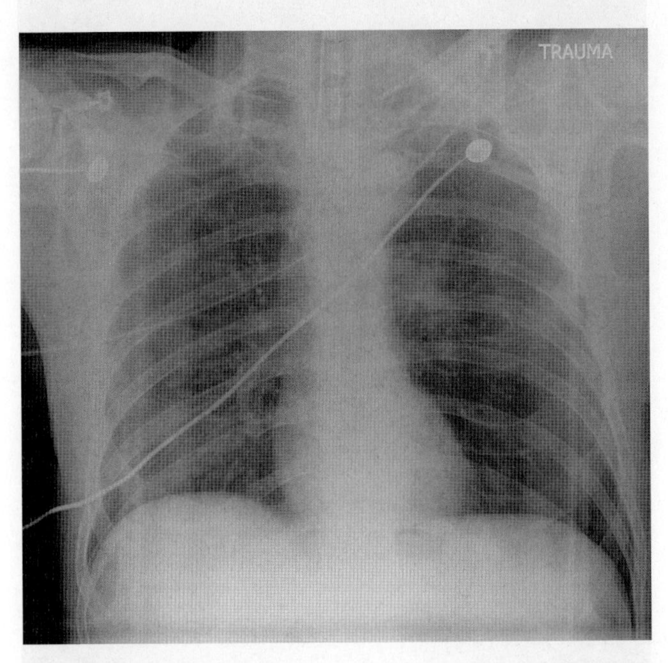

FIGURE 5.52 ■ Deep Sulcus Sign. This frontal radiograph demonstrates a left sided "deep sulcus sign." Note how sharp the left diaphragm appears when compared to the right, and note the increased depth of the left costophrenic angle when compared to the right. These findings imply a left sided subpulmonic pneumothorax.

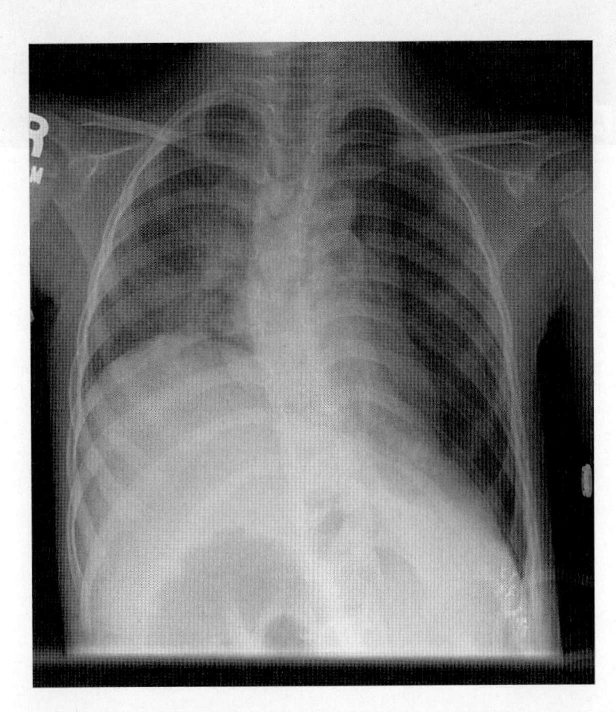

FIGURE 5.53 ■ Deep Sulcus Sign. This frontal radiograph demonstrates a left sided pneumothorax with an associated "deep sulcus sign." Note the increased depth of the left costophrenic angle when compared to the right.

Radiographic Summary

A pleural effusion is the collection of fluid within the pleural space. Pleural effusions appear as dependent radio-opacities on plain radiography. They accumulate in the most dependent portion of the thoracic cavity, and thus layer differently based on the position of the patient. With upright imaging, the lateral view is more sensitive than the PA view for the detection of pleural fluid. Approximately 75 mL of pleural fluid are needed to obscure the posterior costophrenic angle on lateral view, while approximately 175 mL are needed to obscure the lateral costophrenic angle on frontal view. The lateral decubitus view, with the affected side down, is the most sensitive for detecting a small pleural effusion. The lateral decubitus view is also good for differentiating a loculated from a free-flowing effusion. On decubitus views, a small effusion is less than 1.5 cm thick, a moderate effusion is 1.5 to 4.5 cm thick, and large effusions are thicker than 4.5 cm.

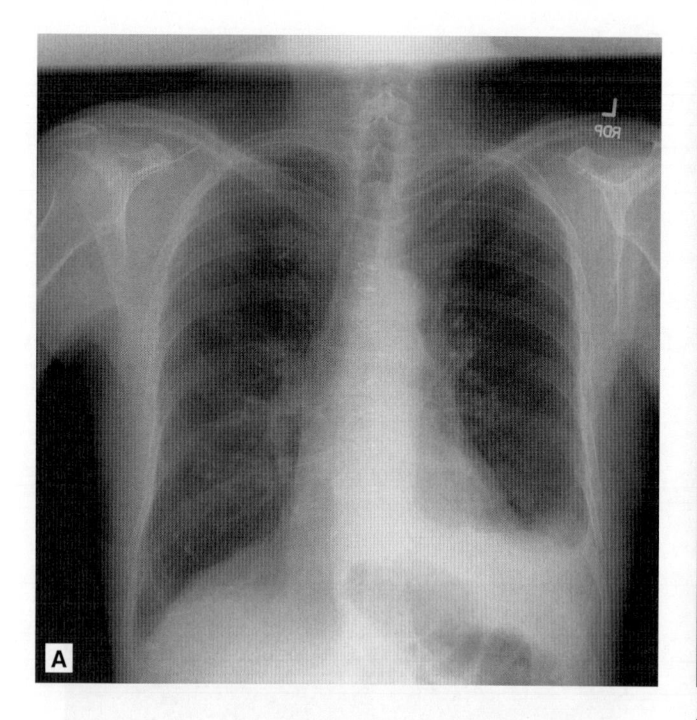

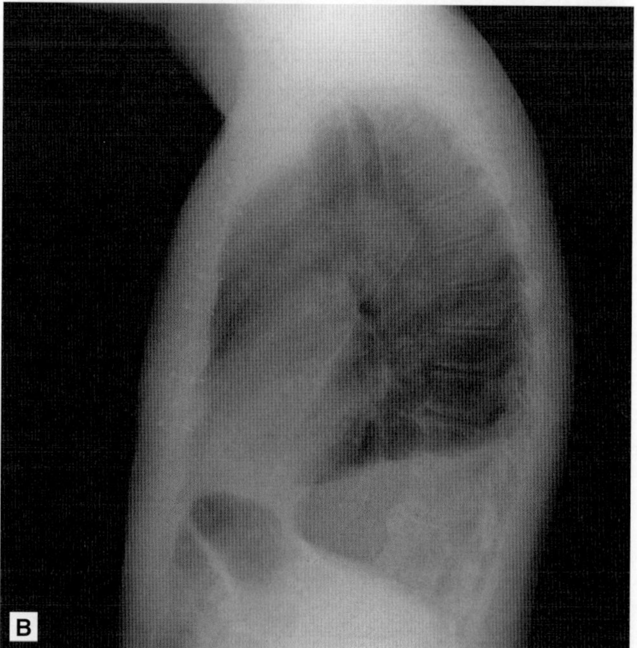

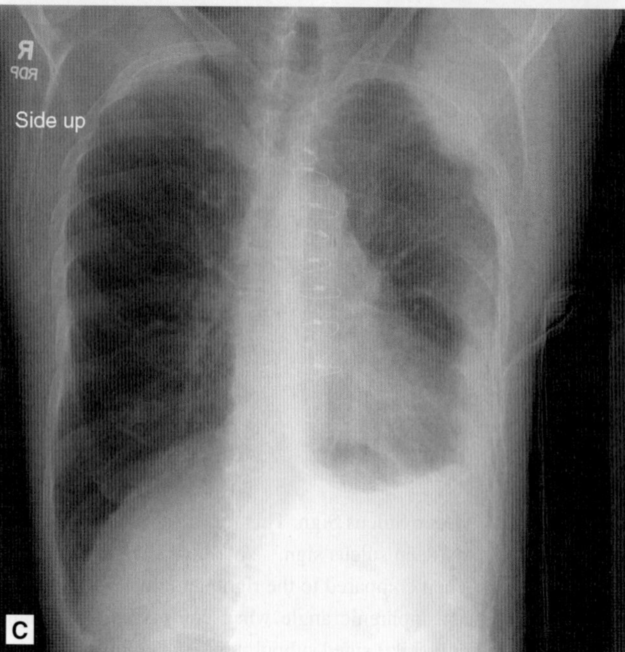

FIGURE 5.54 ■ Pleural Effusion. **A-C:** A left-sided pleural effusion can be seen on the frontal and lateral radiographs. A left lateral decubitus radiograph was performed to demonstrate that the effusion was not loculated but free-flowing.

Large quantities of pleural fluid may accumulate in a subpulmonic location rather than escaping into the general pleural cavity. They can be difficult to detect on chest radiographs because the upper edge of the fluid mimics the contour of the diaphragm. This may be seen as the "lateral peak sign," in which the diaphragm peaks laterally.

Both ultrasound and CT are helpful for detecting small pleural effusions, measuring pleural thickness and characterizing the composition of the fluid. Either can be used to differentiate loculated effusions from solid masses or to facilitate image-guided thoracentesis.

Clinical Implications

The definitive treatment of a pleural effusion is thoracentesis. Pleural fluid should be sent for cell count with differential, gram stain, culture, protein, LDH, amylase and glucose, pH, and cytology. Light's criteria are used to differentiate exudative from transudative effusion. An exudate is probably present if one of the following four criteria are met:

1. Pleural fluid protein/serum protein > 5
2. Pleural fluid LDH > 200 IU/mL
3. Pleural fluid LDH/serum LDH > 0.6
4. Pleural fluid cholesterol greater than or equal to 60 mg/dL

Pearls

1. Large unilateral pleural effusions are suspicious for tuberculosis in young patients and suspicious for malignancy in older patients.
2. Routine use of ultrasound for all diagnostic thoracenteses has been shown to decrease the rate of pneumothorax from approximately 8% to 1%.
3. A lateral radiograph of the chest is much more sensitive and specific for the detection of small pleural effusions than an AP radiograph, especially a portable AP radiograph obtained with the patient supine.

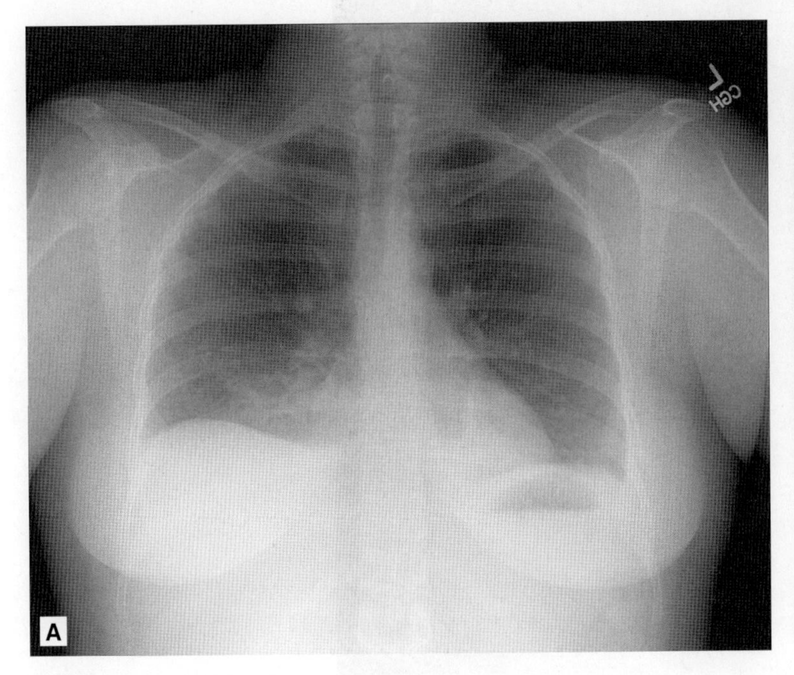

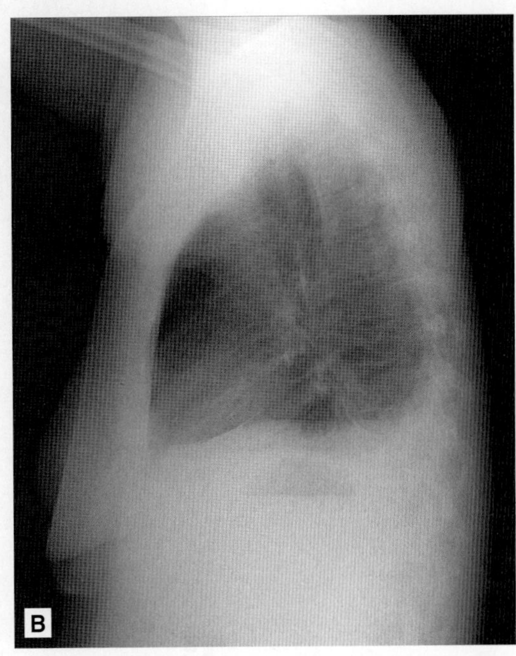

FIGURE 5.55 ■ Pleural Effusion. **A, B:** Note on the frontal radiograph that the peak of the right hemidiaphragm appears to be more prominent with a slight lateral deviation when compared to the left. This is called the "lateral peak sign" and can indicate a subpulmonic pleural effusion. On the lateral view, a pleural effusion is clearly seen.

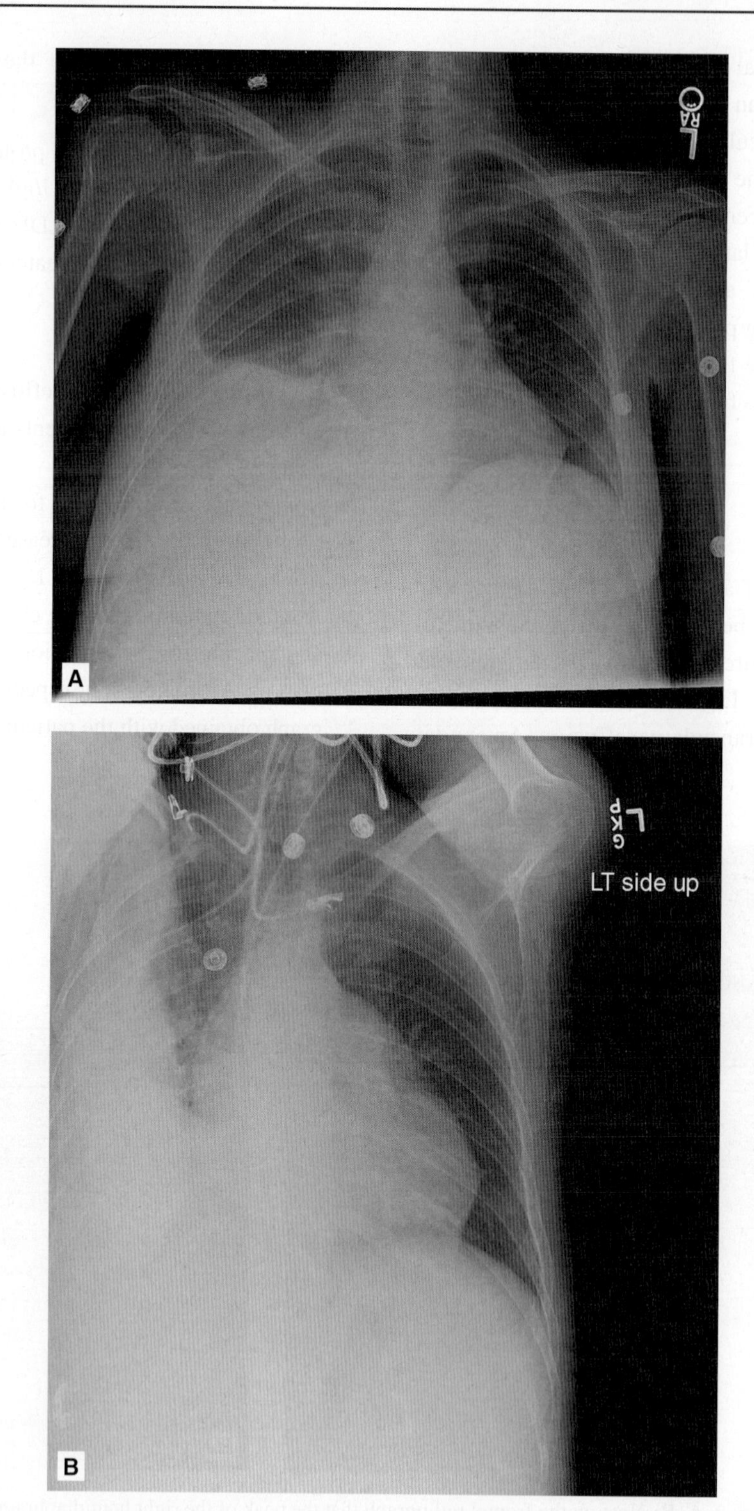

FIGURE 5.56 ■ Pleural Effusion. **A, B:** A right-sided pleural effusion can be seen on the frontal radiograph. A right lateral decubitus radiograph was performed to demonstrate that the effusion was not loculated but free-flowing.

Radiographic Summary

Subcutaneous emphysema is the presence of air beneath the skin surface in the loose subcutaneous tissue and muscle. Air can spread in all directions and may interdigitate with the muscle bundles to produce a characteristic linear streaky pattern, especially in the pectoralis muscles overlying the chest. This may obscure underlying lung pathology such as a pneumothorax.

Clinical Implications

Subcutaneous emphysema can be caused by extension from pneumomediastinum or pneumothorax, necrosis of subcutaneous tissue by gas-forming organisms, or a chest tube malfunction. It is also a seen status post trauma, esophageal rupture, and rarely after medical interventions such as endoscopy, central venous line placement, and bronchoscopy. Clinically, subcutaneous emphysema will present with crepitus, a crackling sensation felt with palpation.

Small amounts of subcutaneous emphysema are usually benign and require no intervention. If large and progressive, massive subcutaneous emphysema can compress the trachea or impede blood flow to the skin causing necrosis. These situations require rapid decompression.

Various approaches have been described, including the use of subcutaneous incisions, needles, or drains to relieve the gas.

Pearls

1. The progression of air spread should be monitored by marking the boundaries on the skin with a pen.
2. Subcutaneous emphysema due to pneumothorax requires chest tube thoracostomy and placement to suction to remove air faster.

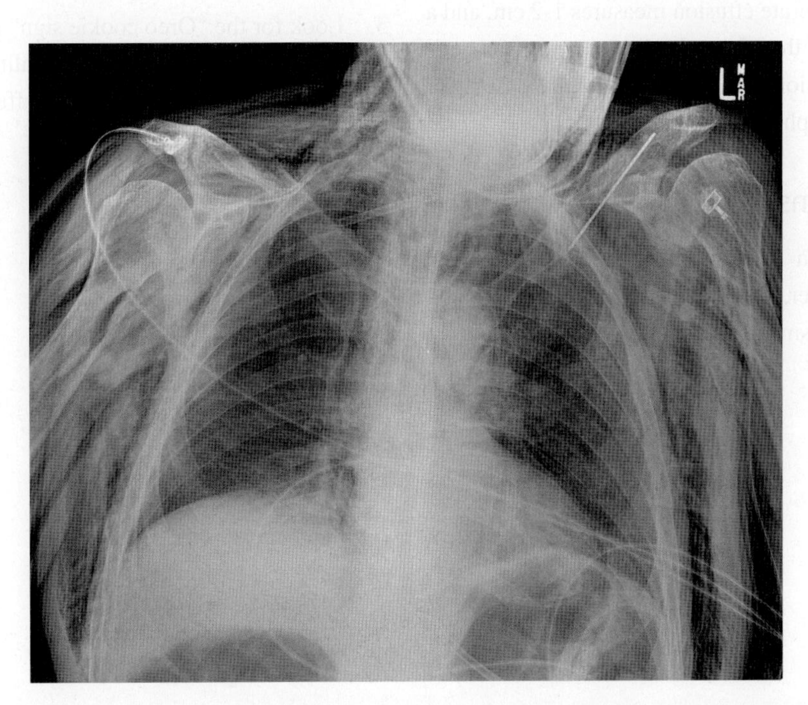

FIGURE 5.57 ■ Subcutaneous Emphysema. Substantial amounts of subcutaneous emphysema can be seen throughout the entire upper body and extremities. Note the striations in the muscles that are outlined by the overlying air. Additionally, pneumomediastinum can be noted with a linear air-interface along the right mediastinum.

Radiographic Summary

A pericardial effusion is the collection of fluid between the pericardium and epicardium. Chest radiographs reveal an enlarged cardiac silhouette with a "water bottle" appearance. This appearance, while suggestive, is not specific and can also be seen with dilated cardiomyopathy. A lateral view of the chest can demonstrate the "Oreo cookie sign" which is white fluid trapped between the pericardial and epicardial fat layers which are more radiolucent, and therefore, darker than the fluid. This sign is best appreciated along the anterior heart border on the lateral view.

The most sensitive and specific imaging modality for the detection of pericardial effusion is echocardiography. On ultrasound, a pericardial effusion will appear as an anechoic area (black stripe) surrounding the heart. The largest pocket should be measured at end-diastole, when the heart is at maximal filling. A thin, <2 mm, rim of pericardial fluid is normal and of no clinical significance. A small effusion on ultrasound measures <1 cm; a moderate effusion measures 1-2 cm, and a large effusion is greater than 2 cm. In the presence of a pericardial pericardial effusion, it is important to also assess for evidence of tamponade physiology.

Clinical Implications

Pericardial effusion can occur as a component of almost any pericardial disorder, including hemorrhagic effusion from trauma or aneurysm rupture, malignant effusion from metastases or postradiation pericarditis, exudative effusion from tuberculosis, viral infection or spread of empyema, and transudative effusion secondary to heart failure, nephrotic syndrome, myxedema or drugs. Small effusions may be completely asymptomatic. As the effusion increases in size, symptoms of chest pain, pressure, or dyspnea can develop.

Treatment depends on both the underlying cause and the severity of cardiac impairment. Most small effusions require either no treatment or treatment of the underlying cause.

Pearls

1. EKG may show electrical alternans, which is beat-to-beat voltage variability secondary to the heart swinging in the larger, fluid-filled pericardial sac.
2. A "water bottle" shape of the cardiac silhouette on chest radiograph is suggestive but nonspecific for pericardial effusion as dilated cardiomyopathy can have a similar appearance.
3. Look for the "Oreo cookie sign" on the lateral view.
4. Echocardiography is the modality of choice and should be performed if a pericardial effusion is suspected clinically or on a chest radiograph.

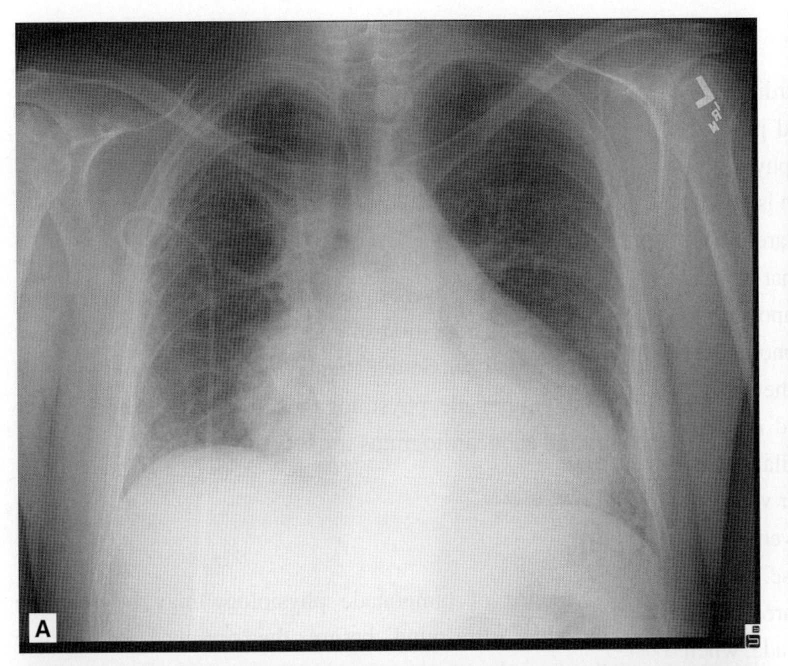

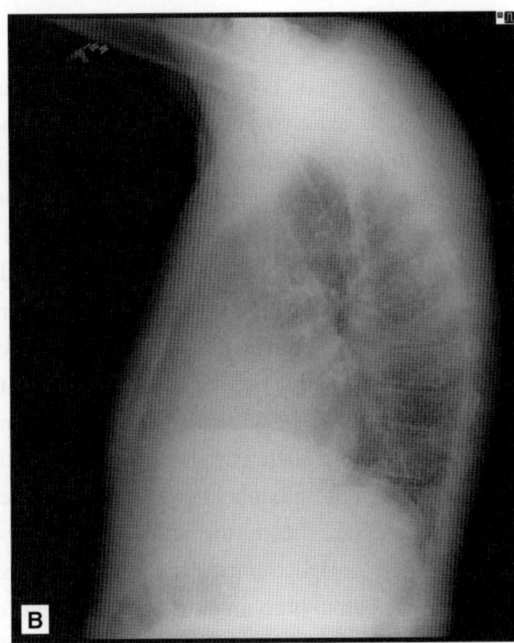

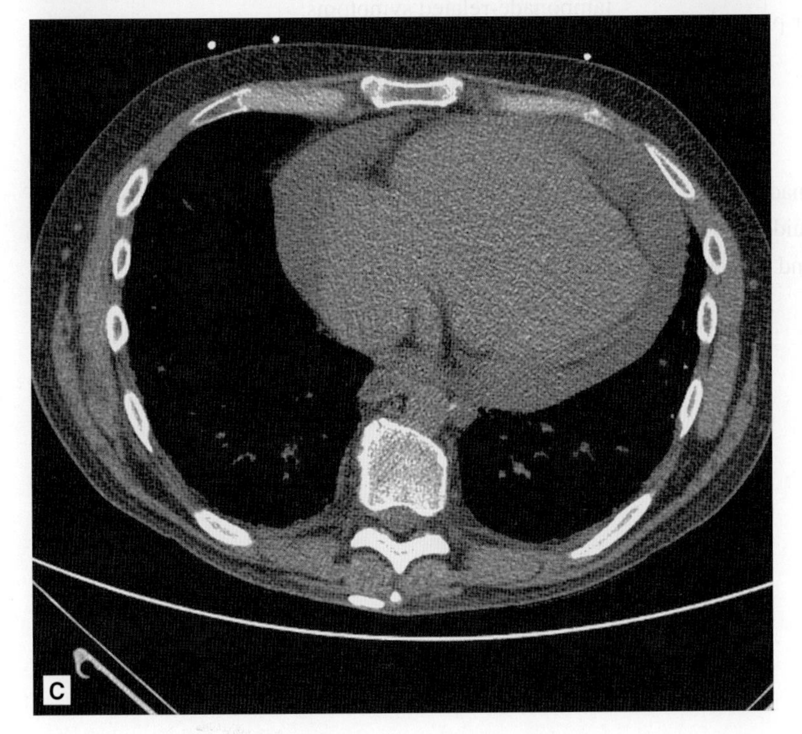

FIGURE 5.58 ■ Pericardial Effusion. **A-C:** Frontal and lateral radiographs demonstrate an enlarged cardiac silhouette, which was a new finding when compared to the patient's previous radiograph. A pericardial effusion was suspected and confirmed on CT. Note the thin rim of pericardial fat surrounded by higher density pericardial fluid on the CT image.

Radiographic Summary

Pericardial tamponade is caused by a large pericardial effusion that exerts external pressure on the heart and prevents complete filling in diastole. Bedside echocardiography can be used to assess the effect that the pericardial effusion is having on cardiac function. Different sonographic findings are visible depending on the stage of tamponade physiology that is present. A pericardial effusion must be present for tamponade to develop. An enlarged and plethoric IVC is the first sonographic evidence that the pericardial effusion is affecting the cardiovascular system. As pericardial pressure rises and exceeds right atrial pressure, there is right atrial systolic collapse that can be best seen on subxiphoid or apical 4-chamber view. As pericardial pressure rises further and exceeds right ventricular pressure, there is right ventricular diastolic collapse. At this point, cardiac output is compromised, and patients are usually tachycardic or hypotensive. In late stages of tamponade, when the pericardial pressure exceeds the left ventricular pressure, this results in an underfilled, hyperdynamic heart.

Clinical Implications

Patients who present with overt cardiac tamponade need emergent bedside pericardiocentesis. Ultrasound-guided pericardiocentesis has demonstrated improved safety and success over a blind approach and should always be used to guide aspiration when available. This should be performed at the site that contains the largest pericardial fluid accumulation that is closest to the chest wall. Approaches include the traditional subxiphoid approach, the left intercostal, parasternal, or apical approaches.

Patients with tamponade physiology via bedside ultrasound, but without overt signs of tamponade require emergent consult for consideration of pericardiocentesis or placement of a pericardial window. Patients with a pericardial effusion without tamponade physiology on ultrasound should have follow-up echocardiograms for surveillance.

Pearls

1. Evidence of tamponade physiology may be seen on bedside ultrasound before the presence of cardiac tamponade-related symptoms.
2. IVC plethora is sensitive but not specific for tamponade physiology. RA and RV collapse are both 100% specific in diagnosing tamponade physiology.
3. Intubation positive pressure ventilation in patients with overt tamponade can lead to acute decompensation. If intubation is necessary, have a pericardiocentesis setup available at the bedside.

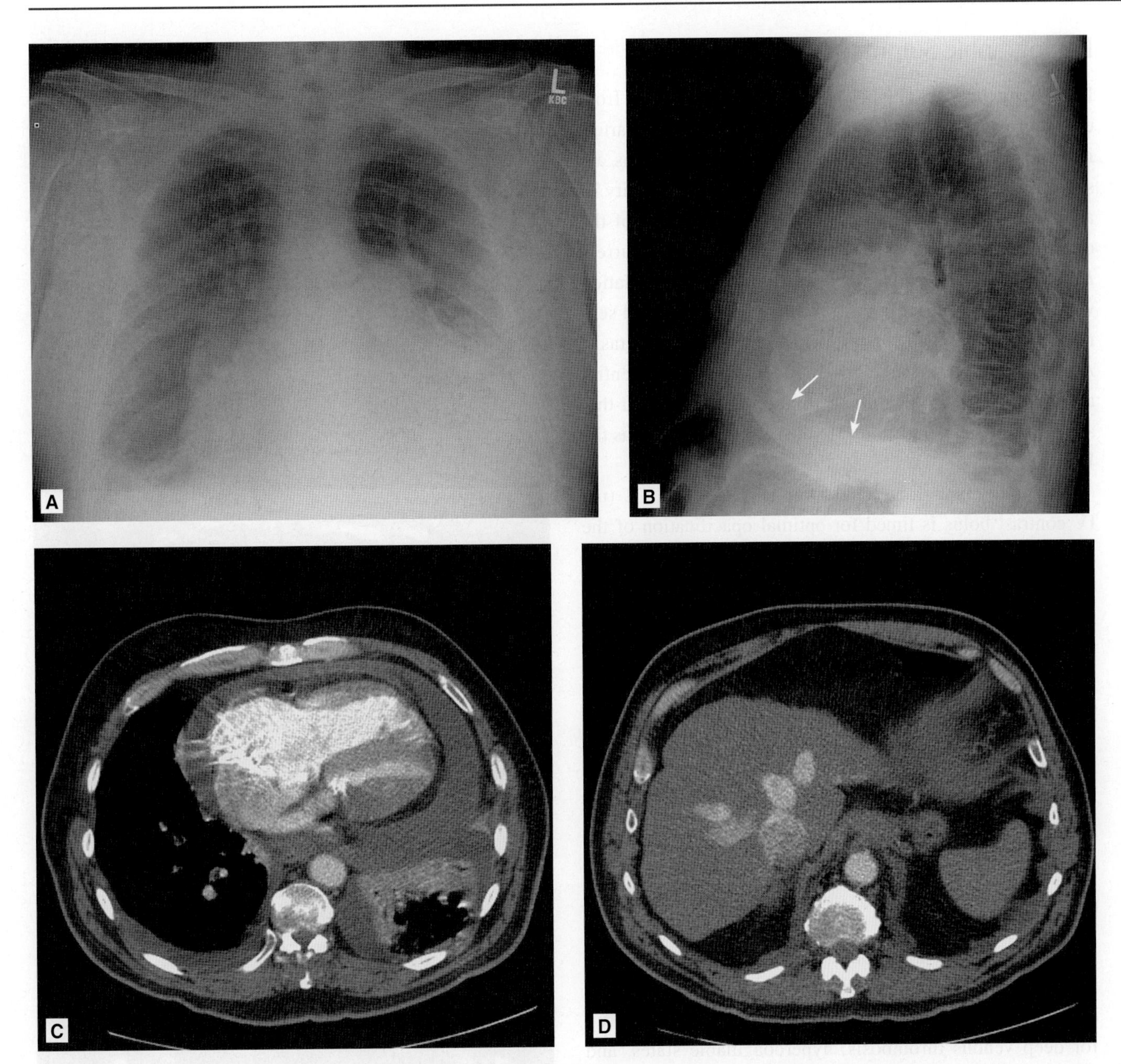

FIGURE 5.59 ■ Pericardial Tamponade. **A-D:** Frontal and lateral radiographs demonstrate an enlarged cardiac silhouette, which was a new finding when compared to the patient's previous radiograph. Note the high attenuation rim of fluid anterior and inferior to the heart on the lateral view (arrows): the "Oreo Cookie sign." A CTA was obtained which nicely demonstrates the pericardial effusion. There is a reflux of contrast into the IVC and hepatic veins, a finding often seen with tamponade physiology due to increased right heart pressures.

Radiographic Summary

Pulmonary embolus (PE) occurs when a vascular clot from elsewhere in the body migrates to the pulmonary arteries, causing occlusion. Plain radiographs radiographs are seldom useful in diagnosing a PE, as the vast majority of acute pulmonary emboli fail to show any evidence of the disease unless lung parenchymal infarction has occurred. *Hampton's hump* is a wedge-shaped area of consolidation with a pleural base which is indicative of an infarcted segment of the lung, and can mimic pneumonia or atelectasis. A large PE can result in relative hypoperfusion of the entire affected hemithorax, resulting in an entire lung field that appears more radiolucent due to the oligemia, known as the *Westermark sign*.

Pulmonary emboli are evident on a PE protocol CT (the IV contrast bolus is timed for optimal opacification of the pulmonary arteries) as filling defects within the normally opacified pulmonary arteries. The classic "saddle embolus" is large enough to be wedged at the initial bifurcation between the two main branches of the pulmonary artery and is usually life-threatening. Smaller segmental pulmonary emboli are discovered by examining flow of contrast through the pulmonary arterial tree in each subsegment, looking for smaller filling defects. Saggital and coronal reformations can be useful in examining the subsegmental branches for smaller emboli.

Clinical Implications

Identification of a PE should prompt anti-coagulation to inhibit further clot formation and identification of the original source of the thrombus. This includes workup for deep venous thrombosis, hypercoagulable states, and neoplastic evaluation. In patients with evidence of decompensation (right heart strain, hypotension, or refractory hypoxia) further therapy may be required, including intravenous thrombolytics, catheter-directed thrombolytics, or thrombectomy.

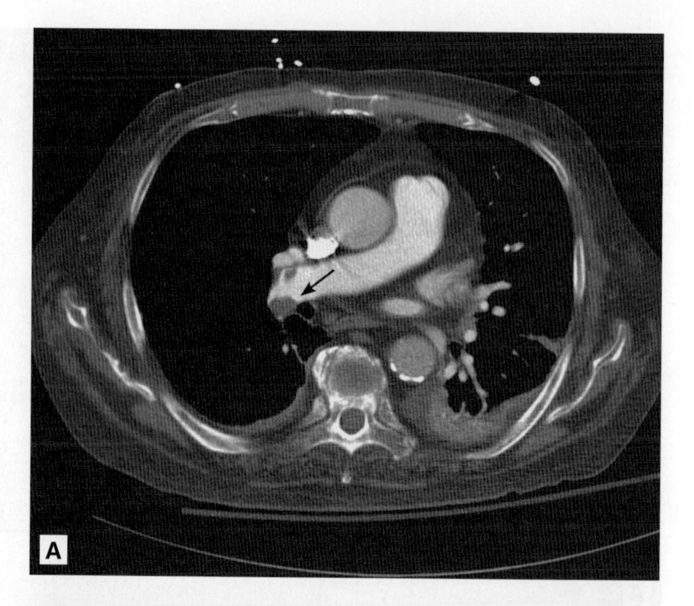

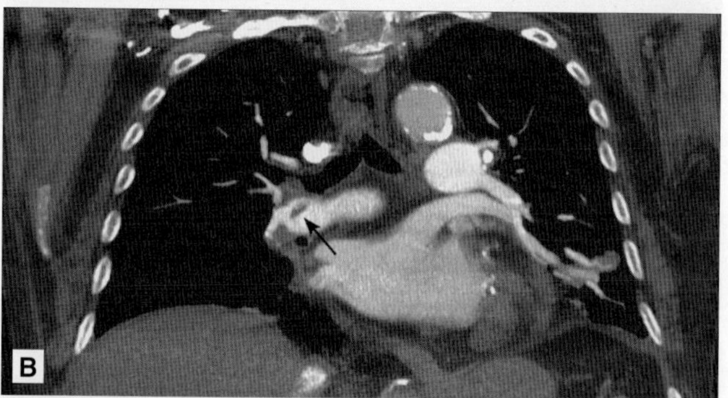

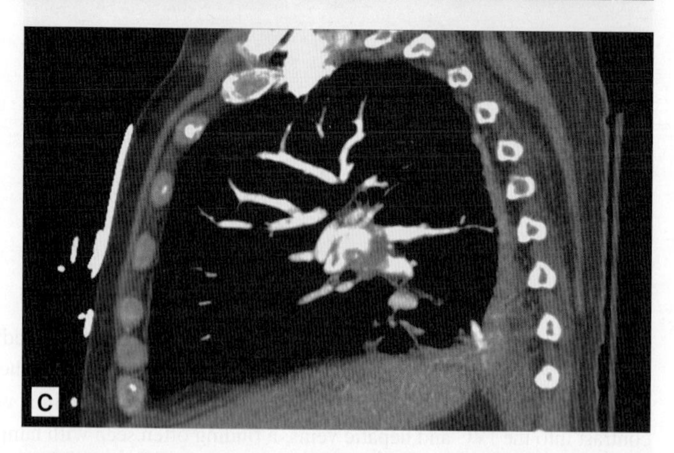

FIGURE 5.60 ■ Pulmonary Embolism. **A-C:** Axial, coronal, and sagittal CTA images demonstrate small filling defects in the distal right main pulmonary artery consistent with pulmonary emboli (arrows).

Pearls

1. Anticoagulation, in the absence of contraindications, should precede diagnostic imaging in patients with symptoms highly suspicious for PE.
2. In a patient with a clinical presentation consistent with PE, Westermark sign is strongly suggestive and reasonably specific; however, this sign lacks sensitivity.
3. Identification of PE by PE protocol CT is highly sensitive, specific, and fast.
4. Identification of a PE should prompt a workup for risk factors for thrombus formation.
5. The most common source is deep venous thrombosis. Ultrasonography of the legs with Doppler should be performed to assess for additional potential clot.
6. IVC filters can prevent further embolization of the clot from the lower extremities to the lungs.

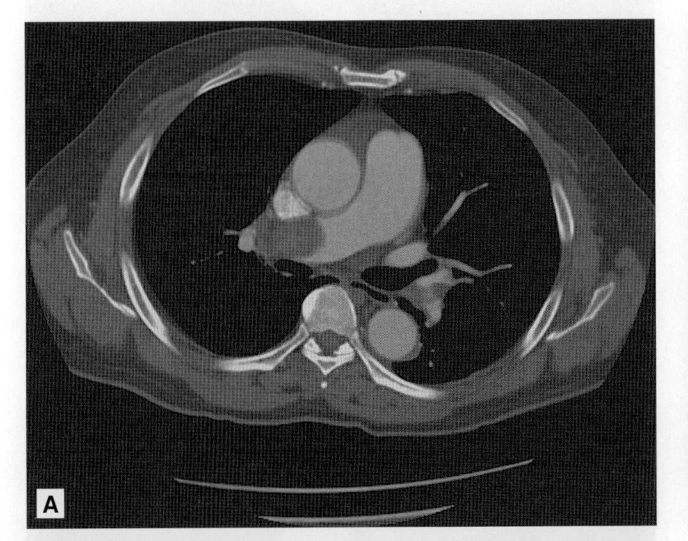

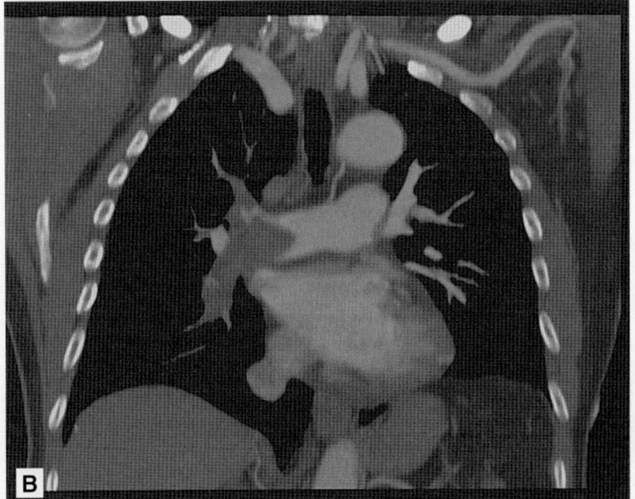

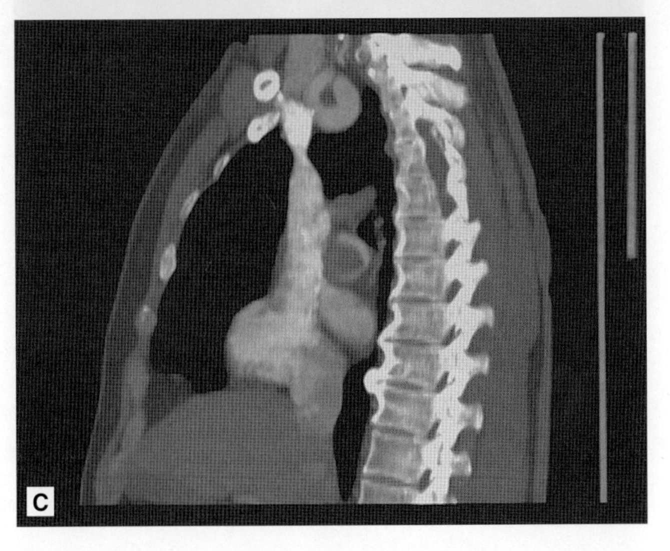

FIGURE 5.61 ■ Pulmonary Embolism. **A-C:** Axial, coronal, and sagittal CTA images demonstrate a large filling defect in the main right pulmonary artery consistent with a large pulmonary embolism.

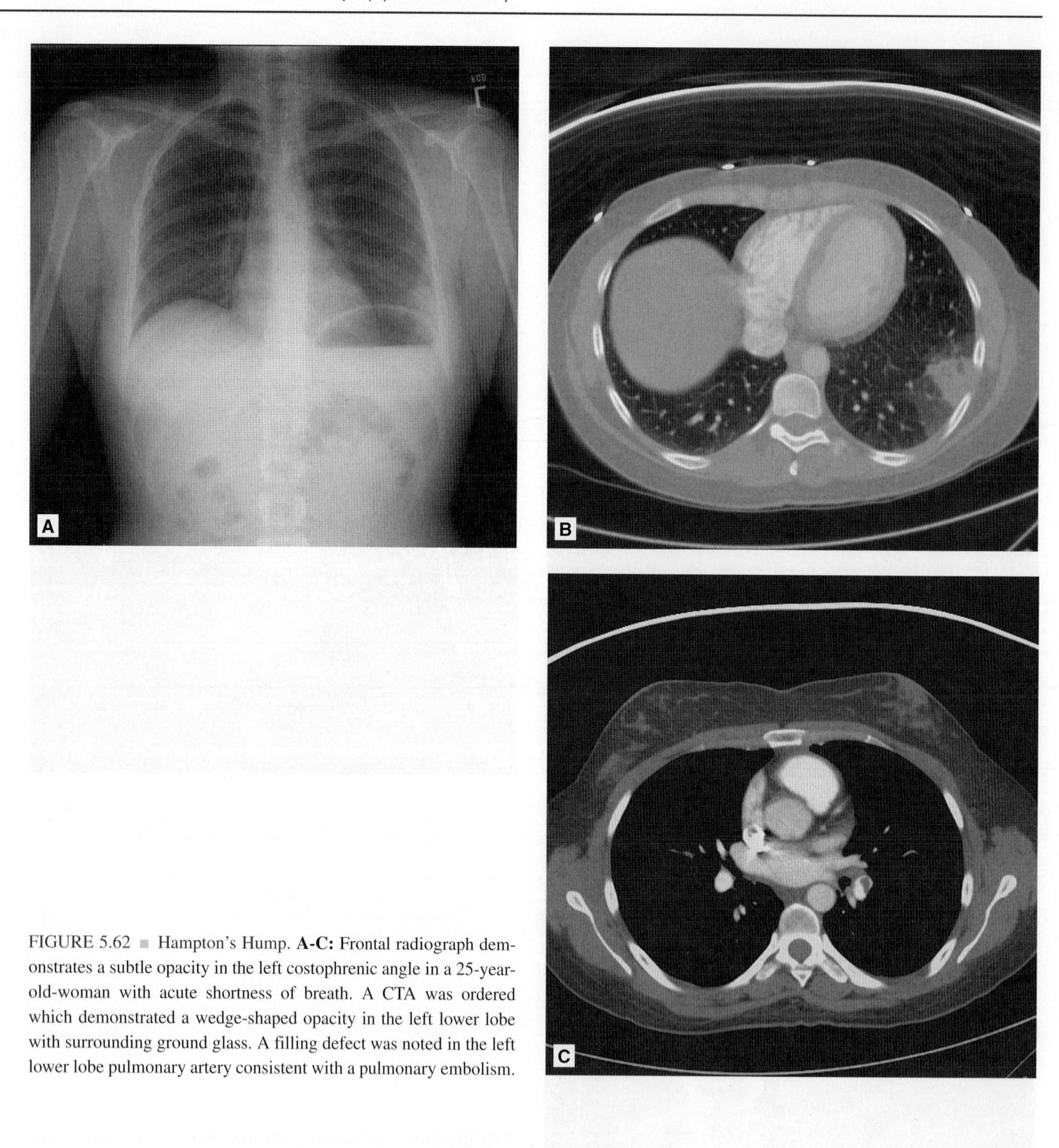

FIGURE 5.62 ■ Hampton's Hump. **A-C:** Frontal radiograph demonstrates a subtle opacity in the left costophrenic angle in a 25-year-old-woman with acute shortness of breath. A CTA was ordered which demonstrated a wedge-shaped opacity in the left lower lobe with surrounding ground glass. A filling defect was noted in the left lower lobe pulmonary artery consistent with a pulmonary embolism.

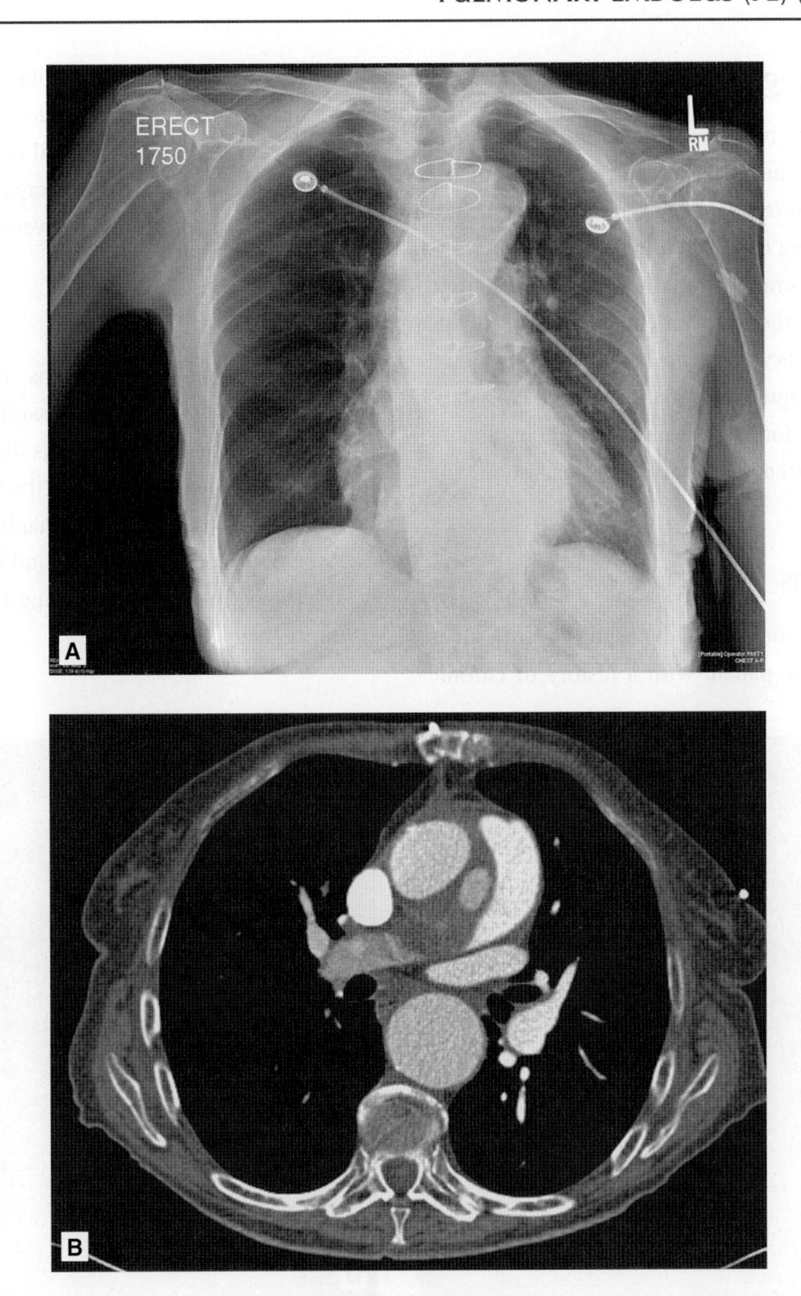

FIGURE 5.63 ■ Westermark's Sign. **A, B:** Frontal radiograph demonstrates decreased vasculature of the right lung when compared to the left lung (the right lung is darker when compared to the left lung). Additionally, the aortic arch is prominent. Axial CTA image demonstrates an aortic pseudoaneurysm with compression and near complete occlusion of the right pulmonary artery.

Radiographic Findings

Asbestosis is the chronic lung disease caused by the inhalation of asbestos fibers and is characterized by gradually worsening pulmonary fibrosis. On plain radiographs, asbestosis appears as thickening of the pleura often with calcifications. Differential considerations for thickened and calcified pleura include prior hemothorax, prior empyema, or prior talc pleurodesis. Clinical history is key in heightening suspicion for the diagnosis. Any suspicion for malignancy due to asbestos exposure requires CT for better evaluation, where pleural-based plaques are seen often with coarse rims consistent with mesothelioma.

Clinical Implications

Chronic high-level environmental exposure to asbestosis is becoming rare, but any patient with a history of chronic exposure with respiratory complaints would benefit form cross-sectional imaging to exclude asbestosis as a diagnosis. Asbestosis can result in increased dyspnea with progression to restrictive lung disease and decreased diffusion of oxygen across the lung parenchyma in severe disease.

Pearls

1. Any patient with pleural "rims" on cross-sectional imaging should be concern for possible mesothelioma.
2. Asbestos exposure typically is discovered when calcified pleural plaques are noted on the frontal and lateral chest radiographs (often over the diaphragms).
3. Asbestosis can present with findings of pulmonary fibrosis, typically favoring the lung bases over the mid and upper lungs.

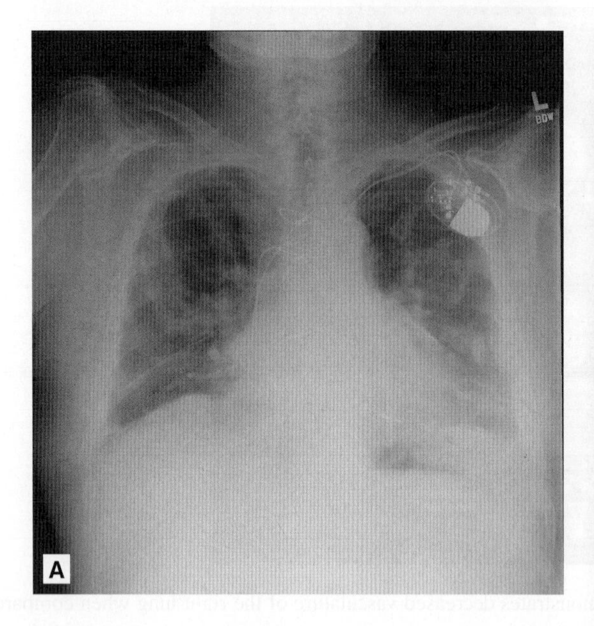

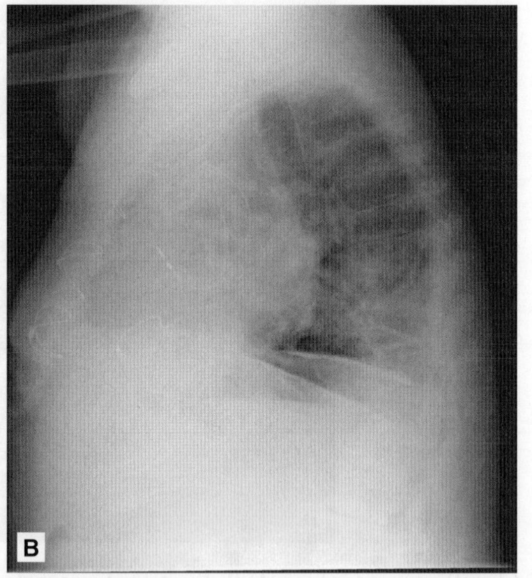

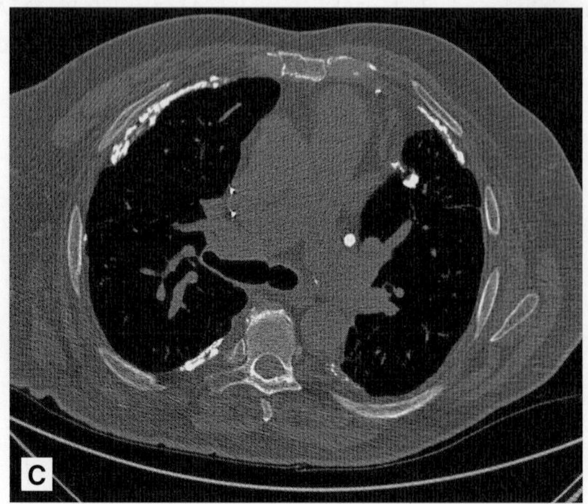

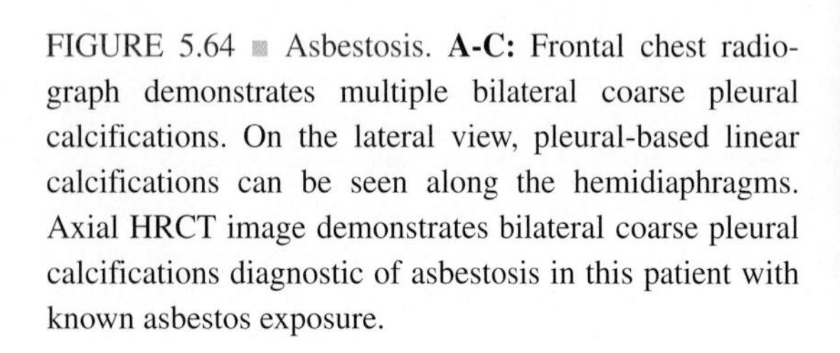

FIGURE 5.64 ■ Asbestosis. **A-C:** Frontal chest radiograph demonstrates multiple bilateral coarse pleural calcifications. On the lateral view, pleural-based linear calcifications can be seen along the hemidiaphragms. Axial HRCT image demonstrates bilateral coarse pleural calcifications diagnostic of asbestosis in this patient with known asbestos exposure.

Radiographic Summary

Congestive heart failure (CHF) results from the heart's inability to effectively pump blood through the cardiovascular system. This results in fluid "backup" or "congestion" within the pulmonary venous system. Increase in the central vascular volume, pulmonary venous engorgement, interstitial edema, and eventually alveolar edema result, in that progression.

The first radiographic sign of CHF is an increase in the central vascular volume. This can be appreciated on an AP view of the chest by widening of the vascular pedicle to more than 6 cm. Relative widening of the vascular pedicle compared to prior examinations is more accurate and relevant than an absolute measurement of the pedicle's width. Pulmonary venous engorgement develops next and can be appreciated on an upright AP view of the chest by noting the increased caliber of the pulmonary veins, as well as a cephalization of flow (the upper lobe pulmonary veins become as thick as or thicker than the lower lobe veins). Please note that this finding is only meaningful on an upright study. Interstitial edema is characterized by bilateral perihilar reticular lines and Kerley B lines (thin, interstitial lines 1-2 cm in length located along the periphery of the lungs, typically at the costophrenic sulci). Finally, alveolar edema is characterized by bilateral symmetric parenchymal consolidation, worse in the lung bases. Cardiomegaly and pleural effusions are typically present as well. Resolution of hydrostatic pulmonary edema occurs in the reverse order.

Clinical Implications

Chest radiography is just one clue in the evaluation of a patient with suspected decompensated heart failure, however, 18% of patients with CHF do not have any radiographic findings described above. A normal chest radiograph does not exclude CHF and other clinical and diagnostic testing should be preformed if CHF is suspected. Historical findings suggestive of CHF include orthopnea, paroxysmal nocturnal dyspnea,

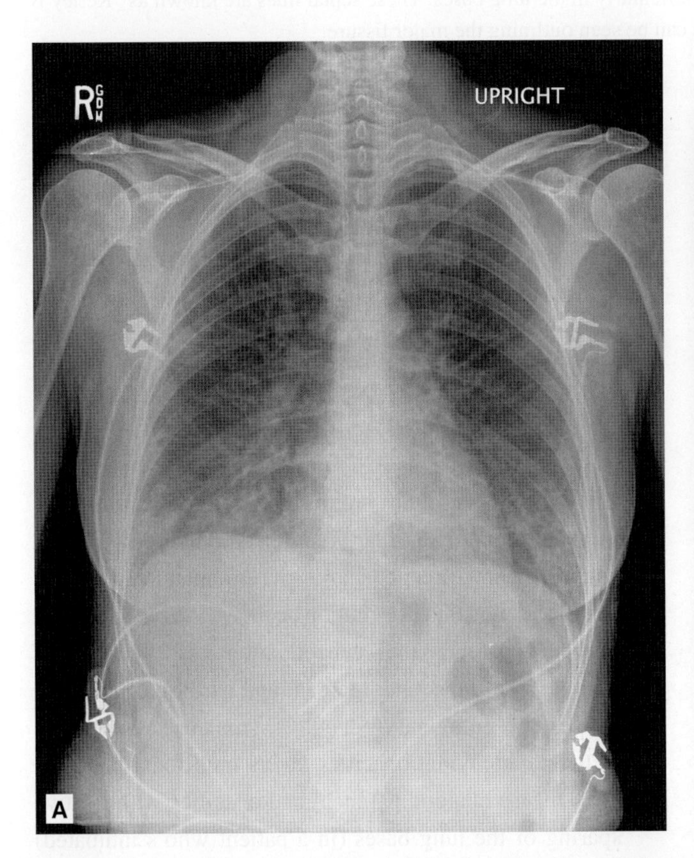

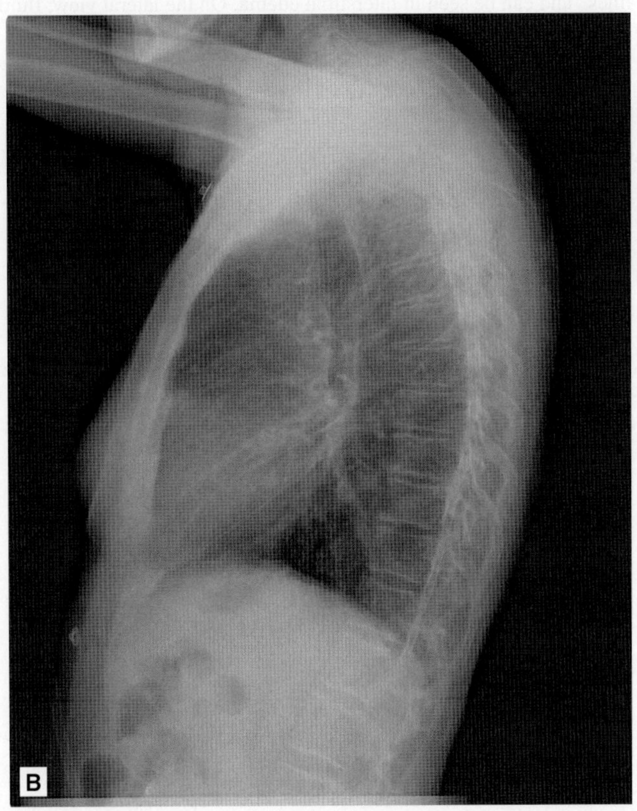

FIGURE 5.65 ■ Interstitial Edema. **A, B:** A frontal radiograph demonstrates a prominent interstitial pattern bilaterally and symmetrically. Interstitial septal lines can be seen in the lung periphery bilaterally, particularly in the lung bases. These septal lines are known as "Kerley's B lines" and can be seen in interstitial edema. This patient does not have cardiomegaly. The combination of interstitial edema and a normal heart size are typically seen in the setting of acute myocardial infarction (or non-cardiogenic causes of edema); the cardiac decompensation leading to edema is acute; cardiomyopathy has not yet developed.

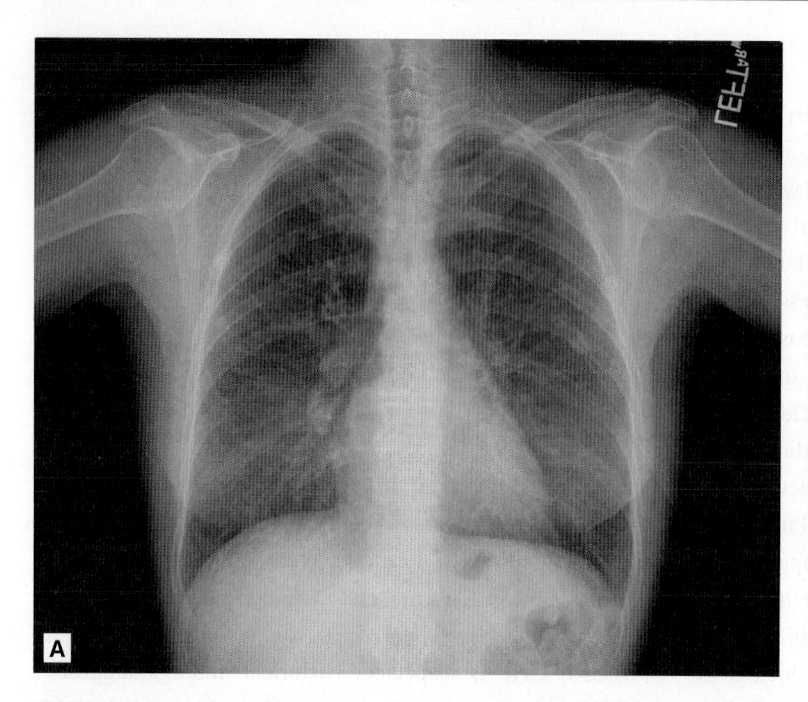

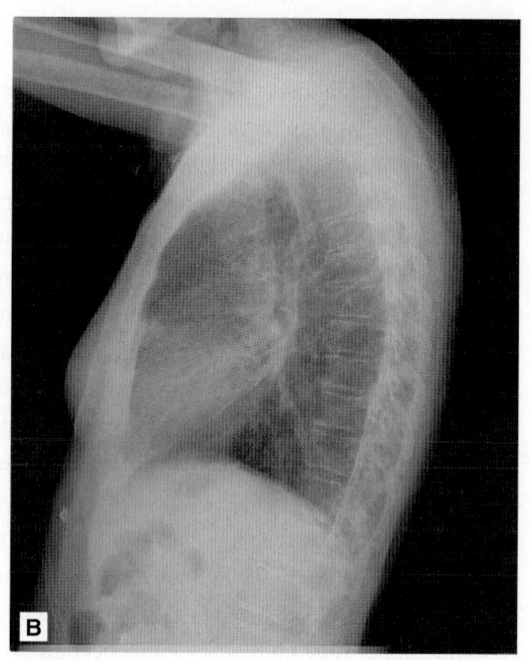

FIGURE 5.66 ■ Kerley B Lines. **A, B:** A frontal radiograph demonstrates a prominent interstitial pattern bilaterally and symmetrically. Interstitial septal lines can be seen in the lung periphery bilaterally, particularly in the lung bases. These septal lines are known as "Kerley B lines" and can be seen in interstitial edema. On the lateral view, fluid can be seen outlining the major fissure.

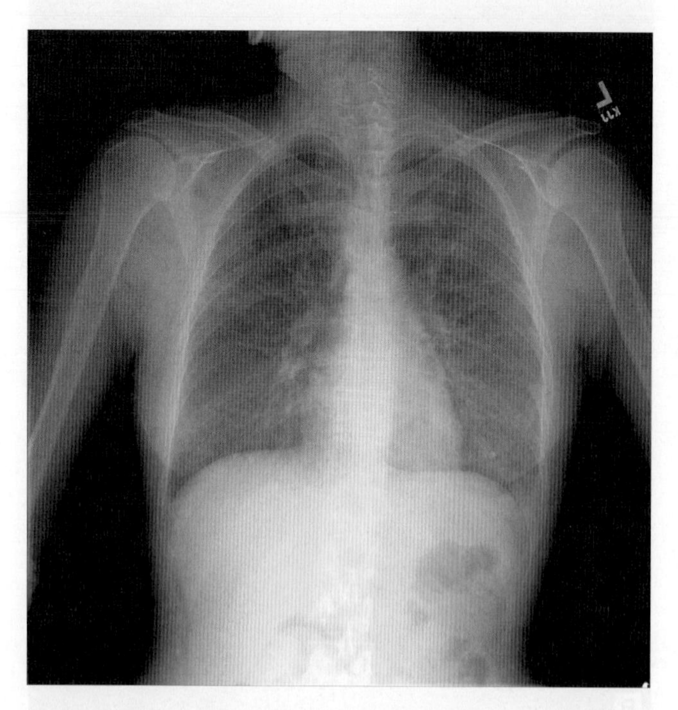

FIGURE 5.67 ■ Interstitial Edema with Cephalization. Frontal radiograph demonstrates a prominent interstitial pattern with Kerley's B lines in this patient with interstitial edema. Note the prominence of the upper lobe vessels, a finding known as cephalization.

shortness of breath, weight gain, abdominal distension, exercise intolerance, and generalized weakness. Examination findings of basilar crackles, S3, peripheral edema, and jugular venous distention are additional clues. Prior myocardial infarction as seen on ECG, elevated brain natriuretic peptide (BNP), and elevated liver enzymes due to hepatic congestion may also provide evidence supporting a diagnosis of CHF.

Pearls

1. CHF decompensation progresses in a typical pattern: increased central vascular volume and pulmonary venous engorgement with cephalization of flow, interstitial edema, and alveolar edema. Resolution occurs in the reverse order.
2. Bibasilar parenchymal consolidation with features of pulmonary venous engorgement and cardiomegaly favor hydrostatic pulmonary edema. Asymmetric distribution of the parenchymal opacities favors multifocal pneumonia. Diffuse bilateral parenchymal opacities with relative sparing of the lung bases (in a patient who's intubated) favor ARDS.
3. Initial management of acute CHF includes oxygen (may require BiPAP), afterload reduction with nitrates, and diuresis.

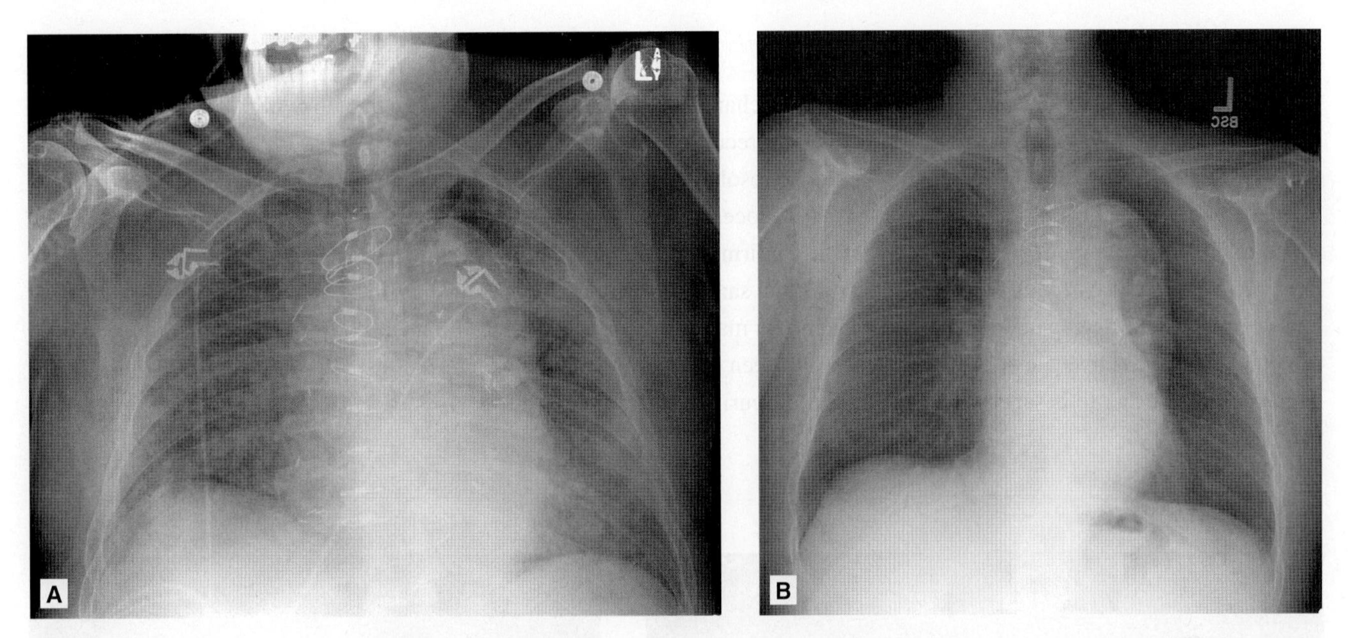

FIGURE 5.68 ■ Alveolar Pulmonary Edema. **A, B:** Frontal radiograph demonstrates bilateral and symmetric airspace opacities in this patient with hydrostatic pulmonary edema. The patient's follow-up radiograph one month later demonstrates resolution of the pulmonary edema. The patient has had a sternotomy and has a thoracic aortic aneurysm.

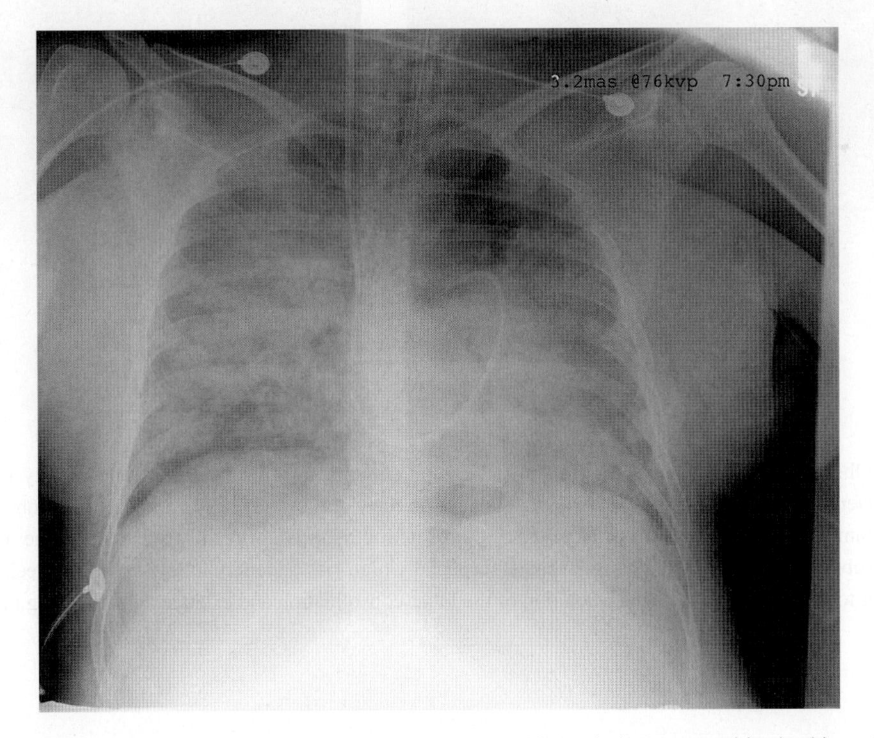

FIGURE 5.69 ■ Florid Pulmonary Edema. Frontal radiograph demonstrates bilateral airspace opacities in this patient with frank pulmonary edema.

Radiographic Findings

Post-obstructive pneumonia is a process in which a mechanical obstruction to a bronchus results in prolonged or recurrent infection. Lobar pneumonia that does not resolve within 6 weeks is concern for a post-obstructive process. Radiographic resolution of a pneumonia should be confirmed in any patient with recurrent disease, particularly if the same lung segment is affected on multiple visits. Suspicion for mass prompts CT imaging to evaluate for a mass that is not seen on plain radiograph due to a superimposed infiltrate obscuring the mass.

Clinical Implications

Pneumonia is frequently treated without repeat radiograph to document resolution, but in elderly patients or those with risk factors for malignancy, repeat radiographs are prudent to exclude an underlying malignancy. Radiographic findings of a lobar pneumonia may persist for as long as six weeks, but should resolve over that time period. If there is concern for recurrent disease, bronchoscopy or CT can provide further illumination as to the cause.

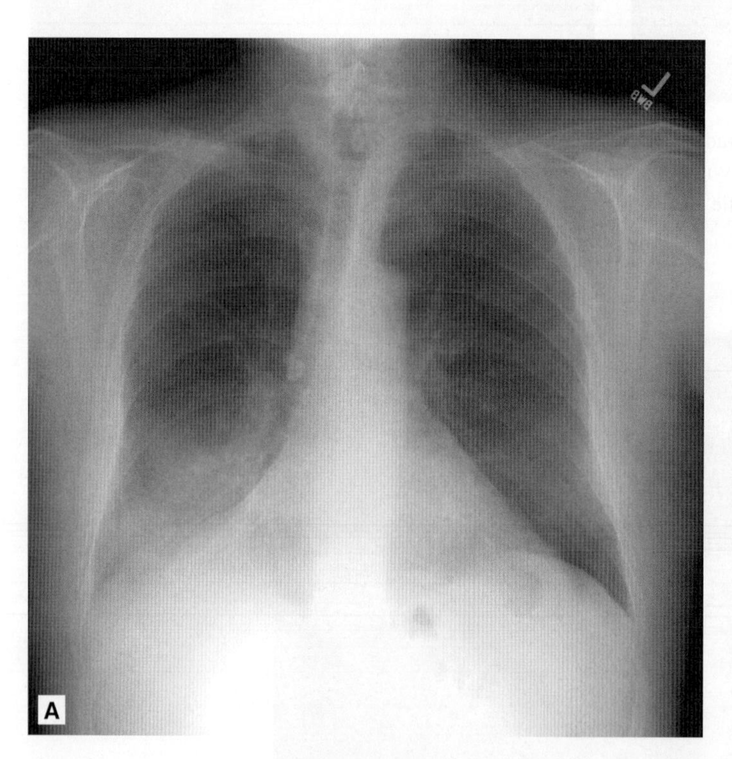

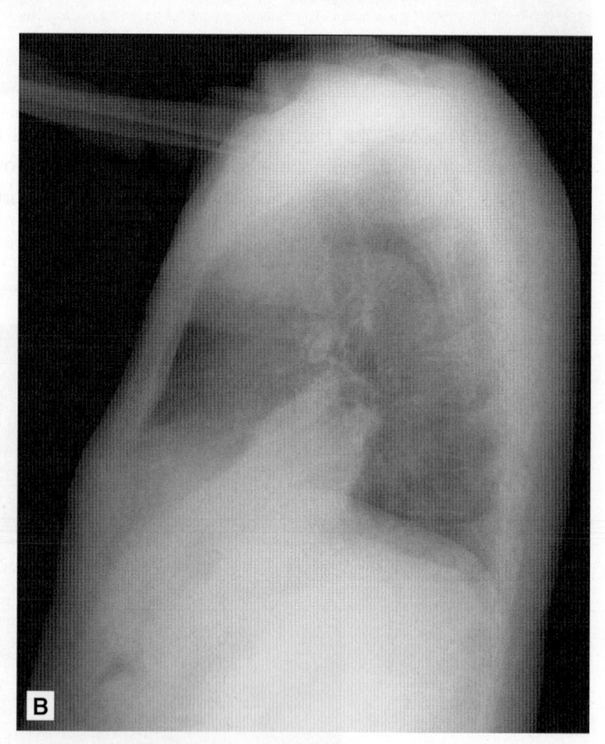

FIGURE 5.70 ■ Post-Obstructive Pneumonia. **A-C:** Frontal radiograph demonstrates a right lower lobe opacity which projects over the posterior heart on the lateral view. The CT image shows consolidation in the right lower lobe. This right lower lobe consolidation was due to a more proximal squamous cell carcinoma mass. Note that the obstructing mass is not readily apparent on the initial radiographs. This underscores the need to obtain radiographic follow-up. In adults (especially high-risk patients), follow-up in 4-6 weeks after the resolution of the acute illness in order to document radiographic resolution of the lobar consolidation and exclude an underlying mass.

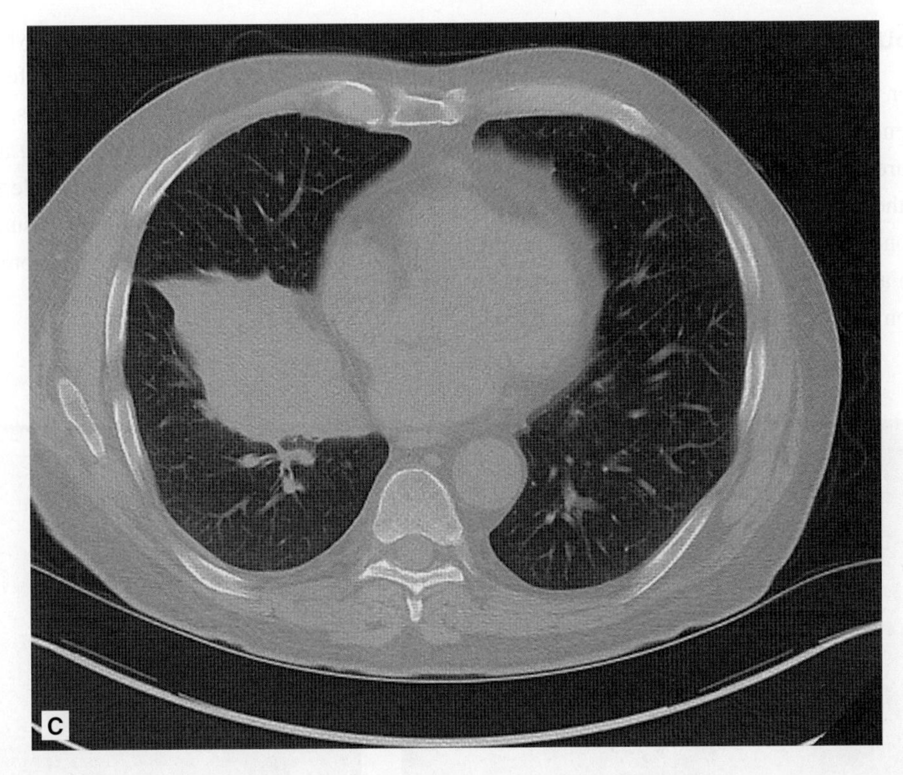

FIGURE 5.70 ■ (*Continued*)

Pearls

1. Pneumonia that recurs in the same segment or does not improve on appropriate therapy should prompt evaluation with CT to search for an obstructive process.
2. It is prudent to obtain radiographic follow-up in adults with lobar pneumonia to document radiographic resolution and exclude and underlying mass. Since the radiographic resolution trails the clinical resolution, follow-up radiographs are best obtained 4-6 weeks after clinical resolution. This is particularly important in high-risk patients.

Radiographic Summary

Primary lung cancer refers to malignancies that originate in the pulmonary parenchyma or airways. Ninety-five percent of all lung cancers are either squamous cell or non-squamous cell lung cancer. In the emergency department or primary care setting, the suspicion for lung cancer is triggered by finding a solitary nodule on a chest radiograph. A pulmonary nodule is defined as a lesion less than 3 cm in diameter that is both within and surrounded by lung parenchyma. If greater than 3 cm, the lesion is called a mass. Nodule features highly suspicious for lung cancer include solitariness, >8 mm in size, lack of calcification, spiculated appearance, and a more central location. Any new or suspicious nodule or mass should be evaluated with CT. Calcifications are usually associated with benign nodules, such as healed granulomatous infections or hamartomas.

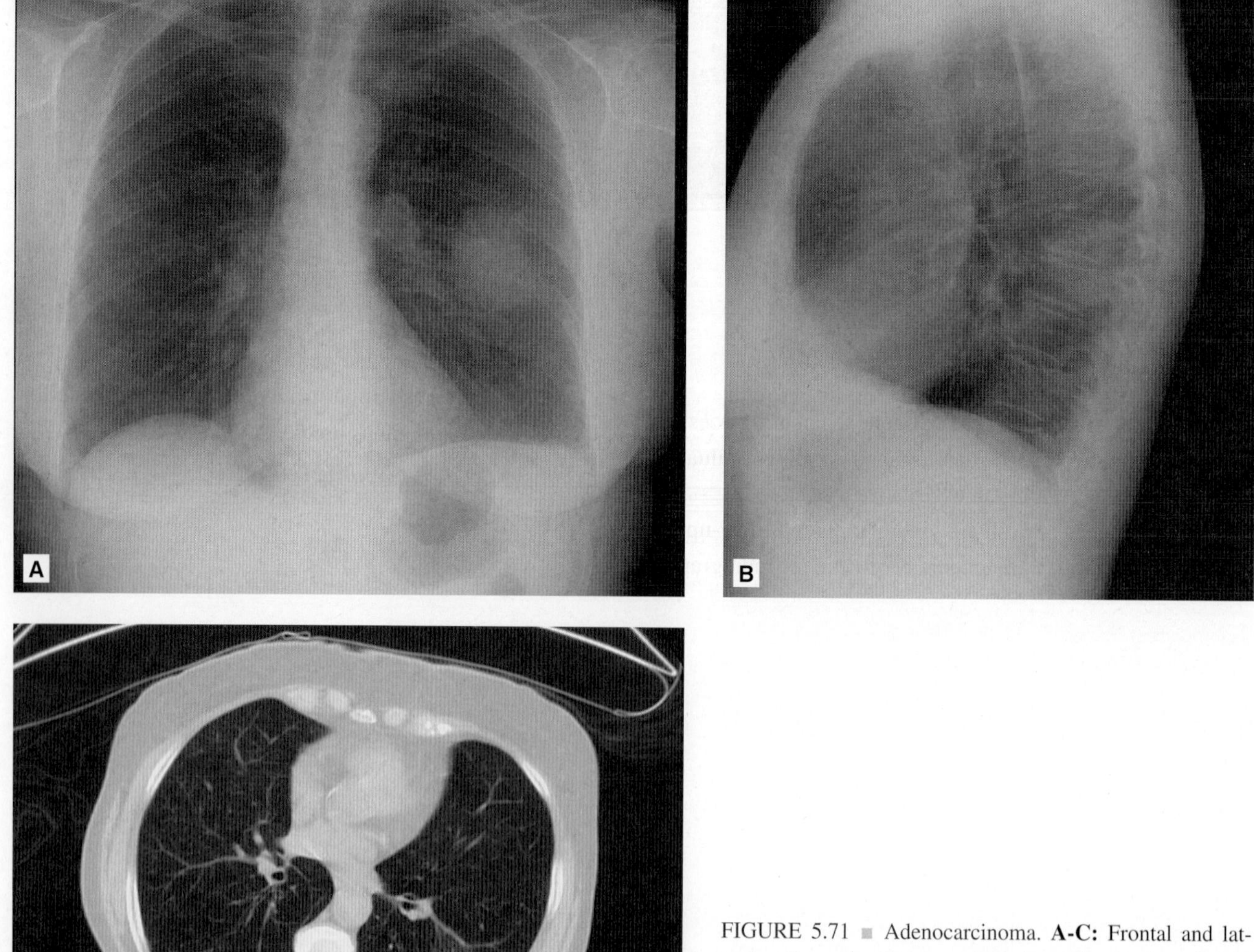

FIGURE 5.71 ■ Adenocarcinoma. **A-C:** Frontal and lateral radiographs show a rounded opacity in the left mid lung which projects posteriorly over the spine on the lateral view. The CT image shows a lobulated mass in the left lower lobe. This was mass biopsied and adenocarcinoma was diagnosed.

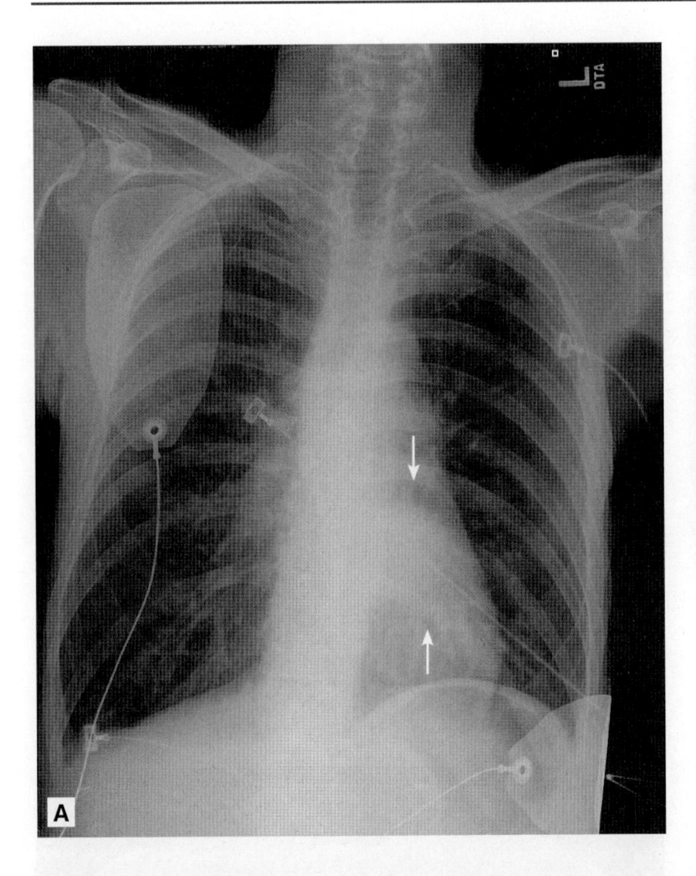

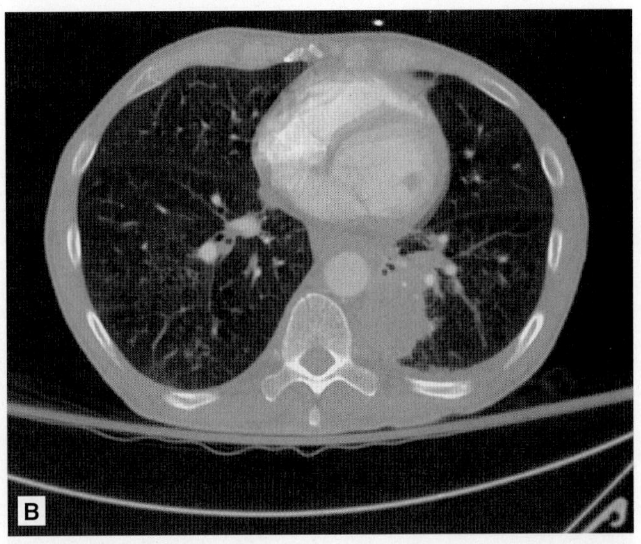

FIGURE 5.72 ■ Adenocarcinoma. **A, B:** Frontal radiograph reveals a subtle rounded retrocardiac mass in the left lower lobe (arrows). A CT scan was ordered which shows a pleural-based mass medially. This mass was biopsied and adenocarcinoma was diagnosed.

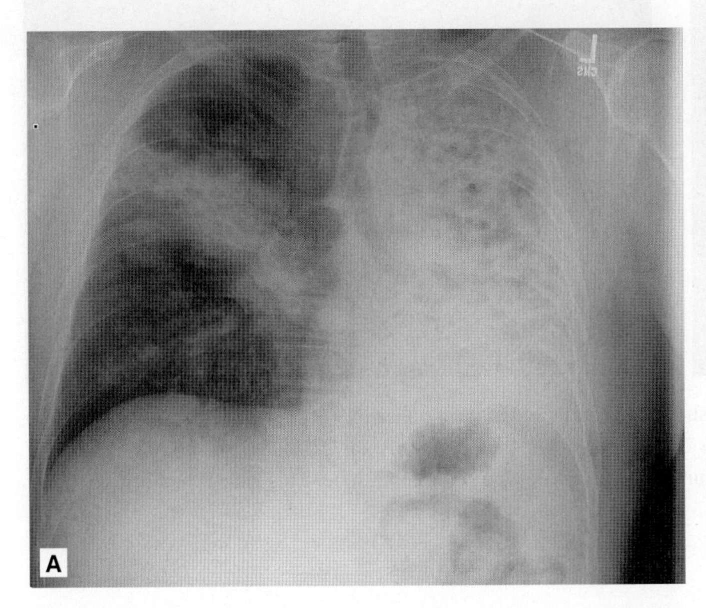

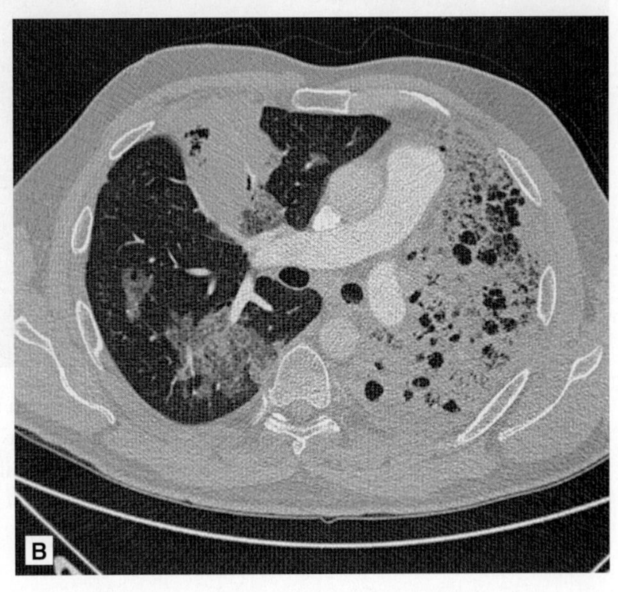

FIGURE 5.73 ■ Bronchioalveolar Cell Carcinoma. **A, B:** Frontal radiographs demonstrate complete opacification of the left lung and a right mid-lung opacity. A CT scan was ordered which showed consolidation throughout the left lung and areas of consolidation and ground-glass in the right lung. A biopsy was performed and bronchioalveolar cell carcinoma was diagnosed.

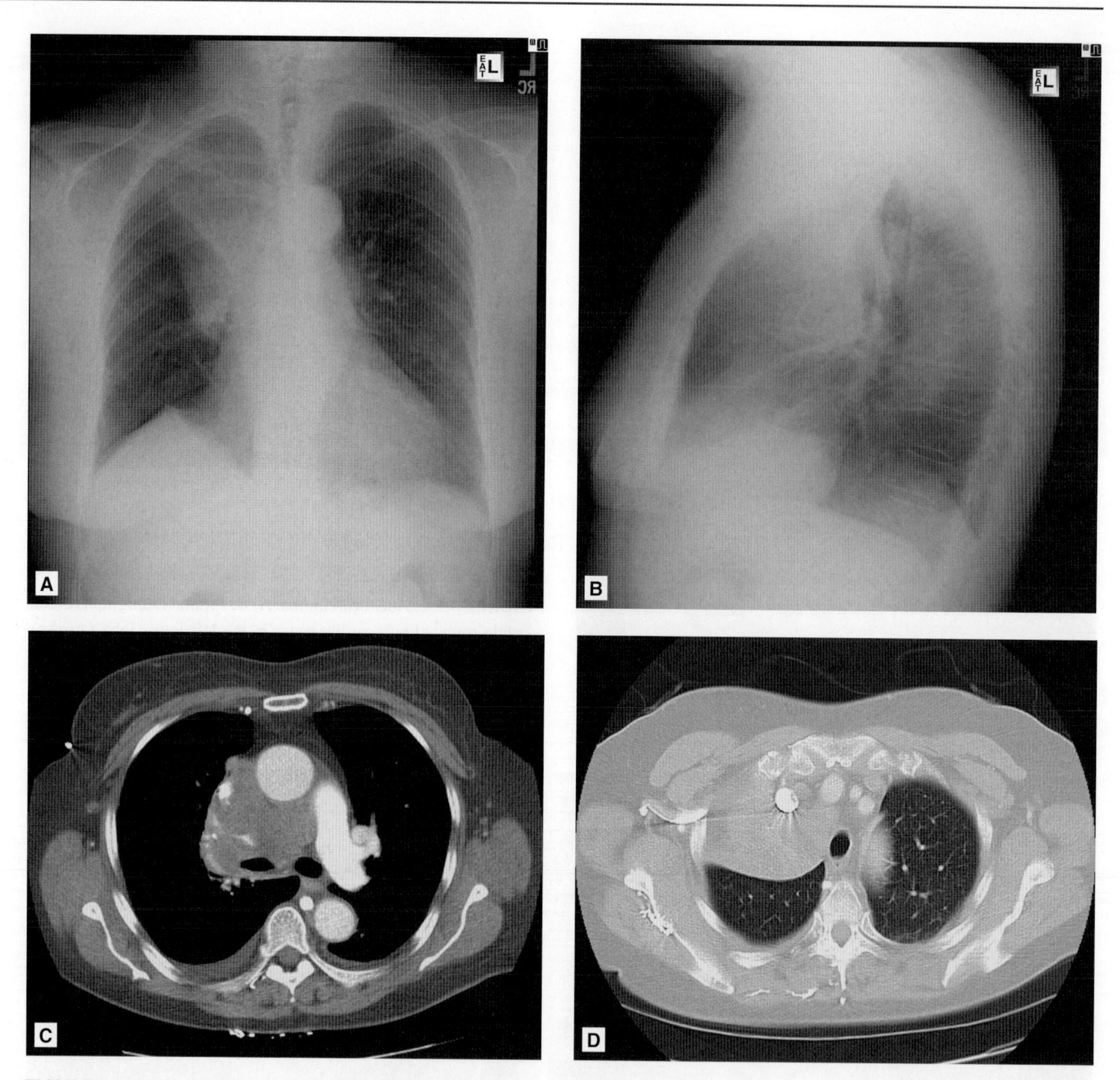

FIGURE 5.74 ■ Primary Lung Cancer. **A-D:** Frontal radiograph shows atelectasis of the right upper lobe (the so-called S sign of Golden) and a right hilar mass. The right upper lobe collapse and hilar mass can be seen on the lateral view. Axial CT images of soft tissue and lung windows show a large mediastinal mass extending to the right hilum with collapse of the right upper lobe. This patient had bronchogenic cancer.

Clinical Implications

Patients must be notified of all nodules found on chest radiograph as follow-up with additional imaging is necessary. Patients can be risk stratified by Fleischner guidelines based on the size of the nodule and the risk level of the patient—patients with a history of smoking or exposure to known lung pathogens (such as silicon or asbestos) are considered high risk and prompt earlier follow-up to determine if the lesion is growing. Any lesion greater than 8 mm on CT requires follow-up immediately for either biopsy or PET scanning to evaluate for malignancy.

Frequently, nodules are found incidentally during ED workups for unrelated complaints. It is important in these instances to alert both the patient as well as the primary care provider to the findings of the radiograph so that outpatient follow-up can be arranged. Large nodules or evidence of metastatic disease may prompt inpatient evaluation and workup.

Pearls

1. Pulmonary nodules >8 mm are concern for malignancy and should prompt an immediate workup.
2. Smaller nodules should be communicated to patients and providers for outpatient monitoring based on risk factors.
3. Nodules that have been stable for more than 2 years (based on prior radiographic studies) can be considered benign.

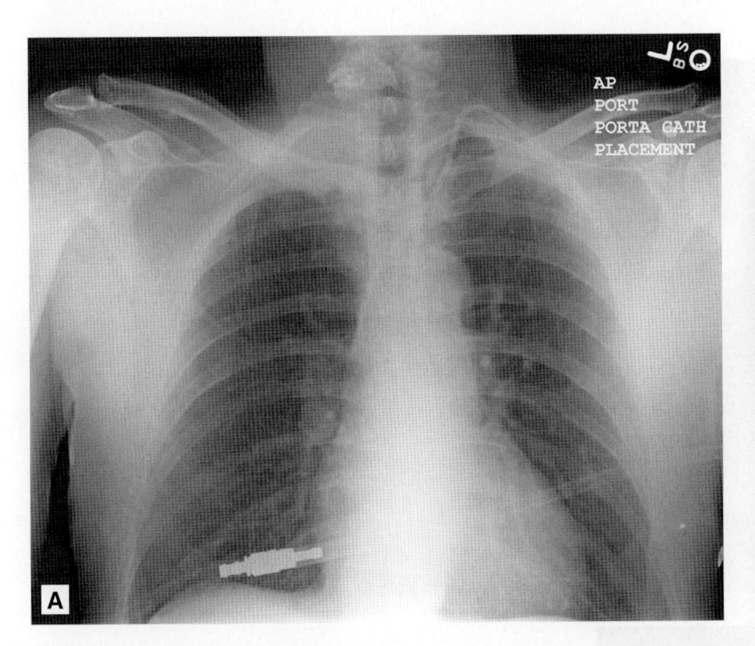

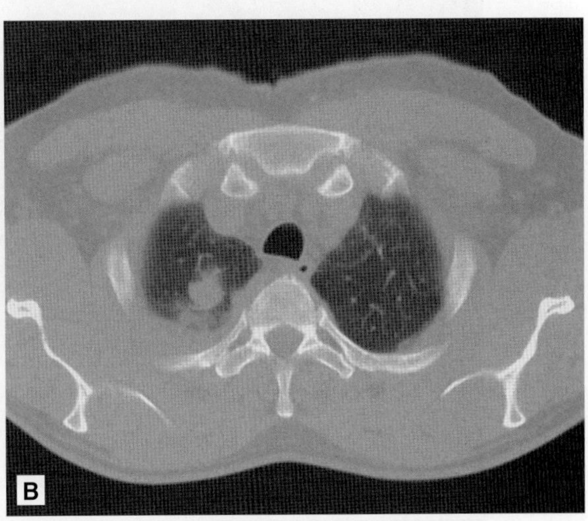

FIGURE 5.75 ■ Pancoast Tumor. **A, B:** Frontal radiograph shows an opacity in the right lung apex (note the destruction of the right second rib posteriorly). A CT scan was ordered which shows a mass with adjacent pleural thickening in the right upper lobe. This patient had a pancoast tumor from adenocarcinoma.

Radiographic Findings

Metastatic disease to the lung is typically seen on chest radiograph as multiple rounded opacities diffusely distributed within the lung parenchyma. Metastatic disease to the lung rarely presents as a solitary lesion. Other radiographic findings of metastatic disease include lymphadenopathy, bony erosions or lytic lesions, and pathologic compression fractures. Cancers that have a propensity to metastasize to lung include choriocarcinoma, osteosarcoma, renal, thyroid, melanoma, breast, and prostate cancer.

Clinical Implications

Multiple nodules or masses on chest radiography should prompt subspecialist evaluation. If the primary tumor is unknown, cross-sectional imaging may be useful to further differentiate the type of primary and possibly discover a source; however, ultimately the diagnosis will likely require biopsy. Lung metastases allow for identification through bronchoscopic biopsy. Treatment of underlying symptoms, such as pain and hypoxia are essential prior to further workup.

Pearls

1. Nodules or masses in more than one lobe of the lung suggest metastatic disease.
2. Metastatic nodules tend to favor lung bases rather than apices.

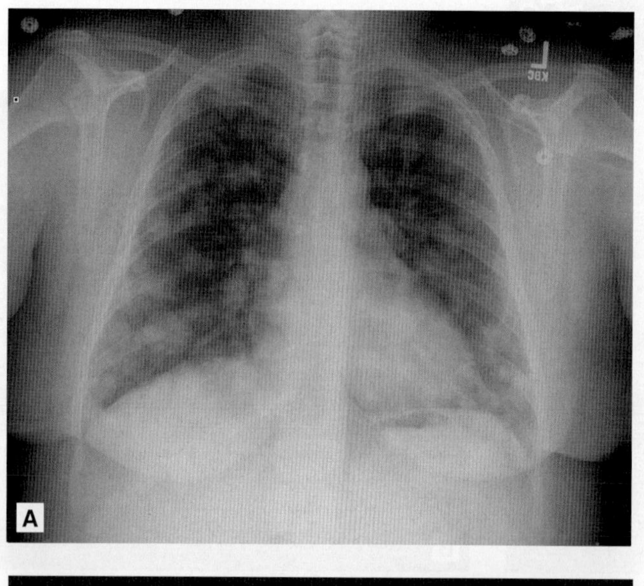

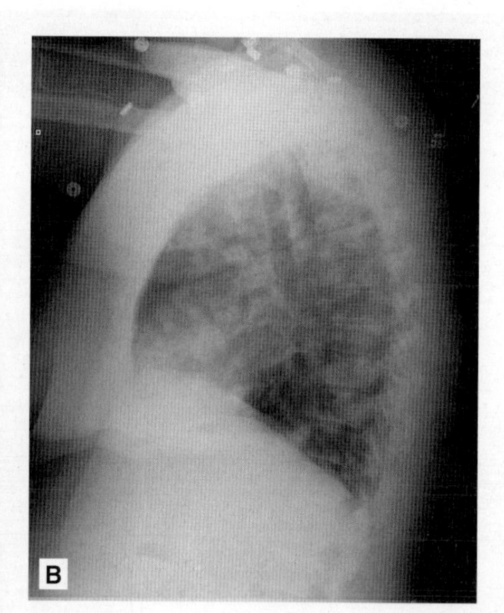

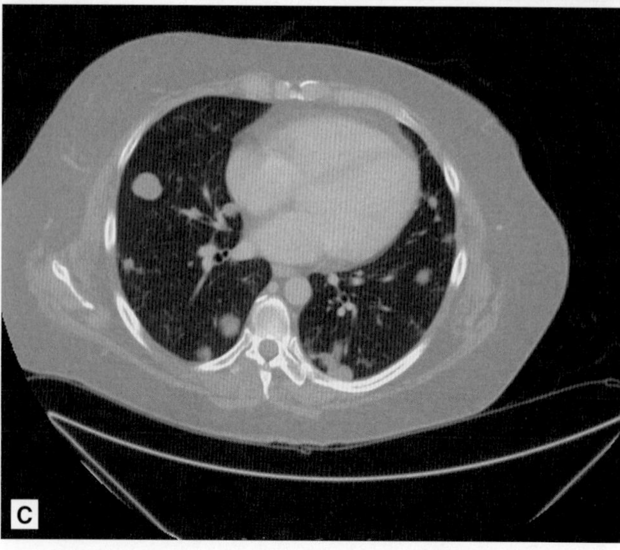

FIGURE 5.76 ■ Pulmonary Metastases. **A-C:** Frontal and lateral radiographs demonstrate innumerable metastatic pulmonary nodules in this patient with choriocarcinoma. The metastatic lesions are clearly seen on the accompanying CT image.

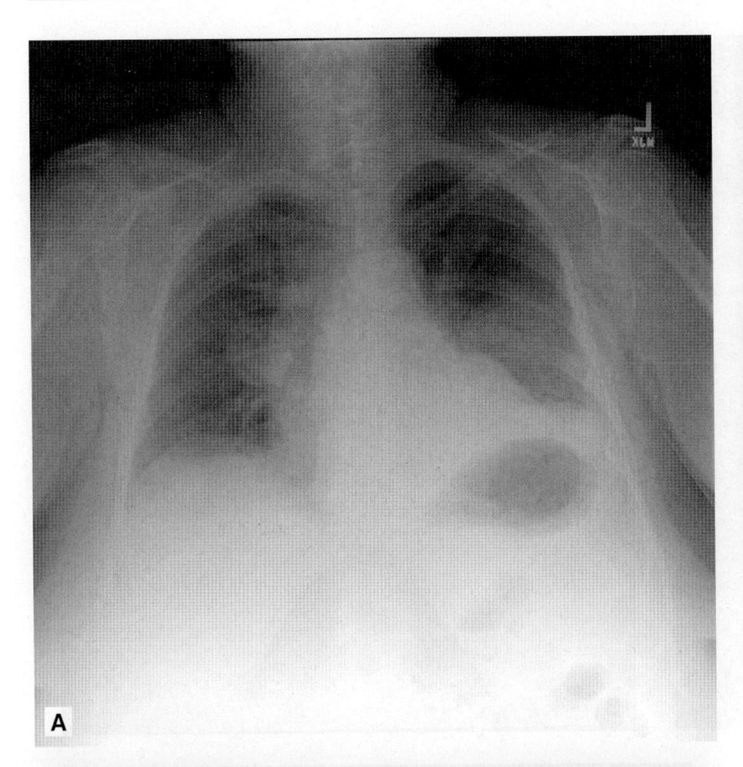

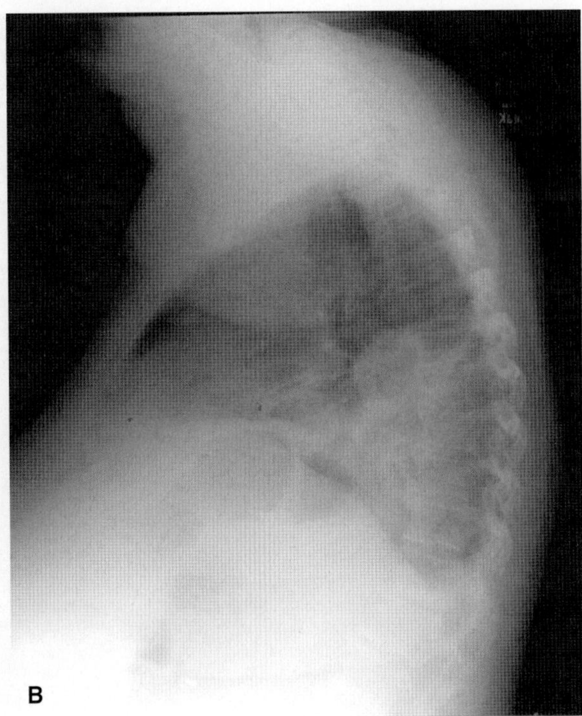

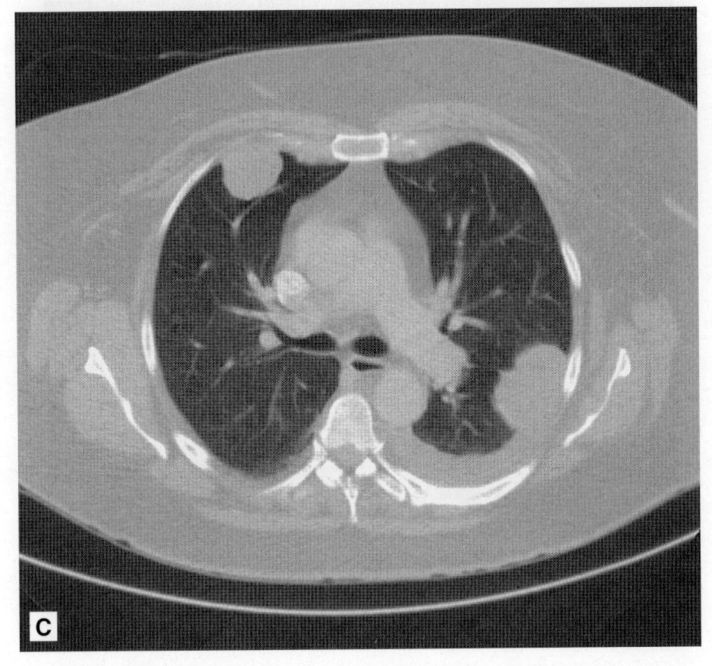

FIGURE 5.77 ■ Pulmonary Metastases. **A-C:** Frontal and lateral radiographs demonstrate bilateral perihilar masses and a left pleural effusion in this patient with an abdominal leiomyosarcoma. The CT image demonstrates large pleural-based masses anteriorly in the right upper lobe and posteriorly in the left upper lobe with a left pleural effusion.

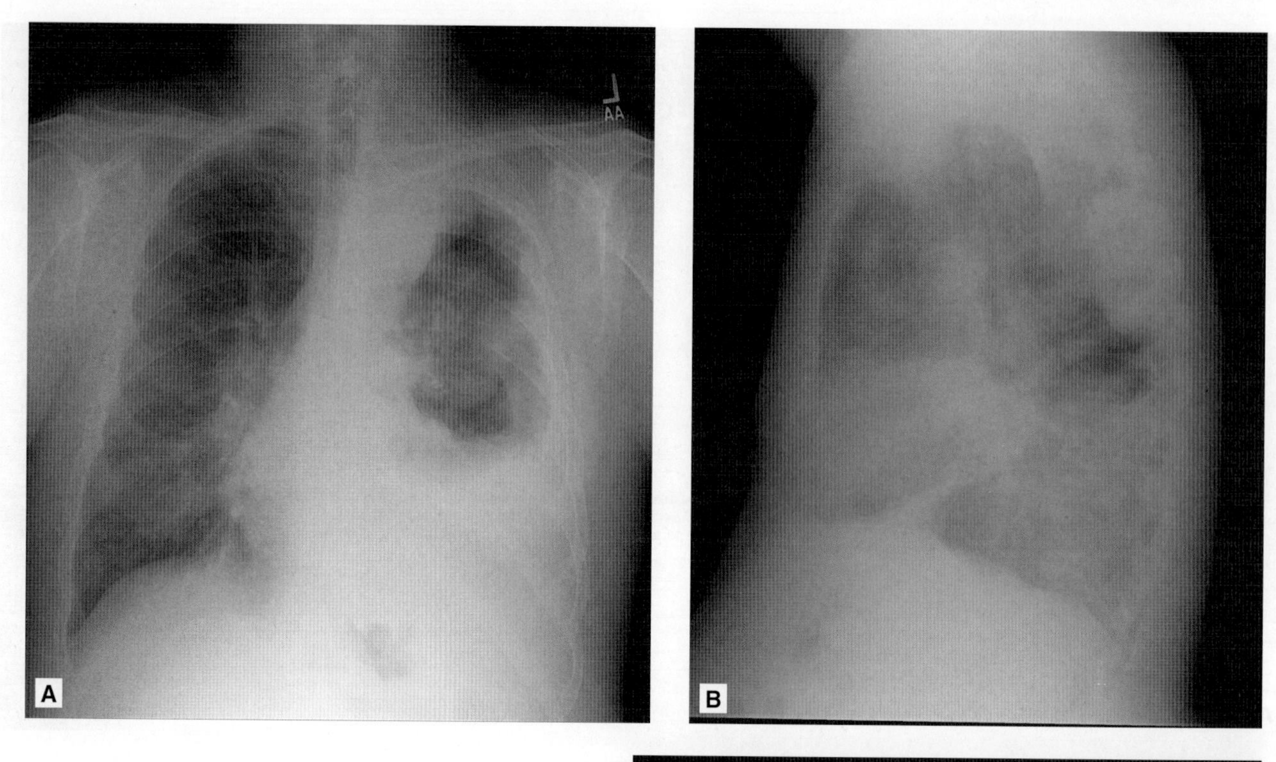

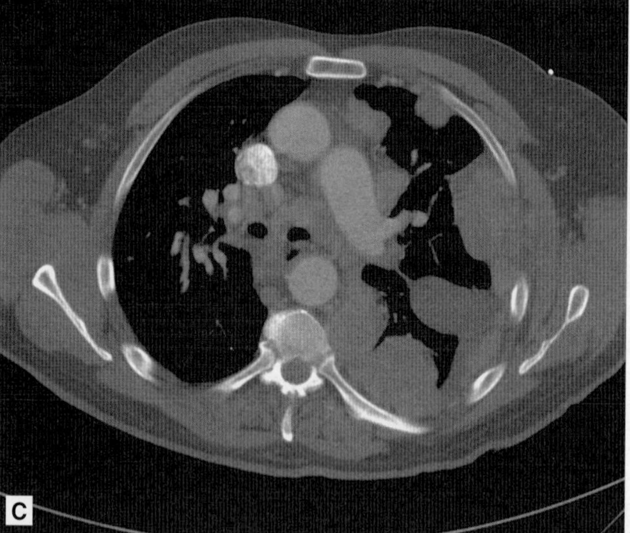

FIGURE 5.78 ■ Pulmonary Metastases. **A-C:** Frontal and lateral radiographs demonstrate nodular and circumferential left-sided pleural thickening. The CT image demonstrates numerous large pleural-based masses. Primary mesothelioma was the favored diagnosis initially, but on biopsy the patient was found to have metastatic renal cell carcinoma.

Radiographic Findings

Pulmonary fibrosis is a chronic inflammation of the tissue surrounding the alveoli due to unknown causes (though thought to be autoimmune) and results in prominent interstitial markings and architectural distortion. Comparison to prior radiographs is useful as most forms of pulmonary fibrosis show gradual progression over time and serve to highlight what is classically a chronic disease process from acute lung disease. Cross-sectional imaging can reveal ground-glass opacities and honeycombing.

Clinical Implications

Interstitial pulmonary fibrosis (IPF), also called Usual Interstitial Pneumonitis, results in a restrictive lung disease that diminishes lung compliance and restricts diffusion of oxygen across the tissue to the blood. Over time, the disease leads to impaired exercise tolerance, chronic hypoxia, and cough. Treatment is aimed at immunomodulation through steroids and cytotoxic agents to halt disease. While late IPF is easily identified on chest radiographs, early disease is difficult to distinguish from other interstitial processes, such as CHF.

Pearls

1. Pulmonary fibrosis has a classic appearance of interstitial markings more prominent at the bases.
2. If pulmonary fibrosis is suspected, further evaluation should be done via high-resolution protocol chest CT to further determine the etiology.

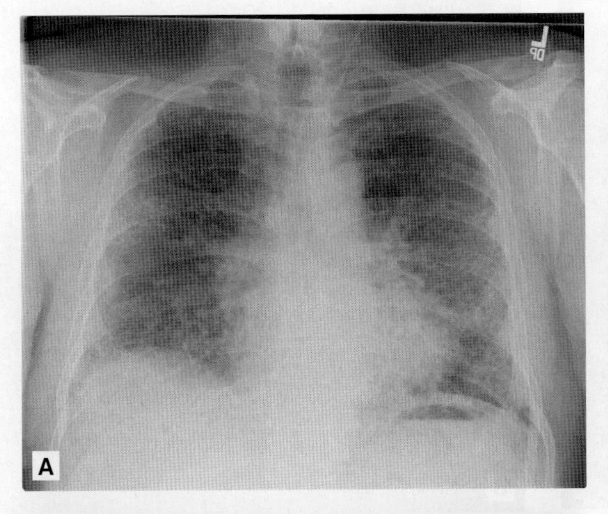

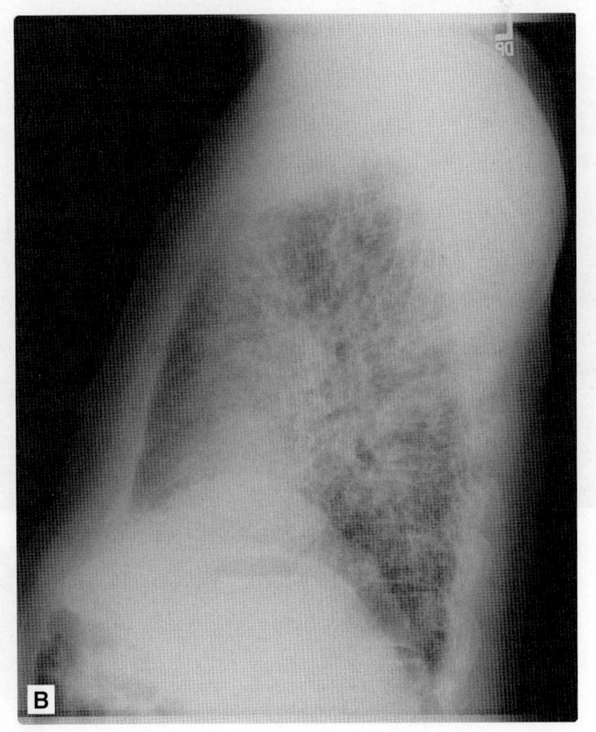

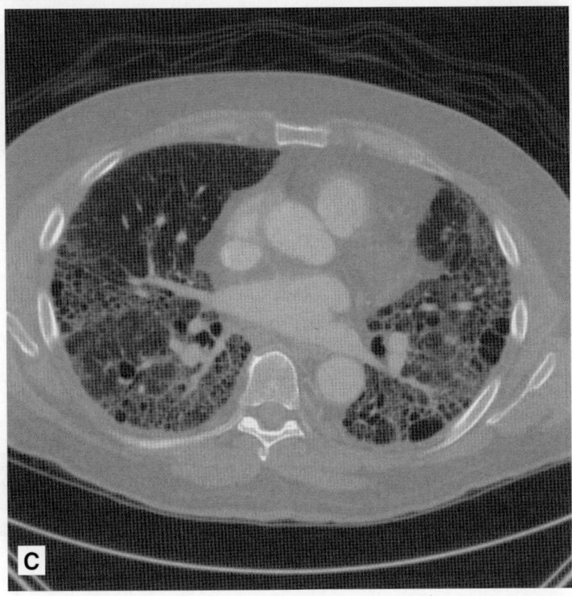

FIGURE 5.79 ■ Pulmonary Fibrosis. **A-C:** Frontal and lateral radiographs demonstrate coarse interstitial changes bilaterally and symmetrically in this patient with pulmonary fibrosis from usual interstitial pneumonitis (UIP). Accompanying chest CT image demonstrates changes of fibrosis with subpleural septal lines as well as subpleural clusters of thin-walled cystic spaces consistent with honeycombing.

Radiographic Findings

COPD is a chronic destructive process in the lung parenchyma resulting in increased compliance and inflammatory broncho-constriction resulting in restricted ventilation. The hallmark of COPD is chronic hyperexpansion. Conventional radiographs reveal flattened diaphragms and an increased antero-posterior diameter of the chest. The lungs appear hyperlucent and the pulmonary vessels appear attenuated and splayed due to bullae. The cardiac silhouette may appear smaller relative to the chest or more vertical due to lowering of the diaphragm. Hyperexpansion often results in an enlarged retrosternal clear space. Large bullae may mimic pneumothorax due to the loss of vascularity in the parenchyma, unlike a pneumothorax, they appear as round areas devoid of vessels and there is no visceral pleural white line. Cross-sectional imaging reveals displaced septae; bullae are frequently seen at the apices.

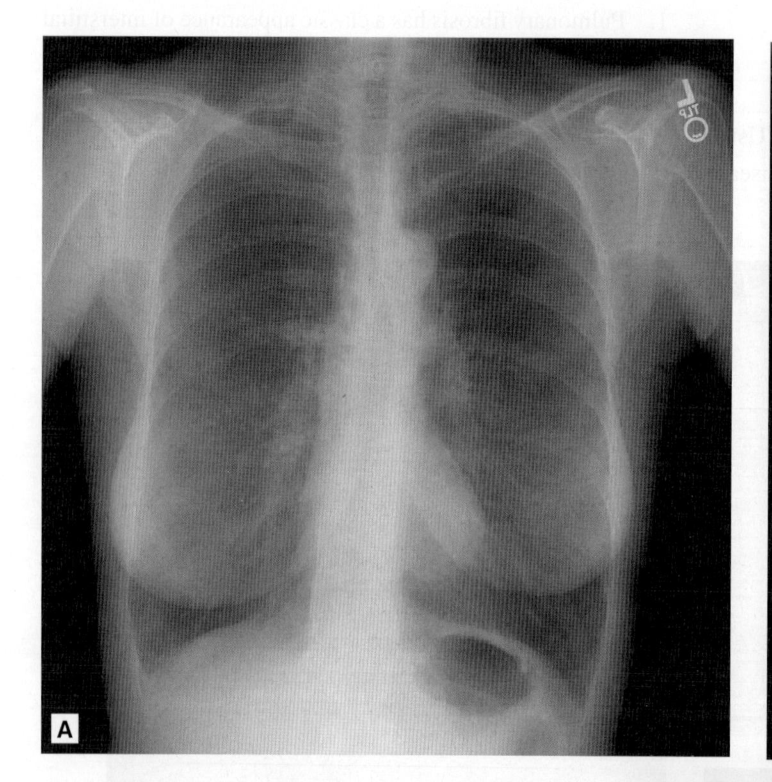

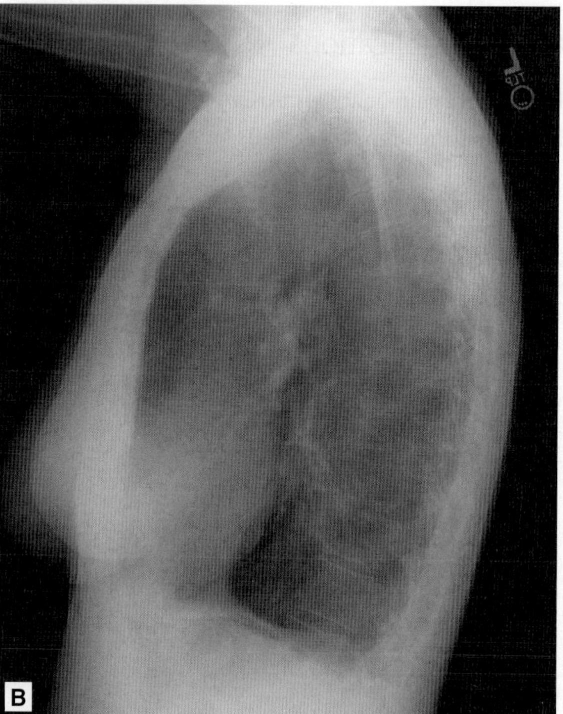

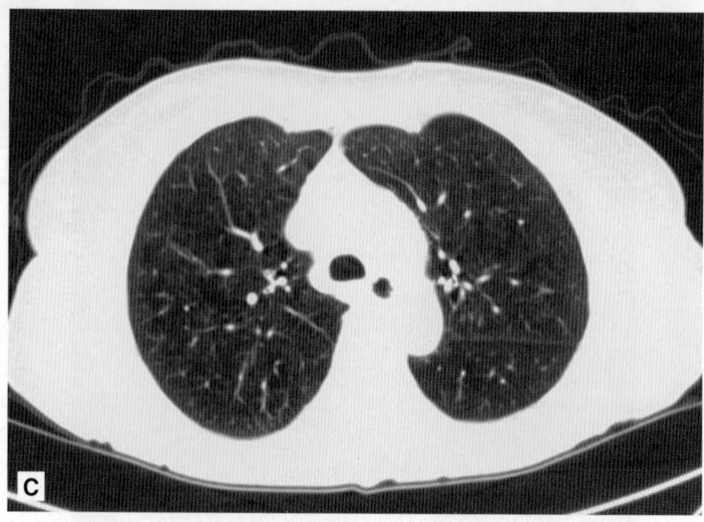

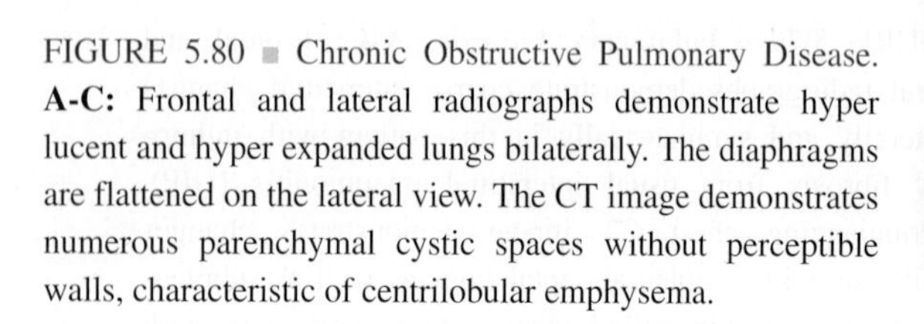
FIGURE 5.80 ■ Chronic Obstructive Pulmonary Disease. **A-C:** Frontal and lateral radiographs demonstrate hyper lucent and hyper expanded lungs bilaterally. The diaphragms are flattened on the lateral view. The CT image demonstrates numerous parenchymal cystic spaces without perceptible walls, characteristic of centrilobular emphysema.

Clinical Implications

Radiographic findings of COPD are not due to acute illness, but rather due to chronic disease over years of obstructive lung processes. Patients with dyspnea and findings of COPD on chest radiograph should be treated empirically with beta-agonists, ipatropium, and steroids to aid in bronchodilation and reduction of inflammation. They are at increased risk for morbidity and mortality due to infection, and therefore a low threshold for antibiotic use is generally preferred, with antibiotic administration during COPD exacerbations resulting in diminished duration of hospitalization.

Pearls

1. Radiographic findings of COPD show evidence of the chronic process rather than acute findings.
2. The lungs are typically hyperinflated and hyperlucent in patients with COPD.
3. Emphysematous changes of COPD tend to favor the apices.

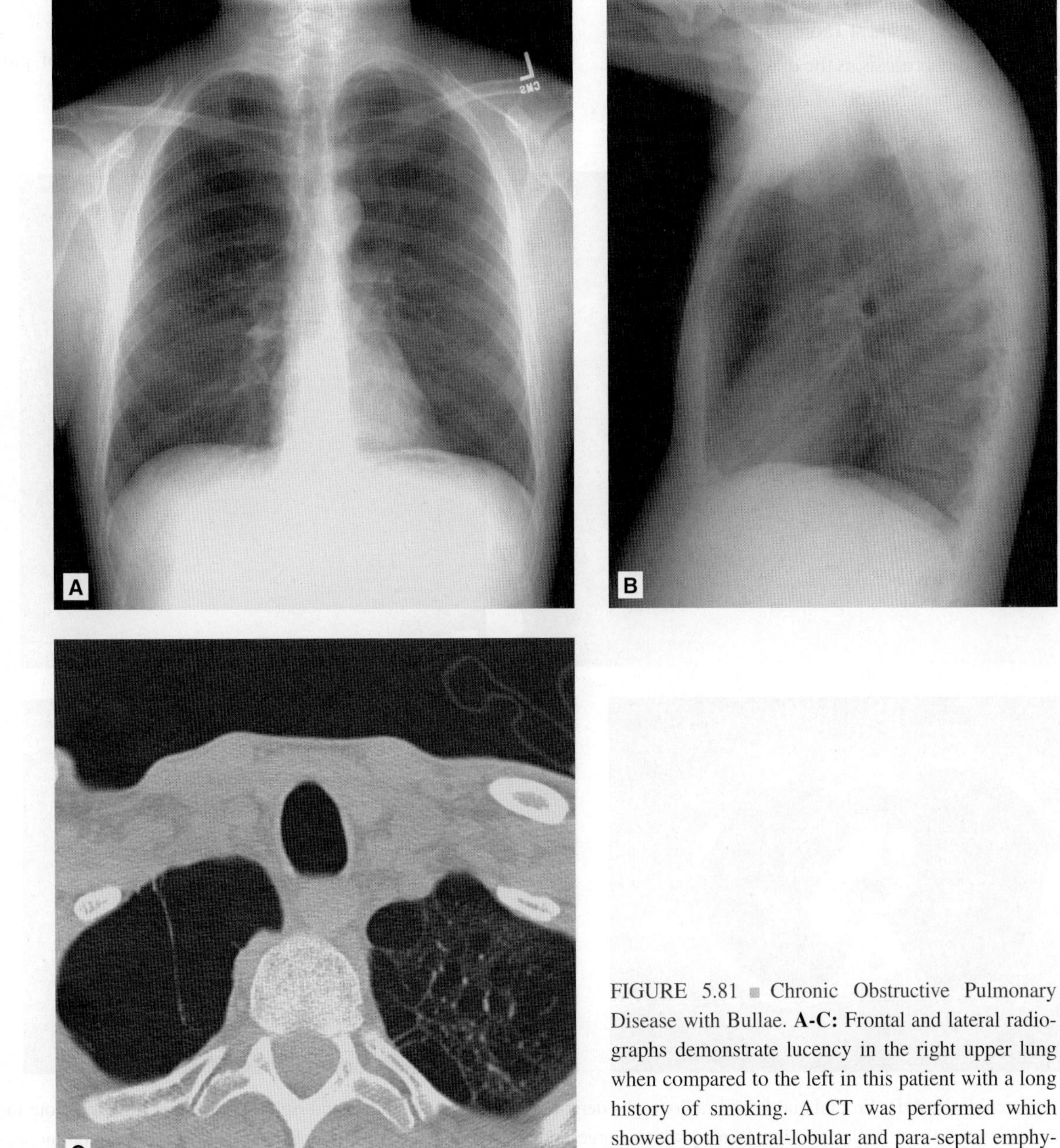

FIGURE 5.81 ■ Chronic Obstructive Pulmonary Disease with Bullae. **A-C:** Frontal and lateral radiographs demonstrate lucency in the right upper lung when compared to the left in this patient with a long history of smoking. A CT was performed which showed both central-lobular and para-septal emphysematous changes.

Radiographic Findings

Sarcoidosis is an idiopathic, multisystem, granulomatous disease that involves the lungs in 90% of those who have it. Hilar and right paratracheal lymphadenopathy are the classic radiographic findings for the disease. Differential considerations include lymphoma and primary tuberculosis. Sarcoidosis can also cause increased interstitial markings and interstitial fibrosis.

Clinical Implications

Sarcoidosis is a difficult diagnosis and requires a biopsy for the definitive diagnosis. Patients with respiratory complaints and isolated lymphadenopathy on chest radiography suggest sarcoidosis, lymphoma or tuberculosis as the diagnosis. In patients with known sarcoidosis, progression of disease seen on chest radiographs over time may prompt more aggressive treatment with steroids or anti-neoplastic agents to prevent sequalae.

Pearls

1. A subcarinal density on the PA and lateral views is due to subcarinal lymphadenopathy and is suggestive of sarcoidosis. The lateral view is particularly helpful.
2. On the frontal chest radiograph, right peri-tracheal fullness and bilateral peri-hilar fullness is commonly referred to as the "1-2-3" sign and is a classic sign for sarcoidosis, however, this sign is not pathognomonic: lymphoma and primary tuberculosis should also be considered.
3. Patients with sarcoidosis can also have changes of pulmonary fibrosis (favoring the mid and upper lungs).

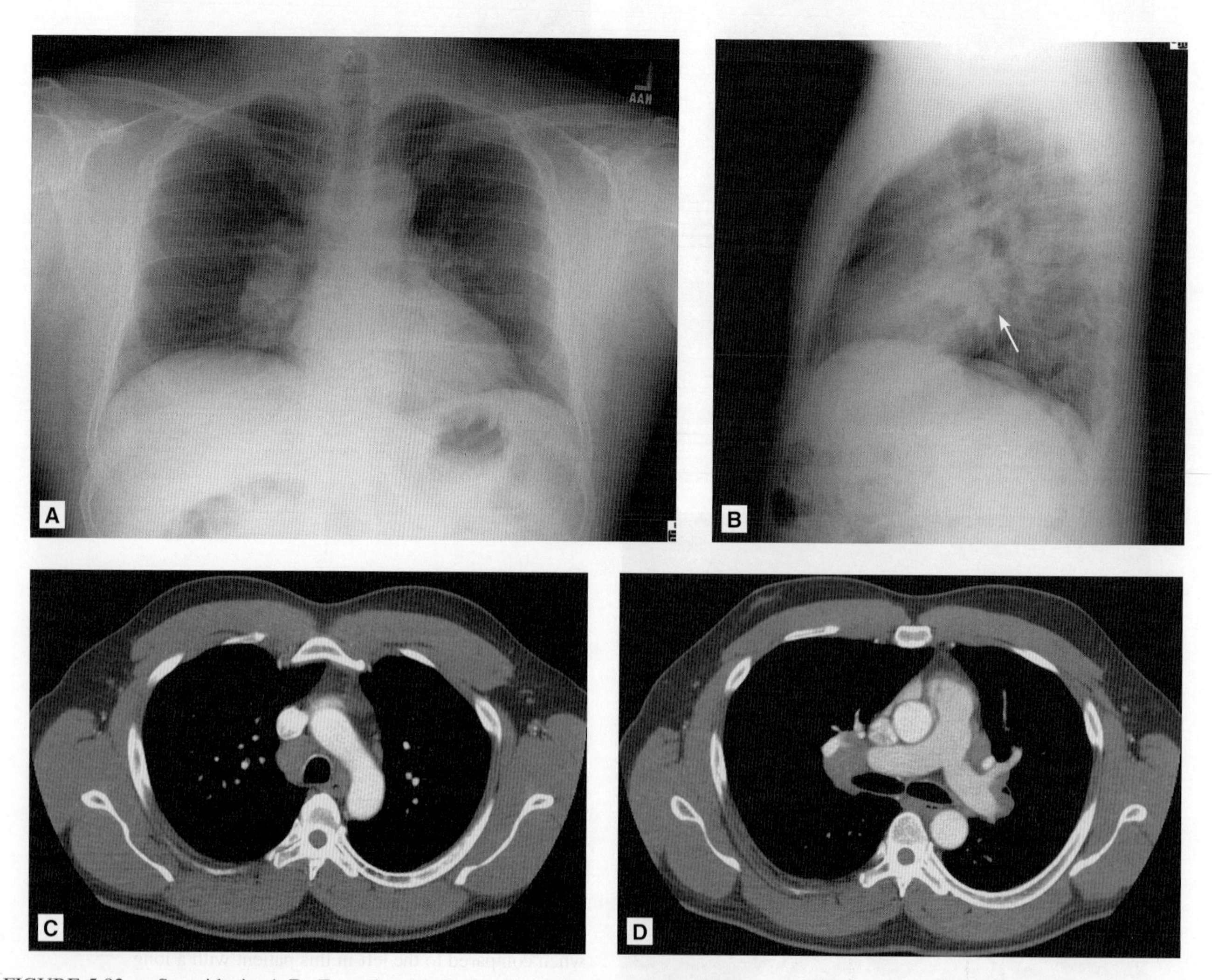

FIGURE 5.82 ■ Sarcoidosis. **A-D:** Frontal and lateral radiographs demonstrate bilateral perihilar and right paratracheal fullness. Note the filling of the infrahilar window on the lateral view (arrow) which suggests these findings are from lymphadenopathy rather than pulmonary hypertension. The contrast-enhanced CT images nicely show the right paratracheal and perihilar lymphadenopathy.

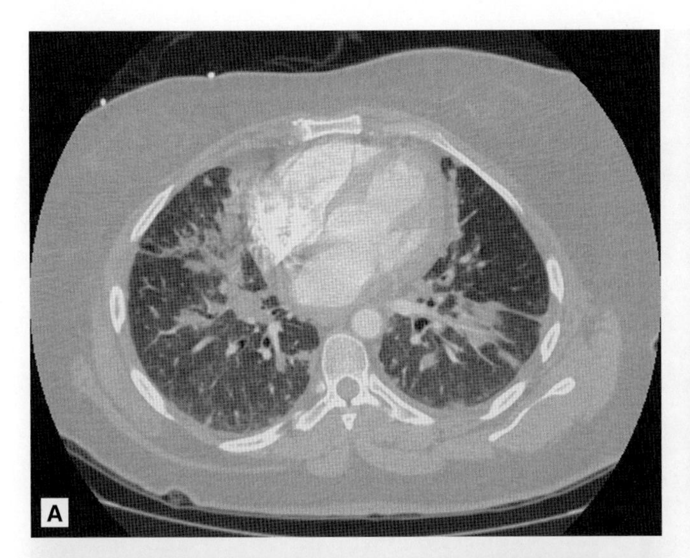

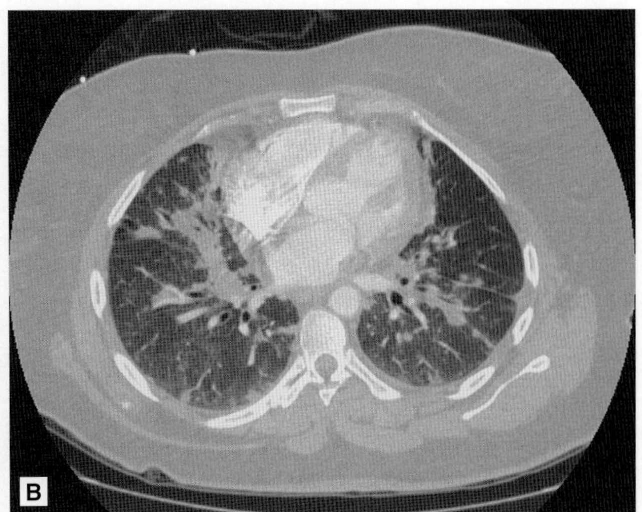

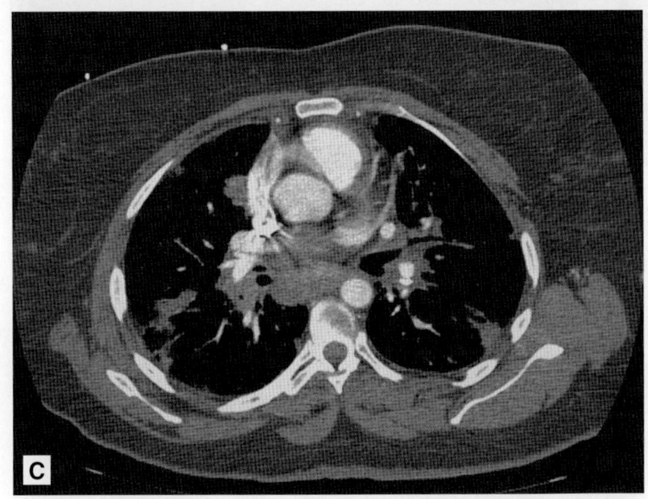

FIGURE 5.83 ■ Sarcoidosis. **A-C:** CT images on lung windows demonstrate bilateral peribronchovascular thickening in this patient with sarcoidosis. Also note the associated mediastinal and hilar lymphadenopathy on the more superior slice with mediastinal windows.

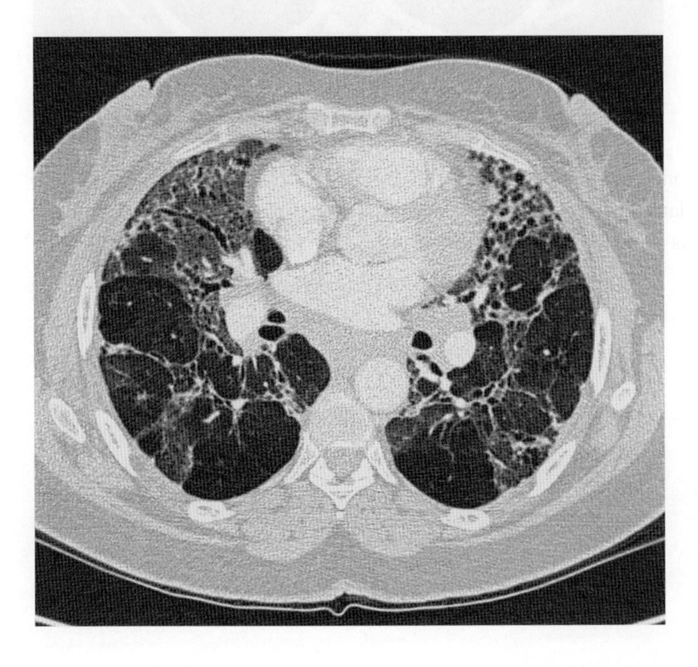

FIGURE 5.84 ■ Sarcoidosis with Pulmonary Fibrosis. Single high-resolution CT image of a patient with pulmonary fibrosis from sarcoidosis. Note the interlobular and intralobular septal lines along with traction bronchiectasis in the right middle lobe. Honeycombing can be seen anteriorly in the lingula. These findings are typical of late-stage pulmonary sarcoidosis.

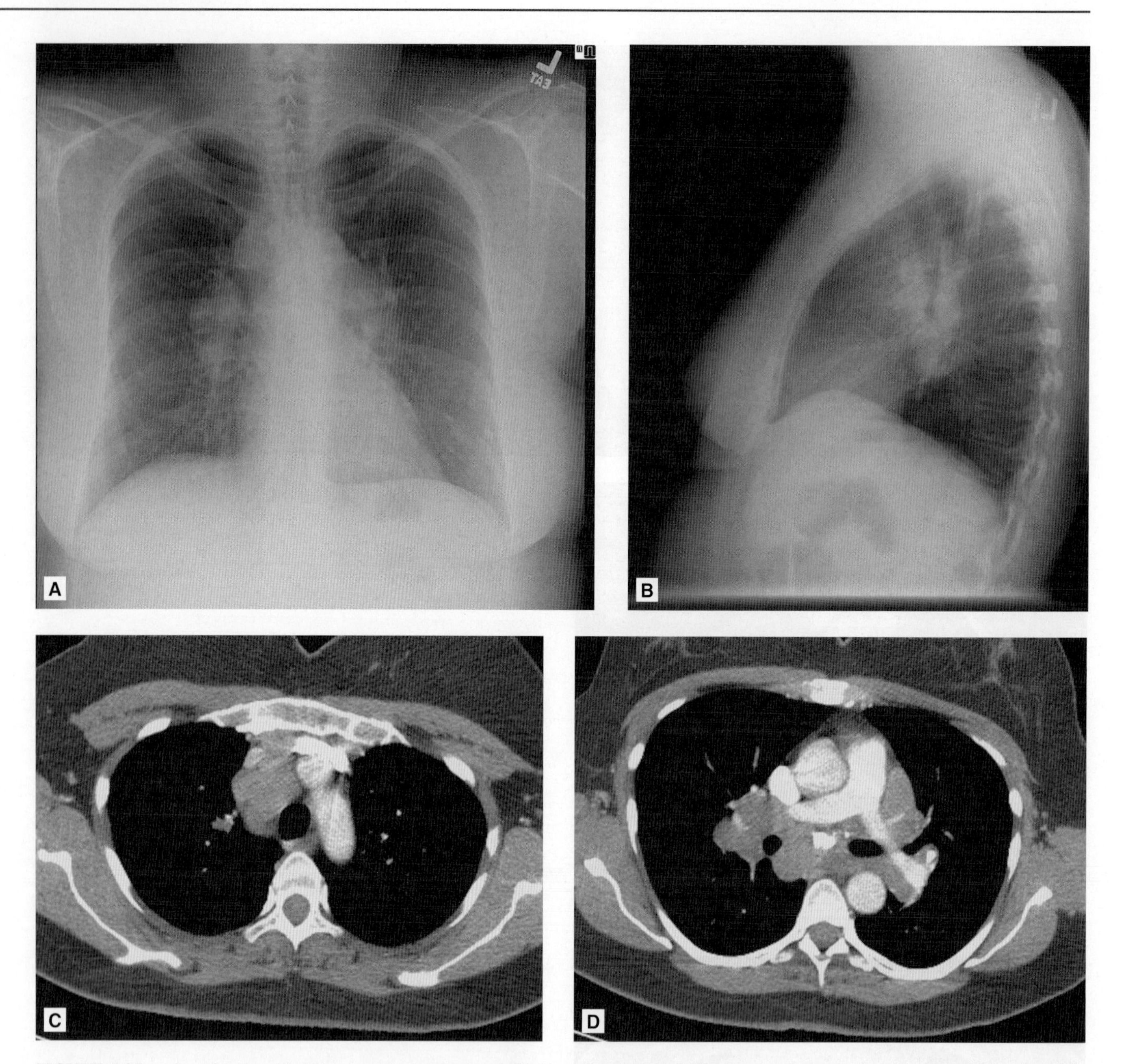

FIGURE 5.85 ■ Sarcoidosis with Hilar Lymphadenopathy. **A-D:** Frontal and lateral radiographs demonstrate bilateral perihilar and right paratracheal fullness. Note the filling of the infrahilar window on the lateral view which confirms these findings are from lymphadenopathy rather than pulmonary hypertension. The contrast-enhanced CT images show the right paratracheal and perihilar lymphadenopathy.

Radiographic Findings

Cystic fibrosis (CF) is a genetic disorder that results in abnormal transport of sodium and chloride across the epithelial cells causing thickened and viscous secretions. In the lungs, this leads to mucous plugging, chronic infection, and bronchiectasis. Mucous plugging may result in varying regions of atelectasis, more commonly in the upper lobes. Chronic infection and scarring cause interstitial markings. Bronchiectasis may be evident as "tram-tacking" markings of parallel linear opacities representing enlarged segmental bronchi that have been widened by chronic infection. Diffuse infiltrates tend to be prominent apically due to the increased frequency of infection in this area, but can be diffuse. Evaluation requires comparison to prior radiographs to evaluate progression as well as to evaluate for subtle new areas for consolidation due to pneumonia and mucous plugging.

Clinical Implications

CF results in thickened mucoid secretions of the respiratory epithelium and impaired evacuation of contaminants in the respiratory tree. Over time, this leads to colonization with respiratory pathogens and scarring from chronic disease. Mucous plugs can result in impaired ventilation and pneumonias which frequently harbor multidrug resistant organisms. Fever and respiratory complaints in a CF patient should result in the careful selection of broad-spectrum antibiotics and hospitalization as the duration and severity of illness are higher than in the general population.

Pearls

1. CF results in scarring, with interstitial infiltrates, "tram tracking," and atelectasis due to mucous plugging.
2. CF tends to favor the upper lung fields over the bases.
3. When reviewing the chest radiograph of a CF patient, it is especially important to look at the old studies to determine if there is a new opacity, which may represent an acute infection on top of chronic lung findings.

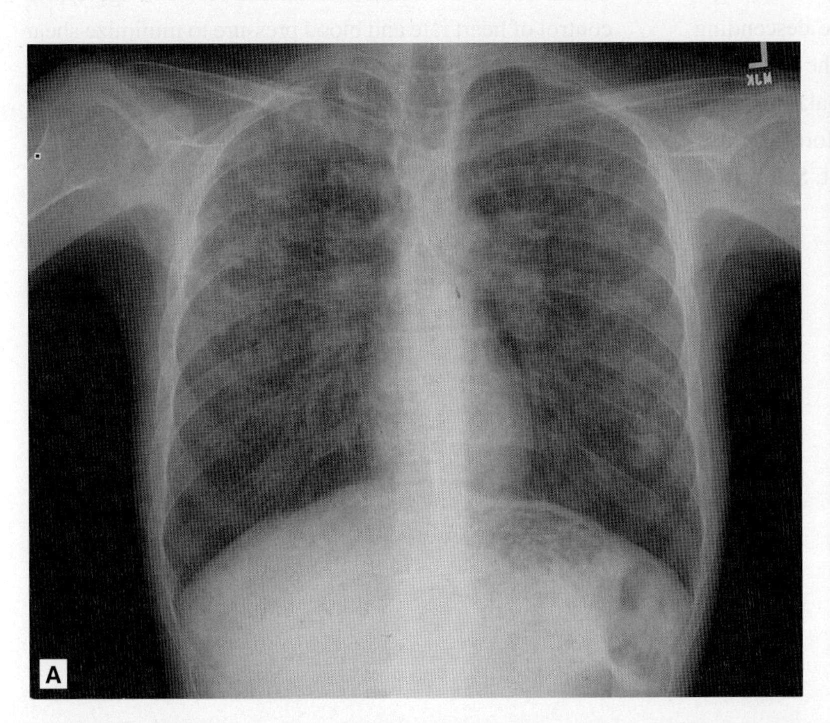

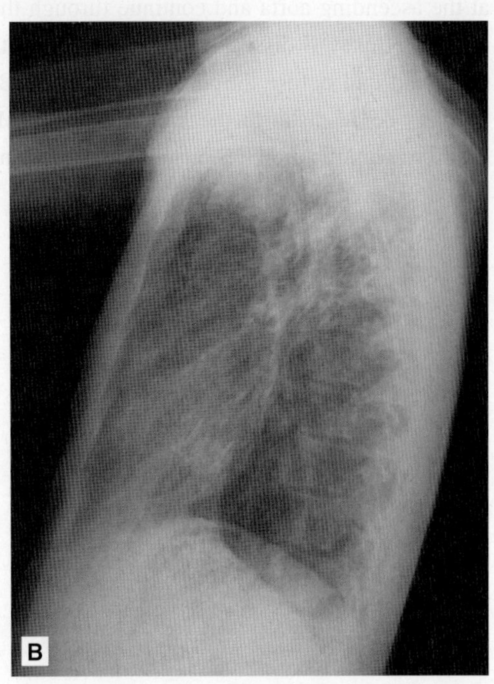

FIGURE 5.86 ■ Cystic Fibrosis. **A, B:** Frontal and lateral chest radiographs demonstrate coarse interstitial markings and bronchiectasis predominantly in the mid and upper lungs with relative sparing of the lung bases in this patient with cystic fibrosis. Note the ring shadows as well as tram-tracking in the upper lungs commonly seen with cystic fibrosis.

Radiographic Findings

Aortic dissection is an acute aortic syndrome characterized by a tear in the intima or adventitia layers creating a false lumen and is propagated by the shear force of an expanding column of blood. Dissections may extend distally, proximally, or in both directions, from the original tear. Nontraumatic aortic dissection may occur with preceding aneurismal dilation, which can be seen on conventional radiography. A dilated aorta (>3 cm) is suspicious for dissection. Suspicion should prompt immediate imaging with cross-sectional imaging provided the patient is stable. To differentiate dissection best, a contrast load should be utilized to better identify the intimal flap and thrombus from normal aortic flow. With contrast each image needs to be evaluated for any evidence of active extravasation as well as identification of the hypodense intimal flap between the dissection and true lumen of the aorta.

Clinical Implications

A thoracic aortic dissection is a medical emergency that requires immediate treatment and traditionally are subdivided based on their origin. DeBakey I dissections begin at the ascending aorta and continue through the descending aorta. DeBakey II dissections are confined to the ascending aorta and end before the left subclavian; DeBakey III dissections begin distal to the left subclavian. More recently, Stanford classification has dictated management. Stanford A dissections (originating in the ascending aorta, regardless of where they end) require surgical management while Stanford B (originating distal to the left subclavian) often respond well to medical management.

Management of an aortic dissection focuses on reducing shear stress on the vessel walls, which requires aggressive blood pressure and heart rate control. Titratable beta-blockers, used in combination with nitrates are the mainstay of therapy.

Aortic dissections may extend into the carotid arteries and may impede blood flow to the brain, cause altered mental status, and stroke. Dissection through intercostal arteries in the descending thoracic aorta can result in severe back pain or ripping chest pain going through to the back and can be a clue to aid in the diagnosis. Dissection proximal to the coronary arteries can occur as well and precipitate myocardial infarction, which is usually a poor prognostic omen.

Pearls

1. Clinical suspicion for aortic dissection requires prompt CT with contrast, as conventional radiographs have limited specificity for dissection.
2. Identification of a dissection should result in aggressive control of heart rate and blood pressure to minimize shear forces on the vessel to prevent further dissection.
3. Any chest pain with altered mental status should prompt evaluation for aortic dissection with carotid extension.

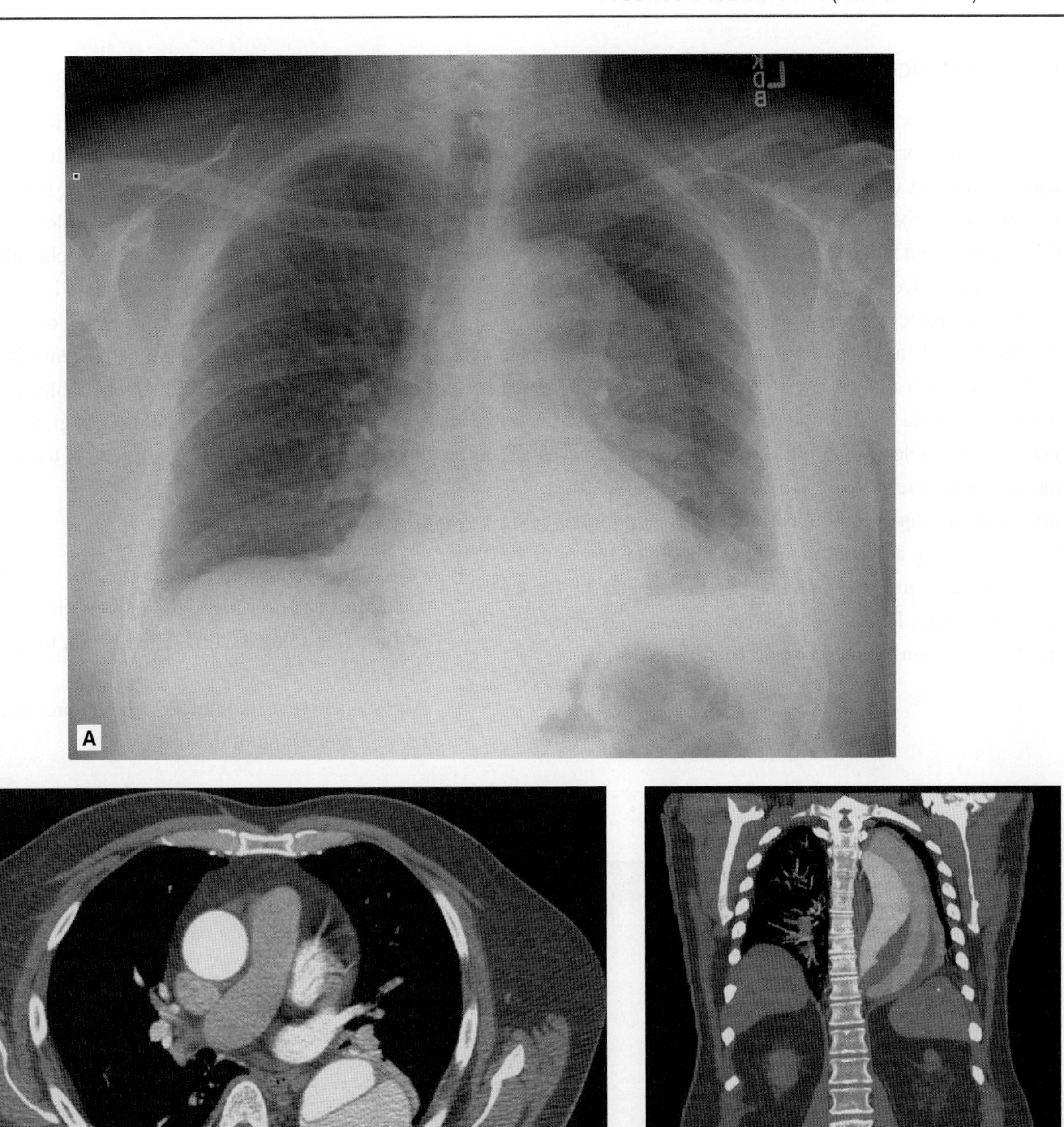

FIGURE 5.87 ■ Aortic Dissection. **A-C:** Frontal radiograph demonstrates prominence of the descending thoracic aorta, concern for aneurysm or dissection. Axial and coronal contrast-enhanced CTA images demonstrate a Stanford type B aortic dissection of the descending thoracic aorta. Note the higher density contrast in the smaller true lumen and the lower density contrast in the larger false lumen.

Radiographic Summary

An aneurysm is dilation of the arterial wall greater than 1.5 times its normal diameter. A thoracic aortic aneurysm can be apparent on plain radiograph, but definitive evaluation requires cross-sectional imaging by contrast-enhanced CT. Aneurysmal dilation of the ascending aorta results in aortic prominence extending to the right and anteriorly into the retrosternal clear space. Dilation of the arch results in enlargement of the aortic knob at the superior aspect of the mediastinum on the PA view. Aneurysmal dilation of the descending aorta can be appreciated on the AP and lateral views. Atherosclerotic calcification of the aorta makes the radiographic detection of aneurysmal dilatation easier. CT imaging relies on specific measurements, with normal being less than 2.9 cm at the aortic annulus, less than 3.9 cm at the mid sinus, 2.9 cm at the sinotubular junction, and 3.9 for the ascending aorta. Distal to the ascending aorta, any measurement greater than 4 cm is considered aneurysmal.

Clinical Implications

Identification of a thoracic aortic aneurysm in the presence of any symptoms of chest pain should result in cross-sectional imaging with contrast to look for dissection. In the absence of symptoms, measurements should be made along with subspecialist referral to determine a surveillance schedule as well as decide when and what interventions should be made.

Medical therapy focuses on management of blood pressure and heart rate over the long term to prevent dissection and further dilation. This is achieved with beta-blockade, calcium channel blockade, and ACE inhibitors/angiotensin receptor blockers depending on the clinical needs of the patient.

Pearls

1. Aortic aneurysms can be seen on chest radiograph, and in the presence of any symptoms of chest pain, should be further evaluated with CT to rule out the possibility of dissection.
2. Aortic aneurysms require strict blood pressure control to prevent worsening of disease.

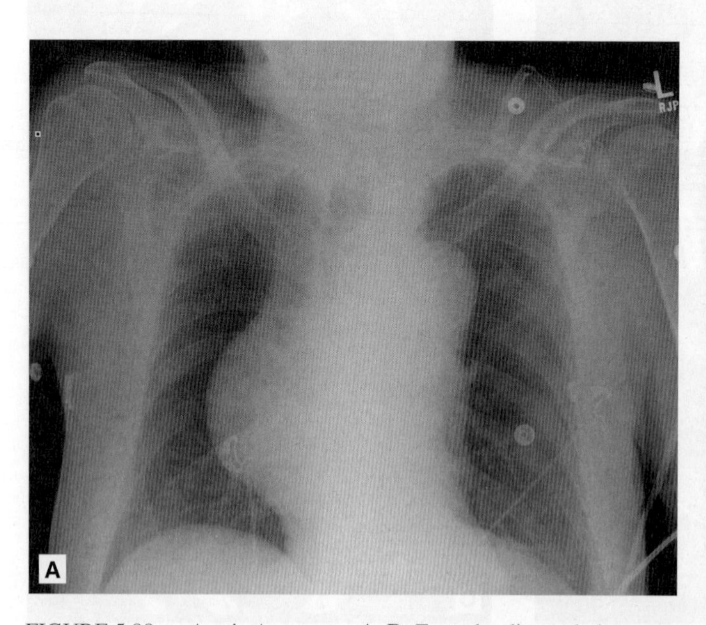

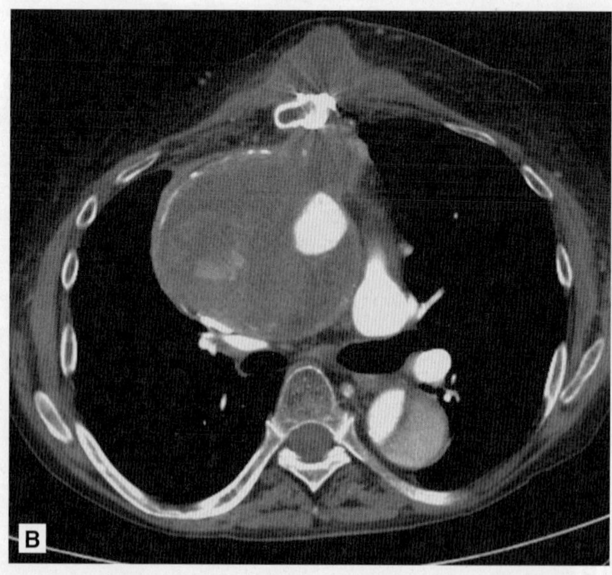

FIGURE 5.88 ■ Aortic Aneurysm. **A, B:** Frontal radiograph demonstrates prominence of the ascending aorta as well as the aortic arch, concern for an aneurysm or dissection. Contrast-enhanced CTA image demonstrates a pseudoaneurysm of the ascending aorta with a hematoma extending into the soft tissues anterior to the sternum. Additionally, there is a dissection of the descending thoracic aorta.

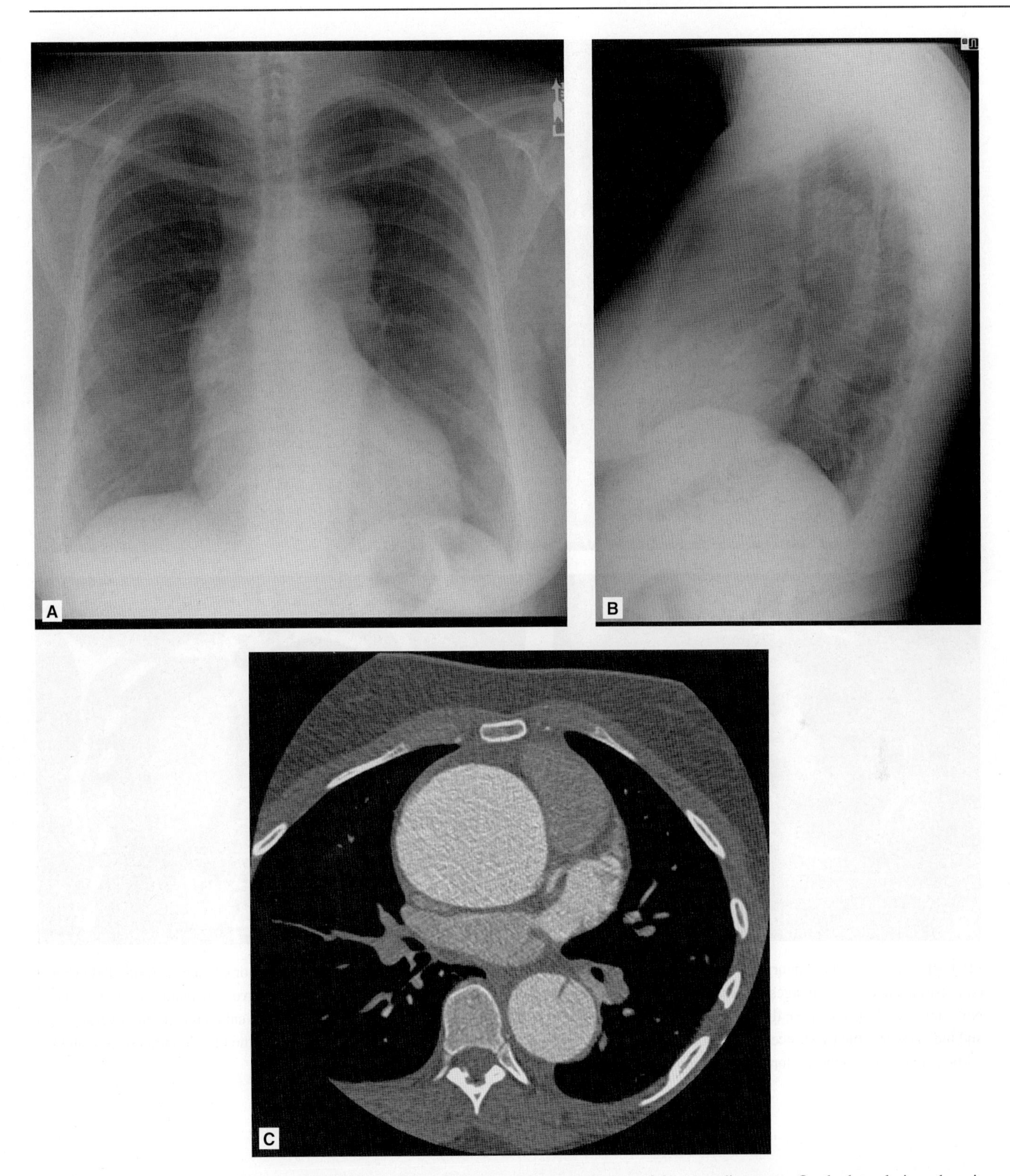

FIGURE 5.89 ■ Aortic Aneurysm. **A-C:** Frontal radiograph demonstrates prominence of the ascending aorta. On the lateral view, there is filling of the retrosternal clear space by the ascending aorta. The contrast-enhanced CTA image demonstrates a large ascending aorta aneurysm measuring 63 mm. Also note a small dissection flap in the descending thoracic aorta.

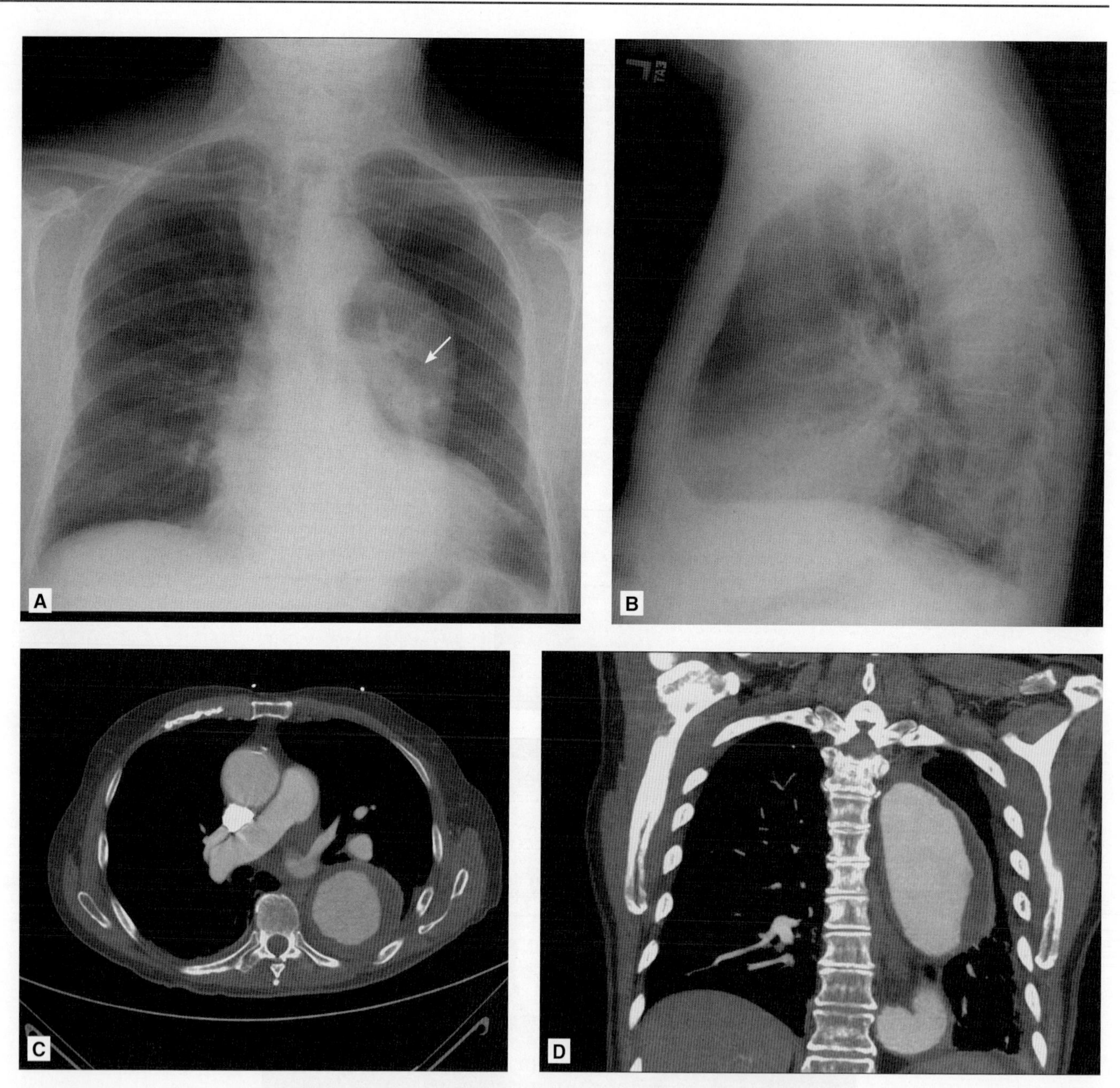

FIGURE 5.90 ■ Aortic Aneurysm. **A-D:** Frontal and lateral radiographs demonstrate prominence of the thoracic aorta. Axial and coronal contrast-enhanced CTA images demonstrate a descending thoracic aorta aneurysm, which contains extensive soft plaque in its periphery. Note how clearly you can see the left pulmonary artery superimposed over the aortic shadow (arrow). This is called the "hilum overlay' sign and indicates that the two processes are in different parts of the mediastinum (i.e., the pulmonary artery is in the middle mediastinum and the aortic aneurysm is in the posterior mediastinum).

Radiographic Findings

Esophageal intubation is readily identified on conventional radiographs with the endotracheal tube not in the trachea. The untrained observer can be misled by radiolucency around the tube which is mistaken for the trachea that is actually air in the esophagus due to ventilation. Every post-intubation chest radiograph should be carefully evaluated to identify the carina and trachea and confirm that the tube is correctly placed. Secondary signs of esophageal intubation include a distended gastric air bubble and pneumomediastinum if the endotracheal tube is outside the esophagus.

Clinical Implications

Intubation outside the trachea is best avoided via direct or indirect observation of the endotracheal tube passing though the vocal cords. However, tubes can be shifted during patient transport and manipulation, and any suspicion of extubation should prompt a chest radiograph to confirm placement.

Pearls

1. All intubations, changes in ventilation status, or large manipulations of the patient should be followed up with a radiograph to confirm appropriate tube placement within the trachea.
2. The distal tip of the ET tube should reside between the clavicular heads when optimally positioned within the trachea.
3. Tube positioning based on a spine landmark is less reliable than using an anterior landmark (clavicular heads) due to variability of patient position and beam direction.

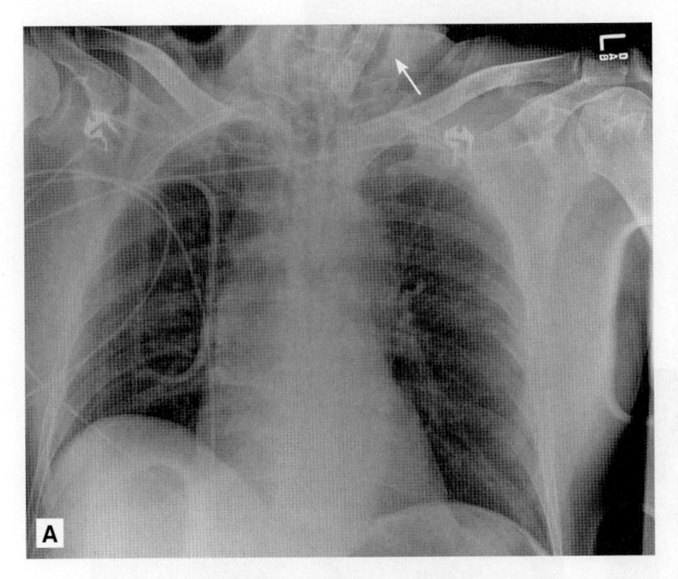

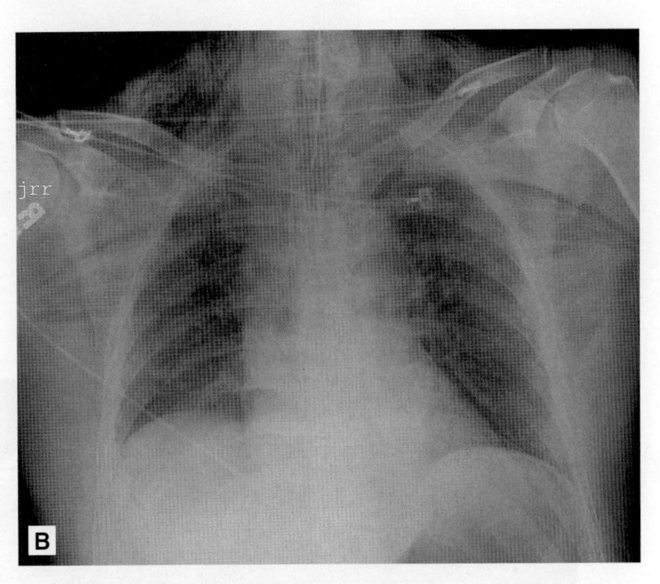

FIGURE 5.91 ■ Esophageal Intubation. **A, B:** Frontal radiograph demonstrates endotracheal tube placement to the left of the trachea in this trauma patient (arrow). Esophageal intubation was suspected and the endotracheal was replaced. The follow-up radiograph demonstrated adequate placement of the endotracheal tube, however, subcutaneous emphysema could be seen in the soft tissues of the neck and thorax from iatrogenic esophageal perforation. (Images courtesy of Ed Donnelly, MD)

Radiographic Findings

Superior vena cava (SVC) syndrome is the result of external compression of the SVC by a tumor impairing venous return. Conventional chest radiography may reveal an obstructing mass, but most frequently will not reveal the cause of the clinical findings. Cross-sectional imaging with a contrast bolus in the venous phase is the best diagnostic study for determining the location and degree of impingement on venous return. Frequently collateral circulation around the SVC is dilated in response to the gradually increasing impairment of venous return through the SVC.

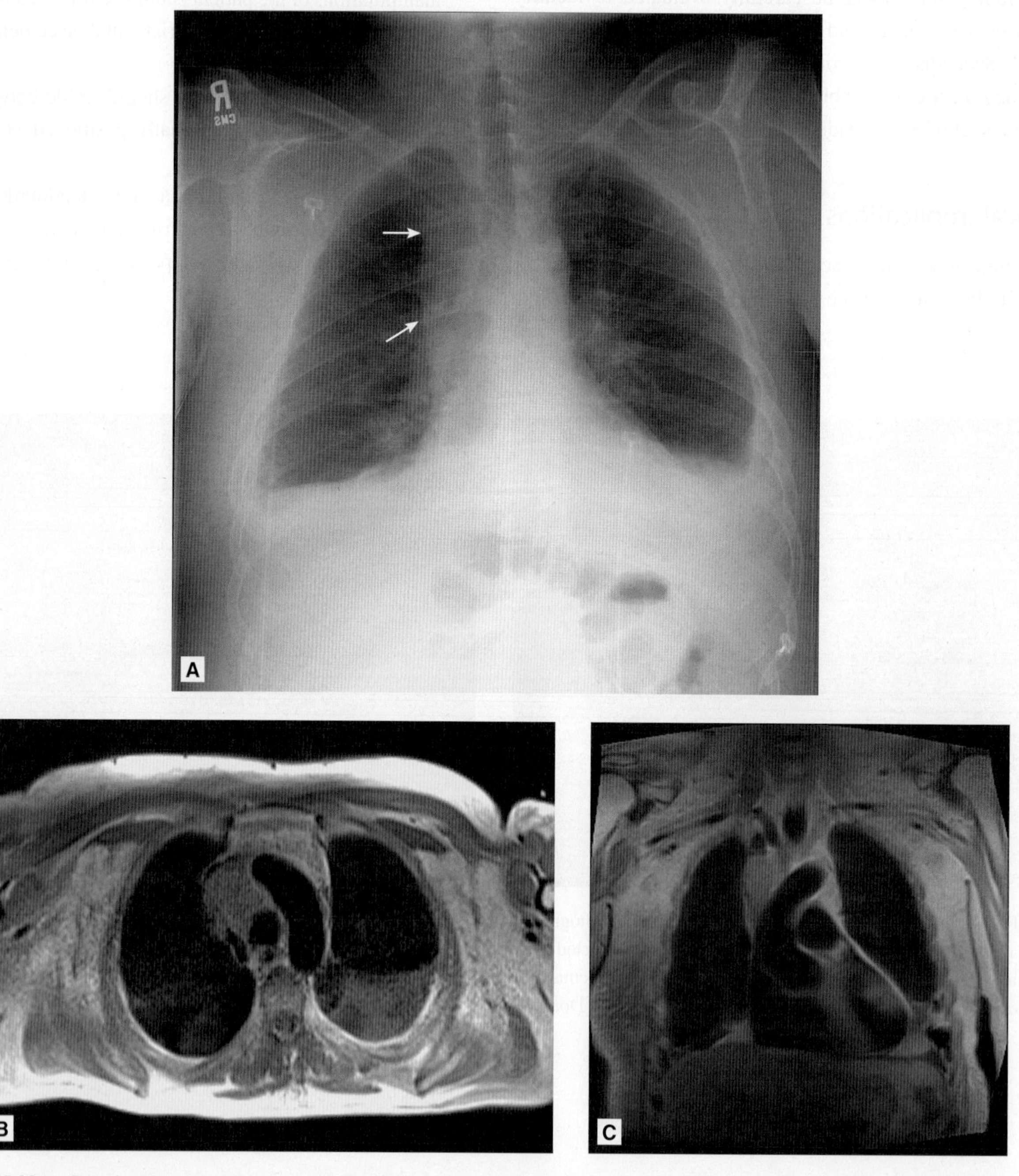

FIGURE 5.92 ■ Superior Vena Cava Syndrome. **A-E:** Frontal chest radiograph demonstrates fullness of the right paratracheal stripe (arrows) in the patient with face, neck, and upper extremity swelling from suspected SVC syndrome. Bilateral pleural effusions are also noted. Axial and coronal dark blood T1-weighted images demonstrate extensive tumor thrombus in the SVC from an adjacent mediastinal tumor. Axial and coronal 2-D time-of-flight images show near-complete occlusion of the SVC.

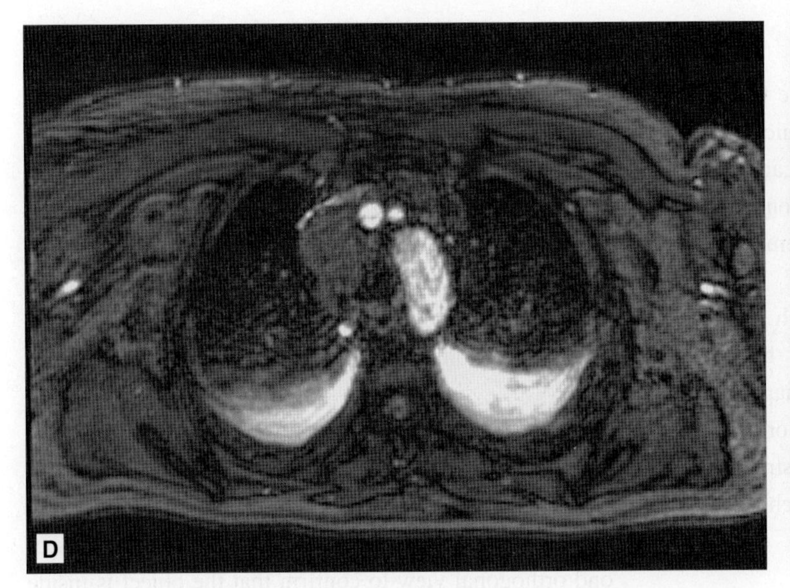

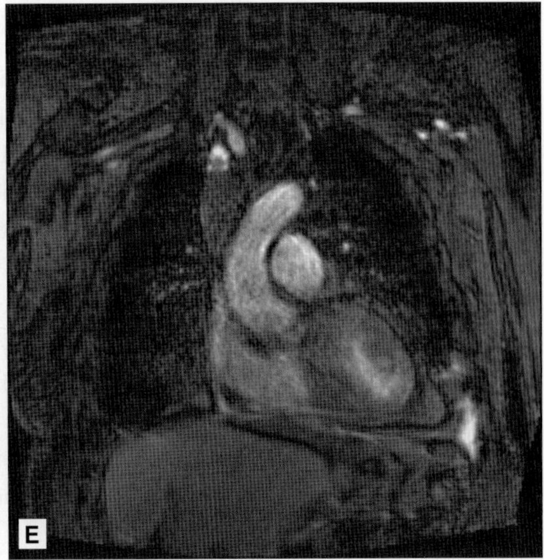

FIGURE 5.92 ■ *(Continued)*

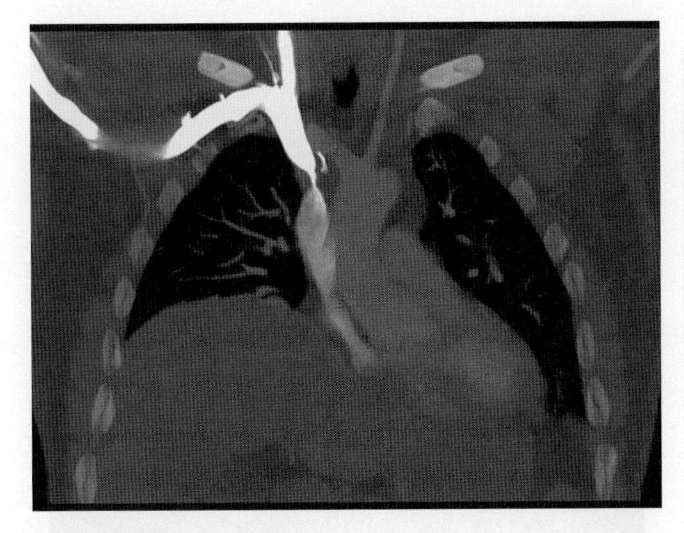

FIGURE 5.93 ■ Superior Vena Cava Syndrome. Coronal CTA image demonstrates critical stenosis of the SVC from an adjacent adenocarcinoma in this patient with face, neck, and upper body swelling from SVC syndrome.

Clinical Implications

The historical features of headache, cough, shortness of breath, and chest pain combined with facial and upper-extremity plethora, dilated superficial veins should prompt a search for SVC obstruction. Management of SVC syndrome depends on the type of the obstructing mass, but frequently relies on radiation therapy to reduce the tumor burden around the SVC to improve venous return.

Pearls

1. Findings of SVC syndrome are predominantly clinical, and should be investigated with venous phase angiography or CT angiography for confirmation.
2. Efforts should be made to elevate the head of the affected patient to allow gravity to assist venous return.

Radiographic Findings

Aspiration of a radio-opaque foreign body into the trachea or bronchopulmonary tree requires two radiographic views orthogonal to each other to determine its location. Large foreign bodies typically cause some degree of obstruction resulting in pneumonitis or pneumonia due to impaired removal of mucus and bacteria.

Non-radio-opaque foreign bodies present a much greater challenge. Inspiratory and expiratory views may be performed to evaluate whether relaxation of the diaphragm results in appropriate deflation of lung parenchyma or if unilateral expansion persists secondary to airway obstruction. Often such foreign bodies are discovered on bronchoscopy performed in patients with recurrent pneumonia.

Clinical Implications

Aspirated foreign bodies are a nidus for inflammation and infection and can be potentially life-threatening if large enough to impede air flow through the larger airways. Removal usually requires bronchoscopy. Unilateral wheezing can often be a clinical sign of airway impairment and foreign-body aspiration in children, and should be evaluated with radiographs. In children too young to cooperate with inspiratory and expiratory radiographs, bilateral decubitus radiographs may aid in diagnosis.

Pearls

1. Any object seen in the chest on one view requires a second orthogonal view to confirm that the object is inside the thorax.
2. Inspiratory and expiratory radiographs may be useful in identifying non-radio-opaque foreign-body aspirations.

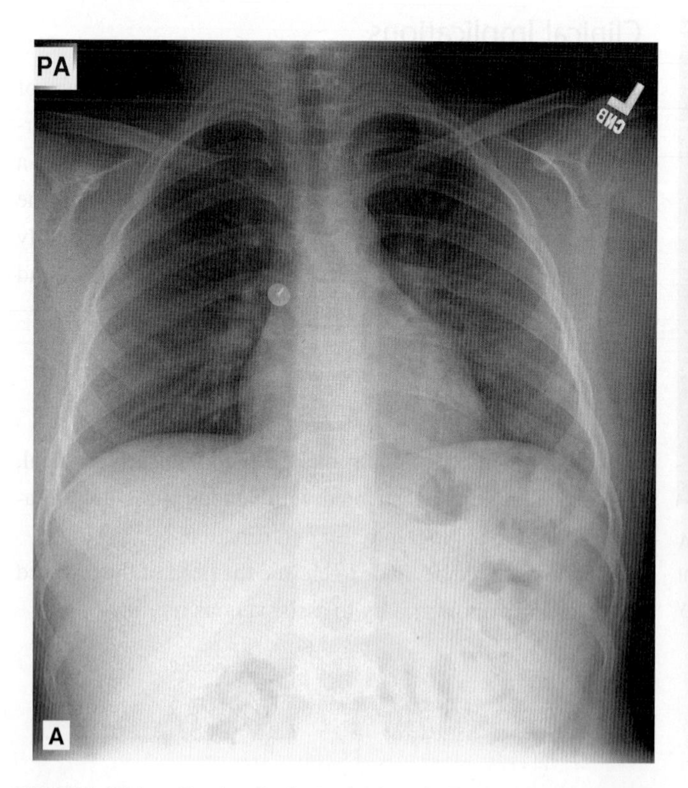

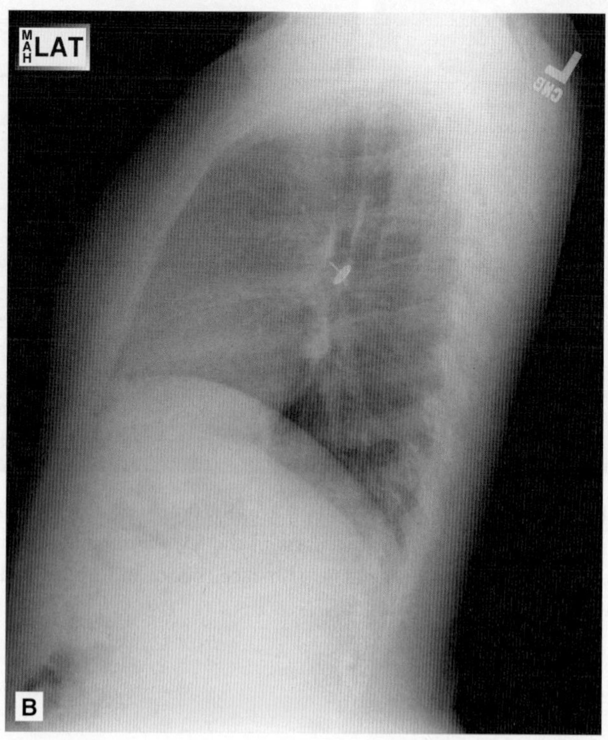

FIGURE 5.94 ■ Foreign Body Aspiration. **A, B:** Frontal chest radiograph demonstrates a metallic foreign body in the right bronchus intermedius. On the lateral view, the foreign body is more readily recognizable as a tack. This tack was successfully removed with bronchoscopy.

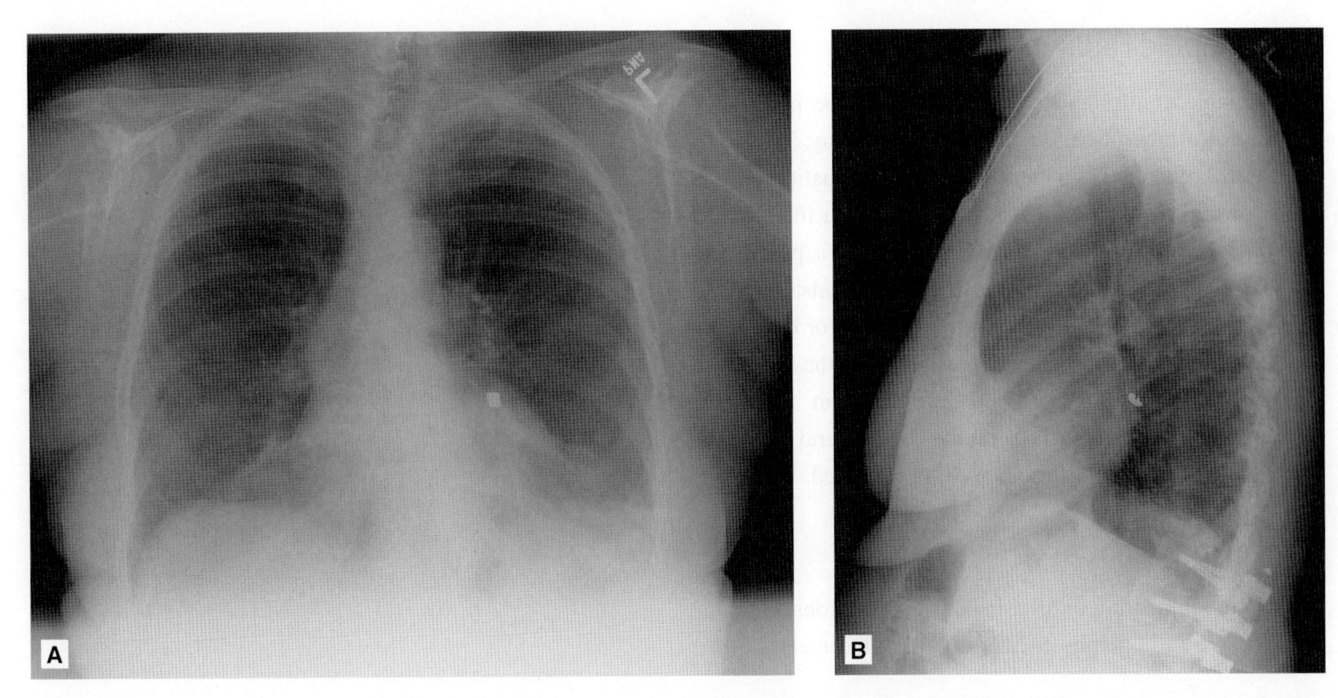

FIGURE 5.95 ■ Foreign Body Aspiration. **A, B:** Frontal and lateral radiographs demonstrated a metallic foreign body in the left infrahilar region. On the lateral view, there is a subtle opacity in the posterior basal segment of the left lower lobe consistent with post-obstructive pneumonitis. Bronchoscopy was performed and a gold crown from one of the patient's teeth was removed.

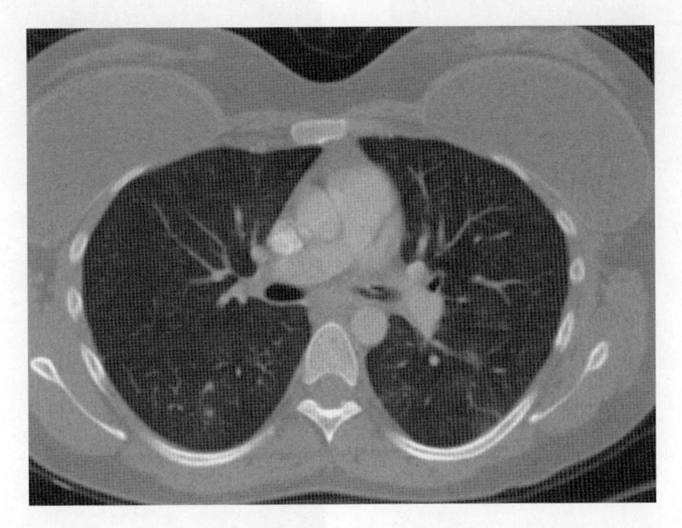

FIGURE 5.96 ■ Foreign Body Aspiration. Axial CT image just below the level of the carina demonstrates a foreign body in the left mainstem bronchus. Bronchoscopy was performed and a chicken bone was successfully removed.

Radiographic Findings

Radiographic confirmation of endotracheal tube placement may reveal a tube placed too deep in the airway. The right mainstem bronchus is an almost direct continuation of the trachea while the left mainstem bronchus has a more acute take-off. Therefore, when the endotracheal tube is placed too distally, it typically advances into the right mainstem bronchus. This can be identified by always looking for the carina and then comparing the endotracheal tube to the carina to determine if it is too deep. Prolonged mainstem intubation frequently results in atelectasis on the contralateral side, and can eventually lead to lung collapse if uncorrected.

Clinical Implications

After initial intubation or after major manipulations, patients should have radiographs to identify the placement of the endotracheal tube. This is particularly relevant in pediatric patients who have wide variance in the length of their trachea and frequently may have an endotracheal tube secured deeper than is necessary. Mainstem intubation can also be clinically identified by asymmetric chest rise during ventilation and absence of breath sounds over the contralateral hemithorax.

Pearls

1. Tube placement should be confirmed radiographically to avoid mainstem intubations.
2. Right mainstem intubation can result in left lung atelectasis.

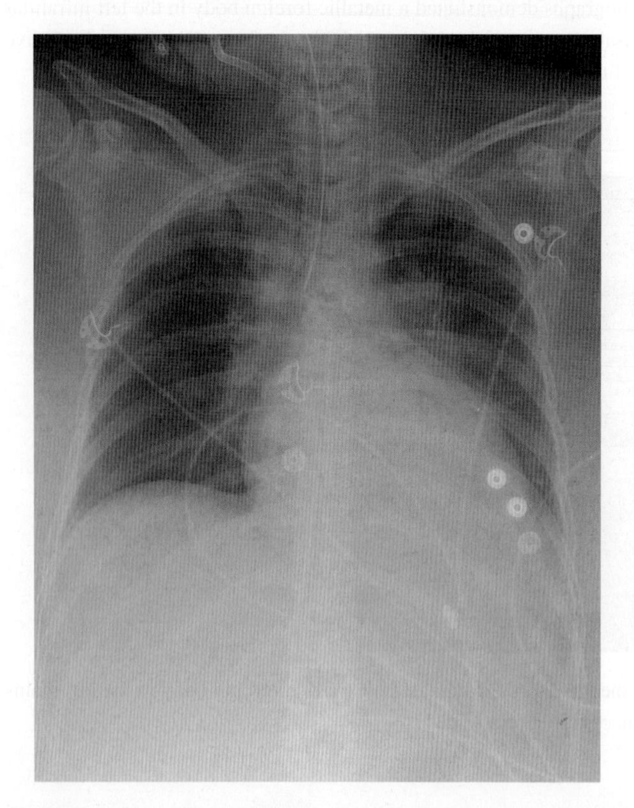

FIGURE 5.97 ■ Right Mainstem Intubation. Frontal radiograph demonstrates the tip of the endotracheal tube terminating in the right mainstem bronchus. Additionally noted is silhouetting of the left hemidiaphragm from left lower lobe atelectasis.

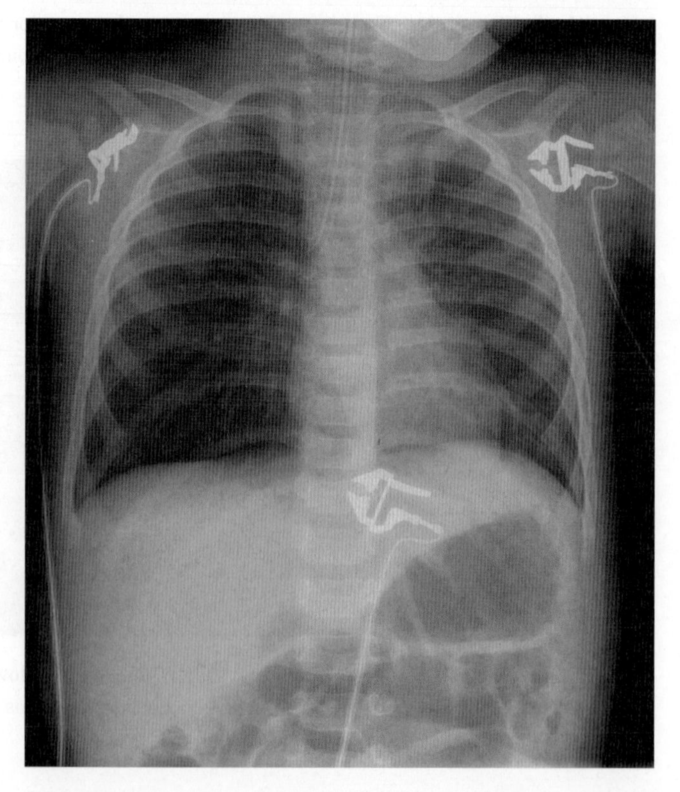

FIGURE 5.98 ■ Right Mainstem Intubation. Frontal radiograph demonstrates the tip of the endotracheal tube terminating below the carina in the right mainstem bronchus. Additionally noted is an opacity in the left lung apex due to subsequent left upper lobe atelectasis.

Radiographic Summary

Coronary artery stenosis is the partial occlusion of the coronary arteries secondary to atherosclerosis. CT cardiac assessment consists of calcium scoring or contrast-assisted angiography. Gated cross-sectional imaging is used to obtain high-resolution slices through the heart during diastole. Quantification of calcium within the coronary vessels is compared with standards and then scored. Since calcium is only present on some atherosclerotic plaques (often older, more stable plaques), it provides only a reference point—lack of calcium is somewhat reassuring for low plaque burden. High calcium burden (scores in the top 25th percentile) is strongly associated with risk of cardiac events. Scanning performed with IV contrast can be used to perform angiography to look at stenoses and flow through the coronaries similar to conventional angiography. Assessments of flow can be made both subjectively as well as objectively by comparing measurements at a stenotic lesion to the downstream diameter of the vessel. 3D reconstructions can also made to better identify the location of major stenoses.

Clinical Implications

CT angiography adds another instrument to the arsenal of tests to risk stratify chest pain to identify patients at risk for acute coronary syndrome and unstable angina. Calcium scoring has been shown to correlate well with risk for future coronary events, but has not been shown to prospectively improve outcomes when used as a screening test. It is useful as a risk-stratification tool for patients with intermediate probability of disease to further stratify their risk and high calcium scores may prompt further evaluation with angiography. CT angiography provides a more definitive view of blood flow through the coronaries, but conventional angiography remains the gold standard. CT angiography has the benefits of being faster and less invasive.

Pearls

1. CT calcium scoring is used to risk-stratify patients with acute coronary syndrome, but has relatively lower sensitivity in higher risk patients.
2. CT angiography has become a non-invasive alternative to conventional angiography.

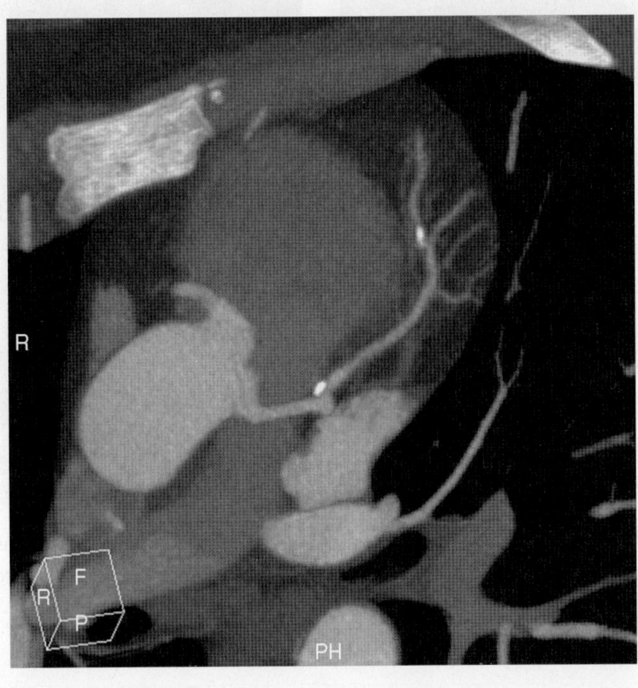

FIGURE 5.99 ■ Coronary Artery Stenosis. Curved multiplanar maximal intensity projection of the left main coronary artery and left anterior descending artery demonstrates calcific atherosclerotic plaques at the origin of the LAD and in the mid-LAD at the origin of the third diagonal branch. At cardiac catheterization, the more proximal plaque was 50% stenosed and the more distal plaque was 90% stenosed; a stent was subsequently placed.

Radiographic Summary

Opacities overlying the cardiomediastinal silhouette may be parenchymal or mediastinal. The "silhouette sign" refers to obliteration of a well-defined boundary; when a perimediastinal opacity exhibits this feature, it is either within the mediastinum or immediately adjacent to it. A lateral view is helpful to further delineate the location of the opacity. Ultimately, cross-sectional imaging (typically contrast-enhanced CT) may be required for definitive localization.

Clinical Implications

In young children, the thymus is quite large and overlies the mediastinum anteriorly. Since the thymic and cardiomediastinal silhouettes are continuous in young children, the term "cardiothymic" silhouette is sometimes used. The large thymus can mimic or obscure a mass or parenchymal consolidation.

Pearls

1. Use PA and lateral views to localize abnormalities. Cross-sectional imaging (typically CECT) may be required for definitive localization and characterization of the abnormality.
2. The differential diagnosis depends on the location of the mediastinal mass. See Table 5.1.
3. The thymus of children is very large and can mimic or obscure a consolidation or mass.

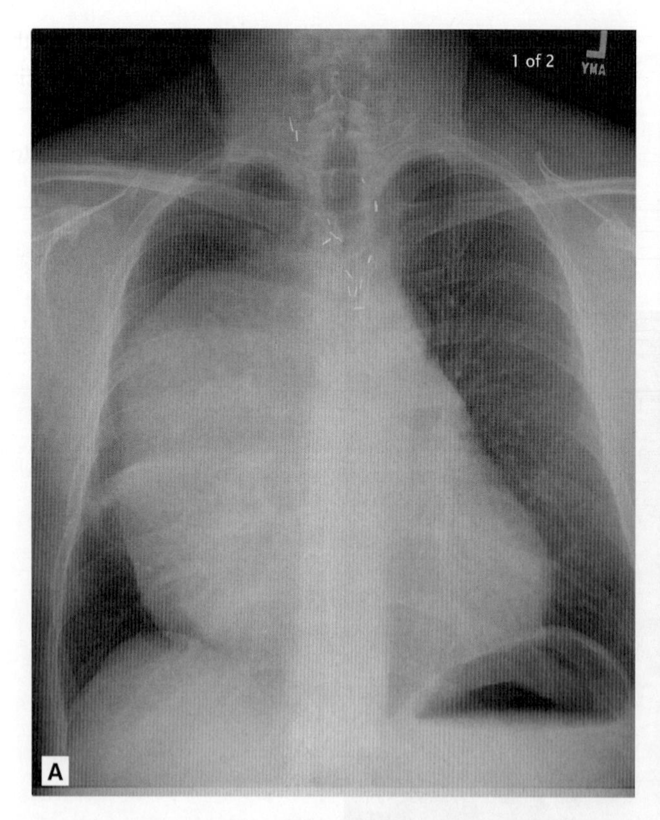

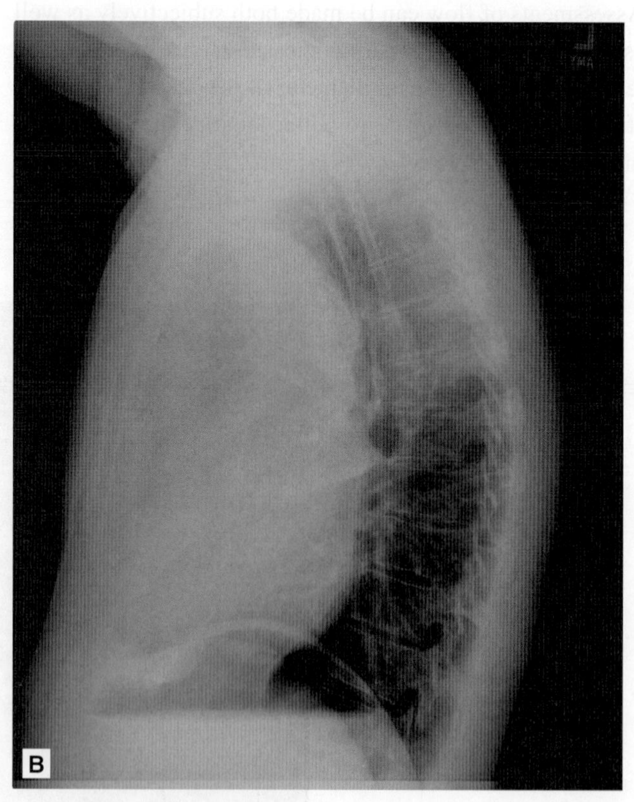

FIGURE 5.100 ■ Anterior Mediastinal Mass. **A, B:** Frontal chest radiograph demonstrates a large mass in the right chest. On the lateral view, this mass is clearly located in the anterior mediastinum. This mass was a biopsy proven thymic carcinoma.

TABLE 5.1 ■ MEDIASTINAL MASSES BASED ON LOCATION

Location	Differential Diagnosis
Anterior	Thyroid goiter Teratoma (germ cell tumor) Thymoma Lymphoma
Middle	Hilar or subcarinal lymphadenopathy or mass Bronchogenic lesions (cyst, neoplasm) Esophageal lesions (dulplication cyst, cancer)
Posterior	Neurogenic tumors Pleural-based tumors Descending aortic aneurysm Extramedullary hematopoiesis Paraspinal hematoma, mass, abscess

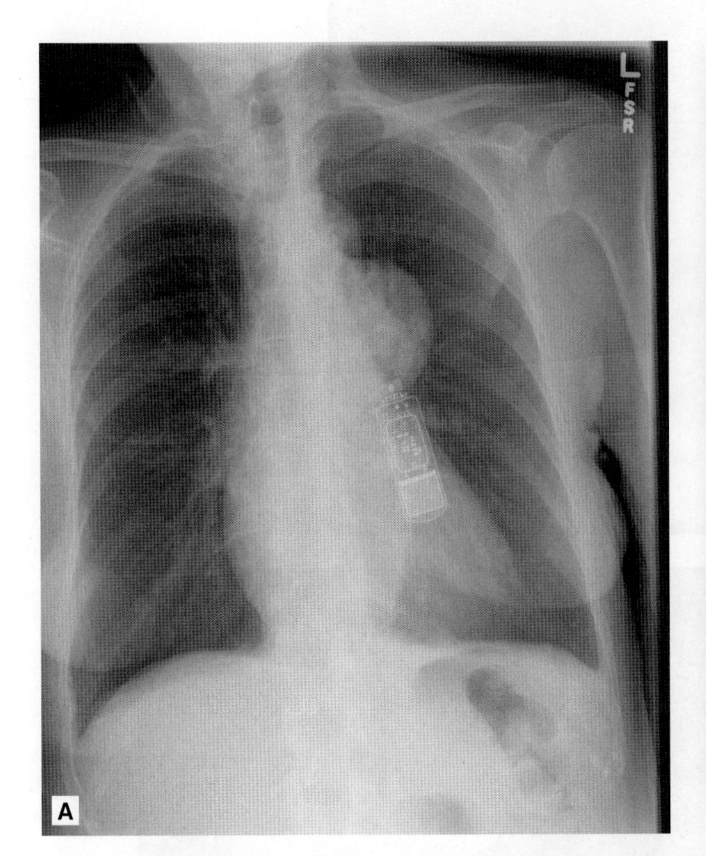

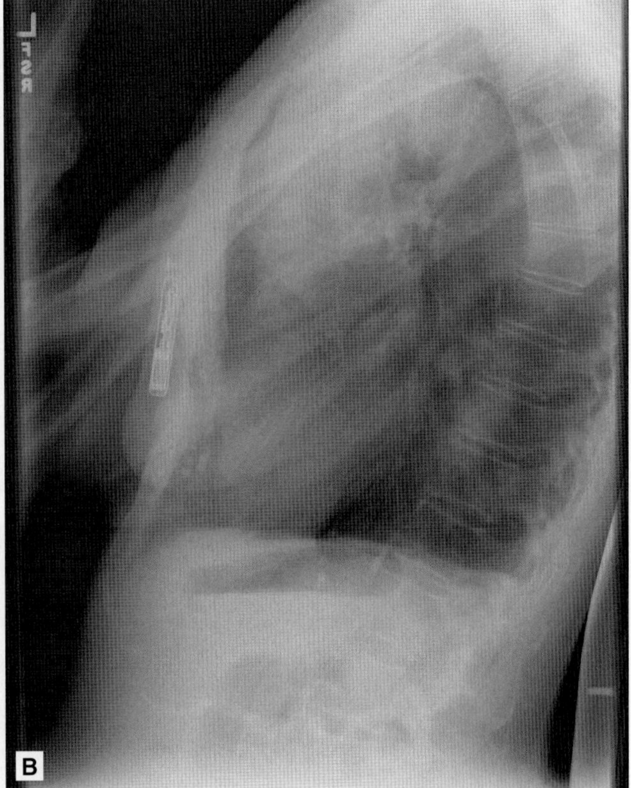

FIGURE 5.101 ■ Posterior Mediastinal Mass. **A, B:** Frontal chest radiograph demonstrates a left perihilar mass. Note how clearly you can see the left pulmonary artery through this mass. This is called the "hilum overlay" sign and indicates that the two processes are in different parts of the mediastinum (i.e., the pulmonary artery is in the middle mediastinum and the mass is in the posterior mediastinum). On the lateral view, the mass can be seen posteriorly projecting over the thoracic spine. This posterior mediastinal mass was a schwannoma.

Radiographic Findings

A cardiac aneurysm is an outpouching of an abnormally thin heart wall and may be difficult to distinguish from chamber enlargement or mediastinal mass. Transthoracic or trans-esophageal echocardiogram have limited definitive diagnostic accuracy but are good initial choices if aneurysm is suspected. Cross-sectional imaging is usually required to provide a definitive diagnosis.

A cardiac pseudoaneurysm is created when a heart wall rupture is contained by myocardial adventitia, adherent pericardium, or scar. A pseudoaneurysm does not contain any myocardial cells and is prone to rupture.

Clinical Implications

In the setting of recent myocardial infarction or blunt trauma, any new mass identified on imaging should raise concern for aneurysmal dilation and prompt echocardiography or cross-sectional imaging.

Left ventricular aneurysms are most commonly caused by anterior wall MI but are also seen in Chagas disease and

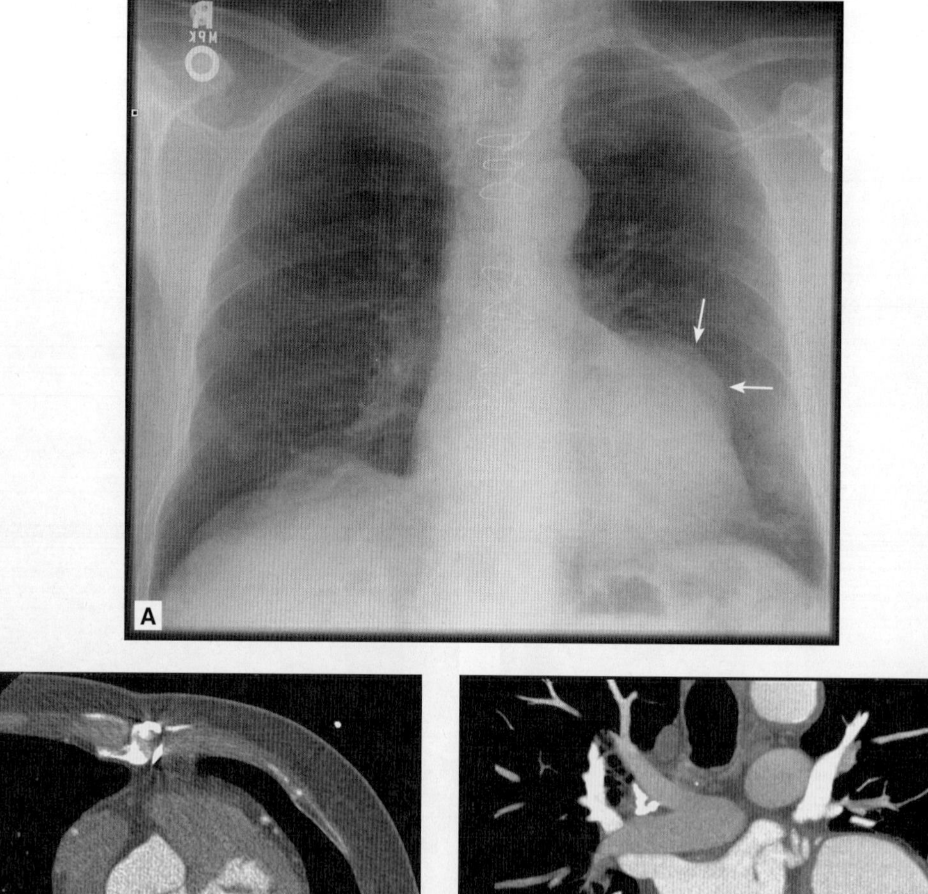

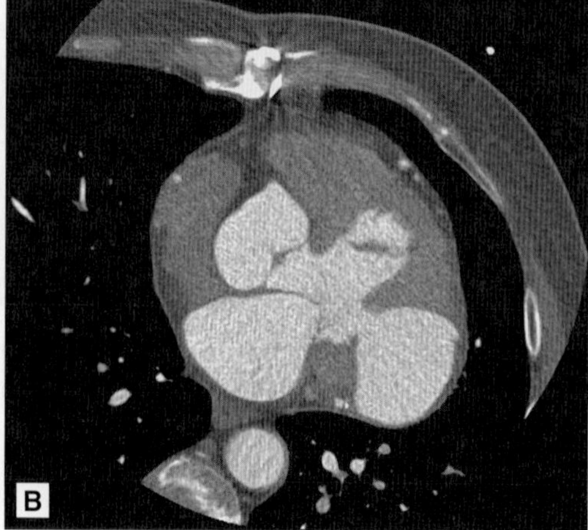

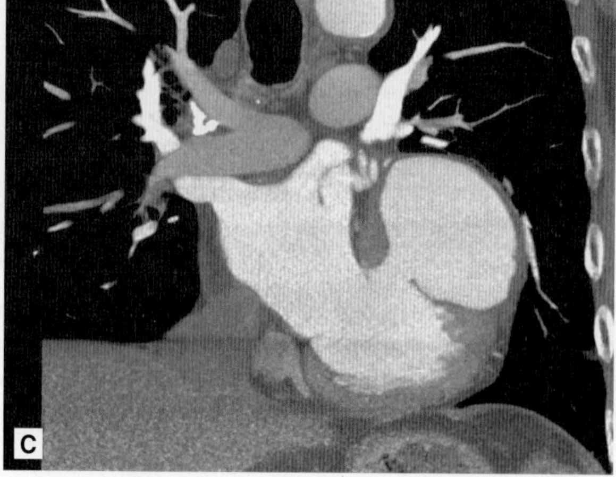

FIGURE 5.102 ■ Cardiac Pseudoaneurysm. **A-C:** Frontal chest radiograph demonstrates an opacity projecting over the left superior heart border (arrows). This mass was concerning for a left ventricular aneurysm in this patient with a recent myocardial infarction and a CTA was ordered. Axial and coronal CTA images demonstrate a large pseudoaneurysm originating from the antero-lateral wall of the left ventricle.

hypertrophic cardiomyopathy. Fifty percent of ventricular aneurysms contain a clot that may embolize.

Pearls

1. Over time, cardiac aneurysms may calcify and be clearly evident on conventional radiography.
2. True cardiac aneurysms will have a wide neck and result from a previous myocardial infarct, typically occurring at the left ventricular apex.
3. False cardiac aneurysms (also known as pseudoaneurysms) will have a narrow neck and are usually the result of previous infection or trauma. Pseudoaneurysms are only contained by the adventitia of the cardiac wall. These usually necessitate emergent surgical intervention.

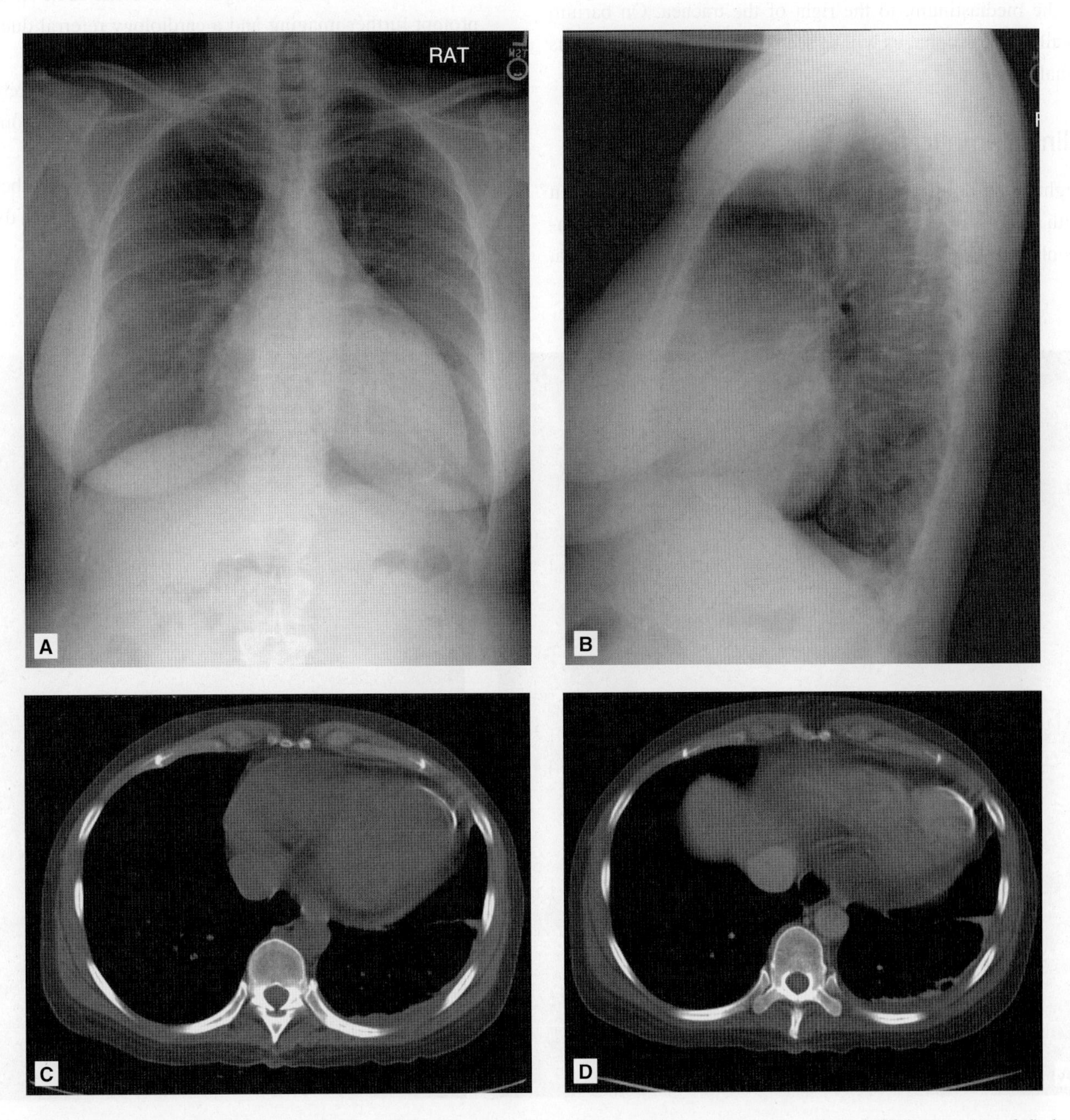

FIGURE 5.103 ■ Cardiac Aneurysm. **A-D:** PA and lateral views of the chest (a and b) and two selected axial CT images (c and d) demonstrate a curvilinear calcification within the left ventricular wall at the cardiac apex. This is a calcified ventricular aneurysm from a prior myocardial infarction.

Radiographic Findings

The aortic arch typically resides on the left. On a PA chest radiograph, the normal left aortic arch is visualized as the first mediastinal "knob" along the left mediastinum from superior to inferior. While this can be displaced by masses or aneurysm, these will usually show associated mass effect and tracheal deviation. Right-sided arch will present as an otherwise normal radiograph with the aortic arch seen in the right aspect of the mediastinum, to the right of the trachea. On barium swallow the esophagus will be seen displaced to the left of its usual position.

Clinical Implications

Right-sided aortic arches are rare, and almost always seen with more serious congenital cardiac anomalies, most commonly tetralogy of Fallot, truncus arteriosis, tricuspid atresia, and transposition of the great vessels. Asymptomatic patients are rare and this is usually an incidental finding in a patient who has known disease and is status post repair in adults. Right-sided arches in children and infants should be referred to a pediatric cardiologist for echo and evaluation.

Pearls

1. Discovery of a possible right-sided aortic arch should prompt further imaging and a cardiology referral due to the high rate of associated cardiac anomalies.
2. The best diagnostic clue to the presence of a right arch is deviation of the trachea to the left, which should prompt closer inspection as to the course of the aortic arch.
3. A right aortic arch coupled with an aberrant left subclavian artery is called a vascular ring and can result in dysphagia from esophageal narrowing.

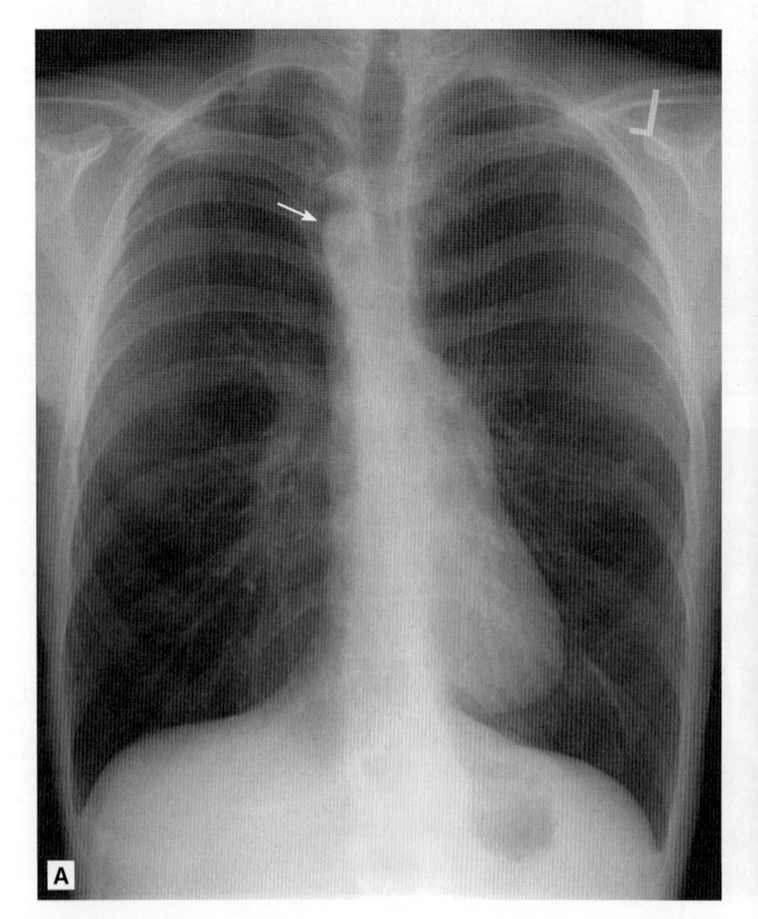

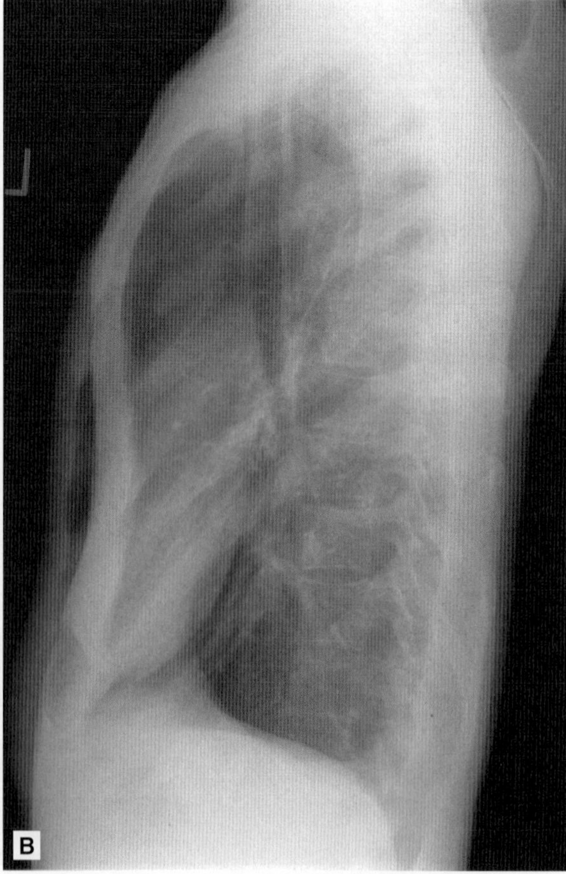

FIGURE 5.104 ■ Right Aortic Arch. **A, B:** Frontal chest radiograph shows a right sided aortic arch (arrow) with tracheal deviation to the left. The right heart border is not visible because there is displacement of the heart into the left chest due to a pectus excavatum deformity, which is seen on the lateral view.

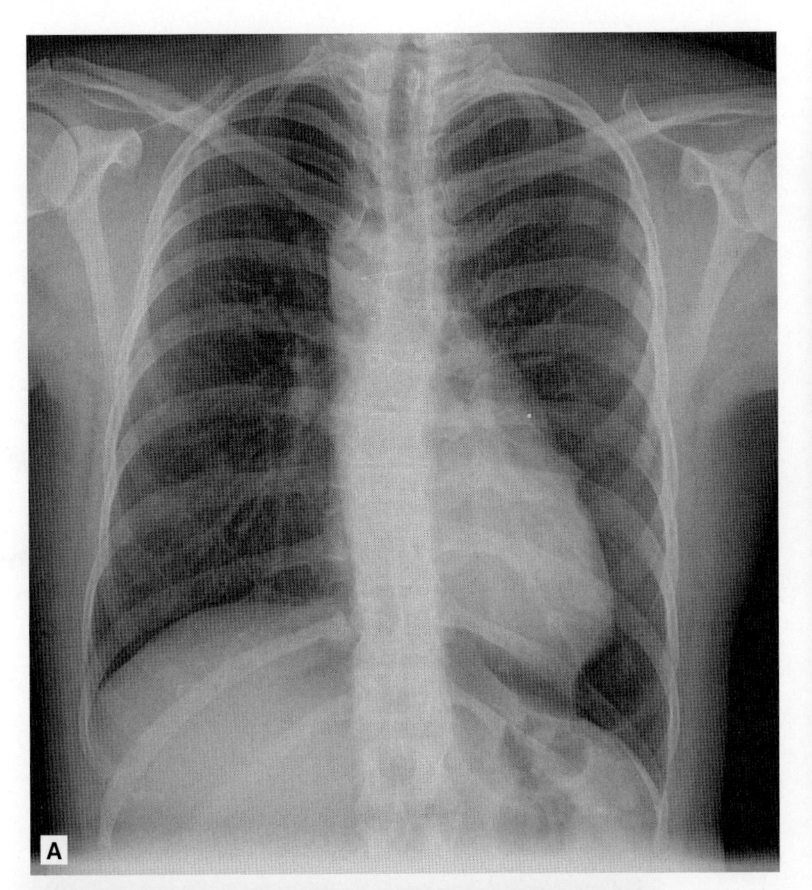

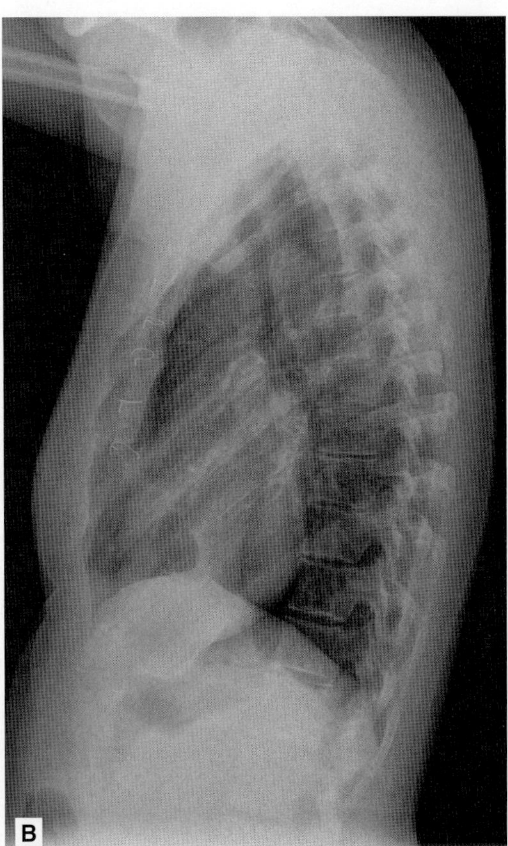

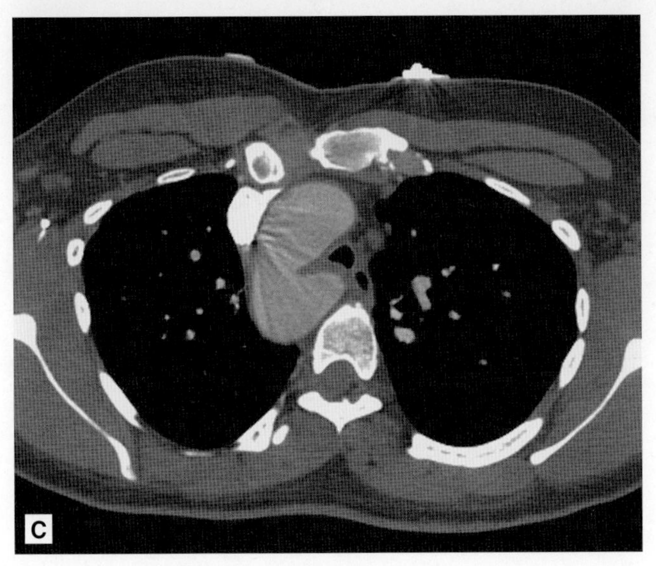

FIGURE 5.105 ■ Right Aortic Arch. **A-C:** Frontal chest radiograph demonstrates a right-sided aortic arch with secondary tracheal deviation to the left. On the lateral view, an oval opacity can be seen between the trachea and the spine. This is an aberrant left subclavian artery with an abnormally large origin (termed a diverticulum of Kommerell) and can be seen on the axial CTA slice.

Chapter 6

TRAUMATIC CONDITIONS OF THE ABDOMEN

Jake Block
Gary Schwartz
R. Jason Thurman

Radiographic Summary

Contrasted CT scan is the preferred method to emergently evaluate patients with suspected liver injury. Liver lacerations are graded per the American Association for the Surgery of Trauma criteria according to their severity based on radiographic features. Grade I liver lacerations feature subcapsular hematomas measuring no greater than 1 cm at their greatest thickness, capsular avulsion, superficial parenchymal lacerations less than 1 cm deep, and isolated periportal blood tracking. Grade II injuries are characterized by parenchymal laceration 1–3 cm deep and parenchymal or subcapsular hematomas 1–3 cm thick. Those injuries demonstrating parenchymal laceration more than 3 cm deep, or subcapsular hematomas more than 3 cm in diameter are considered

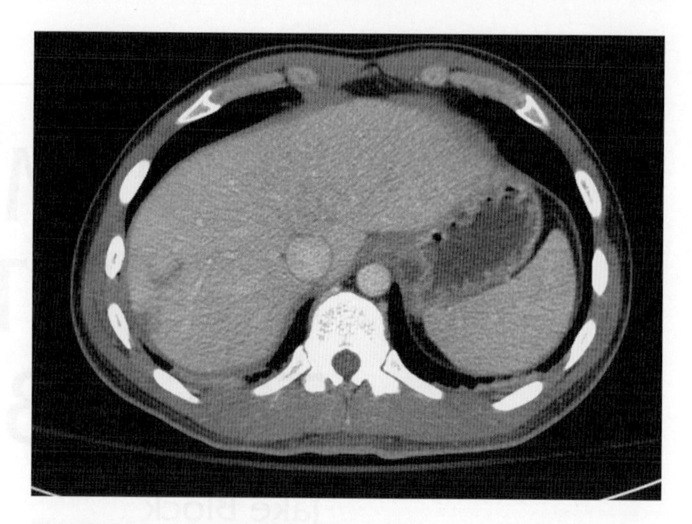

FIGURE 6.1 ■ Grade II Liver Laceration. A small peripheral low-density region is seen in the right hepatic lobe superiorly.

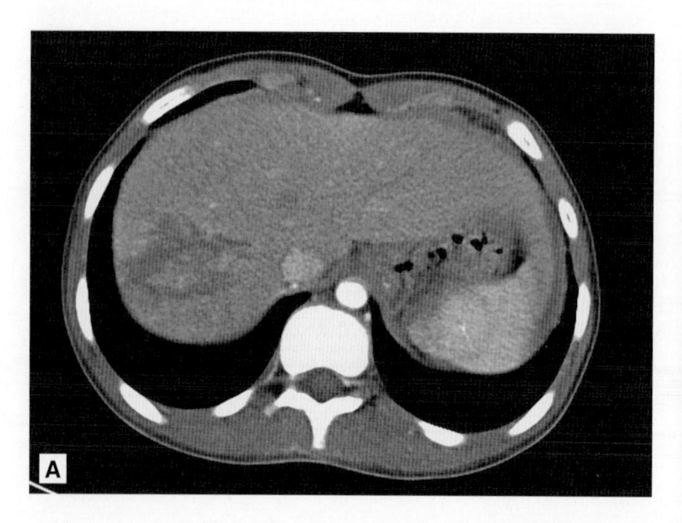

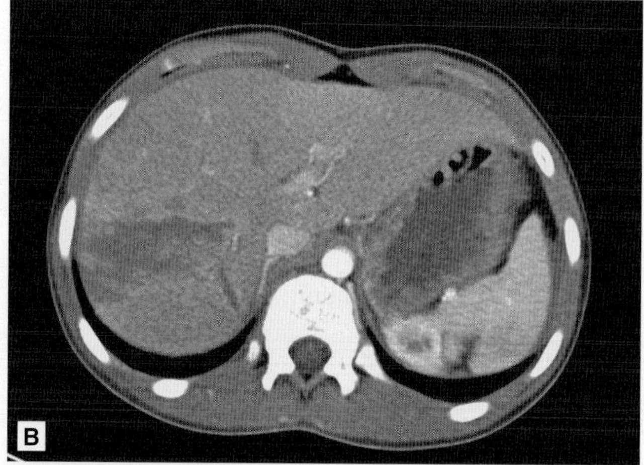

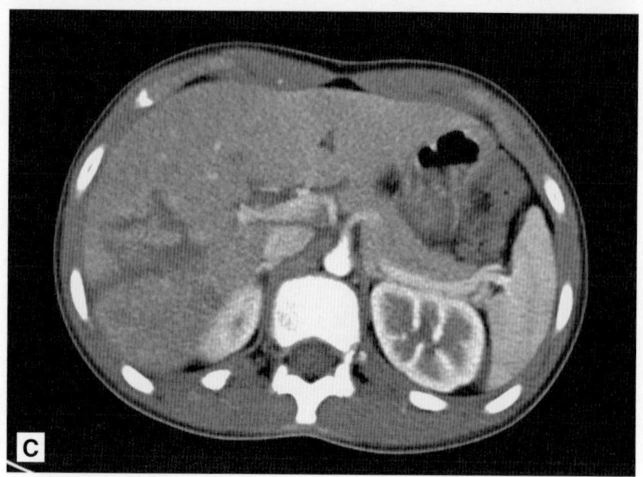

FIGURE 6.2 ■ Grade III Liver Laceration. **A-C:** Extensive branching lacerations are seen in the right hepatic lobe.

Grade III lacerations. Grade IV injuries are recognized by parenchymal or subcapsular hematoma more than 10 cm in diameter, lobar destruction, or devascularization of the liver, while Grade V injuries demonstrate global destruction of the liver parenchyma. Complete hepatic avulsions (Grade VI) may also occur.

Subcapsular hematomas are generally identified between the liver capsule and the enhancing liver parenchyma on contrasted CT, and are most commonly located anterolateral to the right hepatic lobe. Liver parenchymal lacerations are seen as nonenhancing linear or jagged lesions typically observed in the periphery of the organ and may enlarge over time. Acute liver hemorrhage features areas of contrast extravasation on contrasted CT scan, while devascularized areas of the liver appear as unenhanced wedge-shaped regions extending toward the liver periphery.

Clinical Implications

The liver is quite vulnerable to blunt trauma and significant hepatic injuries may rapidly cause severe hemorrhagic shock and death. Contrasted CT scan may be very helpful in guiding therapy for patients who have sustained hepatic injury, both in identifying severe injury or active hemorrhage in

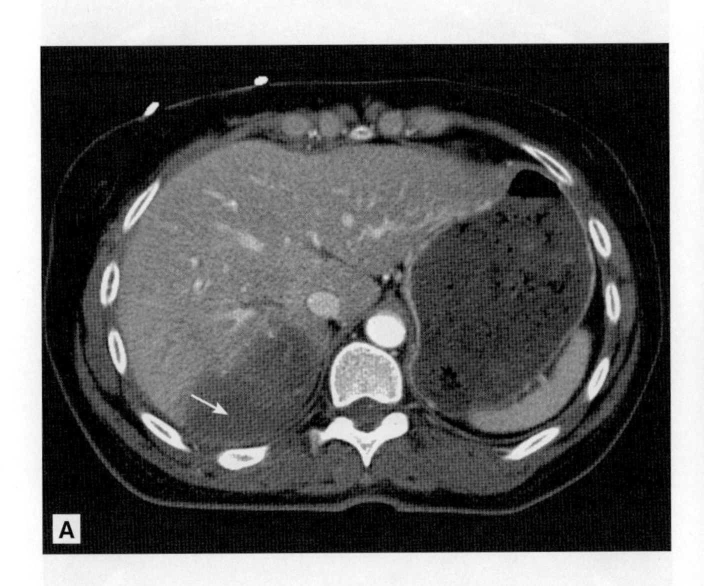

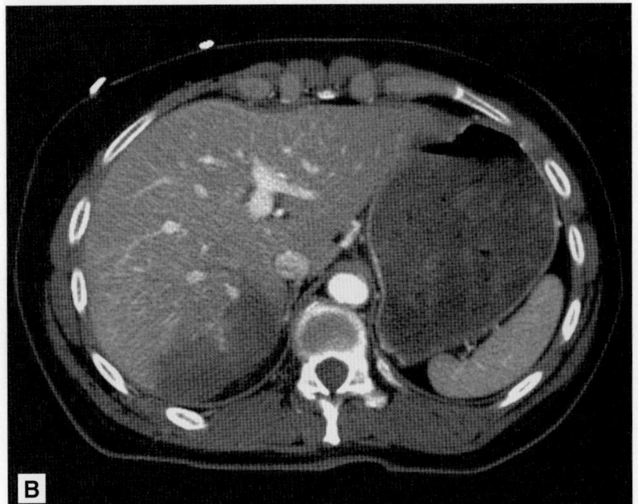

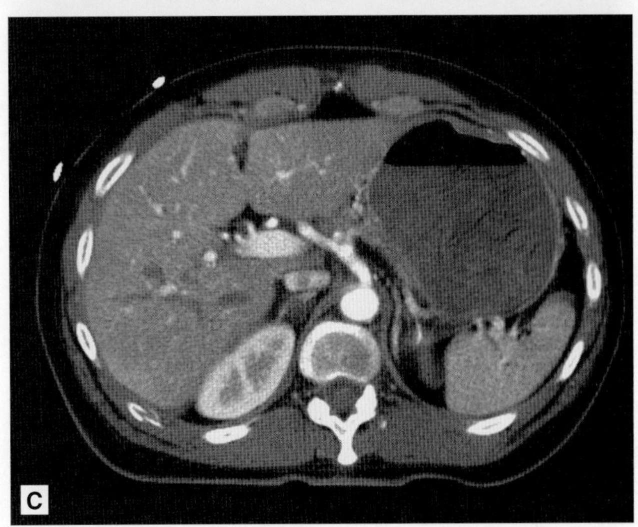

FIGURE 6.3 ■ Liver Laceration with Subcapsular Hematoma. **A-C:** In this case, posterior right hepatic lobe lacerations are visible, with formation of a moderate-sized posterior subcapsular hematoma (arrow).

need of immediate intervention as well as identifying those patients in whom nonoperative management may be appropriate. Hemodynamic stability is the most important factor when considering operative versus nonoperative management regardless of the radiographic features of the injury. Most liver lacerations in stable patients will resolve spontaneously without operative intervention. However, higher-grade liver injuries are associated with a greater incidence of significant vascular injuries and need immediate surgical consultation.

Pearls

1. Treatment options for liver lacerations are frequently guided by the hemodynamic stability of the patient, not necessarily by the imaging findings.
2. Conventional angiography can serve to both identify an active hepatic bleeding source and provide definitive treatment via embolization.

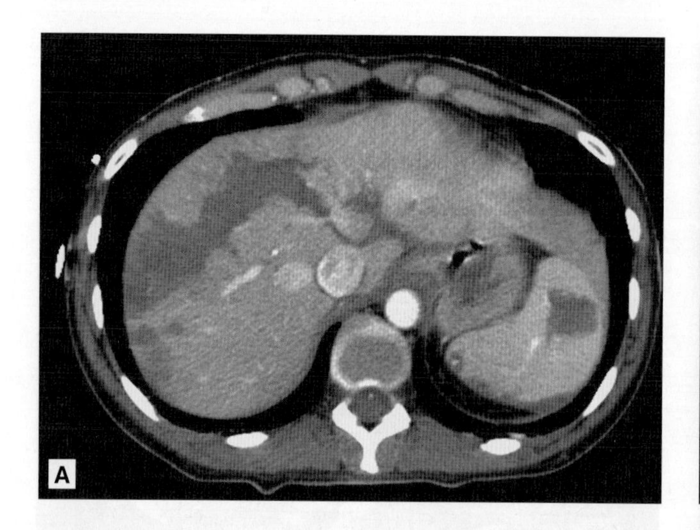

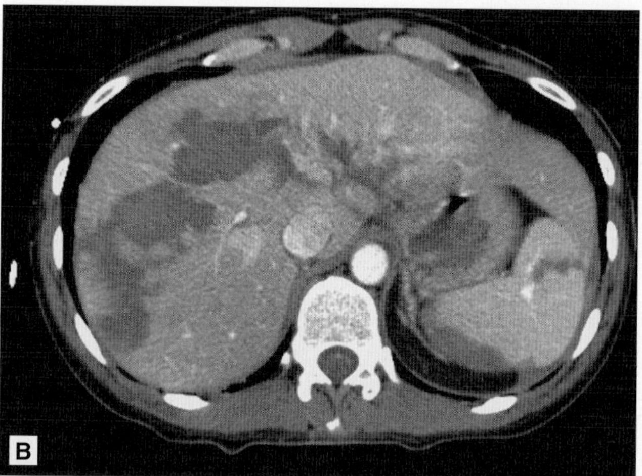

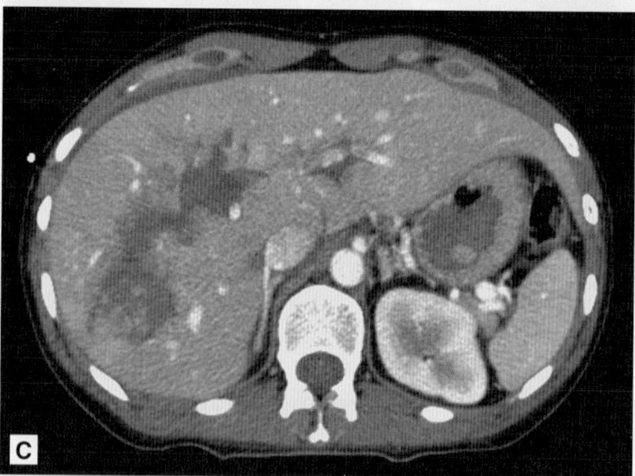

FIGURE 6.4 ■ Liver Laceration. **A-C:** Extensive stellate liver lacerations (Grade V) are seen. Splenic lacerations are also visible.

Radiographic Summary

Contrasted CT scan is the preferred method to emergently evaluate patients with suspected splenic injury. Splenic lacerations are seen as nonenhancing linear or jagged hypodense lesions typically observed in the periphery of the organ. Accompanying subcapsular hematomas are identified as crescent-shaped hypoattenuating fluid collections at the margin of the spleen. Splenic clefts may be confused for lacerations, but generally appear more sharply marginated than true lacerations and may have associated rounded splenic surface contours at the site of the cleft. Intraparenchymal hematomas may also form, and are seen as hypoattenuating areas with mass effect and organ enlargement. Acute splenic hemorrhage is seen as a "blush" of contrast extravasation on contrasted CT scan. Hemoperitoneum is present in a vast majority of splenic injuries.

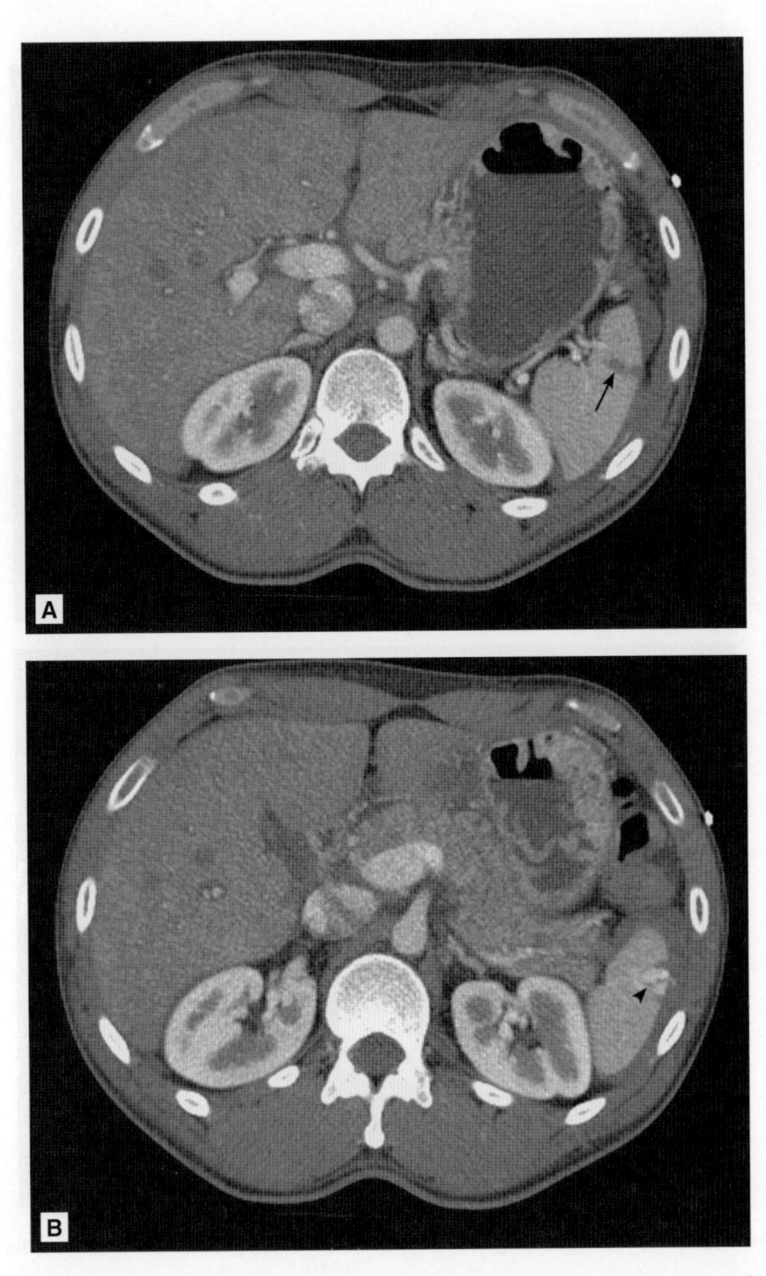

FIGURE 6.5 ■ Splenic Laceration. **A, B:** A small peripheral splenic laceration is seen as a low-density region (arrow). There is a blush of high-density contrast indicating active extravasation from disrupted vasculature (arrowhead). A pericapsular fluid collection is present.

Splenic lacerations are graded per the American Association for the Surgery of Trauma criteria according to their severity based on radiographic features. Grade I splenic lacerations feature subcapsular hematoma measuring less than 10% of the organ surface area or capsular tear of less than 1 cm depth. Those injuries with subcapsular hematoma comprising 10-50% of the organ surface area, intraparenchymal hematoma of less than 5 cm in diameter, or laceration of 1-3 cm in depth without involvement of trabecular vessels are considered Grade II. Grade III lacerations are differentiated from Grade II by the presence of subcapsular hematoma greater than 50% of the organ surface area, expanding subcapsular or parenchymal hematoma, intraparenchymal hematoma of greater than 5 cm, or laceration of greater than 3 cm in depth or involving trabecular vessels. Grade IV injuries feature lacerations involving segmental or hilar vessels with devascularization of greater than 25% of the spleen, while Grade V injuries involve shattered splenic parenchyma or hilar vascular injury.

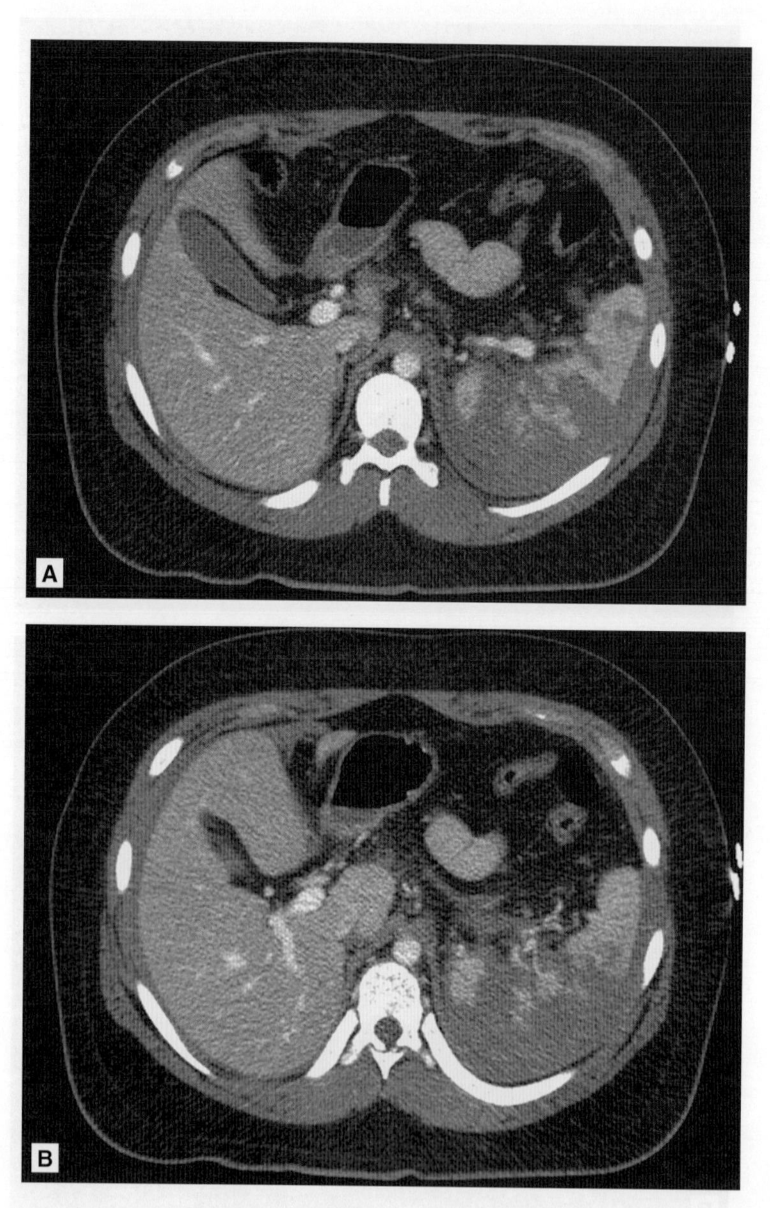

FIGURE 6.6 ■ Splenic Laceration (Grade IV). **A, B:** Large stellate lacerations and regional areas of devascularization are present.

Clinical Implications

The spleen is quite vulnerable to trauma and is the most commonly injured abdominal organ by blunt mechanism. The spleen is a highly vascular organ and when significantly injured hemodynamic instability may rapidly develop. Hemodynamic stability is the most important factor when considering operative versus nonoperative management regardless of the radiographic features of the injury. However, higher-grade splenic injuries are associated with a greater incidence of significant vascular injuries, failure of nonsurgical management, remote complications, and the potential for hemodynamic collapse.

Pearls

1. Hemodynamic stability or lack thereof, not the grade of splenic injury, is the primary compass used to guide the initial management of splenic lacerations.
2. Distinguish normal parenchymal clefts from peripheral lacerations by the lack of surrounding pericapsular hematoma, and rounded or "infolded" surface contours at the site of cleft. Lacerations tend to be more indistinct or jagged in their appearance.

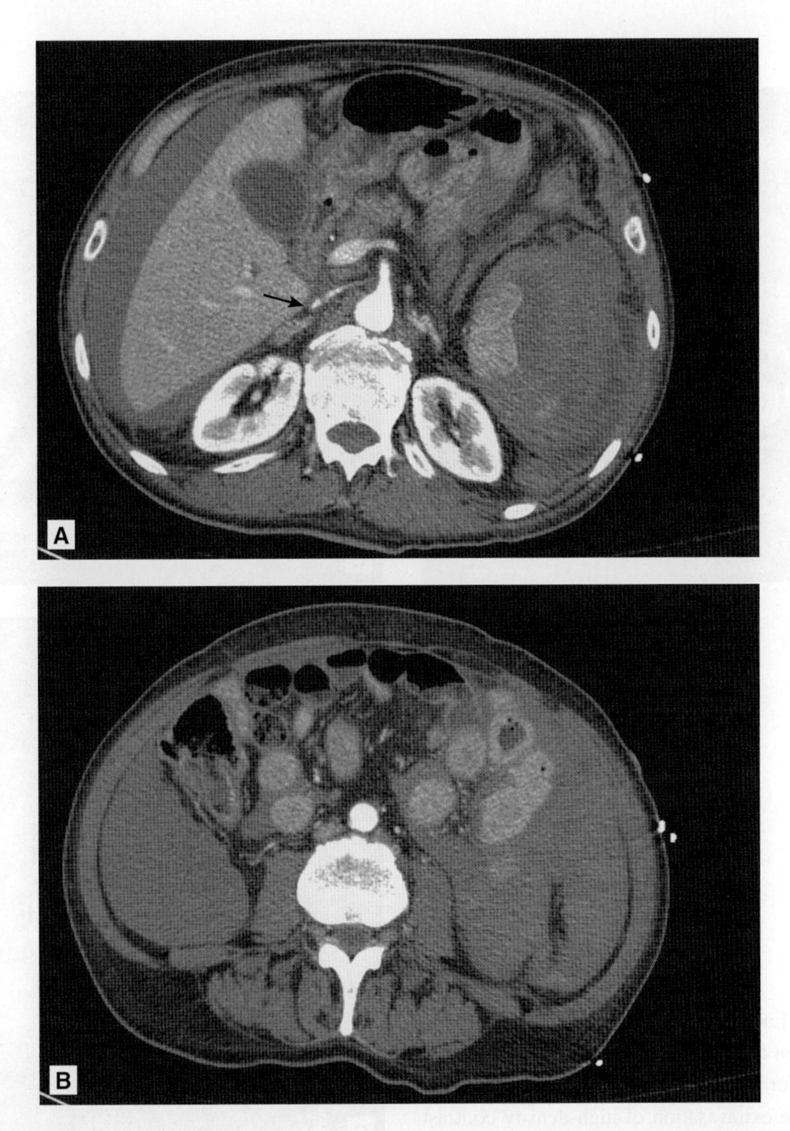

FIGURE 6.7 ■ Splenic Laceration. **A, B:** Extensive hemoperitoneum accompanies the splenic rupture in this case. The spleen is devascularized (Grade V). Intravascular volume loss is present with a slit-like Inferior Vena Cava (arrow). Enhancing loops of small bowel in the lower quadrants are seen consistent with "shock bowel."

Radiographic Summary

Contrasted CT scan is the preferred method to emergently evaluate patients with suspected pancreatic injury unless penetrating trauma mandates an immediate operative intervention and direct exploration. When indications of pancreatic injury are present, they are generally divided into direct and indirect signs of injury. Direct signs of pancreatic injury include detection of parenchymal injury or laceration, pancreatic enlargement or hematoma, fluid separating the splenic vein and pancreas, increased peripancreatic fat attenuation, and active hemorrhage from the pancreas. Indirect signs of injury may include retroperitoneal hematoma, extraperitoneal or intraperitoneal fluid, and peripancreatic fluid. Pancreatic injuries are further graded by AAST classification according to severity. Grade I pancreatic injuries are characterized by superficial contusion with or superficial laceration with no ductal injury. Grade II injuries feature major contusion or laceration of the pancreas without ductal injury. Those injuries where the distal pancreas sustains parenchymal damage or transecting trauma including ductal injury are considered Grade III, while Grade IV injuries are parenchymal injuries or transecting lesions of the proximal pancreas involving the ampulla. Grade V injuries feature massive disruption of the pancreatic head.

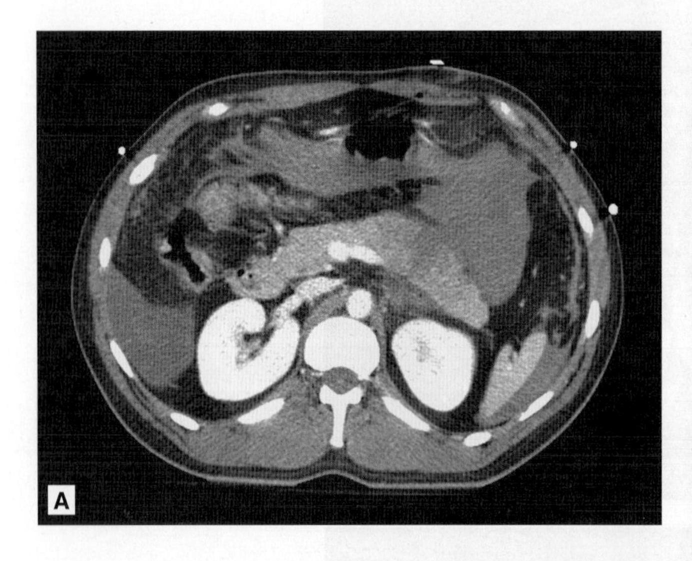

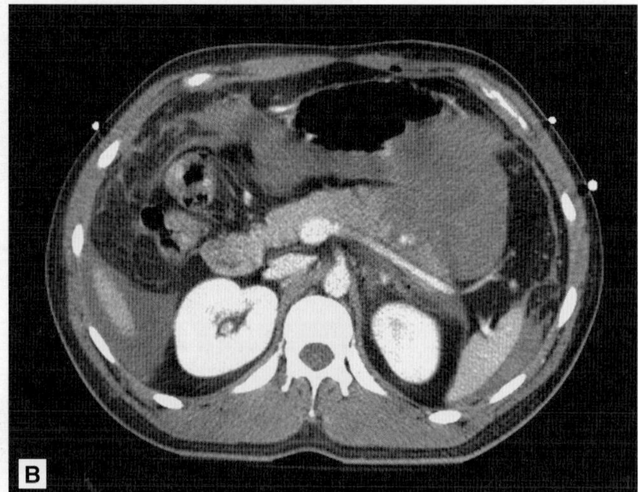

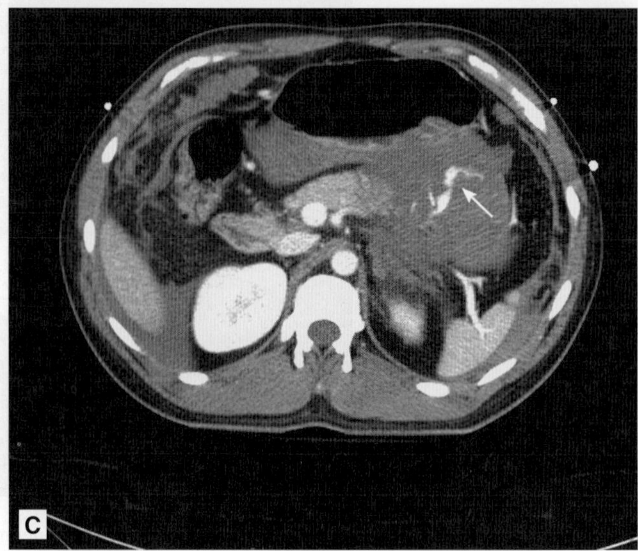

FIGURE 6.8 ■ Pancreatic Laceration. **A-C:** Near-complete transaction of the pancreas is seen at the junction of the pancreatic body and tail. A large hematoma formation is present anterior to the site of pancreatic injury with active extravasation of high-density contrast material (arrow).

Clinical Implications

The pancreas is relatively well protected anatomically and thus blunt pancreatic injuries are less common than other intra-abdominal injuries. Isolated pancreatic injuries are rare. Subtle nonspecific or delayed presentations and the lack of sensitivity of CT scan for injury make this diagnosis difficult. Penetrating injuries to the pancreas are somewhat more common and may arise from wounds from anterior or posterior approach. Contrasted CT scan is often helpful in guiding therapy for patients who have sustained pancreatic injury, both in identifying severity of injury and any active hemorrhage in need of immediate intervention. CT also helps distinguish those patients with less severe injuries in whom nonoperative management may be appropriate. CT scanning is limited however in its ability to identify pancreatic ductal injuries. Due to the prognostic importance of ductal injury, dedicated evaluation with endoscopic retrograde pancreatography (ERP, the gold standard for evaluating pancreatic ductal integrity), or magnetic resonance cholaniopancreatography is often required.

Pearls

1. CT scanning is relatively insensitive for pancreatic injury. This is especially true for pancreatic ductal injuries where MR cholangiopancreatography or ERP are the studies of choice.
2. Isolated pancreatic injuries on CT are uncommon.

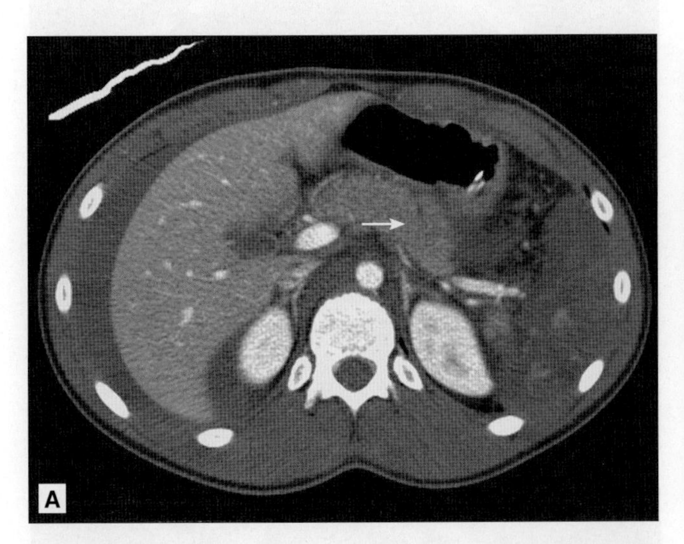

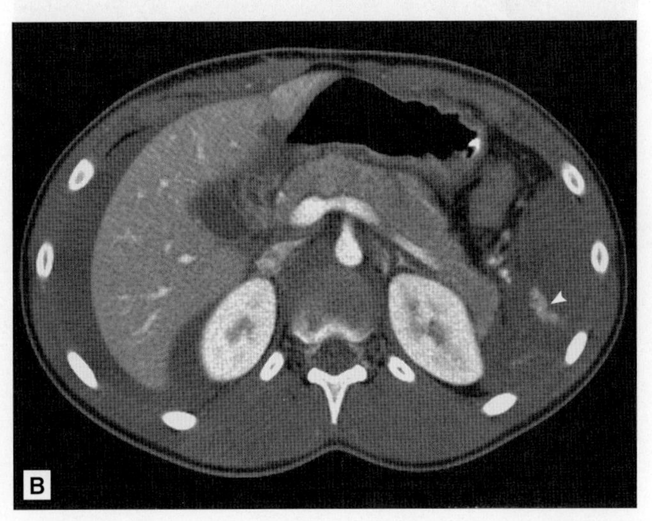

FIGURE 6.9 ■ Pancreatic Laceration. **A, B:** A small laceration is seen in the pancreatic body (arrow). There are additional features of hemoperitoneum and a severe (Grade V) splenic laceration with active extravasation (arrowhead).

Radiographic Summary

An IV contrast CT scan is the preferred method when evaluating a patient with possible hollow viscus injury. In the past, oral and IV contrast was frequently given, but the use of oral contrast has been found to be unnecessary in the majority of cases and adds the potential for aspiration. Intestinal injuries may be either intraperitoneal, retroperitoneal, or both. Radiographic findings may include free air in the abdomen or extravasation of intestinal contents if there is a perforation of the viscus. If there is a transmural injury or a vascular injury with disruption of arterial or venous blood flow to the intestine, bowel wall thickening may be seen. Vascular injuries may also present as mesenteric infiltration or stranding. Hemoperitoneum is a common finding in abdominal trauma from either solid organ or intestinal origin. Therefore, if no solid organ injury is identified, a bowel or mesenteric source of the bleeding should be considered. Unlike intraperitoneal bleeding, the sources of retroperitoneal hematomas are easier to identify since the hematoma typically resides near the area of injury. For example, a retroperitoneal hematoma identified near the duodenum is usually indicative of a duodenal injury.

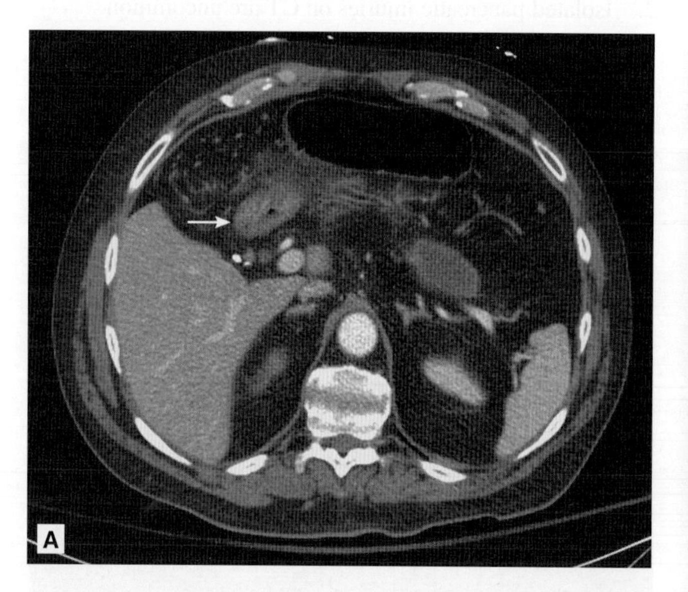

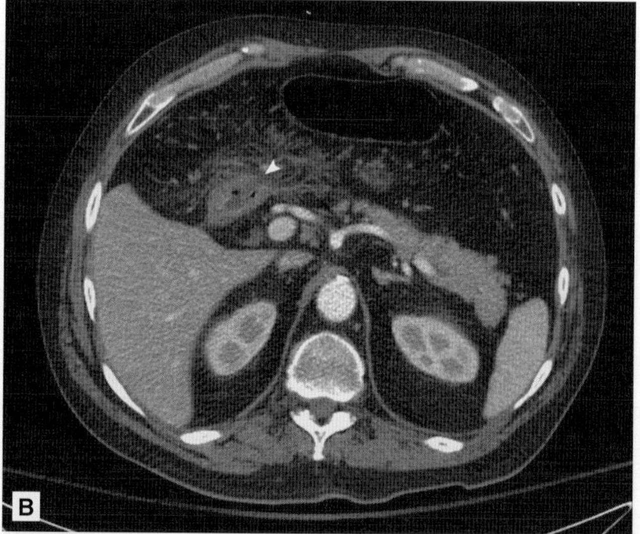

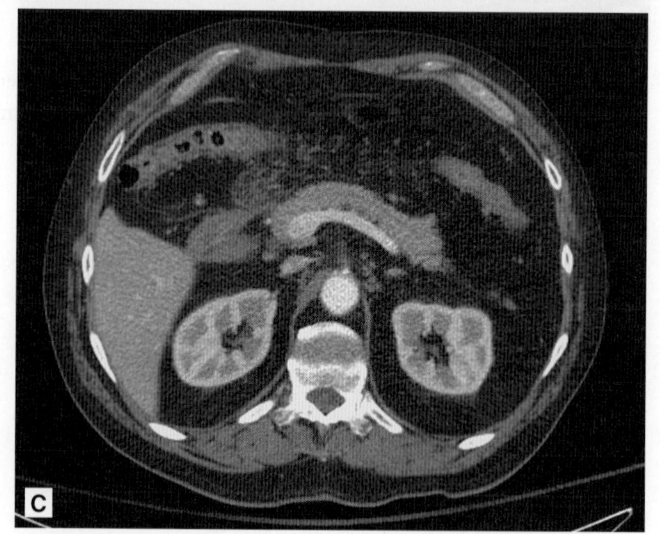

FIGURE 6.10 ■ Duodenal Hematoma. **A-C:** The thickened descending portion of the duodenum is seen (arrow). Surrounding fat stranding is highly suggestive of bowel injury and hematoma formation. Disruption of the duodenal wall is suggested in one of the images (arrowhead).

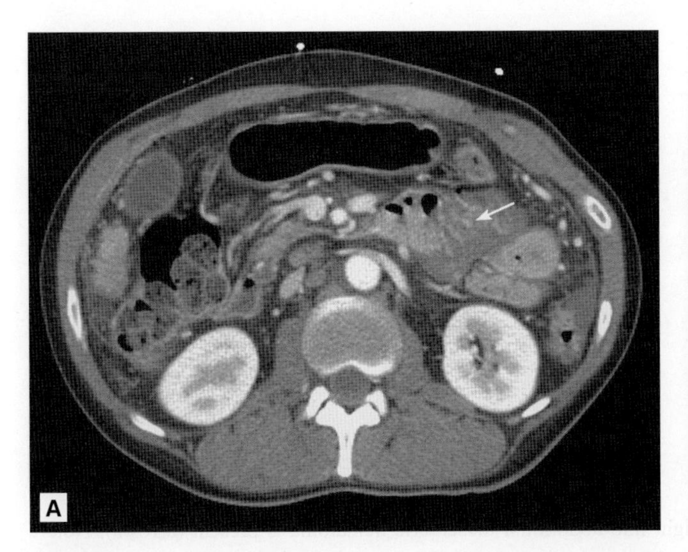

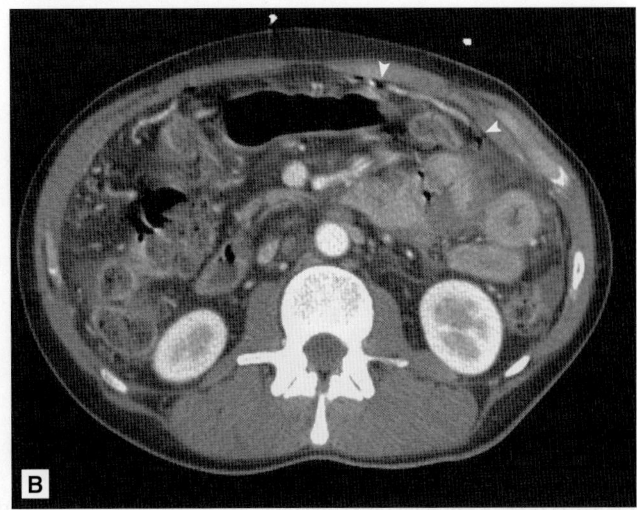

FIGURE 6.11 ■ Duodenal–Jejunal Disruption. **A, B:** Disruption of the bowel wall is identified at the level of the Ligament of Treitz (arrow). There is abundant surrounding fluid/hematoma. A few foci of free air are seen as further evidence of bowel perforation (arrowheads).

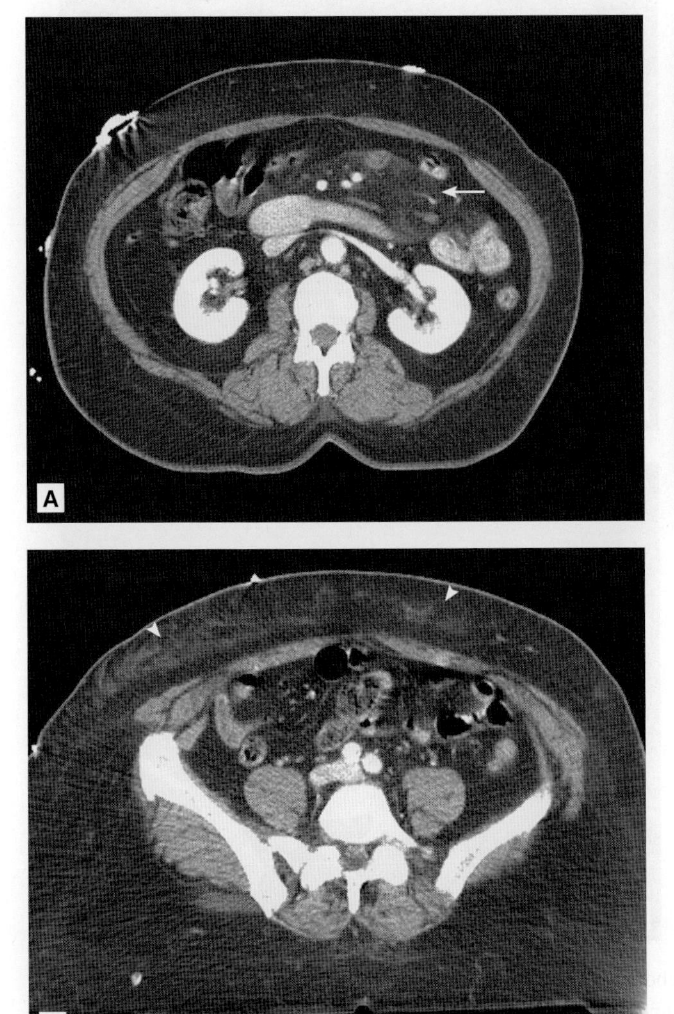

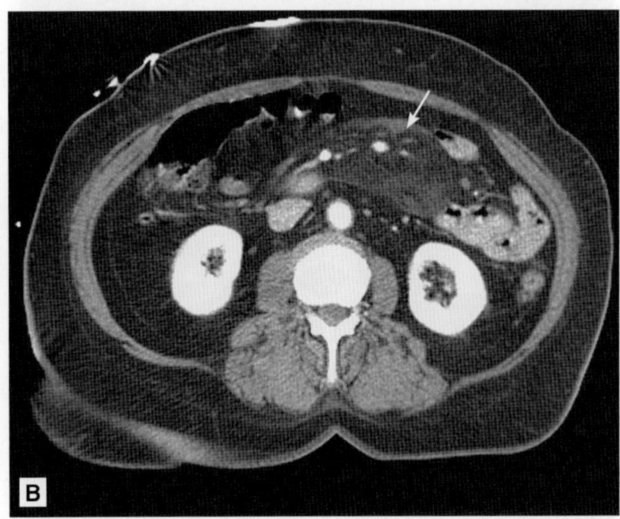

FIGURE 6.12 ■ Mesenteric Hematoma. **A-C:** A subtle region of left upper quadrant fat standing and hematoma formation is seen (arrows) indicating an injury to the mesentery. The inferior image demonstrates a "seat belt" sign, with subcutaneous hematoma formation (arrowheads).

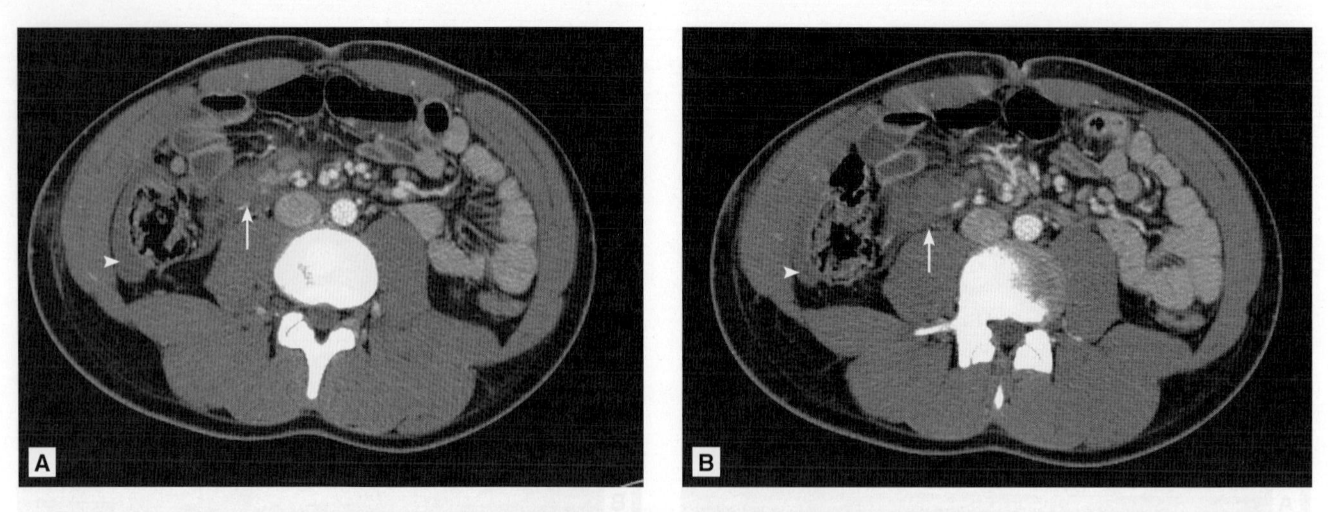

FIGURE 6.13 ■ Mesenteric Hematoma. **A, B:** A moderate-sized right mid-abdominal mesenteric hematoma is present (arrows). Note a small hemoperitoneum within the right paracolic gutter (arrowhead).

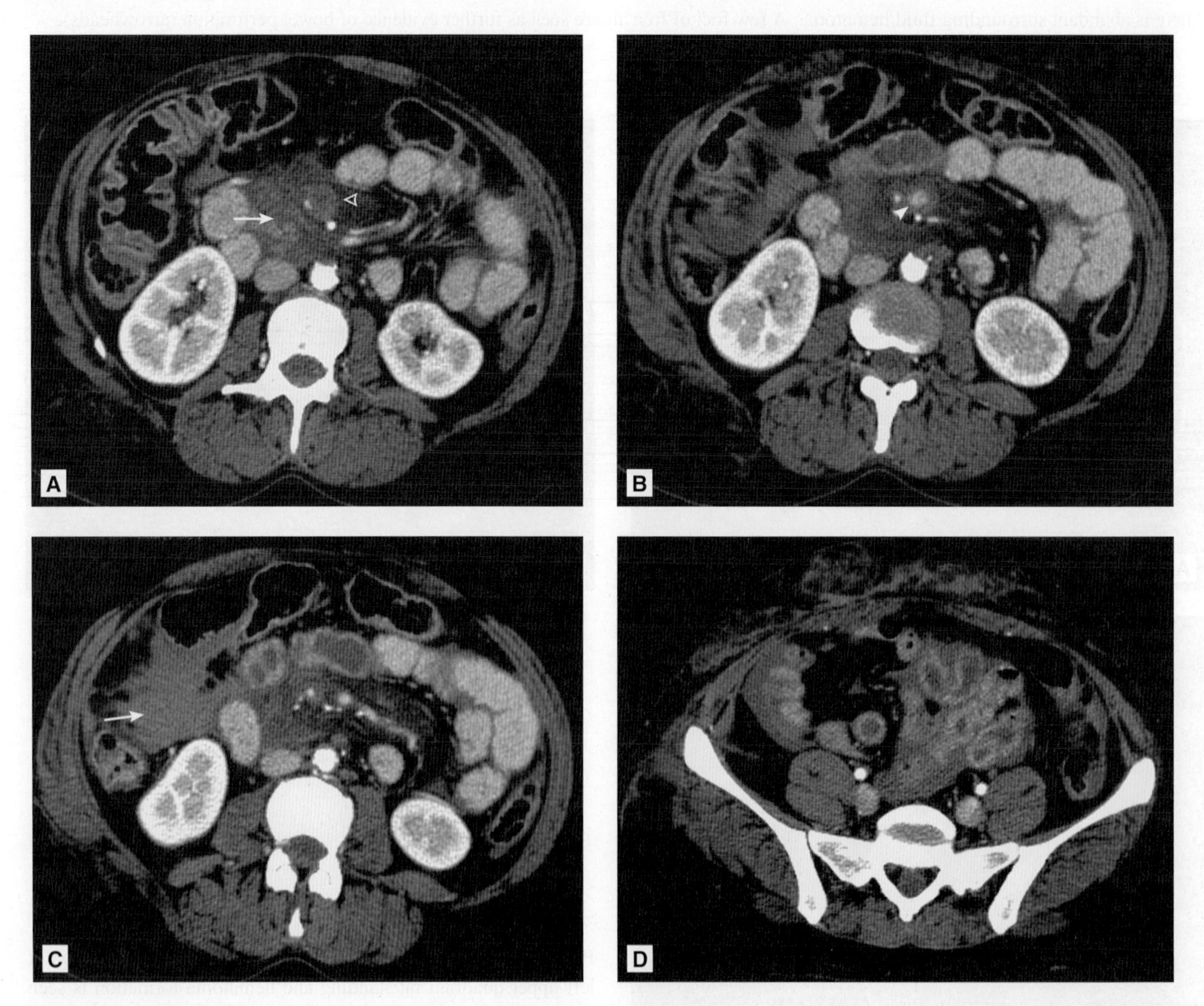

FIGURE 6.14 ■ Superior Mesenteric Vein Disruption. **A-D:** A deep abdominal hematoma formation is seen (arrows). The SMV is identified on the inferior images (arrowheads), but becomes poorly defined superiorly and is discontinuous (open arrowhead). Additional findings include hemoperitoneum and an extensive "seat belt" hematoma.

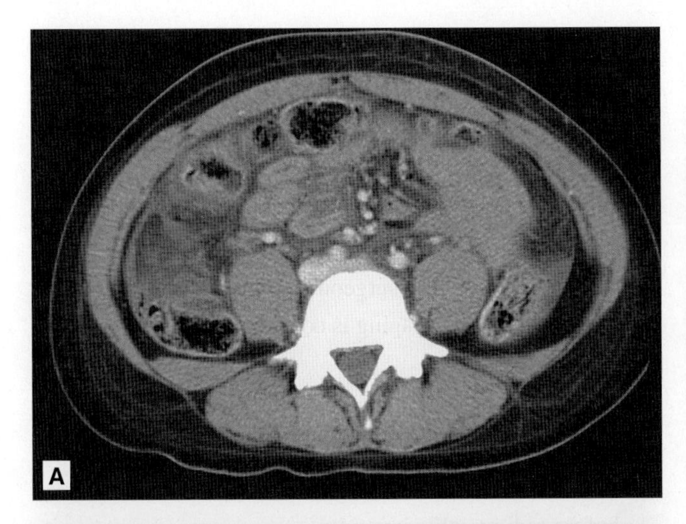

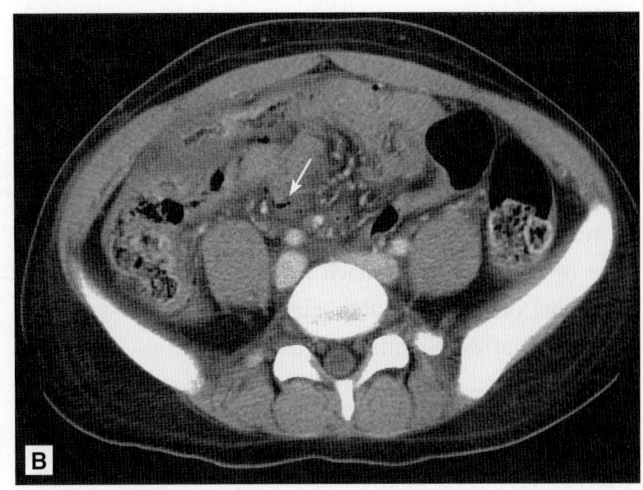

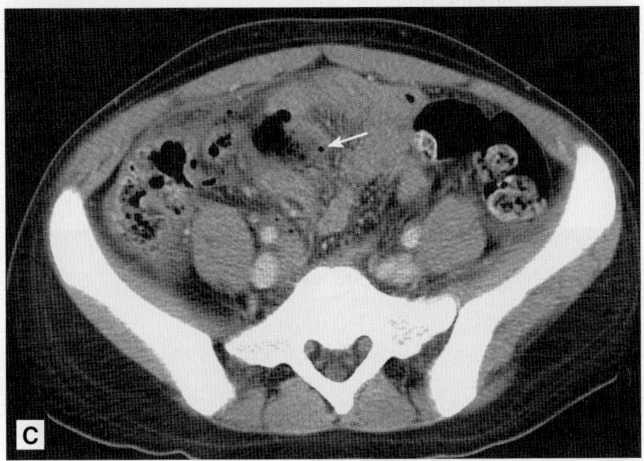

FIGURE 6.15 ■ Colonic Injury. **A-C:** Ill-defined soft tissue stranding and hematoma formation is seen surrounding the ascending colon in the right lower and mid abdomen. Gas foci are seen adjacent to the colonic wall within the mesentery indicating bowel perforation (arrows).

Clinical Implications

Intestinal injuries should be considered in all patients involved in significant blunt force trauma and all penetrating abdominal trauma. Immediately after the trauma, physical examination findings may seem deceptively benign. CT imaging with IV contrast should be performed without delay. Surgical consultation is indicated in all cases of bowel and mesenteric injuries identified on CT. If the patient presents in shock with abdominal tenderness or distention or obvious bowel injury with evisceration, surgical consultation should be obtained immediately.

Pearls

1. On CT, bowel wall thickening in the setting of trauma maybe indicative of a mesenteric vascular injury.
2. Retroperitoneal bleeding is commonly localized near the injury site. This is not necessarily true for intra-abdominal bleeding.

Radiographic Summary

There is a large variety of radiographic findings that may result from penetrating trauma to the abdomen, relating to potential injuries of solid organs, vasculature or hollow viscus. Ballistic injuries to the liver, kidney, spleen or pancreas are readily seen on CT scan. Free air is usually present if there is intestinal or stomach penetration, and mesenteric hematoma or free intra-abdominal fluid can be seen with vascular injuries. Significant vascular injuries can cause bowel ischemia, which can manifest as bowel wall thickening on CT. While CT imaging with IV contrast can commonly define the extent of injury, obtaining an upright abdominal or chest radiograph may be a more expedient method to detect free air. The FAST ultrasound exam is also a quick method that may help to determine if there is free fluid in the pelvis.

Clinical Implications

Any penetrating trauma that is confirmed to have entered the abdomen should be considered a surgical emergency. These patients frequently present with hypotension and tachycardia although may initially appear very stable. Generally, there is no need to exactly define the extent of injury, instead immediate consultation with a surgeon or trauma center should be obtained even before imaging is considered.

Pearls

1. Penetrating abdominal injuries are surgical emergencies so consultation with a surgeon should be obtained even before radiographic imaging.
2. Active vascular extravasation appears as a "blush" of contrast on CT. Some isolated intra-abdominal extravasations can be effectively managed with conventional angiography-guided embolization.

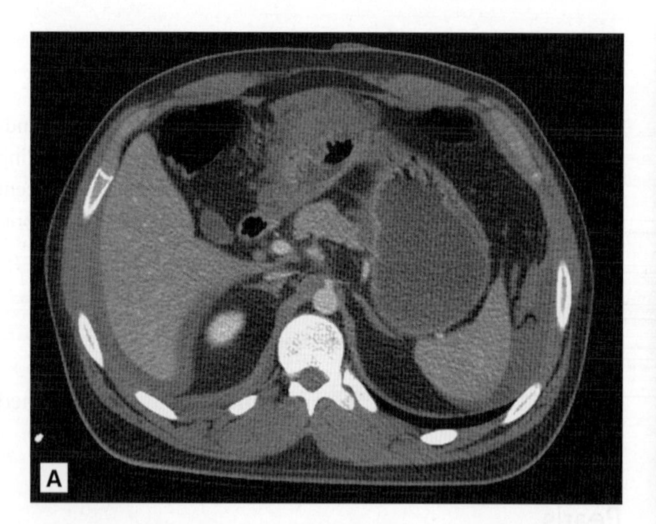

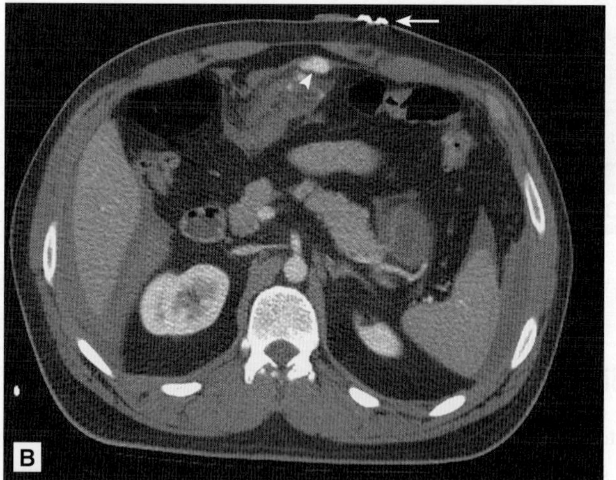

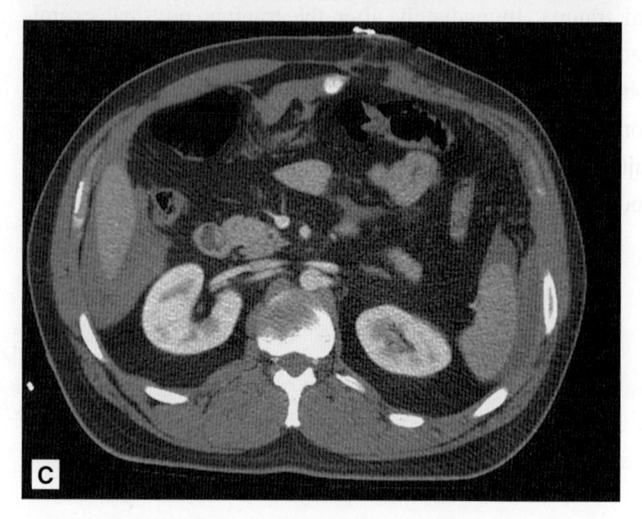

FIGURE 6.16 ■ Penetrating Injury (Stab Wound). **A-C:** The site of injury is marked on the patient's skin with a paperclip (arrow). Underlying this, a gastric injury with associated mesenteric hematoma is visible. Active extravasation of contrast material is identified as a high-density "blush" (arrowhead).

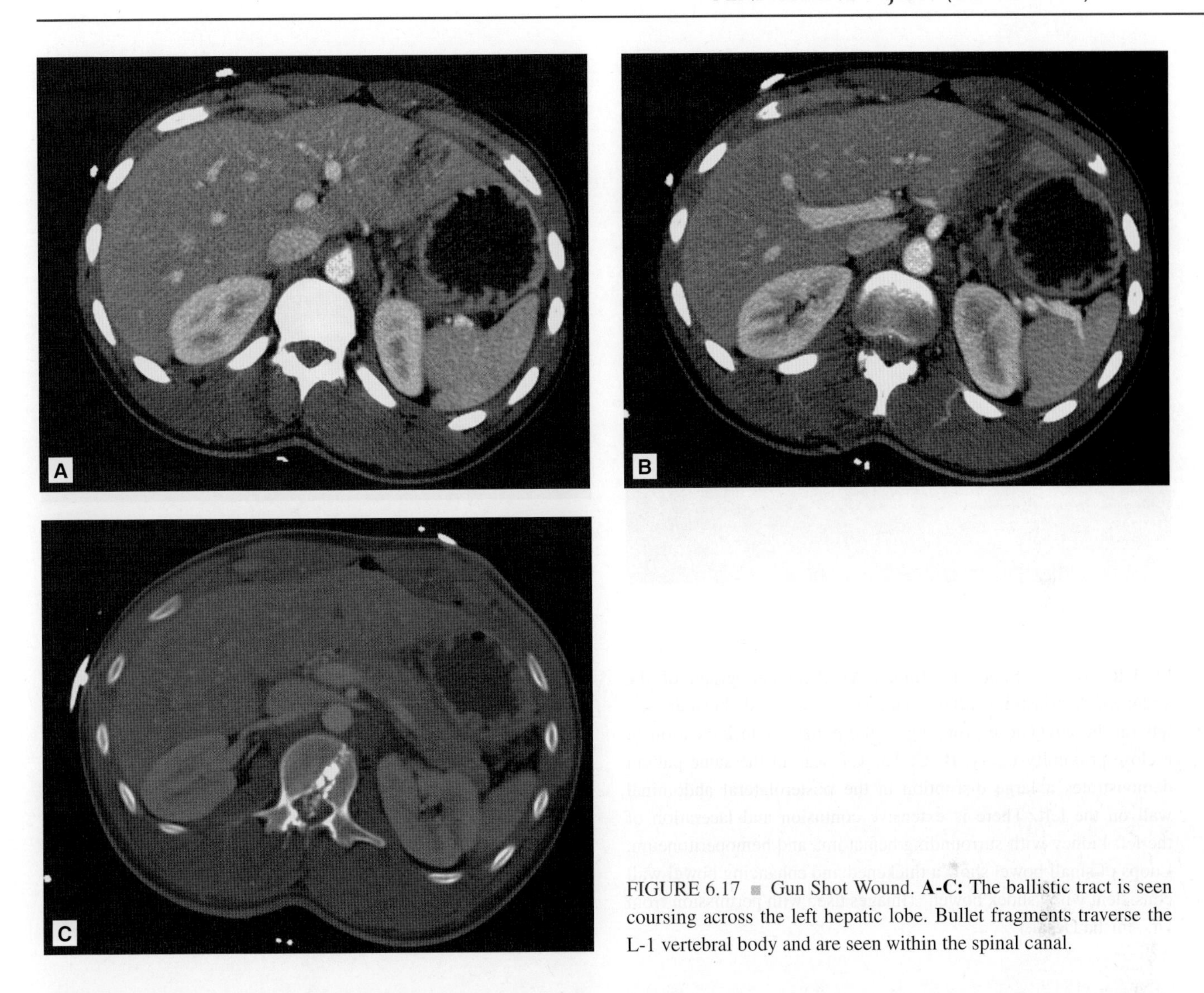

FIGURE 6.17 ■ Gun Shot Wound. **A-C:** The ballistic tract is seen coursing across the left hepatic lobe. Bullet fragments traverse the L-1 vertebral body and are seen within the spinal canal.

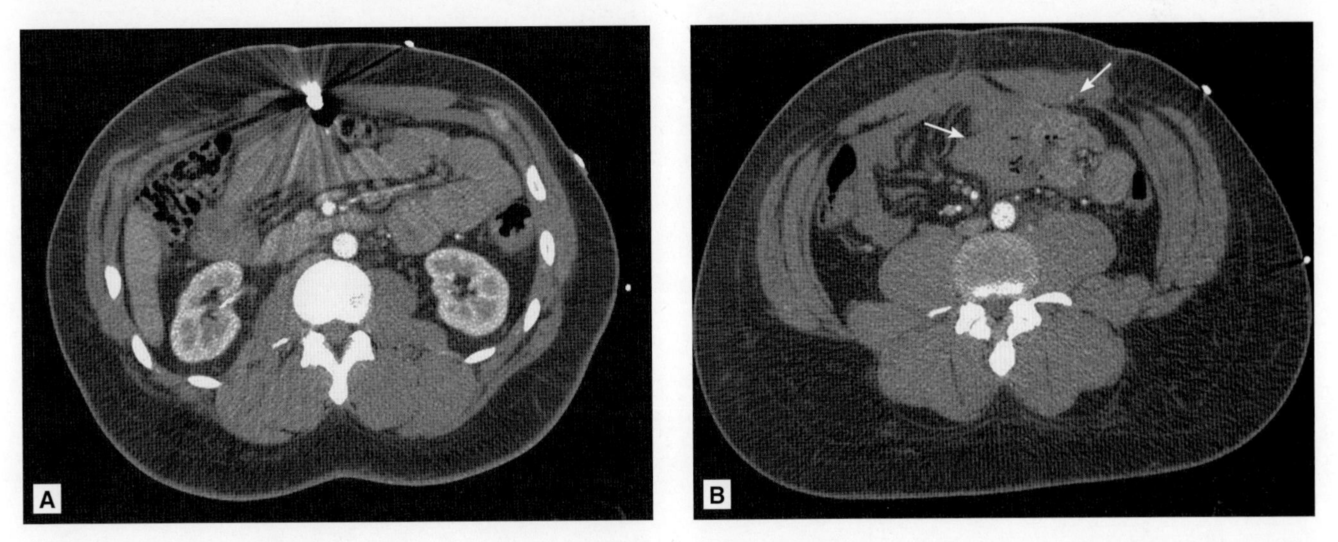

FIGURE 6.18 ■ Gun Shot Wound. **A, B:** A central mesenteric hematoma (arrows) is seen in proximity to the large bullet fragment. The posterior entry wound is not well seen.

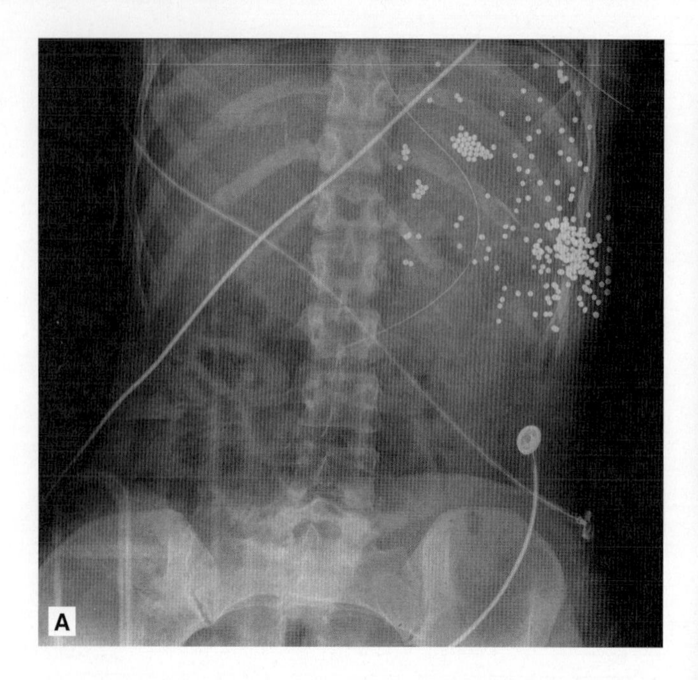

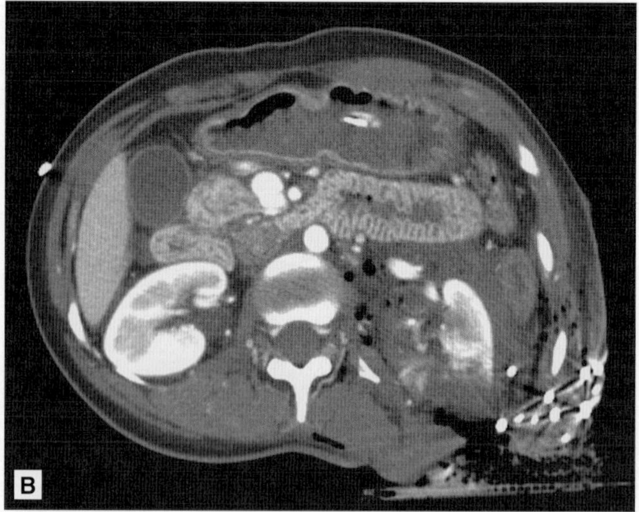

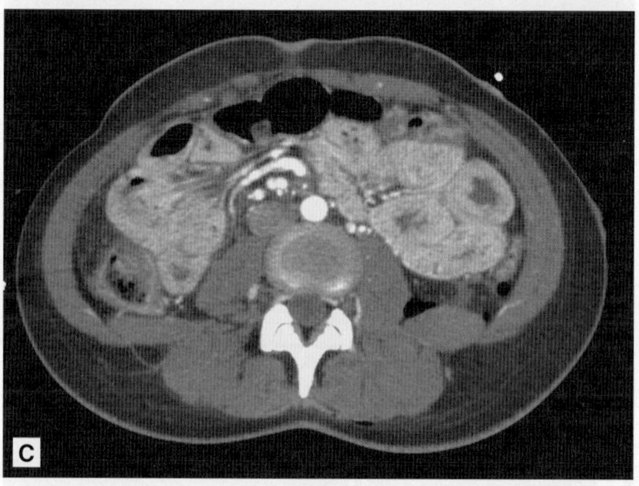

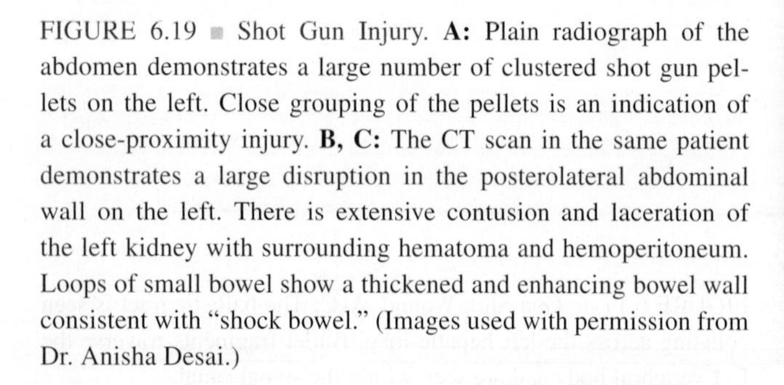

FIGURE 6.19 ■ Shot Gun Injury. **A:** Plain radiograph of the abdomen demonstrates a large number of clustered shot gun pellets on the left. Close grouping of the pellets is an indication of a close-proximity injury. **B, C:** The CT scan in the same patient demonstrates a large disruption in the posterolateral abdominal wall on the left. There is extensive contusion and laceration of the left kidney with surrounding hematoma and hemoperitoneum. Loops of small bowel show a thickened and enhancing bowel wall consistent with "shock bowel." (Images used with permission from Dr. Anisha Desai.)

Radiographic Summary

CT scan with contrast is the preferred method of identifying adrenal hemorrhage and associated injuries. Ultrasound, non-contrast CT, and MRI can also be used to image the adrenals but are not as accurate as contrasted CT. Adrenal hemorrhage should be considered in the post-traumatic patient when the adrenal gland is either enlarged or its typical chevron shape is distorted by a round or oval hematoma. In addition, there may be inflammatory stranding of the periadrenal fat or a posterior pararenal hemorrhage mimicking a thickened diaphragmatic crus.

Clinical Implications

Often a unilateral adrenal hemorrhage has no significant clinical impact on the patient. However, bilateral hemorrhage can result in life-threatening adrenal insufficiency. The bigger problem for patients with unilateral adrenal hemorrhage is the frequency of associated abdominal injuries and the risk of hemodynamic instability. As it is uncommon to have isolated adrenal hemorrhage, one must consider the high potential for other injuries. Most patients with an adrenal hemorrhage, even unilateral hemorrhage, will need evaluation by a trauma surgeon and admission to the hospital. If adrenal insufficiency is suspected, anACTH (cosyntropin) stimulation test is indicated to evaluate adrenal function. Dexamethasone should be considered for any patient under physiologic stress who may have adrenal insufficiency.

Pearls

1. Adrenal hemorrhage is rarely an isolated injury—look for other injuries.
2. Enlarged or distorted adrenal glands with periadrenal fat stranding are indicative of a hemorrhage.
3. Adrenal adenomas are common, and may simulate an adrenal hemorrhage. Adenomas may be low density on CT, and lack the adjacent fat stranding typical of hemorrhage.

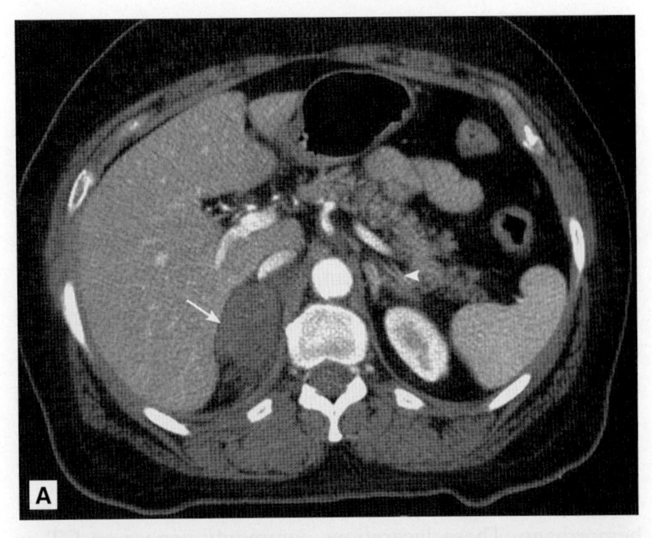

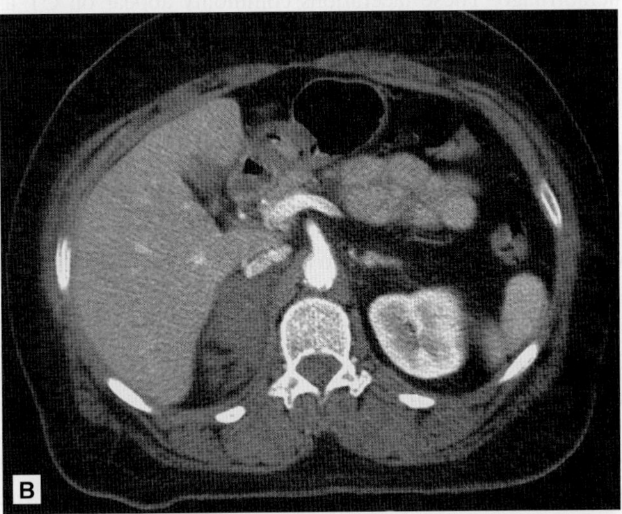

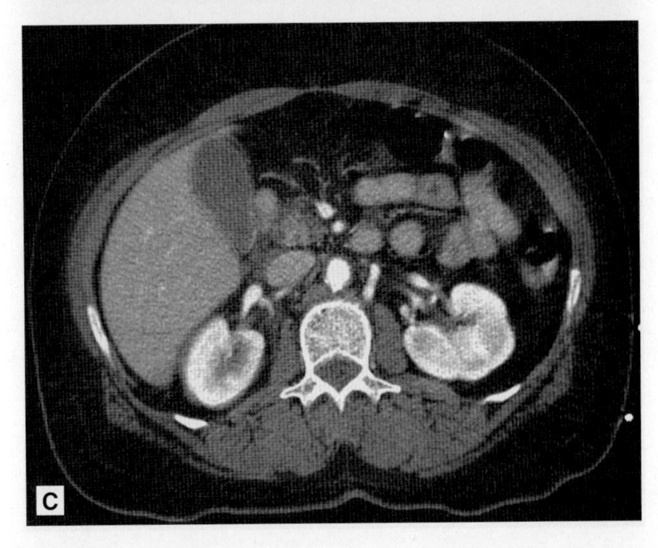

FIGURE 6.20 ■ Adrenal Hematoma. **A-C:** The right adrenal gland is enlarged, with rounded hematoma formation evident (arrow). Some surrounding fat stranding is evident. The normal left adrenal gland is identified (arrowhead).

Radiographic Summary

Contrast CT scan is the preferred method used to emergently evaluate patients with suspected renal injury. Renal injuries are graded as per AAST criteria based on imaging features. Grade 1 renal injuries feature parenchymal contusion or non-expanding hematoma and will appear as ill-defined areas of hypoattenuation on a CT scan. Grade 2 injuries are characterized by a non-expanding, perinephric hematoma confined to the retroperitoneum, or superficial cortical lacerations less than 1 cm without collecting system involvement. Lacerations greater than 1cm indicate Grade 3 injury. Grade 4 injuries involve a renal parenchymal laceration into the collecting system, or injury to the main renal artery/vein with contained hemorrhage. These lacerations commonly appear on CT as parenchymal clefts and if they involve the collecting system, extravasation of contrast may be seen. A shattered or devascularized kidney, ureteropelvic avulsion, or complete laceration or thrombus of the main renal vasculature constitutes Grade 5 injuries. These types of injuries can be seen as a nonenhancing kidney if there is devascularization. Extravasation of contrast may be visible due to disruption of the vasculature or collecting system.

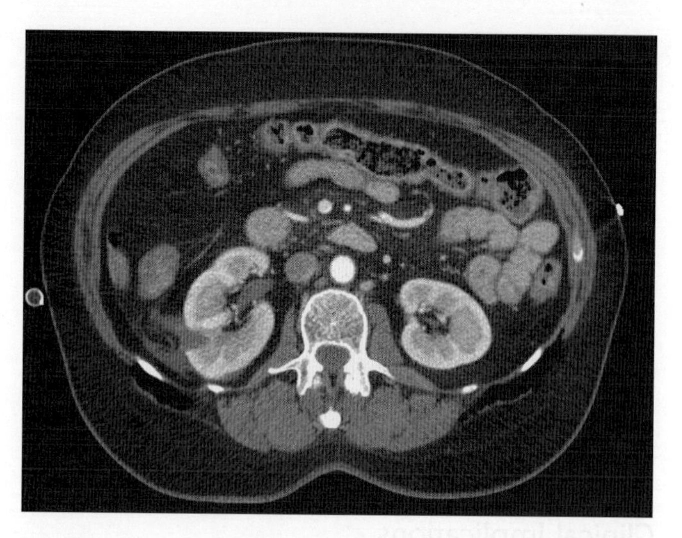

FIGURE 6.21 ■ Renal Laceration. A moderate-sized laceration is identified in the interpolar region of the right kidney. There is perinephric stranding/hematoma extending into the retroperitoneal fat adjacent to the site of injury.

Clinical Implications

Most renal injuries are due to blunt abdominal trauma with sudden deceleration, such as an automobile crash. The kidneys are located high in the retroperitoneum and are protected by surrounding structures—therefore, kidney injuries are frequently not isolated injuries. Although hematuria is very common with a renal injury, significant injuries may be present without this sign.

The vast majority of blunt trauma renal injuries are minor renal contusions that can be treated conservatively. The only absolute indication for emergent surgical exploration is life-threatening bleeding. Surgery may also be needed for

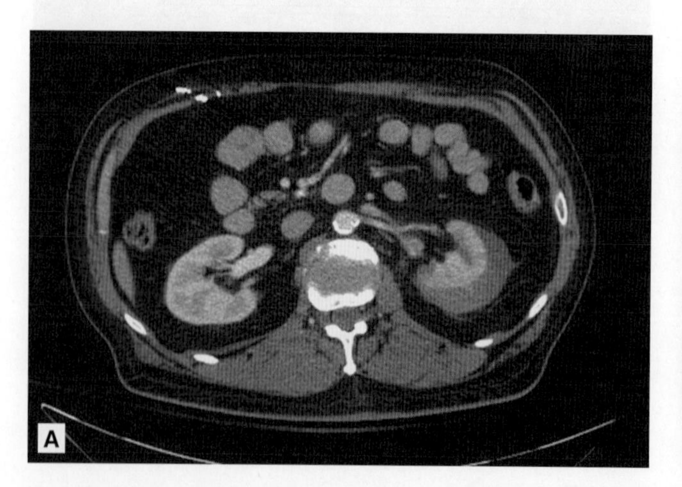

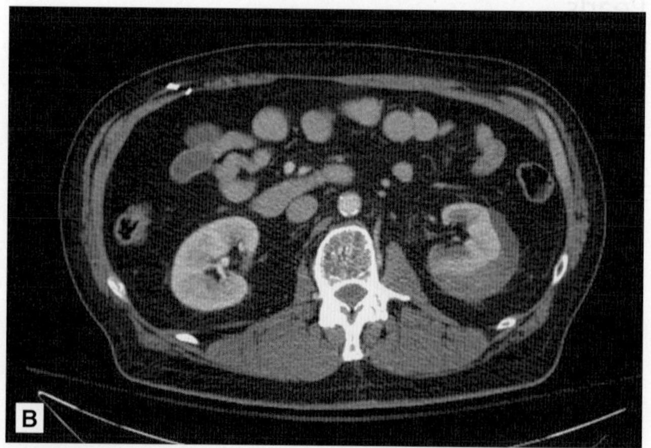

FIGURE 6.22 ■ Subcapsular Hematoma. **A, B:** On the left, a crescentic subcapsular fluid collection is seen. There is subtle diminished enhancement of the left kidney when compared to the right, an indication of decreased perfusion to the injured kidney.

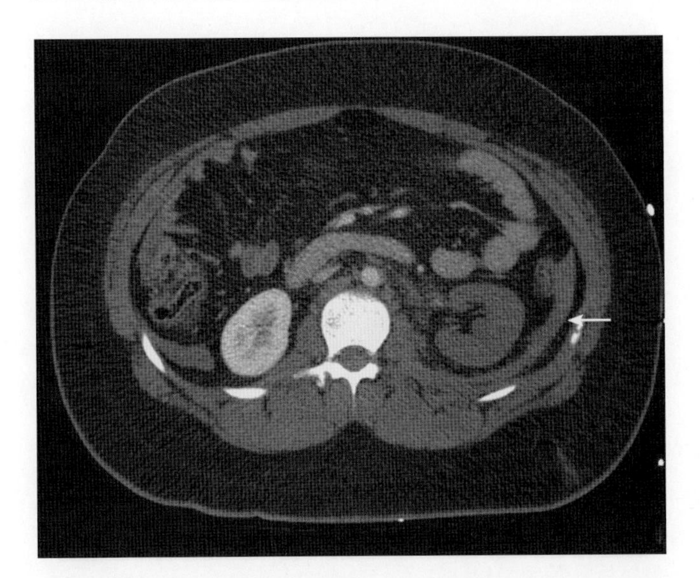

FIGURE 6.23 ■ Renal Pedicle Injury. A complete lack of contrast enhancement is seen within the left kidney, indicating an injury to the renal vasculature. A subtle region of retroperitoneal fat standing is seen, along with some hematoma tracking along the perirenal fascia (arrow).

patients with extensive devitalized tissue, or urinary extravasation not controlled by conservative measures. Although not nearly as common, penetrating trauma can also cause renal injuries. These are almost always associated with other abdominal trauma and require immediate surgical evaluation.

Pearls

1. In the setting of trauma, a nonenhancing kidney is due to a significant vascular injury and requires emergent surgical consultation.
2. Low-attenuation fluid adjacent to the renal hilum may represent a developing urinoma in the setting of renal collecting system laceration. Delayed CT imaging following IV contrast administration may be useful for detecting urine leaks.

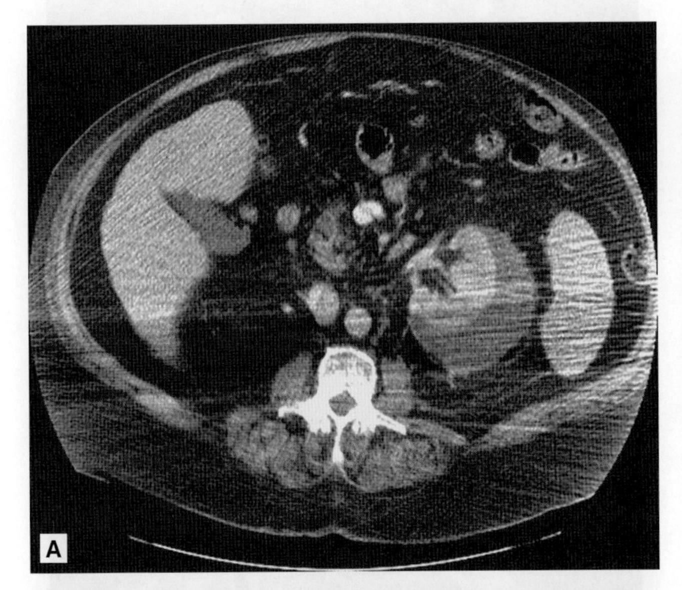

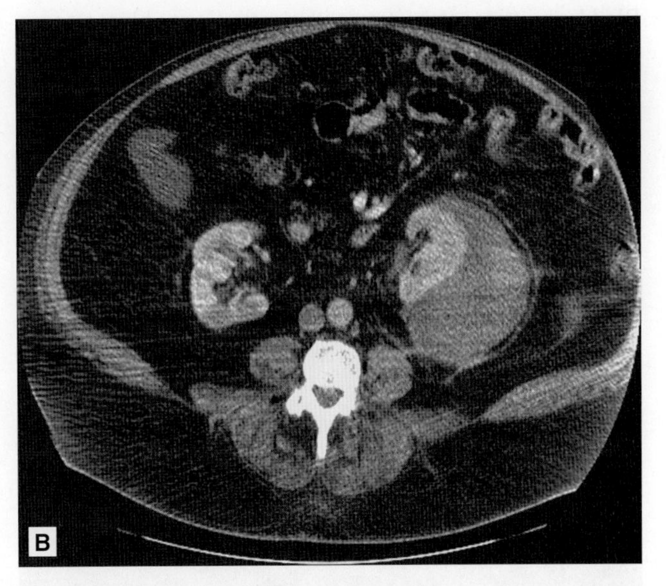

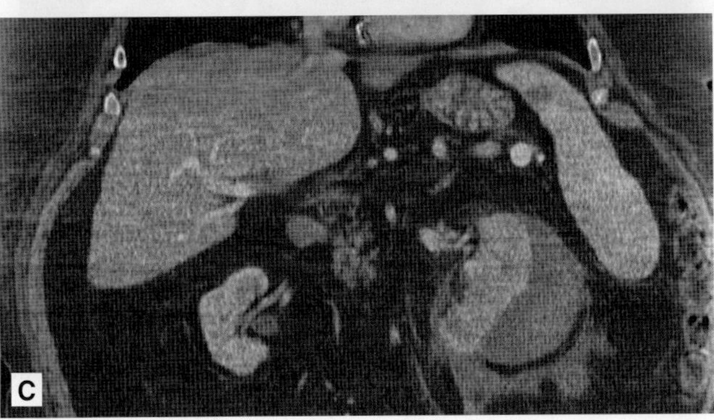

FIGURE 6.24 ■ Page Kidney. **A-C:** This patient developed hypertension in the weeks following an MVA. The CT scan obtained at the time of injury demonstrates a large subcapsular hematoma with compression of the renal parenchyma.

Radiographic Summary

The imaging test of choice for bladder injuries has traditionally been conventional cystography, but CT cystography is playing an expanding role in the diagnosis. The choice between these two options is institution dependent. There are five types of bladder injury patterns. Type 1 (incomplete tear of the bladder mucosa) and Type 3 (intramural bladder lacerations) do not demonstrate extravasation of contrast on imaging. Type 2 injuries involve intraperitoneal rupture, with cystography demonstrating contrast material around the bowel loops, mesenteric folds, or paracolic gutters. Extraperitoneal bladder ruptures (type 4) are the most commonly imaged bladder injury. Radiographic features include extravasation confined to the perivesicular space, but can extend out from this space in complex cases. Combined intraperitoneal and extraperitoneal bladder ruptures (Type 5) may also be encountered.

Clinical Implications

Bladder injuries can be seen with penetrating or blunt trauma, with patients commonly presenting with pelvic pain, hematuria, or an inability to void. Hematuria is found in almost all

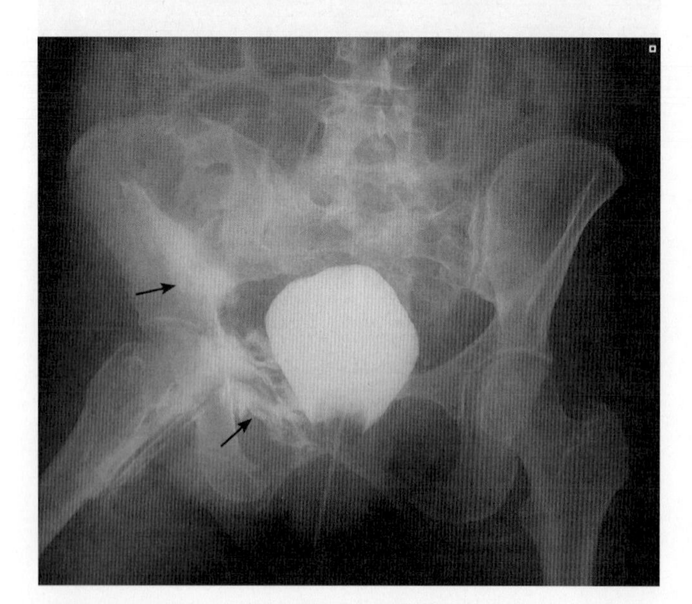

FIGURE 6.25 ■ Extraperitoneal Bladder Rupture. Cystogram image demonstrates "flame-shaped" extravasation of contrast from the bladder, extending to the right-sided extraperitoneal soft tissues (arrows). Bowel loops are seen in the lower abdomen, without surrounding intraperitoneal contrast. Note extensive osseous pelvic trauma with right sacroiliac joint diastasis.

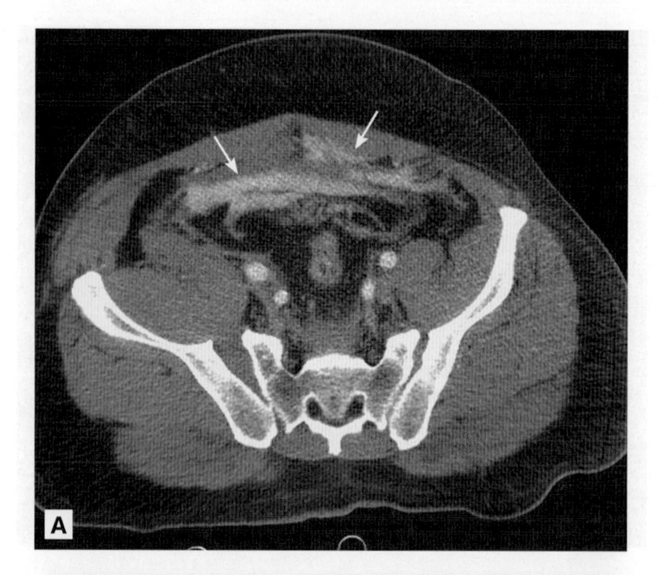

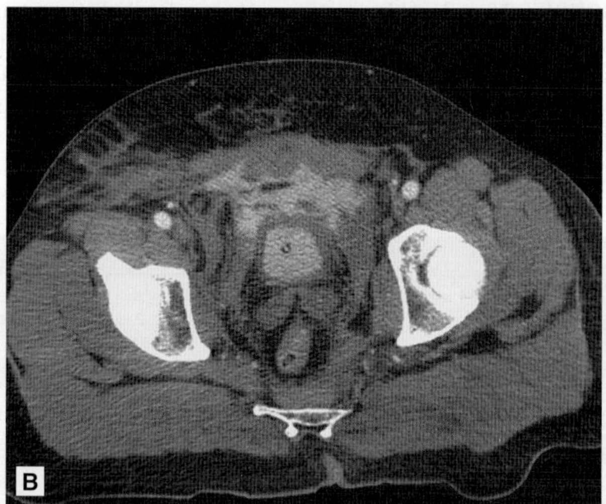

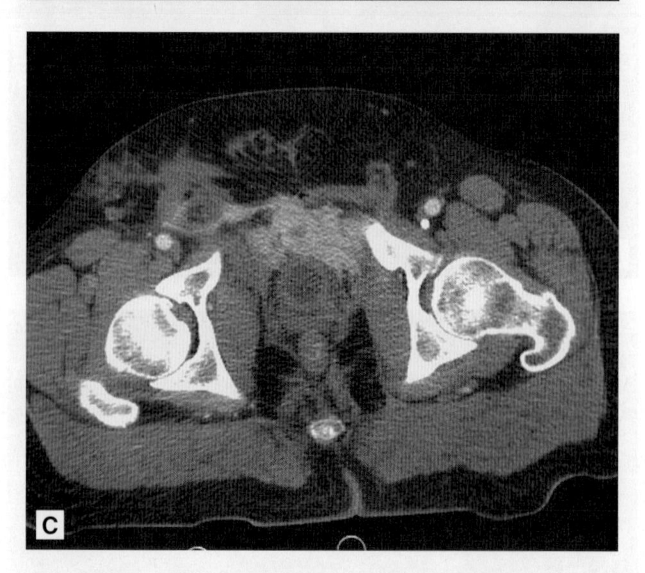

FIGURE 6.26 ■ Extraperitoneal Bladder Rupture. **A-C:** CT scan demonstrates contrast material and hematoma extending along the anterior abdominal wall within the space of Retzius (arrows).

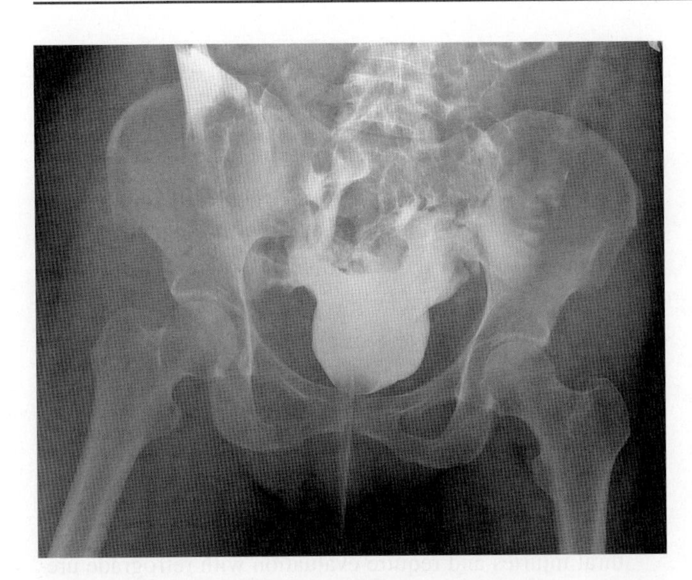

FIGURE 6.27 ■ Intraperitoneal Bladder Rupture. Image from cystogram demonstrates an irregular superior bladder contour with spillage of contrast into the peritoneum. Bowel loops are outlined by high-density contrast material.

bladder injuries. Pelvic pain may be related to pelvic fractures, which are frequently associated with bladder injuries. On exam, a high-riding prostate may be present with a urethral or bladder injury. Bladder injuries must be identified as early as possible before uroperitoneum and resulting sepsis occurs.

Most Type 1 bladder injuries will resolve without any treatment. Most extraperitoneal injuries will resolve with placement of a Foley, but if there is extensive extravasation, surgical repair may be necessary. Injuries involving intraperitoneal rupture require surgical exploration.

Pearls

1. In addition to extravasation of contrast, look for associated pelvic bone injuries.
2. Dedicated CT cystogram is being used in place of conventional cystogram in some hospitals.

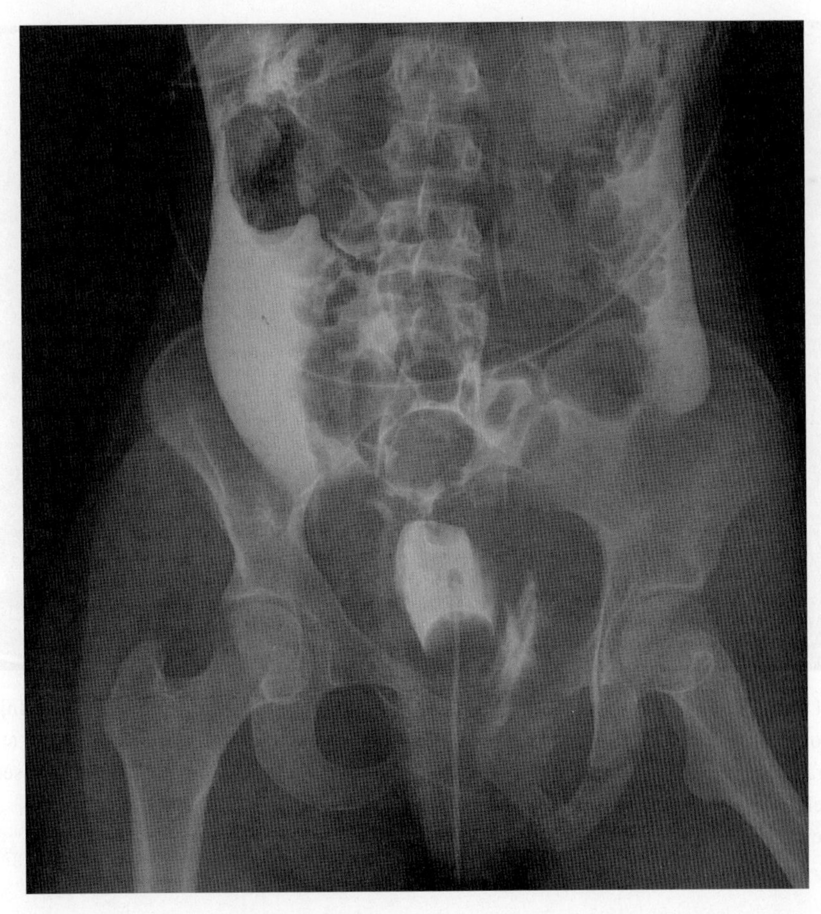

FIGURE 6.28 ■ Bladder Rupture. Evidence of both intraperitoneal and left-sided extraperitoneal bladder rupture (Type 5) is seen on this cystogram image.

Radiographic Summary

Patients with urethral injuries will typically present after significant abdominopelvic trauma. While CT scans are frequently obtained to evaluate for injuries to this region, CT lacks adequate sensitivity for detection of urethral injury and therefore retrograde urethrography is required to rule out injuries of the urethra. Minor urethral injuries may include a simple contusion, or a stretch injury with urethral elongation. These injuries do not demonstrate extravasation on urethrography. Partial urethral disruptions demonstrate extravasation of retrograde contrast injection with some contrast continuing to reach the bladder. Complete disruptions of the urethra will demonstrate extravasation of contrast without any visualization of the bladder.

Clinical Impression

Any patient with significant pelvic trauma is at risk for a urethral injury. History and physical examination findings may include an inability to void, blood at the urethral meatus, high riding prostate and perineal bruising. For these patients, it is important not to place a Foley catheter until a urethral injury is ruled out. Passage of a Foley can change a partial urethral disruption into a complete disruption.

Pearls

1. Inability to void, blood at the urethral meatus, perineal bruising and high riding prostate are associated with urethral injuries and require evaluation with retrograde urethrography prior to placing a Foley.
2. CT scan of the pelvis is not adequate to fully evaluate for a urethral injury.

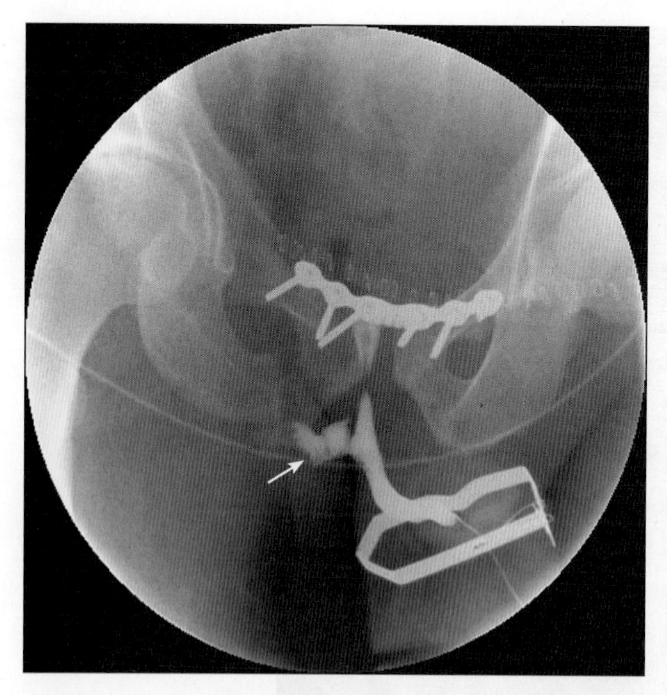

FIGURE 6.29 ■ Penile Urethra Injury. Retrograde urethrogram demonstrates leakage of contrast from the penile urethra (arrow) in this patient following a straddle-type pelvic trauma event. Metallic densities related to prior pelvic fixation and the "penile clamp" used for this type of imaging are visible.

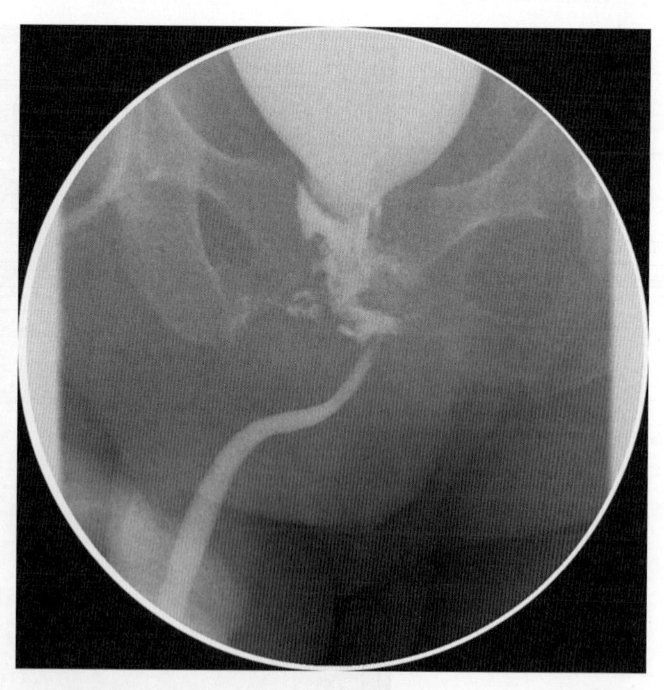

FIGURE 6.30 ■ Membranous Urethra Injury. In this case, there is near-complete disruption of the urethra at the level of the bladder base. Extensive contrast extravasation is seen at the pelvic floor.

Radiographic Summary

Scrotal ultrasound with Doppler, using a linear probe, is the most accurate means of imaging testicular trauma. A normal testicular ultrasound should reveal a homogeneous pattern free of internal irregularities. A testicular fracture may appear as a jagged linear or curvilinear hypoechoic fracture line coursing though the testicle. The contour of the testicle may remain smooth if the integrity of the tunica albuginea is not affected. Acute bleeding in the testicle will appear as hyperechoic areas in the parenchyma. A testicular rupture is diagnosed when there is a break in the echogenic tunica albuginea, resulting in an irregular contour on ultrasound and possibly extruded material.

Clinical Implications

Testicular trauma can be divided into blunt trauma, penetrating trauma and degloving injury. These latter two types of trauma require consultation for surgical exploration. Most blunt trauma to the testicles results in minor injuries and require only conservative treatment. Surgical intervention may be required if the testicle is ruptured or shows signs of an expanding hematoma. Delays in definitive management may lead to testicular infection, atrophy, or necrosis.

Pearls

1. On ultrasound with Doppler, a normal appearing testicle with good blood flow will exclude significant testicular injuries.
2. Ultrasound with Doppler should be performed in any patient with testicular pain and evidence of trauma.

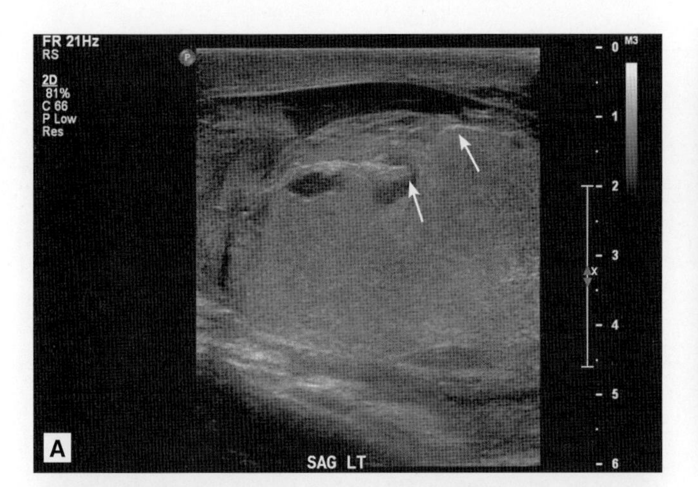

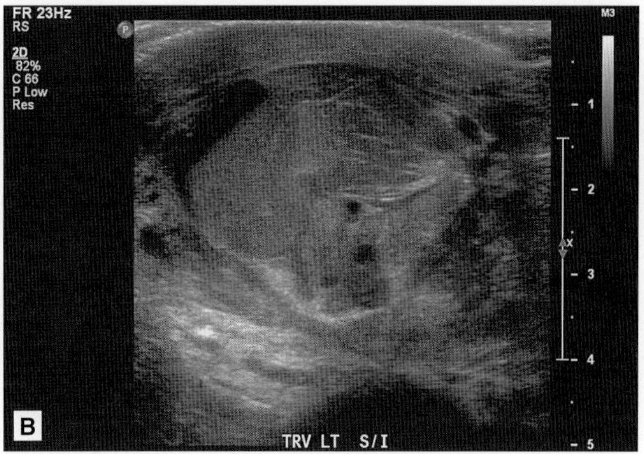

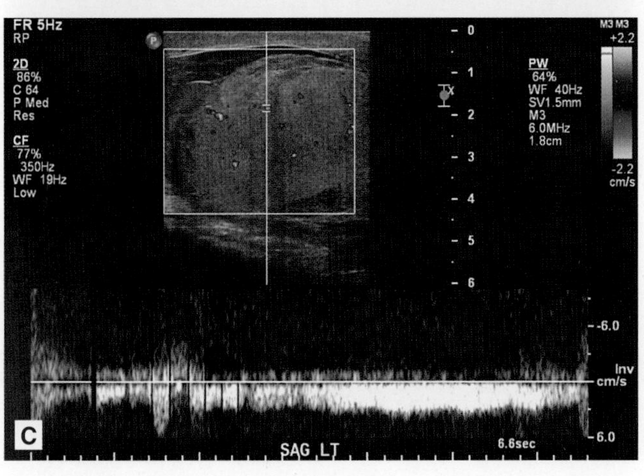

FIGURE 6.31 ■ Testicular Fracture. **A-C:** Following an athletic injury, grayscale sonography demonstrates a deformed left testicle with extruded material visible. The disrupted tunica albugenia is seen (arrows). Doppler imaging demonstrates preserved internal blood flow. (Images used with permission from Dr. Anisha Desai.)

Chapter 7

ATRAUMATIC CONDITIONS OF THE ABDOMEN

Jake Block
Laurie M. Lawrence
Robinson M. Ferre

Radiographic Summary

An abdominal aortic aneurysm (AAA) is a focal dilation of the aortic wall measuring greater than 1.5 times the normal diameter of the aorta. An aortic diameter of 3 cm at the level of the renal arteries meets the definition of an AAA. Most aneurysms produce little to no symptoms unless they rupture.

CT can accurately detect an AAA, mural thrombosis, aneurysmal leakage, and rupture. CT findings of a ruptured aneurysm include anterior displacement of the kidney, indistinct aortic wall, free intraperitoneal fluid, or a retroperitoneal hematoma in the presence of an aneurysm. Leakage and rupture of an AAA can be visualized without the use of IV contrast; however, contrast is necessary to delineate a patent aortic lumen from a mural thrombus and can provide anatomic information about the shape and location of the aneurysm. A normal aortic diameter on CT excludes the diagnosis of an AAA.

ED bedside ultrasonography is very accurate in establishing the presence of an AAA; however, it cannot reliably detect leakage or rupture. In a hemodynamically unstable patient, a ruptured AAA is presumed when it is visualized by ultrasonography.

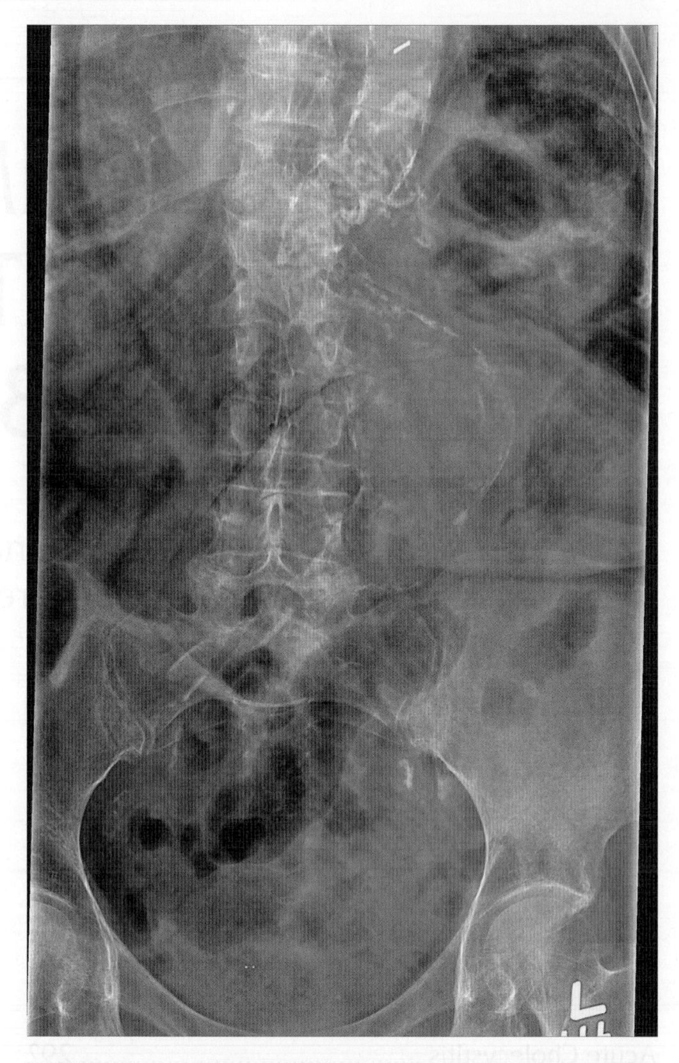

FIGURE 7.1 ■ Abdominal Aortic Aneurysm. Atherosclerotic calcifications delineate the extensive abdominal aortic aneurysm on this plain radiographic image.

Clinical Implications

An asymptomatic aneurysm may be detected during the evaluation of an unrelated medical problem, and can be followed closely as an outpatient. A leaking or ruptured AAA is a true emergency. Clinically stable patients should undergo CT scanning with IV contrast. If the patient is unstable, a bedside ultrasound can be obtained to determine if an aneurysm is present.

Pearls

1. When performing bedside ultrasonography be careful to measure the aortic diameter from outer wall to outer wall. If the aneurysm contains a thrombus, take care not to mistake the edge of the thrombus for the aortic wall. Measuring the inner rim of the thrombus will result in a smaller measurement and may lead to the incorrect conclusion that an aneurysm is not present.
2. Aneurysms measuring greater than 5 cm, or demonstrating an increase in size of greater than 1 cm over a period of 6 months are at increased risk of rupture.

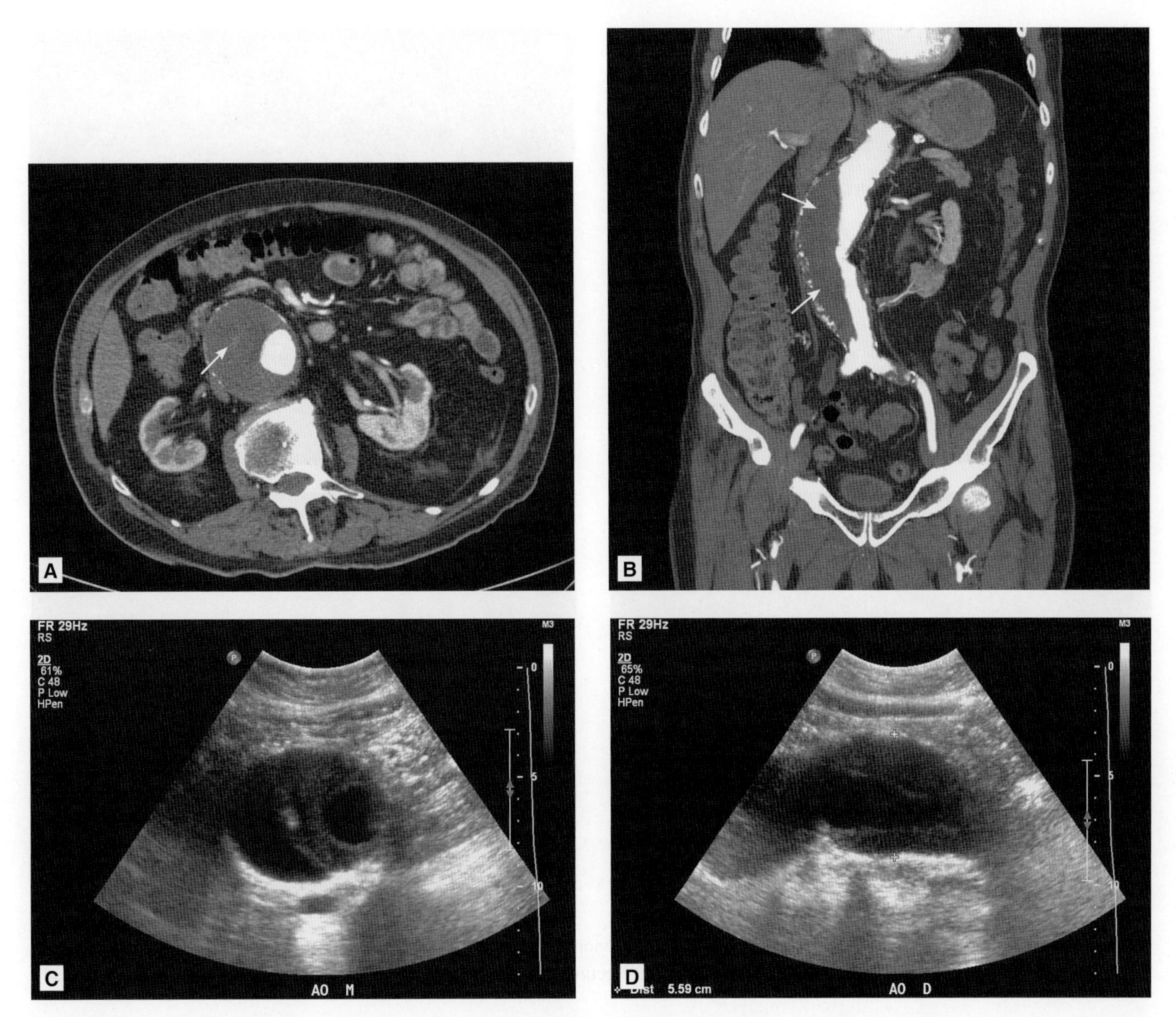

FIGURE 7.2 ■ Abdominal Aortic Aneurysm. **A, B:** Contrast-enhanced CTA demonstrates the extent of mural thrombus visible as low density (arrows) adjacent to the enhanced lumen of the vessel. The aneurysm extends throughout the suprarenal and infrarenal portions of the abdominal aorta. **C, D:** Transaxial and sagittal ultrasound images in the same individual. Mural thrombus is seen as echogenic material within the vessel.

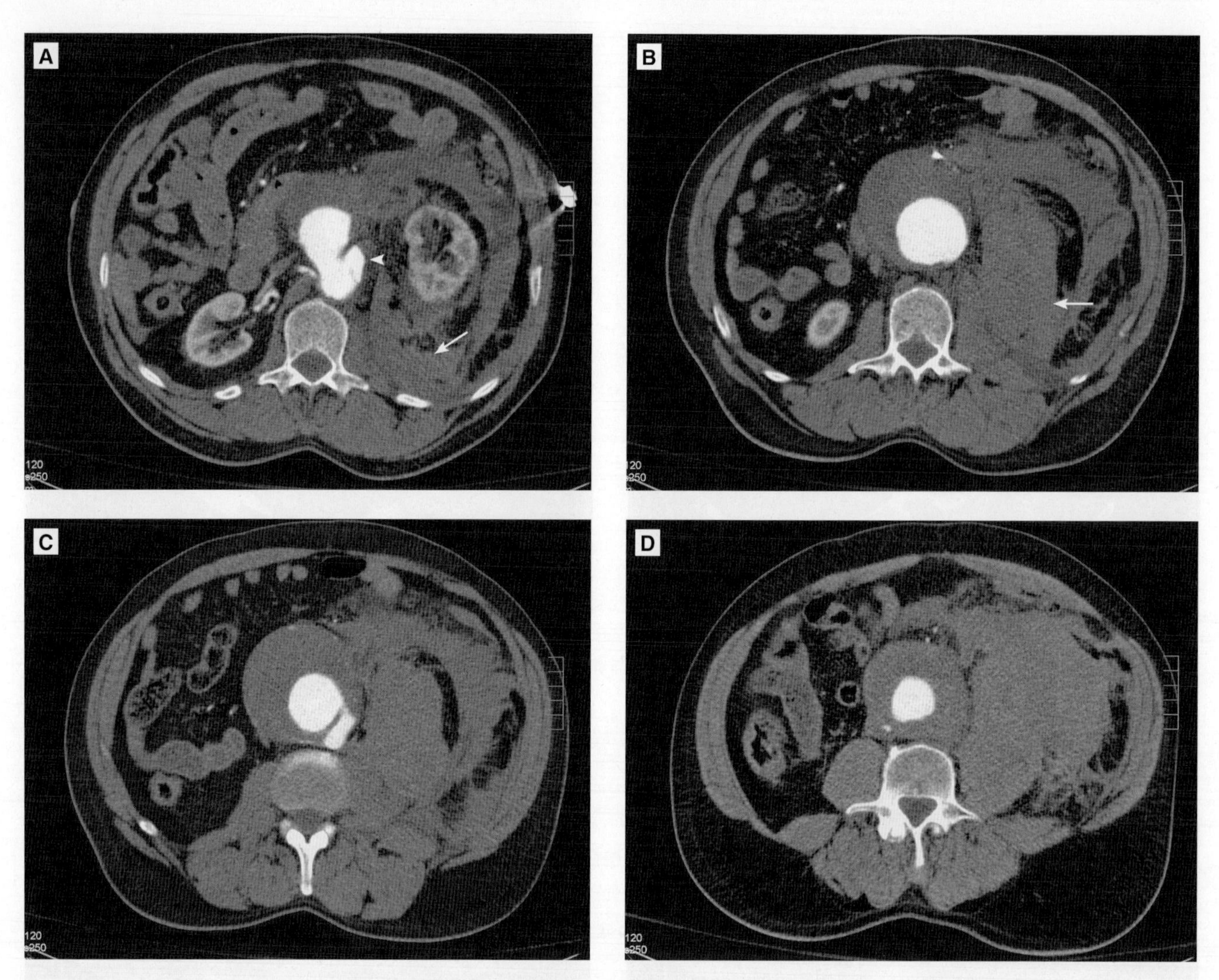

FIGURE 7.3 ■ Ruptured Abdominal Aortic Aneurysm. **A-D:** An abnormal vessel contour is seen with findings of para-aortic stranding and retroperitoneal hematoma (arrows). Intravenous contrast is seen dissecting beyond the expected location of the aortic vessel wall (arrowhead).

Radiographic Summary

Emphysematous cholecystitis is an acute infection of the gallbladder by gas-forming organisms. It is diagnosed radiographically by air within the gallbladder wall or the gallbladder lumen. Gallstones may or may not be present. Other evidence of gallbladder wall inflammation will likely be present, such as a thickened gallbladder wall (>3 mm) and pericholecystic fluid.

Emphysematous cholecystitis can be detected with ultrasound as a comet tail artifact seen within the gallbladder wall or as air artifact within the lumen. On CT, emphysematous cholecystitis will appear as radiolucent areas (gas) within the gallbladder wall or lumen.

Clinical Implications

Emphysematous cholecystitis occurs as a result of an ischemic and gangrenous gallbladder infected with gas-forming organisms. Emphysematous cholecystitis is uncommon and occurs in only about 1% of cases of acute cholecystitis. It is most often found in elderly men with diabetes mellitus. Patients are often febrile, ill appearing, and have a marked leukocytosis with a left shift. They may have evidence of sepsis or septic shock and require fluid resuscitation and vasopressor support.

Overall mortality rates for emphysematous cholecystitis are five times greater than those of nonemphysematous cholecystitis and range from 15 to 25%. Patients should receive early broad-spectrum antibiotics that cover anaerobic and gram-negative rod bacteria. Patients should be treated aggressively if signs of sepsis exist. Emergent surgical consultation for cholecystectomy should also be obtained.

Pearls

1. Occasionally, asymptomatic gallstones may contain internal stellate collections of nitrogen gas (the Mercedes Benz sign). This should not be confused with emphysematous cholecystitis.
2. Cases require surgical consultation and operative management. In some instances, percutaneous drainage and IV antibiotics can serve as a temporizing measure in high-risk surgical candidates.

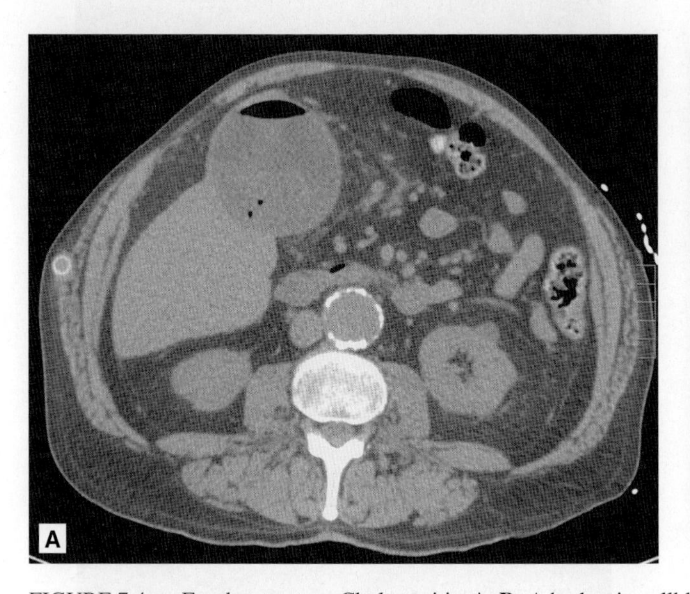

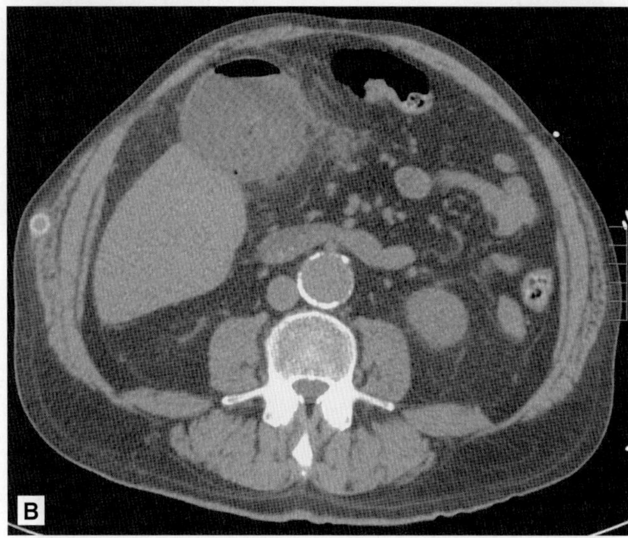

FIGURE 7.4 ■ Emphysematous Cholecystitis. **A, B:** A hydropic gallbladder with intraluminal foci of gas is seen. Pericholecystic fat stranding is present on this noncontrast CT of the abdomen.

Radiographic Summary

Patients who have orally ingested a foreign body or inserted a foreign body into the rectum or vagina will frequently seek medical care in the Emergency Department. Conventional abdominal radiographs can be used to locate the object if it is radiopaque, such as metal and glass. Wood and plastic are generally not radiopaque. CT and MRI may be used with variable success.

"Mules" or "body packers" transport illegal drugs by ingesting drug-filled packets or inserting packets into the rectum or vagina. The packets are often condoms or balloons filled with heroin or cocaine, and vary in their imaging characteristics. On plain abdominal radiographs, the packets may appear as multiple objects of varying radio-opacity throughout the GI tract. A crescent-shaped collection of air may surround condom-wrapped packets, and is described as the "double condom sign."

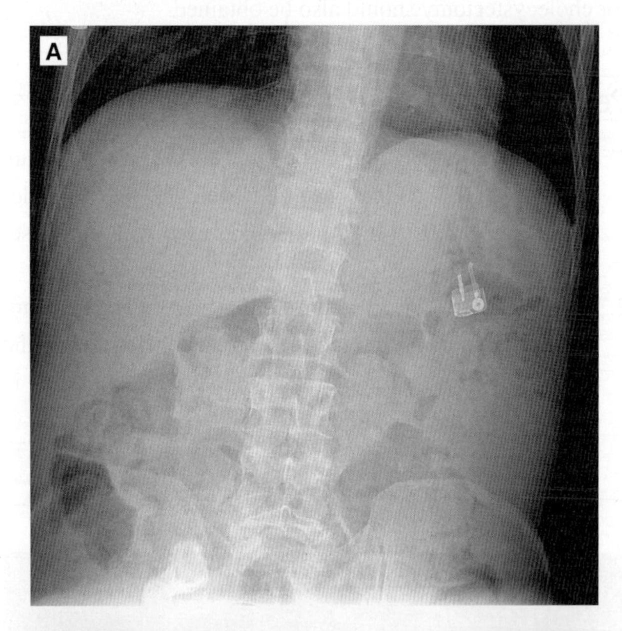

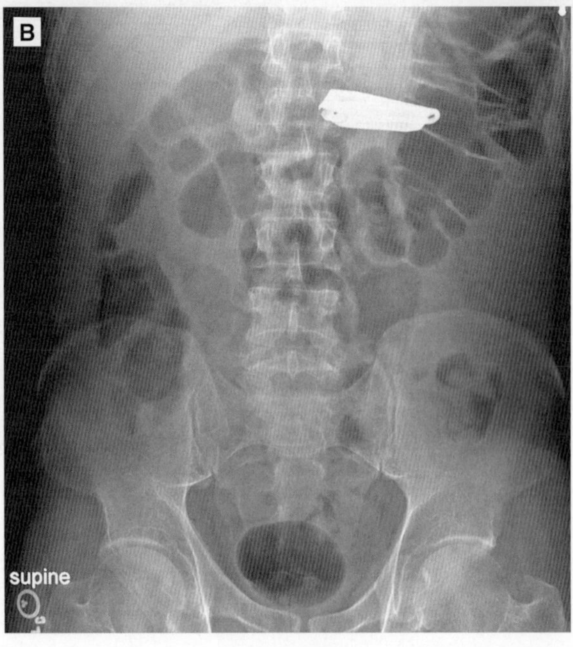

FIGURE 7.5 ■ Ingested Foreign Body. **A, B:** Two abdominal plain radiographs from different dates on this psychiatric patient demonstrate ingested foreign bodies (cigarette lighter and toenail clipper).

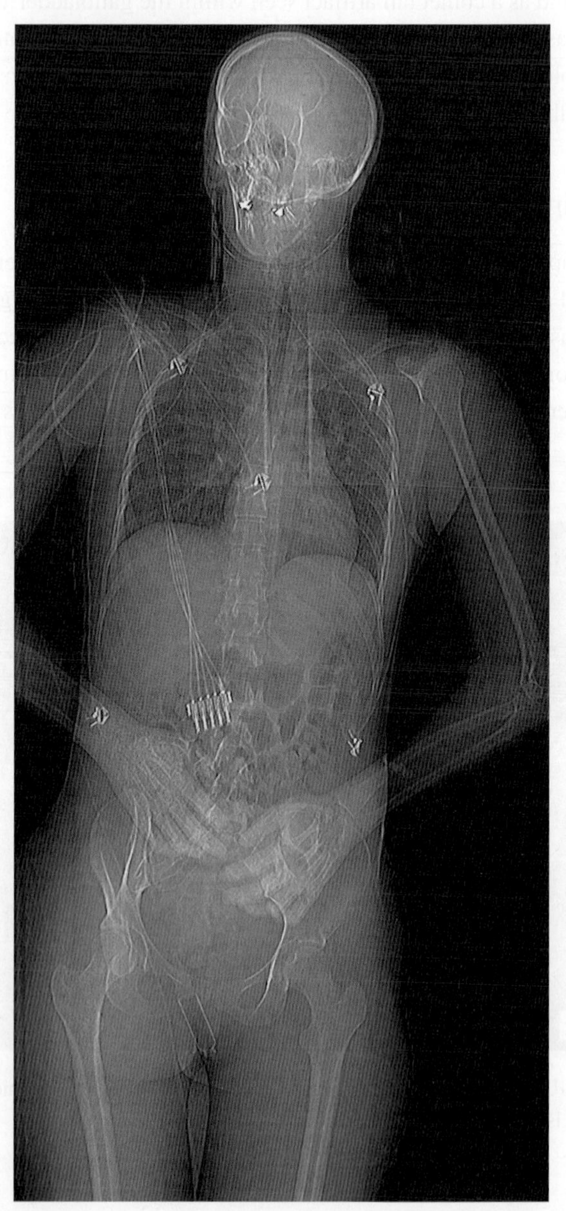

FIGURE 7.6 ■ Vaginal Foreign Body. CT "scout image" obtained in a trauma patient demonstrates a foreign body within the lower pelvis. Physical exam produced a pill bottle containing illegally obtained prescription medication.

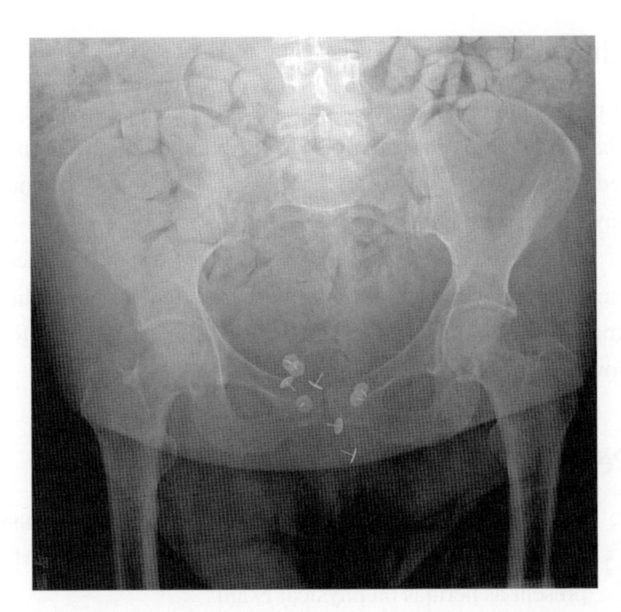

FIGURE 7.7 ■ Vaginal Foreign Bodies. Thumbtacks placed by a mentally ill patient as an attempt to prevent unwanted intercourse.

Clinical Implications

Abdominal foreign bodies that are smooth and less than 2 cm in width and 6 cm in length will generally pass without incident. Large or sharp objects located in the stomach should be referred for endoscopic removal. If such an object has already passed into the duodenum, progress through the GI tract should be followed by serial radiographs. Sharp, long objects can lodge in the GI tract at sites of anatomic sharp angulations, such as the duodenal loop, duodenal–jejunal junction, appendix, and ileocecal valve.

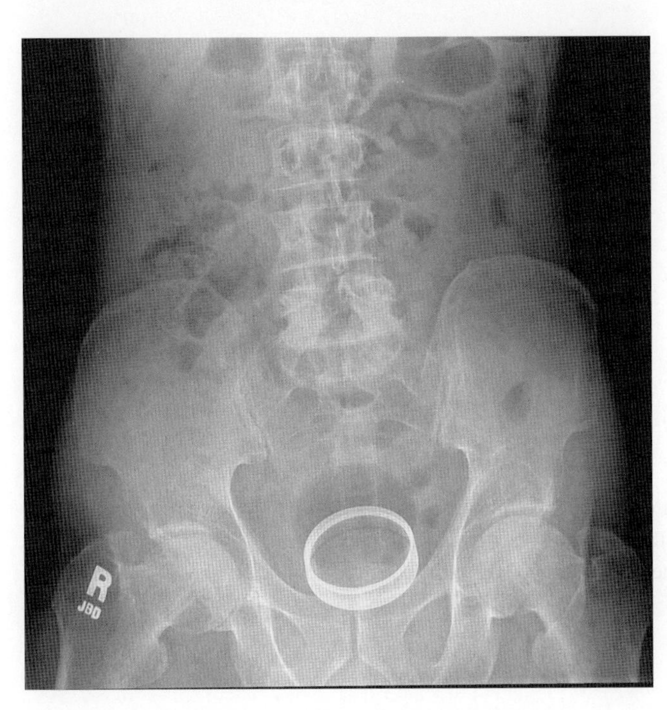

FIGURE 7.8 ■ Rectal Foreign Body. "Cold cream" Jar.

Patients who have swallowed packets of drugs are at risk for fatal overdose if one of the packets ruptures. Removal of the drug packets in the ED should be expedited by whole bowel irrigation.

The presence of blood seen on rectal or vaginal exam indicates laceration and possible perforation, and necessitates a surgical consultation.

Pearls

1. The majority of ingested foreign bodies will pass spontaneously through the gastrointestinal tract without any intervention. Subsequent radiographs are not needed unless the patient develops abdominal pain, fever, vomiting, or constipation.
2. Rectal foreign bodies found on abdominal radiographs to be more than 10 cm from the anal verge are more likely to require surgical intervention for removal.
3. Rectal exam should not be performed on patients complaining of a rectal foreign body until an imaging study has excluded the presence of a sharp object, which could harm the examiner.

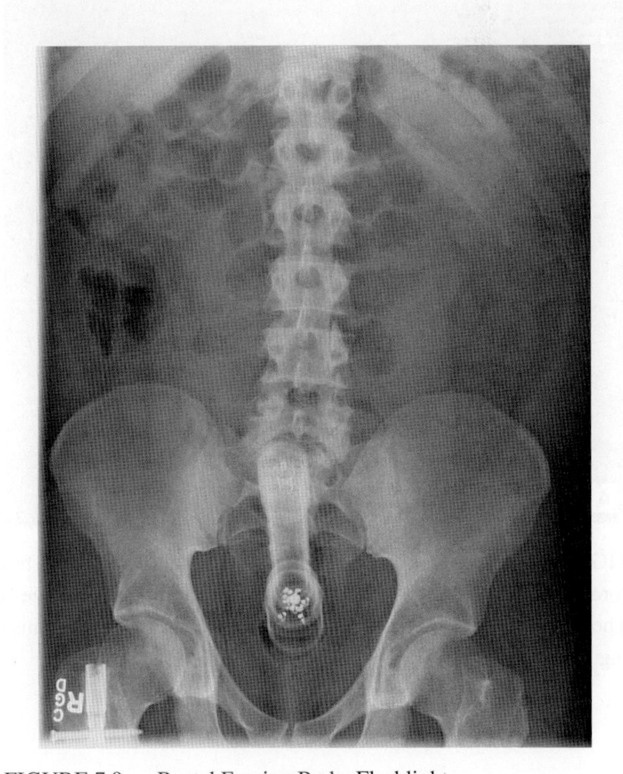

FIGURE 7.9 ■ Rectal Foreign Body. Flashlight.

Radiographic Summary

An abdominal wall hernia is defined as an abnormal protrusion of peritoneal contents through a fascial defect in the abdominal wall. Plain abdominal radiography is generally nondiagnostic of an abdominal wall hernia unless the patient has a complication such as a bowel obstruction, pneumatosis intestinalis as a result of bowel strangulation and infarction, or pneumoperitoneum as the result of a bowel perforation. Plain radiographs may visualize loops of bowel projecting into scrotum or over the obturator foramen.

CT is the test of choice for evaluation of an abdominal wall hernia as it provides accurate detail of the abdominal wall and hernia contents. CT allows visualization of bowel and omentum protruding through the peritoneum. An incarcerated hernia can be identified by fat stranding around the hernia sac. CT findings of a strangulated hernia include bowel wall thickening, extraluminal fluid, marked fat stranding, and engorged mesenteric vessels suggesting vascular compromise.

Ultrasound can also be used to evaluate hernias, and has the added benefit of avoiding ionizing radiation. Color Doppler flow can help differentiate between an incarcerated or strangulated hernia.

Clinical Implications

A patient may be discharged to home if the hernia is reducible *and* if the patient has minimal to no symptoms after hernia reduction. These patients can be referred to a surgeon without any further imaging.

Patients with suspected incarcerated or strangulated hernias should undergo prompt surgical evaluation. Radiographic imaging should be obtained if there is clinical concern for bowel obstruction, ischemia, and perforation.

Pearls

1. An ultrasound can be used to differentiate masses in the abdominal wall and inguinal canal, which do not clearly present as hernias on physical exam.
2. Ultrasound may be used as an aid to hernia reduction. The ultrasound probe can visualize the abdominal fascial defect, allowing the clinician to directly guide the hernia back through the fascial opening into the abdominal cavity.

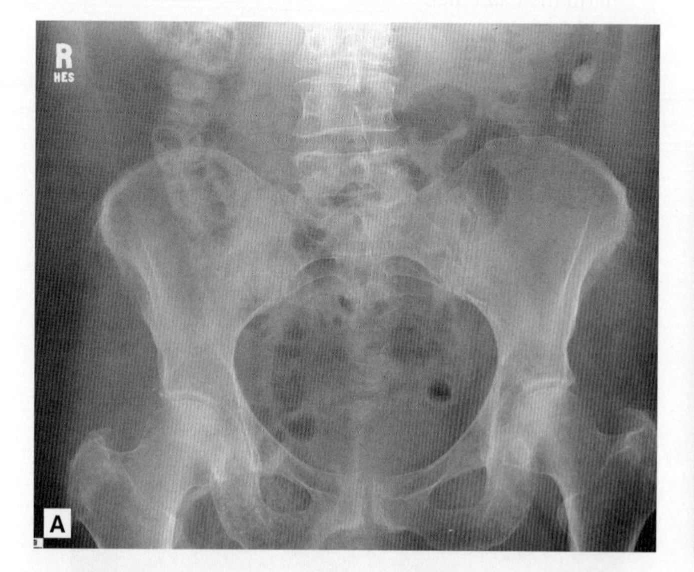

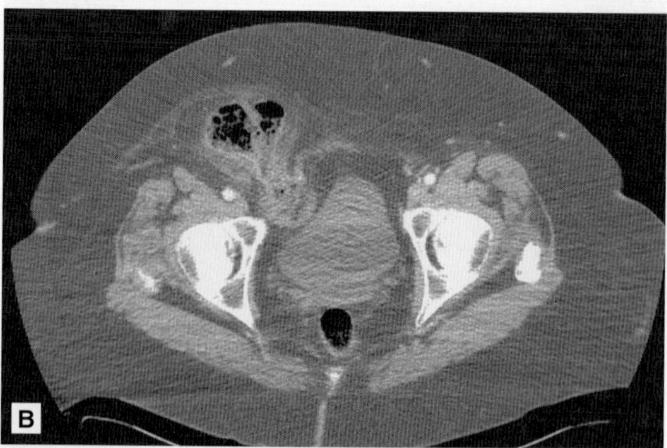

FIGURE 7.10 ■ Inguinal Hernia. **A:** On this plain radiograph, bowel containing fecal material is seen projecting over the right obturator foramen. This location is outside of the expected normal confines of the abdominal cavity and is highly suggestive of an inguinal hernia. There are no distended loops of bowel to suggest obstruction at this time. **B:** CT scan on the same patient demonstrates the bowel-containing inguinal hernia.

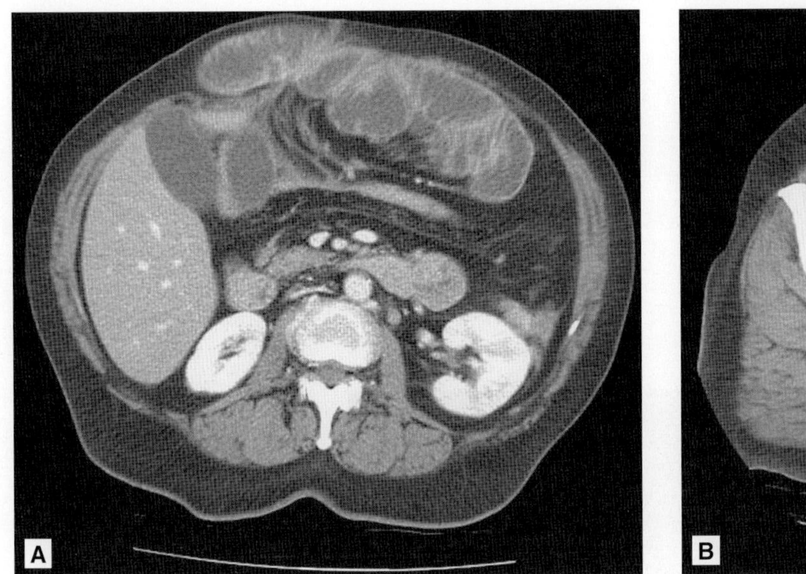

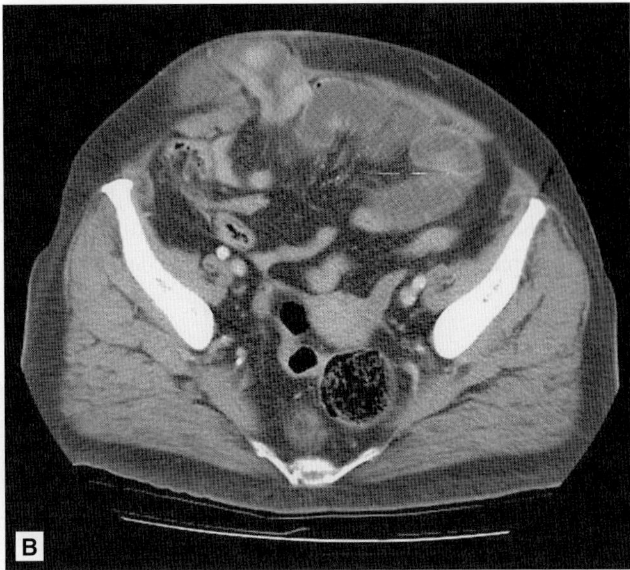

FIGURE 7.11 ■ Abdominal Wall Herniation with Small Bowel Obstruction. **A, B:** Bowel loops are seen extending through a defect in the anterior abdominal wall producing a high-grade obstruction. Note decompressed loops of distal small bowel in the right lower quadrant.

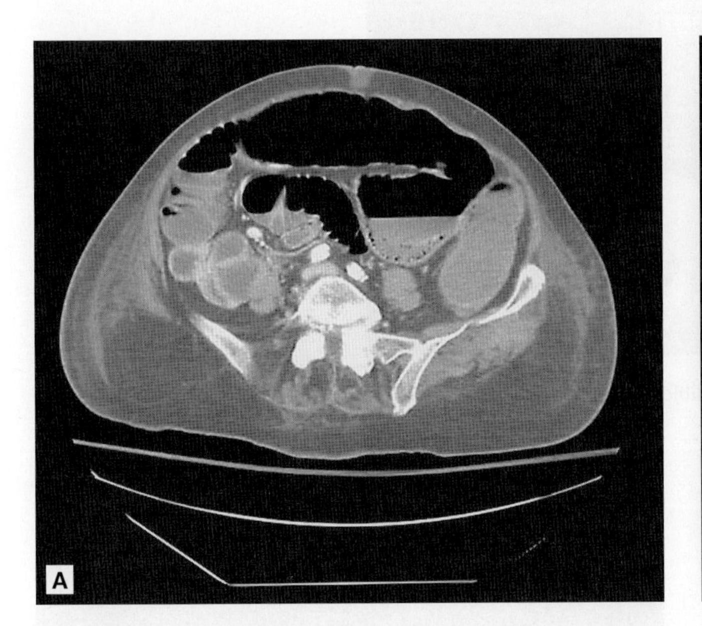

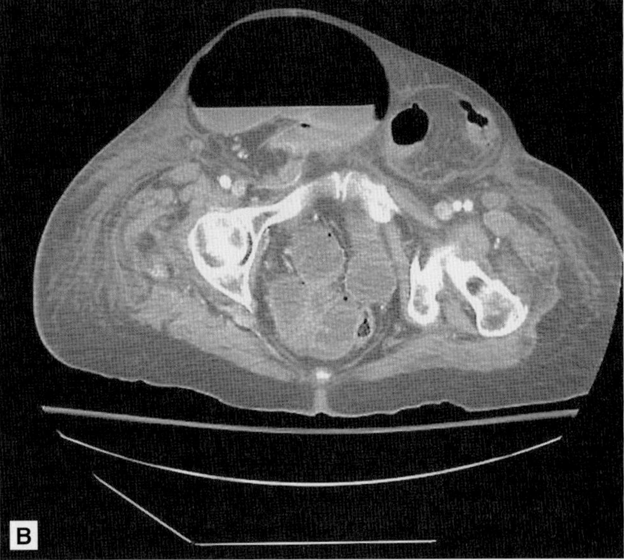

FIGURE 7.12 ■ Inguinal Hernias with Small Bowel Obstruction. **A, B:** Bilateral inguinal hernias containing bowel loops and mesenteric fat are evident. The majority of small bowel loops demonstrated are significantly dilated.

Radiographic Summary

Cholelithiasis is the presence of gallstones within the gallbladder. Sonographically, gallstones greater than 2-3 mm will appear as bright echogenic structures within the gallbladder with an anechoic area just underneath them as a result of acoustic shadowing. Mobile gallstones are differentiated from an impacted stone or gallbladder mass by demonstrating that they are freely mobile when the patient is rolled to the lateral decubitus or prone position. CT is less sensitive than ultrasound in detecting gallstones, which will appear as radio-opaque round structures within the gallbladder.

A contracted gallbladder with multiple stones may appear sonographically as wall-echo-shadow sign. Because little to no bile is present in the gallbladder, a bright, echogenic area representing both the wall and the gallstone with subsequent

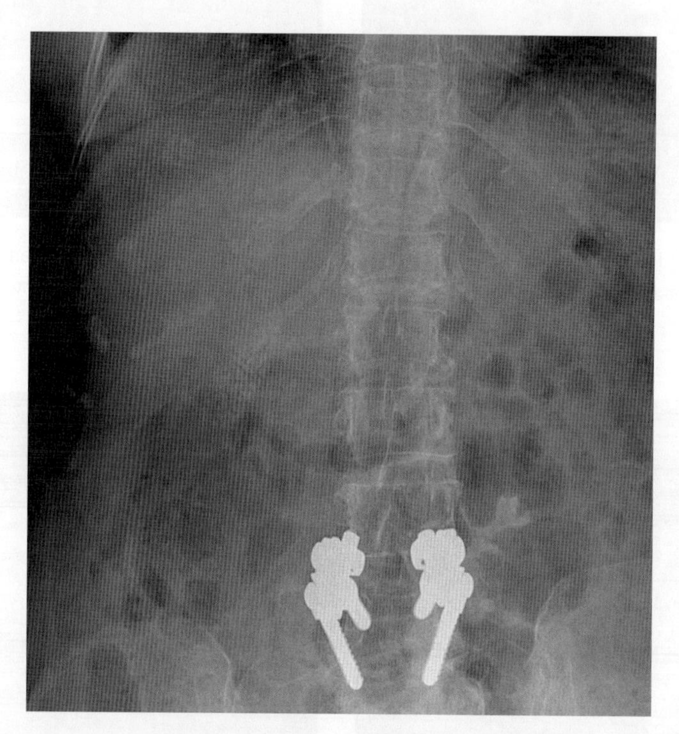

FIGURE 7.13 ■ Cholelithiasis. Multiple calcified gallstones are visible in the right upper quadrant on this plain radiograph.

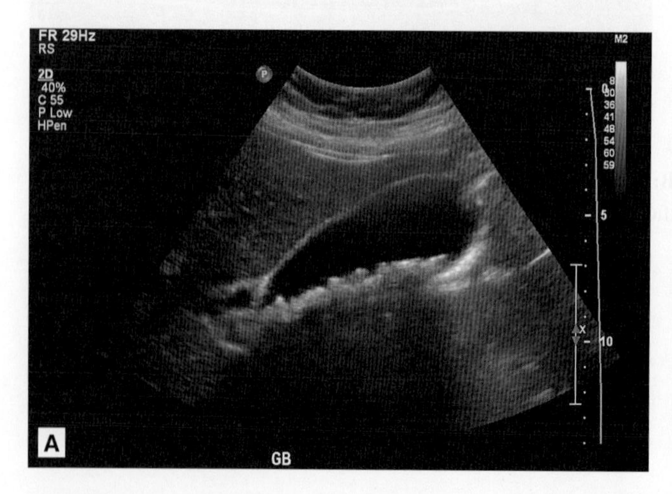

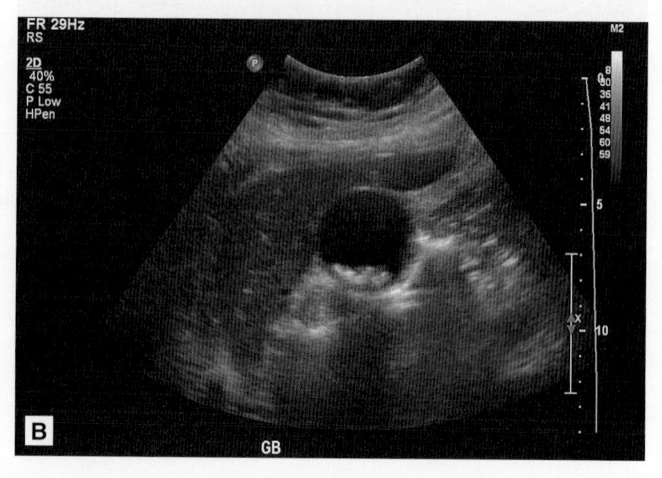

FIGURE 7.14 ■ Cholelithiasis. **A, B:** Multiple gravity-dependent gallstones are visible on longitudinal and short-axis ultrasound images. There is prominent posterior acoustic shadowing. The gallbladder wall is thin with no signs of inflammation.

acoustic shadowing will occur. In patients with wall-echo-shadow complex it is not possible to ascertain whether a gallstone may be impacted in the neck of the gallbladder and may be difficult to ascertain for other signs of gallbladder wall inflammation.

Clinical Implications

While gallstones are present in approximately 15% of the population, most are asymptomatic and require no treatment or intervention. Each year, approximately 3% of patients with gallstones will have an episode of biliary colic with 20% of these patients eventually developing acute cholecystitis. Smaller gallstones (3-4 mm) are less likely to cause acute cholecystitis, but may pass through the cystic duct and into the common bile duct where they can cause obstruction. Depending on the location of that obstruction, these small stones lodged within the common bile duct can lead to gallstone pancreatitis or cholangitis.

Pearls

1. Gallstones require no treatment if they are asymptomatic, but may be a marker of hemolytic diseases if found in children or adolescents.
2. Biliary colic lasts less than 6 hours; if symptoms persist greater than 6 hours a diligent search should be made for an impacted stone in the neck of the gallbladder, cystic duct, or common bile duct.

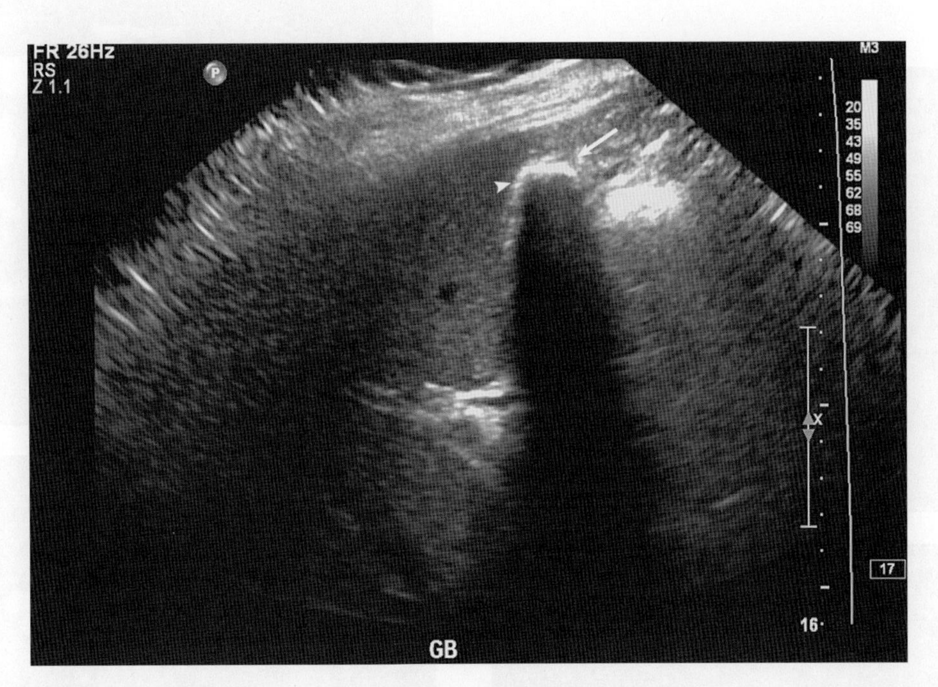

FIGURE 7.15 ■ Cholelithiasis. A "Wall-Echo-Shadow" complex is seen, demonstrating the visible gallbladder wall (arrow), echogenic barrier created by innumerable stones filling the gallbladder (arrowhead), and dark posterior acoustic shadowing.

ACUTE CHOLECYSTITIS

Radiographic Summary

Acute cholecystitis is the rapid development of inflammation of the gallbladder. It is manifested on ultrasound and CT by inflammation and thickening of the gallbladder wall and pericholecystic fluid. In calculous disease, an impacted stone is seen in the gallbladder neck or cystic duct. In acalculous disease, no stones are present. Biliary sludge may be present in either calculous or acalculous cholecystitis and is evidence of biliary stasis from gallbladder dysfunction. Gallbladder wall inflammation is present if the wall measures more than 3 mm in thickness, has surrounding pericholecystic fluid, or is tender with direct compression of the ultrasound probe (sonographic Murphy's sign). However, these findings take time to develop. In early acute cholecystitis, the only sonographic manifestation may be an immobile gallstone lodged within the neck of the gallbladder and a sonographic Murphy's sign.

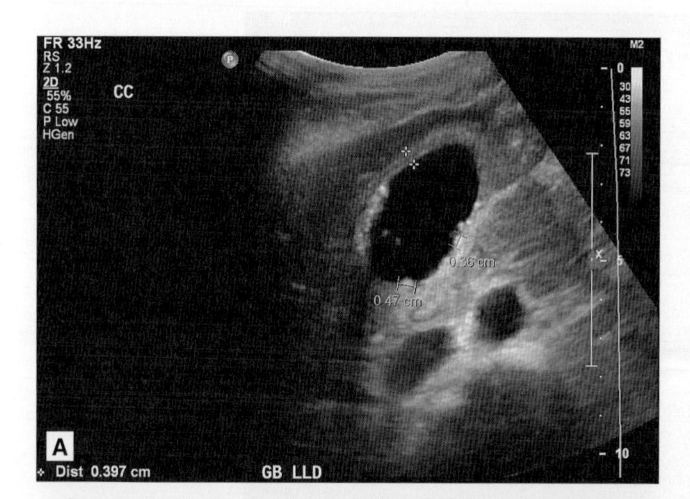

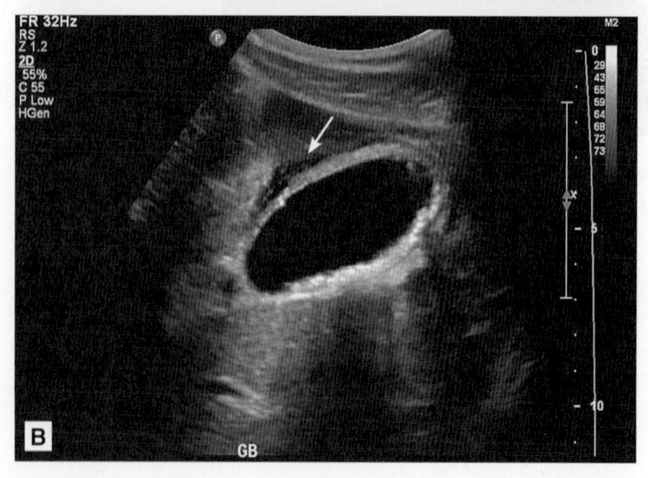

FIGURE 7.16 ■ Acute Cholecystitis. **A, B:** Luminal distension, gallbladder wall thickening, wall edema, and pericholecystic fluid (arrow) is present. Several echogenic gallstones are seen dependently.

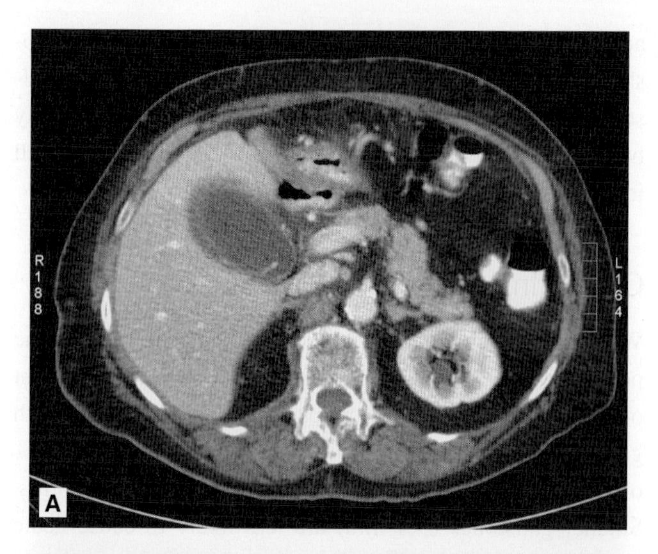

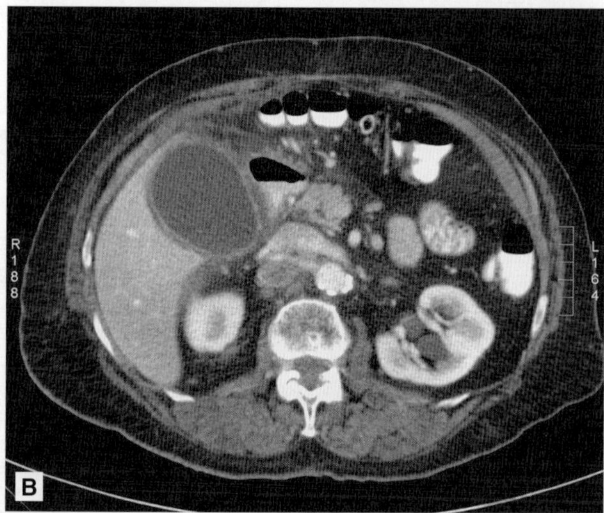

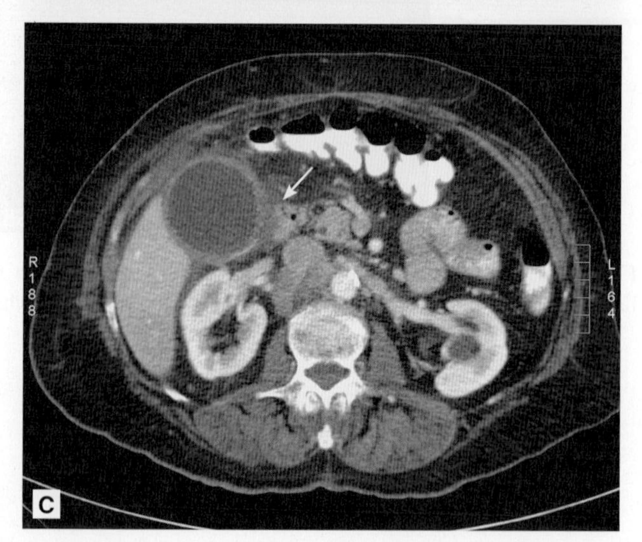

FIGURE 7.17 ■ Acute Cholecystitis. **A-C:** Contrast-enhanced CT demonstrates a hydropic gallbladder with wall thickening and enhancement. Pericholecystic fluid (arrow) and fat stranding is present as an indication of acute inflammation.

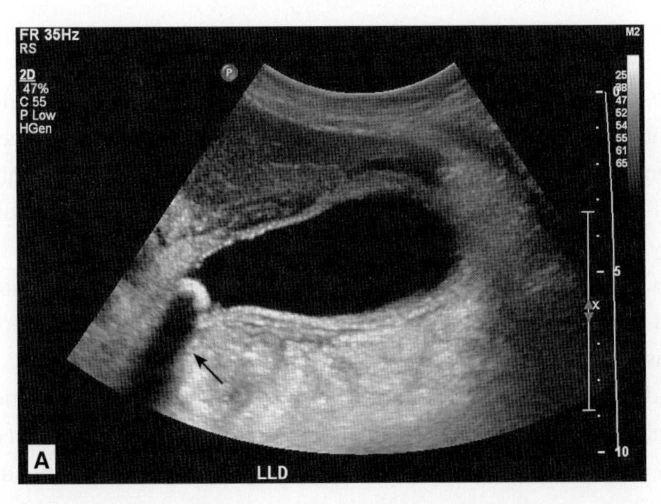

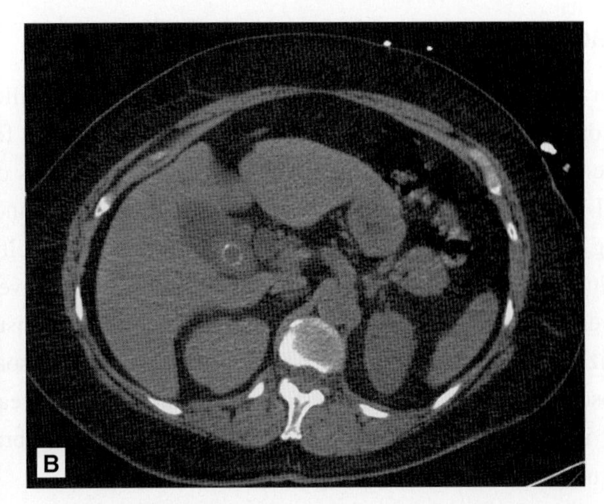

FIGURE 7.18 ■ Acute Cholecystitis. **A, B:** Ultrasound and nonenhanced CT demonstrate a single large gallstone impacted in the neck of the gallbladder. Note the prominent acoustic shadowing (arrow).

In acalculous disease, a large distended gallbladder with a transverse diameter measurement >4 cm is also indicative of acute cholecystitis.

Clinical Implications

Acute cholecystitis is a clinical diagnosis supported by sonographic or radiographic findings. The majority of cases (>90%) are the result of an impacted gallstone in the neck or cystic duct of the gallbladder. Acute cholecystitis is first differentiated clinically from symptomatic cholelithiasis by symptoms that persist for more than 6 hours.

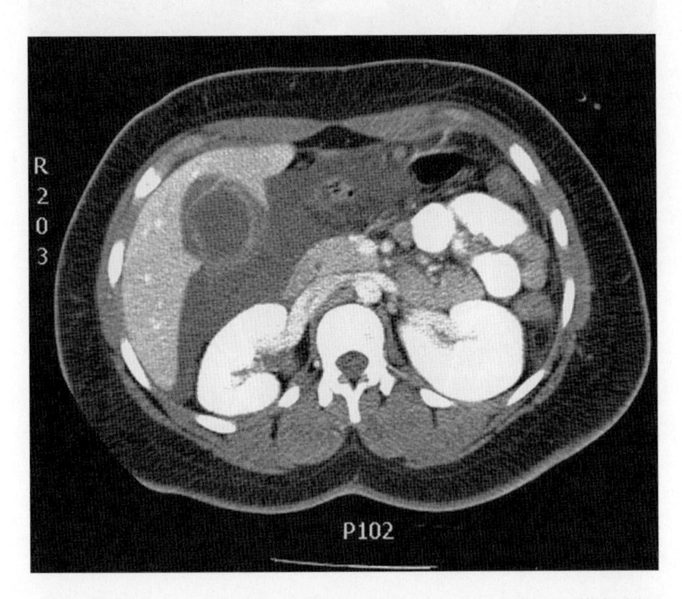

FIGURE 7.19 ■ Ruptured Gallbladder. An irregular gallbladder wall is seen, with abundant pericholecystic fluid indicating rupture and bile leak.

Patients often present with right upper quadrant abdominal pain that radiates to the back, nausea, and vomiting. Laboratory values will often be normal in patients with early acute cholecytitis. As time and inflammation progress, a leukocytosis and mild transaminase elevation will occur reflecting the inflammatory process.

Patients with acute cholecystitis should receive broad-spectrum antibiotics that cover gut microorganisms. A surgeon should be consulted for cholecystectomy. Patients who are high-risk surgical candidates may be candidates for percutaneous gallbladder drainage.

Pearls

1. Acute cholecystitis frequently occurs in patients who are fair, female, fat, and fertile.
2. Can occur in younger patients with sickle cell disease, spherocytosis, G-6PD deficiencies, and other hemolytic disorders.
3. A small and contracted gallbladder (commonly seen after eating a fatty meal) may have a gallbladder wall that appears >3 mm in thickness only because it is contracted. In these cases, the gallbladder wall will have three distinct layers representing the adventitia, muscular layer, and mucosa.

Radiographic Summary

An iliopsoas abscess is a collection of pus located in the iliopsoas muscle compartment. CT is the modality of choice for the evaluation of a suspected iliopsoas abscess. Findings on CT include a focal hypodense lesion, infiltration of surrounding fat, and gas or air fluid levels within the muscle belly. Ultrasound may be diagnostic in up to 50% of cases; however, overlying bowel gas and the pelvic bones may prevent visualization of the abscess. In cases of long-standing iliopsoas abscesses, MRI should be performed to rule out the spread of infection to, or from adjacent soft tissue and vertebral structures.

Clinical Implications

The iliopsoas muscle has a rich blood supply and may develop an abscess as the result of hematogenous or lymphatic seeding from a distal infection. In addition, the iliopsoas muscle lies in close proximity to the sigmoid colon, appendix, pancreas, and kidney and an abscess may develop from the direct spread from one of these contiguous organs. Iliopsoas abscesses may develop as a complication of infectious spondylitis or sacroilitis.

Common bacterial organisms implicated in the formation of iliopsoas abscess are *Staphylococcus aureus*, Streptococci, or *E. coli*, although infections spreading from contiguous

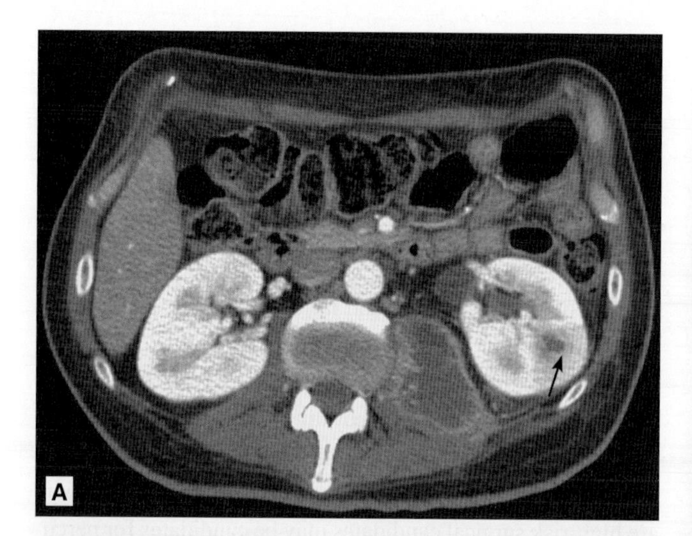

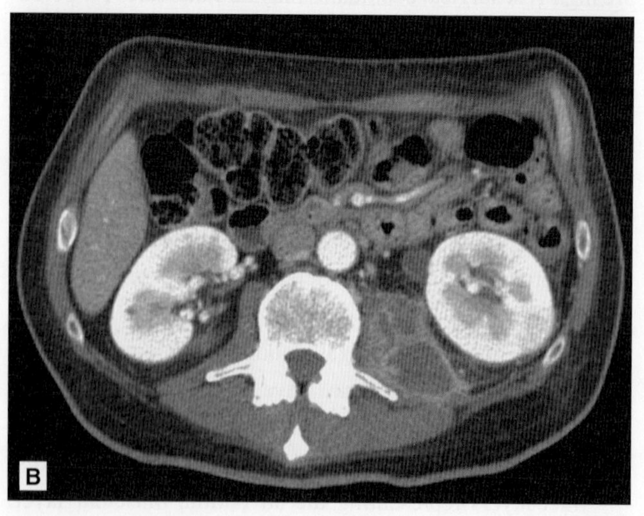

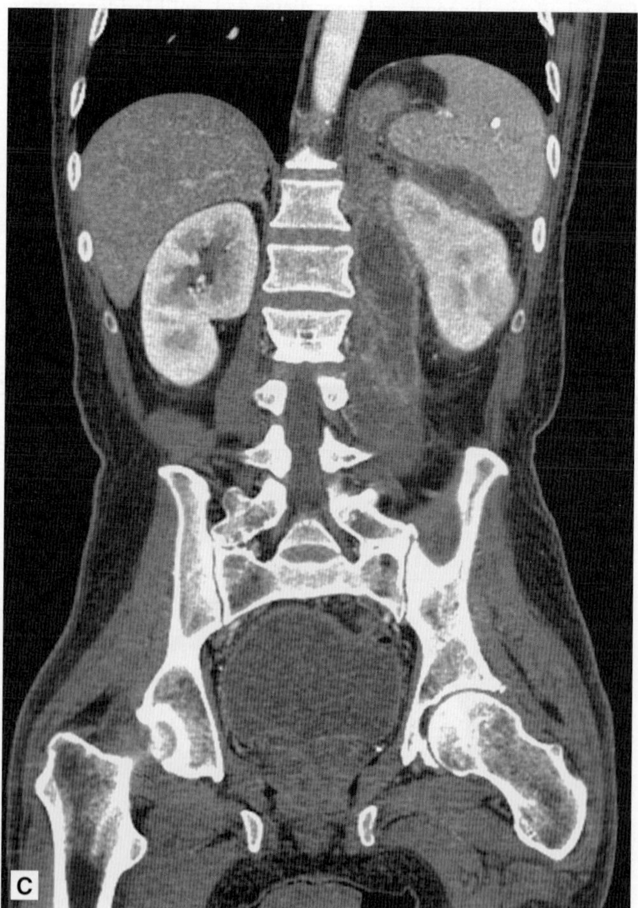

FIGURE 7.20 ■ Iliopsoas Abscess. **A-C:** On both axial and reformatted coronal images, an irregular low-attenuation collection with an enhancing wall is seen in the left psoas muscle. A renal abscess (arrow) is also present in this patient with sequelae of bacterial endocarditis.

organs may be polymicrobial. *Mycobacterium tuberculosis* may cause an iliopsoas abscess in regions of the world where TB infections are endemic. Management of iliopsoas abscesses includes initiation of broad-spectrum antibiotics to cover *Staphylococcus aureus* and enteric organisms as well as abscess drainage.

Pearls

1. CT-guided aspiration may be used to confirm the diagnosis and guide therapy.
2. Tuberculous iliopsoas abscesses may show marked abscess wall thickening, rim calcification, and multiple cavities with the muscle belly when visualized by CT scanning.
3. Ultrasound can miss a small phlegmon or abscess of the iliopsoas muscle.

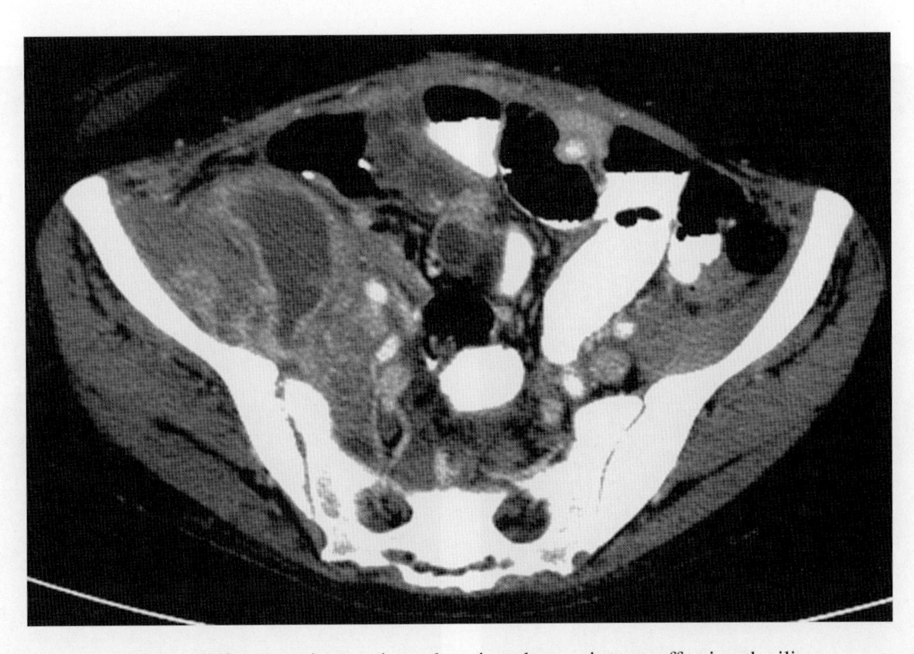

FIGURE 7.21 ■ Iliopsoas Abscess. In a different patient, a rim-enhancing abscess is seen affecting the iliopsoas musculature on the right.

Radiographic Summary

Acalculous cholecystitis is inflammation of the gallbladder in the absence of gallstones. Sonographically or on CT, it appears as a large gallbladder with a transverse diameter measuring greater than 4 cm with evidence of a gallbladder wall inflammation. Gallbladder wall inflammation is manifested by a gallbladder wall thickness greater than 3 mm and/or the presence of pericholecystic fluid. Pericholecystic fluid is more likely to be present with advanced disease but may not be present early in the disease process. In some cases, biliary sludge can be seen layering in the dependent portions of the gallbladder as a result of biliary stasis and gallbladder dysfunction.

In patients with persistent right upper quadrant pain and no evidence of gallstones on sonography, hepatobiliary scan (Tc-99m HIDA) may have utility in establishing the diagnosis of acalculous cholecystitis. Failure to visualize the normal gallbladder on hepatobiliary imaging is consistent with the diagnosis.

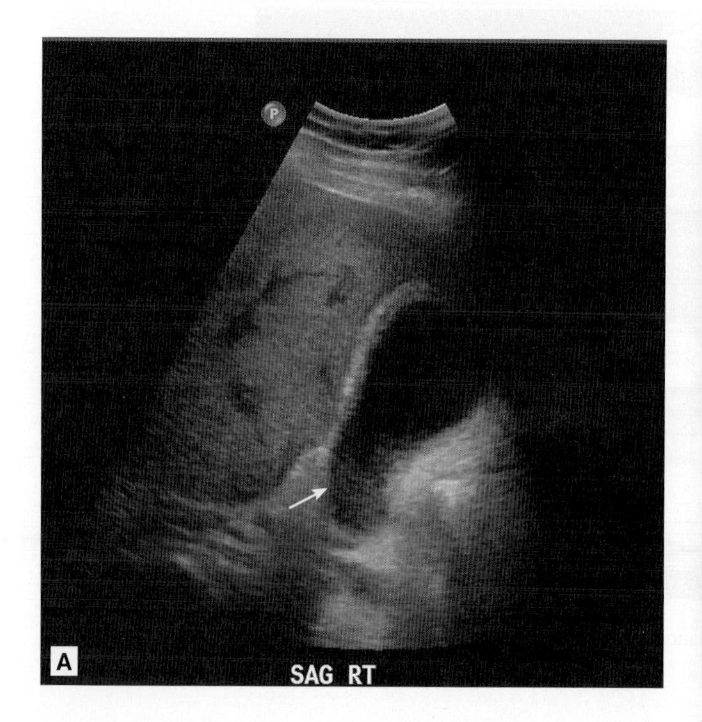

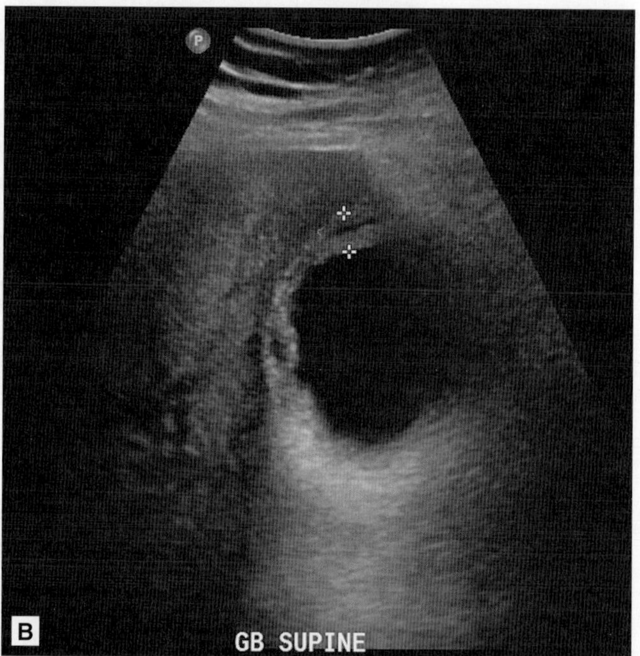

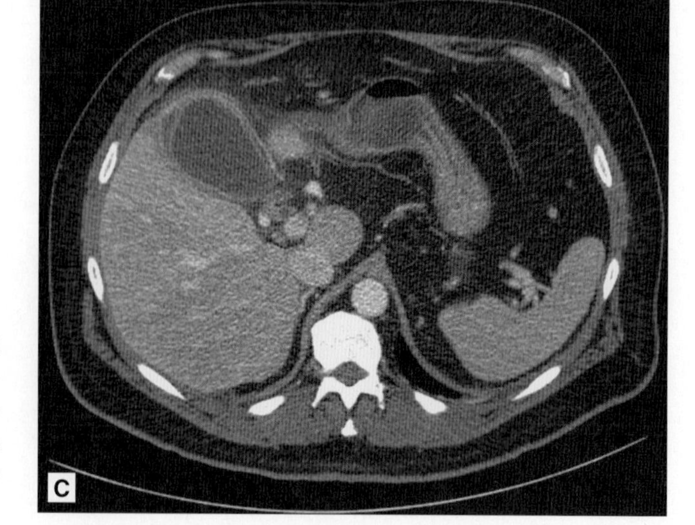

FIGURE 7.22 ■ Acalculous Cholecystitis. **A, B:** Longitudinal and transverse ultrasound images demonstrate gallbladder wall thickening and dependent sludge (arrow). There is distension of the gallbladder lumen. There are no calculi present. **C:** CT scan in the same patient demonstrates gallbladder wall thickening and pericholecystic stranding.

Clinical Implications

Acalculous cholecystitis accounts for approximately 5% of cases of acute cholecytitis and most often occurs in elderly or debilitated patients. It is often a complication of other severe illnesses and most notably occurs in the ICU or in patients receiving TPN. Acalculous cholecystitis is associated with higher mortality (10-50%) and has a higher incidence of gangrene and perforation.

Surgical cholecystectomy is preferred; however, percutaneous drainage may be the only option in patients who are poor surgical candidates. Regardless, patients with suspected acalculous cholecystitis should receive broad-spectrum antibiotics that cover gut flora and have emergent surgical consultation for definitive management.

Pearls

1. Consider acalculous cholecystitis in debilitated elderly patients who present with sepsis without an identifiable source.
2. Treat acalculous cholecystitis with IV antibiotics that cover anaerobic and gram-negative bacteria.

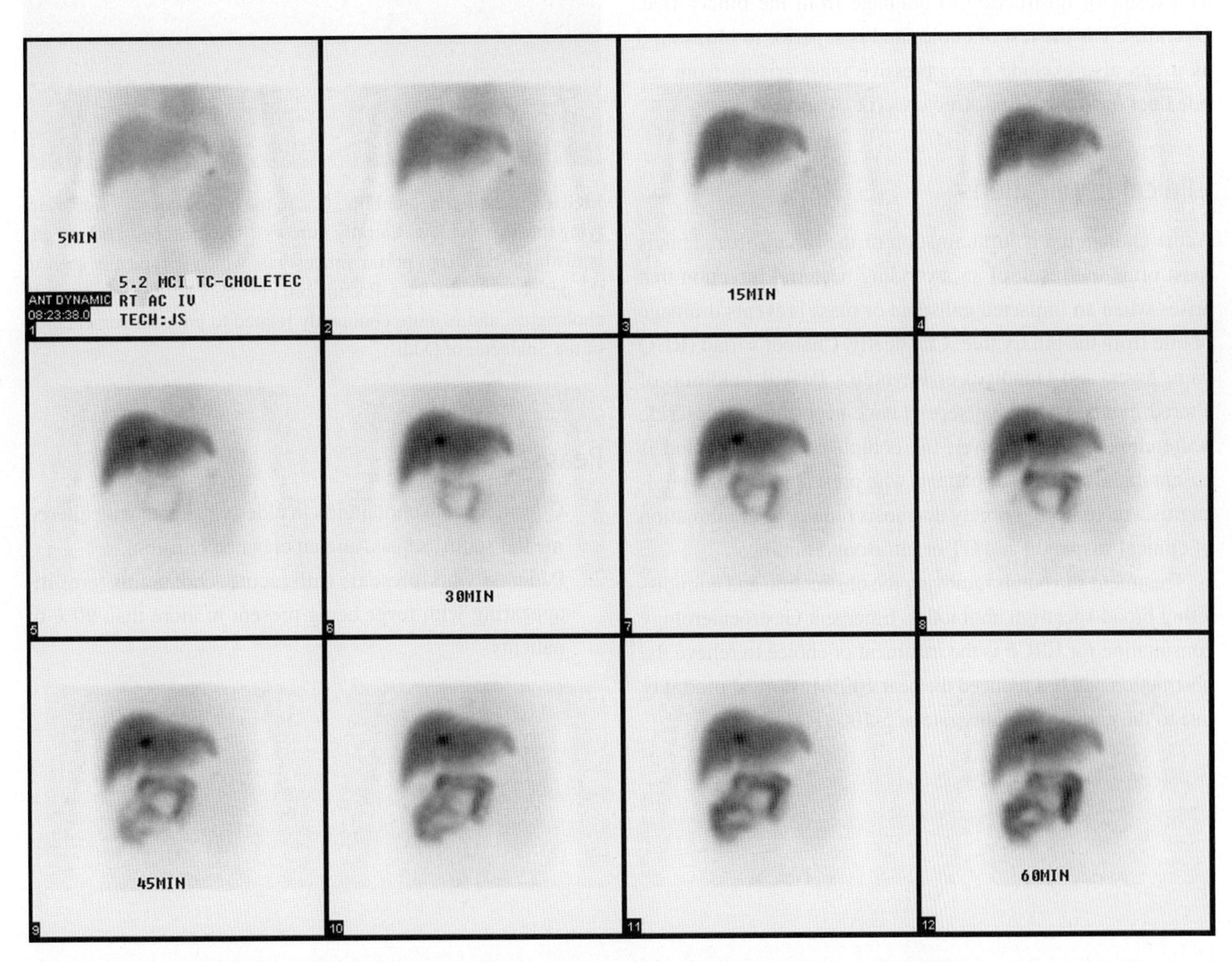

FIGURE 7.23 ■ Acalculous Cholecystitis. Hepatobiliary nuclear medicine (HIDA) scan with nonvisualization of the gallbladder due to cystic duct obstruction. Hepatic activity and excretion of the radiopharmaceutical into the intestines is visible.

Radiographic Summary

Acute cholangitis is a bacterial superinfection of the biliary tree caused by distal bile duct obstruction. It is manifested on CT or ultrasound as intrahepatic biliary duct dilation with associated distal bile duct obstruction. Evidence of intrahepatic abscess formation or air within the biliary tree (pneumobilia) may also be present.

Ultrasound and CT will show bile duct dilation and at times a gallstone within the lumen of the common bile duct. Rarely, common hepatic duct compression as a result of a large intraluminal gallstone or an impacted stone in the cystic duct (Mirizzi syndrome) can also lead to acute cholangitis as a result of obstruction to drainage from the biliary tree. Overall, CT is the test of choice and is superior to ultrasound as it can also exclude a compressive mass arising from the bile duct or surrounding structures (i.e., pancreas).

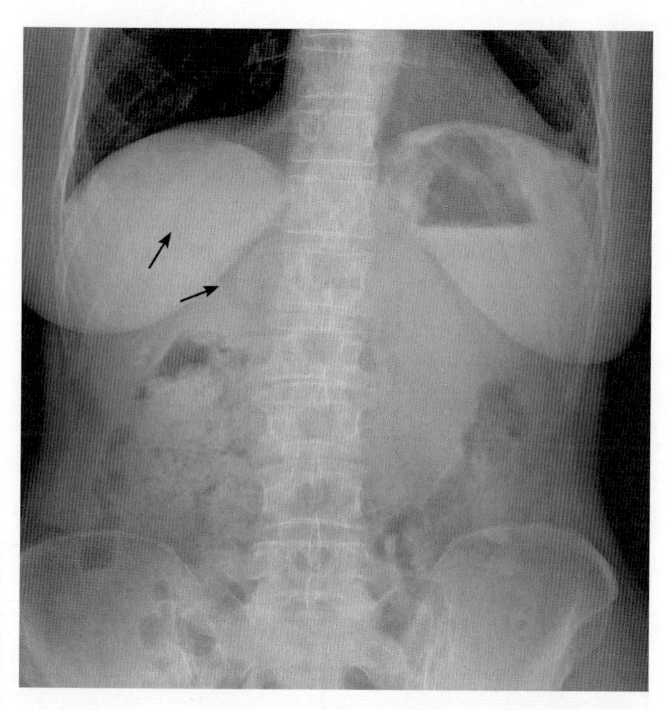

FIGURE 7.24 ■ Pneumobilia. Gas in the biliary ducts is seen overlying the liver shadow centrally (arrows). The location of biliary gas is distinguished from portal venous gas, which is typically seen in the periphery of the liver. Pneumobilia is rarely attributable to acute cholangitis, and is more commonly related to prior instrumentation of the Sphincter of Oddi.

Clinical Implications

Acute cholangitis is inflammation of the biliary tree. This is most often the result of an ascending bacterial infection that arises when an impacted gallstone or mass prevents drainage of bile from the biliary tree. Classically, Charcot's triad (RUQ pain, fever, and jaundice) or Reynold's Pentad (addition of altered mental status and sepsis) have been used to describe acute cholangitis. However, the complete triad or pentad is absent in the majority of patients who present with acute cholangitis. Accurate and timely diagnosis requires a combination of clinical suspicion and CT or ultrasound findings.

Treatment surrounds removing the obstruction and administering broad-spectrum antibiotics. Emergent Gastroenterology consultation for ERCP is the treatment of choice to relieve the obstruction and has reduced the near 100% historical mortality rate to the current mortality rate of 5-10%.

Pearls

1. Consider acute cholangitis in elderly patients with altered mental status, sepsis, and an elevated bilirubin.
2. Patients who present with acute cholangitis are ill-appearing with fever being present in more than 90% of patients.

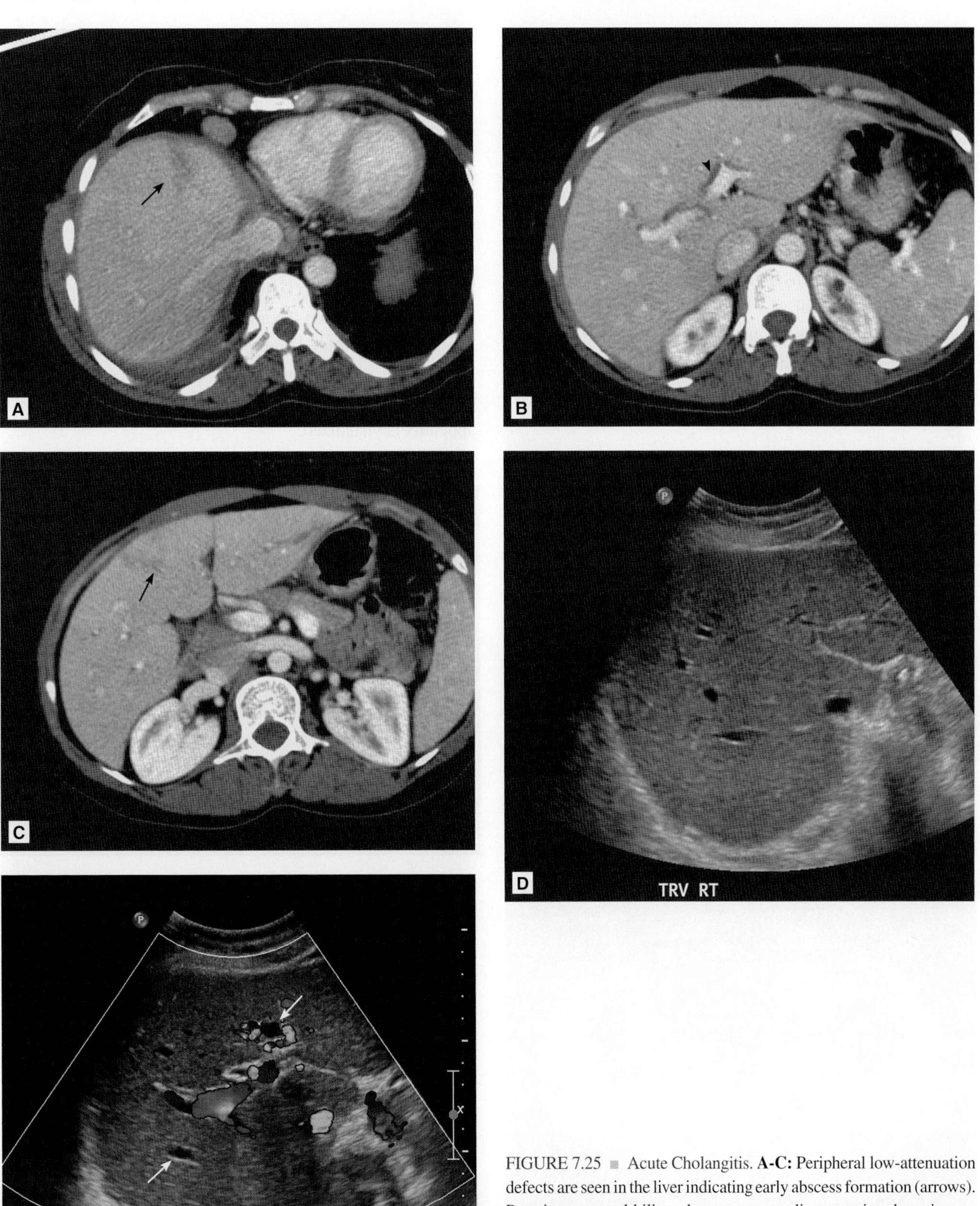

FIGURE 7.25 ■ Acute Cholangitis. **A-C:** Peripheral low-attenuation defects are seen in the liver indicating early abscess formation (arrows). Prominent central biliary ducts are seen adjacent to intrahepatic portal vein branches (arrowhead). **D, E:** Ultrasound of the same patient shows dilation of intrahepatic ducts. The ducts are distinguished from intrahepatic vasculature by lack of flow on color Doppler imaging (arrows).

Radiographic Summary

Appendicitis is the inflammation of the vermiform appendix generally caused by obstruction of the appendiceal lumen. Acute appendicitis is the most common reason for emergency abdominal surgery.

CT has become the gold standard for the radiographic evaluation of acute appendicitis. CT findings suggestive of acute appendicitis are enlarged appendiceal diameter >6 mm with an occluded lumen, appendiceal wall thickening >2 mm, pathologic appendiceal wall enhancement, and periappendiceal fat stranding. Appendicitis is not present if the scan does not demonstrate appendiceal enlargement, obstruction, and abnormal enhancement. A nonvisualized appendix does not rule out acute appendicitis.

Ultrasonography has proven to be reliable in the evaluation of acute appendicitis as well. Ultrasonography is particularly useful when avoidance of ionizing radiation is desirable, especially in children and women of childbearing age.

Ultrasound findings suggestive of acute appendicitis are noncompressible blind-ended tubular structures arising from the cecum, appendiceal diameter >6 mm, presence of an appendicolith, periappendiceal fluid collection, and echogenic prominent pericecal fat. The challenge with ultrasound is finding the appendix. Ultrasound diagnosis of appendicitis is very accurate when the appendix is completely visualized, compressed, measured and the surrounding tissue is scanned to detect any inflammation of the periappendiceal fat. As with CT scanning, appendicitis cannot be ruled out unless a normal appendix is visualized.

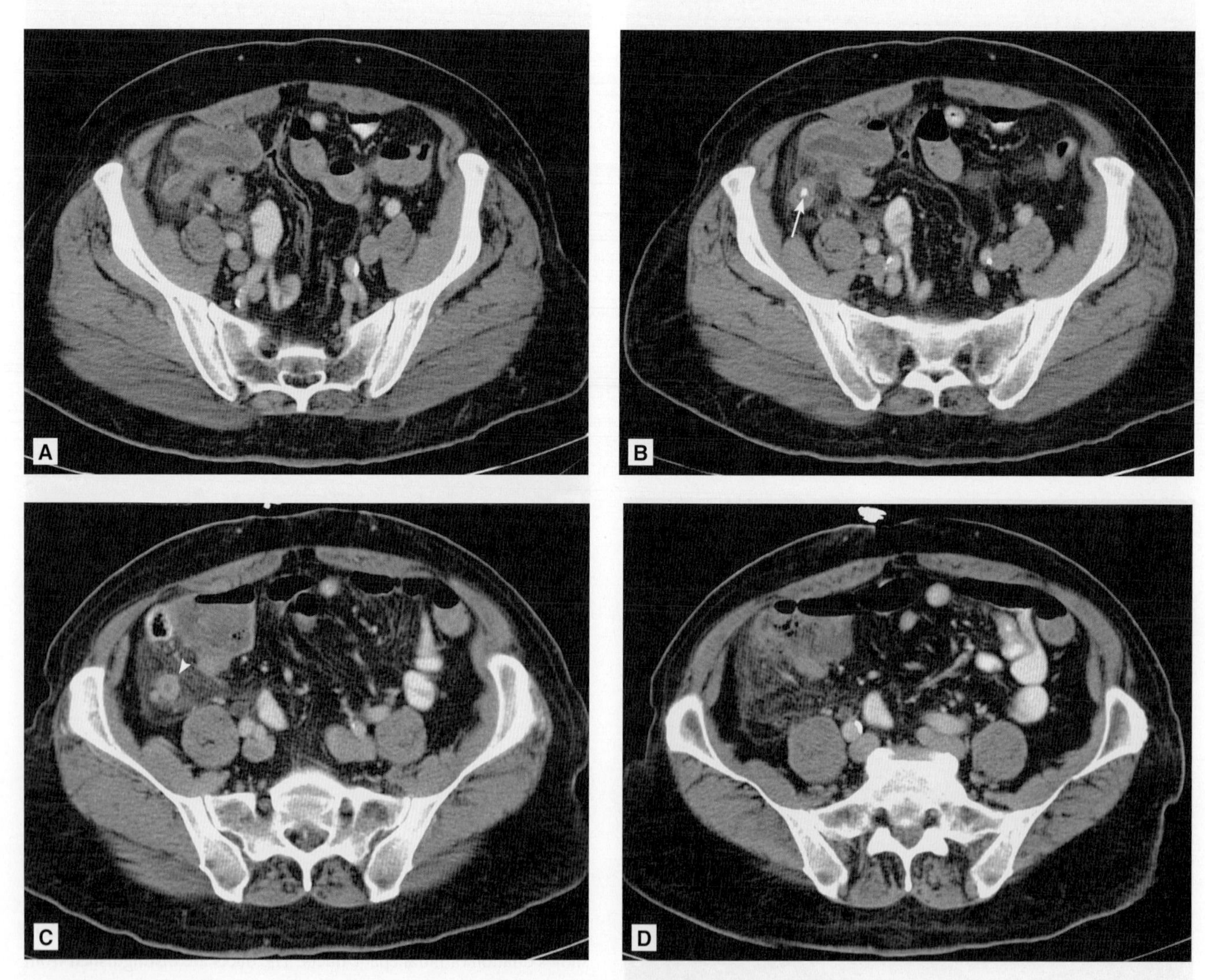

FIGURE 7.26 ■ Acute Appendicitis. **A-D:** The appendix measures 1.5 cm in short axis, and enhances prominently. A calcified appendicolith is present within the lumen (arrow). Note the blind-end of the appendix (arrowhead) and prominent stranding of adjacent fat.

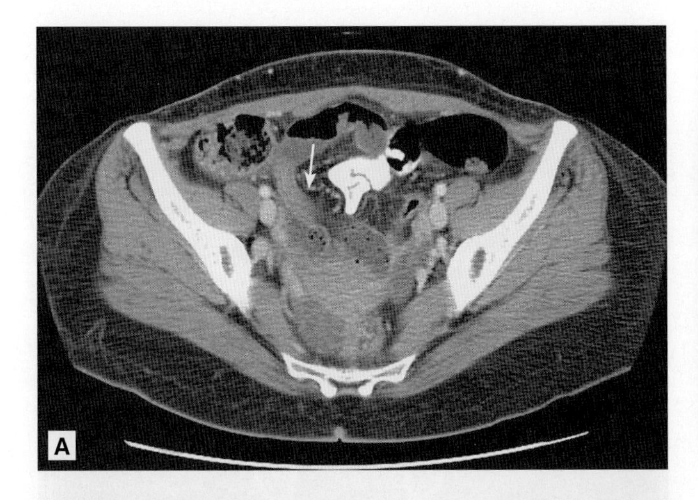

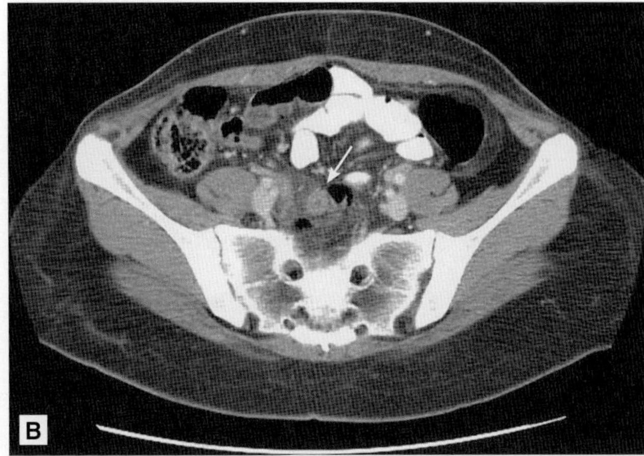

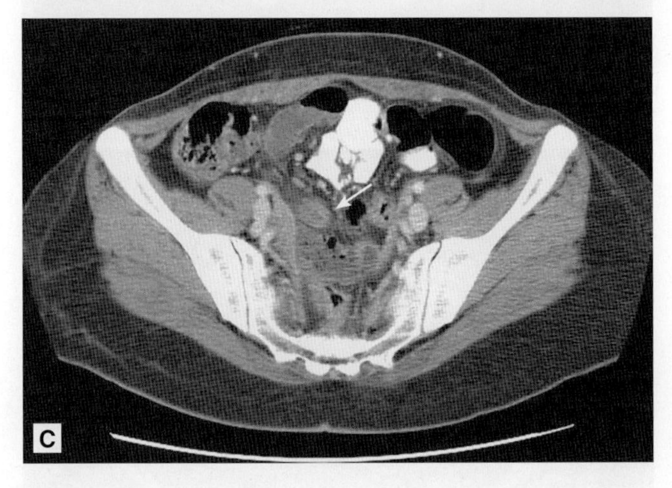

FIGURE 7.27 ■ Acute Appendicitis. **A-C:** The enlarged and enhancing appendix in this case extends towards the midline of the pelvis (arrows). No visible appendicolith is present in this case.

Clinical Implications

The correct diagnosis of appendicitis can occasionally be made from history, physical exam, and laboratory studies, without the aid of radiographic studies. Radiographic studies have decreased the rate of false-negative exploratory surgery from 20% to 3% and proven beneficial when the cause of the abdominal pain is not clear, and in those populations prone to atypical presentations of appendicitis such as young children, elderly, women of childbearing age, diabetics, obese, and immunocompromised patients.

CT remains the preferred study for the detection of appendicitis. Ultrasound has the advantage of imaging without ionizing radiation and is useful for the detection of gynecologic pathology.

Pearls

1. A nonvisualized appendix on CT scan or ultrasound does not rule out appendicitis.
2. Among experienced radiologists, MRI without gadolinium has been found to be extremely accurate in the diagnosis of appendicitis, and may be used in pregnant patients to avoid ionizing radiation.
3. 10% of adults presenting with appendicitis will have an appendolith visualized by plain abdominal radiographs. When present, an appendicolith has a 90% positive predictive value for acute appendicitis.

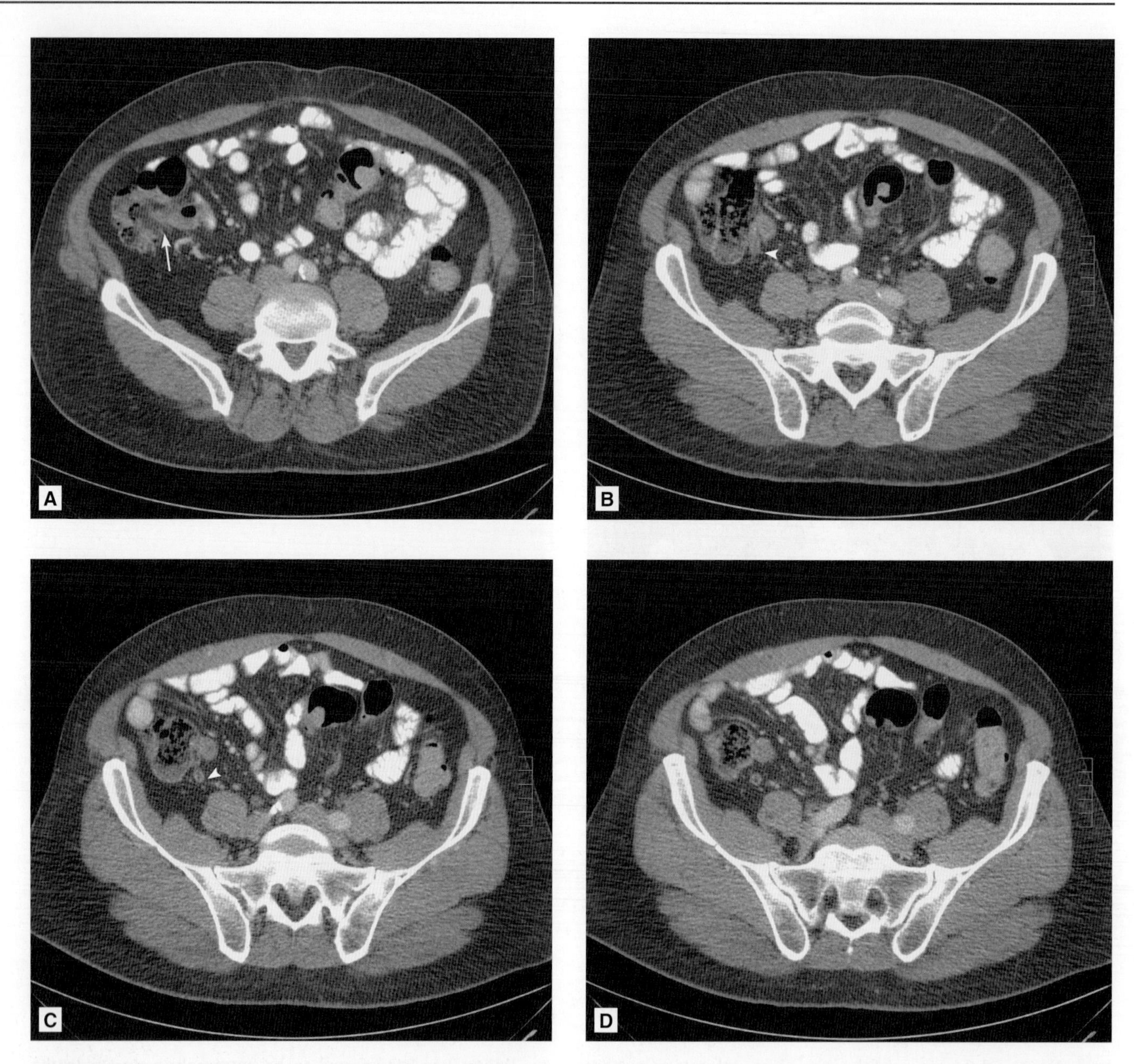

FIGURE 7.28 ■ Normal Appendix. **A-D:** The terminal ileum is identified at its junction with the cecum (arrow). Inferiorly, a blind-ended tubular structure is seen arising from the cecum (arrowheads). In contrast to the prior two cases, there is no surrounding standing, enlargement or enhancement of the normal appendix.

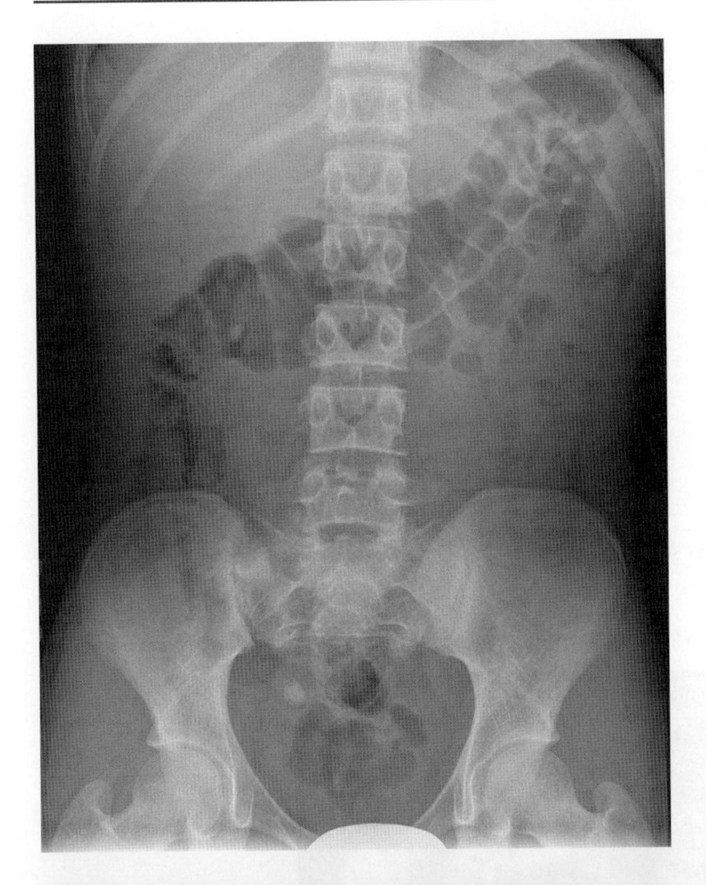

FIGURE 7.29 ■ Appendicolith in Appendicitis. Calcified lamellated appendicolith is seen in the right lower quadrant on this plain radiograph of the abdomen. The abdominal bowel gas pattern is normal.

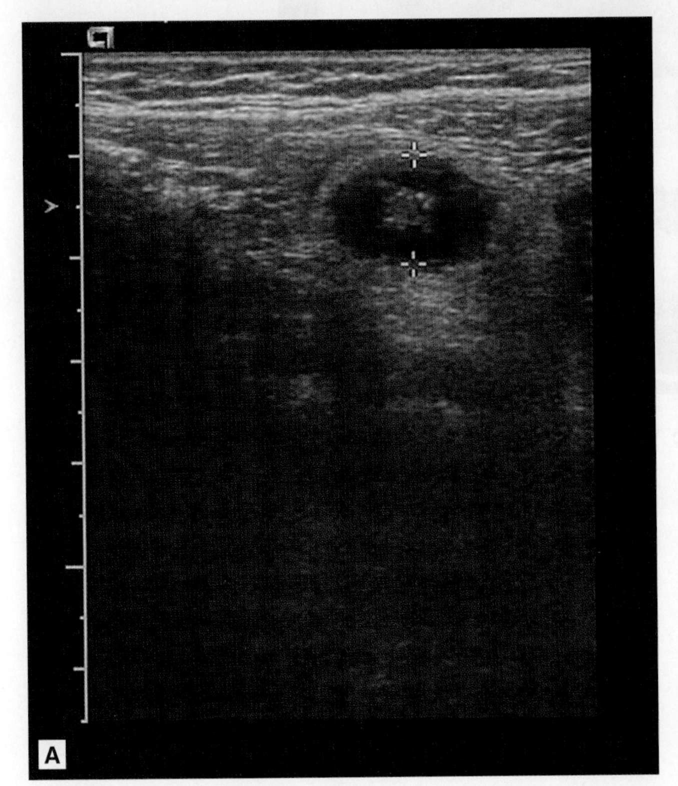

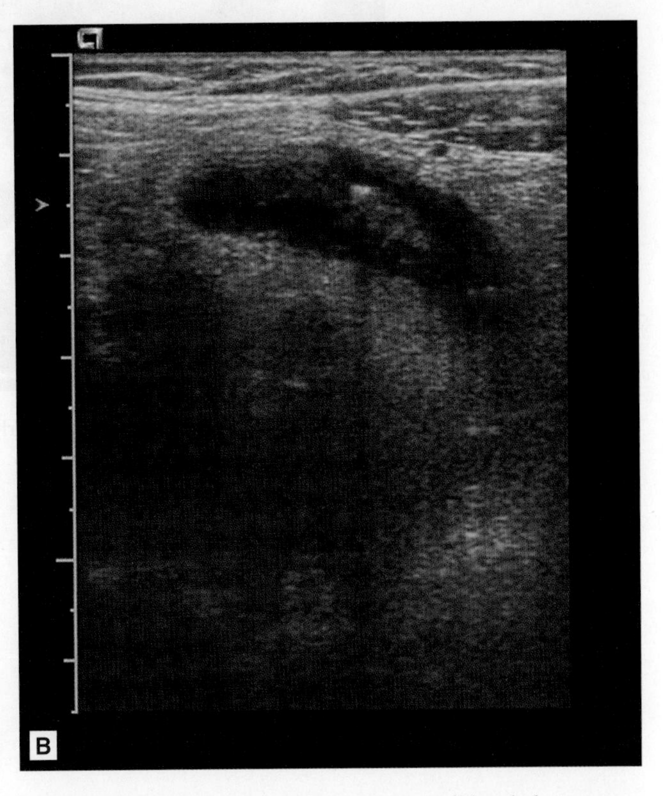

FIGURE 7.30 ■ Appendicitis. **A, B:** On ultrasound, the abnormally enlarged appendix is seen as a 1 cm noncompressible tubular structure in the right lower quadrant. High-density debris is seen within the lumen and produces some acoustic shadowing.

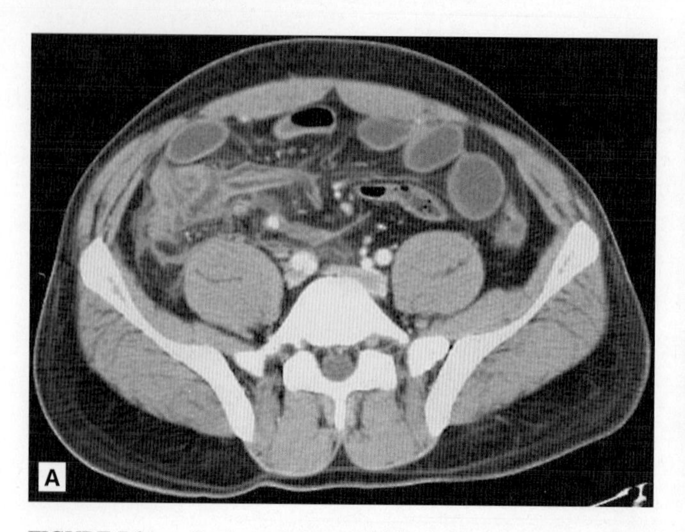

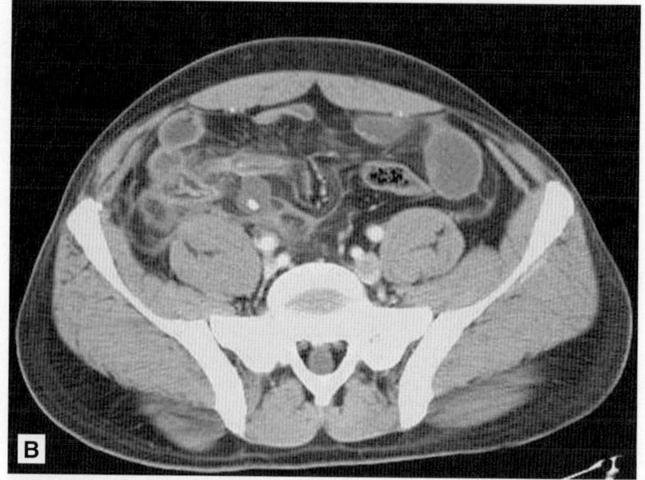

FIGURE 7.31 ■ Perforated Appendicitis. **A, B:** An enhancing tubular structure is seen in the right lower quadrant. There is free fluid and an uncontained appendicolith present, suggesting rupture of the appendix.

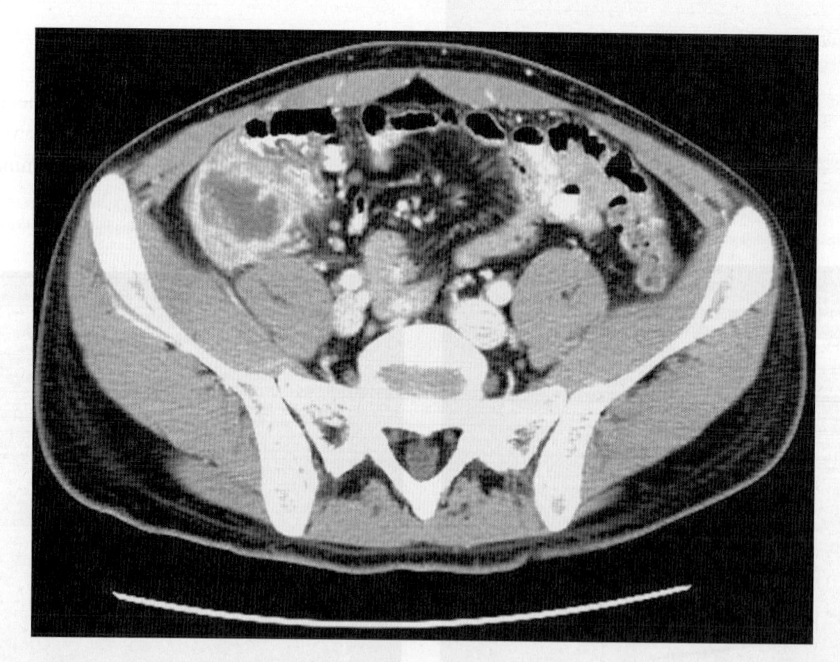

FIGURE 7.32 ■ Ruptured Appendicitis with Abscess. An irregularly shaped abscess is seen in the right lower quadrant, with prominent enhancement of the abscess wall.

Radiographic Summary

Diverticulitis occurs when colonic diverticula become inflamed or infected. In the United States, the majority of cases are located in the sigmoid colon.

CT scan of the abdomen is the preferred radiographic imaging modality for the diagnosis of diverticulitis. Diverticula are identified on CT scan as gas-filled outpouchings of the colonic wall. The CT diagnosis of diverticulitis is contingent on colonic inflammation in the presence of diverticula. CT will show stranding of pericolic fat due to inflammation, bowel wall thickening >1 cm, and pathologic colonic wall enhancement. Intramural abscesses may be identified as small fluid collections within the bowel wall. Extramural intraabdominal abscesses may occur if a diverticulum perforates.

CT of the abdomen can detect complications of diverticulitis including abscess formation, perforation, fistula, and sinus tract formation. An unenhanced CT scan is generally

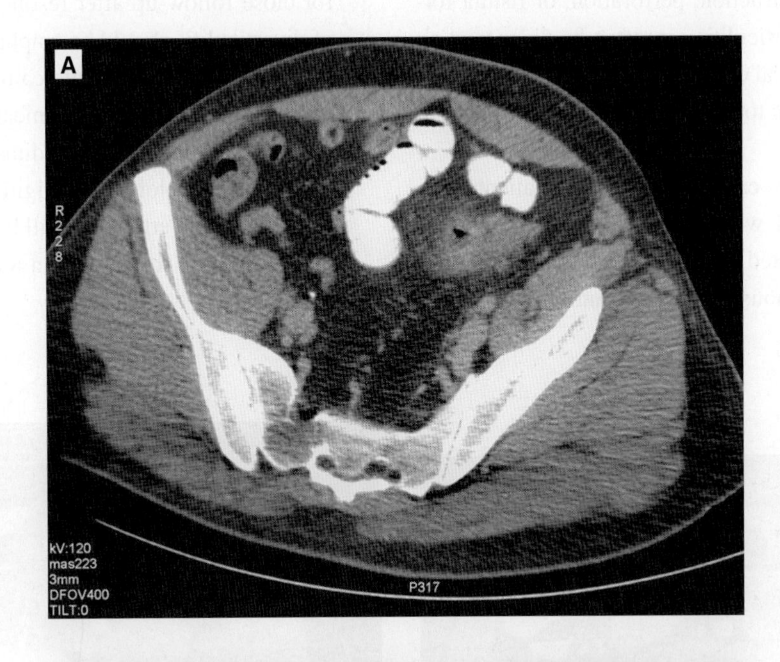

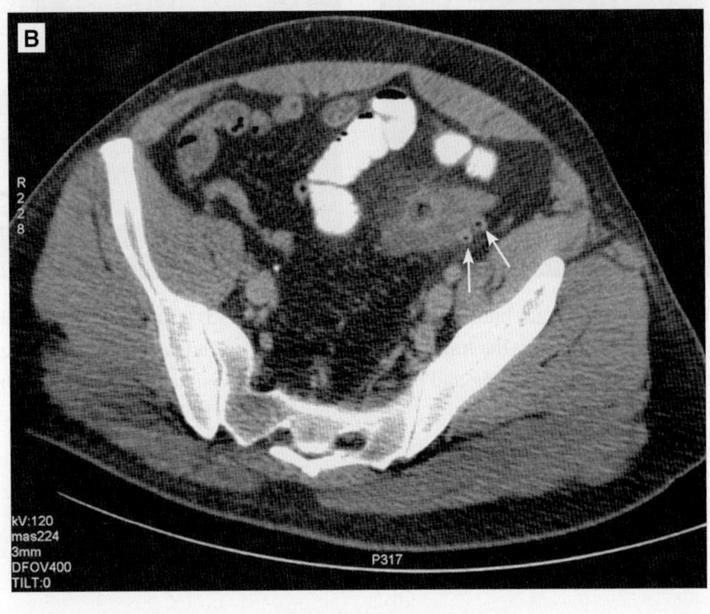

FIGURE 7.33 ■ Diverticulitis. **A, B:** A region of colonic wall thickening and pericolic fat stranding is identified in the left lower quadrant. Nearby colonic diverticula are visible (arrows).

sufficient to allow for the diagnosis of uncomplicated diverticulitis. Addition of IV contrast is necessary to detect the presence of diverticular abscesses, fistulas, and colonic wall inflammation. CT can also be used to guide percutaneous drainage of localized diverticular abscesses.

Clinical Implications

Acute diverticulitis can be classified as complicated or uncomplicated. Complicated diverticulitis occurs when there is abscess formation, obstruction, perforation, or fistula formation. While acute diverticulitis can often be diagnosed on the basis of history, physical exam, and laboratory exam, consideration should be given to obtaining a CT scan to rule out complicated disease.

Findings on CT scan can predict which patients can be successfully managed without the need for procedural intervention. Uncomplicated acute diverticulitis is managed with bowel rest, intravenous fluids, and antibiotic therapy. CT findings that are classified as mild, that is, localized bowel wall thickening and stranding of the pericolic fat, predict a high success rate with medical management alone. ED patients with complicated diverticulitis should be evaluated by a surgeon.

Pearls

1. In 10% of patients, CT scan alone cannot differentiate diverticulitis from colon carcinoma; therefore, the need for close follow-up after resolution of the acute episode of diverticulitis should be emphasized to each patient.
2. Infarcted appendage epiploica or "epiploic appendigitis" may mimic diverticulitis clinically and on CT. Both will demonstrate pericolic stranding adjacent to the bowel. In cases of epiploic appendigitis however, a fat density, rather than a diverticulum will be seen in association with the pericolonic inflammation and nearby diverticula are often absent.

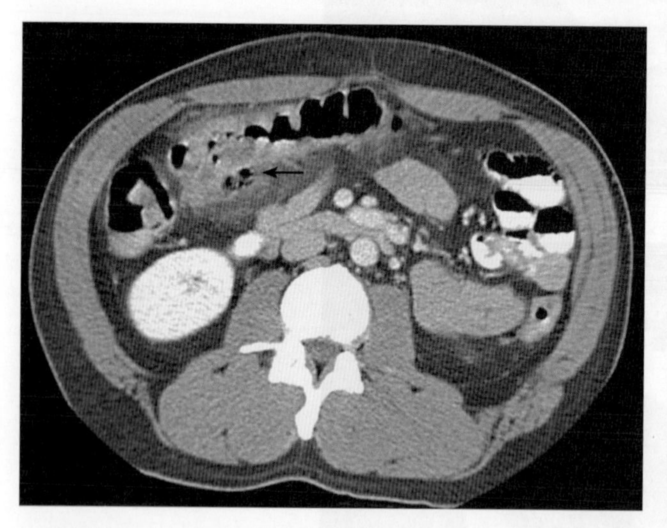

FIGURE 7.34 ■ Diverticulitis. In this individual, gas bubbles representing inflamed diverticula are identified adjacent to the transverse colon (arrow). There is associated colonic wall thickening and pericolic fat stranding.

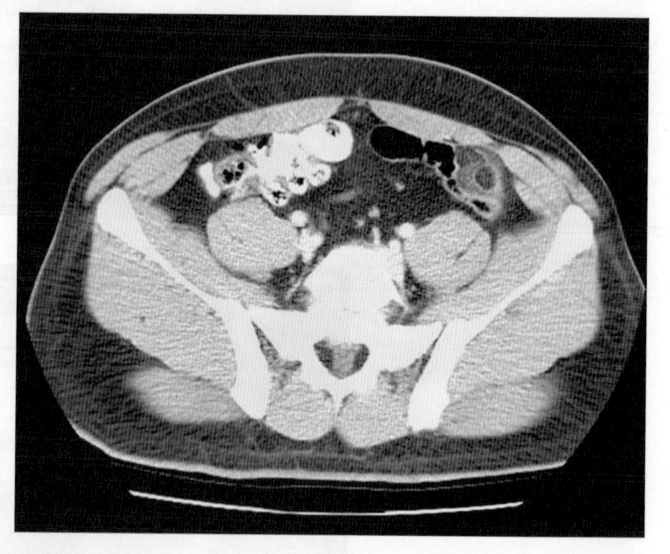

FIGURE 7.35 ■ Infarcted Appendage Epiploica. Rather than a bubble of gas adjacent to the colon, a fat globule with surrounding stranding is visible. This entity is commonly mistaken for diverticulitis. Note the lack of nearby diverticuli.

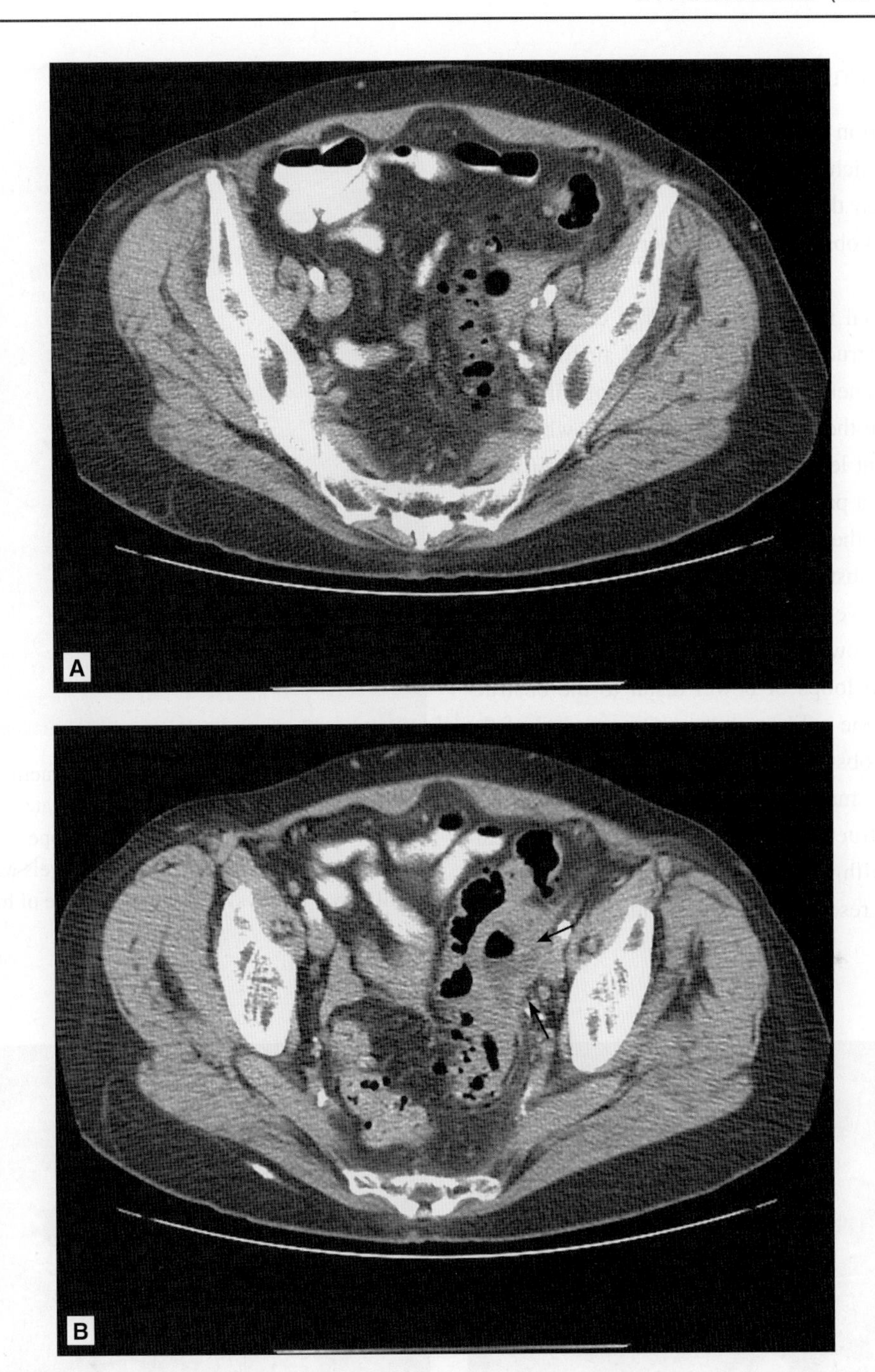

FIGURE 7.36 ■ Diverticular Abscess. **A, B:** Multiple colonic diverticula are present. A well-defined abscess cavity is seen adjacent to the sigmoid colon (arrows). Note the thick enhancing abscess wall.

Radiographic Summary

Small bowel obstruction is the result of a mechanical or functional obstruction, which does not allow passage of the intestinal contents through the small bowel. The most common causes of small bowel obstruction are postoperative adhesions and hernias.

On plain abdominal radiographs, findings characteristics of a small bowel obstruction include dilated air-filled small bowel >3 cm in diameter and the presence of differential air-fluid levels within the same small bowel loop whose levels are separated by at least 2 cm. The presence of air in the distal bowel denotes a partial or early complete small bowel obstruction, whereas the absence of gas in the distal bowel indicates a complete obstruction.

On CT a small bowel obstruction will appear as dilated, fluid-filled loops of bowel proximal to the obstruction, and nondilated, collapsed loops of bowel distal to the obstruction. The change in the caliber, or "transition point" of the bowel at the site of obstruction can often be quite marked. The presence of the "small bowel feces sign" indicates stasis and small bowel obstruction. This sign describes the appearance of gas mixed with stagnant fluid within the obstructed small bowel lumen, resembling feces normally seen in the large bowel only.

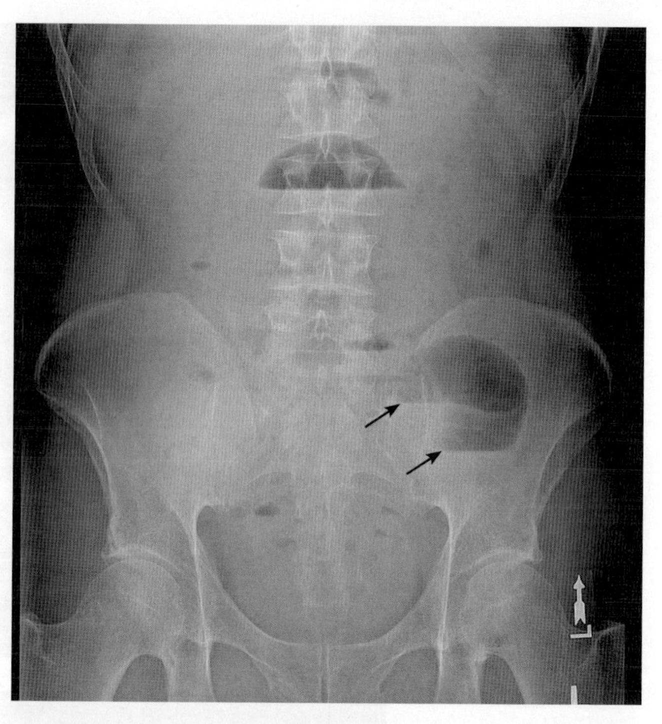

FIGURE 7.37 ■ Small Bowel Obstruction. An upright plain radiograph of the abdomen demonstrates disproportionate distension of small bowel loops in the upper mid-abdomen and left lower quadrant. Differential air-fluid levels within the same loop of small bowel (arrows) is highly predictive of high-grade mechanical obstruction.

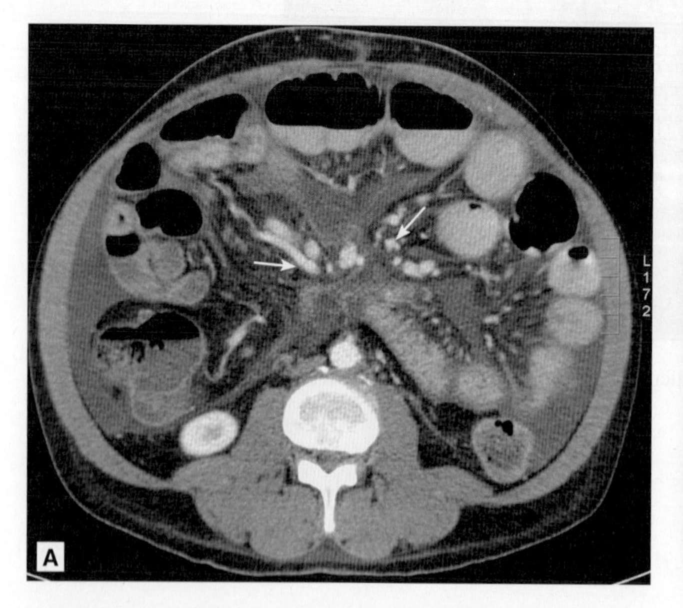

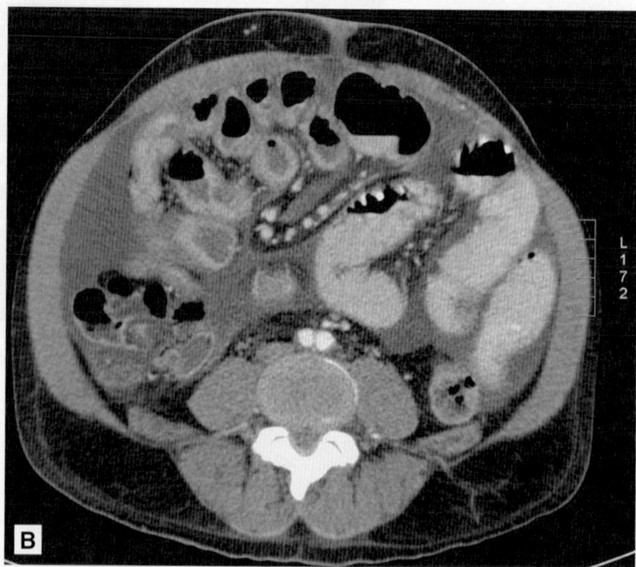

FIGURE 7.38 ■ Small Bowel Obstruction (Adhesions). **A, B:** In this patient with a history of abdominal surgery distended loops of small bowel are seen proximally, and some decompressed loops are visible in the right lower quadrant. This suggests the presence of a transition point. Angular "beak-like" configurations centrally (arrows) are a feature of intraabdominal adhesions.

Clinical Implications

Plain abdominal radiographs have about 50% sensitivity for the detection of small bowel obstruction. CT has a much higher sensitivity and specificity for the detection of small bowel obstruction and the added advantage of being able to identify the exact level of the obstruction and its cause. CT can delineate hernias, tumors, gallstone ileus, and other causes of small bowel obstruction that may not be detected on plain abdominal radiographs alone. The etiology of the obstruction is assumed to be an adhesion if no cause of the obstruction can be identified on the CT scan.

Pearls

1. The majority of patients with *partial* small bowel obstruction seen on CT scan will resolve the obstruction with supportive care, and will not require operative intervention.
2. Oral contrast is often not easily tolerated by patients with a small bowel obstruction and is not necessary to detect a small bowel obstruction on CT scan.

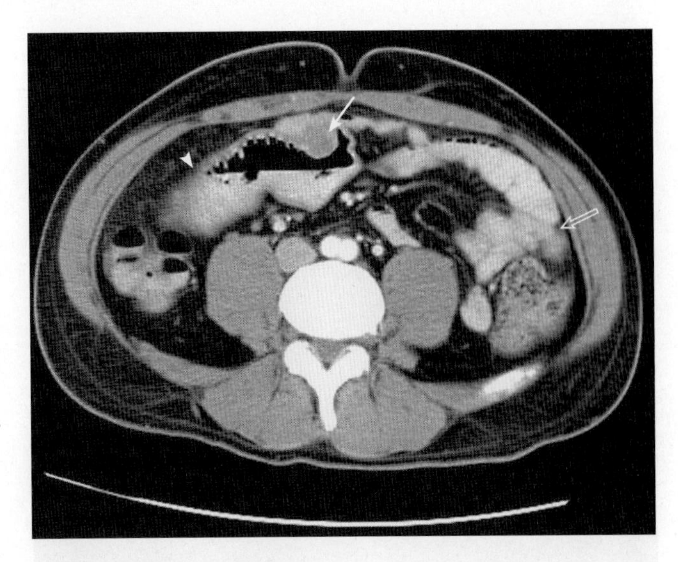

FIGURE 7.39 ■ Small Bowel Obstruction (Adenocarcinoma). A rounded intraluminal mass lesion (arrow) creates a transition point with dilated loops of small bowel proximal to the mass (arrowhead), and decompressed loops distally (open arrow).

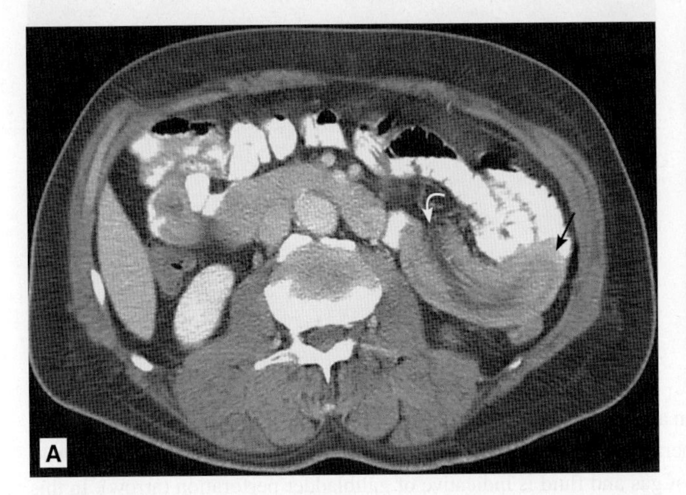

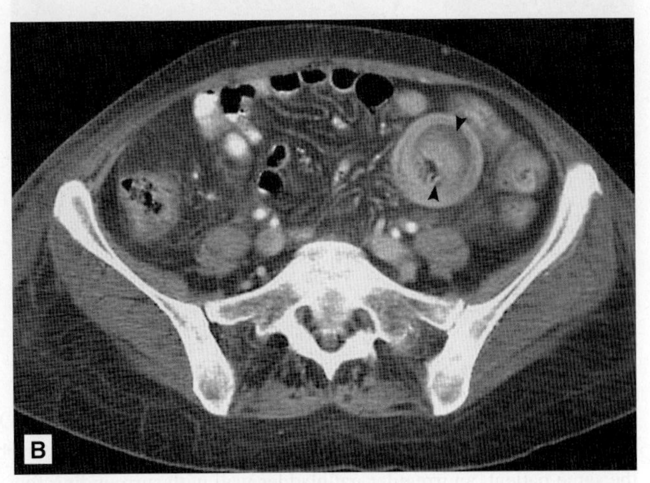

FIGURE 7.40 ■ Small Bowel Obstruction (Intussusception). **A, B:** The rounded leading edge of this ileo-ileal intussusception is visible (arrow). The telescoping bowel loop is identified along with mesenteric fat pulled inside (curved arrow). In cross-section, a "target sign" is seen due to the multiple layers of bowel wall and mesenteric fat (arrowheads).

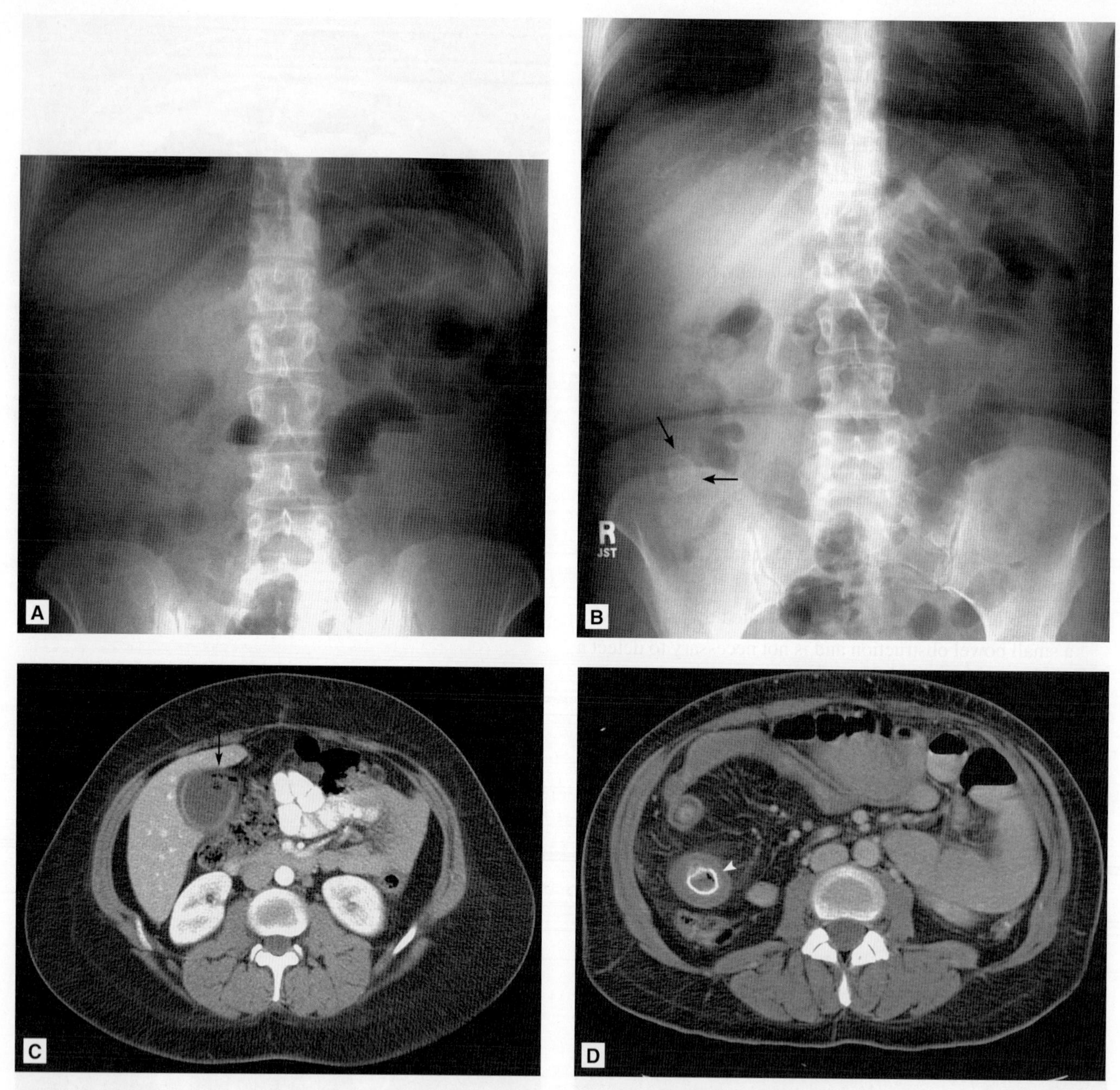

FIGURE 7.41 ■ Small Bowel Obstruction (Gallstone Ileus). **A, B:** On abdominal radiographs, distended loops of small bowel are seen with differential air-fluid levels on the upright view. Note the large peripherally calcified density in the right lower quadrant (arrows). **C, D:** In the same patient, an irregular gallbladder wall with surrounding foci of gas and fluid is indicative of gallbladder perforation (arrow). In this case, the large stone perforated into the duodenum, and is identified as a source of high-grade obstruction at the terminal ileum (arrowhead). Distended loops of small bowel are seen throughout.

Radiographic Summary

Typhlitis is a life-threatening necrotizing enterocolitis arising in the cecum. It was originally described in association with neutropenic patients undergoing treatment for leukemia and lymphoma, but now has been recognized in a variety of immunocompromised conditions including AIDS, solid tumor malignancies, and organ transplants. Complications of typhlitis include perforation, gastrointestinal bleeding, and death.

CT with IV contrast is the study of choice for the diagnosis of typhlitis. The CT scan can exclude appendicitis, ischemic colitis, and pseudomembranous colitis, all of which may present with a similar clinical picture. Findings on abdominal CT scan include cecal distention, thickening of the cecal wall, submucosal bowel wall edema, pneumatosis intestinalis, and pericolonic fluid and stranding.

Typhlitis may be diagnosed with ultrasound as well. Ultrasonograpic features of typhilitis include thickened hypoechoic bowel wall, pericecal fluid, and diminished or absent peristalsis. The patient may complain of pain upon palpation with the ultrasound transducer.

Clinical Implications

The diagnosis of typhilitis should be considered in any neutropenic patient (total neutrophil count < 500/mL) complaining of right lower quadrant abdominal pain. Typhlitis most commonly occurs 10-14 days after the initiation of chemotherapy. CT scan of the abdomen with IV contrast is the ideal study for the evaluation of these patients. Patients presenting with peritonitis, perforation, or clinical instability should undergo prompt surgical consultation.

Pearl

1. For those patients too unstable to undergo CT scanning, bedside ultrasound of the abdomen can assist in the diagnosis of typhlitis.

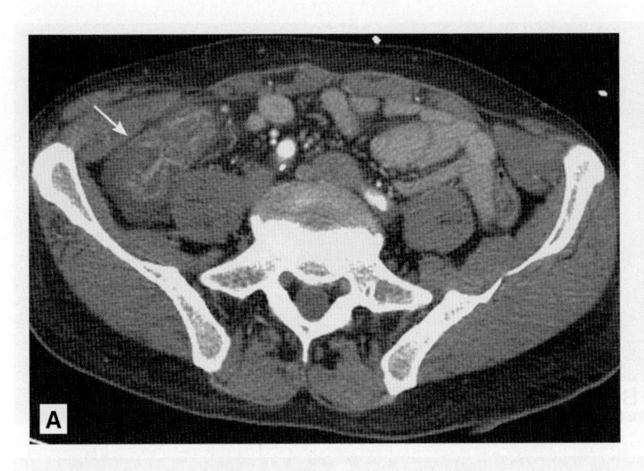

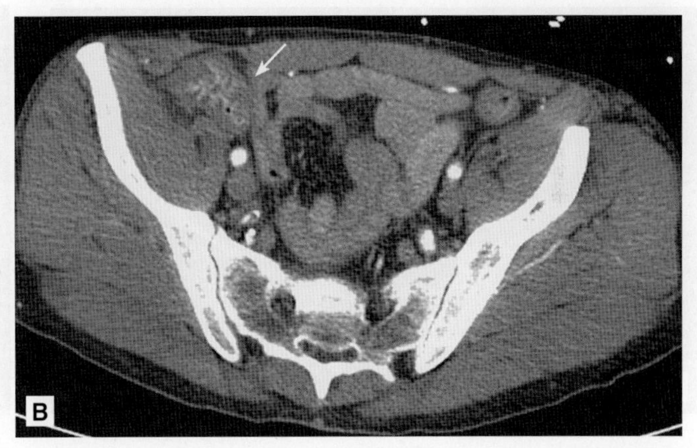

FIGURE 7.42 ■ Typhlitis. Marked bowel wall thickening of the cecum is present in this neutropenic patient (arrows).

Radiologic Summary

Inflammatory bowel disease refers to a group of chronic inflammatory disorders of the gastrointestinal tract. The two major types of inflammatory bowel diseases are ulcerative colitis and Crohn's disease.

Conventional plain radiography is not helpful in the diagnosis of the disease but can be useful to rule out complications such as bowel obstruction, pneumoperitoneum from bowel perforation, or toxic megacolon. Criteria for the diagnosis of toxic megacolon are dilatation of the colon greater than 6 cm, loss of colonic haustrations, and thumbprinting. Thumbprinting is the term used to describe the appearance of mucosal edema, which resembles "thumbs" protruding into the intestinal lumen.

Advanced ulcerative colitis may cause loss of the colonic haustra; radiographically, this finding is described as a "lead-pipe colon."

CT is the preferred study for the evaluation of inflammatory bowel disease. CT scans can assess the extent of bowel involvement and detect abscess formation, obstruction, and fistula formation. The hallmark finding in inflammatory bowel disease is bowel wall thickening. Pathologic enhancement, strictures, and periadventitial stranding are frequently seen as well. The normal bowel wall thickness is 3-5 mm; in ulcerative colitis the bowel wall thickness ranges between 7 and 8 mm. In Crohn's disease, the bowel wall thickness may increase to 30 mm.

Clinical Implications

It is important that the emergency physician rule out life-threatening complications of inflammatory bowel disease including toxic megacolon, bowel obstruction, abscess, or fistula formation. Plain radiographs may rule out obstruction and toxic megacolon, but abdominal CT should be used if there is a concern for perforation, fistula, or abscess formation. Inflammatory bowel disease is a chronic medical condition; discussion with the patient's gastroenterologist can

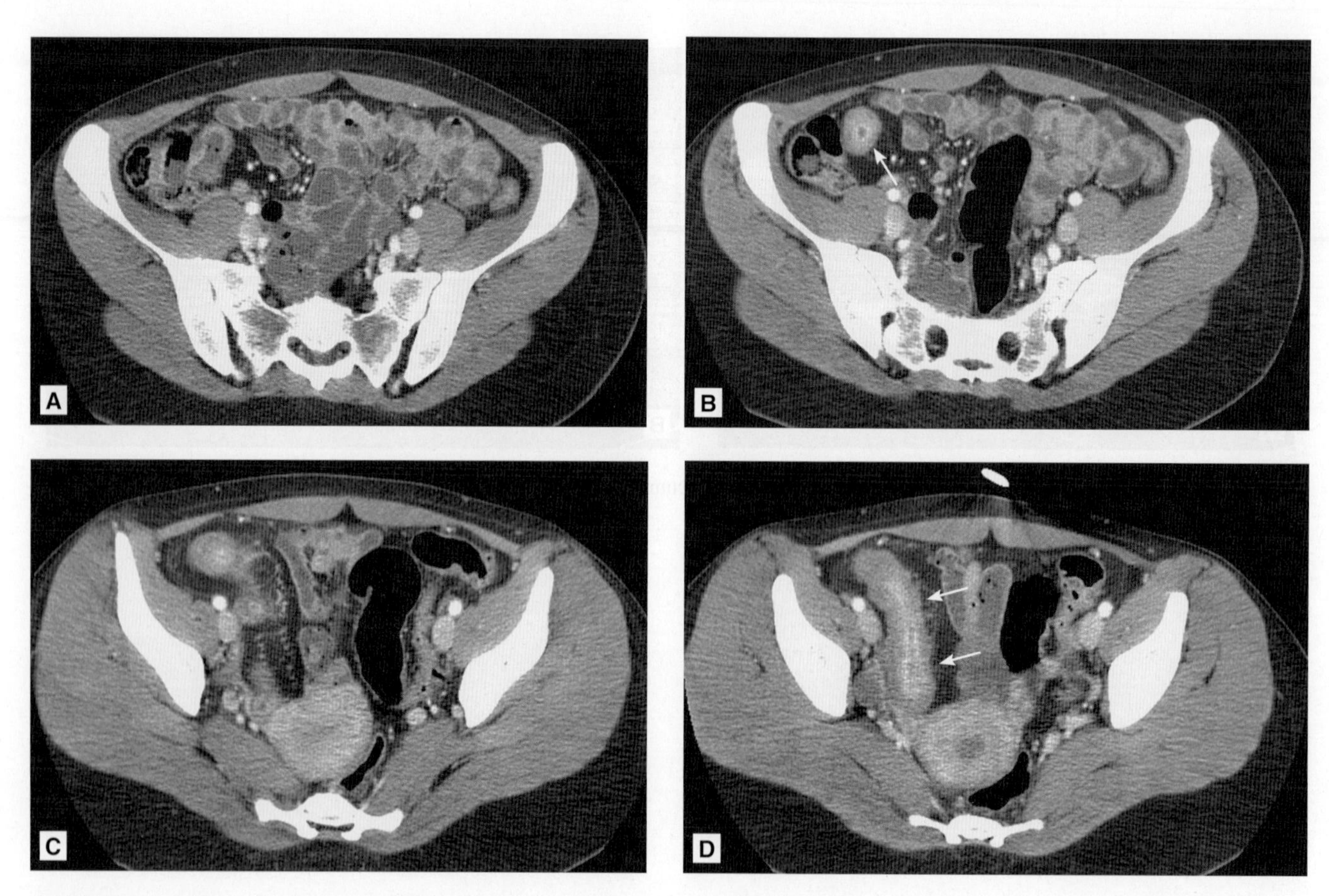

FIGURE 7.43 ■ Crohn's Disease. **A-D:** Prominent bowel wall thickening and inflammatory mesenteric fat stranding (arrows) is visible affecting the terminal ileum. Prominent mucosal enhancement is visible.

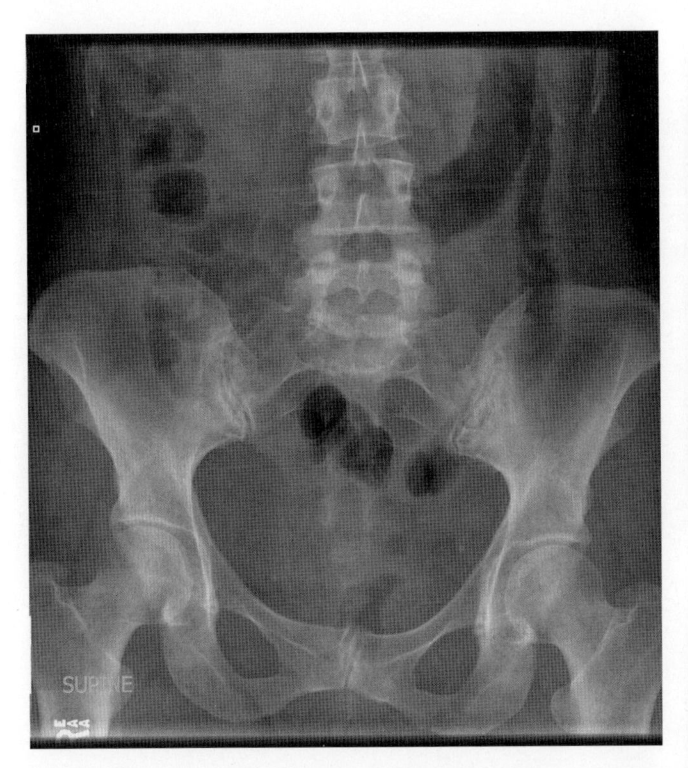

FIGURE 7.44 ■ Ulcerative Colitis. A plain radiograph in a patient with ulcerative colitis demonstrates a portion of the transverse colon and splenic flexure with a lack of distinct haustral markings. This is referred to as a "lead pipe" appearance of the colon.

be invaluable in guiding emergency-department evaluation, therapy, and arranging follow-up.

Pearls

1. In all likelihood, patients suffering from inflammatory bowel disease have undergone prior CT scans of the abdomen and have been exposed to multiple doses of ionizing radiation. In an effort to avoid further exposure to radiation, discuss alternative imaging modalities with a radiologist.
2. Ultrasound may be beneficial in detecting extra-intestinal manifestations of ulcerative colitis such as cholelithiasis, and sclerosing cholangitis.
3. A small bowel follow-through study may be performed as well to evaluate for terminal ileitis, strictures, and fistula formation. A barium enema is an alternative way to evaluate the colon.

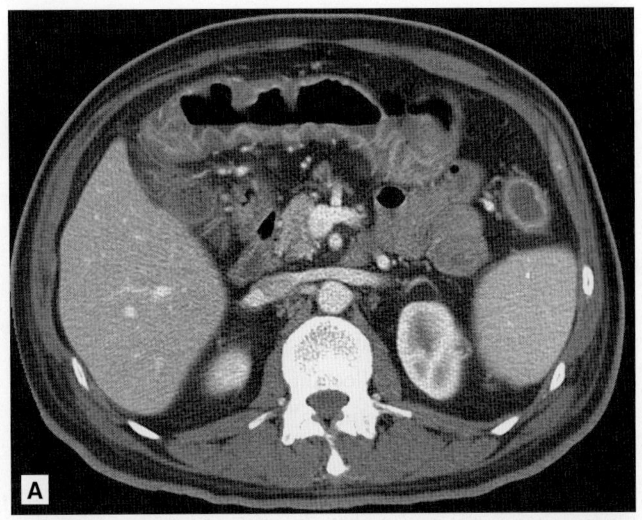

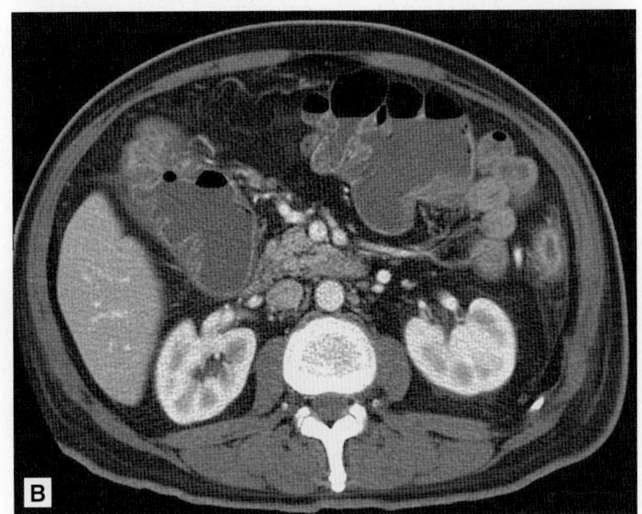

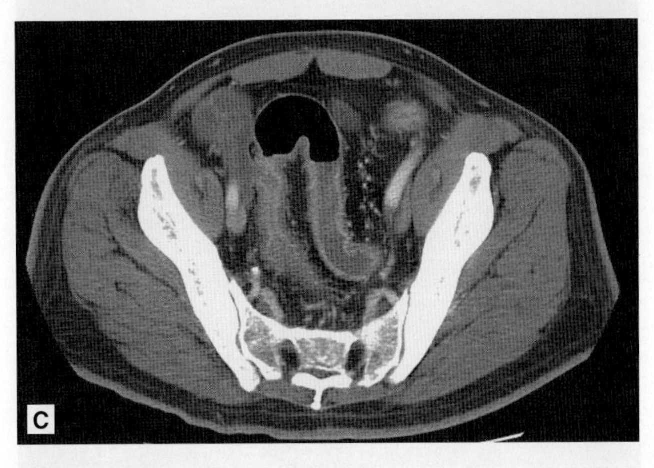

FIGURE 7.45 ■ Ulcerative Colitis. **A-C:** A pattern of abnormally increased mucosal enhancement is seen throughout the colon. The colonic wall is thickened with continuous involvement throughout the entirety of the colon.

Radiographic Summary

Ischemic bowel occurs when the vascular supply to the bowel is disrupted. The end result is bowel ischemia and infarction resulting in bowel wall injury ranging from superficial muscosal involvement to full thickness bowel wall necrosis. Ischemic bowel can be caused by atherosclerosis, emboli, vasculitis, aortic aneurysm, arterial and venous thrombosis, or low flow states as a result of shock or dehydration.

The most common finding on plain radiographs is a nonspecific ileus pattern. Collection of gas in the bowel wall, termed "pneumatosis intestinalis," may be seen along with air in the portal venous system.

CT is very helpful in the evaluation of ischemic bowel because it establishes the diagnosis and excludes alternative causes of abdominal pain. The CT scan not only shows changes in the bowel wall but helps to detect the etiology of the vascular insult. The most common finding on CT scan is thickening of the bowel wall. The most specific finding is decreased enhancement of the bowel wall. Other

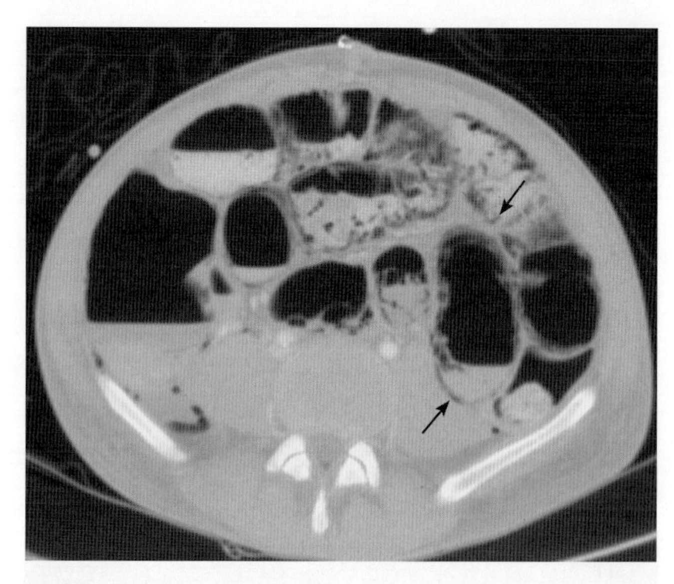

FIGURE 7.47 ■ Pneumatosis Intestinalis. A nonenhanced CT scan of the abdomen demonstrates small gas bubbles nearly circumferentially within the wall of the small intestine. Gas entrapped in the bowel wall (arrows) is seen dependently and separate from the normal intraluminal gas.

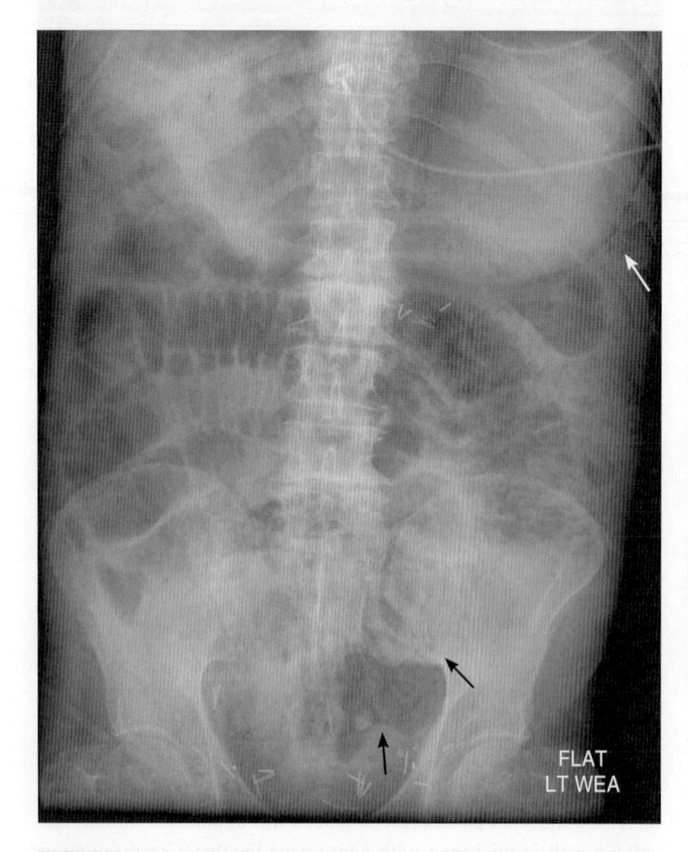

FIGURE 7.46 ■ Pneumatosis Intestinalis. Multiple sites of linear and beaded gas foci are seen in the bowel wall of the stomach and small intestine on this supine plain radiograph (arrows).

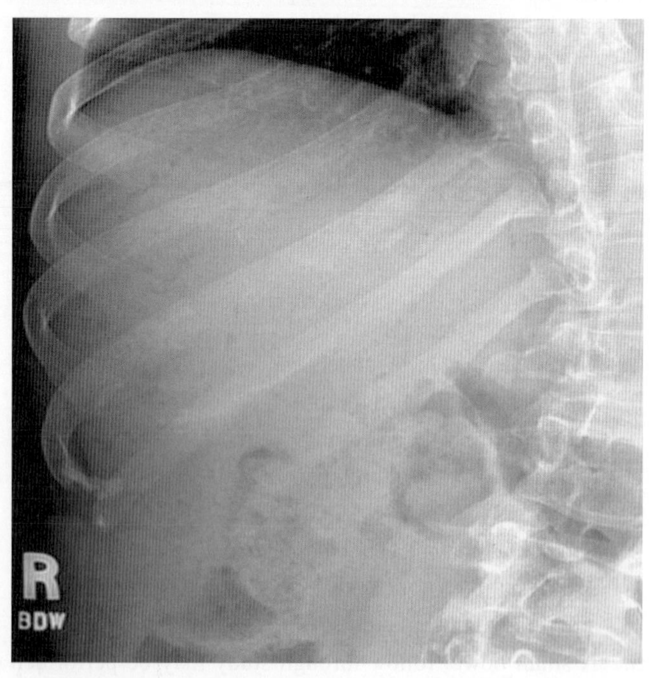

FIGURE 7.48 ■ Portal Venous Gas. Fine linear and branching foci of gas are seen distributed to the periphery of the liver in this patient with necrotic bowel. The peripheral location of the gas distinguishes portal venous gas from pneumobilia.

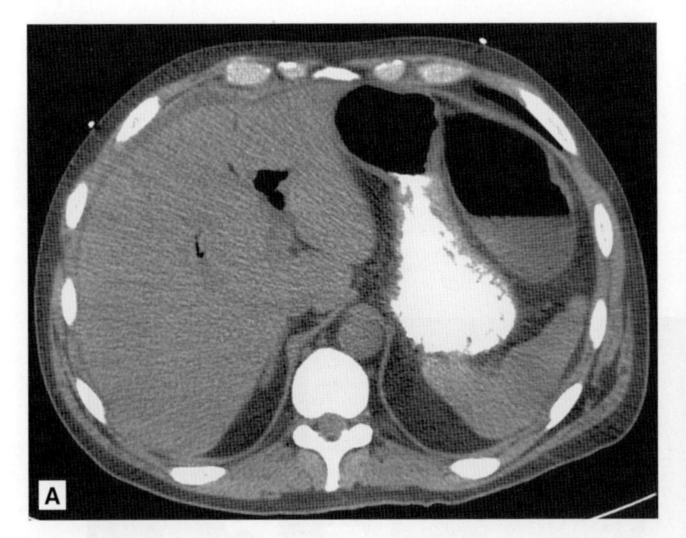

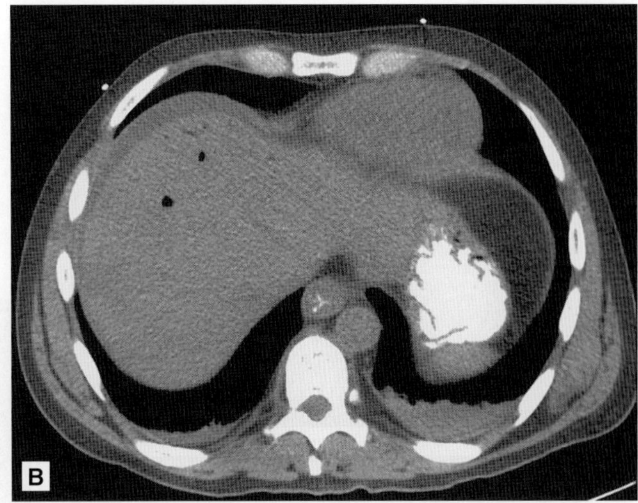

FIGURE 7.49 ■ Portal Venous Gas. **A, B:** Peripheral gas foci are seen in the liver on nonenhanced abdominal CT images.

CT findings include thromboembolism of the mesenteric blood vessels, intramural gas, gas within the mesenteric veins, portal venous gas, thumbprinting due to mucosal edema, and dilatation of the bowel proximal to the ischemic bowel.

Clinical Implications

The classic presentation of ischemic bowel is rapid onset of severe periumbilical abdominal pain in an elderly patient. The patient's complaints are often out of proportion to physical findings, which may seem unremarkable. Patients presenting with signs of peritonitis should undergo urgent surgical evaluation. In stable patients, the most useful study is a CT of the abdomen with IV contrast. The CT can provide information regarding the patency of the mesenteric vessels and the extent of the bowel ischemia.

Pearls

1. MRI is highly sensitive for the diagnosis of mesenteric ischemia, and may be useful in conditions for which iodinated contrast should be avoided such as renal insufficiency and contrast allergy.
2. Conventional angiography of the abdominal vessels can be both diagnostic and therapeutic in that it allows visualization of the vessel as well as permitting administration of vasodilators or fibrinolytic agents.

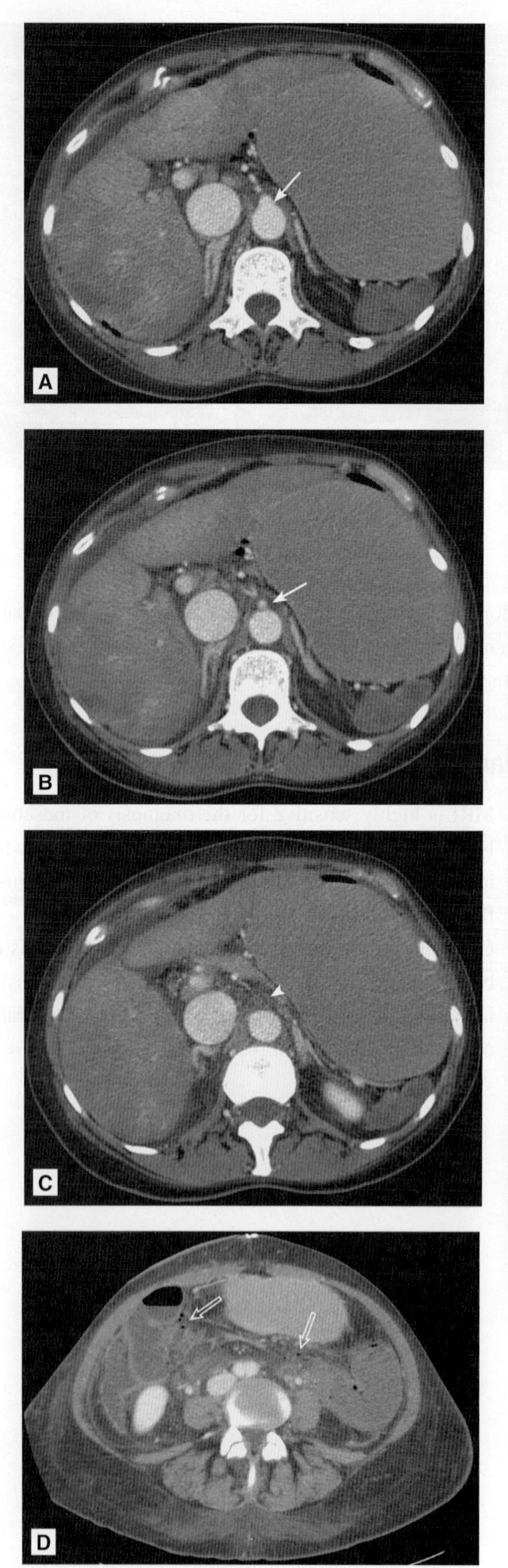

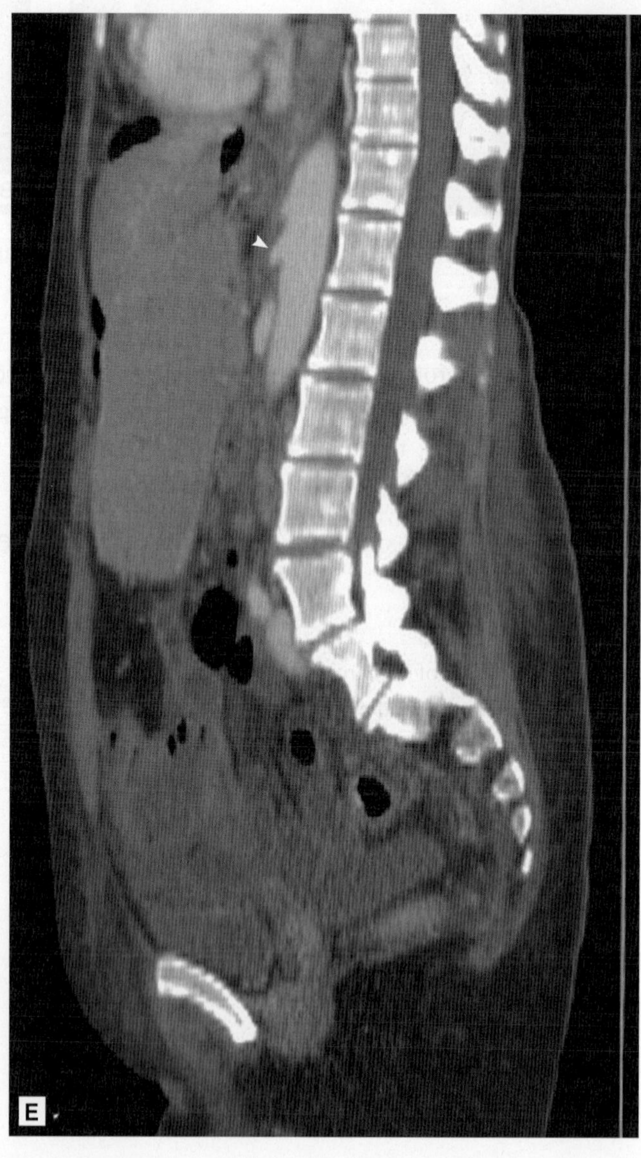

FIGURE 7.50 ■ SMA Occlusion. **A-E:** CT of the abdomen demonstrates the proximal aspect of the SMA (arrows). On subsequent images, the SMA is entirely occluded by clot with no contrast seen in the lumen of the vessel ("C", arrowhead). Gas within the mesentery (open arrow) is a feature of ischemic bowel and necrosis. The sagittal reformatted image again demonstrates truncation of the proximal SMA (arrowhead).

Radiographic Summary

An ovarian teratoma, (dermoid cyst) is a germ-cell tumor that contains a diversity of tissues including hair, teeth, bone, and neural tissue. Ovarian teratomas are best evaluated with a combination of transabdominal and transvaginal ultrasound. Teratomas range in size and echogenicity and often have a mixture of different sonographic patterns reflecting their contents. The two classic dermoid appearances are the "tip of the iceberg" sign and the "dermoid plug" sign. The "tip of the iceberg" sign is characterized by a sonographic pelvic mass in which most of the sonographic beam is absorbed at the top of the mass preventing visualization of the contents of the mass. The "dermoid plug" sign is characterized by one or more hyperechoic rounded areas within the mass. These "dermoid plugs" represent solid tissue components (teeth, hair, bone) surrounded by sebaceous material. On CT, teratomas are seen as a pelvic mass with mixed contents reflecting various elements such as sebum, skin, hair, and teeth.

Clinical Implications

Teratomas are asymptomatic until they are large enough to cause pelvic pain from ligamentous irritation or ovarian torsion. Because teratomas are generally asymptomatic, they are often discovered incidentally on routine imaging studies especially during pregnancy.

Teratomas are congenital tumors and are present at birth. Teratomas are generally benign tumors but they do have a small risk of transformation to malignancy and should be surgically removed and pathologically evaluated when discovered.

Pearls

1. Teratomas are benign congenital tumors with a low risk of malignant transformation that should be removed surgically when present.
2. Fat attenuation, measured as negative Houndsfield units, within an adnexal cyst is diagnostic of teratoma on CT scan.

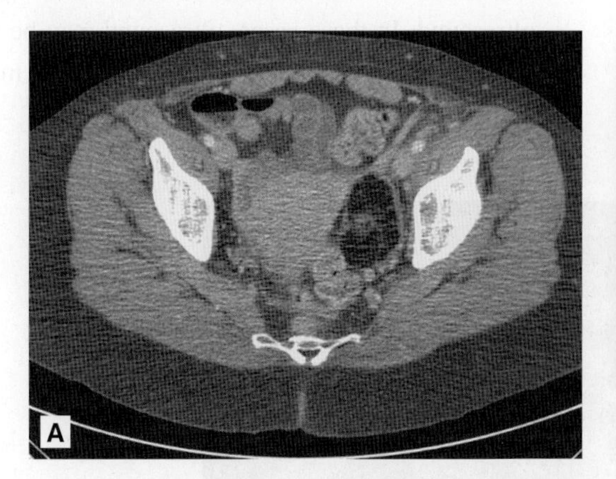

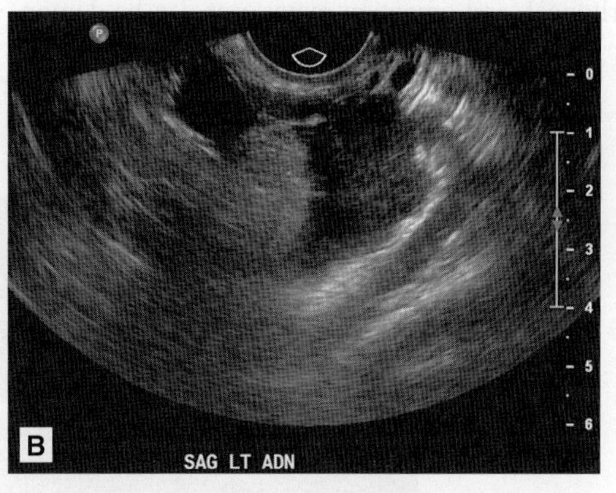

FIGURE 7.51 ■ Ovarian Germ Cell Tumor (Dermoid). **A:** The left adnexal mass seen on CT scan demonstrates varied density, including low-attenuation fatty tissue. Solid elements are also seen within the mass in this 32-year-old female patient. **B:** On ultrasound, the mass shows varied echotexture representing regions of fat and some cystic components.

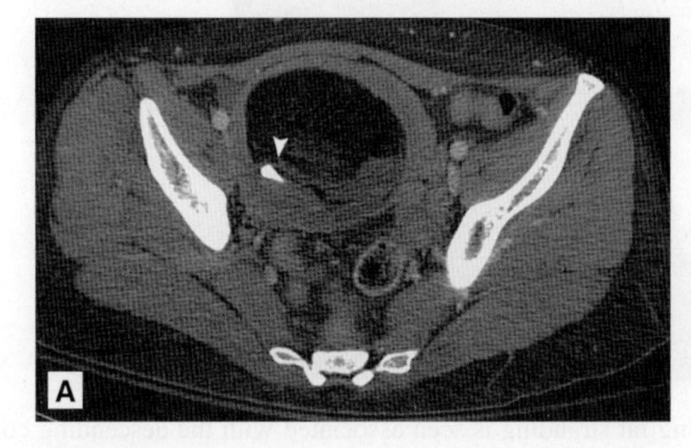

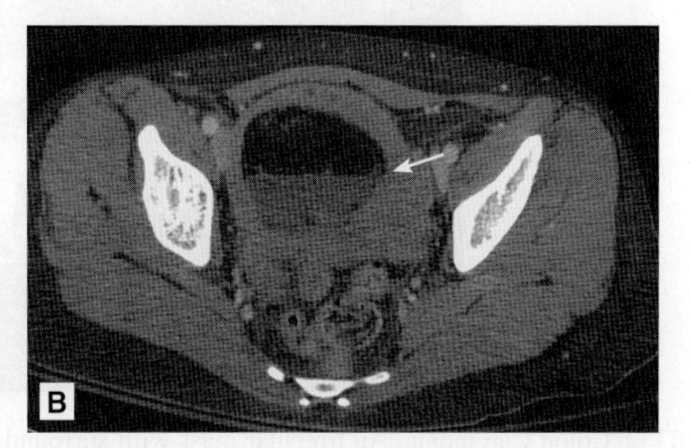

FIGURE 7.52 ■ Ovarian Germ Cell Tumor (Dermoid). **A, B:** CT scan in a different patient demonstrates a right adnexal mass containing varied tissue elements. A fat-fluid layer is visible (arrow). In addition to sebaceous material, a tooth is visible as a densely calcific region (arrowhead).

Radiographic Summary

Adenocarcinoma is the most common colon carcinoma in the United States. Plain abdominal radiographs are not beneficial in the detection of colon carcinomas unless a complication such as bowel perforation or obstruction is present. Rarely, a mucin-producing colon carcinoma will contain calcifications, which can be seen on the plain radiograph. On an abdominal CT scan, a colon carcinoma may be visualized as an intraluminal or intramural mass. Annular carcinomas of the colon produce thickening of the bowel wall and narrowing of the lumen. A CT scan can readily detect obstruction, perforation, and fistula formation caused by the invading tumor. Colonic tumors may act as a leading edge precipitating an episode of intussusception. Intussusception has a targetoid appearance when imaged in cross-section (bowel-within-bowel). A localized perforation as a result of the tumor may present as a collection of fluid and/or gas adjacent to the colon. CT scans may detect enlarged lymph nodes; any lymph node greater than 10 mm is worrisome for a metastatic process. Hepatic, adrenal, peritoneal, and omentum metastases can be demonstrated by CT as well.

Clinical Implications

The emergency physician may identify a colonic mass during the evaluation of a patient presenting with abdominal pain or rectal bleeding. The goal of the clinician is to rule out serious complications such as bowel perforation, obstruction, intussusception, or GI hemorrhage. If the patient is deemed stable for discharge after the discovery of a colonic mass, expeditious follow-up must be arranged.

Pearls

1. CT findings of colon carcinoma are not specific; similar findings such as focal thickening of the bowel wall may be seen with diverticulitis, Crohn's Disease, and ischemic colitis. It is imperative that patients with abnormal CT scan findings are closely followed to rule out colon carcinoma.
2. Generally speaking, colonic masses palpable through the abdominal wall or on rectal exam can be visualized by ultrasound. In these cases, ultrasound may be very beneficial in the evaluation of a colonic or rectal mass.

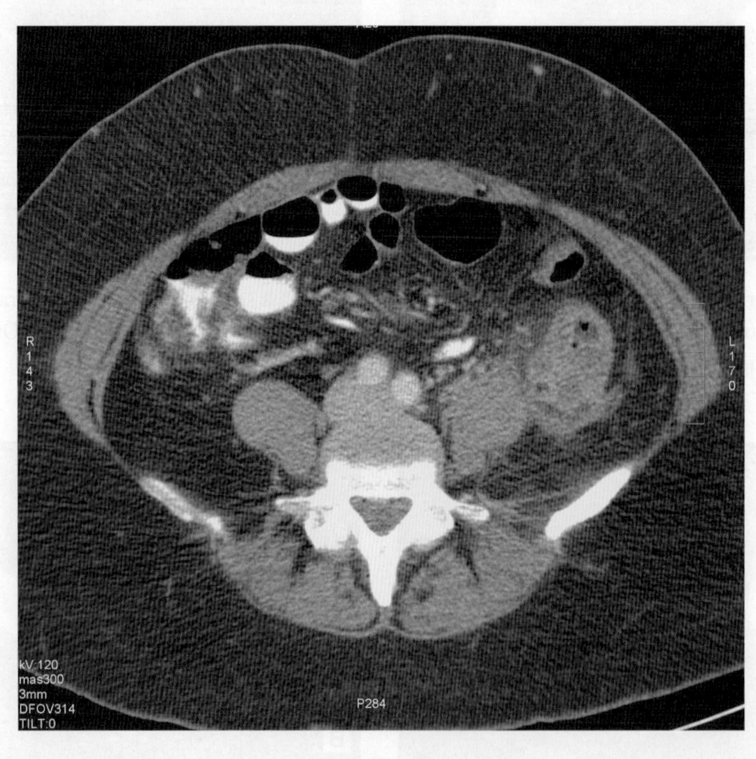

FIGURE 7.53 ■ Colon Carcinoma. An irregular mass with surrounding fat stranding is seen associated with the descending colon on this contrast-enhanced CT. Although diverticulitis has similar radiographic features, the lack of visible diverticula suggests malignancy as the diagnosis.

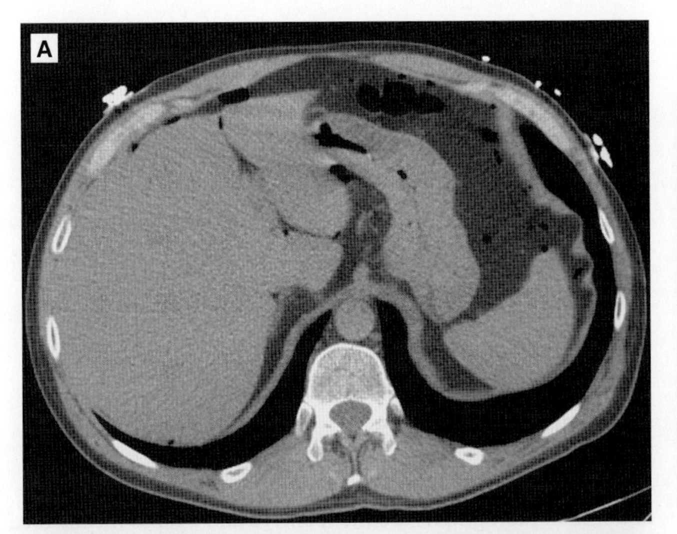

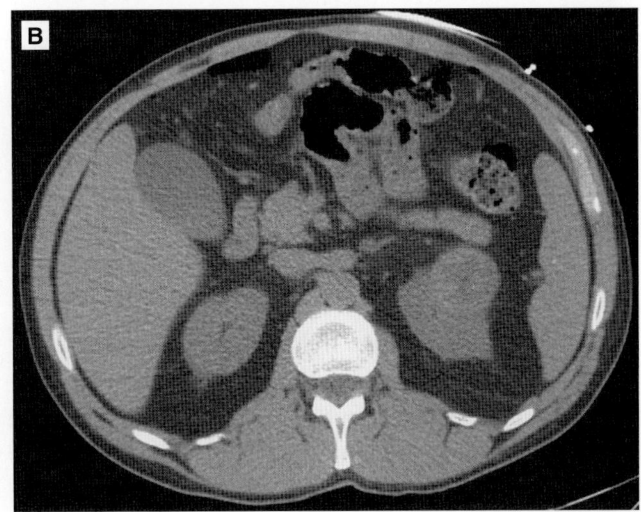

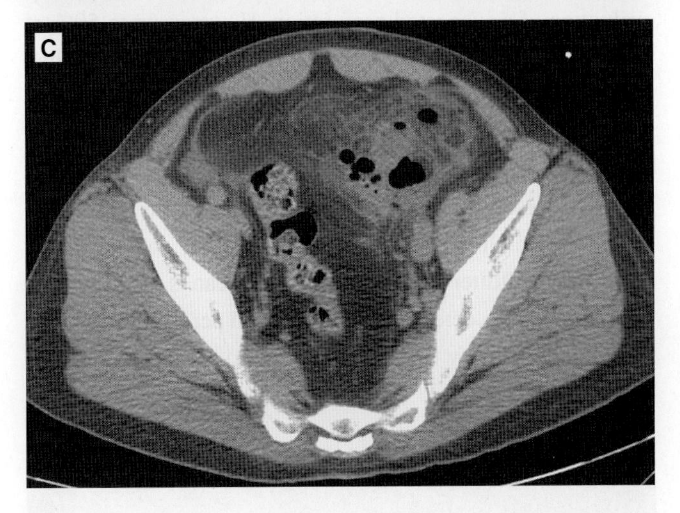

FIGURE 7.54 ■ Colon Carcinoma with Colonic Perforation. **A-C:** Innumerable foci of gas are identified within the mesentery and along the anterior abdominal wall. An irregular mass in the left lower quadrant is identified with surrounding stranding. This proved to represent a perforated colon carcinoma.

Radiographic Summary

Gastrointestinal perforation results when the wall of the gastrointestinal tract is disrupted, resulting in spillage of the intraluminal contents into the abdominal cavity. Perforation permits air to enter the peritoneal cavity, a condition termed as pneumoperitoneum or "free air."

An upright chest radiograph will detect free air as a dark crescent of gas best seen on the right side of the abdomen above the dome of the liver. If the patient is too ill to stand, a left lateral decubitus radiograph will show free air between the liver and the peritoneum. Other signs of free air seen on plain abdominal radiographs include "Rigler's sign"—air outlining both sides of the bowel wall; "Football sign"—large pneumoperitoneum located in the abdominal cavity in which free air may surround the falciform ligament, and will appear as a vertical opaque line outlined with an oval collection of air extending from the right upper quadrant to the umbilicus; and "Telltale triangle sign"—triangular air pocket interspersed between three loops of bowel.

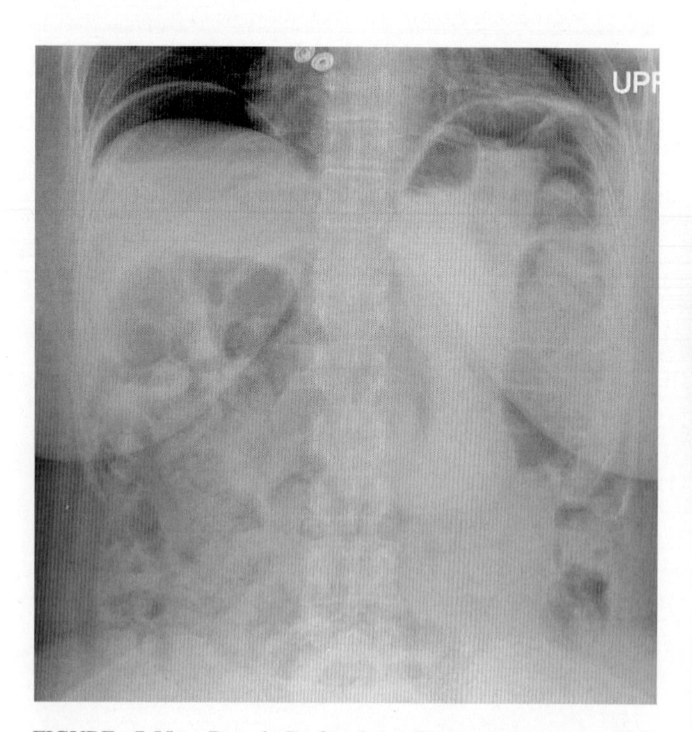

FIGURE 7.55 ■ Bowel Perforation, Pneumoperitoneum. This upright radiograph demonstrates pneumoperitoneum with a gas collection identified between the liver and the right hemidiaphragm. The free air is distinguished by normal colon by the lack of any haustral markings.

CT is an excellent modality for the evaluation of suspected gastrointestinal perforation. Small amounts of free air can be detected on a CT scan; however, the location of the free air may not correlate with the site of perforation. Since a patient undergoes a CT scan in the supine position, free air will most often be visualized beneath the anterior abdominal wall, and overlying the ventral surface of the liver. Administration of water-soluble oral contrast may help to localize the site of the perforation.

Clinical Implications

Upright and lateral chest radiographs and supine and upright abdominal radiographs are inexpensive and a rapid means for evaluation of a suspected perforation. However up to 50% of patients found to have a perforation at the time of surgery had normal plain radiographs. Supine anteroposterior radiographs have an extremely low sensitivity for the detection of free air; very large amounts of free air have to be present to be detectable. Conversely, upright and left lateral decubitus anteroposterior radiographs have an excellent sensitivity and can detect only a few milliliters of free air. The CT scan is the most sensitive tool for the detection of a suspected perforation and can additionally identify the level and cause of the perforation.

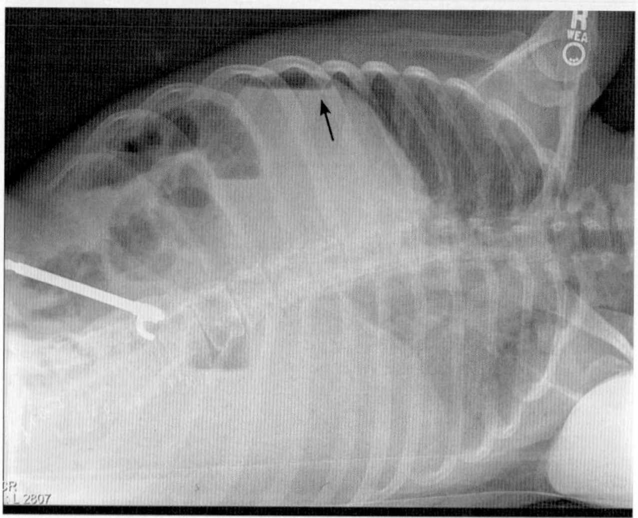

FIGURE 7.56 ■ Bowel Perforation, Pneumoperitoneum. Left lateral decubitus views are utilized to project free intrabdominal air (arrow) over the uniform density of the liver. This view may be utilized for patients in whom upright imaging is not possible.

Pearls

1. Pneumoperitoneum, even when present in large quantities, may be missed on the supine abdominal radiograph. Always obtain an upright or left lateral decubitus along with a supine abdominal radiograph to evaluate for the presence of free air.
2. Viewing the abdominal CT in "lung window setting" may help to detect small amounts of free air.

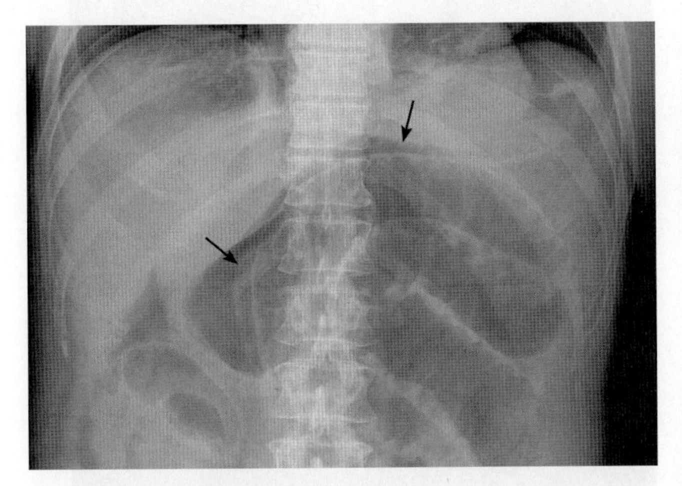

FIGURE 7.57 ■ Bowel Perforation, Pneumoperitoneum. Clear visualization of both sides of the bowel wall (Rigler's sign) is an indication of pneumoperitoneum (arrows). Note the disproportionate distension of small bowel loops in the left mid-abdomen in this patient with small bowel obstruction and perforation. Gallstones incidentally present.

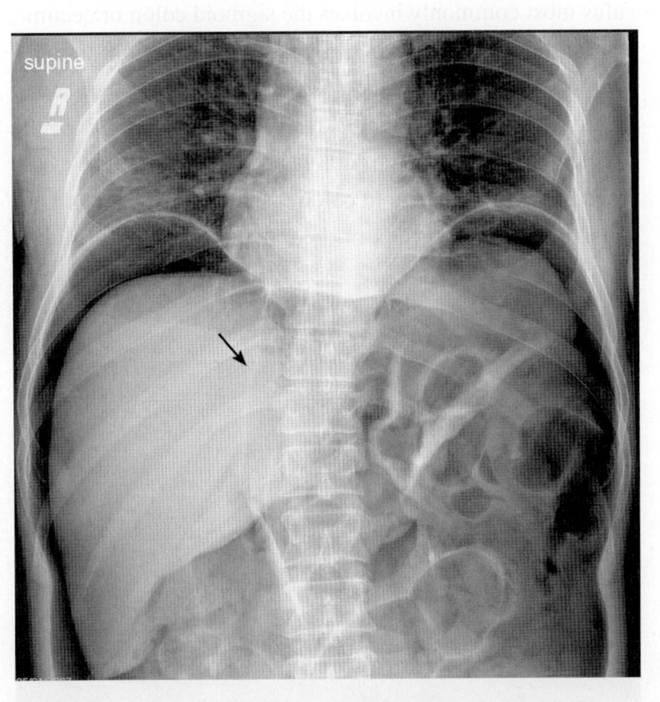

FIGURE 7.58 ■ Bowel Perforation, Pneumoperitoneum. A massive collection of free air is present in the abdomen. The falciform ligament of the liver is outlined by the large pneumoperitoneum (arrow).

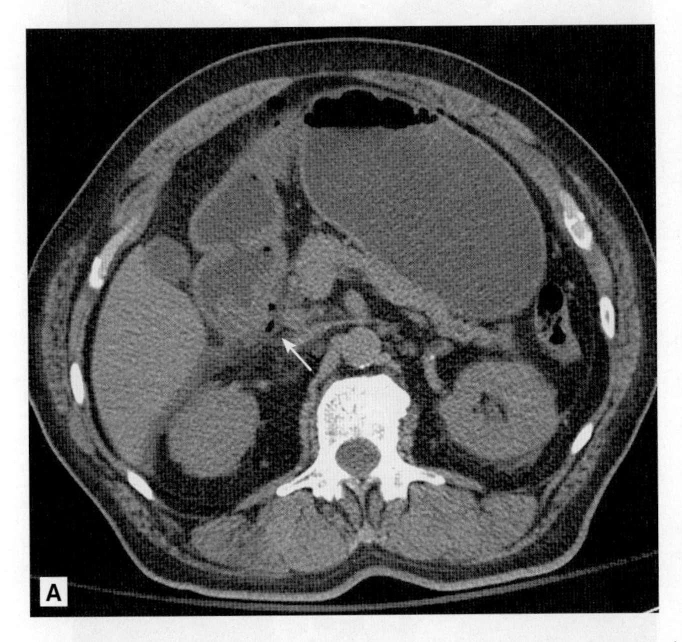

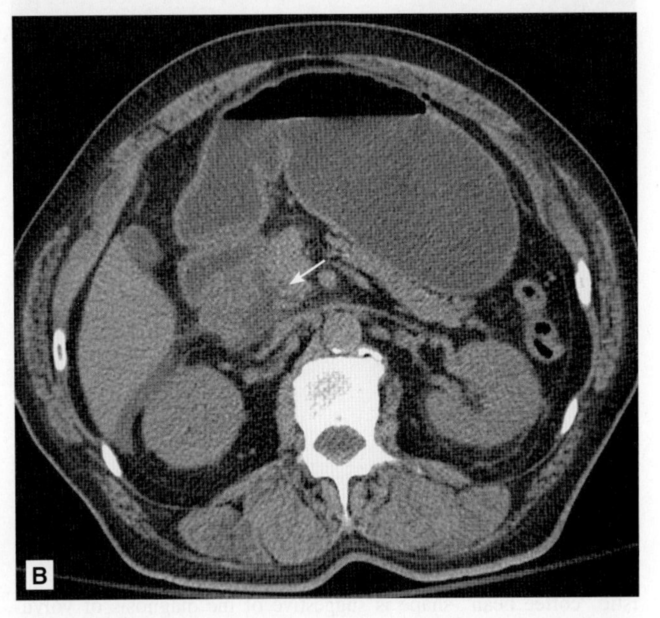

FIGURE 7.59 ■ Duodenal Perforation. **A, B:** Small foci of gas are identified outside of the bowel lumen within the mesentery and along the anterior abdominal wall. The presence of gas and fluid foci adjacent to the first portion of the duodenum (arrows) strongly suggest this as the site of perforation.

Radiographic Summary

Volvulus describes the twisting of a loop of bowel around its mesenteric attachment, resulting in a mechanical bowel obstruction and impaired blood flow to the intestine. A volvulus most commonly involves the sigmoid colon or cecum.

Findings suggestive of a sigmoid volvulus on abdominal radiographs include an inverted U-shaped appearance of the distended sigmoid loop extending from the pelvis to the right upper quadrant. The "coffee bean sign" develops as the closed loop of the sigmoid colon distends with fluid and gas causing the medial walls of the colon to appose forming a

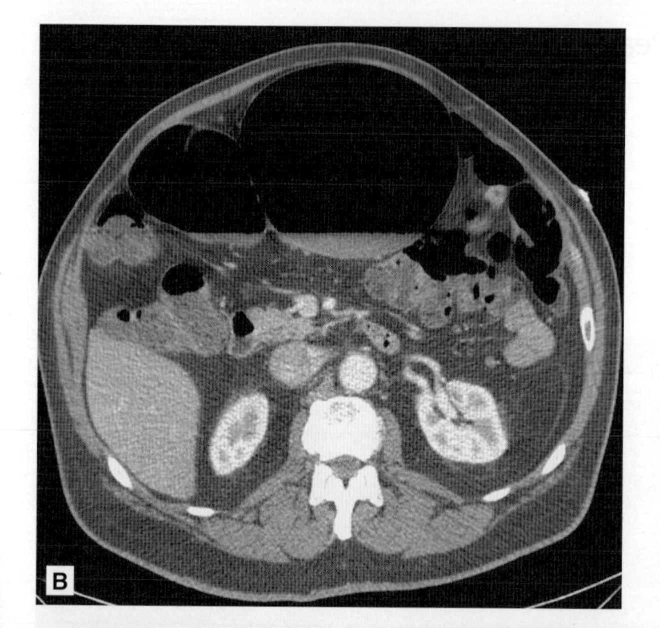

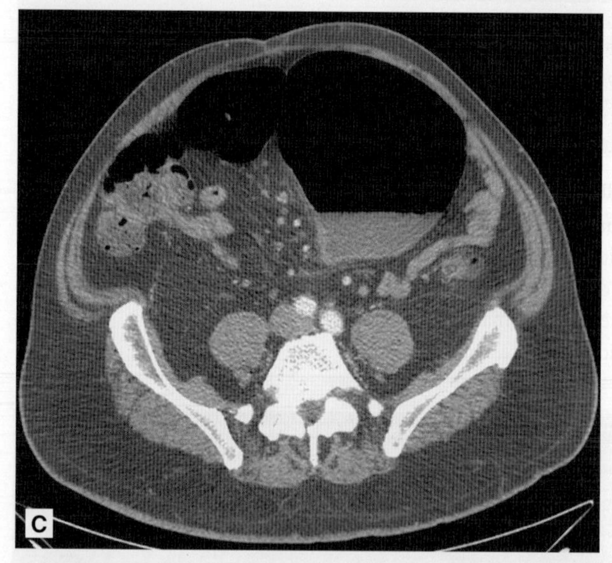

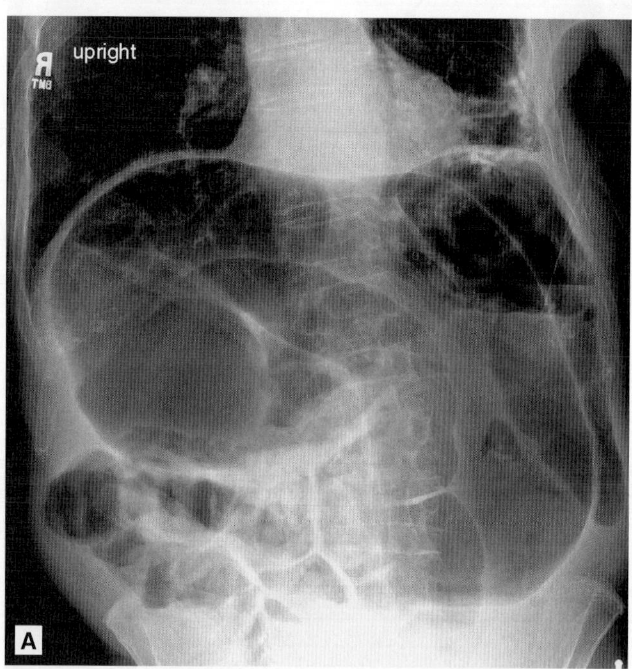

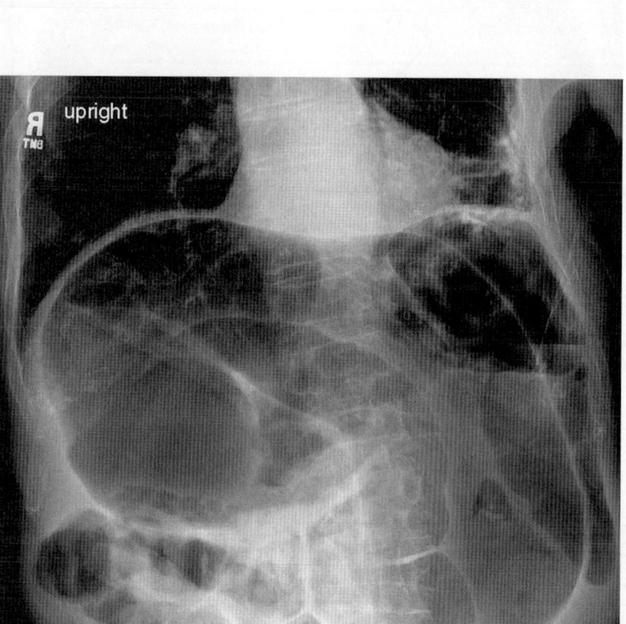

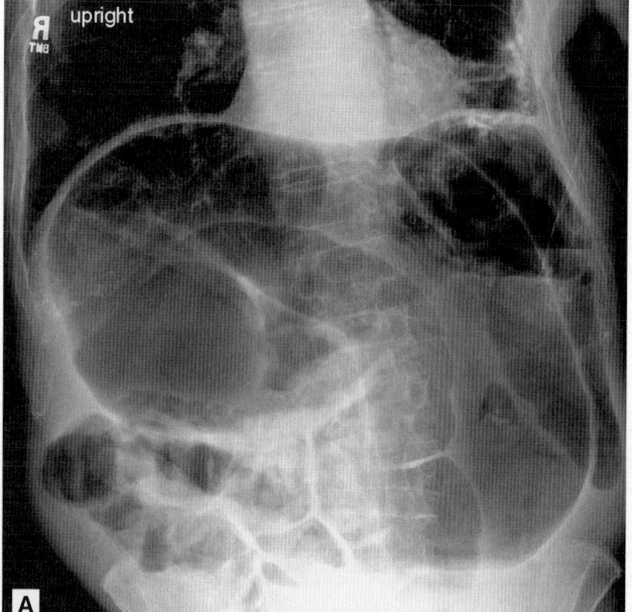

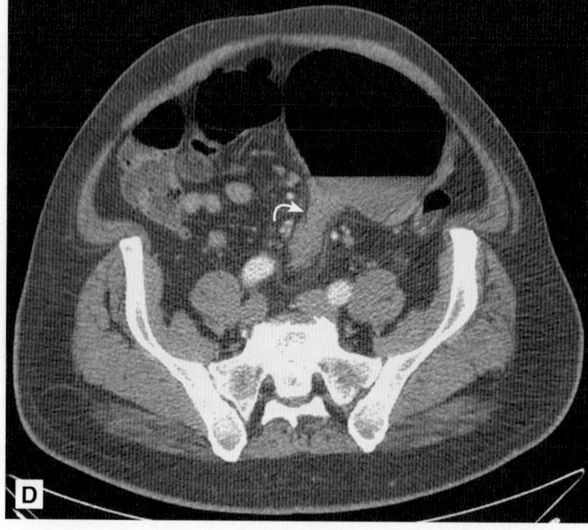

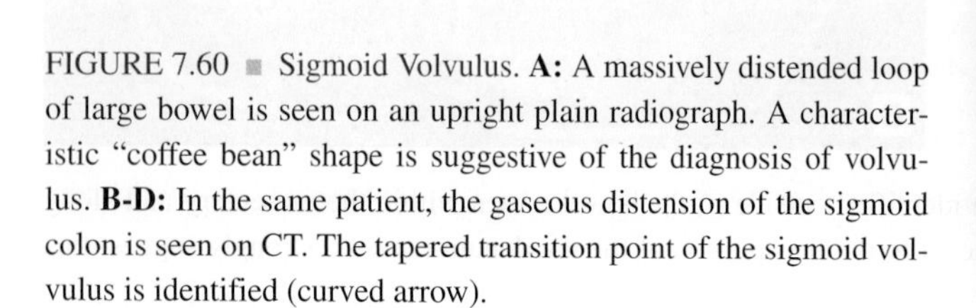

FIGURE 7.60 ■ Sigmoid Volvulus. **A:** A massively distended loop of large bowel is seen on an upright plain radiograph. A characteristic "coffee bean" shape is suggestive of the diagnosis of volvulus. **B-D:** In the same patient, the gaseous distension of the sigmoid colon is seen on CT. The tapered transition point of the sigmoid volvulus is identified (curved arrow).

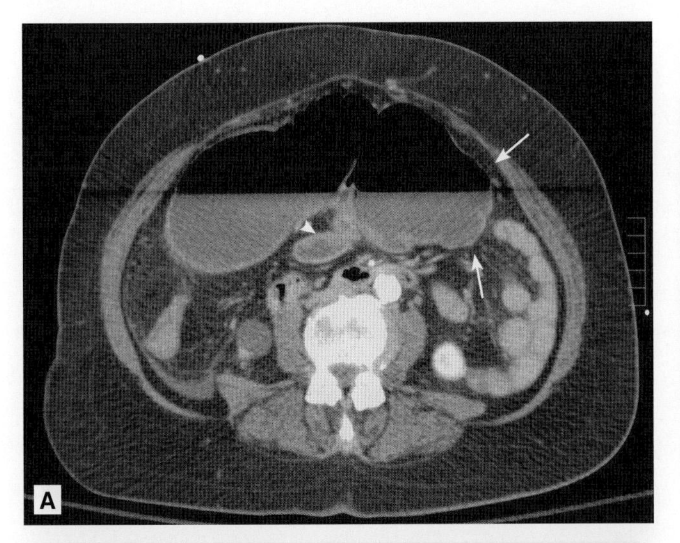

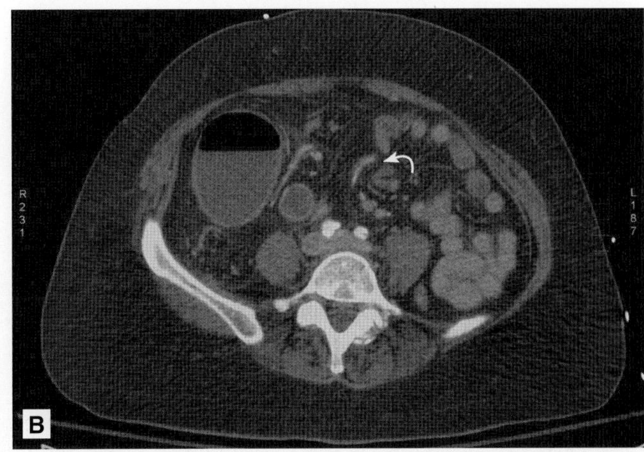

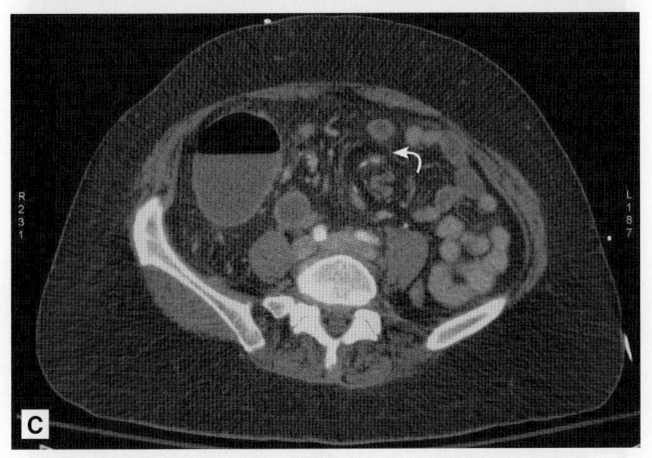

FIGURE 7.61 ■ Cecal Volvulus. **A-C:** On CT, the horizontally oriented cecum can be identified as a blind-ended loop of colon displaced into a transverse orientation within the upper abdomen (arrows). The terminal ileum is seen in the mid abdomen (arrowhead). Twisting mesenteric vessels are a result of the abnormally displaced bowel (curved arrows).

cleft. The resulting shape resembles a coffee bean. A cecal volvulus will appear as a kidney-shaped colonic distention positioned in the left upper quadrant of the abdomen or to the left of the midline. A cecal volvulus generally causes a complete obstruction so there will be very little gas in the distal colon.

A CT scan of the abdomen may show the characteristic "whirl sign" which describes the swirling pattern created by the twisting of the mesentery and vessels. In addition, the edges of the volvulus may show a bird-beak appearance. CT is also useful in the detection of bowel wall ischemia as a result of the volvulus.

Clinical Implications

Sigmoid volvulus can be frequently diagnosed on the basis of plain radiographs alone, whereas the diagnosis of cecal volvulus usually requires an abdominal CT scan. All patients diagnosed as having volvulus need to have a prompt surgical consultation. A sigmoid vovulus may be reduced by the passage of a sigmoidoscope. An elective corrective surgery can be done at a later time. On the other hand, cecal volvulus requires prompt surgical intervention to prevent bowel necrosis.

Pearls

1. Sigmoid volvulus can cause diffuse colonic distention, which may interfere with accurate CT interpretation. Rectal contrast may be needed to make the diagnosis of sigmoid volvulus.
2. In cases of cecal volvulus the cecum will always be displaced—this can be an important clue to diagnosis when the "whirl sign" is not present.

Radiographic Summary

Pancreatitis is an acute inflammatory process of the pancreas. Gallstones and alcohol use account for 80% of the cases seen in the United States. Pancreatic pseudocysts and abscesses are often a complication of acute pancreatitis. Extensive tissue necrosis and liquefaction may result in the formation of a pancreatic abscess. Pancreatic pseudocysts are collections of pancreatic secretions enclosed by fibrous or granulation tissue.

CT is the definitive radiographic study for the diagnosis of acute pancreatitis. Findings of pancreatitis include focal or diffuse enlargement of the pancreas, heterogeneous enhancement of the pancreatic parenchyma, and indistinct pancreatic margins. In addition, infiltration of peripancreatic fat, and

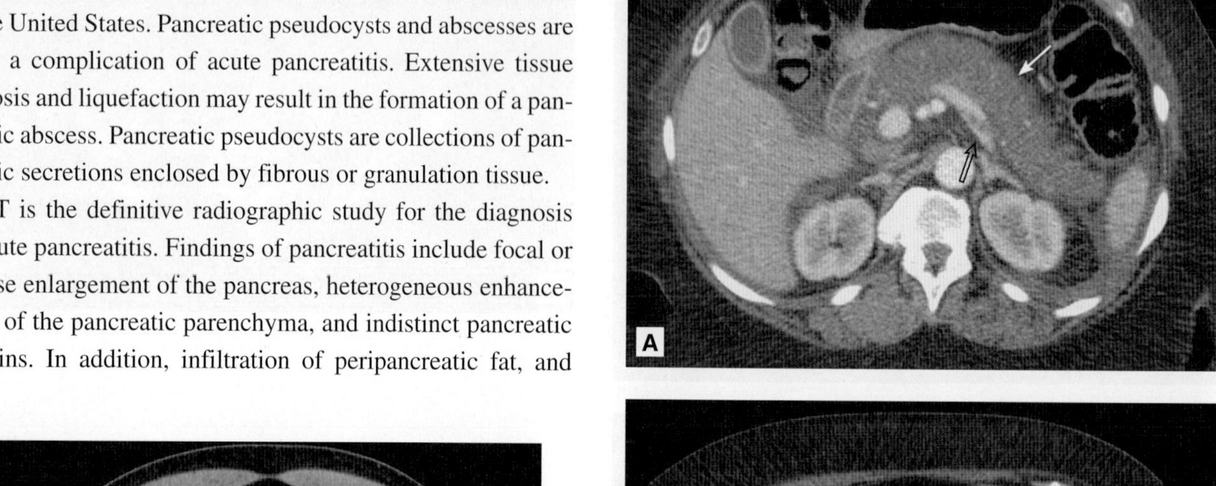

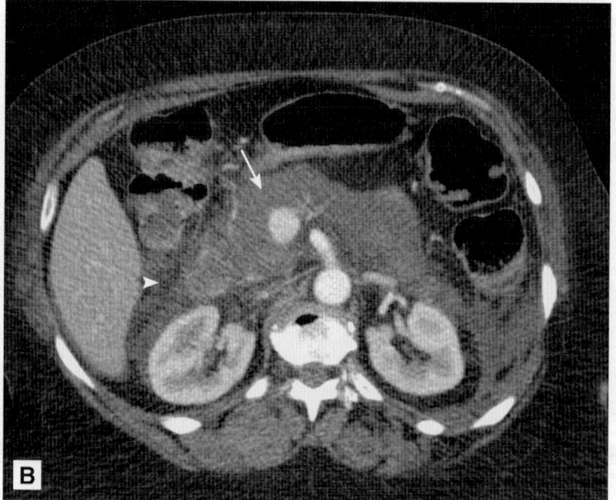

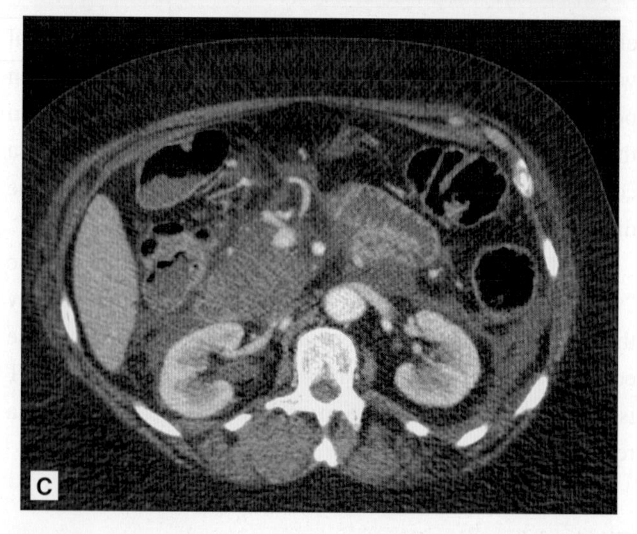

FIGURE 7.63 ■ Pancreatitis. **A-C:** The pancreas appears lower in attenuation with irregular contours in this case of severe pancreatitis (arrows). Intraabdominal and retroperitoneal fluid collections are seen (arrowhead). Low-density streaky thrombus within the splenic vein is visible (open arrow).

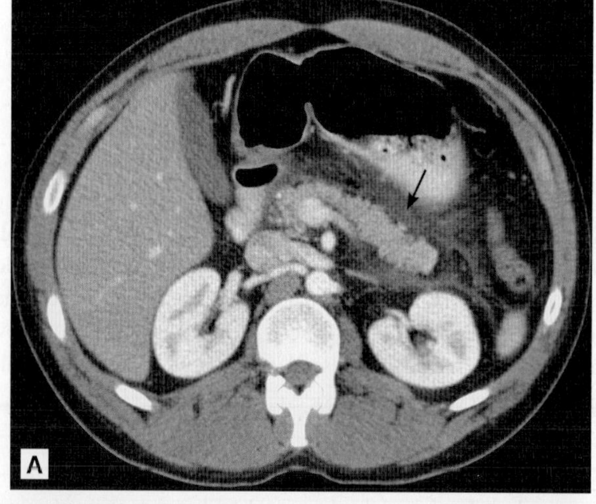

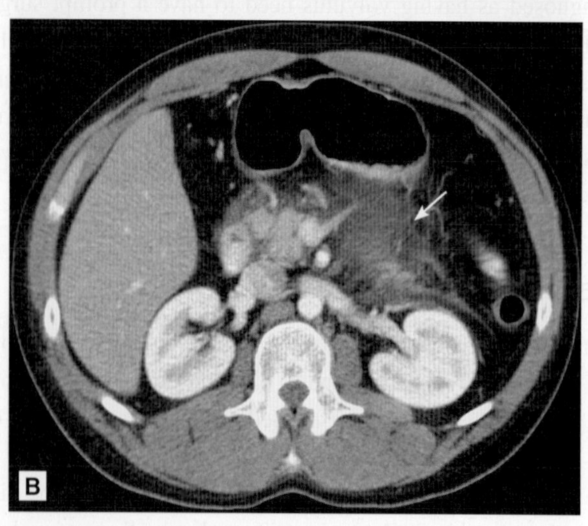

FIGURE 7.62 ■ Pancreatitis. **A, B:** Peripancreatic inflammation is seen on this contrast-enhanced CT of the abdomen (arrows). The pancreatic tissue continues to enhance normally, with no indications of pancreatic necrosis.

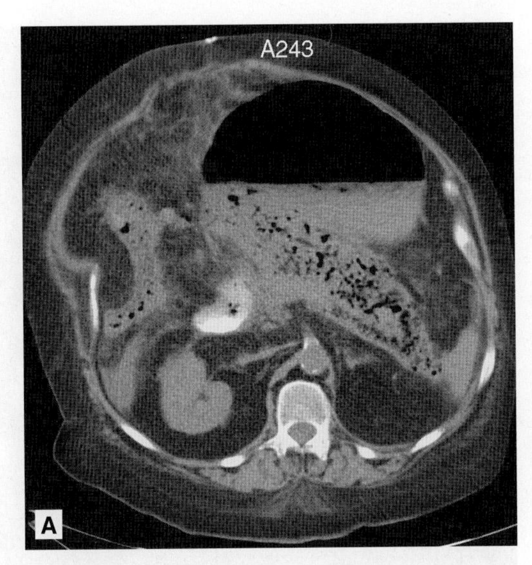

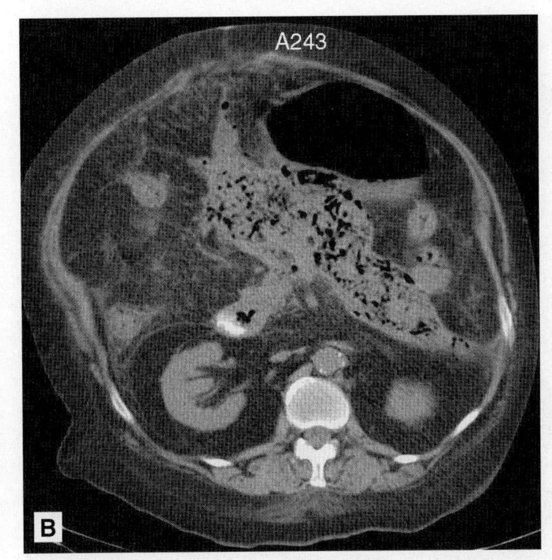

FIGURE 7.64 ■ Necrotizing Pancreatitis. **A, B:** Gas foci are seen throughout the entirety of the pancreas on this nonenhanced CT scan of the abdomen.

fluid collections in the peripancreatic and anterior pararenal spaces may be visualized.

CT can detect complications of acute pancreatitis including pancreatic pseudocysts, abscesses, necrosis, and thrombosis of the splenic or portal veins. Pancreatic pseudocysts will appear on CT scan as round or ovoid fluid collections with a defined wall which may or may not enhance with IV contrast. Pancreatic abscesses will appear as circumscribed thick-walled fluid collections with gas bubbles, or areas of poorly defined fluid collections with heterogeneous attenuation.

On ultrasound, acute pancreatitis will be visualized as an enlarged, hypoechoic pancreas. An ileus may prevent complete visualization due to bowel gas overlying the pancreas. A sonographic examination of the pancreas cannot quantify the extent of pancreatic inflammation or pancreatic necrosis, but is helpful in following pancreatic pseudocysts and the detection of gallstones.

Clinical Implications

The diagnosis of acute pancreatitis can be made on clinical and laboratory studies. Ranson's Criteria and APACHE II can be used to grade the severity of acute pancreatitis. The American College of Gastroenterology recommends that CT scanning with IV contrast be performed for any patient found to have severe pancreatitis. Mild cases of pancreatitis can be managed without a CT scan.

It is important to determine if gallstones are the cause of acute pancreatitis since 30-50% of patients with gallstone pancreatitis will suffer a recurrence if a cholecystectomy is not performed. Many clinicians will perform an ultrasound of the abdomen during a bout of nonalcoholic pancreatitis to rule out cholelithiasis.

Pearls

1. In cases of acute pancreatitis, MRI with gadolinium is equal to CT in diagnostic accuracy, and can be an alternative radiographic modality for the patient in whom iodinated contrast is contraindicated.
2. CT of the pancreas may appear normal in 25% of patients with mild pancreatitis.

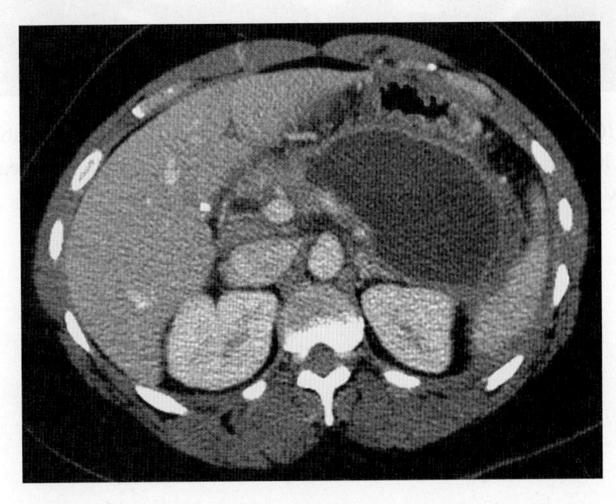

FIGURE 7.65 ■ Pancreatic Pseudocyst. An encapsulated fluid collection is seen associated with the pancreatic body and tail.

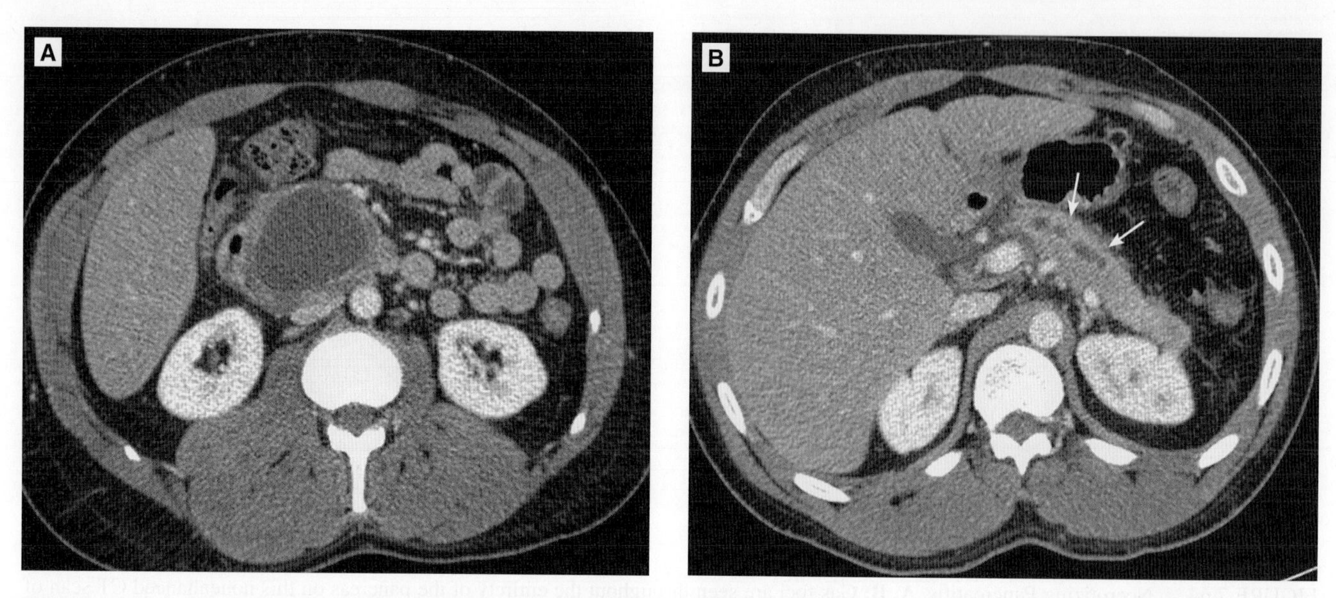

FIGURE 7.66 ■ Pancreatic Pseudocyst. **A, B:** In this patient with sequelae of chronic pancreatitis, a well-defined rounded fluid collection is identified within the pancreatic head. The pancreatic duct is enlarged and demonstrates a "beaded" configuration (arrows) as a result of repeated bouts of inflammation.

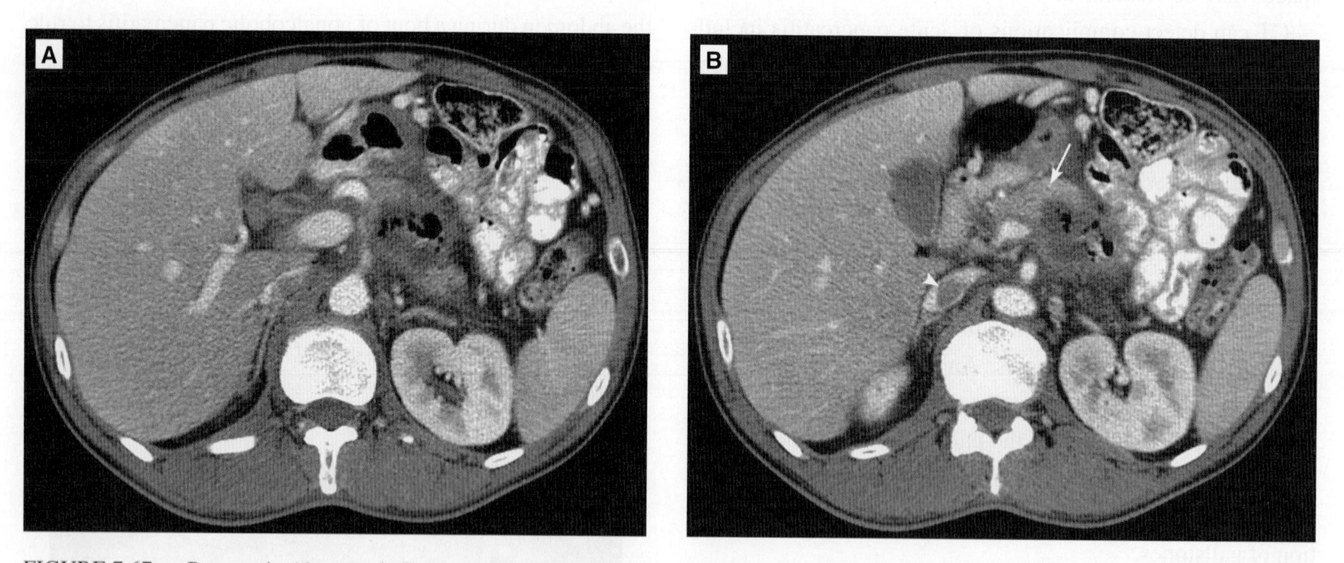

FIGURE 7.67 ■ Pancreatic Abscess. **A, B:** Centrally within the abdomen, a low attenuation necrotic collection with foci of gas is identified within the pancreas. Adjacent non-necrotic portions of the pancreatic body can be seen with normal enhancement (arrow). Clot within the IVC is also visible (arrowhead).

Radiographic Summary

A liver metastasis is a lesion that has spread from the original primary tumor to the liver. The liver is second only to the lymphatic system as a site of metastasis. Colon, gastric, pancreatic, breast, and lung cancers frequently metastasize to the liver. CT and MRI of the abdomen are the most sensitive modalities for the detection of liver metastasis. The majority of liver metastasis are hypovascular and will appear as hypoattentuated lesions on the IV contrasted CT scan. Ultrasound can detect liver metastases as well. The presence of metastasis may distort the shape of the liver, causing its surface to appear nodular or lobular.

Clinical Implications

Liver metastasis may present with a variety of signs and symptoms ranging from no symptoms and a normal exam to abdominal pain, jaundice, hepatomegaly, and ascites. If the clinician suspects liver metastasis, an abdominal CT with IV contrast should be obtained.

In the Emergency Department, liver metastasis may be detected as an incidental finding noted during the evaluation of an unrelated medical complaint. The abnormal radiologic exam may be the first indication that the patient has a malignancy. In the patient known to have a malignancy, the findings of liver metastasis may indicate heretofore-undetected disease progression. It is important to deliver unpleasant information to the patient in a tactful manner, preferably in a quiet, private setting. It should be stressed that the radiographic study is not a tissue diagnosis and that in all likelihood further procedures will be needed to obtain a definitive diagnosis. A reliable follow-up plan should be developed if the patient is discharged.

Pearls

1. Liver metastasis may radiographically resemble other types of lesions that commonly appear in the liver, for instance, multiple hemangiomas and benign cysts may be mistaken for metastasis.
2. On ultrasound examination, multiple hepatic nodules of differing sizes and echogenicity are worrisome for metastasis.

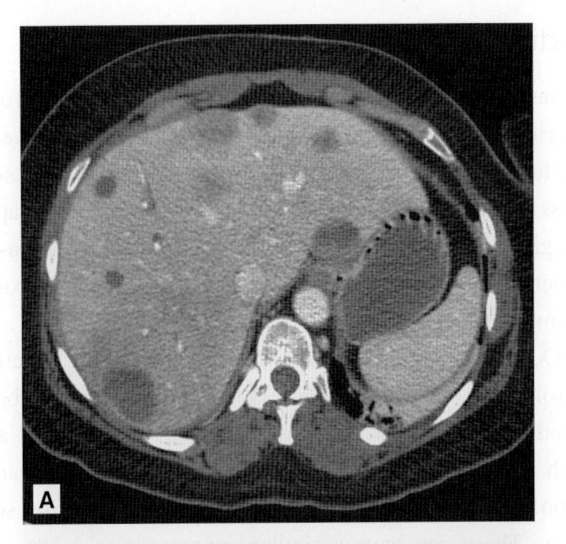

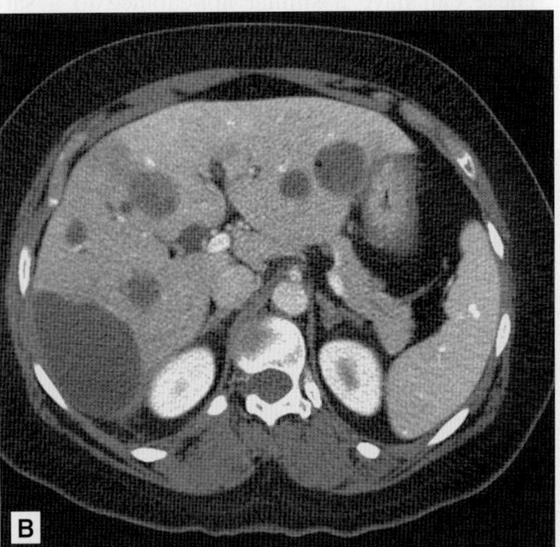

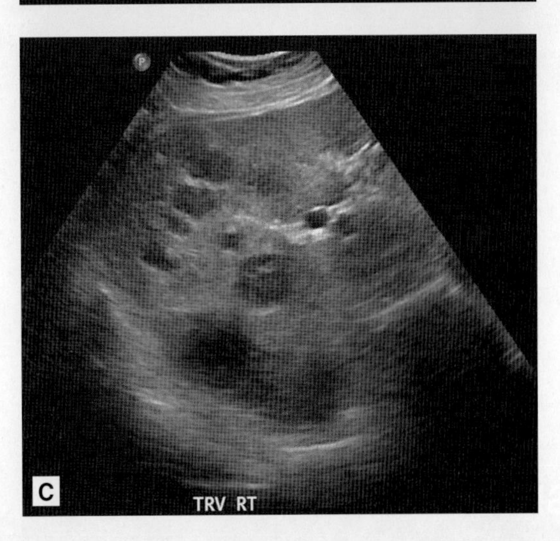

FIGURE 7.68 ■ Liver Metastasis. **A, B:** Rounded low- attenuation lesions are seen throughout all lobes of the liver on contrasted CT of the abdomen in a patient with metastatic colon carcinoma. **C:** In the same patient, ultrasound evaluation demonstrates low echotexture lesions throughout the liver.

Radiographic Summary

Ultrasound is the preferred method to image uterine fibroids. Uterine fibroids are benign smooth muscle and connective tissue tumors that most commonly appear as a hypoechoic solid mass within the muscular layer of the uterus on sonographic imaging. However, they can also appear heterogeneous or hyperechoic and can be found prolapsing into the myometrium or as an exophytic uterine mass.

Occasionally, fibroids may calcify or necrose. Calcified fibroids can be seen on plain radiographs and CT. Fibroid calcifications appear as a well-defined hyperechoic area with acoustic shadowing. Necrotic fibroids will appear as hypoechoic to anechoic spaces within an otherwise solid mass. These can have a similar appearance to a sarcoma, especially if associated with a significant amount of free fluid in the pelvis.

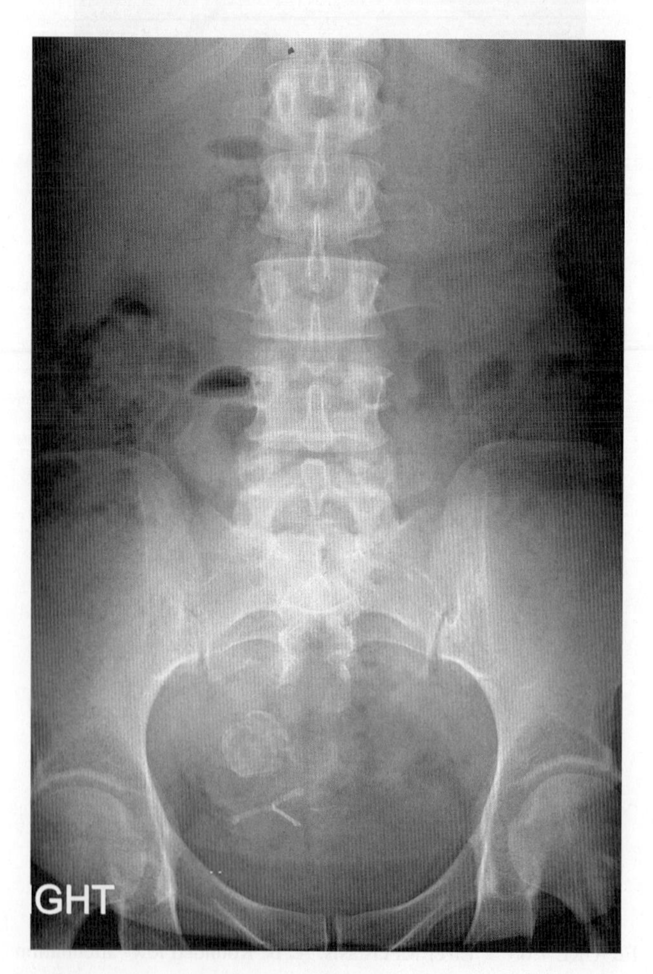

FIGURE 7.69 ■ Uterine Fibroid Tumor. A peripherally calcified rounded mass is seen in the right hemipelvis on this plain radiograph. This fibroid tumor in this patient is seen in proximity to an intrauterine device.

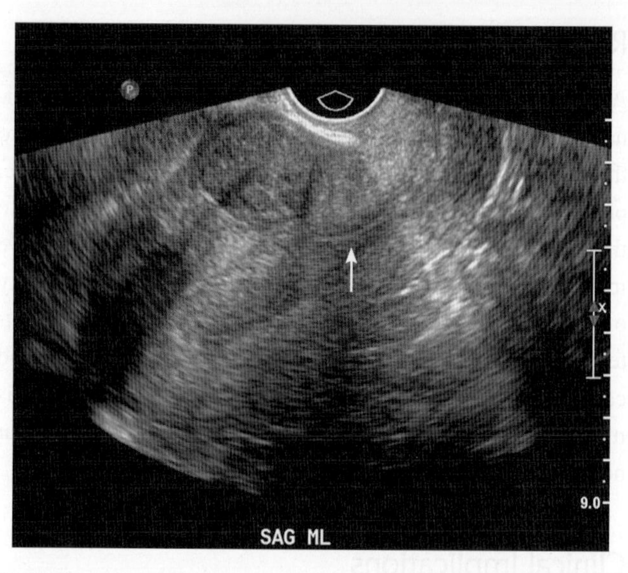

FIGURE 7.70 ■ Uterine Fibroid Tumor. An anterior myometrial and subserosal fibroid tumor is seen as a mixed echotexture mass on this sagittal sonographic image. The endometrial stripe (arrow) is not affected by this anterior mass.

Uterine fibroids usually have a straightforward sonographic appearance. However, they have been termed the "pelvic mimicker" as they can mimic many other pathologic pelvic conditions such as adnexal masses, uterine duplication, adenomyosis, ectopic pregnancy, and other pregnancy-related conditions. On CT, noncalcified uterine fibroids are isodense to hypodense as compared to the uterine wall.

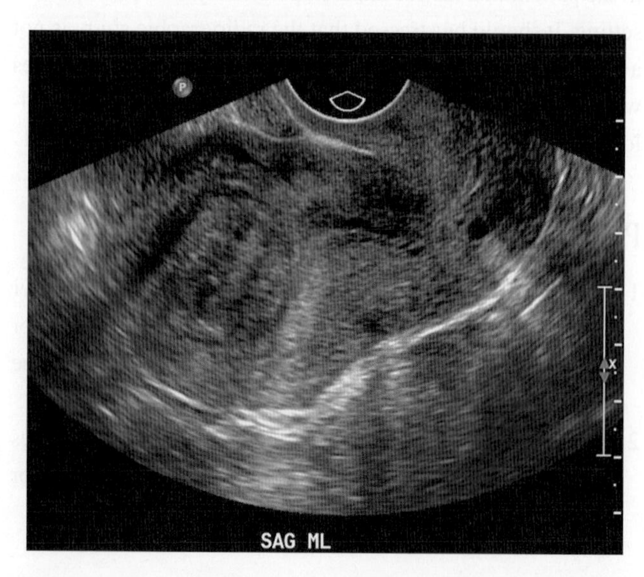

FIGURE 7.71 ■ Uterine Fibroid Tumor. A mixed echotexture rounded fibroid tumor is seen in the fundus, measuring nearly 3 cm in size. The mass extends to the submucosal region superiorly.

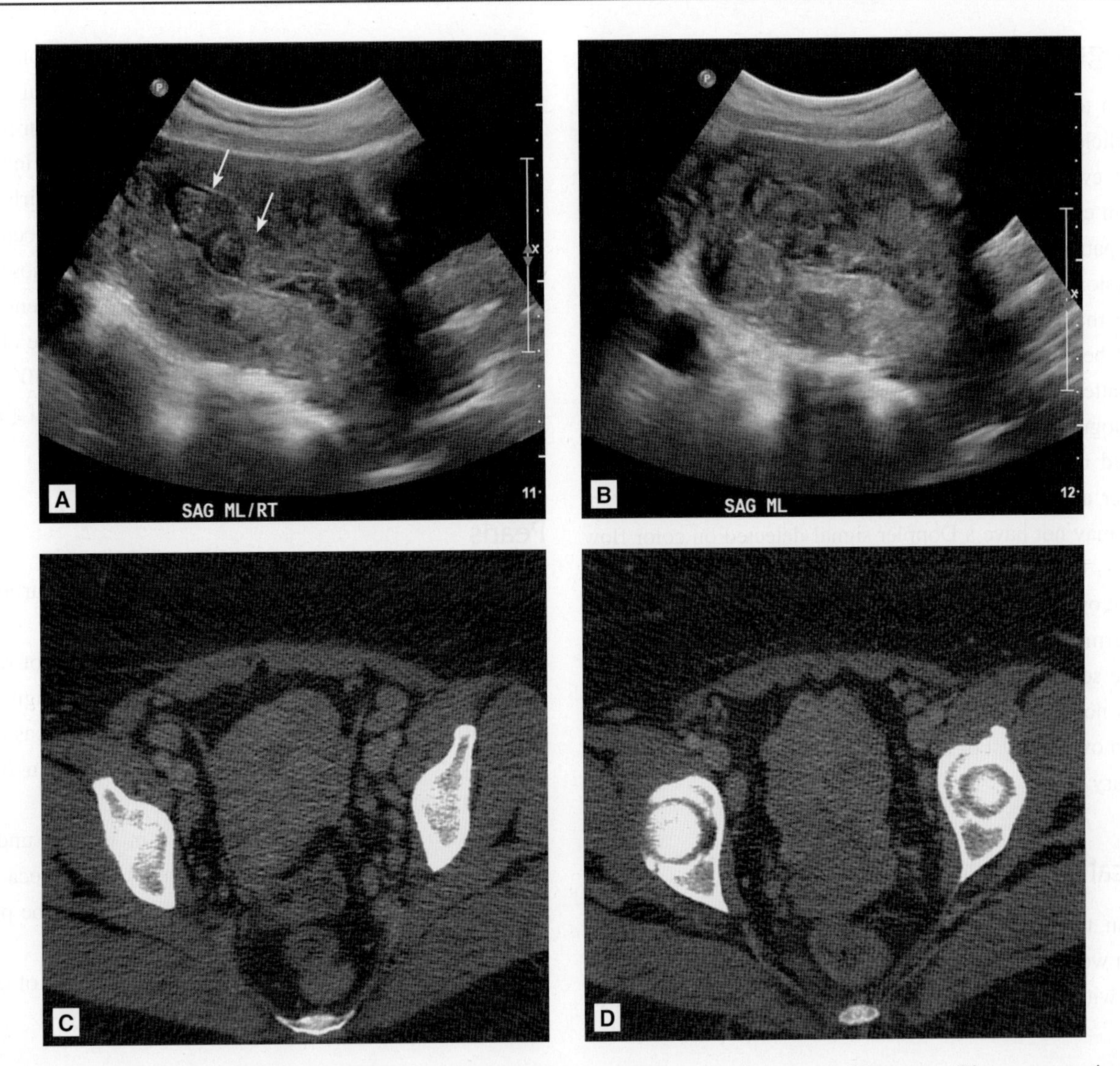

FIGURE 7.72 ■ Uterine Fibroid Tumor. **A, B:** Numerous fibroid tumors alter the normal contours of the uterus. There are prominent submucosal fibroids distorting the endometrium (arrows). **C, D:** In the same patient, CT scan demonstrates the enlarged fibroid uterus in the midline of the pelvis.

Clinical Implications

Fibroids are benign soft tissue tumors that arise from smooth muscle. They occur more frequently in African American women and those over the age of 30. They are usually asymptomatic and discovered incidentally on ultrasound examination.

Patients presenting to the ED with menorrhagia or metromenorrhagia may have fibroids that impair the ability of the uterus to effectively contract and stop menstrual bleeding. These patients may also have significant pain as a result of uterine contraction.

Patients with menorrhagia and metromenorrhagia should be referred to a gynecologist for further treatment. Definitive treatment is a hysterectomy, however more treatment options are currently available including myomectomy, embolization, and high frequency, focused ultrasound.

Pearls

1. Although rare, uterine leiomyosarcomas may appear similar to benign fibroid tumors on ultrasound. A rapidly enlarging uterine mass should be considered suspicious for sarcoma.
2. Large and exophytic fibroid tumors may be a cause of ureteral compression and hydronephrosis. Be sure to image the renal collecting systems during ultrasound examination in these patients.

Radiographic Summary

Ovarian torsion occurs when the ovary twists on its vascular pedicle causing acute ovarian ischemia. Ovarian torsion is best evaluated by transvaginal ultrasound with Doppler. Ovarian enlargement is the most common sonographic finding in patients with ovarian torsion. Most patients with ovarian torsion will have an ovarian mass or cyst that measures greater than 4 cm. Color flow and spectral Doppler analysis should be performed to assess for both arterial and venous flow patterns.

Sonographically, it is often impossible to differentiate a torsed ovary from other adnexal masses. In these cases, Doppler analysis is not always helpful as normal ovaries at times, may not have a Doppler signal detected on color flow analysis. Furthermore, a detectable Doppler signal does not rule out ovarian torsion as the interruption of blood flow may be intermittent. In these cases, a "hyperemic" flow pattern may be seen as the diastolic flow is increased when the torsion is not present. CT may demonstrate an enlarged ovary with an ovarian cyst or mass, but cannot assess blood flow to the ovary.

Clinical Implications

Ovarian torsion classically presents with unilateral pelvic pain in women of childbearing age. It is almost always associated with a pathologically enlarged ovary due to a cyst or mass measuring greater than 4 cm. Ovarian torsion is possible with smaller masses or cysts or even in normal ovaries. Approximately 20% of cases of ovarian torsion occur in pregnancy as a result of a large corpus luteum cyst and increased ligamentous laxity in the pelvis. In prepubescent girls, ovarian torsion often presents with normal ovaries and occurs as a result of a long fallopian tube or absence of the mesosalpinx.

Patients with ovarian torsion should have emergent evaluation by a gynecologist in an attempt to salvage the affected ovary. Although the ovarian salvage rate is low (<10%), earlier diagnosis allows for laparoscopic treatment and a reduction in complications.

Pearls

1. Ovarian torsion is very unlikely in normal appearing ovaries without a cyst or mass.
2. Sonographic Doppler signal findings should not replace clinical suspicion to rule in or rule out the diagnosis of ovarian torsion as Doppler signal may on occasion, be undetectable in normal ovaries and present in ovaries with intermittent torsion.
3. Ovarian torsion is more common in women undergoing ovarian stimulation. In these cases, large theca lutein cysts may alter the position of the fallopian tube predisposing to ovarian torsion.
4. Ultrasound with Doppler is the imaging study of choice to evaluate the ovaries and uterus.

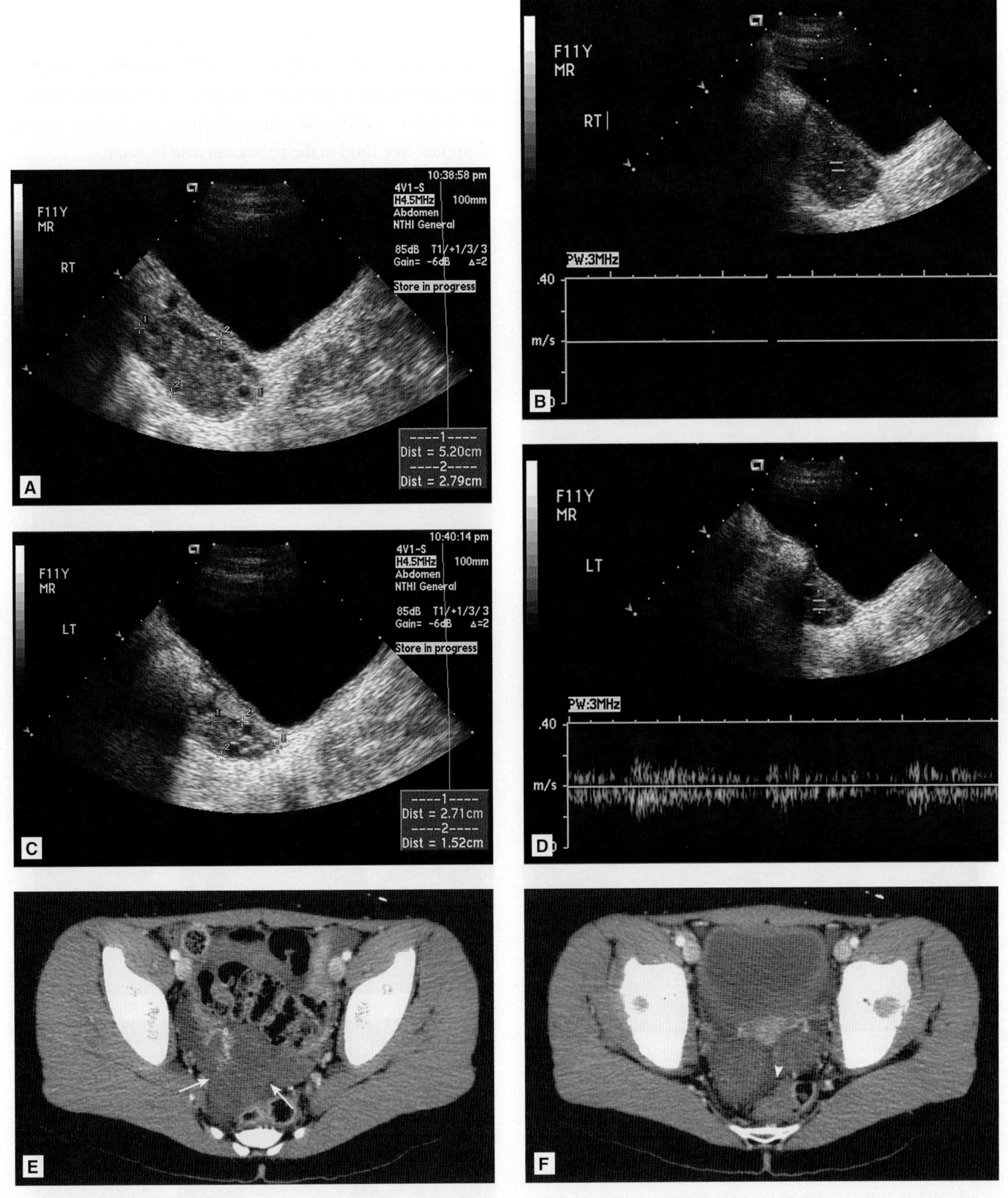

FIGURE 7.73 ■ Ovarian Torsion. **A-D:** The enlarged right ovary is seen with multiple peripheral follicles. Color Doppler evaluation and m-mode imaging reveals no internal flow. For comparison, the normal left ovary is imaged. **E, F:** On the CT of the same patient, the enlarged right ovary is demonstrated (arrows), with a small amount of free fluid in the pelvis (arrowhead). CT scan alone is rarely (if ever) diagnostic of ovarian torsion.

TUBO-OVARIAN ABSCESS

Radiographic Summary

A tubo-ovarian abscess (TOA) is an inflammatory mass of the fallopian tube, ovary, and adjacent structures. Ultrasound is the test of choice to evaluate for TOA or other findings consistent with PID but may be limited in some patients due to pain and tenderness.

On ultrasound, hydrosalpinx with an associated complex adnexal mass with a central hypoechoic area is suggestive of a TOA. While a hydrosalpinx is a fluid-filled fallopian tube, a pyosalpinx has the appearance of a thick-walled tube, absence of Doppler signal, and internal echoes suggesting debris. Complex free fluid in the pelvis can also be seen.

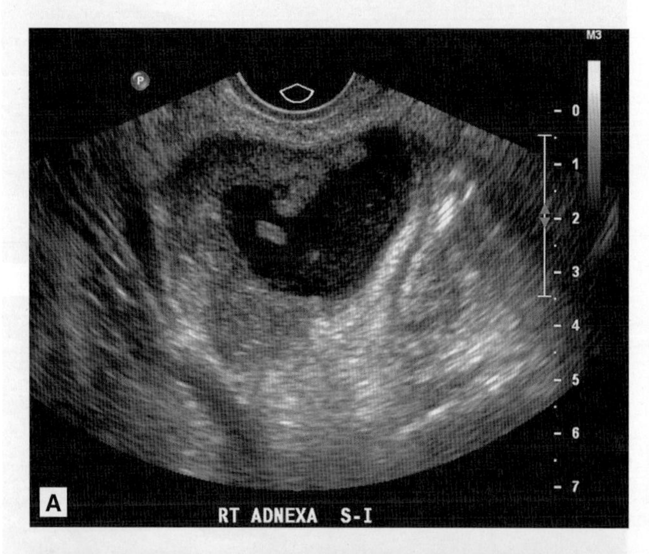

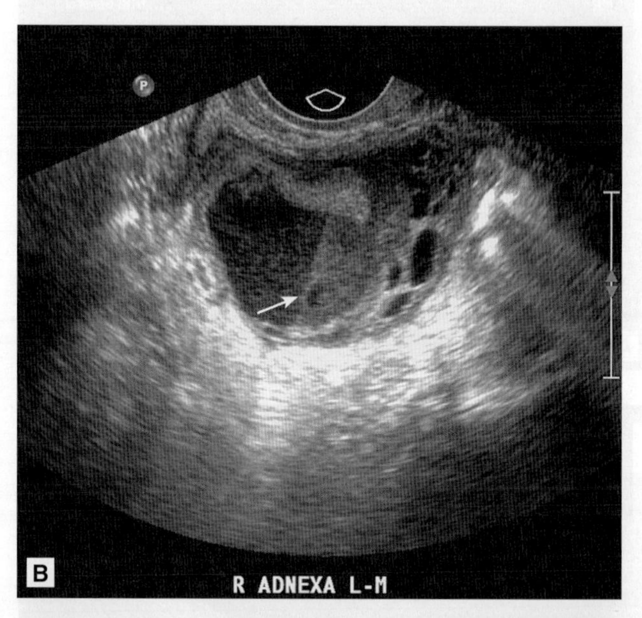

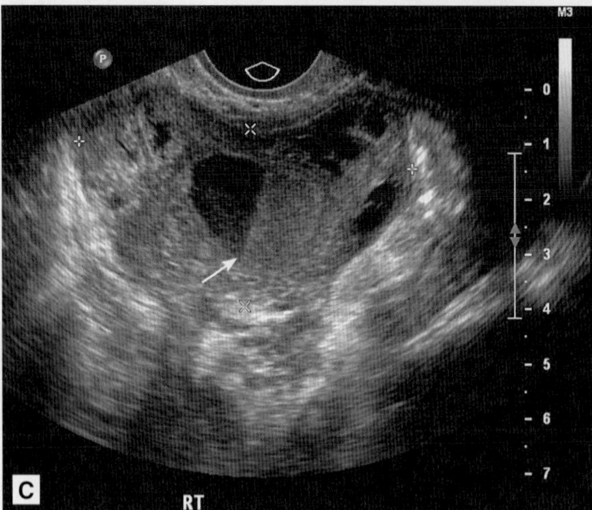

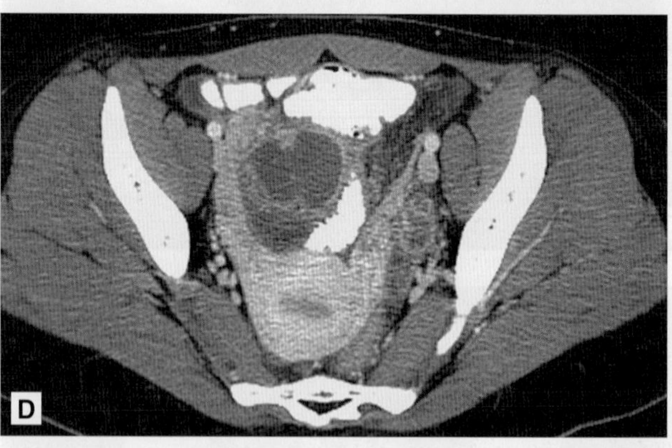

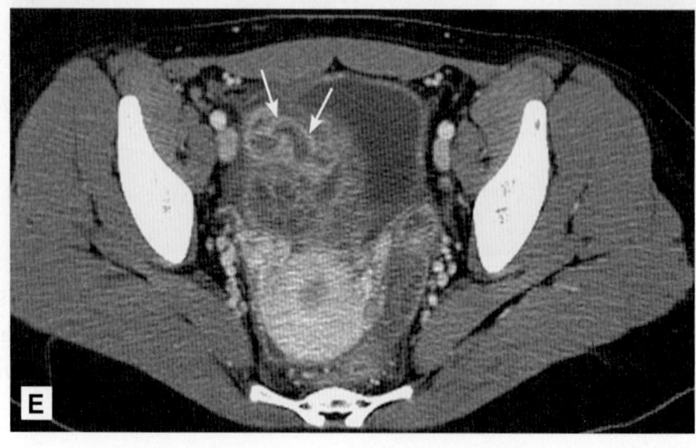

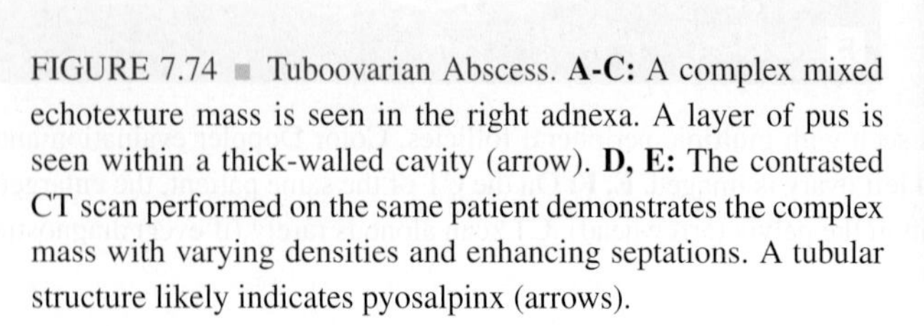

FIGURE 7.74 ■ Tuboovarian Abscess. **A-C:** A complex mixed echotexture mass is seen in the right adnexa. A layer of pus is seen within a thick-walled cavity (arrow). **D, E:** The contrasted CT scan performed on the same patient demonstrates the complex mass with varying densities and enhancing septations. A tubular structure likely indicates pyosalpinx (arrows).

The sonographic appearance of a TOA is nonspecific and can appear similar to several other conditions including ectopic pregnancy, ovarian tumors, endometriomas, hemorrhagic ovarian cysts, and abscesses in adjacent bowel. On a CT, a TOA appears as a complex pelvic mass with regular margins that contains debris. It may appear similar to an endometrioma or hemorrhagic ovarian cyst. An associated low-attenuation area representing a fluid-filled fallopian tube may also be present.

Clinical Implications

Pelvic inflammatory disease (PID) is caused by an ascending infection from the vagina and cervix. Patients with PID rarely develop a TOA and routine imaging is not indicated. In patients who appear toxic or have evidence of sepsis, imaging is extremely helpful as patients with a TOA, in addition to receiving antibiotics that cover *Nisseria gonorrhea* and *Chlamdyia trachomatis*, should receive antibiotics that cover gram-negative organisms, anaerobes, and Streptococci. Patients with TOA should have emergent gynecologic evaluation and should be admitted to the hospital for IV antibiotics and close surveillance.

Up to 80% of patients with evidence of a TOA will improve with antibiotics alone and do not require surgical drainage. However, patients that do not respond to treatment within 72 hours or have evidence of a ruptured TOA need surgical exploration and drainage.

Pearls

1. Evaluate for TOA in patients with PID and sepsis or failure to improve within 72 hours of antibiotics administration.
2. Patients with TOA should be admitted for IV antibiotics. Most patients improve without the need for surgical drainage.

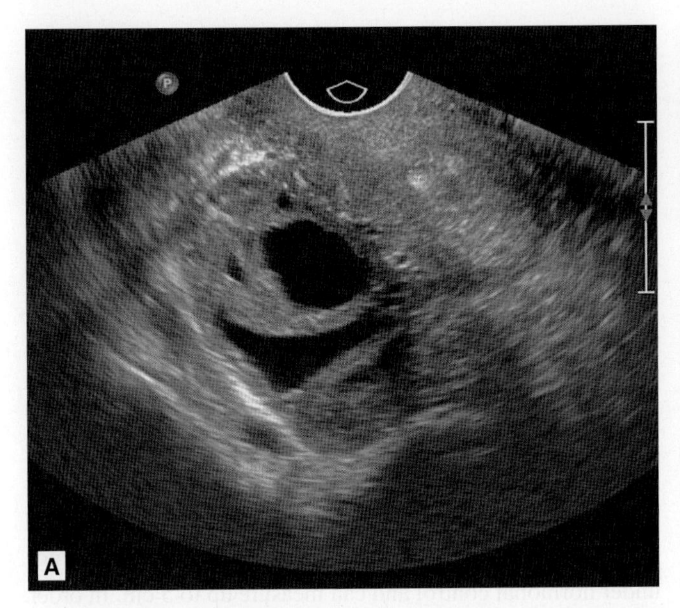

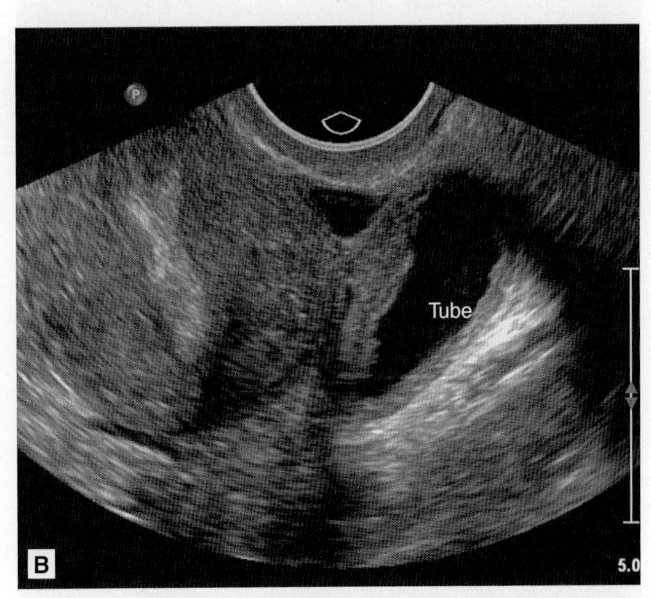

FIGURE 7.75 ■ Tuboovarian Abscess. **A, B:** A complex mass with thick echogenic septations is present in the right adnexa. The enlarged fallopian tube is identified.

Radiographic Summary

An ovarian cyst is a fluid-filled sac within the ovary. Transabdominal and transvaginal sonography are the tests of choice to evaluate and characterize ovarian cysts. CT offers no additional benefit, except in identifying other potential causes of pelvic pain or bleeding. Simple ovarian cysts have thin (<3 mm) smooth walls, are anechoic and usually measure up to 2.5 cm, but can measure as much as 5 cm. Simple ovarian cysts are either functional or nonfunctional and are almost always benign.

Complex ovarian cysts have thick, irregular walls with septa or internal echoes. Complex ovarian cysts have a wide differential diagnosis including hemorrhagic cyst, teratoma, endometrioma, ovarian torsion, abscess, or cystic neoplasm.

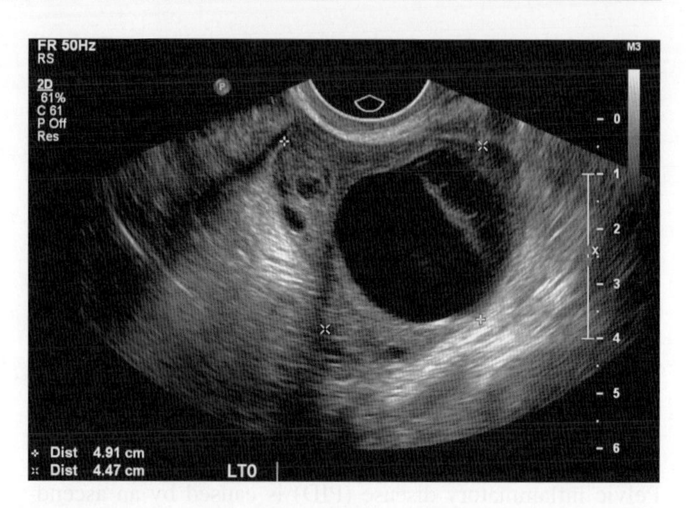

FIGURE 7.77 ■ Hemorrhagic Corpus Luteum Cyst. A thick-walled cyst is seen with complex internal echoes within the left ovary.

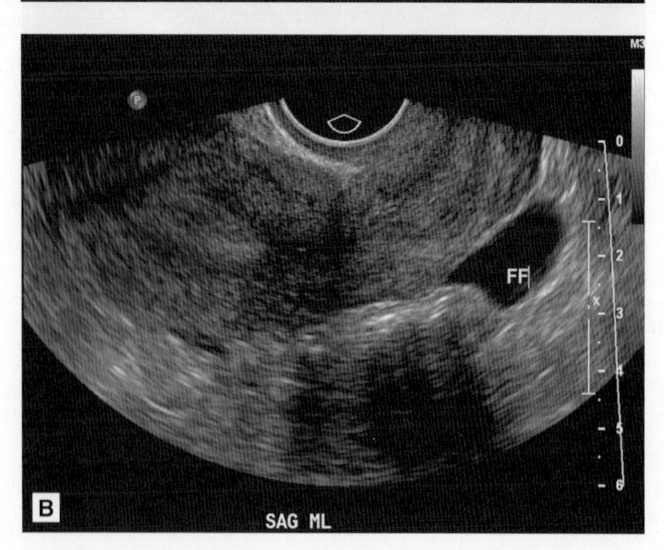

FIGURE 7.76 ■ Functional Ovarian Cyst. **A, B:** Grayscale sonographic images demonstrate a 2 cm thin-walled ovarian cyst, typical of a mature follicle. Note smaller peripheral follicles in the left ovary. A physiologic quantity of free fluid is noted in the cul-de-sac.

Clinical Implications

Ovarian cysts can be divided into functional, nonfunctional, and neoplastic. Functional cysts are always benign and are most common in women of reproductive age arising from the normal process of ovulation. They are under hormonal control and vary in size throughout the menstrual cycle. Each month a dominant follicle known as the Graafian follicle ruptures and releases an oocyte. This ruptured follicle then becomes the corpus luteum and at maturity usually measures up to 2 cm. Multiple functional cysts can occur as a result of excessive gonadotropin stimulation and can be seen in patients being treated for infertility, in patients with a molar pregnancy, or rarely multiple or diabetic pregnancy.

Nonfunctional ovarian cysts are simple cysts that are not under hormonal control and can measure up to 5 cm. In order to differentiate functional from nonfunctional cysts a repeat ultrasound may be performed 6 weeks later; a simple cyst that is unchanged in size and shape on follow-up is a nonfunctional cyst. Cysts that are greater than 5 cm are more likely to be neoplastic and warrant further investigation.

Simple ovarian cysts are usually asymptomatic but can cause pain or discomfort as a result of torsion, rupture, hemorrhage, or pressure on adjacent anatomic structures. Complex ovarian cysts require follow-up imaging and referral to a gynecologist.

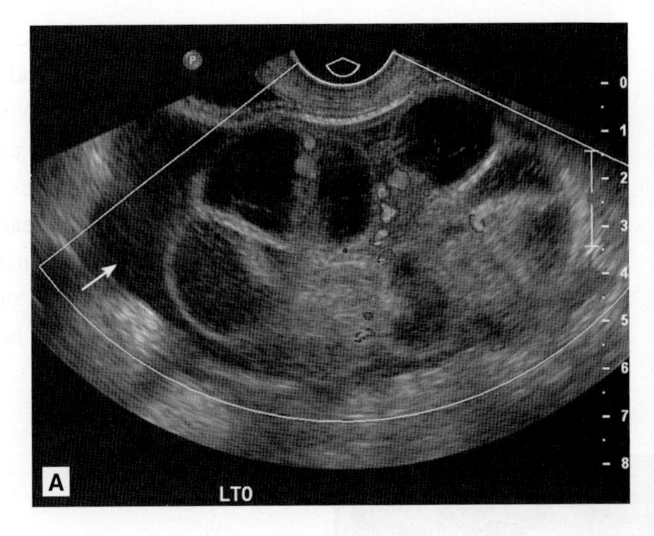

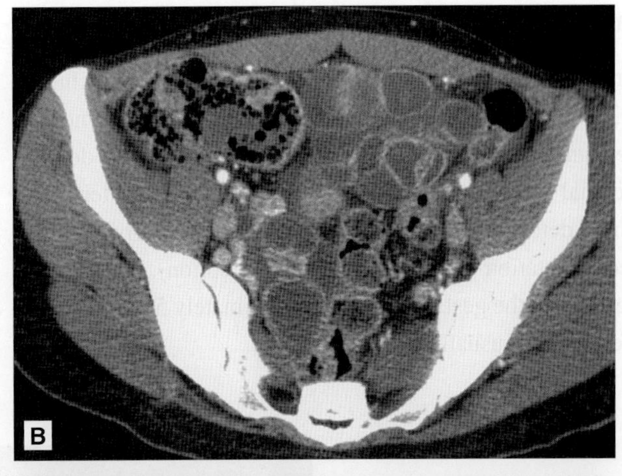

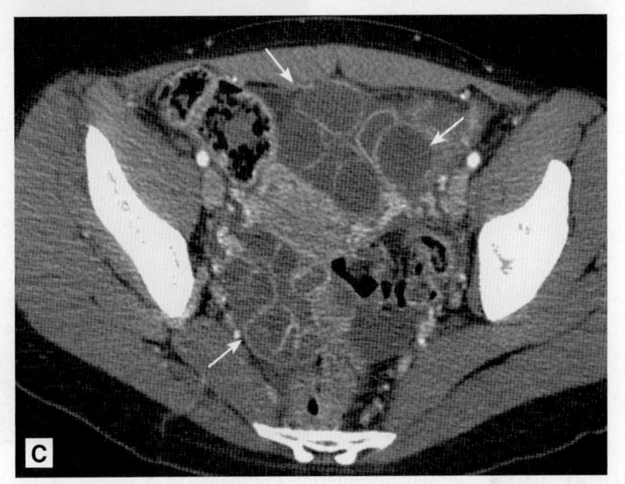

FIGURE 7.78 ■ Ovarian Hyperstimulation Syndrome. **A:** Numerous large ovarian follicles are seen on transvaginal sonogram in this patient receiving clomiphene citrate for infertility treatment. Note the small amount of free fluid adjacent to the enlarged left ovary (arrow). **B, C:** CT scan in the same patient demonstrates the markedly enlarged ovaries with numerous cysts (arrows). The normal uterus is seen in the midline.

Pearls

1. Functional ovarian cysts are always benign, have a simple anechoic appearance, are less than 2.5 cm, and vary in size according to the menstrual cycle.
2. Ovarian cysts that are complex (thick walled, contain internal echoes) should have follow-up imaging in 6 weeks to evaluate for resolution or changes in size.
3. Simple ovarian cysts do not require repeat imaging unless they have mixed internal echoes, are larger than 2.5 cm, or occur in post-menopausal women.
4. Ovarian cysts are most often asymptomatic and a thorough search for other causes of pelvic pain should be excluded before attributing the pain to an ovarian cyst.

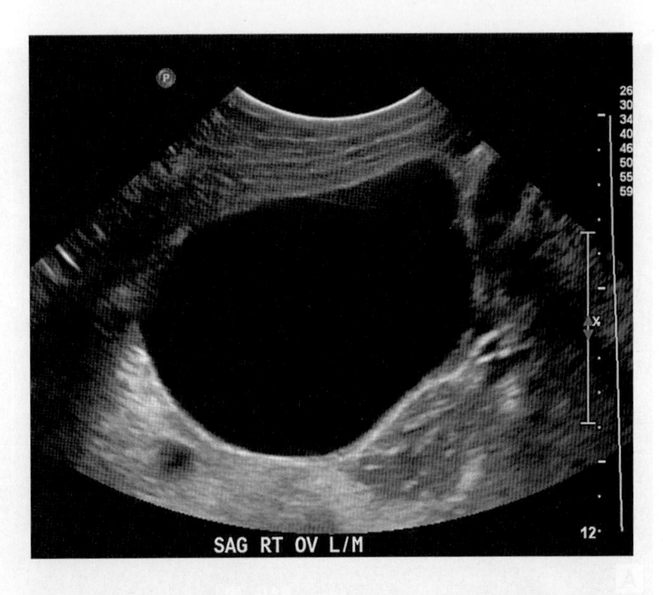

FIGURE 7.79 ■ Ovarian Cyst. A large simple-appearing right ovarian cyst is seen, measuring 10 cm in size. Follow-up imaging in 6 weeks (not shown) demonstrated complete resolution.

Radiographic Summary

Ultrasound is the modality of choice to evaluate and characterize pregnancy. The first sonographic evidence of a normal pregnancy is the gestation sac characterized by a double-decidual reaction within the body or fundus of the uterus and can be detected by transvaginal ultrasound as early as 4 ½-5 weeks gestation (2 ½-3 weeks from conception). A yolk sac is seen within the gestation sac at approximately 5 ½ weeks and a fetal pole is usually seen by 6 weeks.

The location of the gestational sac is important to assess and should be located within the central portion of the body or fundus of the uterus. A gestational sac located in the cervix or cornua of the uterus, while still within the uterus, is an ectopic pregnancy.

A fetal pole or yolk sac is usually present when the mean gestational sac diameter measures 1 cm. A mean gestational sac greater than 16 mm without a fetal pole is diagnostic of an anembryonic pregnancy. Fetal cardiac activity should be

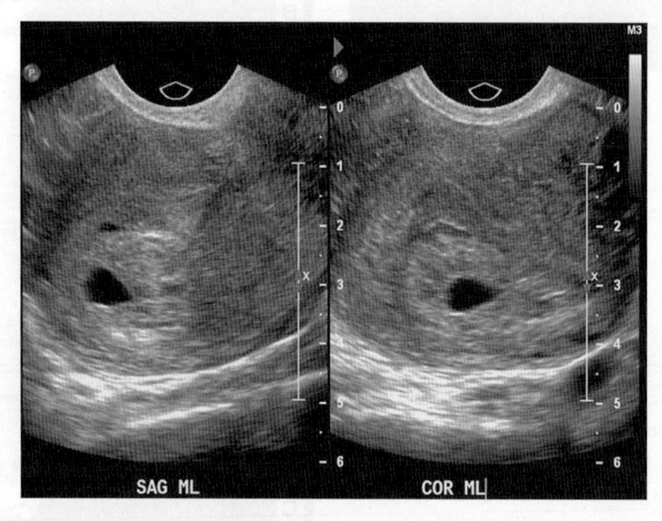

FIGURE 7.80 ■ Normal Intrauterine Pregnancy at 5 Weeks. A normal gestational sac is seen at 5 weeks. The sac has an expected ovoid shape with adjacent decidual reaction. No Yolk sac or fetal pole is seen at this stage.

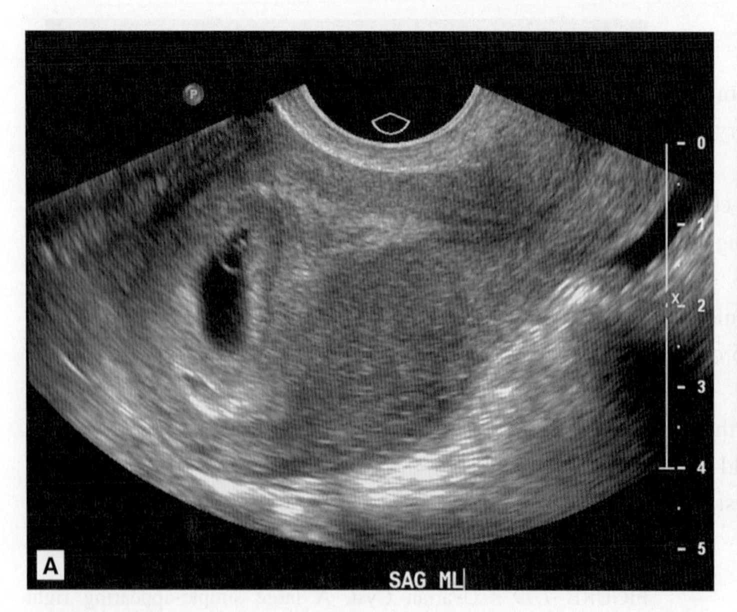

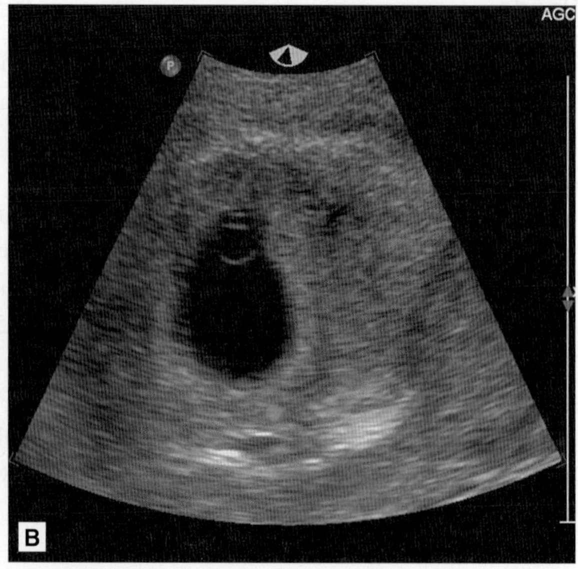

FIGURE 7.81 ■ Normal Intrauterine Pregnancy at 5.5 Weeks. **A, B:** Transvaginal images now demonstrate a rounded yolk sac within the gestational sac.

measured when present and is usually between 120 and 160 beats per minute. Evidence of fetal cardiac activity should be present by the time the fetal pole measures 5 mm and lack of fetal cardiac activity in a fetal pole over 7 mm is indicative of fetal demise.

Clinical Implications

Patients with vaginal bleeding or pelvic pain and a positive pregnancy test should have sonographic imaging to confirm the presence of an intrauterine pregnancy. While a gestational sac is the first evidence of a normal intra-uterine pregnancy, a pseudogestational sac may mimic an intrauterine pregnancy and will measure less than 1 cm in diameter. A definitive intrauterine pregnancy can therefore only be determined by the presence of a gestational sac that measures greater than 1 cm or contains a yolk sac or fetal pole.

Patients with a normal intrauterine pregnancy who are not receiving fertility treatment should be given return miscarriage precautions and can be safely discharged with routine obstetric follow-up. Patients receiving fertility treatment have an increased risk of heterotopic pregnancy and management should be done in conjunction with a gynecologist.

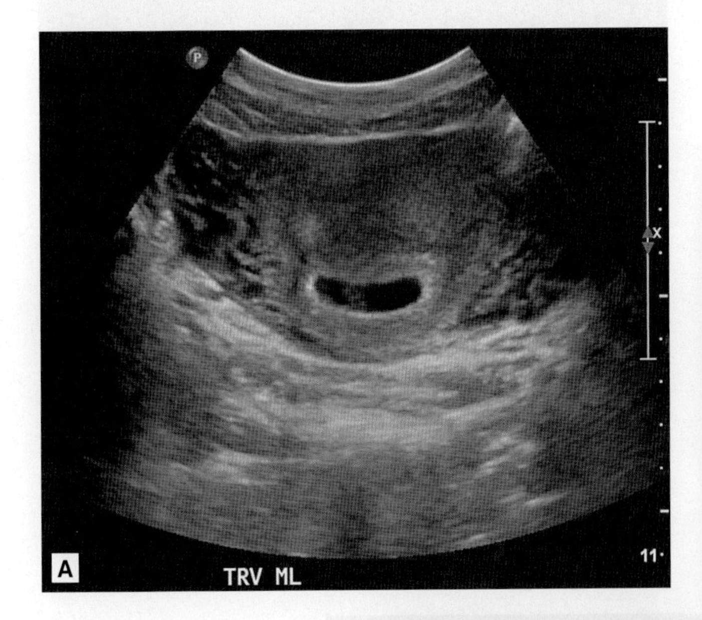

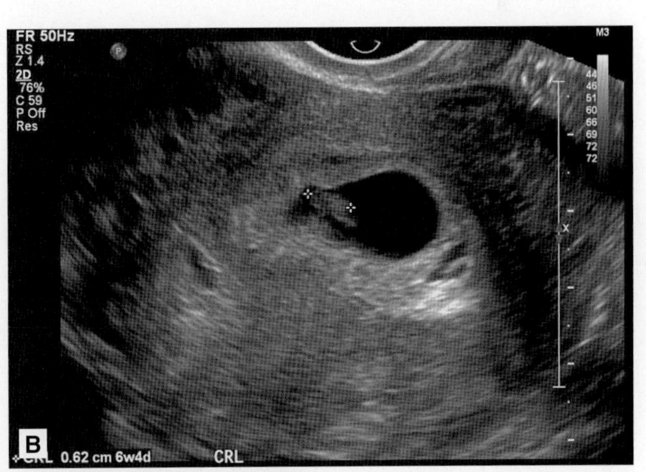

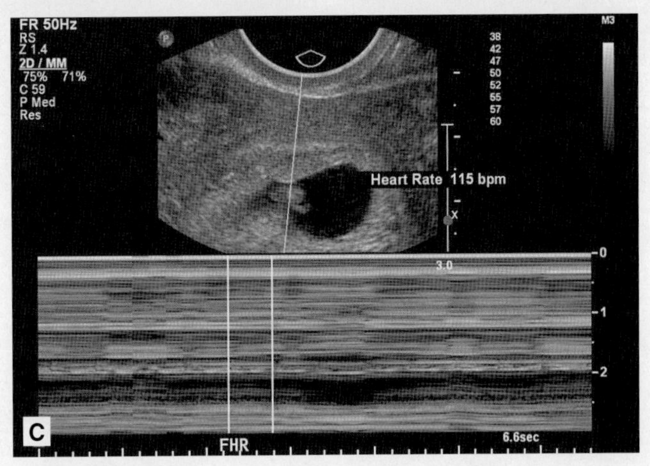

FIGURE 7.82 ■ Normal Intrauterine Pregnancy at 6.5 Weeks. **A-C:** A fetal pole is identified, with an estimated gestational age of 6 weeks, 4 days based on crown-rump-length. The fetal heart rate is detected and measured by m-mode sonography.

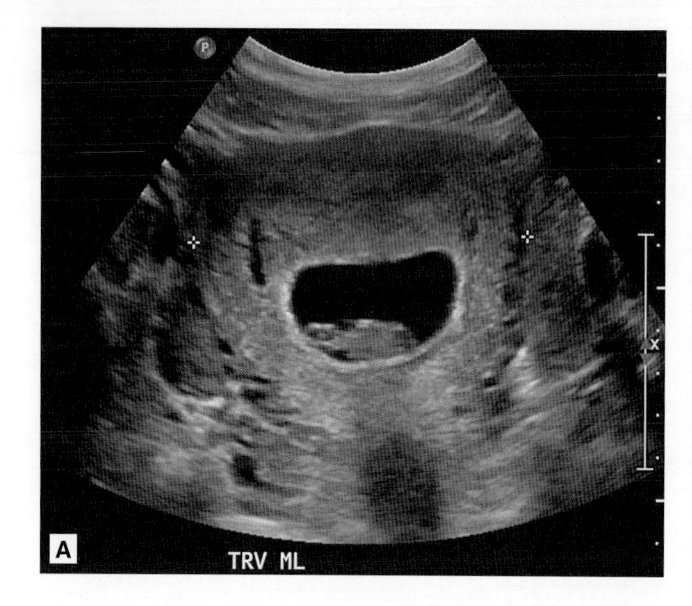

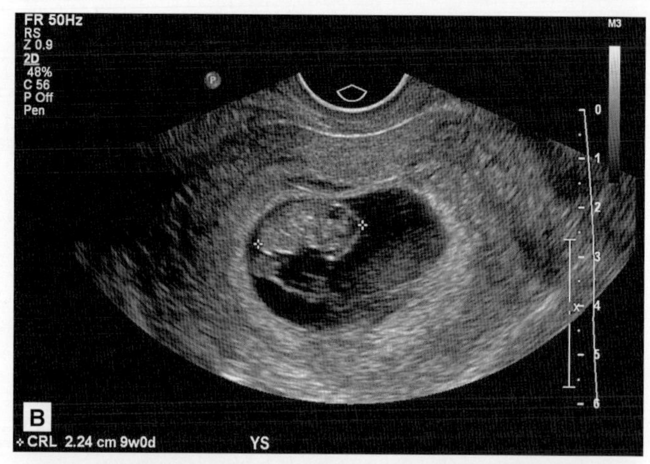

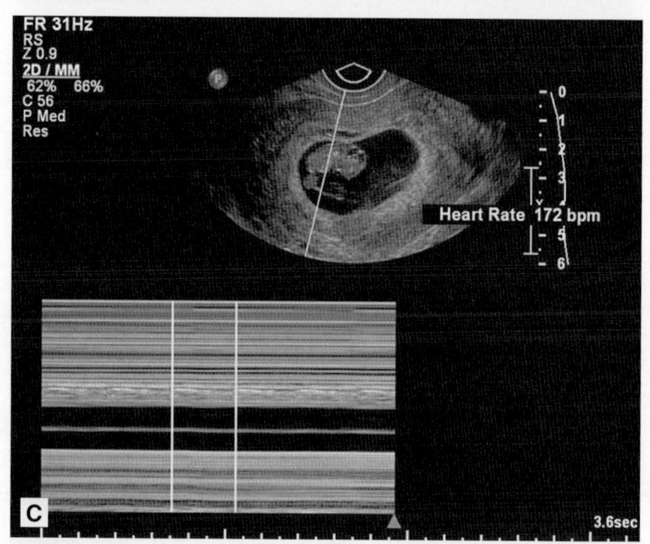

FIGURE 7.83 ■ Normal Intrauterine Pregnancy at 8 Weeks, 5 Days. **A-C.**

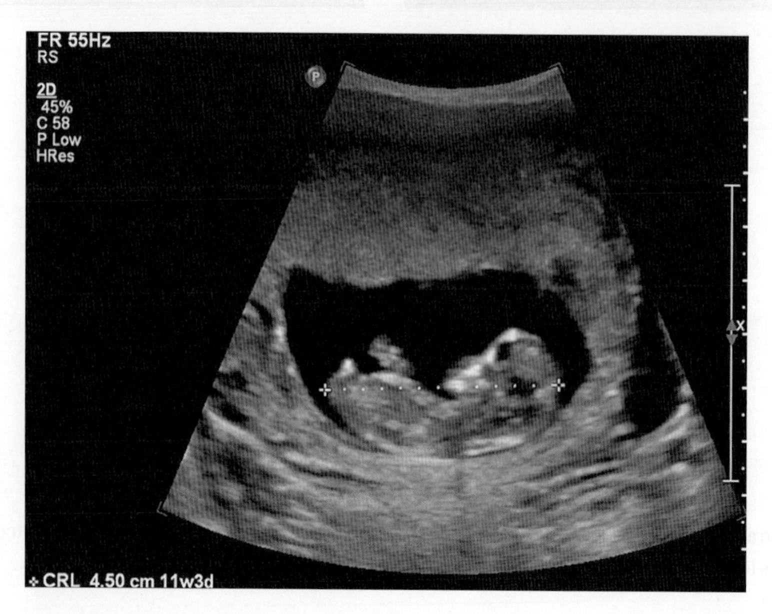

FIGURE 7.84 ■ Normal Intrauterine Pregnancy at 11 Weeks, 3 Days.

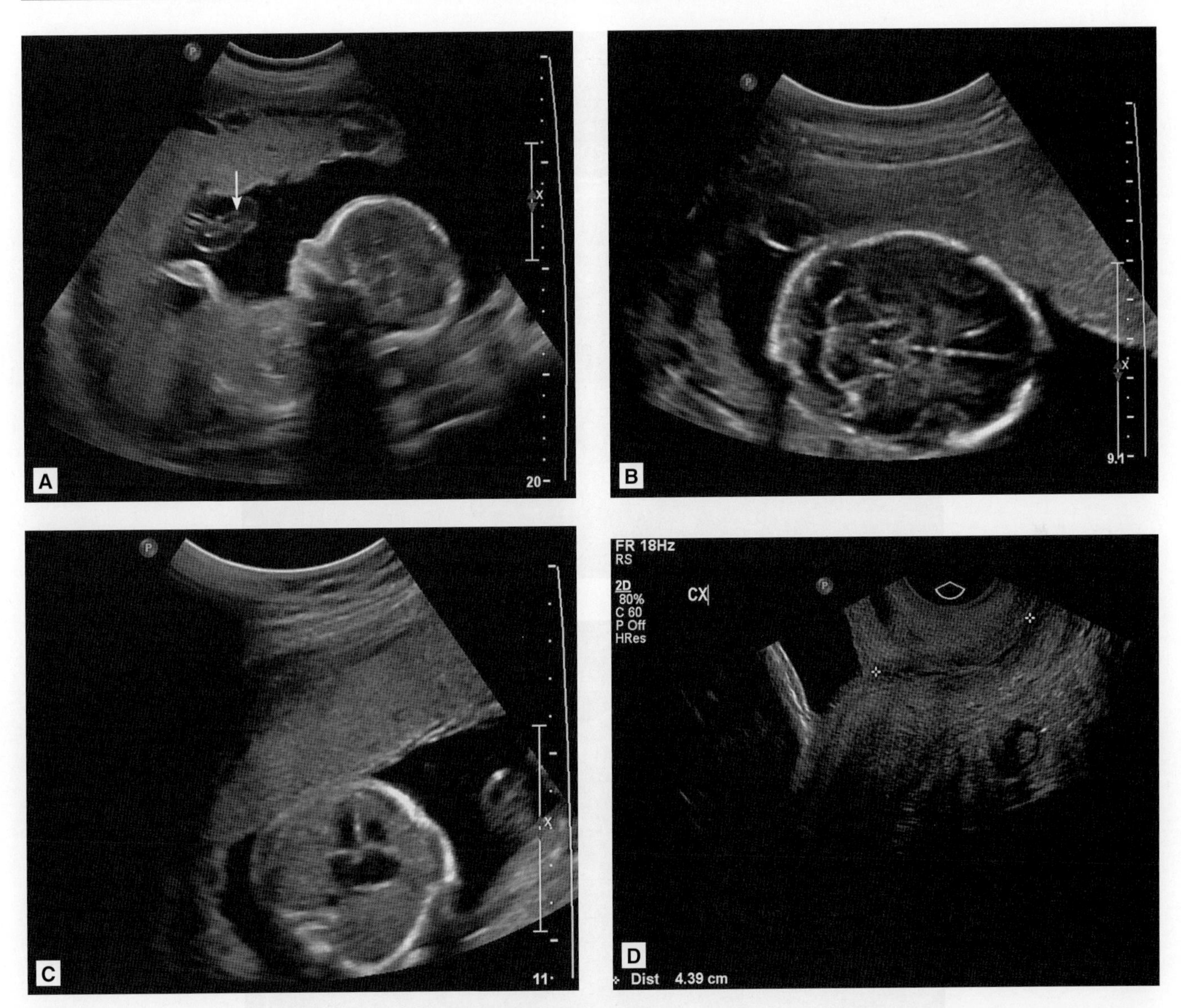

FIGURE 7.85 ■ Normal Intrauterine Pregnancy at 22 Weeks. **A-C:** A complete anatomic survey may be performed at this gestational age. A singleton vertex-presentation pregnancy is seen. A normal three-vessel umbilical cord is present (arrow). An appropriate volume of anechoic amniotic fluid is present. The symmetry of normal brain development and a "four-chamber" view of the fetal heart is seen. **D:** The cervical os is closed, and the length of the normal cervix is measured at greater than 4 cm.

Pearls

1. All pregnant patients who present with vaginal bleeding or pelvic pain should have sonographic imaging to evaluate for an intrauterine or ectopic pregnancy regardless of quantitative beta-HCG.
2. Patients with a normal intrauterine pregnancy, a closed cervical os, and not receiving assisted fertility treatments, can be safely discharged without obstetric consultation.

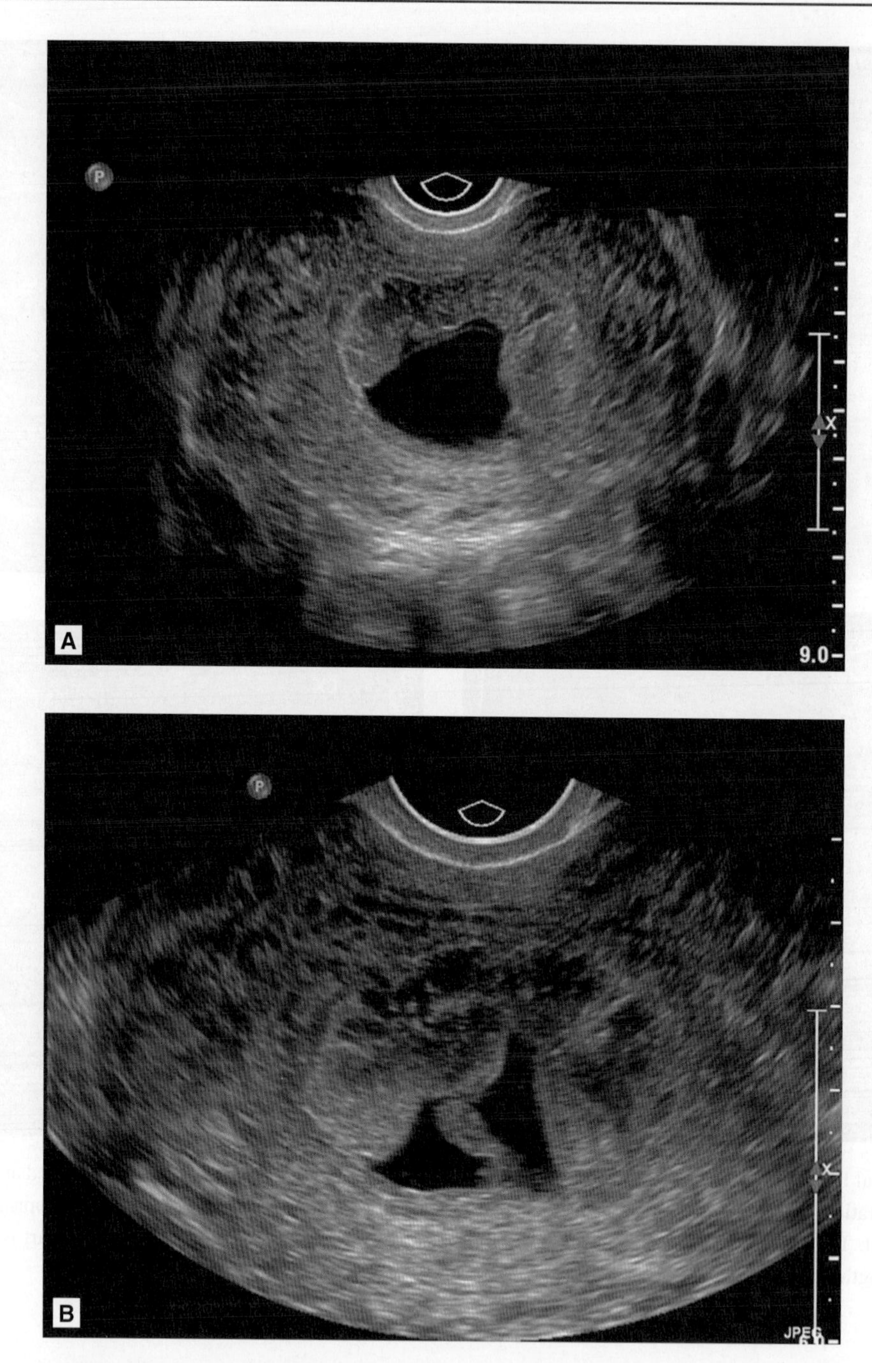

FIGURE 7.86 ■ Intrauterine Embryonic Demise. **A, B:** Transvaginal images demonstrate an irregular gestational sac and the lack of a visible yolk sac in this 7-week pregnancy. The fetal heartbeat could not be detected.

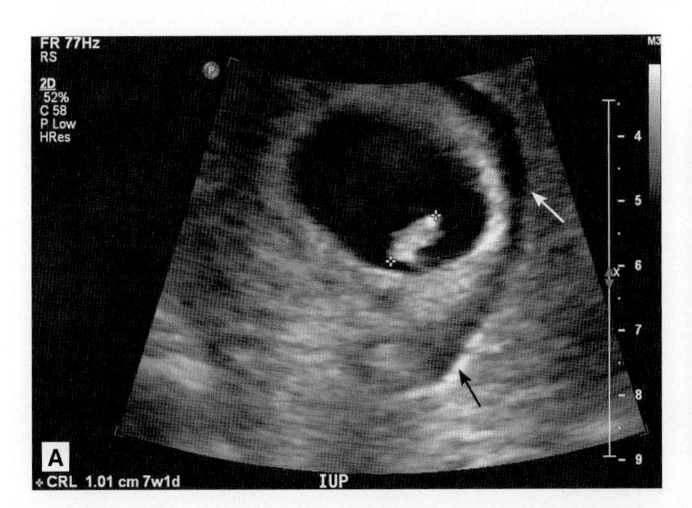

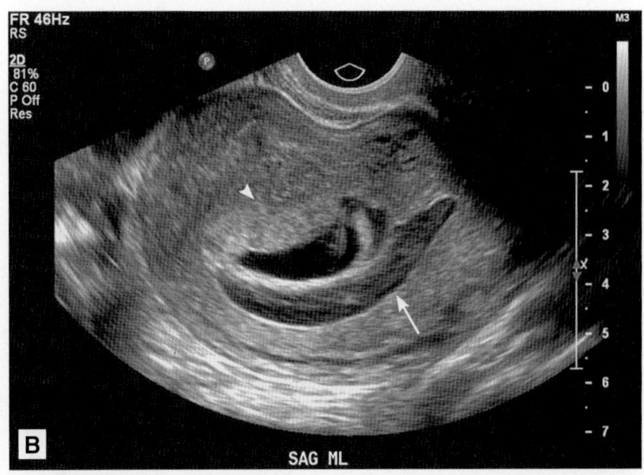

FIGURE 7.87 ■ Subchorionic Hemorrhage. **A, B:** A large region of hypoechoic blood is seen between the chorion and the endometrium (arrows). The location of the placenta is identified opposite from the region of hemorrhage (arrowhead).

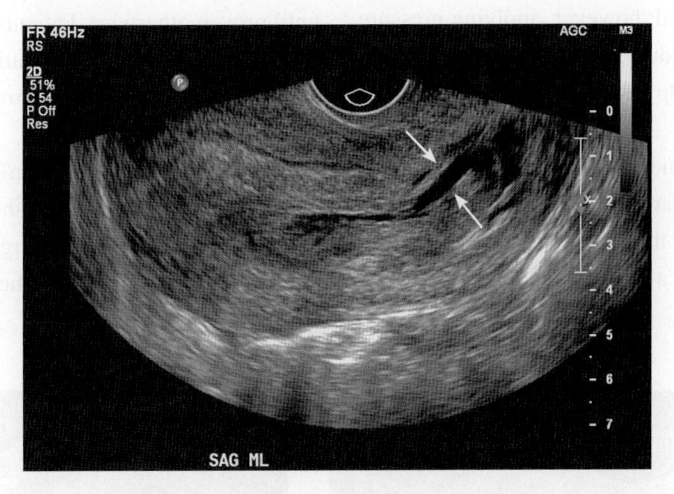

FIGURE 7.88 ■ Spontaneous Abortion (in Progress). Sagittal ultrasound image in a 32-year-old woman believed to be 9 weeks pregnant shows an open cervical os (arrows) with passage of products of conception.

Radiographic Summary

An ectopic pregnancy is a pregnancy that occurs outside of the central portion of the uterine body or fundus. Only 15% of ectopic pregnancies will have an embryo visible outside of the uterus. Sonographic findings suggestive of ectopic pregnancy include a complex adnexal mass, pelvic free fluid, a tubal ring, and an empty uterus with or without a pseudogestational sac.

A complex adnexal mass has mixed echotexture and is the most common sonographic finding in ectopic pregnancy. Increased vascularity by color flow Doppler may be present and has been described as a "ring of fire" representing the vascularity of the developing gestational sac.

A tubal ring is an adnexal mass that is separate from the ovary and appears as an anechoic sac surrounded by a thick echogenic rim of tissue. A corpus luteal cyst can appear similar to a tubal ring on ultrasound; however, applying pressure with a free hand over the transducer to look for separation of the questionable mass can help distinguish between a tubal ring and a corpus luteal cyst.

A small amount of free fluid in the uterine cul-de-sac is normal. However, free fluid that can be seen tracking around more than the bottom third of the uterus, while only moderate in amount, is concern for a ruptured ectopic. Free fluid that is present within Morison's pouch is suggestive of a large amount of intraperitoneal fluid and should be assumed to be a ruptured ectopic pregnancy until proven otherwise.

Clinical Implications

Patients who present with pelvic pain or vaginal bleeding and are pregnant should have sonographic imaging to evaluate for an ectopic pregnancy regardless of the quantitative beta-HCG level. Several studies have shown that approximately 15% of patients with a beta-HCG level less than 1500 IU/L and an empty uterus on ultrasound will have an ectopic pregnancy.

Ruptured ectopic pregnancy is the leading cause of maternal death in first-trimester pregnancy. Women who present with abdominal pain, hypotension, and a positive pregnancy test should be assumed to have a ruptured ectopic pregnancy until proven otherwise. Patients who are unstable should have emergent gynecologic evaluation and ultrasound performed at the bedside to assess for intra-abdominal free fluid and evidence of ectopic pregnancy.

All patients with suspicion for ectopic pregnancy, regardless of hemodynamic status, should have emergent evaluation by a gynecologist in the emergency department for consideration of surgical or medical therapy.

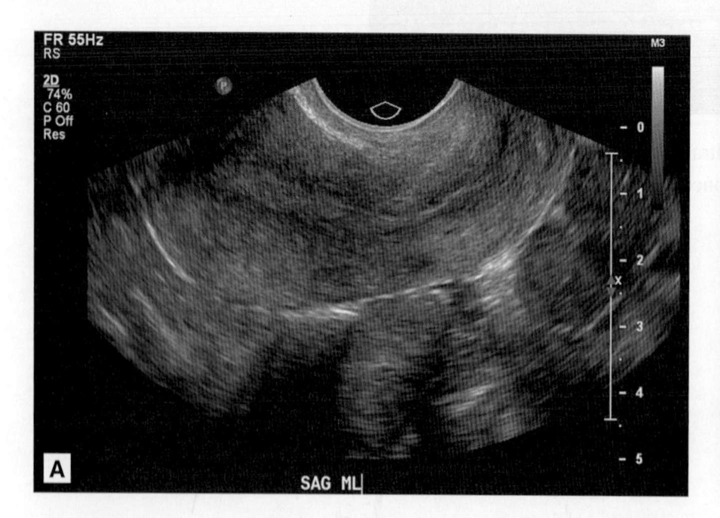

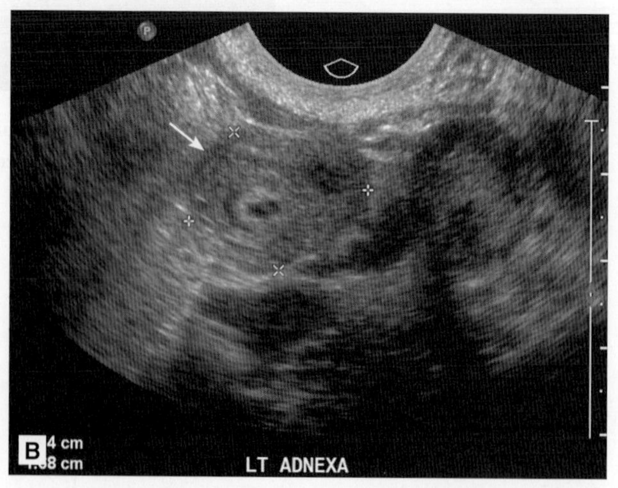

FIGURE 7.89 ■ Ectopic Pregnancy. **A:** Sagittal image of the uterus in a patient with positive BHCG demonstrates thick decidual reaction but the lack of an intrauterine gestation sac. **B:** Transvaginal ultrasound demonstrates an adnexal mass (arrow) separate from the left ovary. An echogenic rim surrounds the unruptured tubal ectopic pregnancy.

Pearls

1. An extrauterine fetal pole and gestational sac is only seen in 15% of ectopic pregnancies.
2. An intrauterine pregnancy in patients receiving in vitro fertilization does not rule out an ectopic pregnancy as heterotopic pregnancy occurs in up to 1% of these patients.
3. The location of an intrauterine pregnancy is important as ectopic pregnancies can occur within the uterus at the cornua and cervix.
4. Patients with a beta-HCG less than 3000, a mean gestational sac less than 3 cm, and present less than 3 weeks from their missed period are excellent candidates for methotrexate therapy.

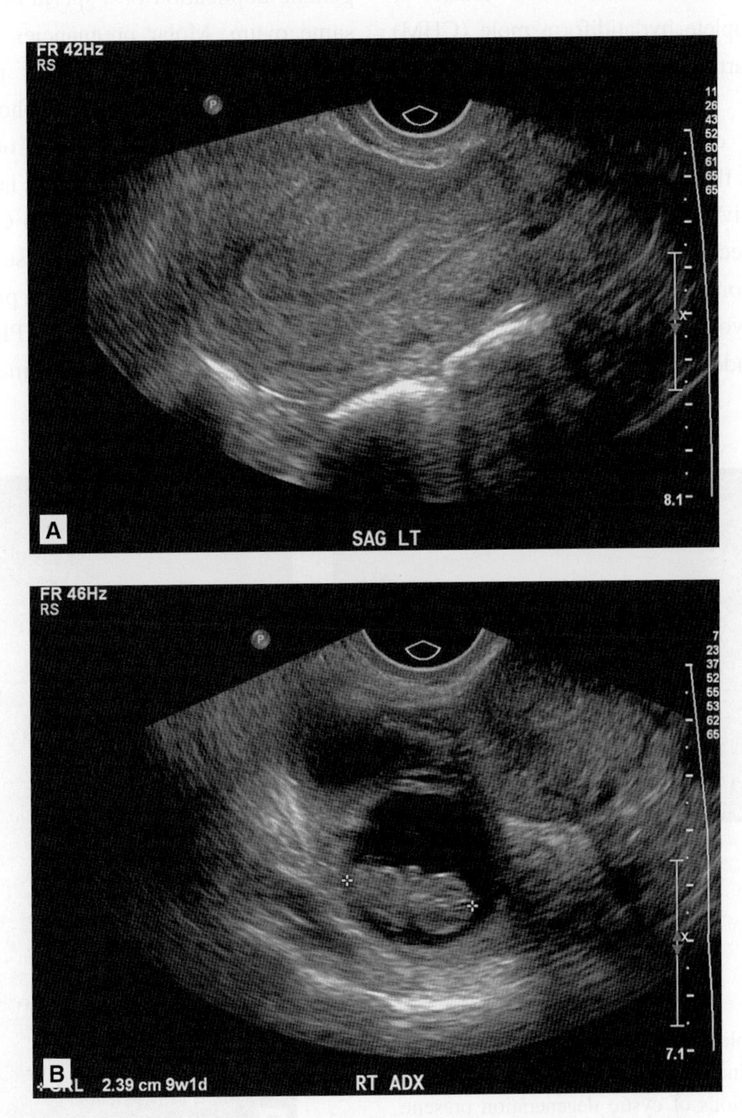

FIGURE 7.90 ■ Ectopic Pregnancy. **A:** Sagittal image of the uterus in a patient estimated to be 9 weeks pregnant by LMP demonstrates thick decidual reaction and the lack of an intrauterine gestation sac. **B:** In the right adnexa, the live embryo is identified within the distended right fallopian tube.

Radiographic Summary

A molar pregnancy is part of a spectrum of gestational trophoblastic tumors that include benign hydatidform moles, locally invasive moles, and choriocarcinoma. It is an abnormal pregnancy where a nonviable fertilized egg implants into the uterus. Molar pregnancies in the second and third trimester appear as multiple innumerable small anechoic cysts within the endometrial canal, sometimes described as a "cluster of grapes." In general, a complete hydatidiform mole (CHM) fills the uterus while a partial mole is associated with an abnormal nonviable fetus.

Molar pregnancies are difficult to detect sonographically in early pregnancy as the sonographic appearance of a hydatidiform mole is relatively nonspecific and can appear as a homogenously hyperechoic endometrial mass similar to an anembryonic gestational sac. Because these findings are similar to an anembryonic pregnancy, a single sonographic exam cannot exclude a molar pregnancy in the first trimester. In up to half of cases, theca lutein cysts will be present in both ovaries and will appear as multiseptated ovarian cysts.

Clinical Implications

Molar pregnancies are the most common form of gestational trophoblastic neoplasms and occur as a result of abnormal genetic duplication of a sperm or two sperms fertilizing the same ovum. Molar pregnancies are divided into complete hydatidiform mole (CHM) or partial hydatidiform mole (PHM). CHM consists of trophoblastic tissue and lacks a fetus whereas a PHM consists of both trophoblastic tissue and an abnormal embryo that is not viable. In rare instances, a twin gestation will result in a CHM and a separate viable embryo, which under careful surveillance may survive to term. A hyaditidiform mole is a premalignant condition with up to 20% of CHMs and 1% of PHMs undergoing malignant transformation to choriocarcinoma.

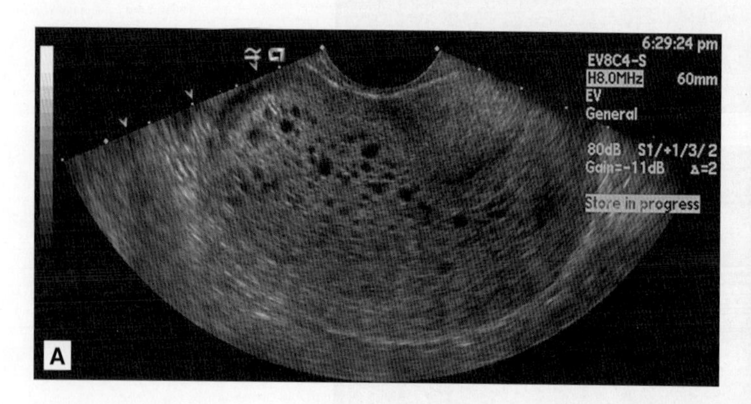

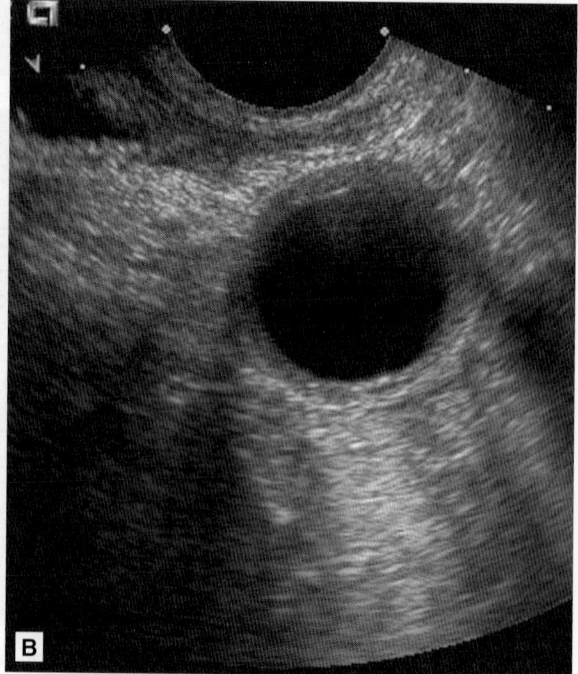

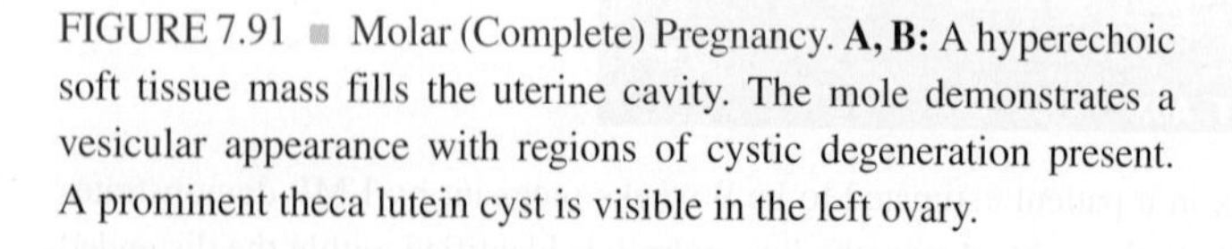

FIGURE 7.91 ■ Molar (Complete) Pregnancy. **A, B:** A hyperechoic soft tissue mass fills the uterine cavity. The mole demonstrates a vesicular appearance with regions of cystic degeneration present. A prominent theca lutein cyst is visible in the left ovary.

Molar pregnancies should be considered in patients with hyperemesis gravidarum, very high levels of beta-HCG, and a uterus larger than expected. Patients may also present with hypertension, proteinuria, and hyperthyroidism. All patients with a molar pregnancy should be evaluated by a gynecologist for definitive evaluation and treatment that consists of suction D&C and serial beta-HCG measurements.

Pearls

1. A molar pregnancy may be indistinguishable from a blighted ovum in early first-trimester pregnancy.
2. In very rare instances, a patient with a CHM may have a normal viable twin gestation that will survive to term.

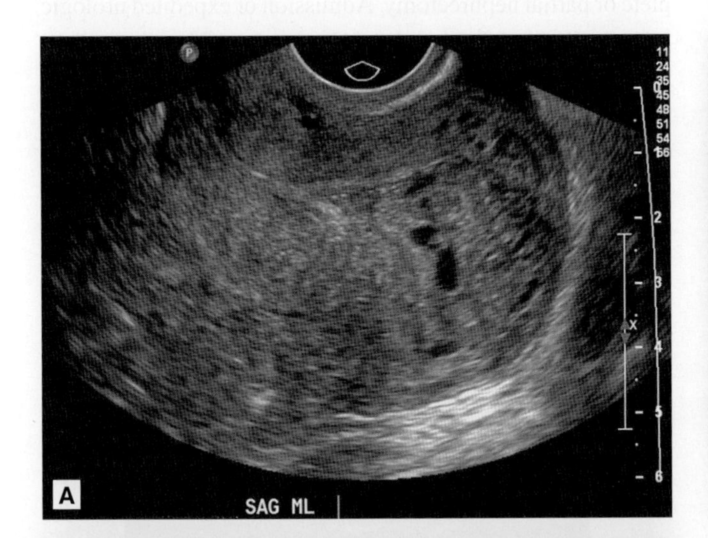

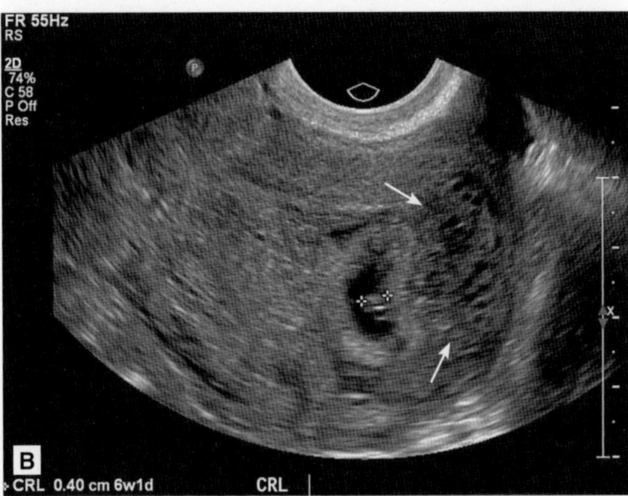

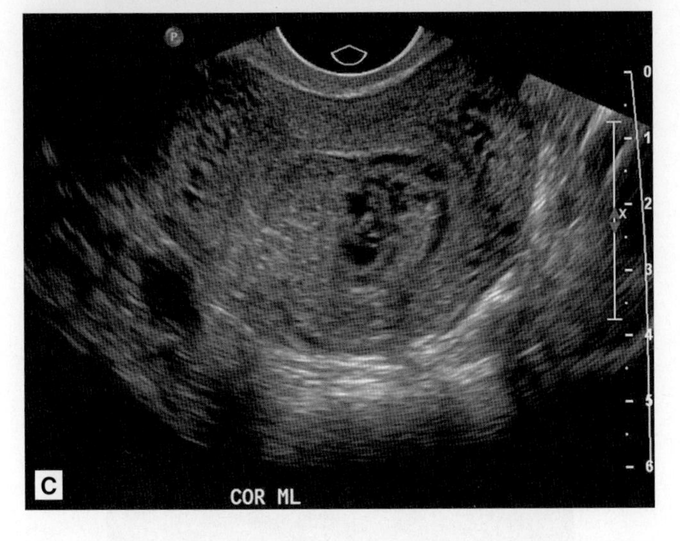

FIGURE 7.92 ■ Partial Molar Pregnancy. **A-C:** In this example, identifiable products of conception are present including a gestational sac and fetal pole. A hyperechoic intrauterine mass is seen adjacent to the gestational sac and exhibits innumerable cystic spaces (arrows).

RENAL CELL CARCINOMA

Radiographic Summary

Renal cell carcinoma is a highly vascular solid tumor that originates from the renal cortex. Sonographically, renal cell carcinoma appears as a solid mass within the renal parenchyma with increased vascularity as demonstrated by color flow or power Doppler. Approximately 50% of lesions are hyperechoic to the surrounding renal parenychma and 10% are hypoechoic. The remainder of the lesions are isoechoic and are detected as an irregularity of the renal contour within an area of the kidney showing increased vascularity.

A contrast-enhanced CT scan is the study of choice to diagnose and stage renal cell carcinoma and shows the tumor as a solid renal mass with increased enhancement. In 10% of cases there will be multiple lesions within the same kidney, and 20% will demonstrate renal vein involvement.

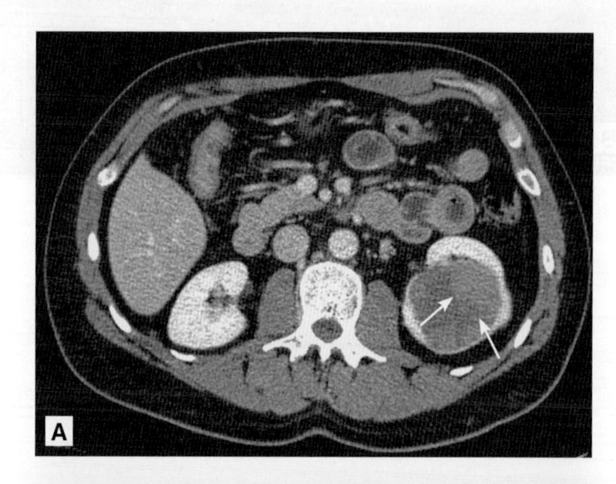

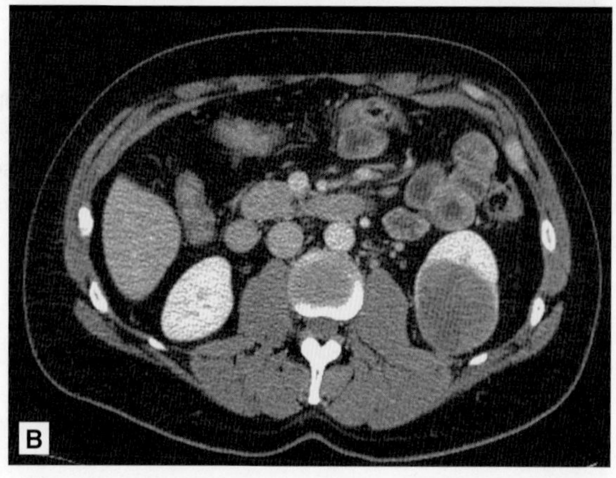

FIGURE 7.93 ■ Renal Cell Carcinoma. **A, B:** A low-attenuation mass is seen within the left kidney. The mass displaces normal renal parenchyma, and demonstrates some internal enhancement. The presence of soft tissue density within the mass (arrows) helps distinguish RCC from common renal cysts.

Clinical Implications

Renal cell carcinoma accounts for 90% of primary renal malignancies. Any solid kidney mass should be assumed to be a renal cell carcinoma until proven otherwise. As many as a third of all renal cell carcinomas are diagnosed as incidental findings on studies performed for other reasons.

The treatment of renal cell carcinoma is surgical with complete or partial nephrectomy. Admission or expedited urologic and oncologic evaluation should be arranged for patients diagnosed with renal cell carcinoma in the emergency department.

Pearls

1. Incidental renal cysts on non-ontrast CT studies that are solid or have a complex cystic component should have follow-up imaging to evaluate for vascularity to exclude renal cell carcinoma.
2. One third of patients diagnosed with renal cell carcinoma will be asymptomatic at the time of diagnosis.

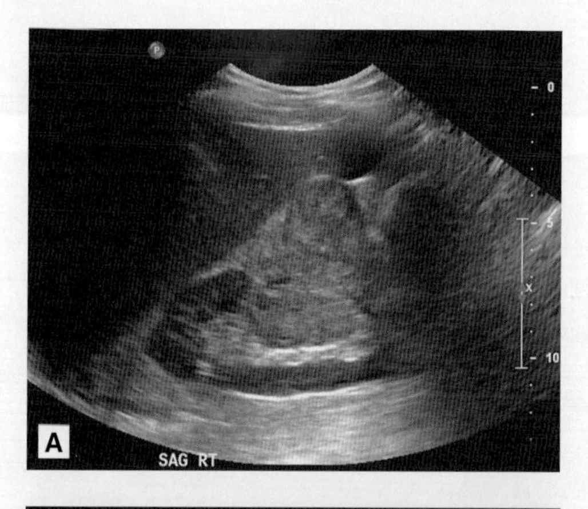

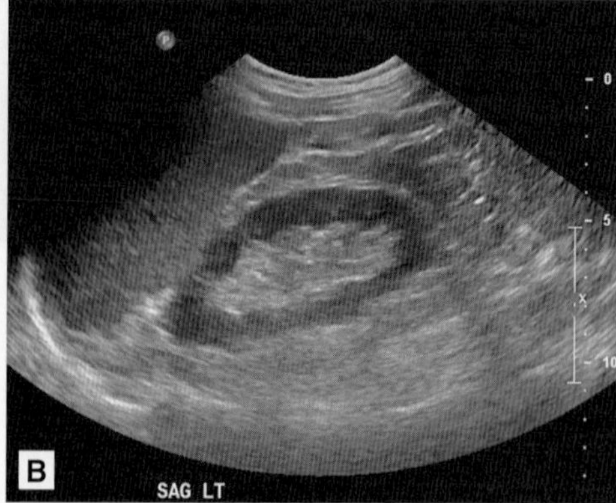

FIGURE 7.94 ■ Renal Cell Carcinoma. **A, B:** A large exophytic mass is seen with increased echotexture, extending throughout the interpolar region of the right kidney. The mass appears to abut the undersurface of the liver. The normal left kidney is demonstrated as a reference.

Radiographic Summary

Epididymitis is an inflammation of the epididymis and is most commonly due to infectious causes. Doppler ultrasonography confirms this diagnosis. The hallmark ultrasonic finding is enlargement and decreased echogenicity of the epididymitis. Inflammation of the epididymis may be diffuse or focal so it is important to scan through the entire structure to avoid missing focal disease. Complex hypoechoic fluid collections within the epididymis represent small abscesses and suggest advanced epididymitis. Color Doppler is helpful when gray-scale findings are equivocal. Hyperemia and increased vascularity of the epididymis suggest epididymitis.

Clinical Implications

The diagnosis of epididymitis can be made clinically, but is often confirmed with ultrasound when testicular torsion is being excluded. Subacute or acute unilateral testicular pain with swelling and tenderness is the typical presentation. Likely cause and therefore treatment depends on age and sexual activity. Children with pyuria should be treated with antibiotics against coliforms. Heterosexual sexually active adolescents should be treated with empiric antibiotics against Gonococcus and chlamydia. Homosexual patients should be treated for Gonococcus, chlamydia, and coliforms.

Pearls

1. Epididymitis is usually confirmed by US while excluding testicular torsion in patients with testicular pain.
2. Epididymitis, orchitis, and testicular torsion are difficult to distinguish on clinical examination alone. One should have a low threshold for ordering an ultrasound in a patient with acute testicular pain.

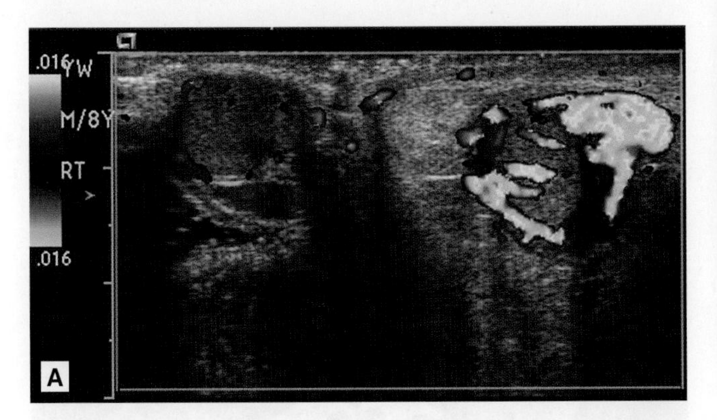

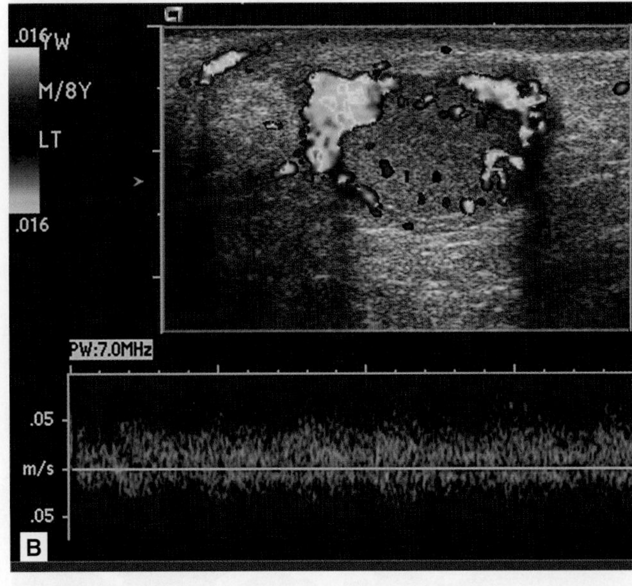

FIGURE 7.95 ■ Epididymitis. **A, B:** Two sonographic images demonstrate that the right epidydimis is enlarged, relatively hyperechoic, and markedly hyperemic compared to the normal left side. Doppler shows normal flow within both testes.

Radiographic Summary

Pyelonephritis is inflammation of the kidney as a result of bacterial infection. It is manifested on renal imaging studies as areas of poor perfusion and renal enlargement. CT with IV contrast is more sensitive than ultrasound in detecting abnormalities caused by renal infection. CT imaging shows an enlarged kidney, with a classic "striated" appearance with administration of IV contrasting reflecting focal areas of poor perfusion as a result of infection. On ultrasound these mixed areas of perfusion of the kidney are manifested as a patchy appearance of the renal parenchyma with loss of the corticomedullary interface. The primary purpose of imaging studies in pyelonephritis is to exclude complicating factors including urolithiasis, urinary tract obstruction, renal abscess formation, and emphysematous pyelonephritis.

Clinical Implications

Pyelonephritis is a clinical diagnosis manifested by pyuria, fever, and costo-vertebral angle tenderness. Radiologic imaging is not routinely performed unless there are specific indications or there is a high suspicion for renal abscess or an obstructing urolith.

Imaging with CT or ultrasound is indicated if patients fail to respond to appropriate antibiotics within 72 hours, have severe sepsis or septic shock, have symptoms of renal colic, or have relapse of symptoms after treatment with appropriate antibiotics. Imaging should be considered in men who present with symptoms of pyelonephritis to exclude anatomic abnormalities or presence of a urolith. Imaging should also be considered in diabetics with pyelonephritis due to the high risk of developing emphysematous pyelonephritis, which requires emergent nephrectomy.

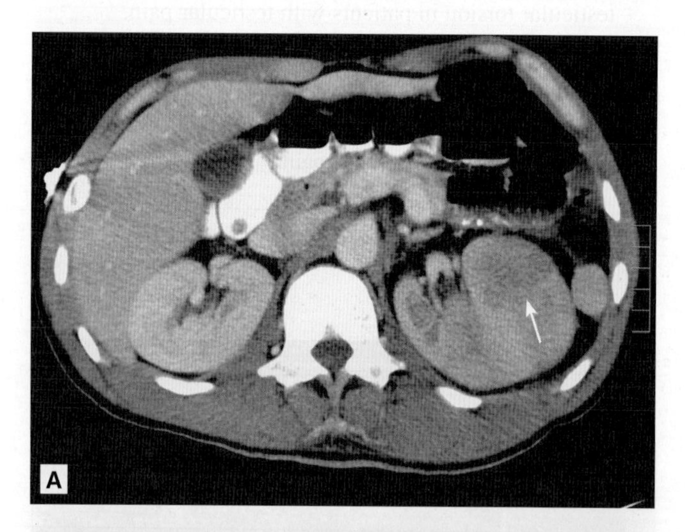

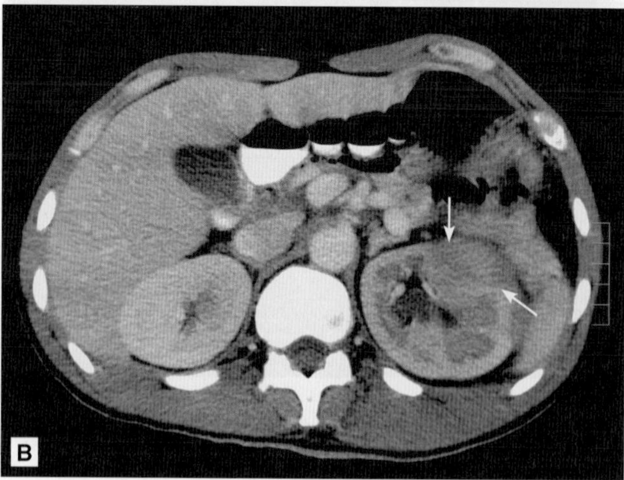

FIGURE 7.96 ■ Pyelonephritis. **A, B:** The left kidney appears enlarged, and enhances more slowly when compared to the right side. There are regions of low attenuation and loss of corticomedullary differentiation (arrows).

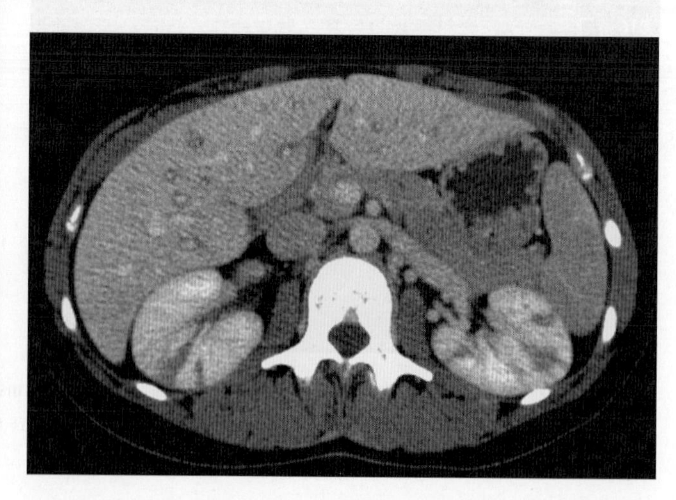

FIGURE 7.97 ■ Pyelonephritis. Bilaterally, there are well-defined focal areas of poor enhancement and low attenuation within the kidneys. This produces the classic "striated nephrogram" appearance.

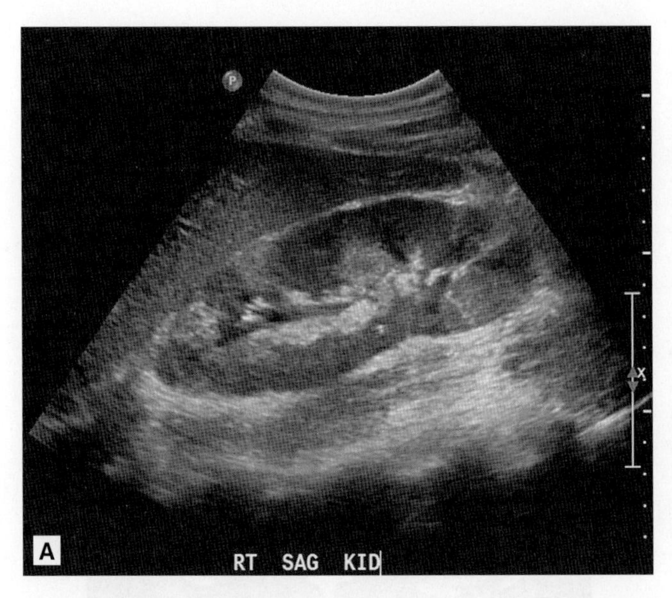

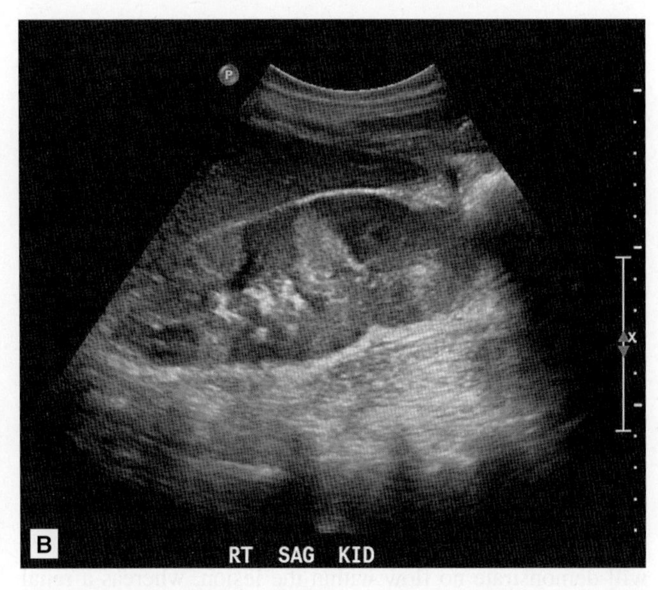

FIGURE 7.98 ▪ Pyelonephritis. **A, B:** On ultrasound, regions of varying echotexture are seen throughout the right kidney. Loss of normal corticomedullary differentiation is seen.

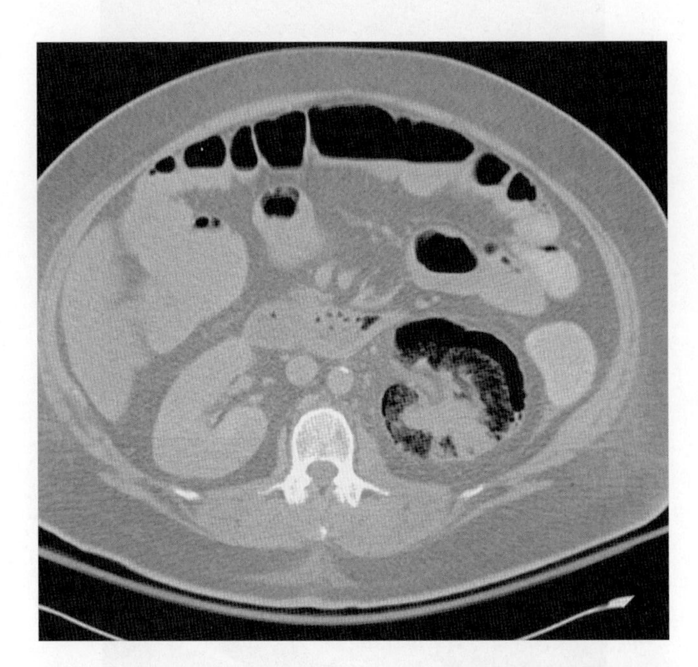

FIGURE 7.99 ▪ Emphysematous Pyelonephritis. Gas is identified within the renal parenchyma and contained within the renal capsule in this patient with immunosuppression and emphysematous pyelonephritis.

Patients with pyelonephritis and a urolith, signs of urinary tract obstruction, renal abscess formation, or other anatomic abnormalities, should have emergent urologic evaluation in addition to appropriate antibiotic therapy.

Pearls

1. Obtain imaging on any patient with pyelonephritis who fails to show clinical improvement within 72 hours after appropriate antibiotic administration.
2. Patients with evidence of an obstructing urolith and pyelonephritis require emergent urology consultation and surgical drainage.
3. Consider imaging men, diabetics, and hypotensive patients who present with pyelonephritis to exclude renal abscess, a urinary tract obstruction, gas forming organisms, and urolith.

Radiographic Summary

A renal abscess is a collection of inflammatory fluid within the renal cortex or corticomedullary parenchyma. Ultrasound and CT are both useful modalities to detect renal abscesses. CT should be performed with and without IV contrast to help characterize any lesions seen. Renal abscesses that are due to hematogenous spread will be isolated to the renal cortex and on CT will appear as a poorly defined, hypodense, wedge-shaped complex lesion within the renal cortex that fails to enhance with IV contrast. On ultrasound, a renal cortical abscess will appear as a hypoechoic lesion isolated to the renal cortex with internal mixed echoes from purulent debris and necrotic tissue. Color-flow Doppler findings are an important diagnostic feature in these lesions as a renal abscess will demonstrate no flow within the lesion, whereas a renal malignancy will show increased flow within the lesion itself.

Renal abscesses that occur due to ascending urinary tract infection will have evidence of abscess formation in the renal cortex and medulla. These corticomedullary abscesses can be visualized with CT or ultrasound; they reside at the corticomedullary junction.

Clinical Implications

Renal abscesses are best divided into those that are cortical and corticomedullary. Abscesses that are corticomedullary are due to ascending spread of bacteria through the urinary tract and are caused by *E. coli* more than 75% of the time. On the other hand, renal cortical abscesses are primarily due to hematogenous spread of bacteria from an extrarenal source and are caused by *Staphylococcus aureus* 90% of the time. Patients with corticomedullary abscesses are likely to have specific risk factors including recurrent urinary tract infections, diabetes mellitus, renal calculi, vesicoureteral reflux, or recent urologic instrumentation.

All patients with renal abscesses need IV antibiotics and emergent urologic consultation. Patients who have septic shock or an abscess greater than 5 cm should undergo percutaneous or surgical drainage of the abscess.

Pearls

1. Coritcomedullary abscesses are due to ascending urinary tract infection and are most often due to gram-negative bacteria.
2. Patients with renal cortical abscesses will usually have a normal urinalysis, a normal urine culture, and absence of dysuria. They will often have a history of a current or recent soft tissue infection and should have a search for additional areas of bacterial seeding.

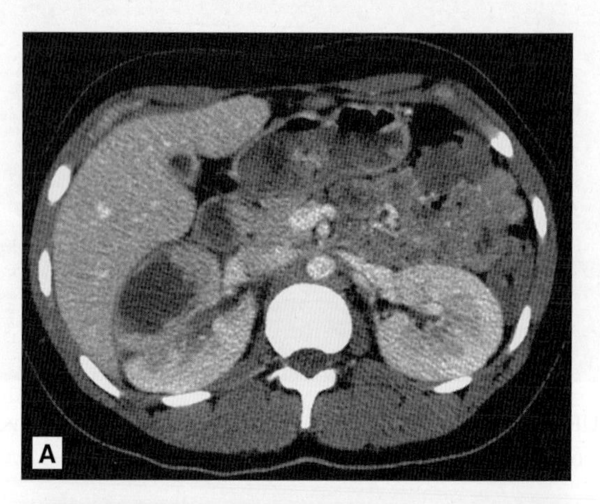

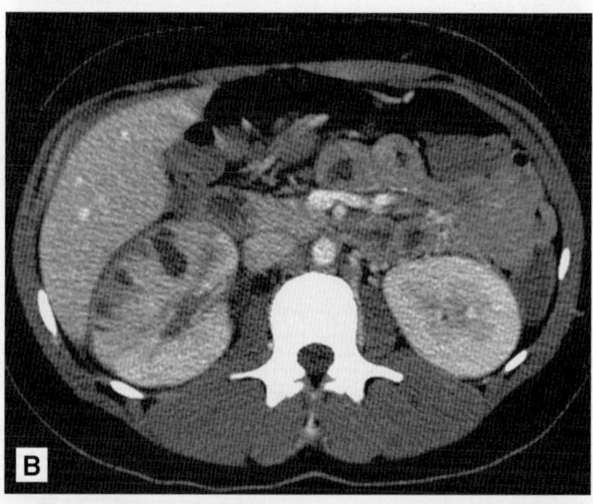

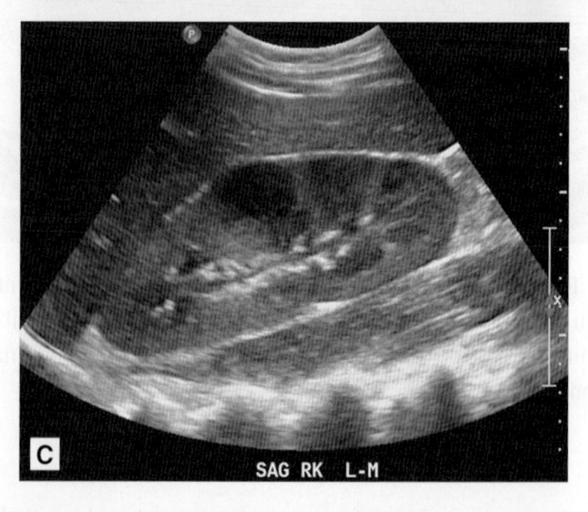

FIGURE 7.100 ■ Renal Abscess. **A, B:** Well-defined regions of fluid attenuation are seen within the right kidney on this contrast-enhanced CT of the abdomen. Multiple renal abscesses are present. **C:** A sonographic image reveals the large region of diminished echotexture within the interpolar region of the right kidney.

Radiographic Summary

Ovarian cancer represents a diverse set of tumors that arise from different types of tissue present in the ovaries. Ovarian cancer can present as either a complex cystic or solid mass. Most tumors are cystic in appearance and as many as 20% will be bilateral at presentation. An exophytic fibroid or a nongynecologic mass can resemble an ovarian neoplasm on initial sonographic examination.

Ovarian cysts that have thick walls, multiple septations, and mixed echogenicity are more likely to be malignant. However complex ovarian cysts, such as hemorrhagic cyst, dermoid, cystadenomas, and TOAes can also have a similar appearance. Masses smaller than 5 cm are likely to be benign, whereas masses greater than 10 cm are more likely to be malignant. In advanced stages, malignant ascites may also be present.

Clinical Implications

Ovarian cancer is the 9th most common type of cancer in women, but causes 5% of cancer deaths in the United States. Most patients with ovarian cancer are asymptomatic until late in the disease course. Metastatic disease is often present throughout the peritoneum due to local spread.

Most ovarian masses are benign. However, patients with ovarian masses suspicious for ovarian cancer, especially in postmenopausal women, should have a follow-up arranged with a gynecologist and repeat sonographic imaging in 6 weeks. Surgery is the treatment for all stages of ovarian cancer. Chemotherapy may be used to treat the remaining disease if present.

Pearl

1. Repeat sonographic imaging of complex ovarian cysts and simple cysts greater than 5 mm in 6 weeks is recommended in all patients to help differentiate benign from pathologic masses.

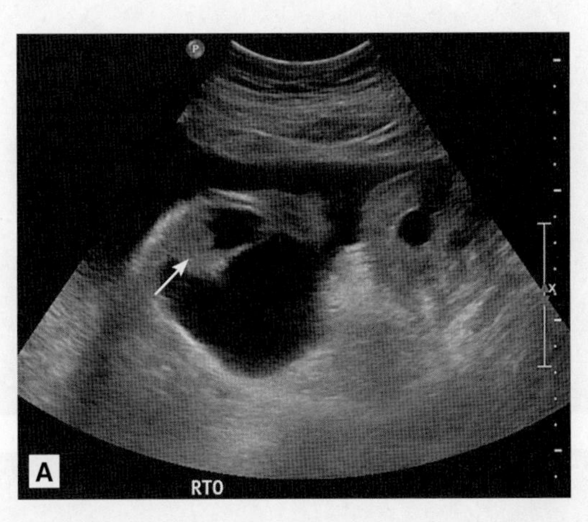

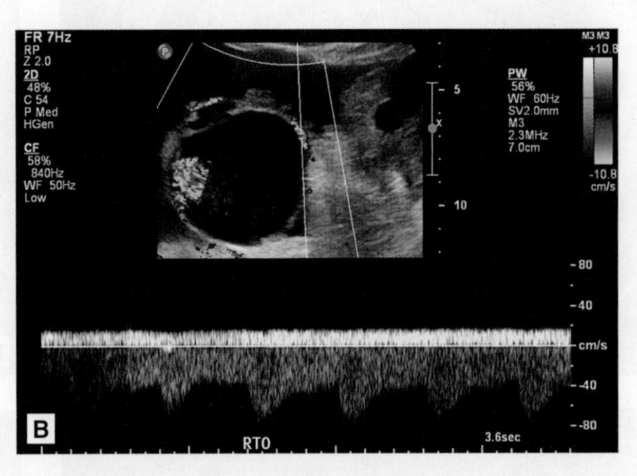

FIGURE 7.101 ■ Ovarian Cancer. **A, B:** A right-sided adnexal mass is seen with irregular thickened septations and a prominent mural nodule (arrow). Tumor vascularity is demonstrated on color Doppler imaging.

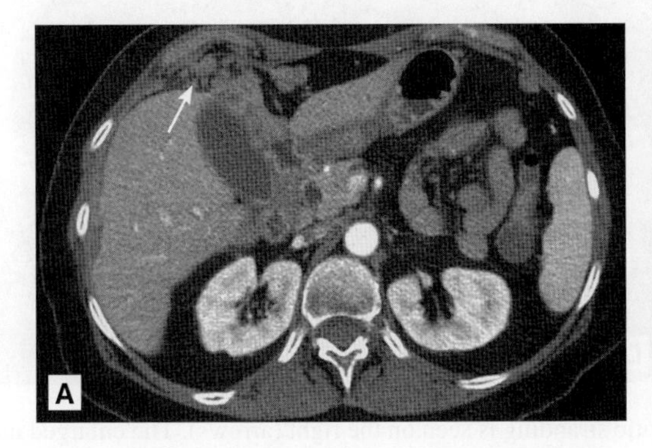

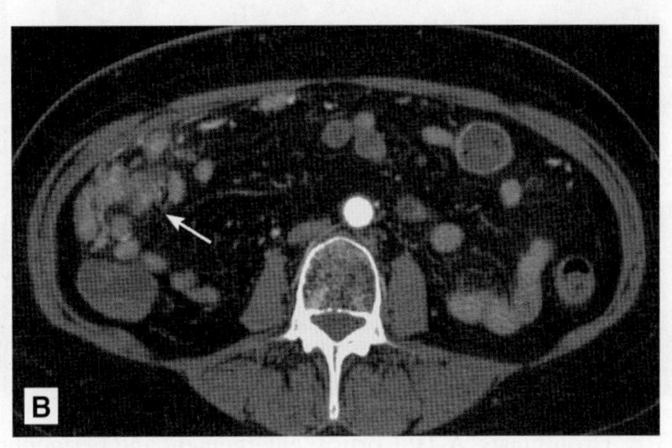

FIGURE 7.102 ■ Ovarian Cancer. **A, B:** Numerous enhancing omental implants are present in this ovarian cancer patient, indicating metastatic spread of malignancy within the peritoneal cavity (arrows).

Radiographic Summary

Urolithiasis is a stone anywhere in the urinary tract from the kidney to the urethra. CT scan is the study of choice and is more than 95% sensitive and specific for urolithiasis. All stones are opaque on CT except for pure matrix and indinavir stones. Other findings on CT that suggest a urolith within the ureter include, hydronephrosis, peri-nephric stranding, ureteral dilation, or soft-tissue rim sign (rim of soft tissue around the urolith).

Phleboliths are calcifications within the veins of the pelvis and can be mistaken for uroliths. Phleboliths will often appear hollow, have a comet tail appearance, and lack a soft tissue rim sign.

While ultrasound is less sensitive and specific than CT, it is preferred over CT in young patients and in those who are pregnant. Stones within the ureter are difficult to detect and hydronephrosis may be the only evidence of a urolith within the ureter. Stones within the kidney or uretero-vesicular junction may be identified by acoustic shadowing or "twinkling" artifact on color flow Doppler. An obstructing stone at the UV junction is implied by the absence of the "jet sign" on that side. Ultrasound is also preferable as a follow-up or subsequent imaging modality in patients with recurrent bouts of urolithiasis in whom multiple CT examination would result in significant cumulative radiation exposure and a potentially increased risk for developing a subsequent radiation-induced malignancy.

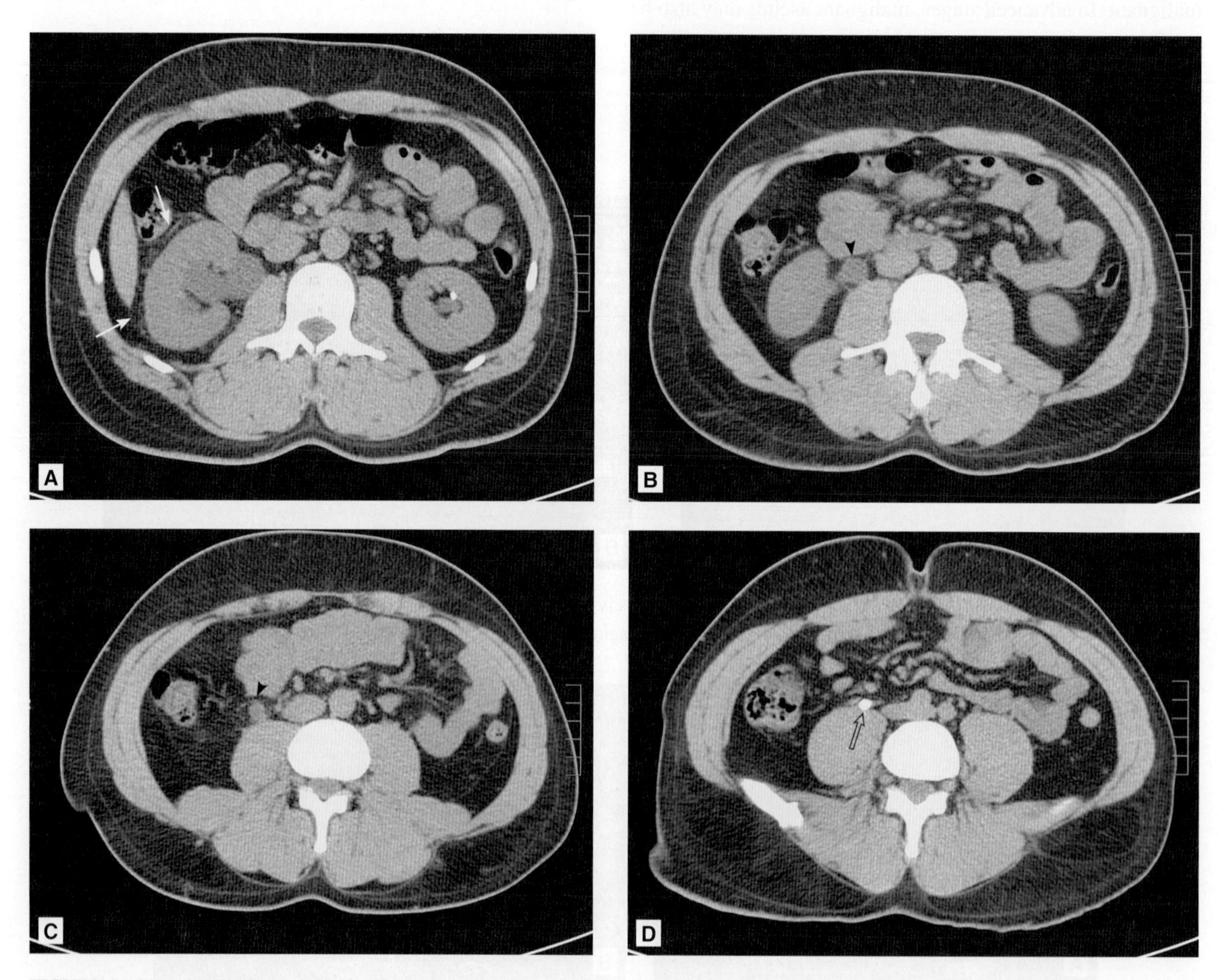

FIGURE 7.103 ■ Urolithiasis. **A-D:** Cortical enlargement and perinephritic stranding is seen on the right (arrows). The enlarged ureter with periureteral inflammation can be seen (arrowheads). An angular 6 mm stone is identified in the mid right ureter (open arrow). Note the small stone within the collecting system of the left kidney.

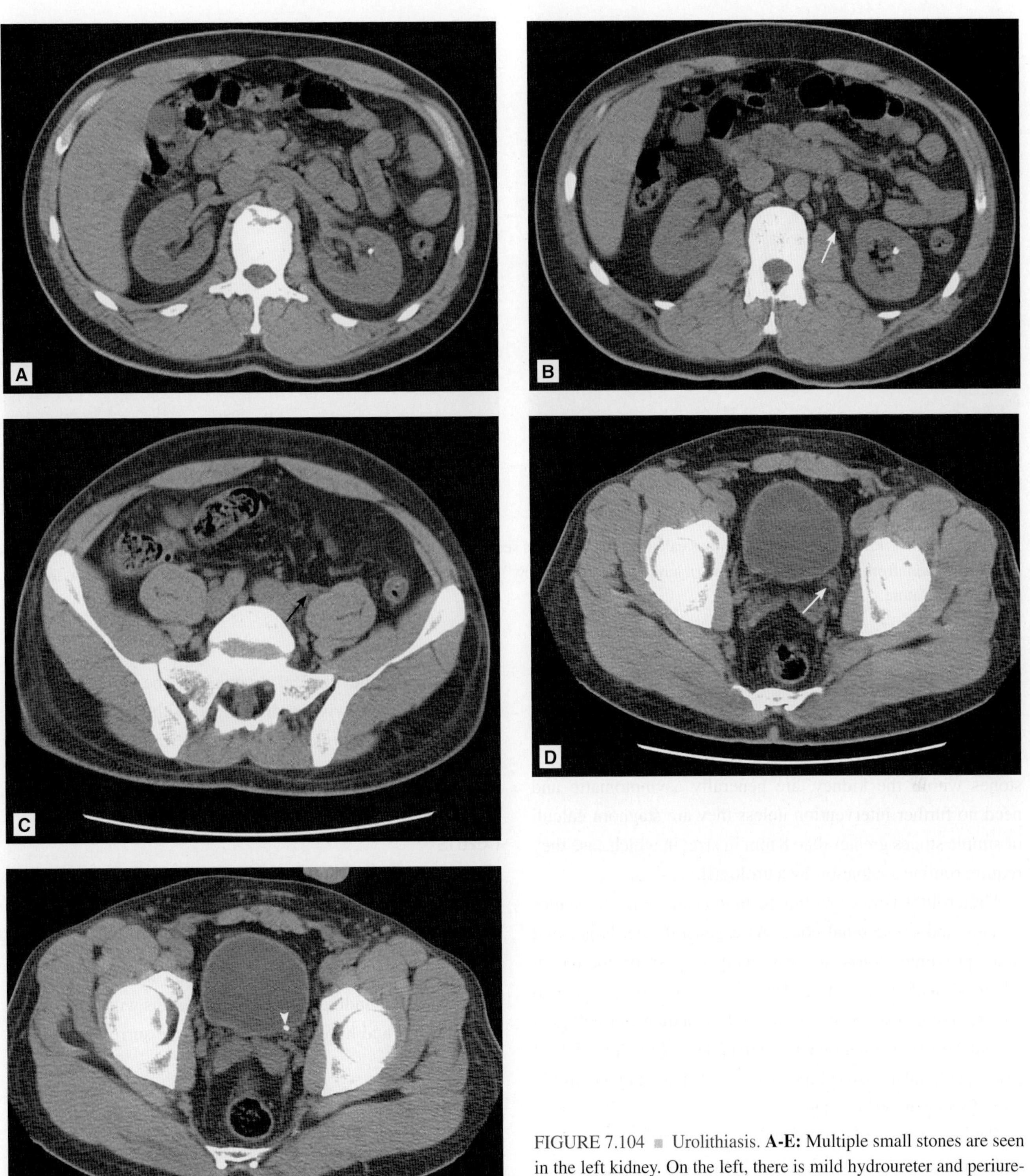

FIGURE 7.104 ■ Urolithiasis. **A-E:** Multiple small stones are seen in the left kidney. On the left, there is mild hydroureter and periureteral stranding (arrows). A 3 mm intramural stone is identified at the left ureterovesicle junction (arrowhead).

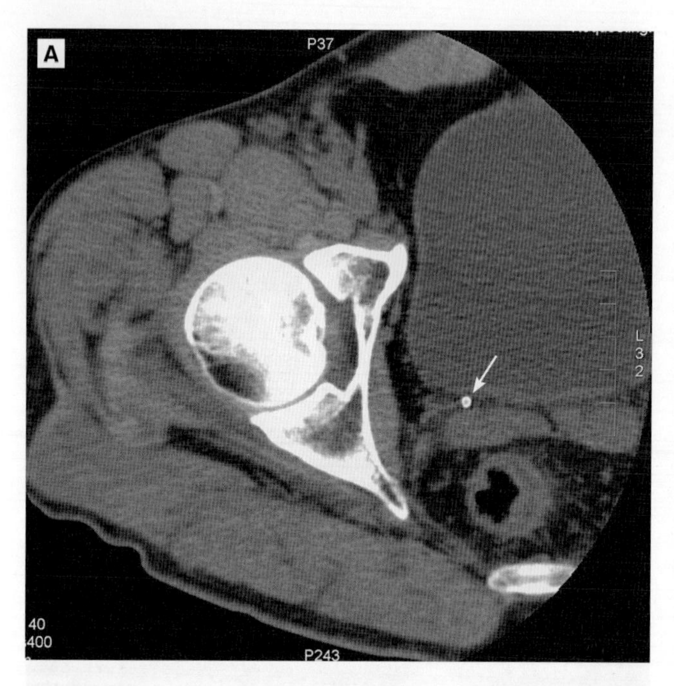

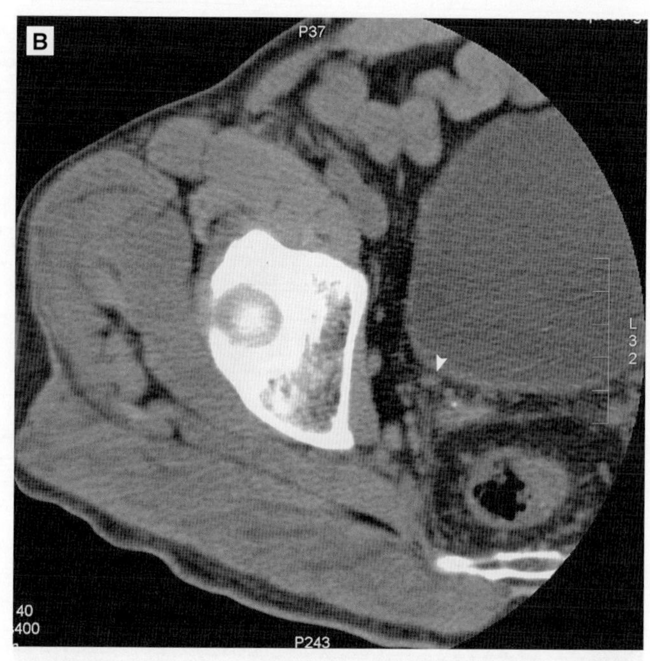

FIGURE 7.105 ■ Phlebolith. **A, B:** A venous calcification (arrow) is seen separate from the normal distal ureter on the right (arrowhead). To distinguish them from stones, phleboliths often have a rounded "hollow" appearance with a "comet tail" configuration representing associated venous vasculature.

Clinical Implications

Urolithiasis may be more specifically classified by the location of the urolith within the urinary tract. Renal calculi, or stones within the kidney, are generally asymptomatic and need no further intervention unless they are staghorn calculi or simple stones greater than 8 mm in size; in which case they require routine evaluation by a urologist.

Ureteroliths (stones within the ureter) are generally symptomatic and cause renal colic. As a general rule, larger and more proximal stones are less likely to pass on their own whereas smaller and more distal stones are more likely to pass spontaneously. Stones 4 mm or less in diameter will pass spontaneously on their own more than 85% of the time. Distal stones, defined as beyond the iliac vessels have a much higher rate of spontaneous passage.

Patients with evidence of an upper urinary tract infection and an obstructing ureterolith should be given broad-spectrum antibiotics and a urologist should be emergently consulted for admission and surgical drainage of the infected kidney. Patients may otherwise be discharged with routine follow-up if their pain is controlled, they are able to tolerate oral fluids and have no evidence of renal failure.

Pearls

1. Stones within the ureter are likely to pass if they are distal to the iliac vessels and less than 4 mm in size.
2. Phleboliths often have a rounded hollow appearance, a comet tail on ultrasound, and do not have a rim of soft tissue surrounding them on CT. Uroliths within the ureter are solid and have a rim of soft tissue surrounding them on CT.
3. An obstructing ureterolith with evidence of an upper urinary tract infection is a true urologic emergency and requires IV antibiotics, admission, and urologic evaluation for surgical drainage.

Chapter 8

PELVIC TRAUMA

David S. Taber
Michael N. Johnston

Radiographic Summary

Fractures may involve the columns, walls, or dome of the acetabulum. They are classified by Letournel and Judet as five *elementary* and five *associated* fractures. Elementary fractures are predominantly single-plane injuries. Associated fractures are combinations of the elementary types, and are multiplane and more complex. The AP pelvis radiograph is typically the first imaging study followed by CT scanning. Some patients may have additional 45° oblique pelvis radiographs, known as Judet views. CT is more sensitive than plain radiographs for detecting acetabular fractures.

Five fracture types in the Letournel–Judet classification account for 80-90% of cases. Posterior acetabular wall fractures are the most common. A portion of the posterior articular surface and rim is sheared from the pelvis by posterior dislocation of the hip. Transverse acetabular fractures divide the hemipelvis through the acetabulum into superior and inferior portions, and do not involve the obturator

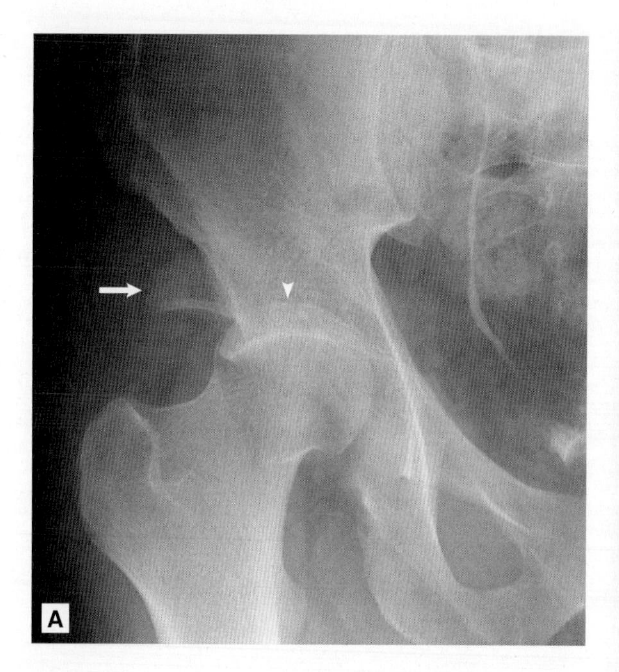

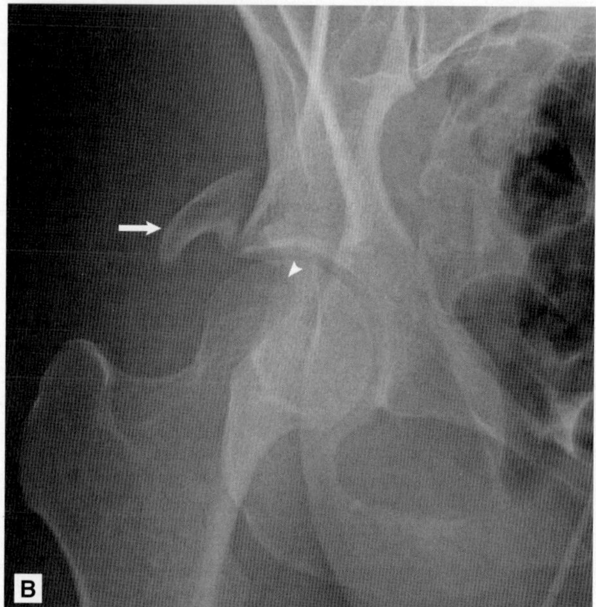

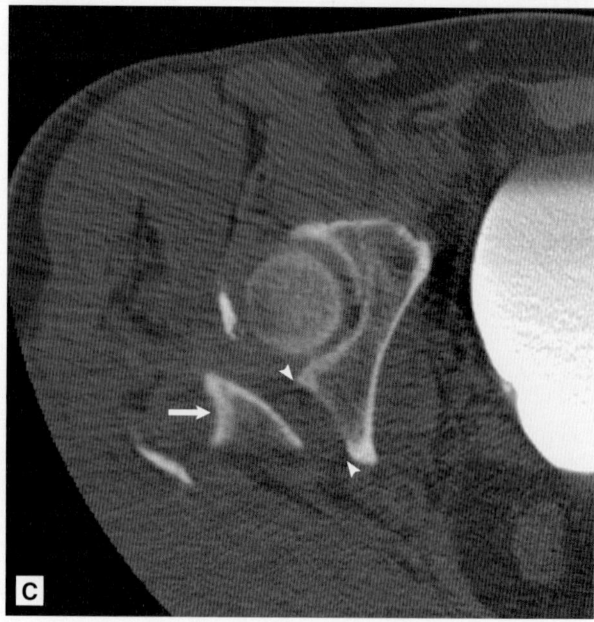

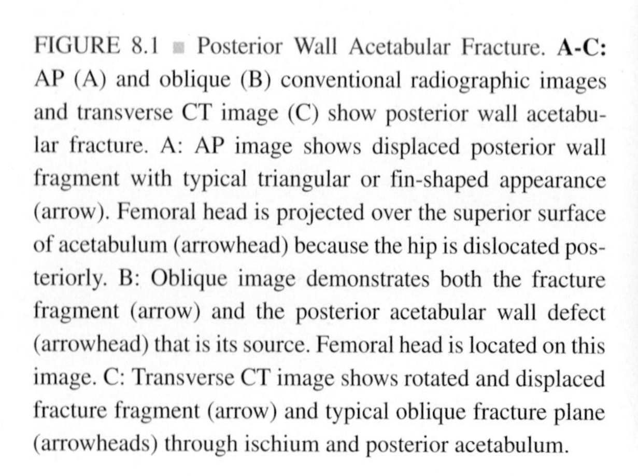

FIGURE 8.1 ■ Posterior Wall Acetabular Fracture. **A-C:** AP (A) and oblique (B) conventional radiographic images and transverse CT image (C) show posterior wall acetabular fracture. A: AP image shows displaced posterior wall fragment with typical triangular or fin-shaped appearance (arrow). Femoral head is projected over the superior surface of acetabulum (arrowhead) because the hip is dislocated posteriorly. B: Oblique image demonstrates both the fracture fragment (arrow) and the posterior acetabular wall defect (arrowhead) that is its source. Femoral head is located on this image. C: Transverse CT image shows rotated and displaced fracture fragment (arrow) and typical oblique fracture plane (arrowheads) through ischium and posterior acetabulum.

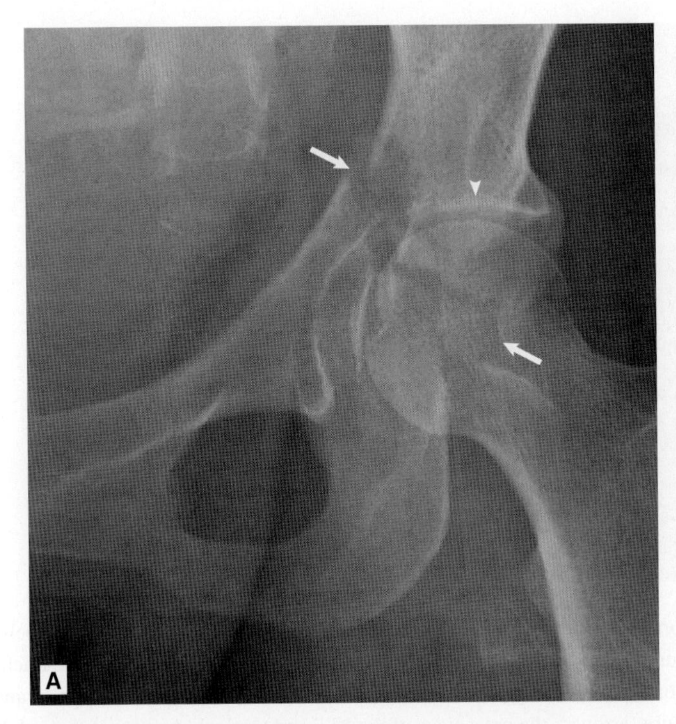

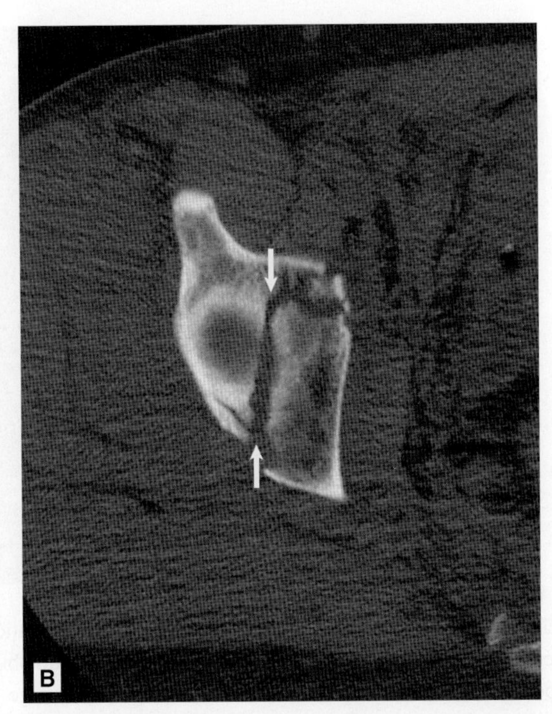

FIGURE 8.2 ■ Transverse Acetabular Fracture. **A, B:** Oblique conventional radiographic image (A) and transverse CT image (B) illustrate transverse acetabular fracture. A: Conventional image shows the fracture plane dividing hemipelvis into superior and inferior portions through the hip socket (arrows). Superior articular surface or "dome" remains attached to superior portion (arrowhead). Note that inferior ischiopubic ramus is intact. (Skin fold artifact simulates ramus fracture.) (B) Transverse CT image at the level of superior articular surface shows predominantly sagittal plane typical of transverse fracture (arrows).

ring. Radiographically, part of the superior articular surface or dome remains attached to the intact ilium. The fracture plane actually is oblique from superomedial to inferolateral. A combination of posterior wall and transverse injuries characterizes the transverse and posterior wall fracture. The T-shaped fracture combines the transverse fracture with a vertical fracture most commonly passing through the acetabular fossa and notch and the inferior ischiopubic ramus. The both-column fracture is a complex injury with no part of the articular surface of the hip socket remaining attached to the axial skeleton. The "spur" sign, representing the edge of intact ilium adjacent to the fracture, is pathognomonic of the both-column fracture.

Clinical Implications

Acetabular fractures result from significant force driving the femoral head into the hip socket, either laterally through the hip (as from a direct blow against the greater trochanter from a fall) or through the femur (as in the "dashboard" mechanism). They are associated frequently with hip dislocation

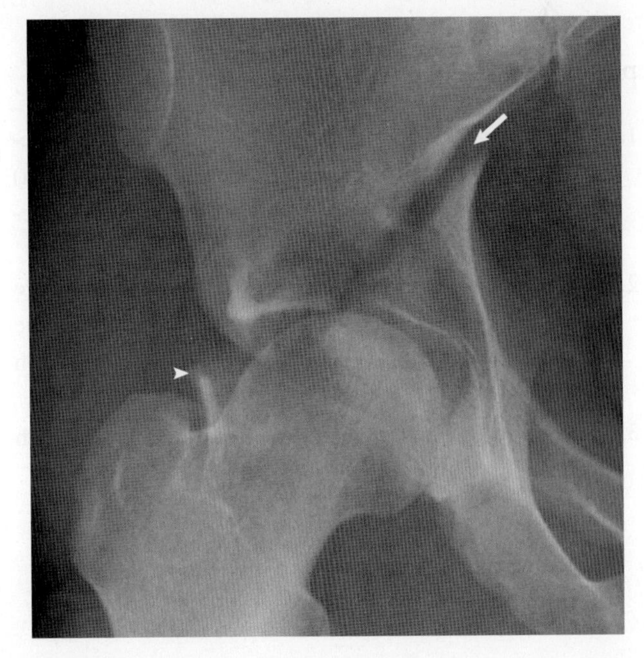

FIGURE 8.3 ■ Transverse and Posterior Wall Acetabular Fracture. Oblique conventional radiographic image shows both a transverse fracture component (arrow) and a displaced posterior wall fracture fragment (arrowhead).

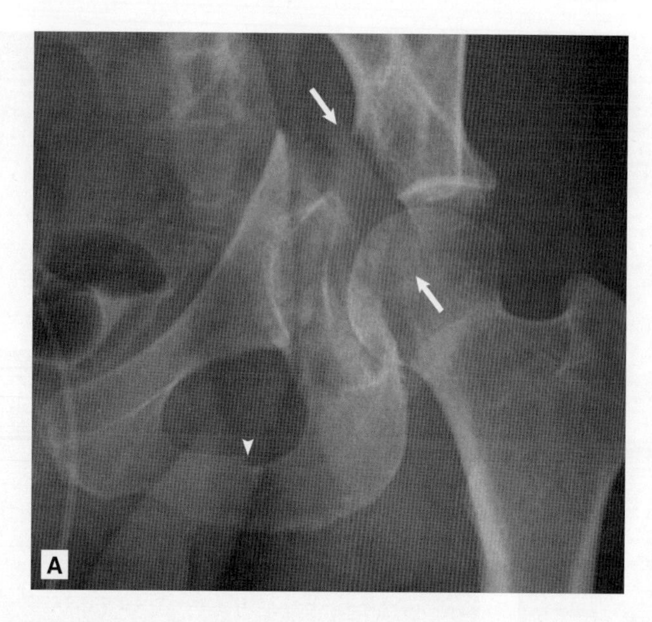

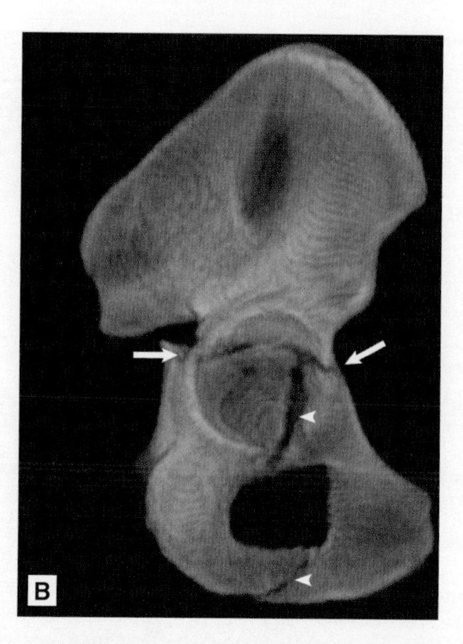

FIGURE 8.4 ■ T-Shaped Acetabular Fracture. **A, B:** Conventional radiographic image (A) and 3D-reformatted CT image of hemipelvis, rotated in coronal plane to fully demonstrate acetabulum and obturator ring (B) show T-shaped fracture. A: In addition to transverse fracture component (arrows), oblique conventional radiographic image of typical T-shaped fracture shows fracture of inferior ischiopubic ramus (arrowhead). B: 3D reformatted CT image shows transverse fracture (arrows), the crosspiece of the "T," and vertical component through hip socket and inferior ischiopubic ramus (arrowheads), the stem of the "T."

and injuries to the femur and knee as well as the sciatic nerve. All patients with acetabular fractures require appropriate analgesia, hospitalization, and orthopedic consultation.

Pearls

1. Due to the overlapping nature of the anterior and posterior components of acetabular anatomy, oblique (Judet) views are often necessary for identification and characterization of acetabular fractures.
2. Acetabular fractures may be associated with sciatic nerve injury, femoral head osteonecrosis, or post-traumatic osteoarthritis and may result in significant long-term disability.
3. Failure to diagnose an associated hip dislocation with acetabular fracture is a medico-legal pitfall.

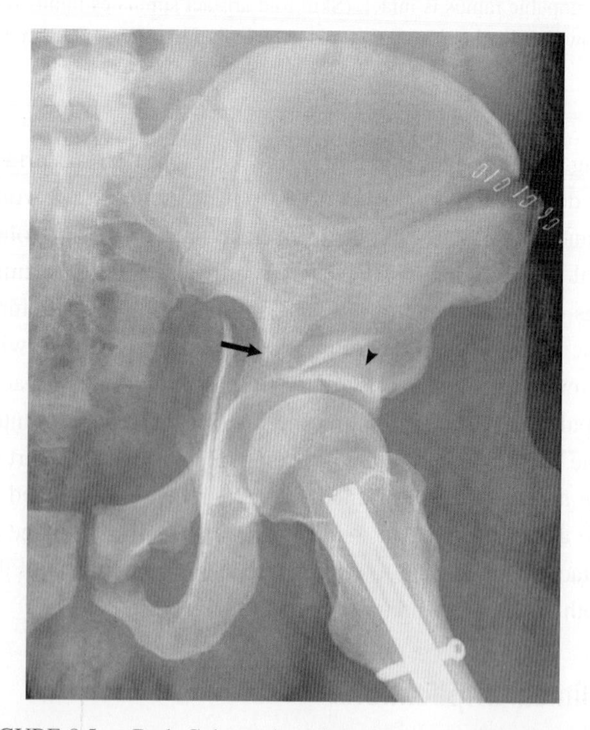

FIGURE 8.5 ■ Both-Column Acetabular Fracture. AP pelvis conventional radiographic image shows comminuted fracture of iliac wing, acetabulum, and obturator ring. Edge of fracture across iliac wing creates spur sign (arrow) pathognomonic of both-column acetabular fracture. Articular dome is itself comminuted and not attached to ilium (arrowhead).

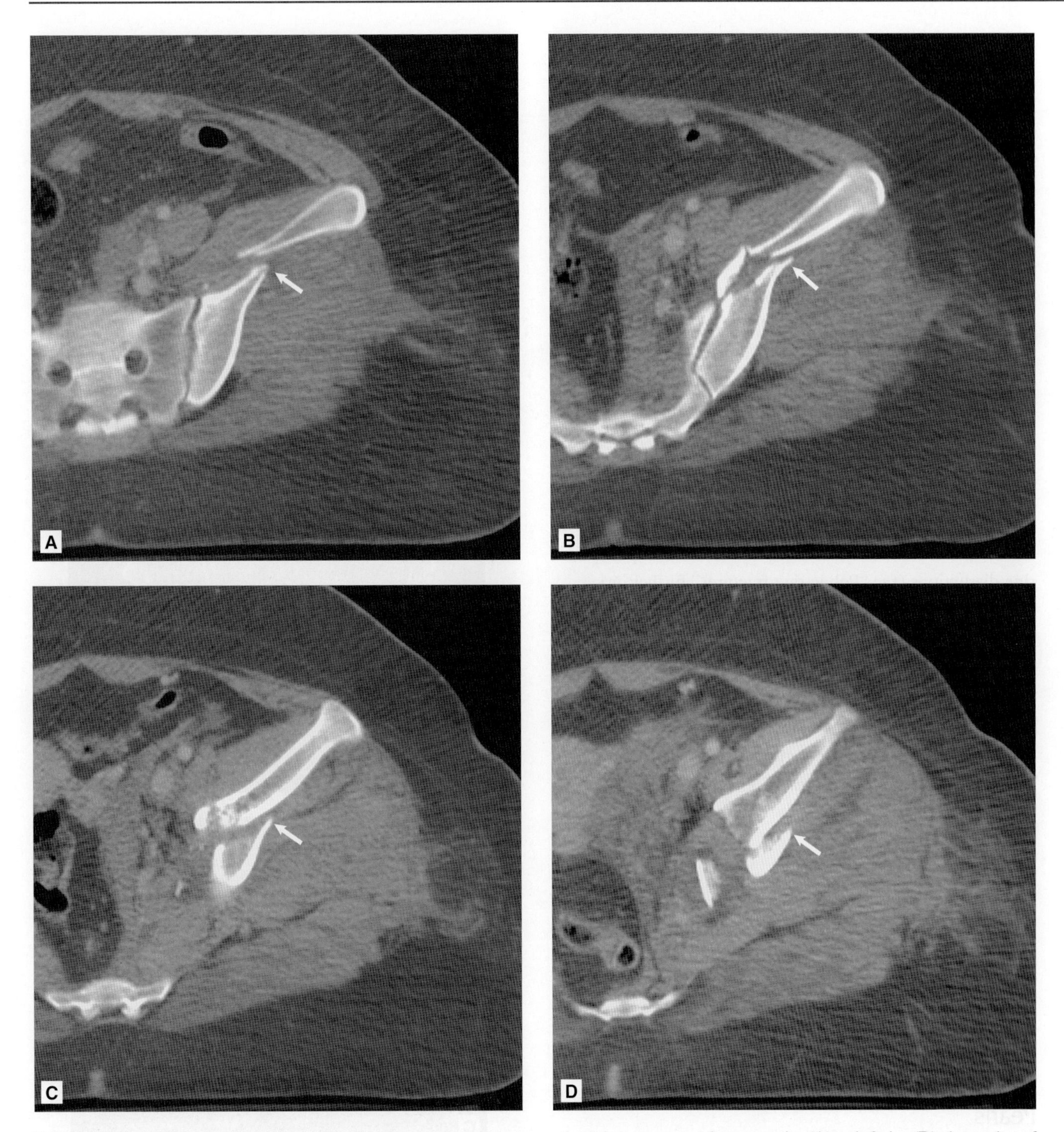

FIGURE 8.6 ■ CT Depiction of Spur Sign. Four transverse CT images of pelvis in sequence from superior (**A**) to inferior (**D**) show edge of ilium adjacent to fracture (arrows) decreasing in size and disappearing before any articular surface is encountered.

Radiographic Summary

Ramus fractures may involve one or both rami. AP pelvis radiographs are the initial study obtained. Superior ramus fractures may be oblique to horizontal and parasymphyseal, more vertical and in the midportion of the superior pubic ramus, or vertical and far laterally near the acetabulum (a "pubic root" fracture). Inferior ischiopubic ramus fractures are usually nearly vertical and may appear incomplete, or may be undisplaced and virtually invisible on conventional radiographs. An ipsilateral incomplete or "buckle" fracture of the anterior sacral wall may accompany pubic ramus fractures. These may be subtle, seen only as a slight irregularity of the contour of the superior edge of one or more sacral neural foramina. Additional inlet and outlet pelvis views can be used to supplement the AP radiograph. These are views of the entire pelvis with the x-ray beam angled caudally through the pelvis (the inlet view) or cephalad through the pelvis (the outlet view). These fractures may be part of more complex pelvic ring disruptions (*see* "Pelvic ring fractures" further on).

CT scan may demonstrate nondisplaced ramus fractures with increased accuracy as compared to radiographs. The extent of ramus fractures and the potential involvement of pubic root fractures at the anterior acetabular articular surface are better characterized on CT scan. CT scan also has utility in assessing intra- and extra-peritoneal injuries (such as bladder ruptures) that may accompany bony pelvic trauma.

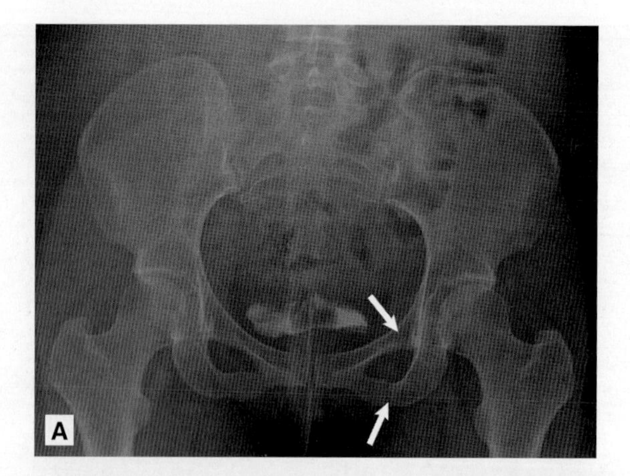

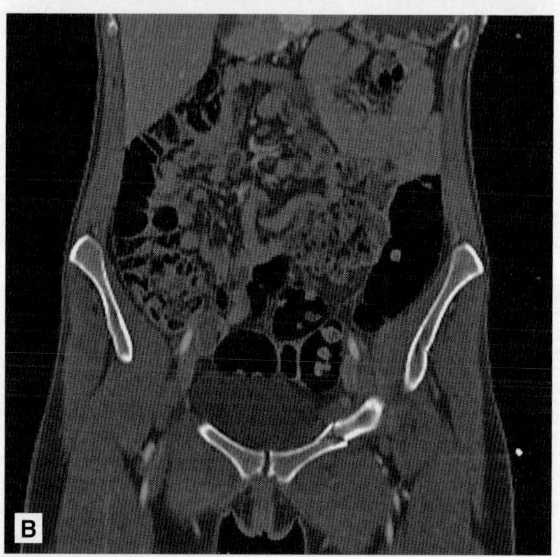

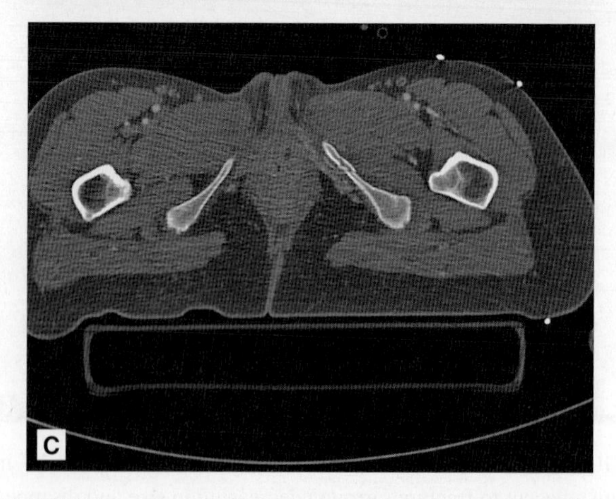

FIGURE 8.7 ■ Unilateral Superior and Inferior Ramus Fractures. Conventional radiograph shows superior pubic ramus and inferior ischiopubic ramus fracture (arrows). Note Foley catheter and contrast in bladder related to prior CT scan. **A:** AP view of the pelvis shows nondisplaced fractures of the left superior and inferior pubic rami (arrows). **B-C:** Coronal and axial CT reformations through the pelvis in a different patient demonstrate nondisplaced left sided superior pubic ramus and inferior ischiopubic ramus fractures.

Clinical Implications

Isolated pubic ramus fractures may be seen in the setting of falls or direct trauma among elderly patients. They can also occur as a stress fracture related to exercise among young patients or in pregnant women. Treatment typically consists of analgesics, crutches to assist with ambulation, and follow-up with orthopedics or primary care within 1-2 weeks.

Pearls

1. Pubic ramus fractures may develop as insufficiency fractures in elderly patients who present with pain concerning for femoral neck fractures and no history of trauma.
2. In osteopenic elderly patients, if plain films do not show a suspected fracture, MR is important to demonstrate the ramus fracture and to exclude hip fracture.

Radiographic Summary

Fractures of the right and left superior pubic and inferior ischiopubic rami are usually readily identifiable on a standard AP radiograph of the pelvis as well as on CT scan. The superior ramus components are usually fractured in a vertical plane when associated with vertical shear (VS) injuries. Other fracture patterns may occur. Orthopedic surgeons will usually obtain inlet and outlet views in addition to the AP radiograph to characterize displacement and plan management. These fractures may be part of a VS pelvic ring disruption (*see* "Pelvic ring fractures" further on).

Clinical Implications

Bilateral pubic rami fractures in isolation are a rare injury, and may be produced by a straddle-type injury or VS mechanisms. They are also seen as part of an injury complex associated with lateral compression (LC) injuries, especially LC type III fractures in the Young–Burgess classification (*see* "Pelvic ring fractures" further on). These fractures have a significant risk of major hemorrhage and concomitant bladder and urethral injury. Interventional radiology may be required to embolize vessels in patients with severe hemorrhage. Retrograde urethrography should be obtained prior to Foley catheter placement to rule out associated disruption of the urinary tract.

Pearls

1. Consider associated genitourinary and retroperitoneal injuries in the setting of bilateral pubic ramus fractures.
2. These fractures may also present as insufficiency fractures in older, osteopenic patients, and if plain films are not diagnostic their presence may be established by using MR if the clinical situation indicates.

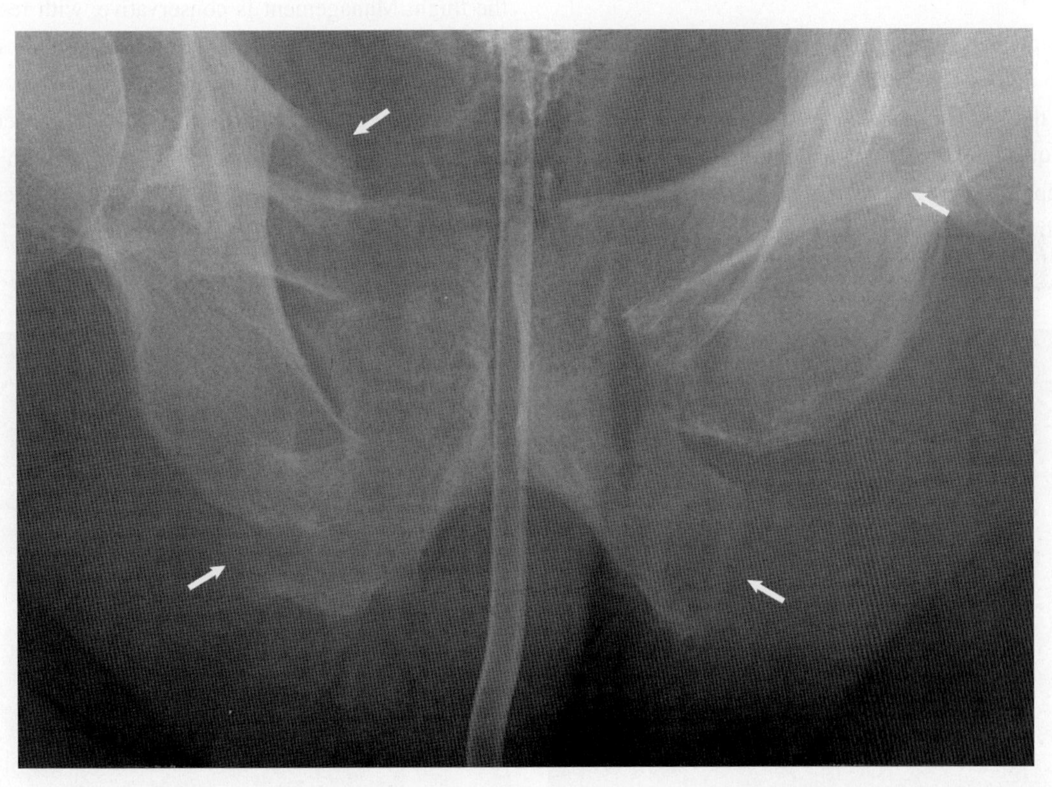

FIGURE 8.8 ■ Bilateral Superior and Inferior Ramus Fractures. Coned-down image from AP pelvis radiographic image shows right and left superior pubic and inferior ischiopubic ramus fractures (arrows).

Radiographic Summary

AP pelvis radiographs demonstrate avulsion fractures as separation of the apophysis of the iliac crest, the anterior superior iliac spine, the anterior inferior iliac spine, or the ischial tuberosity from the underlying normal pelvic bones. Other images are usually not needed, although inlet, outlet, or Judet views may be used to confirm the diagnosis if the AP image is equivocal. CT is not required. It should be noted that some asymmetry in the immature ossification foci (particularly those of the ischial tuberosities) is a common finding in children, and is not necessarily indicative of avulsive trauma.

In younger patients with less bony maturation, only a thin rim of avulsed subchondral bone is visualized at the site of injury on radiographs, with the majority of the avulsion affecting the nonossified cartilaginous apophysis.

Clinical Implications

Apophyseal avulsion fractures are uncommon sport-related injuries seen among 14- to 25-year-olds. Iliac crest avulsions result from the sudden contraction of the external obliques, internal obliques, and transversus abdominus muscles. Patients will often report feeling and hearing a "pop" and have immediate pain, limiting their ability to continue activity.

Avulsion fracture of the anterior superior iliac spine results from forceful contraction of the sartorius muscle, resulting in avulsion of its ASIS origin. This injury is most commonly seen in teenage sprinters and hurdlers due to the need for forceful and sudden hip flexion in these sports. Patients with this injury will have pain on hip flexion and abduction.

Avulsion fracture of the anterior inferior iliac spine results from forceful contraction of the rectus femoris muscle, resulting in avulsion of the AIIS origin of its direct head. This is typically an injury seen in teenage soccer players or other sports that involve kicking. Patients present with pain on hip flexion and tenderness along the AIIS following the injury.

Avulsion fracture of the ischial tuberosity results from forceful contraction of the hamstrings, resulting in avulsion of their origin. This is the most common of the pelvic avulsion fractures. This classically is an injury in a teenage sprinter or hurdler. Patients will complain of pain sitting and flexing the thigh. Management is conservative, with rest, NSAIDS, crutches to assist with ambulation, and primary care follow-up in 1-2 weeks.

Treatment of crest avulsions is generally conservative, with rest and analgesics and non-weight-bearing with crutches for 2-4 weeks, followed by slow resumption of activities over 8-12 weeks.

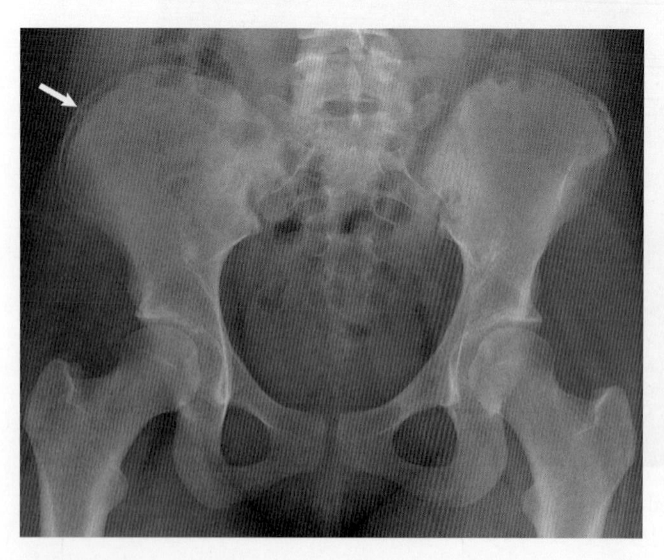

FIGURE 8.9 ■ Avulsion of the Apophysis of the Iliac Crest. AP pelvis image shows a subtle avulsion of the right iliac crest (arrow) in a skeletally immature girl.

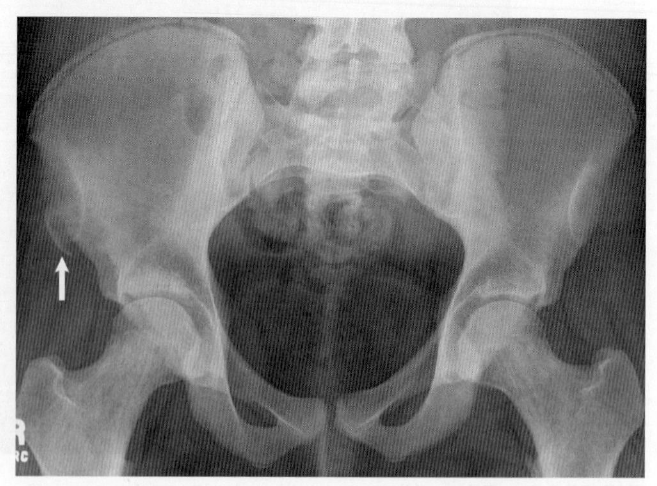

FIGURE 8.10 ■ Avulsion of the Anterior Superior Iliac Spine. AP pelvis in a young male track athlete shows avulsion of the anterior superior iliac spine (arrow).

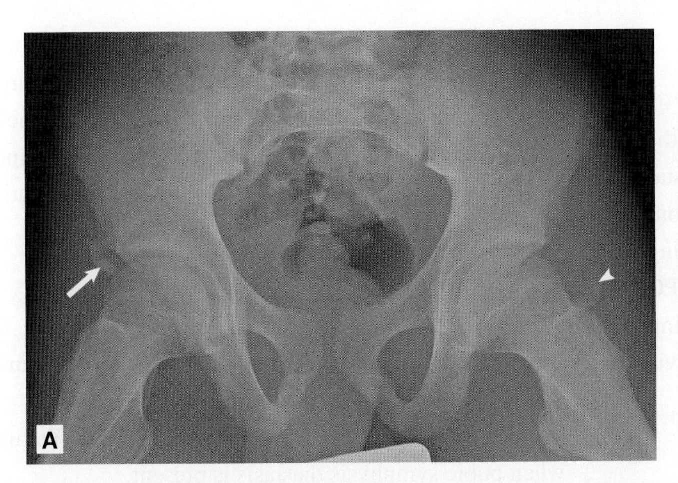

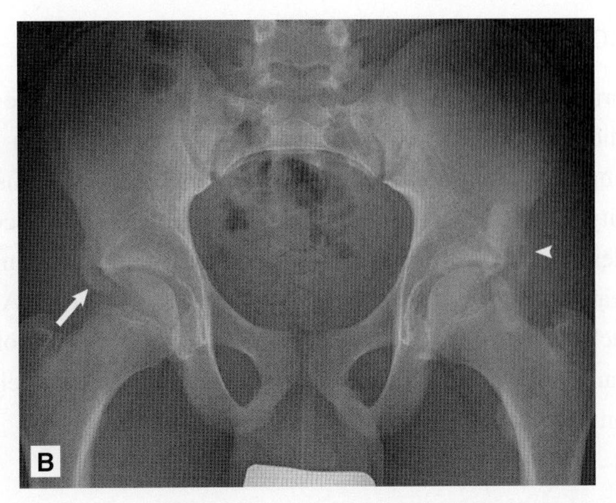

FIGURE 8.11 ■ Avulsion of the Anterior Inferior Iliac Spine. **A, B:** Avulsions of right and left anterior inferior iliac spines in a skeletally immature boy. A: AP pelvis radiographic image obtained at initial presentation shows avulsions of the right (arrow) and left (arrowhead) anterior inferior iliac spines. Mild distraction or displacement, as on the right, is typical of these injuries. A somewhat unusual degree of displacement is seen on the left. B: Follow-up AP pelvis image, obtained four months after image (A). Right (arrow) and left (arrowhead) avulsions are healing. On the left, healing includes retraction of the fragment towards its normal location and abundant heterotopic ossification.

Management of iliac spine avusions is conservative, with rest, NSAIDS, crutches to assist with ambulation, and primary care follow-up in 1-2 weeks.

Pearls

1. Surgery for these injuries is rarely indicated, though it may be required to remove painful fragments or to obtain proper anatomic alignment. Separation of the iliac crest by greater than 3 cm may be an indication for surgical repair.
2. Premature return to sports participation may result in failure of nonoperative management.
3. Suspect iliac spine avulsion in any athlete with pain at the anterior superior or anterior inferior spine following forceful hip flexion, as avulsion fractures are often missed and mistaken for muscle strains.

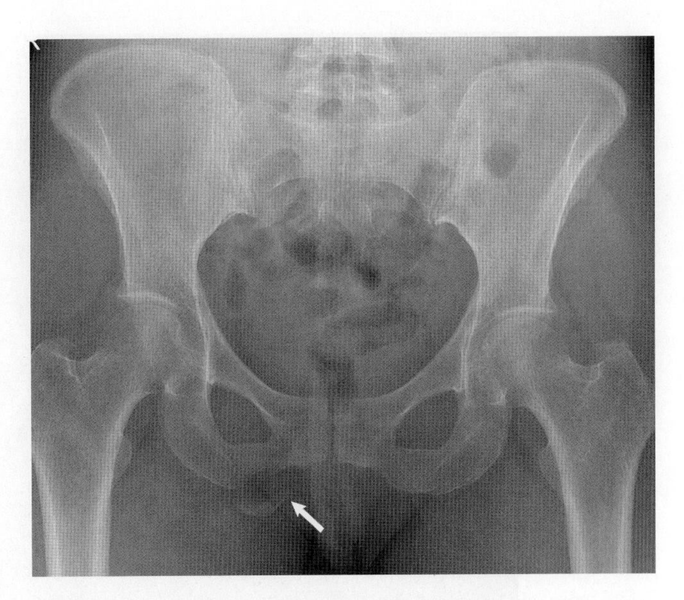

FIGURE 8.12 ■ Avulsion of the Ischial Tuberosity. AP pelvis image shows avulsion of the right ischial tuberosity (arrow) in a skeletally mature woman. This occurred as a result of a running injury with associated hamstring strain.

Radiographic Summary

Normally, the symphysis pubis measures 5-6 mm wide on radiographs. Anterior compression injuries may widen the symphysis to more than 1 cm without posterior pelvic instability. In pregnancy or after childbirth, width of 1 cm is considered normal. In the setting of acute trauma, widening greater than 2.5 cm commonly indicates a significant APC mechanism with associated disruption of a sacroiliac joint, or an extending sacral/iliac fracture separating the hemipelvis from the axial skeleton ("open book" pelvis).

Clinical Implications

Pubic symphysis diastasis can be seen in straddle and APC injuries. The wider the diastasis, the higher is the association with other pelvic injuries including hemorrhage and bladder and urethral injuries. With diastasis, pelvic volume increases dramatically, increasing the potential for large-volume, life-threatening hemorrhage. Pelvic binding helps to lessen pelvic volume in the setting of diastasis and is indicated to curtail blood loss. Emergent orthopedic consultation is indicated.

Pearls

1. Impotence can occur in association with these injuries due to damage to adjacent nerve structures.
2. Look for associated SI joint or sacral or iliac fractures when pubic symphysis diastasis is present.
3. Conventional radiography and CT are equivalent for demonstrating symphyseal diastasis. CT is superior to conventional imaging for depiction of associated sacroiliac and visceral injuries and pelvic hemorrhage.

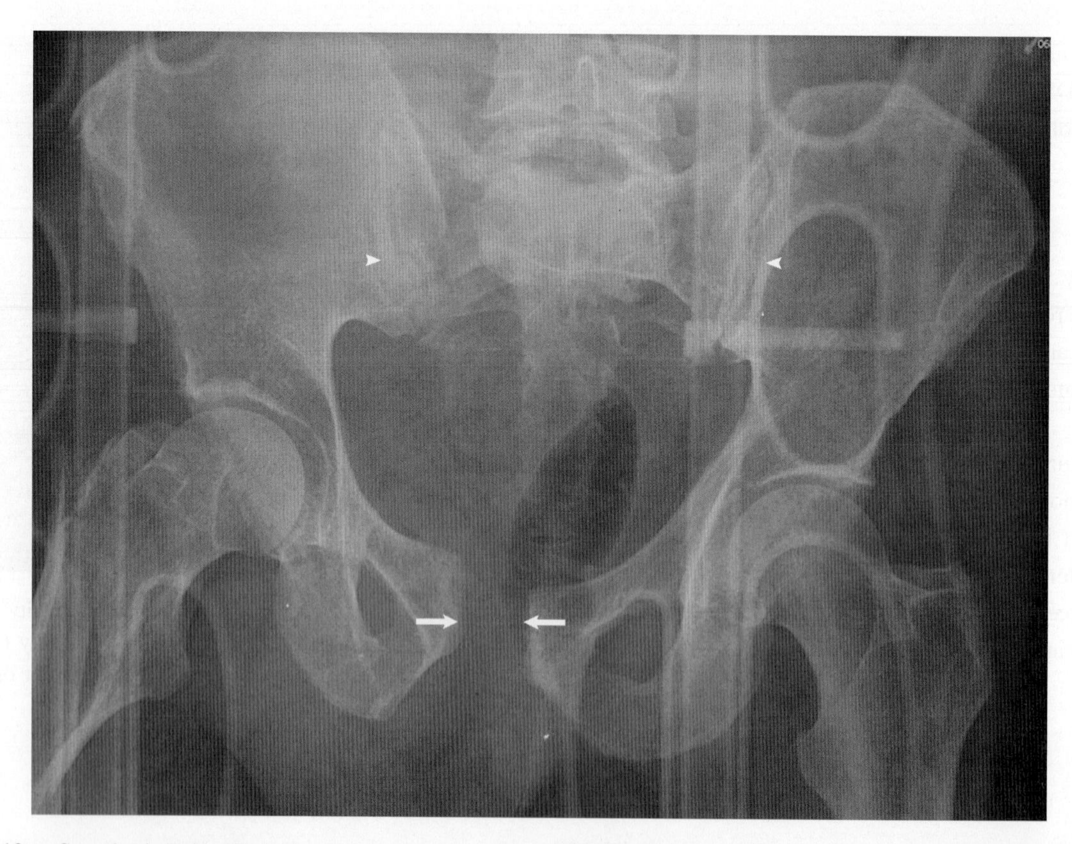

FIGURE 8.13 ■ Symphysis Pubis Diastasis. AP pelvis image shows widening of the symphysis pubis (arrows, measuring 2.4 cm on the original study). Note that the SI joints (arrowheads) are normal width and alignment. However, a vertically oriented sacral fracture can be seen near the midline.

Radiographic Summary

Isolated iliac wing fractures are commonly visible on radiographs as vertical fractures coursing through the iliac crest, although the orientation of the fractures may vary. Duverney fractures may be comminuted, but are rarely significantly displaced. It is common for these fractures to extend to the lateral margin of the pelvis in the immediate supraacetabular region, without involvement of the acetabular articular surface.

Once the fracture is detected, CT or additional conventional radiographs, inlet–outlet or Judet views, may be performed to evaluate for additional injuries. These fractures are commonly associated with lateral compression (LC) mechanism, and may demonstrate concomitant sacral buckle fractures or pubic rami injuries.

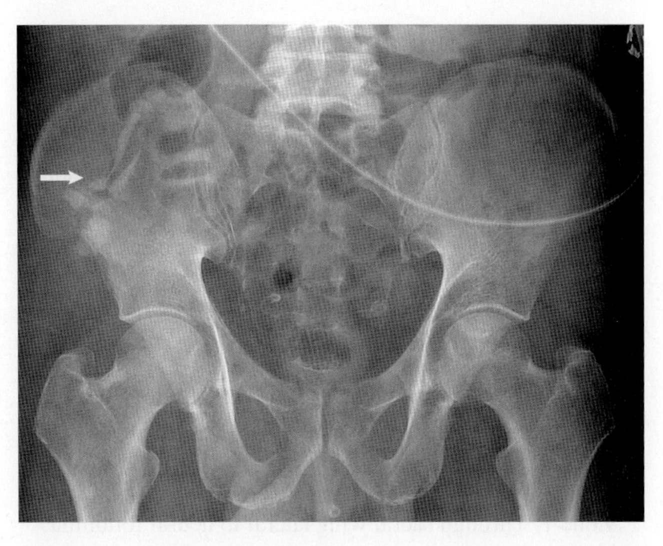

FIGURE 8.14 ■ Isolated Iliac Wing Fracture (Duverney Fracture). AP pelvis radiographic image shows comminuted right iliac wing fracture (arrow). There is no other fracture, subluxation, or dislocation.

Clinical Implications

Iliac wing fractures result from direct trauma, usually directed in a lateral to medial compression fashion. Exam findings include swelling, tenderness, and often bruising over the iliac wing. Significant abdominal pain may be present and associated ileus can occur. As this is not a weight-bearing portion of the pelvis, conservative treatment with analgesics is the norm. Open fractures require surgical treatment.

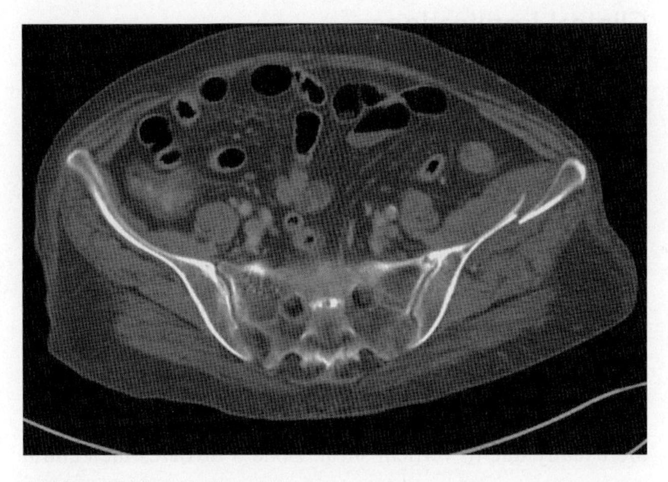

FIGURE 8.15 ■ Isolated Iliac Wing Fracture (Duverney Fracture). Axial CT image in a different patient with an isolated left iliac wing fracture. Note the slight posterior displacement of the fracture typical of these injuries.

Pearls

1. Rare cases of bowel perforation and sepsis have been reported with this injury.
2. Iliac wing fractures are not always isolated, and in addition to LC pelvic ring injuries, they may in fact represent part of both-column or, less commonly, anterior column acetabular fractures.

Radiographic Summary

AP views alone of the pelvis provide limited evaluation of the sacrum because of its shape and orientation and superimposed bowel contents. Inlet views show the sacral spinal canal and superior view of the S1 vertebra, and can be helpful in determining anterior or posterior displacement of the SI joint, sacrum, or iliac wing. The pelvic outlet view provides a true AP view of the sacrum, which is useful for determining vertical displacement of the hemipelvis, widened SI joint, or discontinuity of the sacral foramina. CT is useful for assessing the sacrum and SI joints. Sacral fractures are typically classified by zones:

Zone 1: Through sacral wing lateral to neural foramina
Zone 2: Through neural foramina
Zone 3: Through the central portion or body of the sacrum and canal

Clinical Implications

Transverse fractures may occur from anteroposterior trauma. Upper transverse fractures may result from a fall in a flexed position. All may result in neurologic findings such as urinary retention, perineal numbness, and neurogenic bladder. Transverse fractures are most frequently found between S2 and S3, and less frequently occur at S1 or S2. A detailed genitorectal examination should be conducted to exclude an open fracture. Zone 1 fractures are caused by lateral compression of the pelvis, vertical shear fracture, or sacrotuberous avulsions. Zone 2 fractures involve one or more foramen and are usually due to vertical shear. Zone 3 involves the central canal. Although Zone 3 fractures are less frequent, they have the highest rate of neurological deficits of the three zones. L5 nerve root damage is common in Zone 2 injuries. In Zone 3 injuries, central canal involvement with caudaequina syndrome may occur.

Pearls

1. Early orthopedic consultation and surgery are key for those patients with associated neurologic injury.
2. Observation of asymmetric irregularities in the bony margins of the sacral foramina on radiographs is helpful for detection of subtle Zone 2 sacral fracture.
3. Sacral fractures rarely occur in isolation; look for other pelvic fractures carefully.

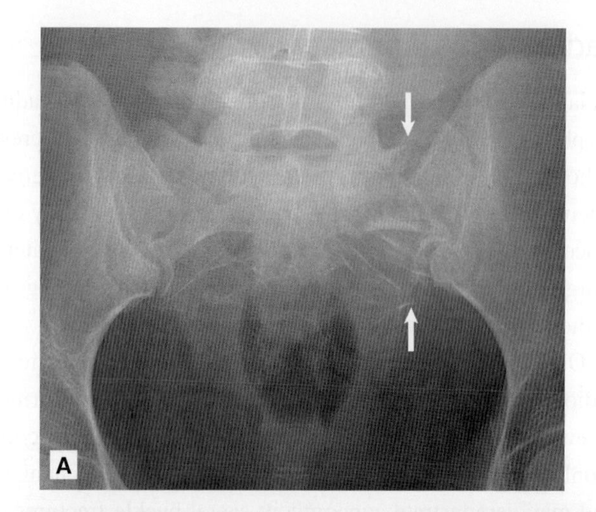

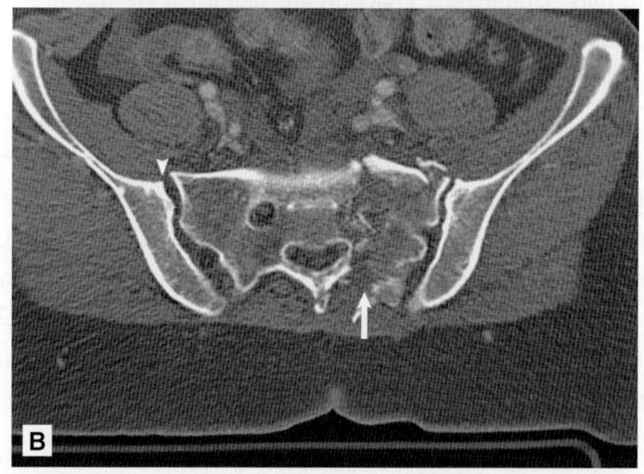

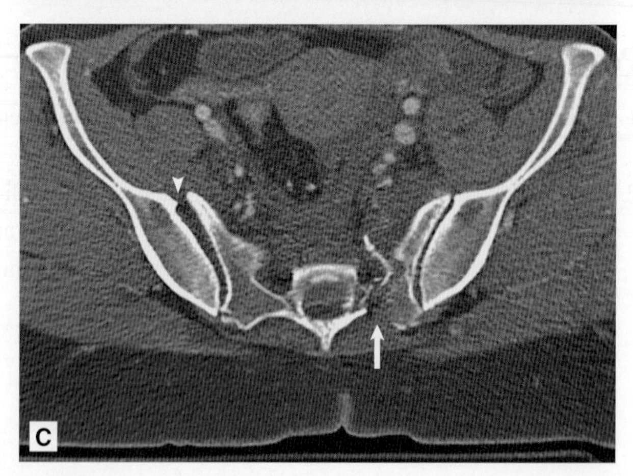

FIGURE 8.16 ■ Sacral Fracture. **A-C:** AP pelvis image and transverse CT images at level of sacrum show Zone 2 fracture of left sacral wing. A: Conventional radiographic image shows vertical fracture of left sacral wing, manifest as fractures of the superior margin of the wing and as fractures of superior edges of several left neural foramina (arrows). B, C: Transverse CT images at level of sacrum show fracture of left sacral wing, predominately extending through Zone 2 from anterior to posterior through the neural foramina (arrows). In addition, the right sacroiliac joint is diastatic anteriorly (arrowheads), a coincidental finding.

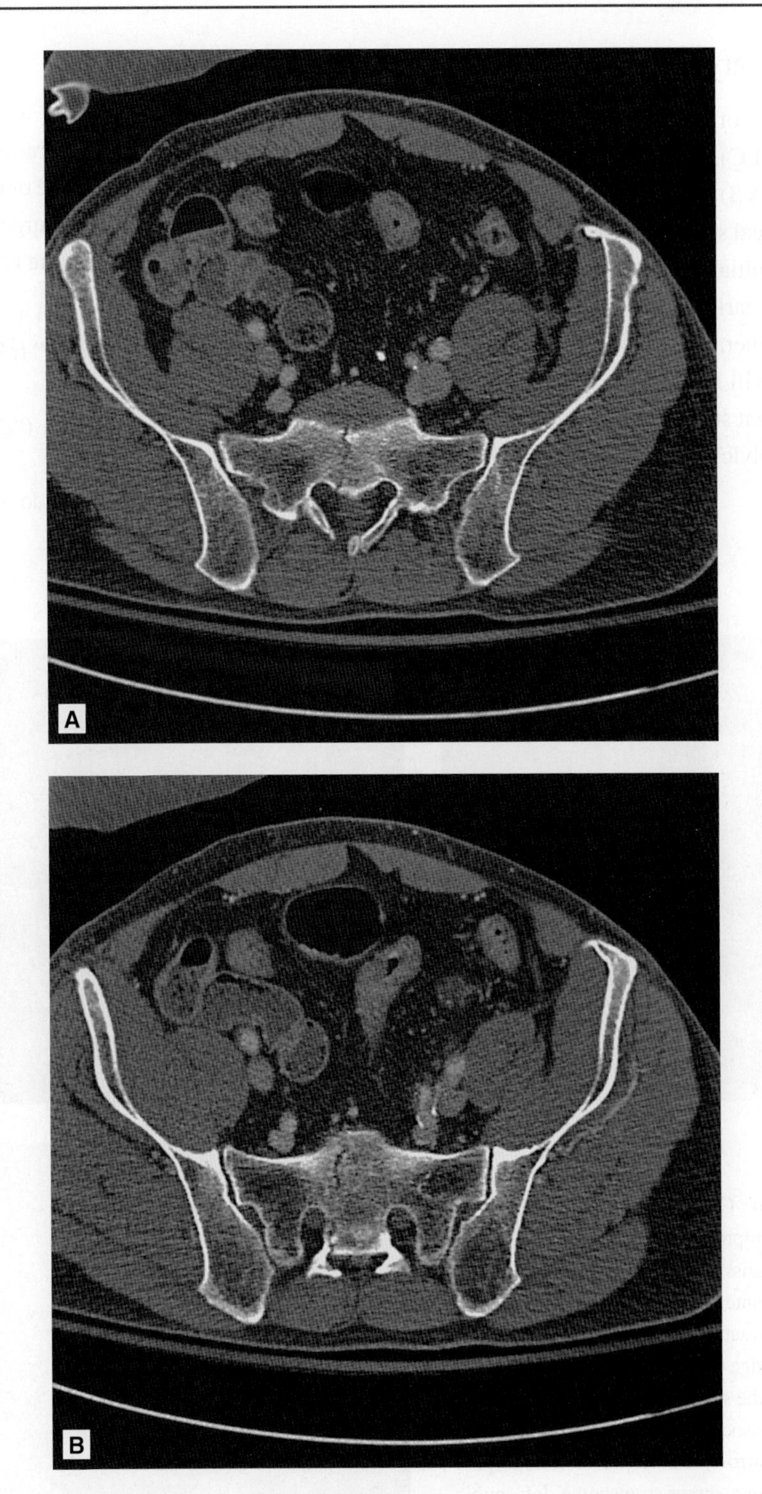

FIGURE 8.17 ■ Sacral Fracture. **A, B:** CT images in a different patient demonstrate a Zone 3 sacral fracture, coursing to the right of midline and medial to the S1 sacral foramina.

Radiographic Summary

Fractures and dislocations of the pelvic ring are classified as lateral compression (LC), anteroposterior compression (APC), or vertical shear (VS) mechanisms of injury. An AP pelvis radiograph is the usual screening x-ray. X-ray is helpful in the unstable patient to initially characterize the type of pelvic fracture and allow for early notification of interventional radiology if embolization therapy is ultimately required. Most severely injured patients will have CT imaging of the pelvis. CT scan is the best emergent study for evaluation of all pelvic anatomy and degree of pelvic, retroperitoneal, and intraperitoneal bleeding.

Lateral Compression

In a LC pelvic fracture, there are fractures of the superior pubic and inferior ischiopubic rami. The superior ramus fracture is characteristically oblique or nearly horizontal and parasymphyseal. The Young and Burgess classification is defined by the injury associated with the ramus fractures:

Type I: Sacral compression fracture on side of impact, an incomplete or "buckle" fracture of the anterior sacral wall.

Type II: Iliac wing fracture ("crescent fracture") on side of impact.

Type III: LC-I or LC-II on side of impact with contralateral APC injury (*see* below).

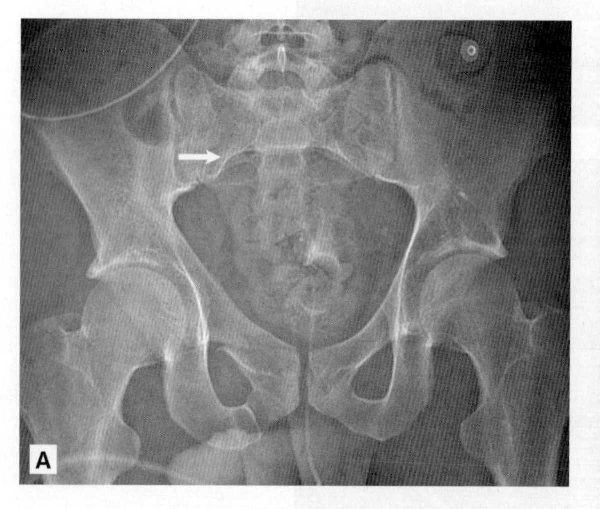

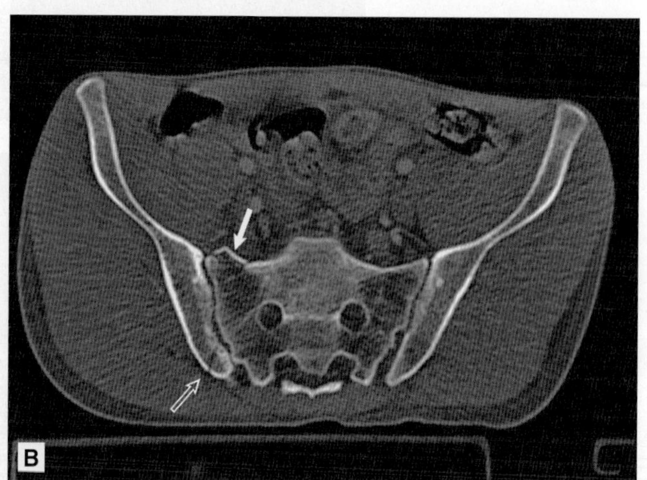

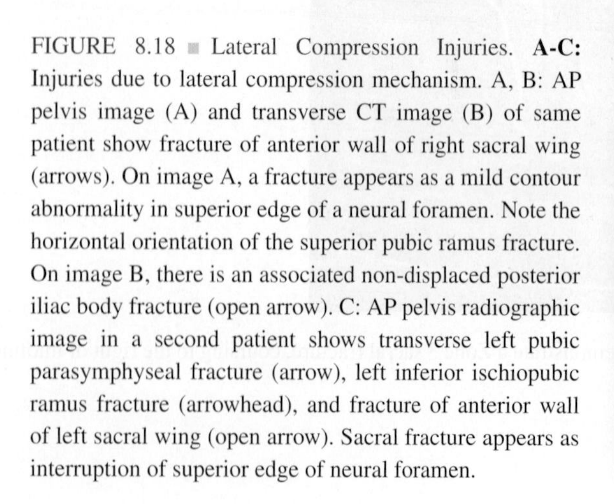

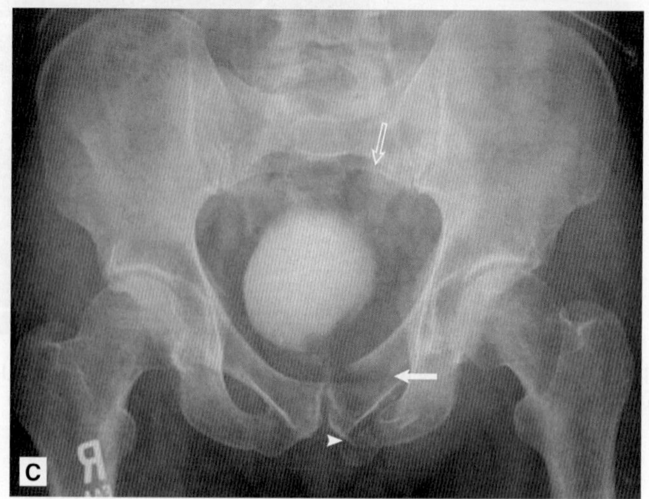

FIGURE 8.18 ■ Lateral Compression Injuries. **A-C:** Injuries due to lateral compression mechanism. A, B: AP pelvis image (A) and transverse CT image (B) of same patient show fracture of anterior wall of right sacral wing (arrows). On image A, a fracture appears as a mild contour abnormality in superior edge of a neural foramen. Note the horizontal orientation of the superior pubic ramus fracture. On image B, there is an associated non-displaced posterior iliac body fracture (open arrow). C: AP pelvis radiographic image in a second patient shows transverse left pubic parasymphyseal fracture (arrow), left inferior ischiopubic ramus fracture (arrowhead), and fracture of anterior wall of left sacral wing (open arrow). Sacral fracture appears as interruption of superior edge of neural foramen.

Anteroposterior Compression

APC pelvic fractures are the second most common types of pelvic ring injury, accounting for approximately 25% of pelvic fractures. Head-on automobile collision is a common mechanism of this injury. The Young and Burgess classification of APC fractures is as follows:

Type I: Symphysis pubis less than 2.5 cm wide; SI joints may look normal.

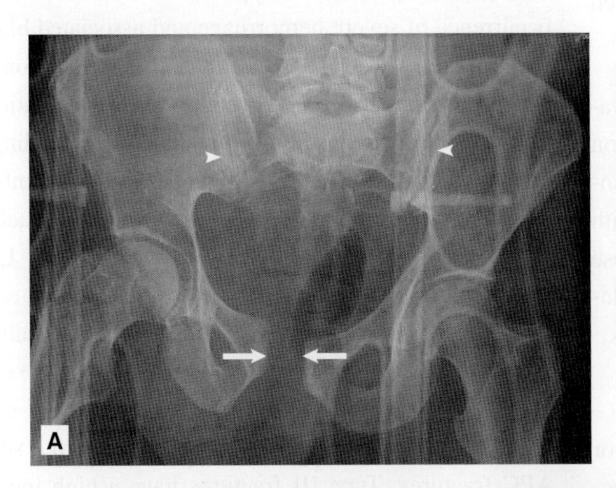

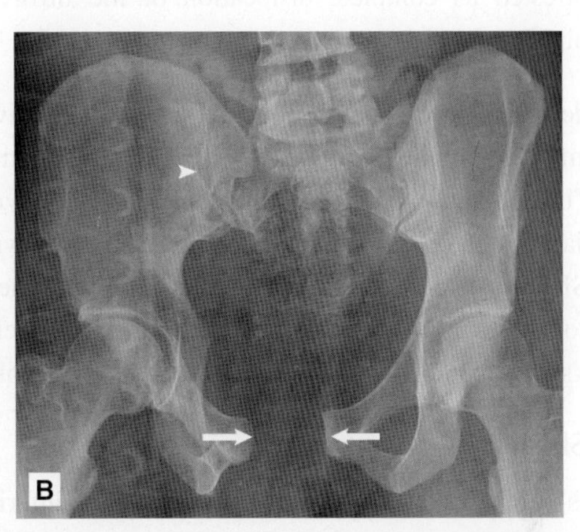

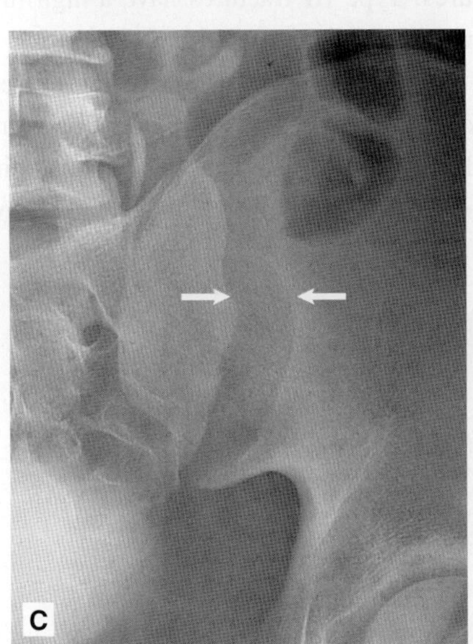

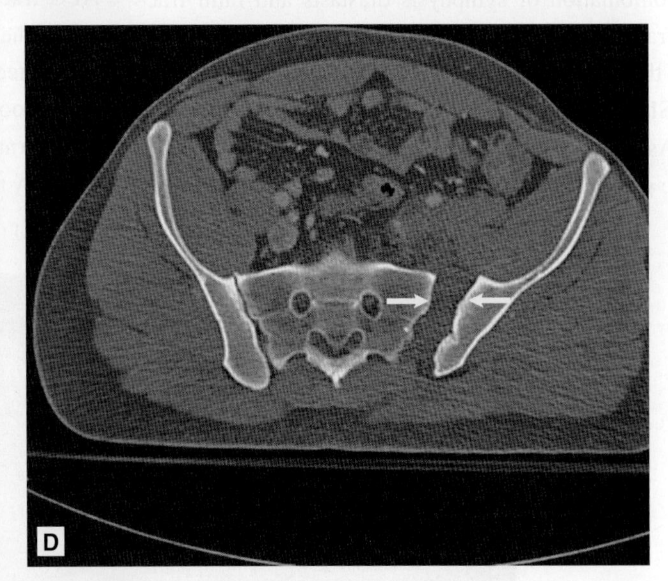

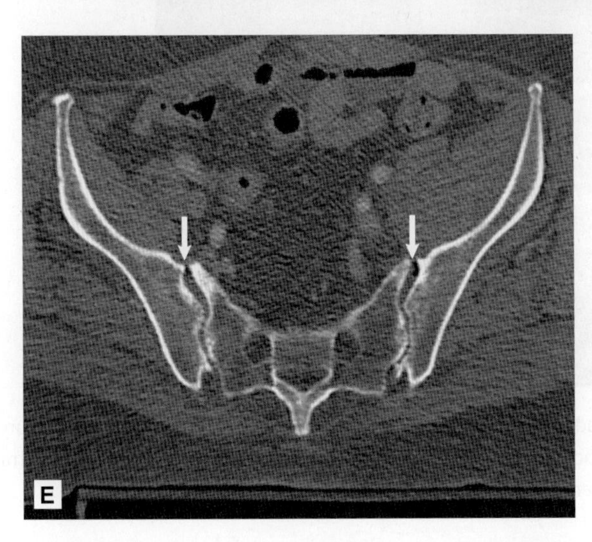

FIGURE 8.19 ■ AP Compression Injuries. **A-E:** Conventional and CT images of anteroposterior compression mechanism injuries. A: Same as Figure 8.13. AP pelvis image shows widening of the symphysis pubis (arrows). Note that the SI joints (arrowheads) are normal width and alignment. A Zone 3 sacral fracture is present, to the left of midline. B: AP pelvis image shows widening of the symphysis pubis greater than 2.5 cm (arrows) and diastasis of the right SI joint (arrowhead). C, D: Conventional AP image and transverse CT image in a different patient show marked widening of the entire left SI joint (arrows), indicating that all anterior and posterior ligaments are disrupted. E: Transverse CT image of pelvis shows mild widening of each SI joint anteriorly (arrows).

Type II: Symphysis width more than 2.5 cm, SI joint anterior widening due to torn sacrospinous and sacrotuberous ligaments.

Type III: Complete symphyseal and SI joint disruptions, manifested as complete dislocation of the involved hemipelvis from the sacrum.

A vertical displaced fracture of a sacral wing is equivalent to complete SI joint disruption in the APC classification scheme. The "open book" injury is the combination of symphyseal diastasis or superior and inferior ramus fracture with bilateral SI joint disruption or sacral wing fractures. These combinations allow the hemipelves to rotate externally relative to the spine, in analogy to opening the covers of a book.

Vertical Shear

Symphysis pubis diastasis, fractures of superior and inferior rami, a combination of symphysis diastasis and rami fractures, or fractures of all four rami are all radiographic presentations of the anterior part of a VS injury. Posteriorly, an iliac fracture, SI dislocation, or sacroiliac fracture-dislocation may be seen. Associated fracture of the ipsilateral 4th or 5th lumbar transverse process is common.

Clinical Implications

Type I LC fractures have a low incidence of severe hemorrhage, and associated bladder or urethral injuries are not commonly seen. In contrast, Type III LC fractures have a high occurrence of severe hemorrhage and associated bladder and urethral injury. Retroperitoneal bleeding is common and may be large volume, requiring aggressive resuscitation. Early reduction of LC pelvis fractures with external binding devices or external fixation may help limit bleeding. Embolization of bleeding arterial vessels may be required to stabilize the patient prior to definitive fixation. Treatment of LC type I injuries consists of a few days of bed rest followed by protected weight-bearing. All other injury types typically require open reduction and internal fixation.

Similarly, significant arterial bleeding and associated injuries of the genitourinary tract vary with the severity of APC fractures. Type III fractures have a high incidence of severe hemorrhage and retroperitoneal bleeding as well as associated bladder and urethral injury. Prompt reduction of open book pelvis fractures with external binding devices or external fixation may help limit life-threatening hemorrhage by reducing pelvic volume. As with other severe pelvic

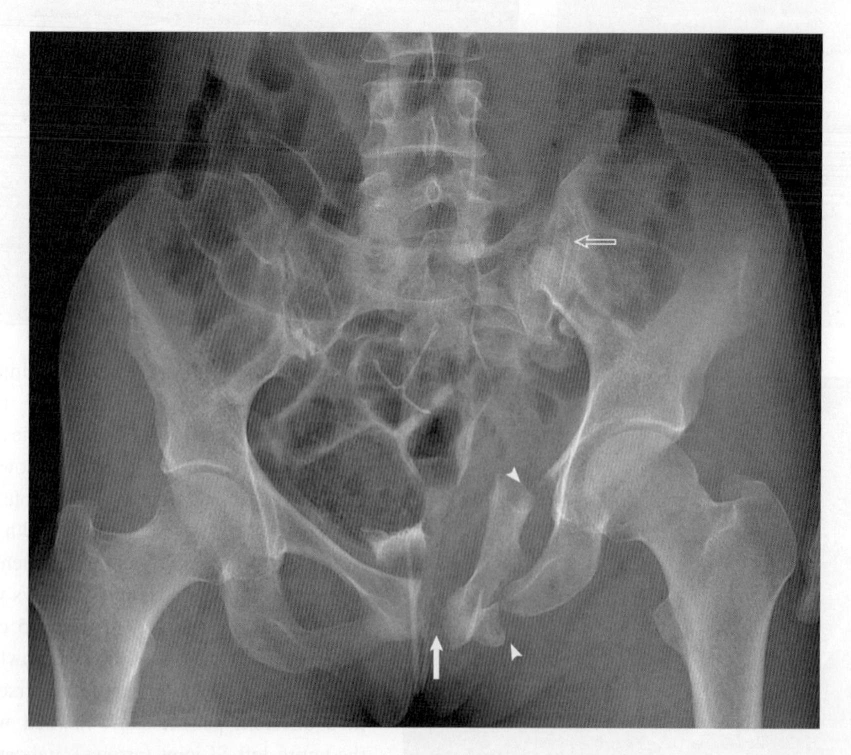

FIGURE 8.20 ■ Vertical Shear Fracture-Dislocation. AP pelvis radiograph shows disrupted symphysis pubis (arrow) and fractures of superior pubic and inferior ischiopubic rami (arrowheads). Note the vertical orientation and displacement of the superior pubic ramus fracture. The left sacroiliac joint is disrupted (open arrow). Injuries result in superior dislocation of left hemipelvis from the sacrum.

fractures, embolization of bleeding vessels may be required to stabilize the patient prior to definitive operative fixation. Treatment of AP compression type I injuries consists of initial bed rest followed by protected weight-bearing. More severe injuries typically require open reduction and internal fixation.

VS fractures have the highest occurrence of severe hemorrhage and shock. Bladder and urethral injuries are commonly associated with VS fractures. Ligamentous injury to the anterior and posterior SI ligaments, the sacrospinous and sacrotuberous ligaments, and the symphysis ligaments may also occur.

Mixed or combined patterns of pelvic injuries often occur with significant trauma, the most common being VS combined with LC. Complex mechanisms of injury result in combinations of these characteristics in a substantial number of patients.

Pearls

1. The orientation of superior pubic ramus fractures may provide a clue to the mechanism of pelvis ring injury, with horizontally oriented fractures typical of LC, and vertically oriented fractures commonly associated with vertical shear.
2. Inlet and outlet views of the pelvis are crucial for assessing anterior-to-posterior as well as vertical displacement of complex pelvic ring fracture components.
3. Be prepared for large-volume crystalloid and blood product resuscitation in patients with several pelvic ring injuries as severe hemorrhage and shock may rapidly develop.
4. Prompt administration of pelvic binding devices (or proper wrapping of the pelvis) may be life-saving by abruptly decreasing pelvic volume and limiting associated hemorrhage.

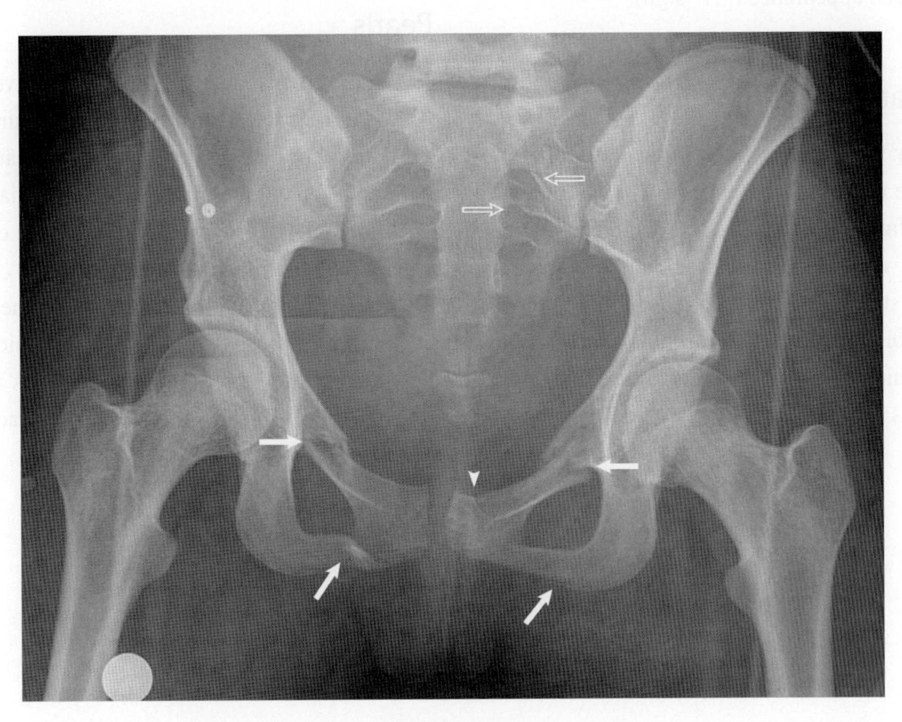

FIGURE 8.21 ■ Combined Mechanism of Injury. AP pelvis radiographic image shows right and left superior and inferior ramus fractures, often associated with a straddle injury (arrows). Additionally, there are left parasymphyseal superior ramus (arrowhead) and "buckle" left anterior sacral wall (open arrows) fractures characteristic of lateral compression forces.

Radiographic Summary

Nondisplaced sacral insufficiency injuries are commonly radiographically occult. Initial radiographs may be normal or show osteopenia. Occasionally subtle irregularities in the bony margins of the anterior sacral foramina may be seen on x-ray. CT also has limited sensitivity for detection of nondisplaced insufficiency fracture in the setting of significant demineralization. Findings include increased density in the sacral wing paralleling the SI joint (unilaterally or bilaterally) indicative of a stress reaction, or superimposed curvilinear lucencies if there is a "completed" fracture. MRI is highly sensitive for detection of these injuries, and will show abnormal signal intensities in the sacral wing paralleling the SI joint, with or without a visible fracture line. Parasymphyseal pubic or pubic root insufficiency fractures commonly accompany these injuries. Bone scan of the pelvis (ordinarily not performed in the ED setting) classically shows increased uptake in both sacral ala and body of the sacrum, showing an H- or butterfly-shaped appearance ("H" sign).

Clinical Implications

Sacral insufficiency fractures are often missed on initial presentation due to the clinician's reliance on x-rays to identify acute fractures or failure to consider the diagnosis. Patients often present with non-specific marked lumbosacral pain, mimicking lumbar strains, but may also present with pain in the buttock, hip, groin, or pelvis. Patients almost always have great difficulty or pain with ambulation if they are able to walk at all. The diagnosis of sacral insufficiency fractures must be considered in patients at risk for osteopenia and osteoporosis, especially in the elderly. However, insufficiency fractures may also be seen in patients who have undergone radiation to the pelvis, have demineralizing bone diseases, have used chronic steroids, or have other conditions that may weaken the bony pelvis. Patients typically present with severe sacropelvic pain that is sudden in onset with no or minimal history of trauma. Although uncommon, sacral insufficiency fracture can present with cauda equina syndrome. Given the diagnostic limitations of x-ray and CT to identify insufficiency fractures, MRI should be performed in patients where clinical suspicion of insufficiency fractures is present. Once identified, most sacral insufficiency fractures can be managed non-operatively with limited weight-bearing, rest, and pain control. Complete healing may take nine to twelve months. Sarcoplasty may be considered in patients with severe intractable pain, and operative fixation may be required in cases of neurological impairment.

Pearls

1. Radiographs and CT are insensitive in the diagnosis of nondisplaced insufficiency fractures of the pelvis in elderly or osteoporotic patients. Because the clinical presentation commonly overlaps with that of occult hip fracture, MRI is often indicated in those cases where there is sufficient clinical concern.
2. Early diagnosis is key for proper therapy and lessening complications. A high index of clinical suspicion in the appropriate patient population leads to appropriate testing and diagnosis of insufficiency fractures.

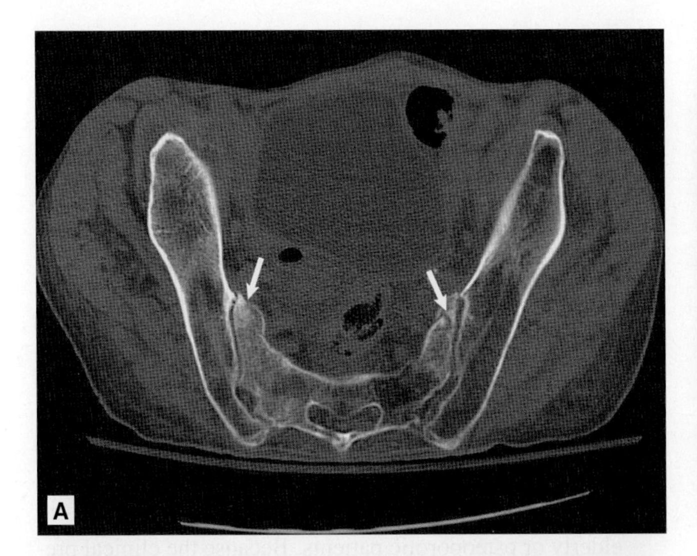

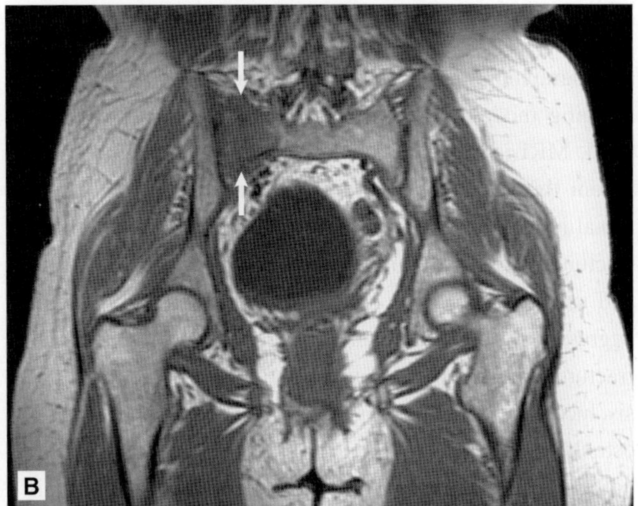

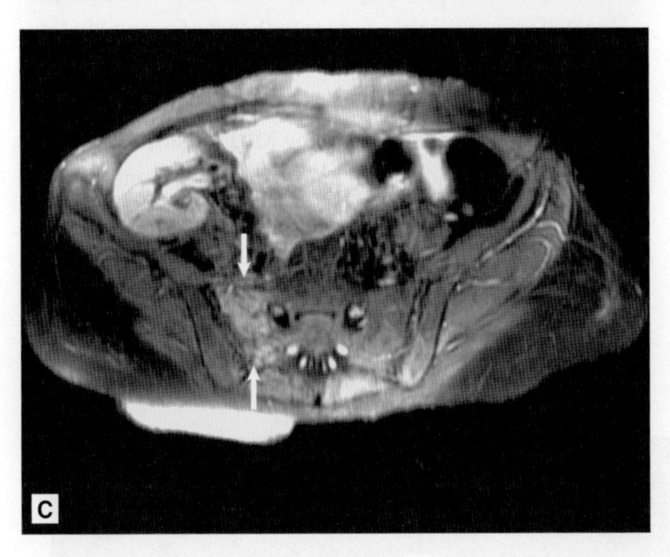

FIGURE 8.22 ■ Sacral Insufficiency Fractures. **A-C:** CT and MR images of sacral insufficiency fractures in elderly woman with no recent trauma. A, B: Transverse CT image (A) and coronal T1-weighted MR images show right sacral wing insufficiency fracture (arrows). Conventional radiographic pelvic images showed osteopenia but were otherwise normal (C) Transverse short-tau inversion recovery (STIR) MR image in second patient shows right sacral wing insufficiency fracture (arrows).

Radiographic Summary

Radiographic findings depend on the site of the fracture. Imaging modalities may include plain radiographs, CT, or MRI. MRI is indicated for high-risk patients or patients in whom the suspicion of injury remains high when conventional images are negative. Parasymphyseal and pubic ramus fractures may have abundant periosteal new bone formation and substantial lucency at the fracture plane, simulating an aggressive or destructive process, depending on the stage of fracture maturity. Radiographic findings may include sclerosis, lucent fracture line, bone expansion, exuberant callus, and osteolysis, although a definite fracture line or cortical break is not essential to the diagnosis. The most common finding is a sclerotic band through the medullary space. Sacral, iliac, and supra-acetabular stress reactions or fractures may accompany the ramus abnormalities.

Clinical Implications

Pubic insufficiency fractures may present in a similar fashion to hip fractures with severe groin and buttock pain and difficulty walking. As with sacral insufficiency fractures, a high index of clinical suspicion is important in making the diagnosis as initial radiographs lack the sensitivity of MRI. Thus, in at-risk patients with the appropriate clinical presentation, especially the elderly and those with osteopenia, MRI should be considered when plain radiographs are unrevealing. Management of pubic insufficiency fractures begins with non-weight-bearing, followed by physical therapy and progressive return to weight-bearing and ambulation. With appropriate therapy most patients recover over a period of weeks to months.

Pearls

1. Plain radiographs and CT are insensitive in the diagnosis of nondisplaced insufficiency fractures of the pelvis in elderly or osteoporotic patients. Because the clinical presentation commonly overlaps with that of occult hip fracture, MRI is often indicated in those cases where there is sufficient clinical concern.
2. Osteopenic patients undergoing MRI for suspected radiographically occult hip fractures may be found to have pubic or ischiopubic ramus stress fractures. Therefore, when examining for occult hip fractures in osteopenic patients, sequences of the whole pelvis should be obtained to rule out associated insufficiency fractures due to the overlap in clinical presentations.

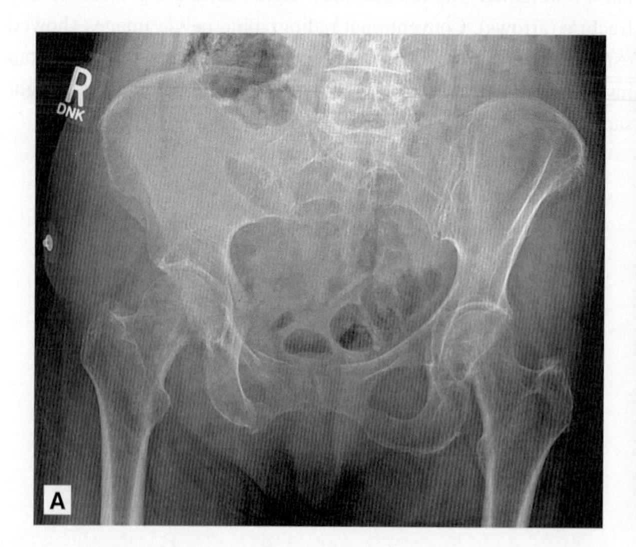

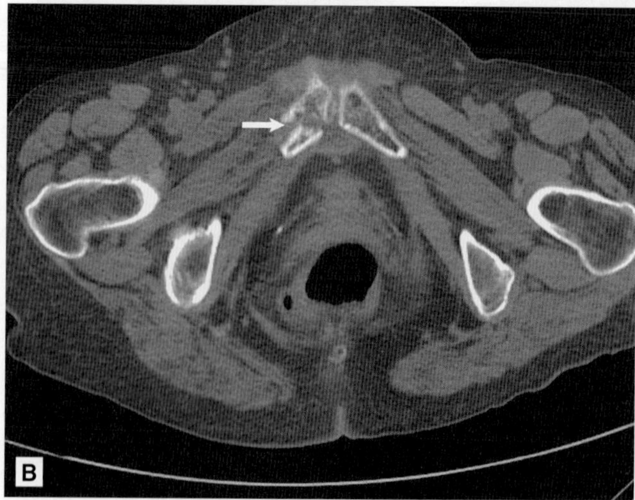

FIGURE 8.23 ■ Pubic Insufficiency Fracture. **A:** AP radiograph of the pelvis in an elderly woman who complained of hip pain while ambulating. The image demonstrates minimally displaced acute superior and inferior pubic rami fractures on the right. The bony structures appear osteoporotic. **B:** Transverse CT image at level of pubic symphysis in elderly, osteopenic woman shows transverse insufficiency fracture of parasymphyseal right pubis (arrow). Conventional radiographic AP pelvis image showed osteopenia.

Radiographic Summary

AP and lateral sacrococcygeal radiographs are not sensitive in the detection of coccygeal fractures in the absence of significant displacement. Normal developmental variations in the general appearance and orientation of the bones of the coccyx (including significant anterior angulation, congenital clefts, and alignment inconsistencies) make these injuries challenging to diagnose on plain films. Occasionally, clearly visible buckling of the anterior cortex of a coccygeal segment is seen in association with transverse coccyx fractures. Coccygeal fractures may appear as incidental findings on CT scans.

Clinical Implications

The typical mechanism for coccygeal injury is a fall in a sitting position, although fractures can occur during childbirth or in contact sports from a direct blow. Pain may be noted on direct palpation of the coccyx and on rectal exam. Rectal exam may also serve to identify associated rectal injury. Management is generally conservative with rest, sitz baths, analgesics, and donut-ring cushion. Orthopedic follow-up is generally not necessary in uncomplicated injury. Surgical excision of a fracture fragment may be required in the setting of chronic pain.

Pearls

1. Physical examination is more informative than radiography in diagnosis of acute, isolated coccyx fractures.
2. Rarely, rectal injuries may result from tearing from coccygeal fracture edges.
3. There is a wide variety of normal variation in the appearance of the coccyx. The presence of significant anterior angulation at the sacrococcygeal junction is not specific for acute injury.

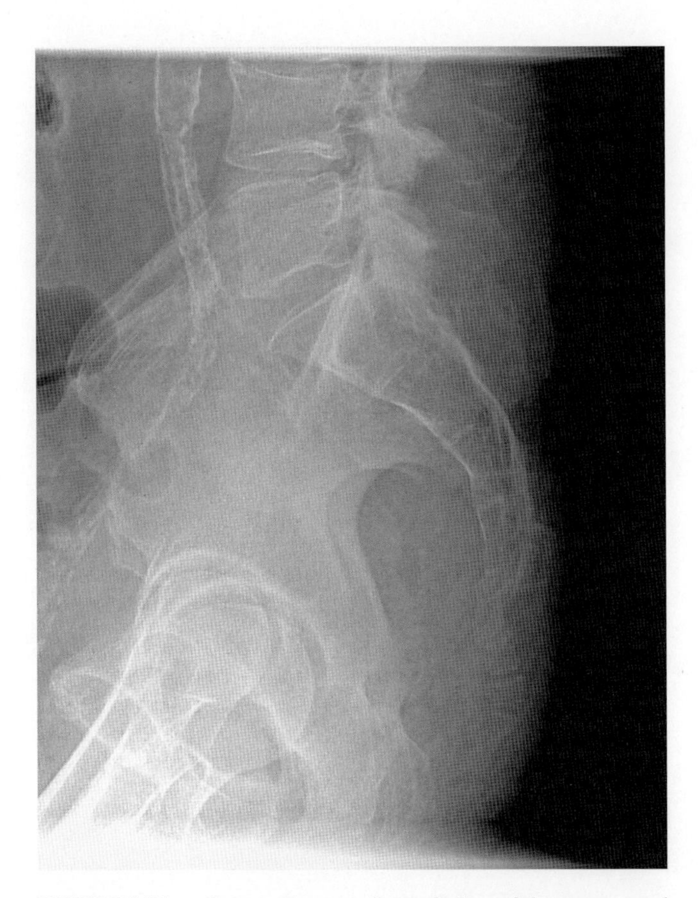

FIGURE 8.24 ■ Coccyx Fracture. Lateral view of the sacrum and coccyx in an elderly patient demonstrates a mildly displaced fracture of the coccyx occurring near the sacro-coccygeal junction.

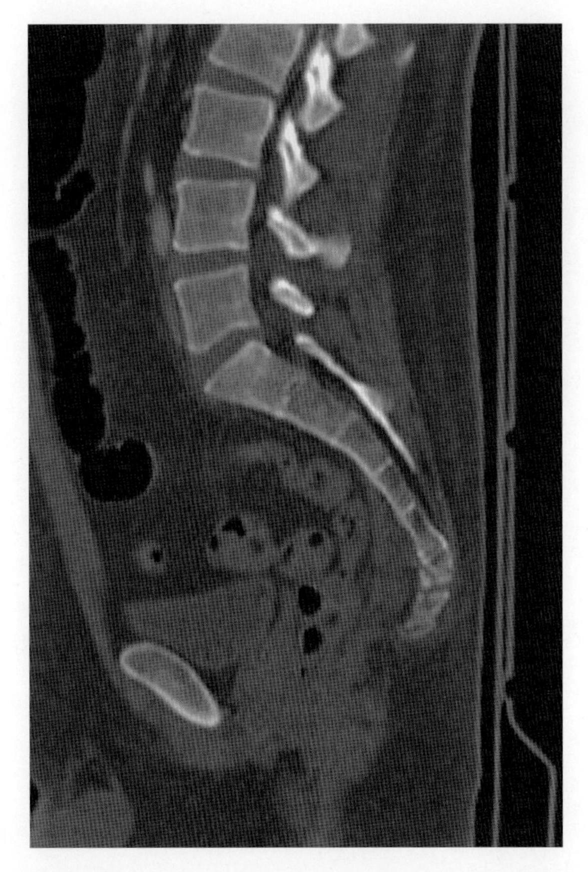

FIGURE 8.25 ■ Coccyx Fracture. Sagittal CT reformation image of pelvis at level of coccyx shows a nondisplaced coccyx fracture. Conventional AP and lateral sacrococcygeal radiographic images (not shown) were normal.

Chapter 9

UPPER EXTREMITY

Martin I. Jordanov
Robert Warne Fitch

Radiographic Summary

Acromio-clavicular (AC) separation is an injury to the ligamentous structures of the AC joint. On AP radiographs of the shoulder, the inferior aspect of the distal clavicle should align with the inferior aspect of the acromion. In type I injuries, there is a sprain or partial tear to the AC ligament and imaging will appear normal. In type II injuries, the AC ligament is torn and the space between the distal clavicle and acromion may appear wider (as compared to the other shoulder) and the distal clavicle may be slightly superiorly displaced in relation to the acromion, but less than 100%. Type III injuries involve a tear of the AC and coraco-clavicular (CC) ligaments and the distal clavicle is 100% displaced superiorly in relation to the acromion. Type IV injuries are rare and occur when the distal clavicle is displaced posteriorly. Type V injuries are severe type III injuries; in these, the distal clavicle punctures the trapezius muscle. Type VI injuries occur when the distal clavicle is inferiorly displaced below the coracoid.

Clinical Implications

AC separation injuries occur when patients fall or sustain a blow to the top of the shoulder. Physical findings include swelling and pain on palpation of the AC joint. Patients will have pain with cross arm testing (reaching from the affected arm to the opposite shoulder). Radiographs can help determine the severity and type of the injury. Type I, II, and III injuries are treated conservatively with a sling for comfort and activity as tolerated. Type IV, V, and VI injuries are rare, and treated surgically on an outpatient basis. Patients with symptomatic arthritis as a result of these injuries may ultimately be treated with a distal clavicle excision (Mumford procedure).

Pearls

1. AP chest radiographs can be helpful in providing a comparative view of the unaffected AC joint.
2. Weighted arm views can aid in the diagnosis but do not change overall management and are not routinely recommended.

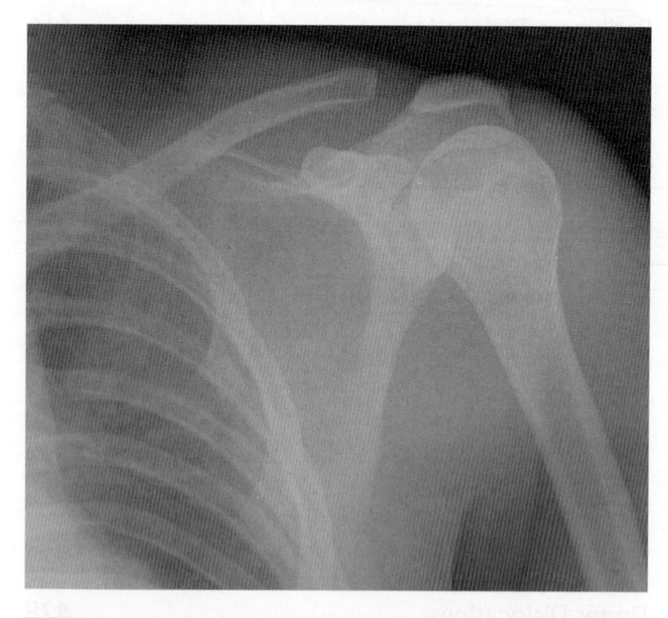

FIGURE 9.1 ■ Grade 2 Acromio-Clavicular Separation. AP view of the left shoulder demonstrates mild widening of the left acromio-clavicular joint (it measured 12 mm; the upper limit of normal is 8 mm). The distance between the coracoid process and undersurface of the clavicle remains normal (upper normal is 13 mm). The findings are consistent with grade 2 acromio-clavicular separation. Grade 1 A-C separation is radiographically occult.

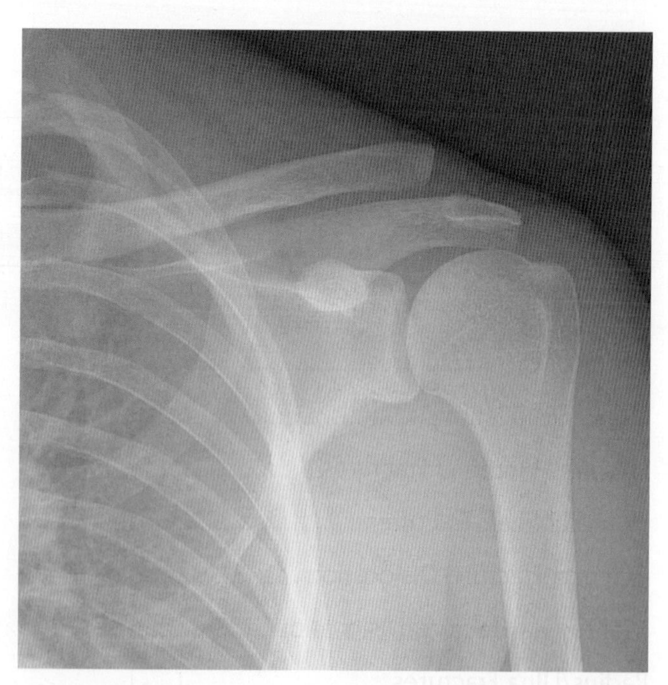

FIGURE 9.2 ■ Grade 3 Acromio-Clavicular Separation. AP view of the left shoulder shows slight widening of the left A-C joint, marked widening of the left CC interval, and superior displacement of the lateral aspect of the left clavicle in relationship to the acromion.

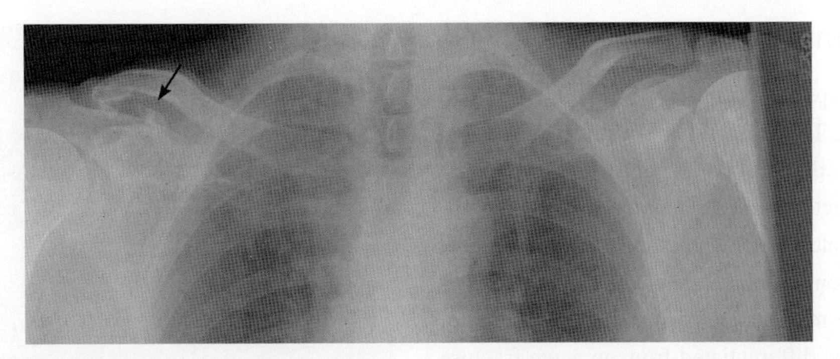

FIGURE 9.3 ■ Remote Right Acromio-Clavicular Separation. An AP view of the upper chest shows linear mature heterotopic ossification between the right coracoid and clavicle (arrow) and an abnormal, foreshortened and mildly irregular appearance of the distal end of the right clavicle. These findings indicate that the patient has had a high grade A-C separation in the past (months or years ago).

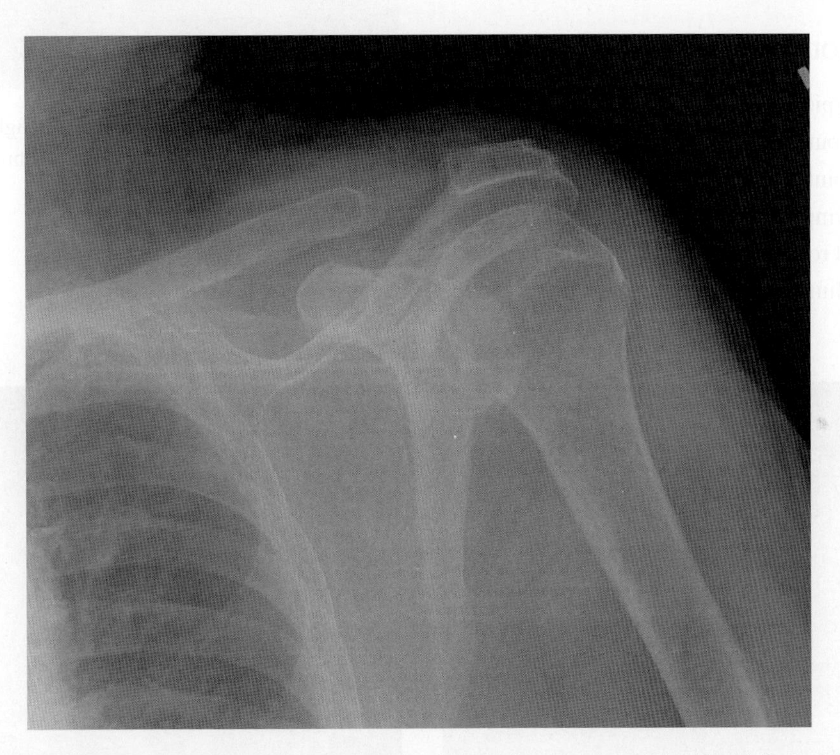

FIGURE 9.4 ■ Mumford Procedure. An AP view of the left shoulder shows prior resection of the distal left clavicle (Mumford procedure). This is done to alleviate or prevent further supraspinatus tendinopathy. Notice the rounded, well-corticated edge of the resected distal left clavicle. This should not be confused with acromio-clavicular separation.

Radiographic Summary

Acromion fractures typically result from direct trauma to the superior shoulder. These fractures are often subtle and are best seen on the axillary and/or scapular Y views of the shoulder. Acromial fractures may be confused with os acromionale. Os acromionale occurs when the ossification center at the tip of the acromion fails to fuse with the rest of the acromion. Os acromionale may be symptomatic and cause pain. An os acromiale can be differentiated from an acute fracture by its sclerotic and rounded edges. CT and MRI can often better illustrate the diagnosis.

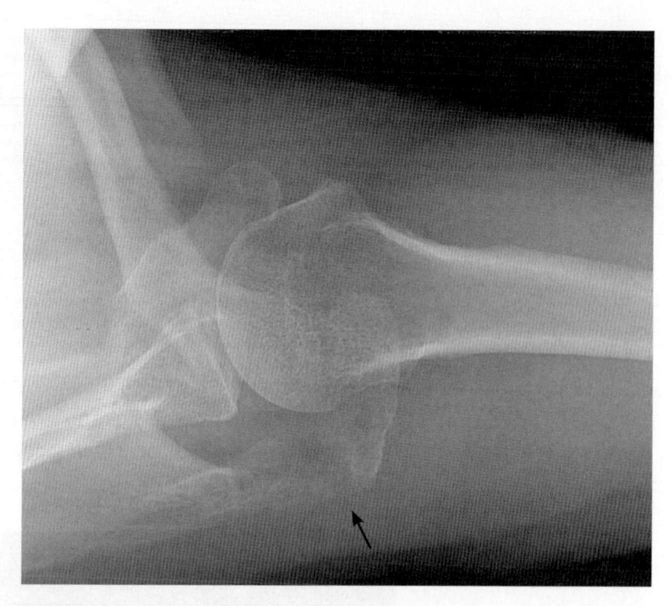

FIGURE 9.5 ■ Acromial Fracture. A single axillary view of the left shoulder shows a nondisplaced fracture through the base of the acromion (arrow).

Clinical Implications

Acromion fractures typically result from a direct downward blow to the shoulder, but may also occur in superiorly dislocated gleno-humeral joint injuries. Patients will be point tender over the acromion. Symptomatic os acrominale may present with impingement and rotator cuff pain. MRI will often show bony edema surrounding the unfused synchondrosis of the

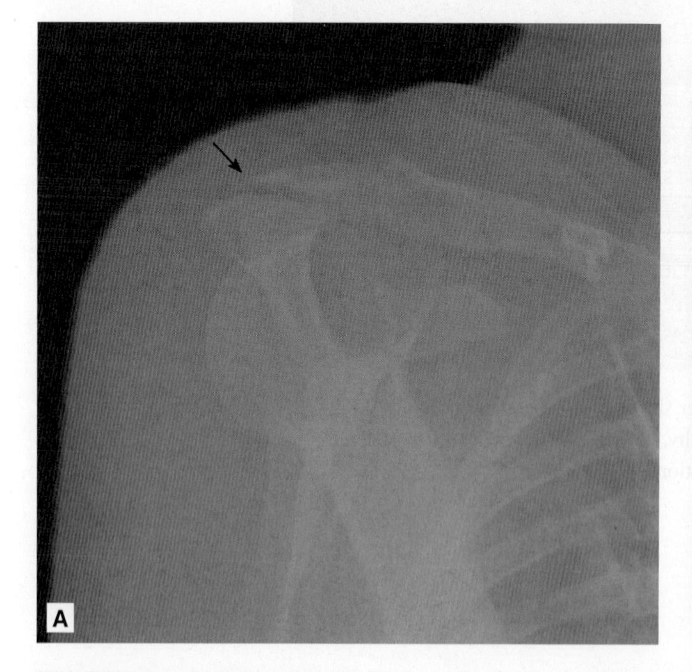

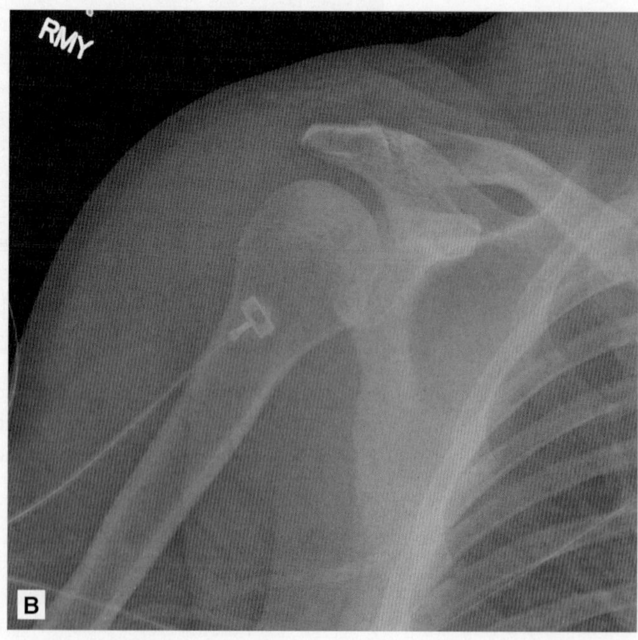

FIGURE 9.6 ■ Right Acromial Fracture. **A, B:** A scapular Y view of the right shoulder (A) shows a fracture of the right acromial process (arrow). Because of the orientation of the fracture plane, the fracture is invisible on the AP view (B). Acromial fractures (and fractures of the scapula in general) can be very subtle and may only be visible on a single view of a radiographic study.

os indicative of shear forces across the region. Hypertrophic changes (osteophytosis, subchondral sclerosis) are frequently seen as well if the os is unstable. Symptomatic patients may require operative treatment if conservative measures fail. Most acromion fractures can be treated conservatively, though displaced fractures may require operative fixation.

Pearls

1. Acromial fractures are often subtle and seen frequently on only one radiographic view.
2. Most patients with os acrominale are asymptomatic. If present, symptoms attributable to an unstable os acromiale are generally mild and can be treated conservatively.
3. An unstable os acromiale can contribute to supraspinatus tendinopathy and tears. These complications are best imaged with shoulder MRI.

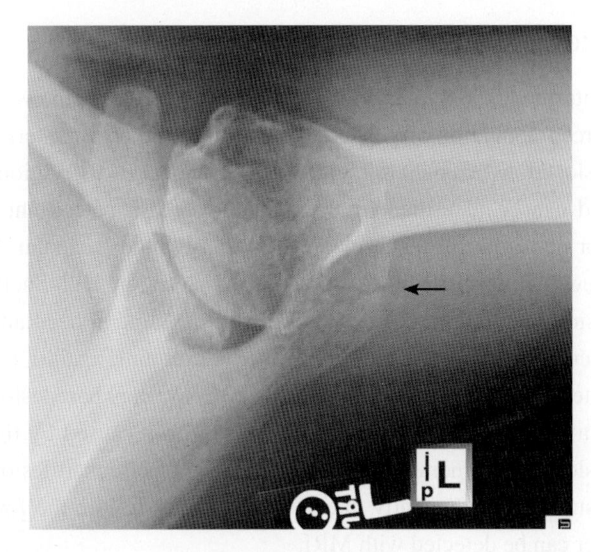

FIGURE 9.7 ■ Left Acromial Fracture. An axillary view of the left shoulder shows a very subtle nondisplaced fracture of the acromion (arrow). This fracture was not visible on the AP view.

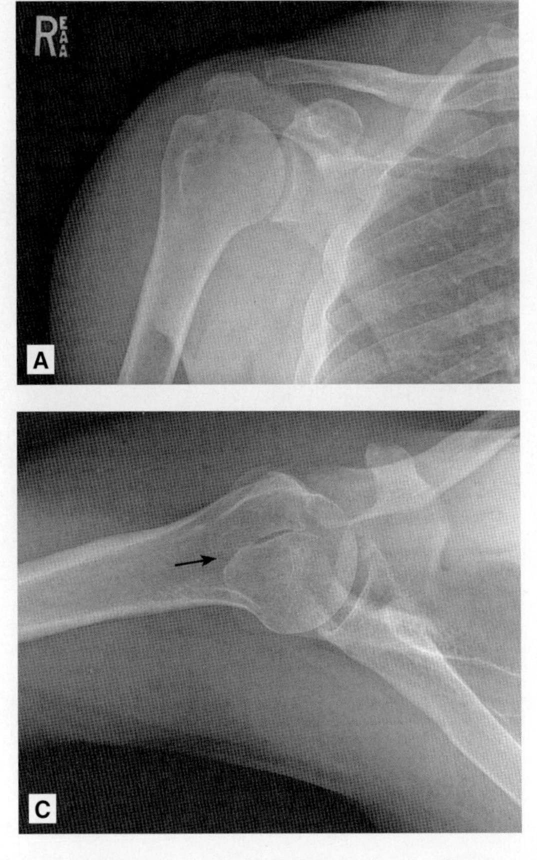

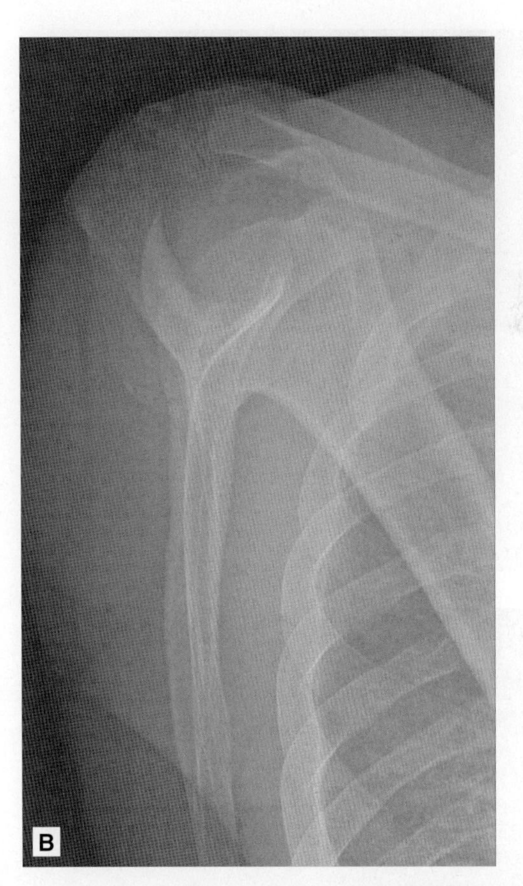

FIGURE 9.8 ■ Os Acromiale. **A-C:** AP, scapular Y and axillary views of the right shoulder show the typical appearance of an os acromiale. This is a normal variant and is caused by failure of fusion of the ossification center of the acromion to the scapular spine. Notice the sclerotic and somewhat rounded edges of the os acromiale (arrow) and compare that to the jagged or straight lines of the fracture planes seen in the acromial fractures. It is important to be able to differentiate between an os acromiale and acromial fractures. An os acromiale may be a cause of pain: motion at the synchondrosis can lead to degenerative and hypertrophic changes about the synchondrosis. This, in turn, can contribute to supraspinatus tendinopathy and tears.

Radiographic Summary

Anterior glenohumeral dislocations typically occur with forced abduction and external rotation to the arm. Anterior dislocations account for 90% of glenohumeral dislocations and can be identified by the humeral head displaced anterior and inferior to the glenoid. Axillary and/or scapular Y views can confirm the direction of the dislocation. Hill–Sachs lesions can be seen as deformation of the humeral head and occur as a result of the humeral head colliding against the anteroinferior rim of the glenoid. A bony Bankhart lesion is a fracture of the anteroinferior glenoid rim caused by the dislocating humeral head. A labroligamentous Bankart lesion results more frequently than a bony Bankart lesion; the former can be detected with MRI.

Clinical Implications

Anterior glenohumeral dislocations are the most common joint dislocations presenting to the emergency department. Radiographs should be obtained when the diagnosis is in question and post reduction radiographs are mandatory to confirm reduction and assess for the presence of fractures. Hill–Sachs and bony Bankart fractures are easier to appreciate on the post reduction radiographs. Pre and post reduction neurovascular exams should be performed as axillary nerve and artery injuries can occur. Patients should be placed in a sling and swathe post reduction and orthopedic follow-up is necessary. Repeat dislocation risk is highest in young athletes. Patients over age 40 are at risk for concomitant rotator cuff injuries associated with their dislocation.

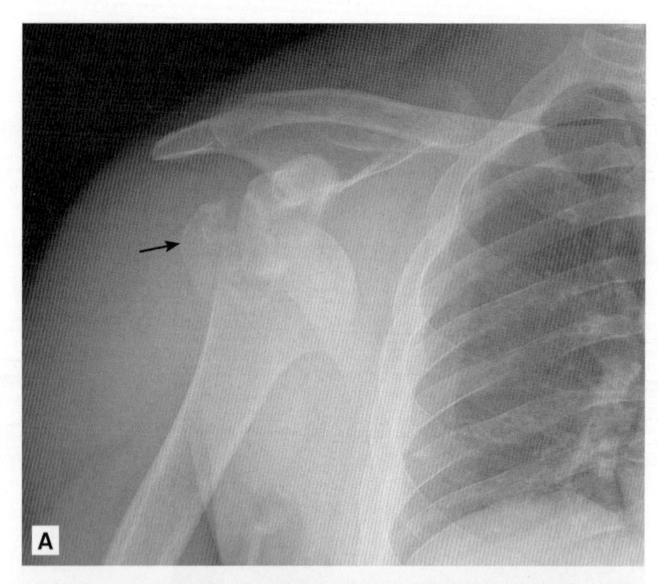

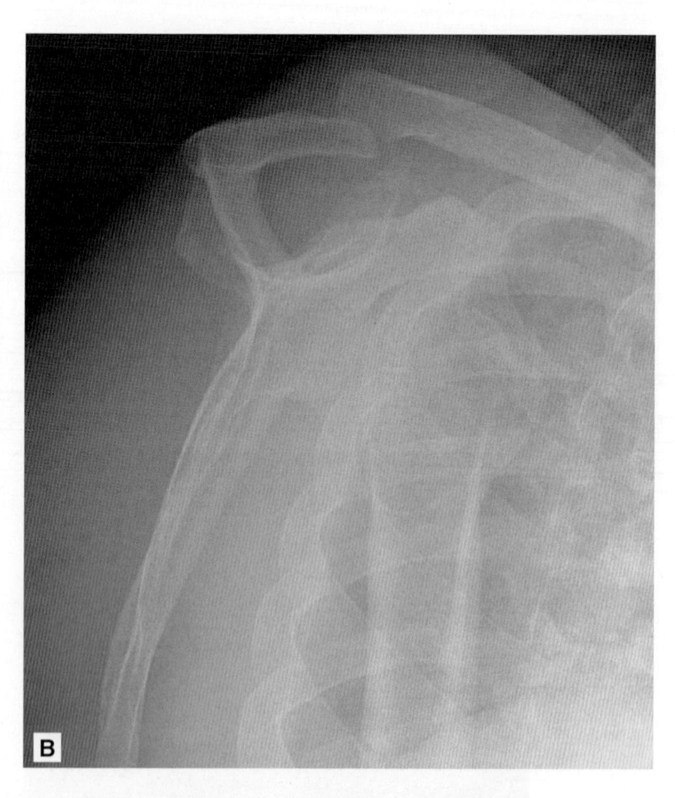

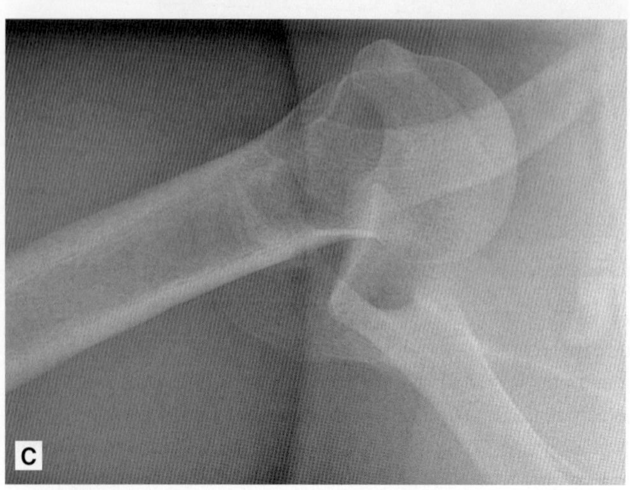

FIGURE 9.9 ■ Anterior Shoulder Dislocation. **A-C:** AP, scapular Y, and axillary views of the right shoulder demonstrate anterior dislocation of the humeral head. There is a large fracture of the greater humeral tuberosity (arrow).

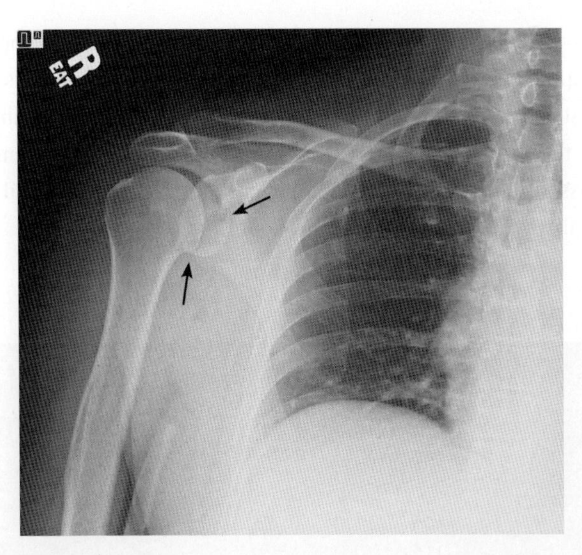

FIGURE 9.10 ■ Bankart Fracture. A single AP view of the right shoulder demonstrates a large bony Bankart fracture (arrows) consistent with a prior anterior dislocation event. The humeral head is located within the glenoid at this time.

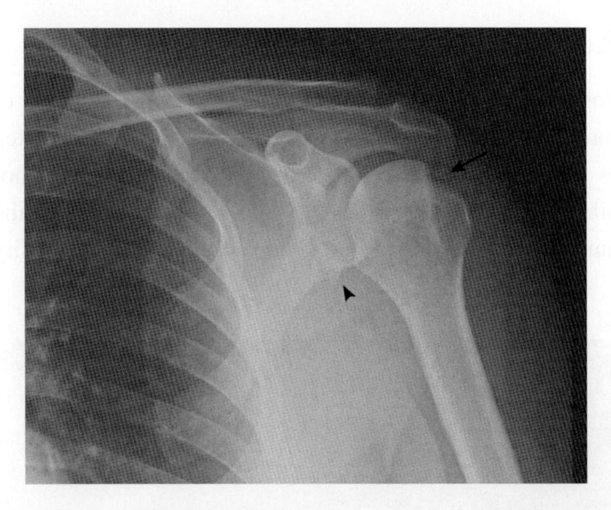

FIGURE 9.11 ■ Hill–Sachs Fracture. AP view of the left shoulder obtained with internal rotation of the left humerus shows a very large Hill–Sachs fracture deformity in the postero-lateral aspect of the left humeral head (arrow). A small bony Bankart fracture is present as well (arrowhead).

Pearls

1. Reduction may be performed without radiographs when the diagnosis is strongly suspected. A successful reduction becomes more difficult the longer the joint remains dislocated.
2. Patients with Bankart fractures are at higher risk for joint instability and recurrent dislocation.
3. Intraarticular lidocaine injections can often be administered instead of procedural sedation for analgesia during reduction. Injections of 20 cc of 1% lidocaine or marcaine into the joint after sterile preparation have been shown to be as effective as procedural sedation and can reduce the cost and the total time spent in the ED by several hours.
4. Reduction can be confirmed clinically by ranging the patient's humerus through full external and internal rotation and flexion/abduction of the glenohumeral joint to 90°.

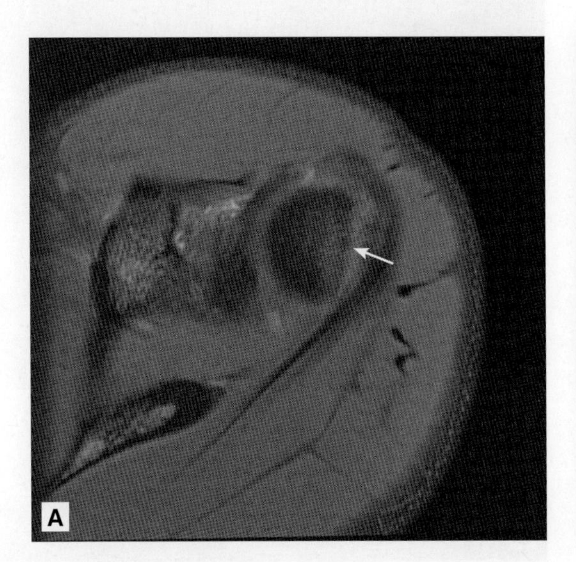

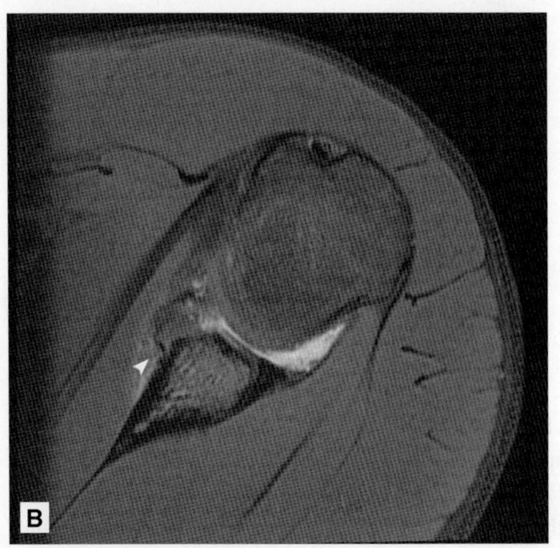

FIGURE 9.12 ■ Hill–Sachs and Bankart Fractures. **A, B:** Axial fat saturated T1-weighted images at the level of the superior aspect of the humeral head (A) and mid glenoid (B) demonstrate a hatchet-like deformity in the postero-lateral aspect of the humeral head consistent with a Hill–Sachs fracture (arrow) and a bony Bankart fracture (arrowhead). These are consistent with a prior anterior shoulder dislocation event. At this time, the humeral head is located within the glenoid.

Radiographic Summary

Posterior glenohumeral dislocations occur as a result of forced posterior and internal rotation of the shoulder, often as a result of seizures, electrocutions, falls, and automobile accidents. The diagnosis should be suspected when the humeral head is internally rotated and the greater tuberosity is not seen on the AP view (light bulb sign). Axillary or Y scapular views must be obtained to confirm the diagnosis as posterior glenohumeral dislocations can be extremely subtle on the anterior–posterior views and are the most frequently missed joint dislocations. CT-scan imaging can be helpful to confirm the diagnosis when in doubt.

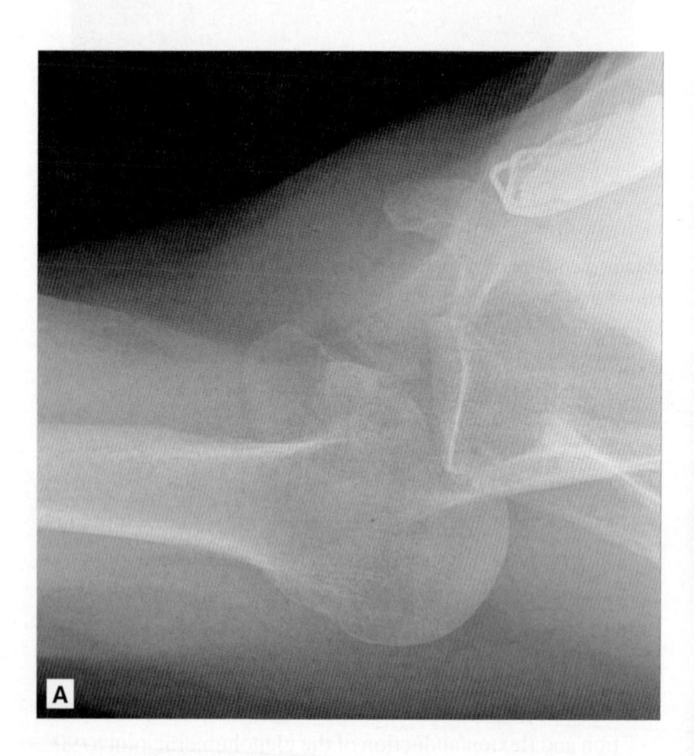

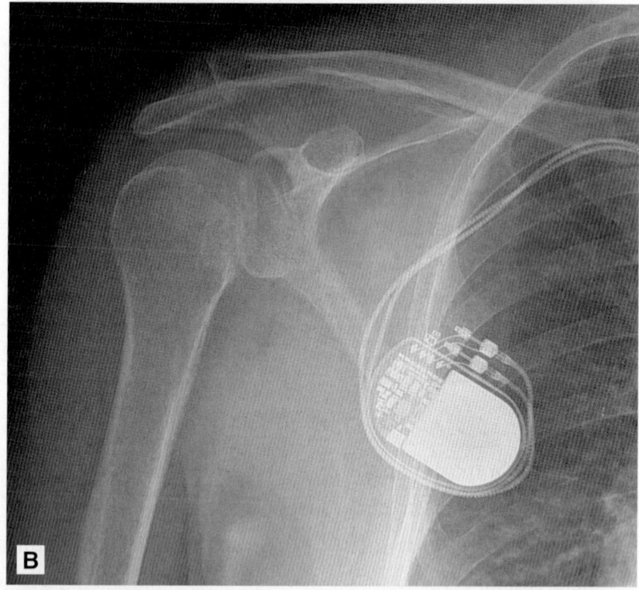

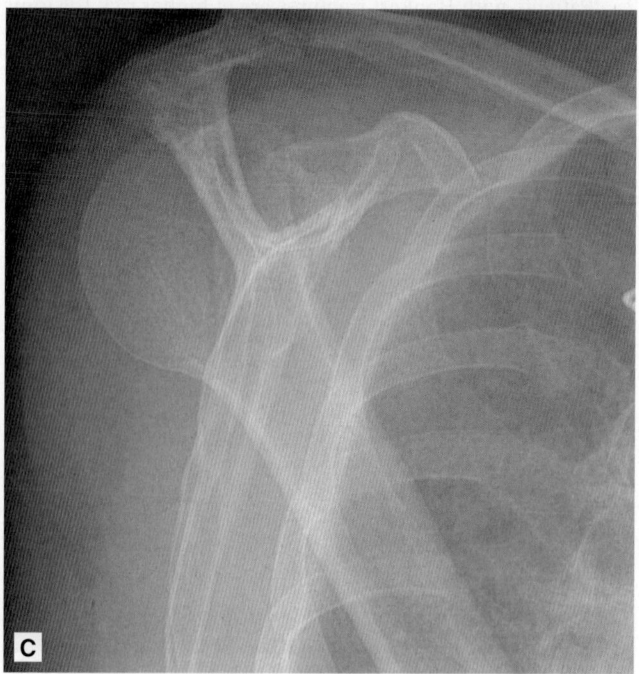

FIGURE 9.13 ■ Posterior Shoulder Dislocation. **A-C:** Axillary, AP, and scapular Y views of the right shoulder demonstrate posterior dislocation of the right humeral head. There is an impaction fracture on the anterior aspect of the humeral head ("anterior trough impaction fracture" or "reverse Hill–Sachs fracture").

Clinical Implications

Axillary or scapular Y views must be obtained in addition to the AP views to evaluate for posterior glenohumeral dislocation. Patients who hold their arm in internal rotation and cannot be externally rotated should be evaluated for posterior dislocation. Fractures of the posterior glenoid rim (reverse Bankart) or anterior humeral head (anterior trough impaction) may make reduction more difficult; posterior glenohumeral dislocations frequently require reduction in the operating room.

Pearls

1. Posterior shoulder dislocations are the most frequently missed joint dislocations. Axillary and/or scapular Y view must be obtained on every patient to adequately evaluate for posterior dislocation. The findings on the AP view are extremely subtle (loss of the normal parallelism between the humeral head articular surface and anterior glenoid rim).
2. The diagnosis can often be excluded clinically if the patient's shoulder can be fully externally rotated with the elbow at the patient's side.

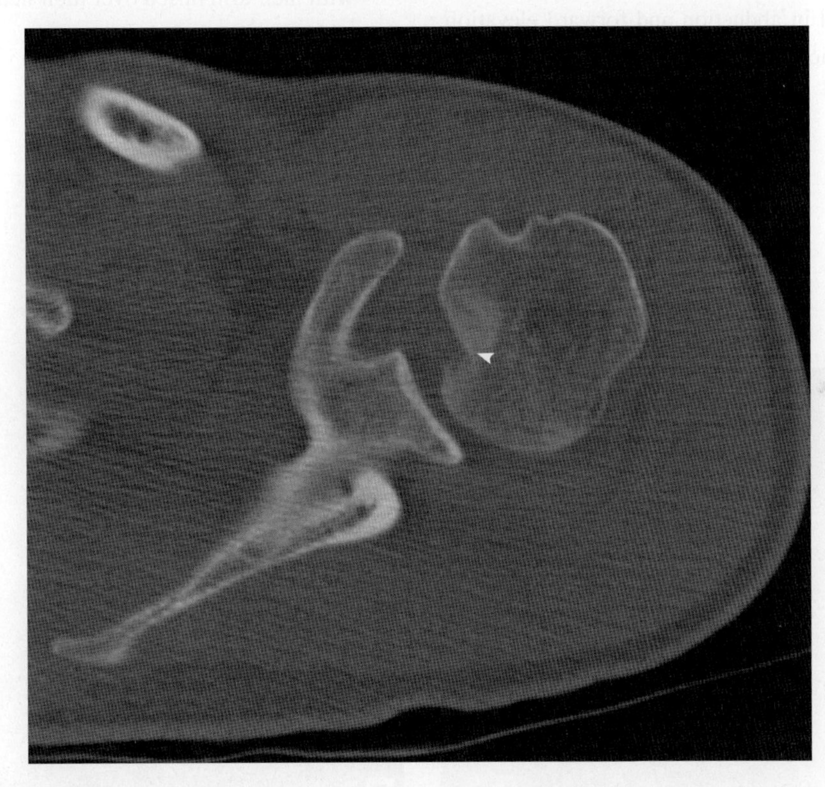

FIGURE 9.14 ■ Posterior Shoulder Dislocation. A single axial CT image through the left shoulder of a different patient demonstrates a prominent anterior trough impaction fracture on the anterior aspect of the left humeral head (arrowhead). This fracture is obtained when the humeral head impacts against the posterior glenoid rim during a posterior dislocation event. At this time, the left humeral head is located within the glenoid.

Radiographic Summary

Luxatio Erecta occurs when the humeral head is inferiorly dislocated from the glenoid. This can easily be identified on AP shoulder views and frequently on AP chest radiographs obtained during initial trauma evaluations.

Clinical Implications

Luxatio Erecta is the least common shoulder dislocation representing only 1-3% of all shoulder dislocations. However, it is commonly associated with neurovascular injury to the axillary nerve and/or artery. Diagnosis can be suspected in patients who present with their arm raised over their heads with the shoulder fixed in abduction and forward elevation. Reduction can be difficult as the humeral head can often become "locked" between the glenoid and ribs. Axial traction and often anterior traction on the humeral head may be necessary to free the humerus from the glenoid rim. CT angiograms can help evaluate for axillary artery injuries when suspected. Orthopedic and vascular surgery consultations should be considered.

Pearls

1. Luxatio erecta is the least common of the shoulder dislocations, but has the highest association with vascular and nerve injuries.
2. Diagnosis should be suspected in patients who present with their arm raised over their heads with the inability to adduct or lower their arms.

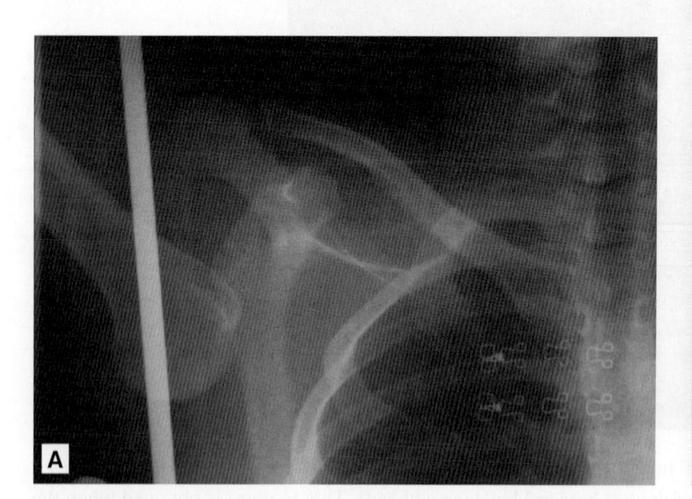

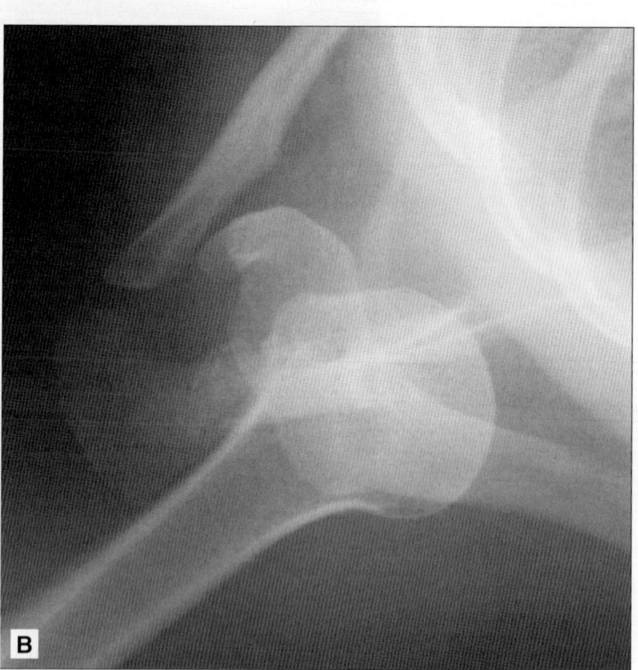

FIGURE 9.15 ■ Luxatioerecta. **A, B:** AP and axillary views of a shoulder demonstrate the typical appearance of luxatioerecta: the humeral head is dislocated inferior to the glenoid and the upper extremity is "stuck" in an abducted position. On the axillary view, the humeral head projects over the glenoid and acromion because the humeral head is dislocated inferior to the glenoid fossa.

Radiographic Summary

Calcific tendonitis is caused by deposition of calcium hydroxyapatite within the tendons of the rotator cuff. These deposits are radiographically apparent. The involved tendon is determined by the location of the calcium hydroxyapatite deposit: the supraspinatus, infraspinatus, and teres minor attach to the greater humeral tuberosity from anterior to posterior while the subscapularis attaches primarily to the lesser humeral tuberosity anteriorly.

Clinical Implications

Calcific tendonitis usually occurs in patients 30-50 years old with a higher incidence in diabetics. While not always painful when seen on radiographs, the calcium deposit can become painful during the resorptive phase. Patients present with acute onset pain that may mimic a rotator cuff tear, gouty attack, or infection. Calcific tendonitis is typically a self-limited condition and resolves on its own with time. Additional treatment options include NSAID, physical therapy, and corticosteroid injections. Image-guided percutaneous aspiration may be performed but does not alter the long-term outcome. Surgical resection is reserved for refractory cases.

Pearls

1. Calcific tendonitis is rarely associated with rotator cuff tears.
2. Calcific tendonitis goes through four clinical stages: The formative stage presents with an unknown trigger and the calcium deposit resembles chalk. The resting phase occurs once the calcific deposit is solidified and typically is not painful. The resorptive phase is painful due to an associated inflammatory reaction caused by the calcium breaking down. The material at this phase resembles toothpaste. The tendon returns to normal in the postcalcific phase.

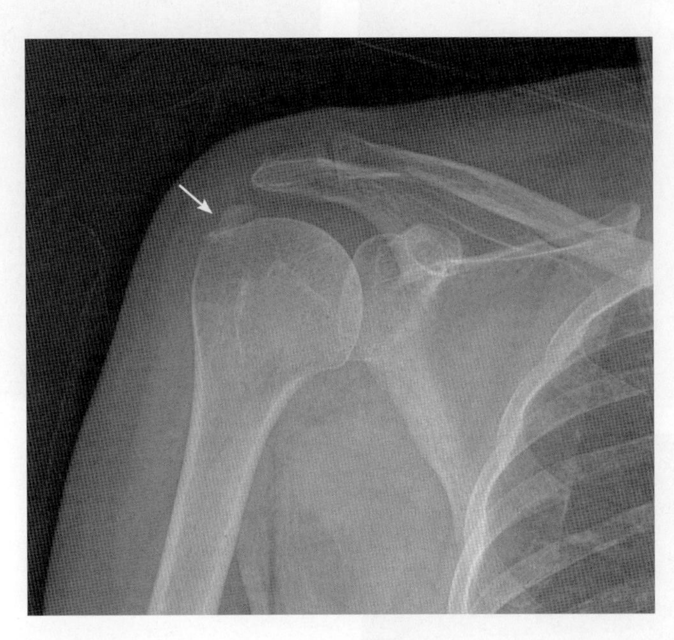

FIGURE 9.16 ■ Calcific Tendonitis. An AP view of the right shoulder obtained with external rotation of the humerus shows an amorphous globular calcification within the expected position of the distal supraspinatus tendon (arrow). The calcification is a focus of calcium hydroxyapatite and this patient has calcific tendinitis.

Radiographic Features

Scapular fractures may be difficult to identify on conventional radiographs. Suspected fractures should be evaluated with AP shoulder radiographs as well as a scapular Y view. Fractures of the scapula are much easier to identify on CT imaging.

Clinical Implications

Scapular fractures can be seen following traumatic injuries such as falls and motor vehicle accidents. When identified, clinicians should have a high index of suspicion for additional thoracic injuries (rib fractures, pneumothorax, lung contusion). A CT scan of the shoulder should be performed if a scapular fracture involves the glenoid. Fractures involving the articular surface of the glenoid may need surgical fixation and orthopedic consultation should be obtained. Most fractures

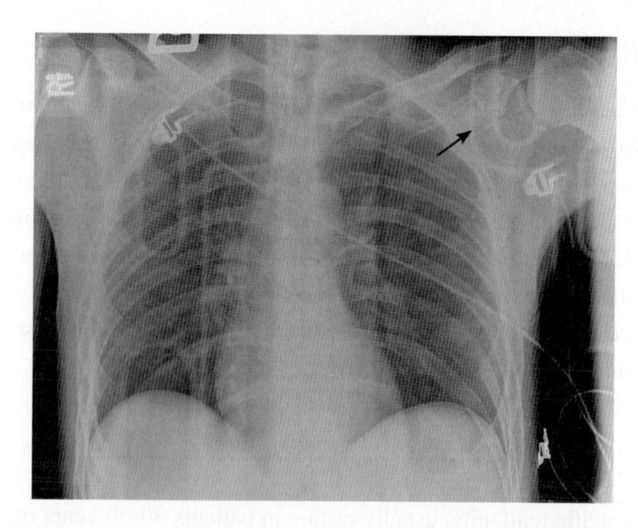

FIGURE 9.17 ■ Scapular Fracture. An AP radiograph of the chest of a trauma victim shows a nondisplaced fracture of the left scapula extending parallel to the scapular spine and through the articular surface of the glenoid fossa (arrow). Multiple left rib fractures are present as well.

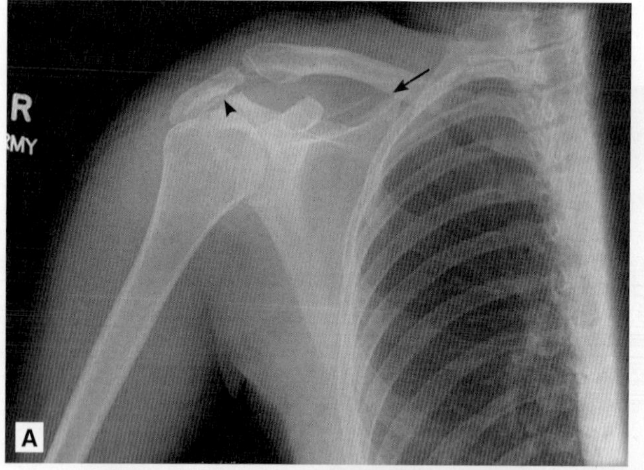

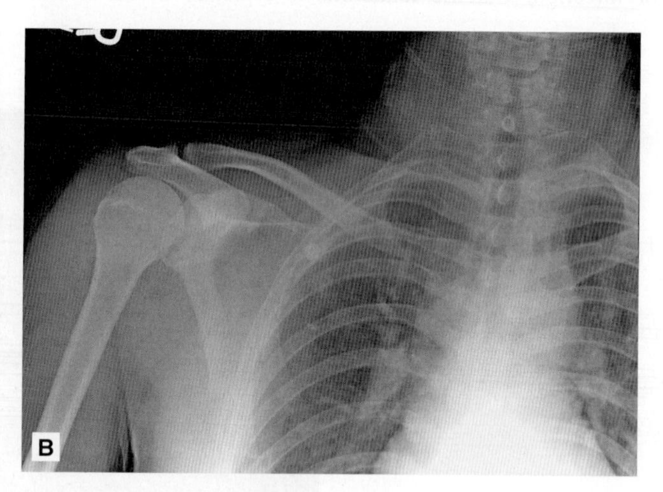

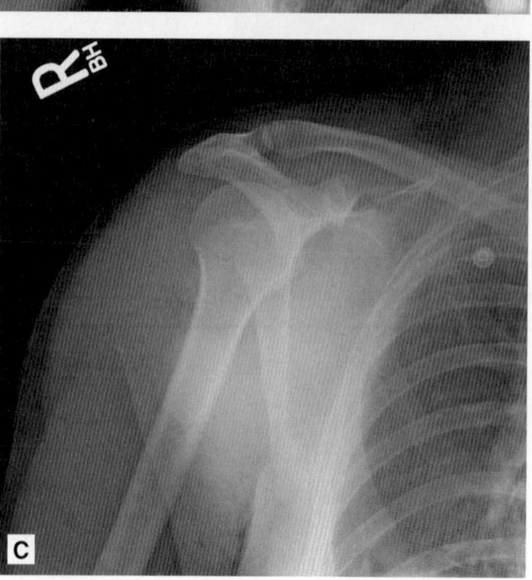

FIGURE 9.18 ■ Scapular Fracture. **A:** An AP view of the right shoulder demonstrates a fracture extending along the superior scapula border (arrow). There is an additional fracture through the acromion as well (arrowhead). There is extensive regional soft tissue edema. **B, C:** An AP view of the right scapula of a different patient (B) shows subtle step-off and disruption of the "scapular X": this may be the only sign of a nondisplaced scapular fracture extending though the scapular spine. An attempted scapular Y view (C) shows the fracture better.

of the scapular spine and body without glenoid involvement can be managed non-operatively with a sling with outpatient orthopedic evaluation.

Pearls

1. Scapular fractures may be difficult to diagnose on conventional radiographs.
2. Non-contrasted CT imaging of the shoulder should be performed if a scapular fracture involves the articular portion of the glenoid. Factures that extend through the articular surface of the glenoid may require operative fixation.

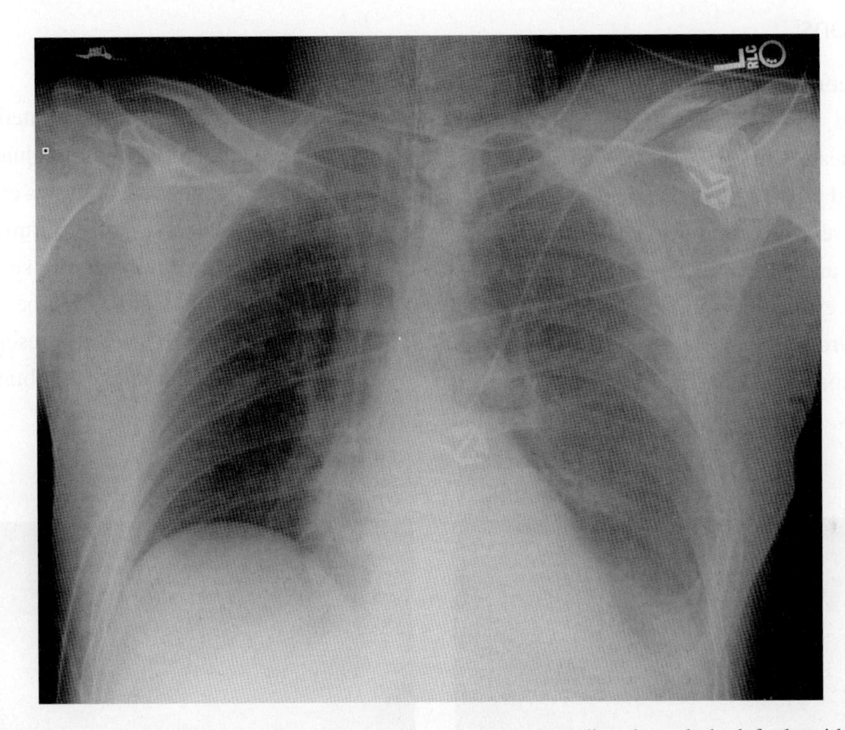

FIGURE 9.19 ■ Glenoid Neck Fracture. AP view of the chest shows a fracture extending through the left glenoid neck. The glenoid is severed from the rest of the scapula and mildly displaced. The fracture does not extend through the glenoid articular surface, however, and the glenohumeral joint alignment is maintained. Left clavicular and left rib fractures are present as well.

Radiographic Summary

Clavicle fractures can typically be identified on AP radiographs of the shoulder. Clavicle fractures can be classified as proximal, middle third, or distal. When AP radiographs do not reveal a clavicular fracture but clinical suspicion remains high, a 45° AP cepahalad view can be helpful. CT imaging may be necessary to further evaluate proximal third fractures, particularly when the sternoclavicular (SC) joint is involved.

Clinical Implications

Clavicle fractures are common and can result from direct and indirect forces applied to the shoulder. Most patients will describe point tenderness at the fracture site and will clinically have bruising and a palpable deformity. Open clavicle fractures are rare, but severe tenting of the skin can be seen in severely angulated and displaced fractures and requires emergent orthopedic evaluation. Most clavicle fractures occur in the middle third of the clavicle. Nondisplaced fractures can be treated conservatively in a sling for comfort. Communited fractures, fractures with foreshortening, and severely displaced or angulated fractures may require surgical fixation. Displaced distal clavicle fractures may indicate injury to the CC and AC ligaments and requires orthopedic follow-up. Proximal third fractures are the least common. They are often associated with severe trauma to the mediastinum and their presence should alert the physician for potential internal injury. CT imaging is usually necessary to fully evaluate the fracture pattern and SC joint involvement, as well as assess for additional trauma to the chest.

Pearls

1. Clavicle fractures with associated tenting of the skin require emergent orthopedic evaluation.
2. The majority of clavicle fractures can be managed nonoperatively; however, severely comminuted, displaced, and angulated fractures may require surgical management.
3. Proximal clavicle fractures can be associated with severe intrathoracic injury. When present, clinicians should assess for additional injury by obtaining a contrasted CT scan of the chest.

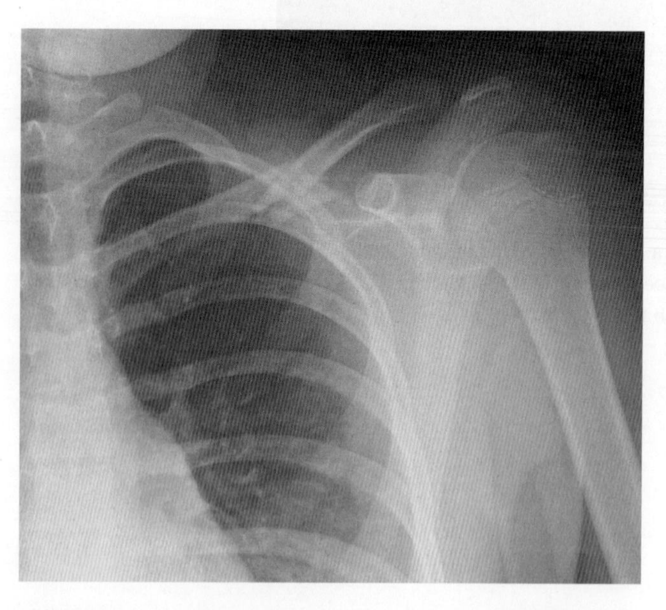

FIGURE 9.20 ■ Clavicle Fracture. An AP view of the left shoulder demonstrates a mildly comminuted and minimally angulated but nondisplaced fracture of the middle third of the left clavicle.

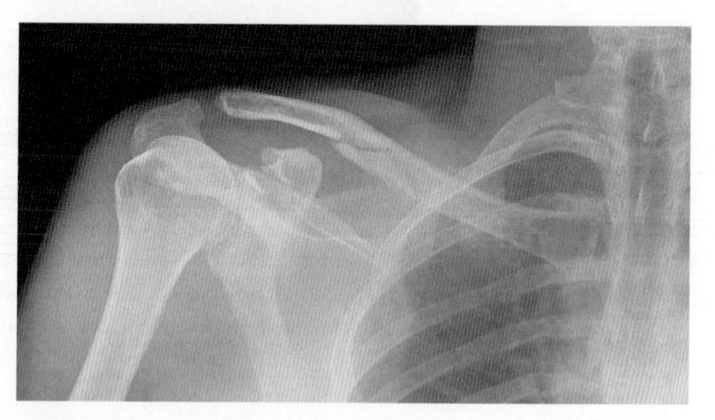

FIGURE 9.21 ■ Right Clavicle Fracture. An AP view of the right shoulder shows a nondisplaced fracture at the junction of the middle and lateral thirds of the right clavicle.

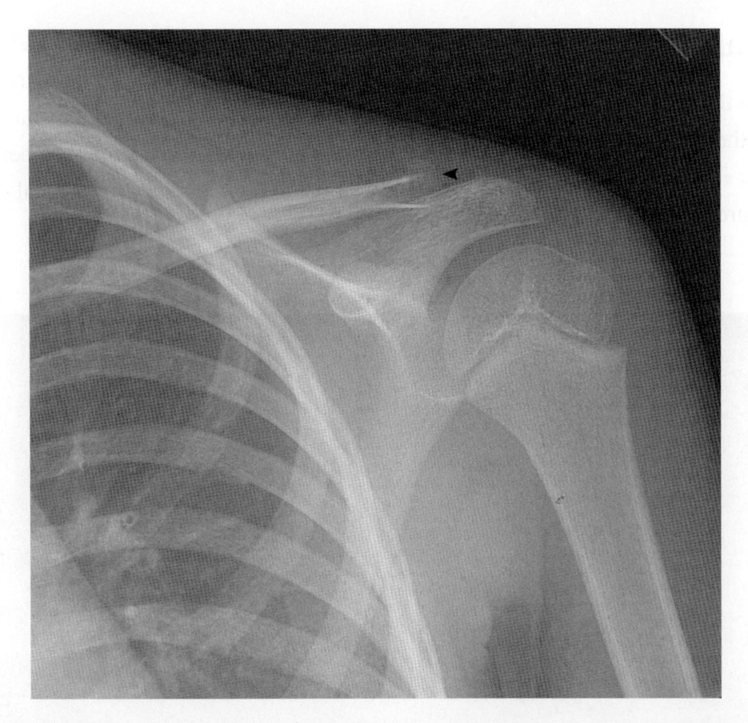

FIGURE 9.22 ■ Left Clavicle Fracture. An AP view of the left clavicle of a young child shows a very subtle fracture of the most lateral aspect of the left clavicle extending into the acromion-clavicular joint (arrowhead). The alignment of the left acromion-clavicular joint is normal.

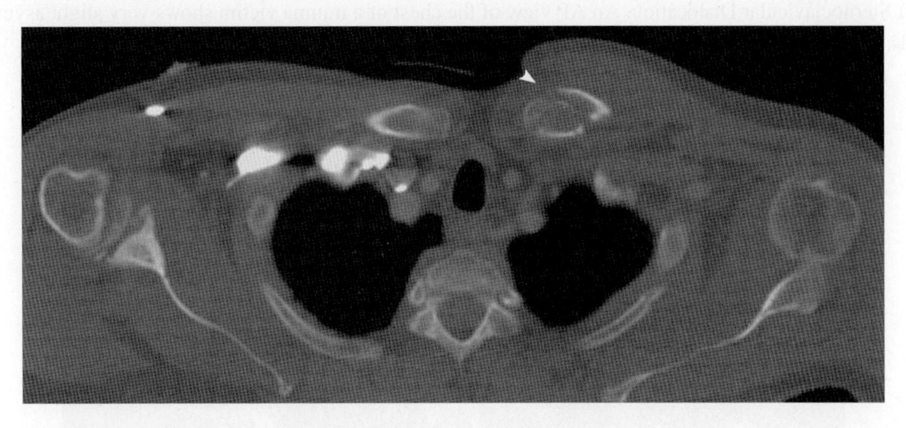

FIGURE 9.23 ■ Left Clavicular Head Fracture. A single axial CT image at the level of the clavicular heads shows a mildly comminuted fracture of the left clavicular head (arrowhead). Medial clavicular fractures are very subtle. This fracture was not visible on the conventional radiographs of the chest, even in retrospect. Look for subtle malalignment of the clavicular heads on AP views of the chest.

Radiographic Summary

SC dislocations occur when the proximal clavicle is displaced anteriorly or posteriorly at the SC joint. Sternoclavicular subluxations can be difficult or impossible to appreciate on conventional radiographs. The greater the clavicular displacement, the higher is the sensitivity of radiographs. Frank SC dislocations can be seen on AP chest radiographs by noting asymmetry in the positioning of the clavicular heads. CT imaging is the gold standard and should be performed with CT angiogram of the chest when there is clinical concern for vascular injury.

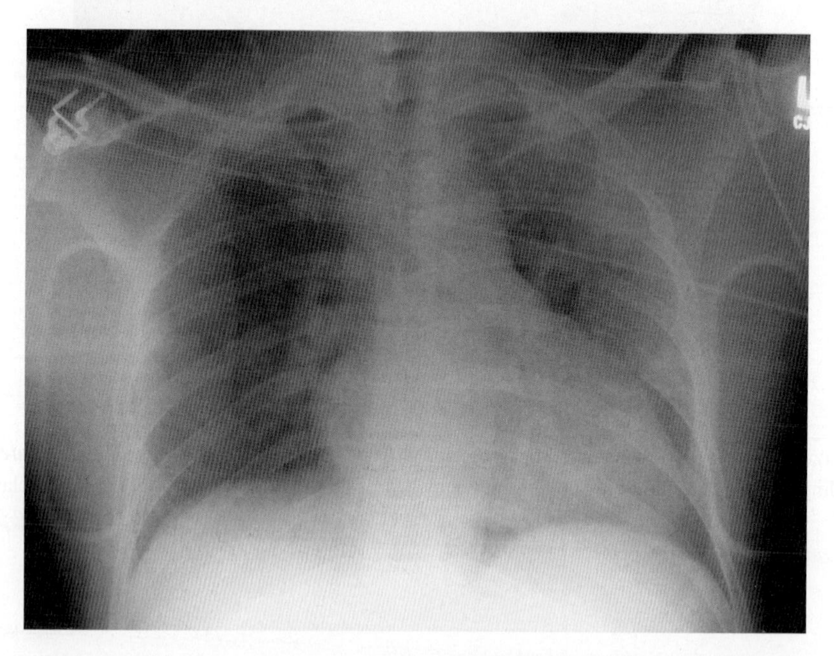

FIGURE 9.24 ■ Left Sternoclavicular Dislocation. An AP view of the chest of a trauma victim shows very slight asymmetry in the position of the clavicular heads. The left clavicular head is positioned slightly more inferiorly than the right.

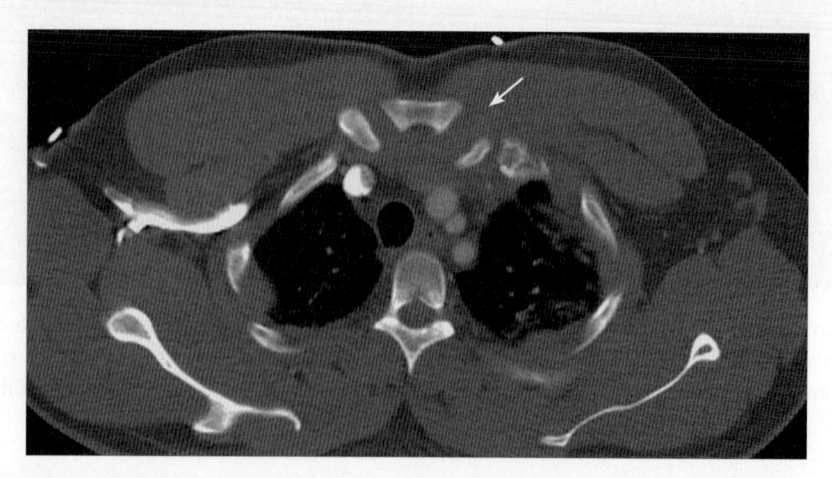

FIGURE 9.25 ■ Left Sternoclavicular Dislocation. An axial CT image at the level of the sternoclavicular joints shows abnormal widening of the left sternoclavicular joint (arrow) consistent with mild dissociation. The density surrounding this abnormal joint and extending into the anterior mediastinum is a hematoma. Notice the normal right sternoclavicular joint.

Clinical Implications

SC dislocations can occur following blunt trauma to the joint or can be seen following a fall onto the lateral shoulder. Clinically, patients will have pain, swelling, and often palpable deformity to the joint. Anterior dislocations often do not require reduction and can be treated nonoperatively. Posterior dislocations may require reduction due to impingement on the underlying vascular structures.

Pearls

1. Reduction should not be performed in the ED due to serious risk of vascular compromise. Reductions should be performed in the operating room with orthopedics and vascular surgery readily available.
2. A serendipity view radiograph can be taken by directing the beam 40° cephalad on AP view. This view should include both medial clavicular heads and allows the viewer to evaluate the SC joints for subtle asymmetry.

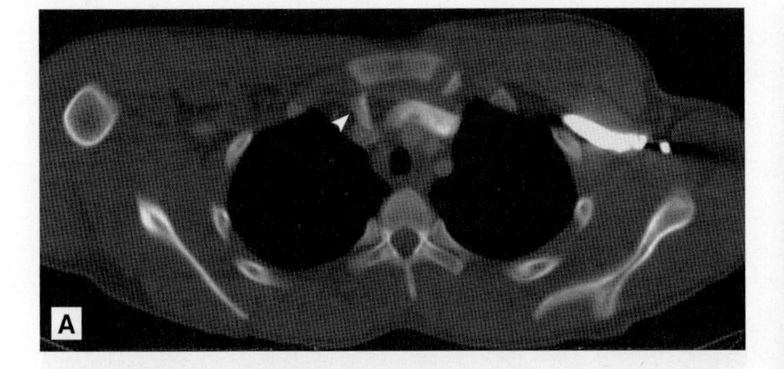

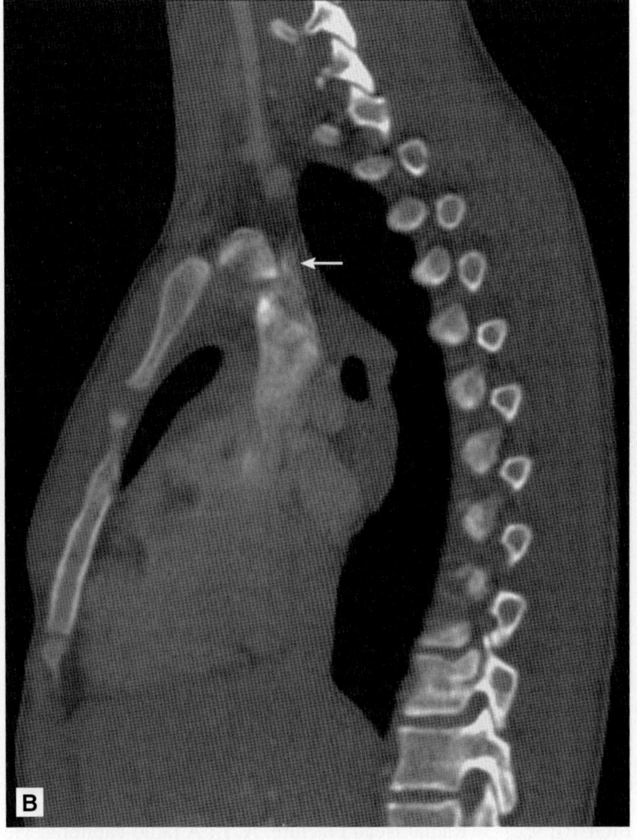

FIGURE 9.26 ■ Right Sternoclavicular Dislocation. **A, B:** Axial and sagittal CT images of a different patient show posterior dislocation of the right clavicular head at the right sternoclavicular joint (arrowhead). The posteriorly displaced clavicle indents the right internal jugular vein (arrow).

Radiographic Summary

Radial head and neck fractures can usually be seen on standard AP and lateral elbow radiographs. An elbow effusion, best seen on the lateral view (posterior fat pad elevation or anterior sail sign) should alert the clinician to the possibility of an occult fracture, if a fracture is not apparent. Radial head views (45° inferior to superior lateral elbow radiographs) are frequently helpful because the ulna no longer overlies the radius.

Clinical Implications

Nondisplaced or minimally displaced fractures (<1-2 mm of step off along the articular surface) of the radial head and neck can be placed in a sling for comfort with early active range of motion allowed, as tolerated. Patients will require close orthopedic follow-up in 1 week for repeat radiographs to ensure no additional displacement. Displaced/depressed radial head fractures with >2 mm depression should have close follow-up with orthopedics for probable surgical fixation. These patients can be managed temporarily in a sling or posterior splint.

Pearls

1. The most common cause of a traumatic joint effusion seen on adult elbow radiographs is a radial head fracture. Patients with the presence of a posterior fat pad despite no definitive fracture should be treated for an occult radial head fracture.
2. A radial head view may be helpful in confirming the diagnosis. Minimally displaced fractures are frequently visible only on this view.
3. CT imaging can aid in assessing the amount of displacement and depression when radiographs are inconclusive.

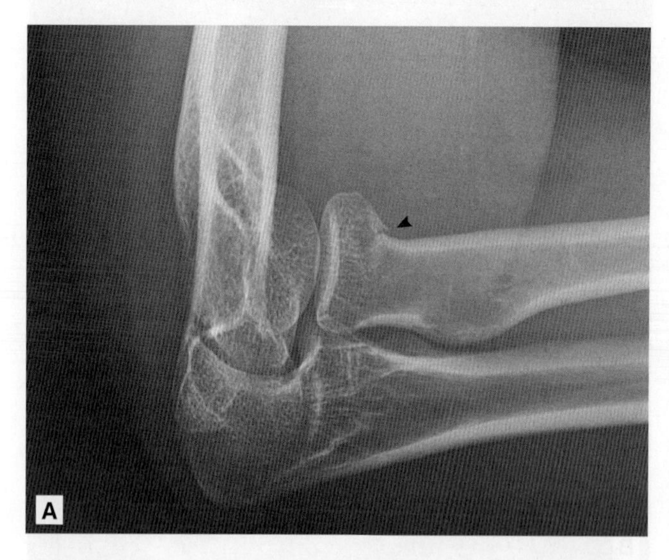

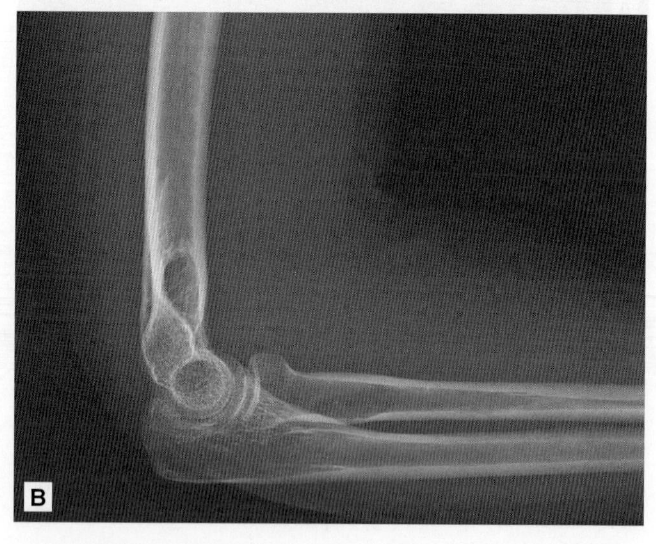

FIGURE 9.27 ■ Radial Head Fracture. **A, B:** A radio-capitellar view shows a subtle fracture of the radial head (arrowhead) which was not visible on the AP or lateral views (only the lateral view is shown here). A moderate joint effusion is visible on the lateral view (B).

Radiographic Summary

Olecranon fractures can be identified on AP and lateral radiographs of the elbow. These can be seen in elderly patients as a result of indirect trauma resulting form the sudden pull of the triceps on its insertion, or may be associated in younger patients with blunt direct trauma to the posterior elbow after a fall.

Clinical Implications

Small avulsion fractures with intact triceps mechanism may be treated conservatively in a sling or with a posterior splint. Fractures extending past the trochlear notch, comminuted fractures, and large or displaced fractures require surgical plate fixation.

Pearls

1. Ulnar nerve injuries can occur with olecranon fractures and should be assessed at the time of evaluation.
2. Open fractures should be suspected with overlying lacerations seen over the olecranon sustained after a fall with direct trauma to the posterior elbow.

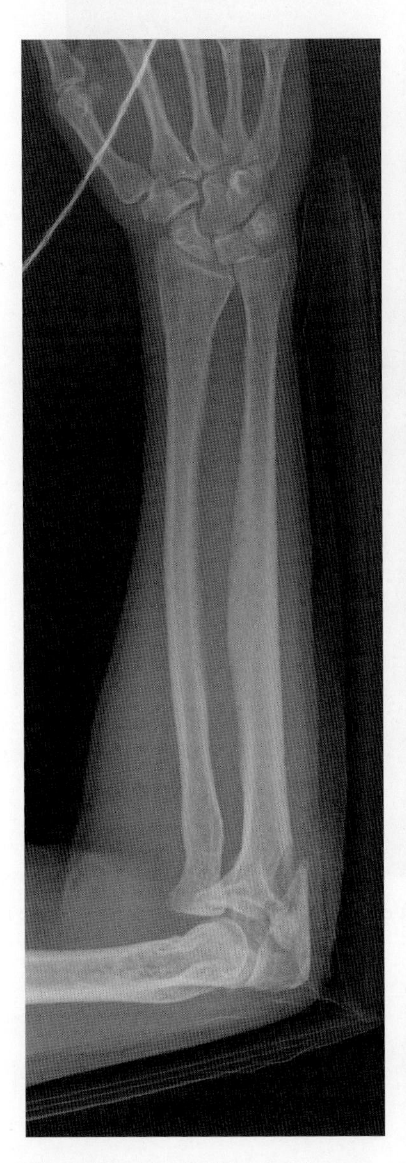

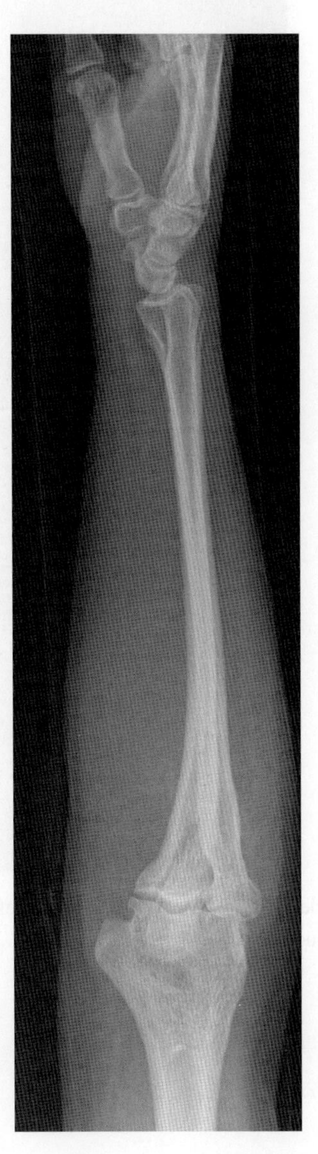

FIGURE 9.28 ■ Olecronon Fracture and Radial Head Dislocation. AP and lateral views of the right forearm show a minimally displaced fracture of the olecranon and volar dislocation of the radial head.

Radiographic Summary

Medial epicondyle avulsion fractures are a common elbow injury during adolescence occurring before fusion of the medial epicondyle ossification center. Throwing athletes will often report a sudden pop with associated pain along the medial epicondyle due to a bony avulsion injury of the ulnar collateral ligament. AP views of the elbow show displacement of the medial epicondyle ossification center. Knowledge of the expected normal order of appearance and fusion of the ossification centers at the elbow is critical in making the diagnosis (Table 9.1). It is important to realize that while the order of appearance is predictable, the exact age is somewhat variable. The ossification centers appear earlier in girls than in boys. They typically fuse between the ages of 14 and 16, except

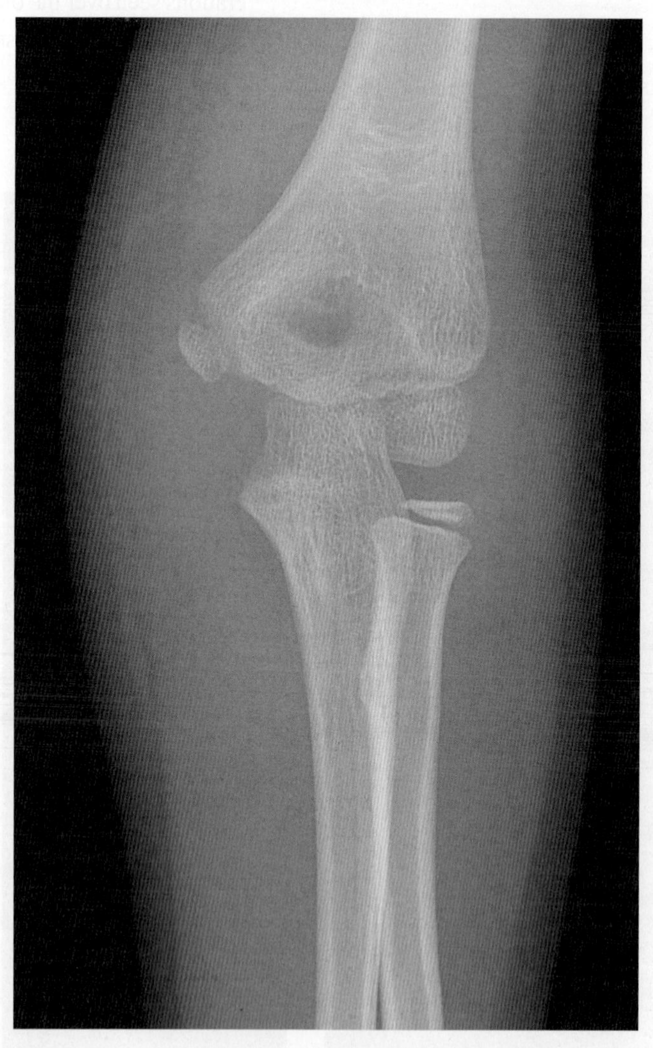

FIGURE 9.29 ■ Medial Epicondyle Fracture. An AP view of the left elbow shows an avulsion fracture of the medial humeral epicondyle. There is extensive regional soft tissue edema.

TABLE 9.1 ■ ORDER AND APPROXIMATE AGE OF APPEARANCE OF THE OSSIFICATION CENTERS AROUND THE ELBOW

Ossification Center	Approximate Age at Which the Ossification Center Appears
C: capitellum	1
R: radial head	3
I: internal (medial) epicondyle	5
T: trochlea	7
O: olecranon	9
E: external (lateral) epicondyle	11

for the medial epicondyle ossification center that is the last to fuse at age 18-19. Perhaps the single most important relationship at the elbow is the order of appearance of the medial epicondyle and trochlea of the humerus: the medial epicondyle normally appears earlier than the trochlea. Therefore, it is not normal for the medial epicondyle ossification center to be absent while an ossification center is observed near the expected position of the trochlea. If this abnormal relationship is observed, an avulsion fracture of the medial epicondyle is present with the center displaced distally in the region of the trochlea. If the findings are equivocal, a comparative radiograph of the contralateral elbow should be obtained to assess for a subtle abnormality of the medial epicondyle. MRI may be helpful to evaluate injury to the ulnar collateral ligament.

Clinical Implications

Little league elbow is a spectrum of injuries to the medial elbow ranging from apophysitis to an avulsion fracture of the medial epicondylar ossification center. Patients will have pain on palpation of the medial epicondyle. Valgus loading of the medial elbow will also elicit pain and instability with fractures and injuries to the ulnar collateral ligament. Avulsion fractures with less than 2 mm of displacement can be treated with a sling or splint immobilization and rest for 4-6 weeks. Avulsion fractures with >2 mm of displacement may benefit from surgical fixation and require orthopedic referral.

Pearls

1. A comparative AP view of the contralateral normal elbow may be helpful to evaluate for subtle avulsion fractures.
2. The medial epicondyle is the last ossification center to close (at age 18-19) and is subjected to increased valgus loads with pitching.
3. Little League baseball has restrictions parents and coaches should be aware of including: total pitches per game, avoidance of breaking pitches until a certain age, and games off between games pitched. Patients and parents should be reminded of these rules when presenting with these injuries.

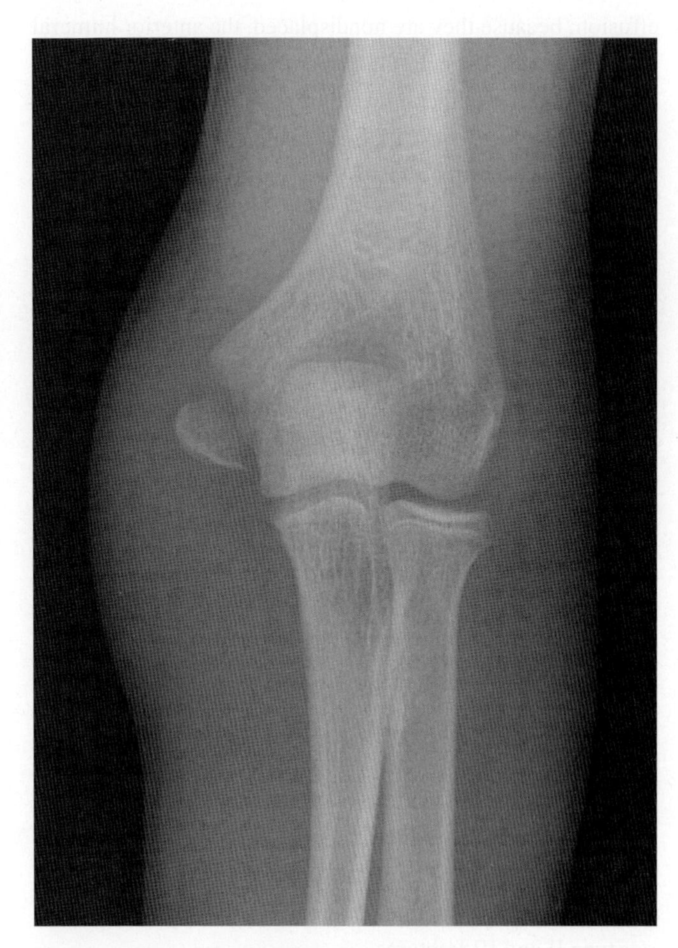

FIGURE 9.30 ■ Medial Epicondyle Fracture. AP view of the left elbow of another child with the same injury.

Radiographic Summary

Supracondylar fractures are the most common elbow fractures in children. They typically result from a fall onto an outstretched hand. AP and lateral radiographs of the elbow should be performed. Forearm radiographs should be obtained as well because associated forearm fractures are common. A lateral elbow radiograph will show a joint effusion presenting as an elevated posterior fat pad or anterior sail sign. Normally, the anterior humeral line (a line drawn down the anterior humerus) bisects the middle third of the capitellum. If, instead, it bisects the anterior third of the capitellum (or projects even further anteriorly), a supracondylar fracture is present. These fractures can be classified as type I, II and III. Type I fractures are nondisplaced with presence of a joint effusion; because they are nondisplaced, the anterior humeral line is normal. Type II injuries involve mild displacement with the anterior humeral line hitting the anterior third or less of the capitellum. Type III fractures are displaced with disruption of the anterior and posterior cortices of the humerus.

Clinical Implications

Supracondylar fractures are a common fracture pattern seen in younger patients following a fall onto an outstretched hand. There is a high association of brachial artery injury as well as injury to median, ulnar, and radial nerves. A thorough neurovascular exam must be performed to assess for these injuries. Type I fractures may be treated in a double sugar-tong splint or posterior splint with an A-frame with sling and orthopedic follow-up. All open fractures, fractures with neurovascular compromise, and type II and III fractures require operative fixation and emergent orthopedic consultation.

Pearls

1. The most common cause of a traumatic effusion without radiographic evidence of fracture in a pediatric patient is an occult supracondylar fracture.
2. Brachial artery injuries are reported in up to 10-20% of all supracondylar fractures and are most common with type II and III fractures.
3. Median nerve injuries are most common with posterior and laterally displaced fractures.
4. Radial nerve injuries are seen in posterior and medially displaced fractures.
5. Ulnar nerve injuries are associated with supracondylar fractures with flexion angulation.

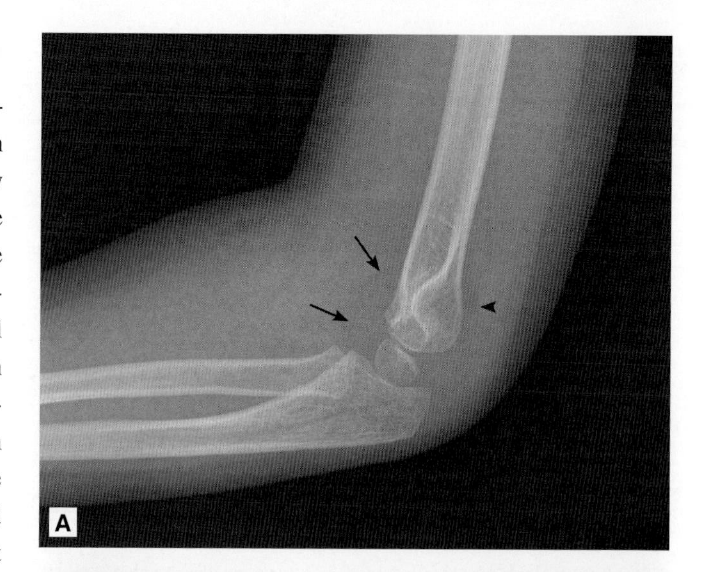

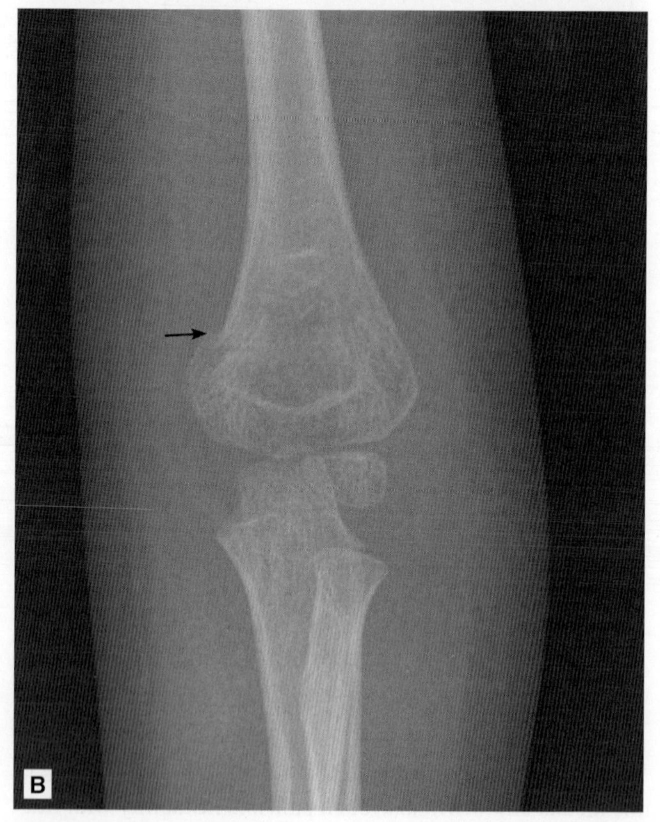

FIGURE 9.31 ■ Supracondylar Fracture. **A, B:** Lateral and AP views of the left elbow demonstrate a very large joint effusion. Notice the enormous "sail sign" anteriorly (arrows) and the prominent posterior fat pad (arrow head). The position of the capitelum is abnormal. A line drawn along the anterior cortex of the humerus should intersect the middle third of the capitelum. In this case, such a line would pass along the anterior cortex of the capitelum. This indicates that the capitelum is displaced posteriorly. Therefore, the patient has a mildly displaced supracondylar fracture. A very subtle fracture line is visible on the AP view (B) through the medial epicondyle (arrow).

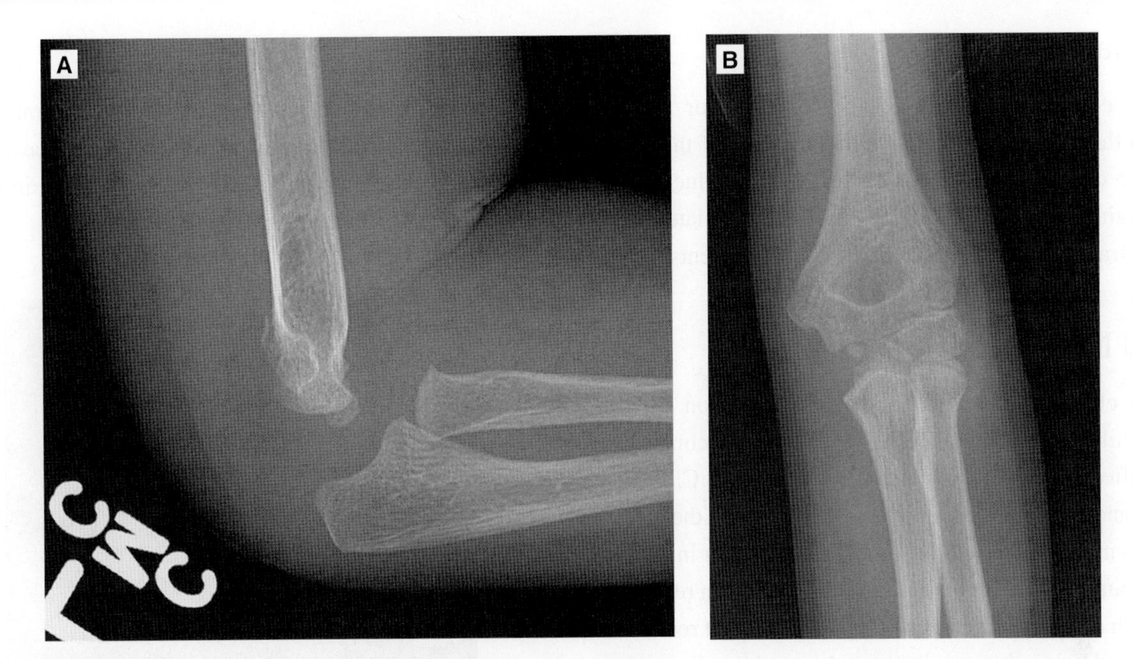

FIGURE 9.32 ■ Supracondylar Fracture. **A, B:** Lateral and AP views of the left elbow of a different child show a mildly posteriorly displaced supracondylar fracture with a very large associated joint effusion. The fracture is very subtle on the AP view.

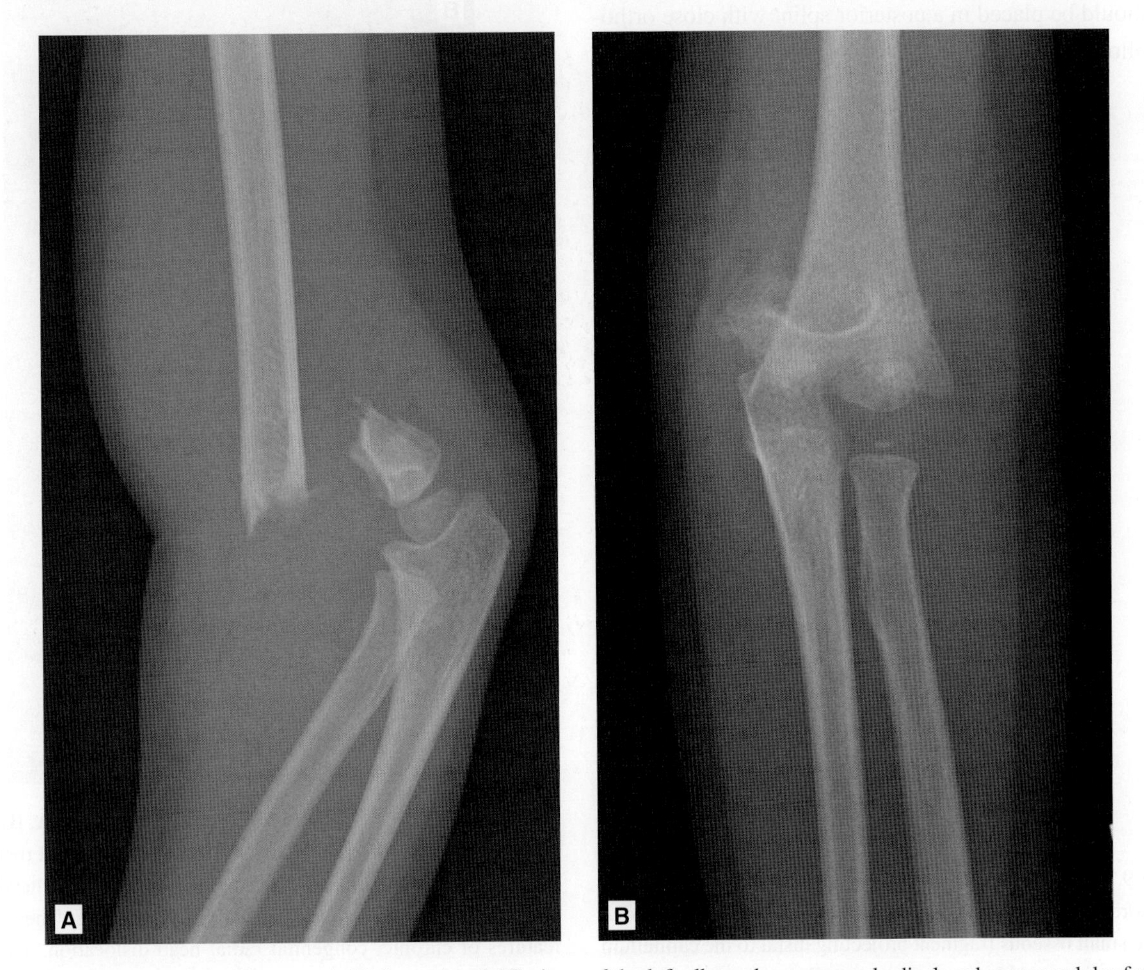

FIGURE 9.33 ■ Supracondylar Fracture. **A, B:** Lateral and AP views of the left elbow show a severely displaced supracondylar fracture.

Radiographic Summary

Posterior elbow dislocations occur with a fall or twisting injury to the elbow. AP and lateral radiographs of the elbow should be obtained to rule out fractures. Post reduction CT scan imaging may be useful in the setting of associated intra-articular fractures to rule out intra-articular fragments.

Clinical Implications

Posterior elbow dislocations are the most common dislocations in children under age 12 and the second most common in adults (after anterior glenohumeral dislocations). Clinically, the olecranon will be prominent on palpation and the patient will resist motion of the elbow joint. Neurovascular injuries to the ulnar and median nerves and brachial artery can result and a thorough exam should be performed pre and post reduction. Neurovascular injuries require emergent orthopedic evaluation. Posterior elbow dislocations can be reduced with analgesia and anesthesia with axial traction. Post reduction, the elbow should be placed in a posterior splint with close orthopedic follow-up for early range of motion exercises.

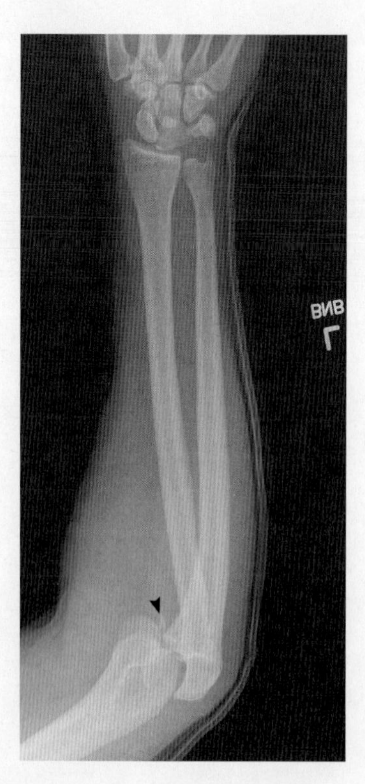

FIGURE 9.34 ■ Posterior Elbow Dislocation. A single AP view of the left forearm shows posterior dislocation of the ulna and radial head. The small osseous fragment projecting distal to the capitellum is the fractured coronoid process (arrowhead).

Pearls

1. Posterior elbow dislocations are the most common joint dislocation in adolescents with a peak incidence at age 12.
2. Early recognition of brachial artery injury is imperative to prevent Volkmann's ischemic contracture.

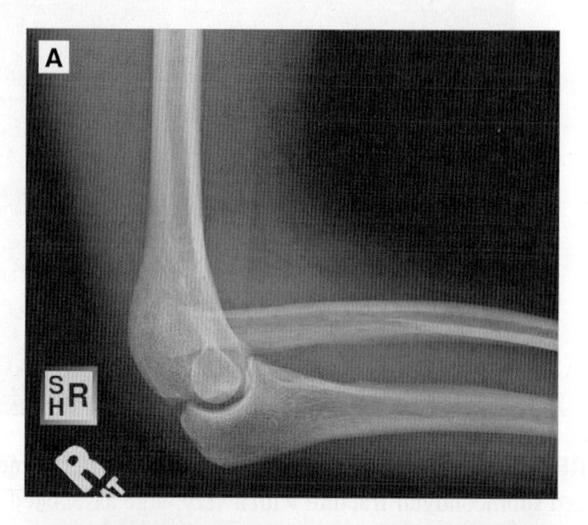

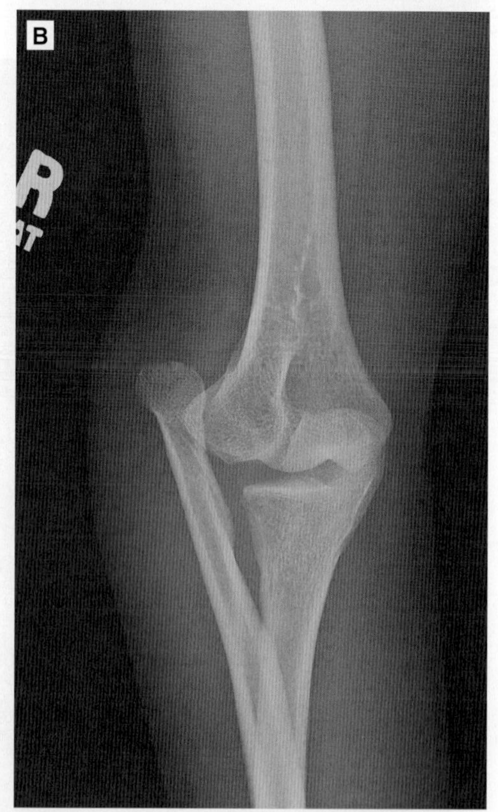

FIGURE 9.35 ■ Congenital Radial Head Dislocation. **A, B:** Lateral and AP views of the right elbow show volar and lateral dislocation of the radial head. Notice that the capitellum and radial head appear dysmorphic and the radius appears unusually long. These are the features of chronic, congenital radial head dislocation. This is not an acute injury.

Radiographic Summary

AP, scapular Y, and axillary views should be obtained to evaluate trauma to the proximal humerus. A Velpeau view (the x-ray beam is oriented superior to inferior while the patient leans backwards with arm in internal rotation) may be obtained if the patient cannot tolerate an axillary view. The proximal humerus can be divided into four parts using the Neer classification system. The anatomical neck is along the junction of the articular surface and capsular attachment of the humeral head. The surgical neck is in the proximal humeral metaphysis, distal to the humeral head and tuberosities. The greater tuberosity is the lateral superior aspect of the humeral head, and the lesser tuberosity is located along the anterior aspect of the proximal humerus. Fractures of the proximal humerus can be classified using the Neer classification system based on the number of segments involved and displaced. One- part fractures are fractures that have no displaced fragments. Two-part fractures have one displaced fragment. Three-part fractures have two displaced fracture fragments but the humeral head remains in contact with the glenoid. Four-part fractures have three or more displaced fragments and an associated glenohumeral dislocation. A CT scan may be helpful to further characterize the amount of displacement or rotation of the fracture fragments and should be obtained in comminuted fractures.

Clinical Implications

Proximal humerus fractures commonly occur in elderly patients after a fall. Patients will have swelling, ecchymosis, and pain on palpation and with attempted range of motion. Displaced fractures may cause axillary of suprascapular nerve injuries and may present with numbness and weakness of the deltoid and supraspinatus/infraspinatus muscles. The majority of nondisplaced and minimally displaced fractures can be treated nonoperatively with a sling for comfort. Most one-part fractures can also be treated nonoperatively. Fractures involving multiple segments and displaced fragments should be evaluated by orthopedics for operative fixation. All open fractures, fractures with dislocation of the humeral head, and fractures with associated neurovascular compromise require emergent orthopedic evaluation.

Pearls

1. Loss of range of motion is a common complication of proximal humerus fractures once they have healed and early range of motion with pendulum exercises may be initiated within the first few weeks.
2. Fractures involving the anatomic neck are at greatest risk for osteonecrosis and close orthopedic follow-up is necessary.

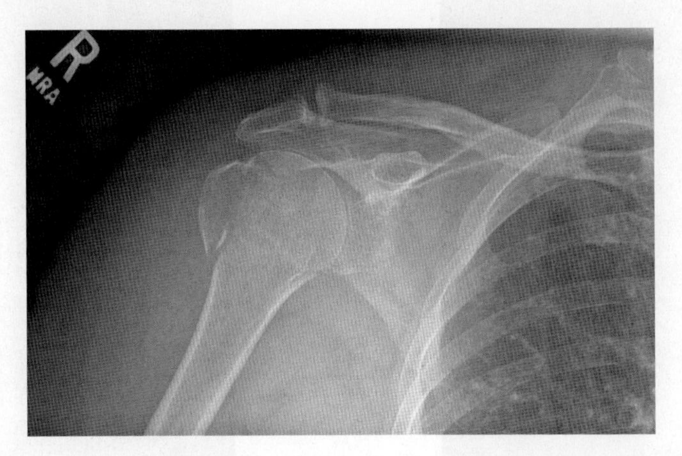

FIGURE 9.36 ■ Proximal Humerus Fracture. AP view of the right shoulder shows a comminuted fracture of the proximal right humerus with fracture planes extending through the surgical neck and undermining the greater tuberosity. There is no significant displacement and the shoulder is located.

Radiographic Summary

AP and lateral views of the humerus can be obtained to evaluate the amount of displacement and angulation of midshaft humerus fractures. Fractures can be classified as spiral, oblique, or transverse, and further classified as being simple, wedge (one fragment), or comminuted (multiple fragments).

Clinical Implications

Humerus shaft fractures typically result from a direct blow to the upper arm. Clinical exam should assess for injury to the radial nerve that may be injured in up to 20% of fractures. Many fractures can be treated nonoperatively with acceptable positioning being less than 20° of anterior/posterior

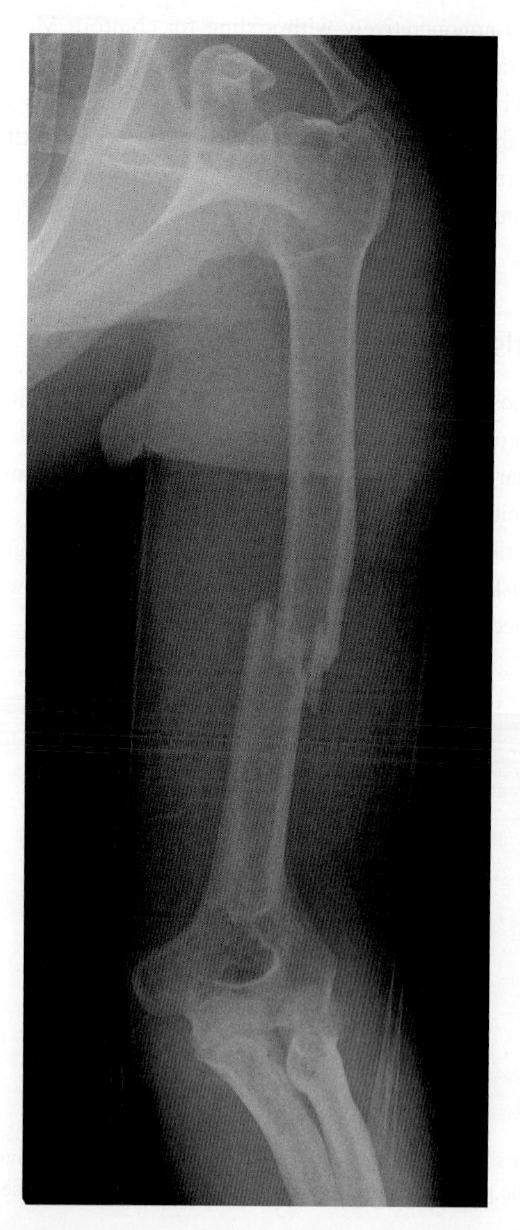

FIGURE 9.37 ■ Midshaft Humerus Fracture. AP view of the left humerus shows a transverse fracture through the mid humeral diaphysis. There is medial displacement of the distal segment by ½ shaft width and no significant angulation deformity.

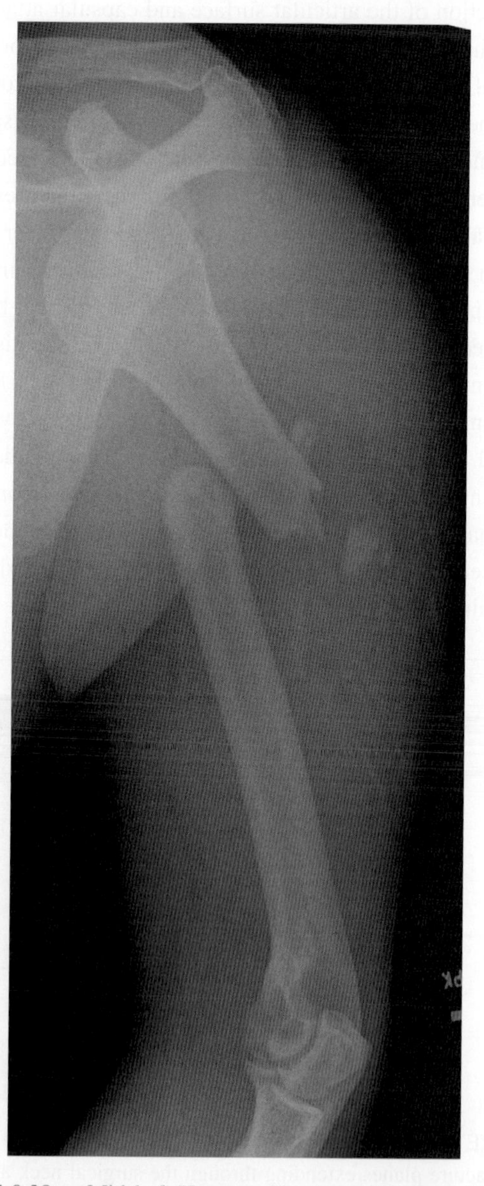

FIGURE 9.38 ■ Midshaft Humerus Fracture. AP view of the left humerus shows a mildly comminuted fracture of the proximal humeral shaft with 2 shafts width medial displacement of the distal humeral segment and some lateral apex angulation. Two small osseous fragments are displaced into the regional soft tissues.

angulation, less than 30° of varus angulation, and less than 1-2 cm foreshortening. Simple transverse fractures may be treated with a sling. Spiral, oblique, and angulated fractures may benefit from placement in a coaptation splint or Sarmiento brace. All open fractures and fractures with associated vascular or radial nerve injury require emergent orthopedic evaluation.

Pearls

1. The radial nerve injury is the most common nerve injury associated with humeral shaft fractures and most frequently occurs with distal humerus fractures.
2. Up to 75% of radial nerve injuries associated with humeral shaft fractures are temporary neuropraxias that may resolve in several months, although all should be emergently assessed by orthopedics at presentation.
3. Pediatric patients less than 3 years old or with an inconsistent mechanism of injury who present with proximal and midshaft humerus fractures should be assessed for possible child abuse.

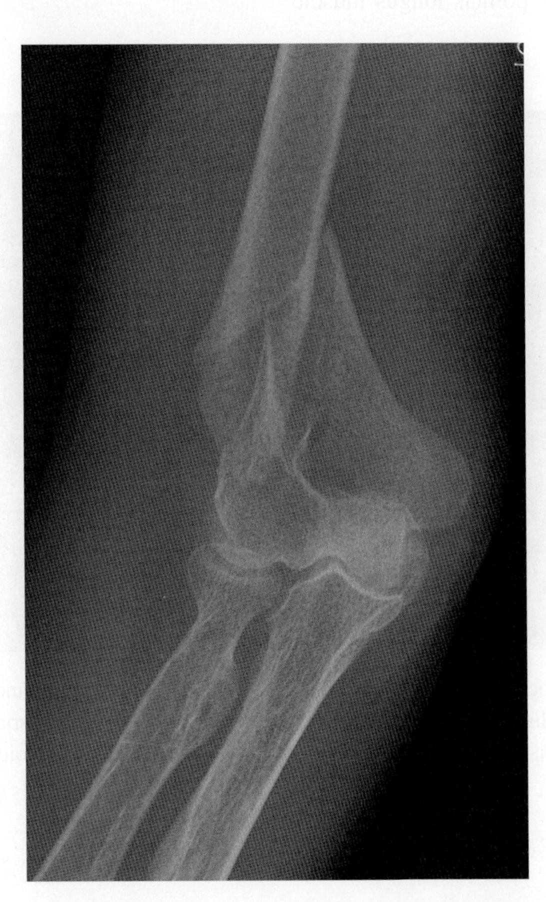

FIGURE 9.39 ■ Distal Humerus Fracture. AP view of the right elbow demonstrates a spiral fracture of the distal humeral shaft. The elbow remains located.

Radiographic Summary

Galeazzi fracture-dislocation can be seen on standard AP, lateral, and oblique radiographs of the wrist and forearm. The injury involves a fracture to the middle to distal third of the radius with associated disruption/dislocation of the distal radioulnar joint (DRUJ). The injury typically results from a fall onto an outstretched and hyperpronated wrist.

Clinical Implications

Galeazzi fracture-dislocations can be associated with compartment syndrome of the forearm and injury to the anterior interosseus nerve. This is a purely motor nerve that can be assessed by exercising the flexor pollicis longus muscle while making the "OK" sign. Galeazzi fractures in adults require operative fixation to stabilize the radial fracture and the DRUJ. Pediatric patients can often be treated with closed reduction and splinting, but should have prompt evaluation by orthopedics.

Pearls

1. The anterior interosseus nerve is a purely motor nerve and injury can be missed unless a thorough neurovascular exam is performed.
2. It is imperative to include imaging of the elbow and wrist when assessing forearm fractures to identify associated injuries and dislocations.

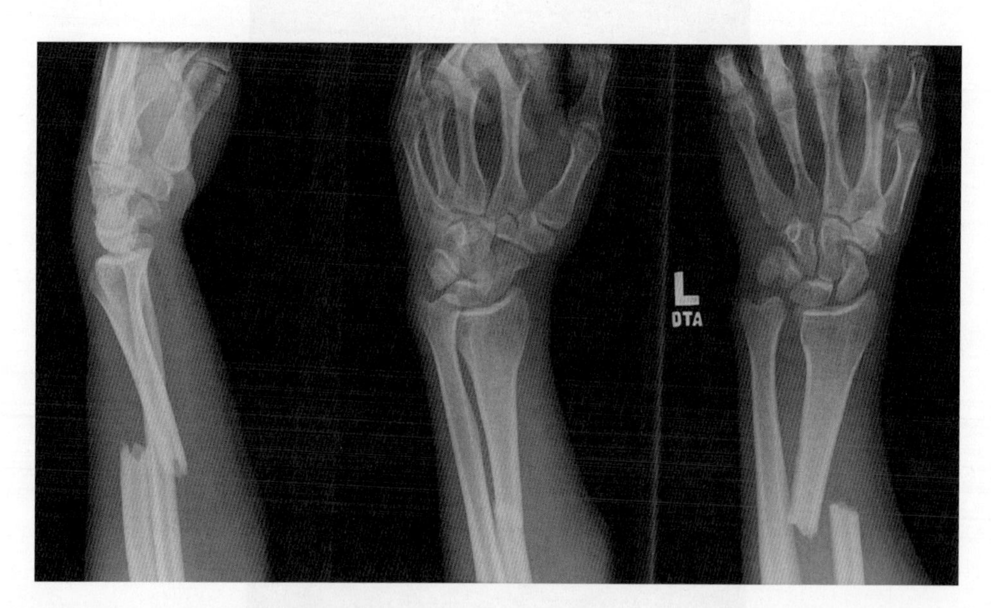

FIGURE 9.40 ■ Galeazzi Fracture-Dislocation. PA, oblique and lateral views of the left wrist demonstrate a displaced fracture of the distal radius and significant widening and malalignment of the distal radio-ulnar joint consistent with disruption of this joint. These are the features of a Galeazzi fracture-dislocation. There is also a tiny avulsion fracture of the tip of the ulnar styloid.

Radiographic Summary

Monteggia fracture-dislocations are proximal third ulnar fractures with associated dislocation of the radial head. AP, lateral and oblique radiographs of the elbow should be obtained to evaluate the injury. The dislocation of the radial head may be difficult to appreciate on a single view. The radio-capitellar line (a line drawn along the midline of the radial shaft) should bisect the capitellum on AP, oblique, and lateral radiographs. If it does not bisect the capitellum, a radial head dislocation or subluxation is present.

Clinical Implications

Monteggia fracture-dislocations are caused by a direct blow to the forearm with associated hyperpronation and hyperextension of the forearm. These injuries can be associated with damage to the radial nerve due to anterior displacement of the radial head. Operative fixation is typically needed, and associated nerve injuries require emergent orthopedic consultation.

Pearls

1. A Monteggia fracture-dislocation can lead to recurrent radial head dislocations even after operative fixation.
2. Fractures involving the forearm must include adequate imaging of the elbow to avoid missing a radial head dislocation.

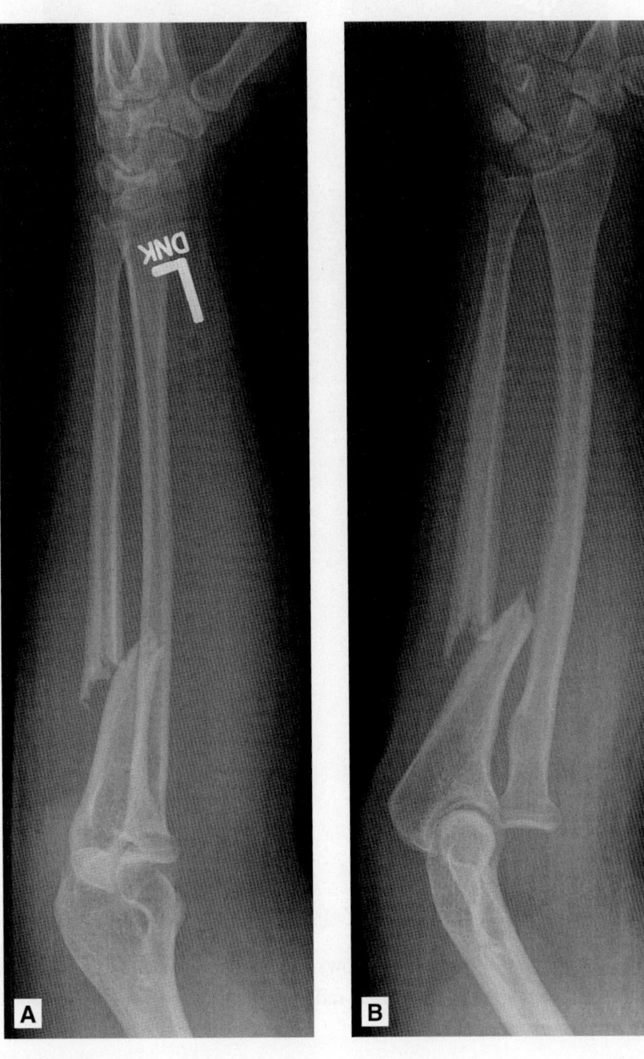

FIGURE 9.41 ■ Monteggia Fracture-Dislocation. **A, B:** Two views of the left forearm show a displaced fracture of the proximal ulna and dislocation of the radial head. These are the features of a Monteggia fracture-dislocation.

Radiographic Summary

Fractures involving both the radius and ulna should be evaluated with AP and lateral forearm radiographs. When only the radius is fractured, the DRUJ should be carefully assessed for subtle subluxation or dislocation on dedicated AP wrist radiographs.

Clinical Implications

All open fractures and the majority of adult both bone forearm fractures should undergo open reduction internal fixation. Unlike adults, children with both bone forearm fractures may be treated conservatively following adequate closed reduction and splinting. Younger patients have the potential to remodel the fracture site up to age 13. Younger patients will tolerate more angulation and rotation of the fractures, however after age 10-12, less angulation is tolerable as remodeling potential becomes more limited.

Pearls

1. Imaging should include the wrist and elbow to verify no additional injury or dislocation has occurred to the DRUJ or radial head.
2. Both bone forearm fractures in patients over age 13 require operative fixation when any angulation or rotational deformity is present.

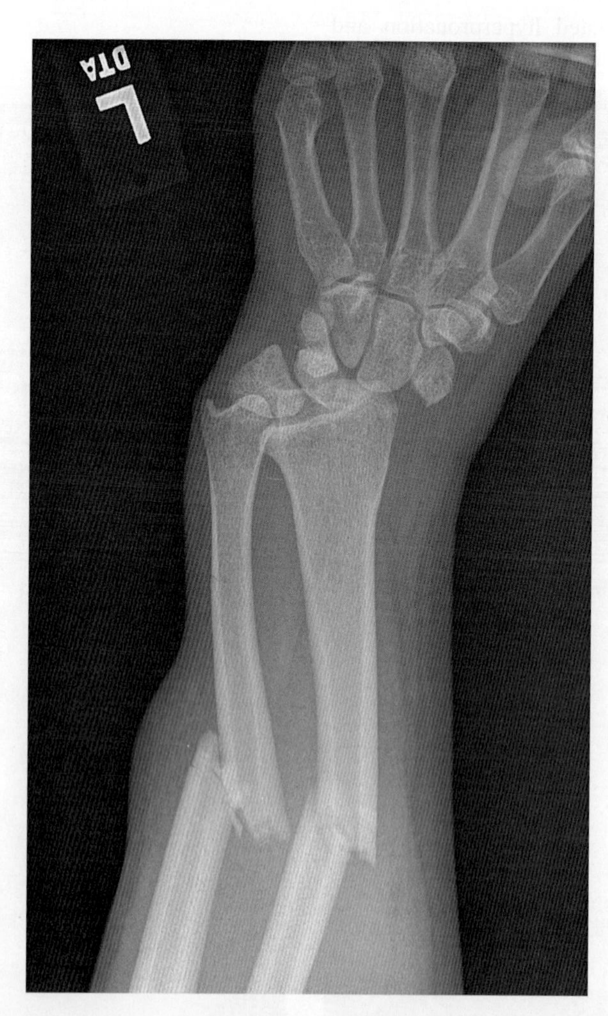

FIGURE 9.42 ■ Radius–Ulna Fracture. PA view of the left wrist shows mildly displaced and angulated fractures of both the radial and ulnar shafts. The patient also has an unusual lunate dislocation, as well as radial dislocation of the carpal bones and disruption of the distal radio-ulnar joint.

Radiographic Summary

Colles' fractures are fractures of the distal radial metaphysis with dorsal displacement and angulation. They occur typically due to a fall onto an outstretched hand with forced dorsiflexion. Tension fractures occur on the volar radius while the dorsal radius is compressed. AP, lateral and oblique images of the wrist should be obtained to fully evaluate the injury. Associated ulnar styloid fractures may indicate additional injury to the triangular fibrocartilage complex. Scapholunate ligament injuries and DRUJ injury may also be present and can be identified on the AP images.

Clinical Implications

Colles' fractures are common injuries in older patients after a fall onto an outstretched hand. Patients will present with pain and swelling over the distal radius with dorsal angulation of the wrist and hand in relation to the forearm ("dinner fork deformity"). Open fractures and medial nerve injury mandate emergent orthopedic evaluation. Displaced fractures should be reduced with hematoma block or procedural sedation and placed in a sugar-tong splint. Most fractures will benefit from operative fixation and stabilization.

Pearls

1. Colles' fracture patterns are referred to as "dinner fork deformity" because of the dorsal angulation of the hand/wrist in regards to the radius.
2. Acute carpal tunnel syndrome can occur with Colles' fractures due to compression of the median nerve.

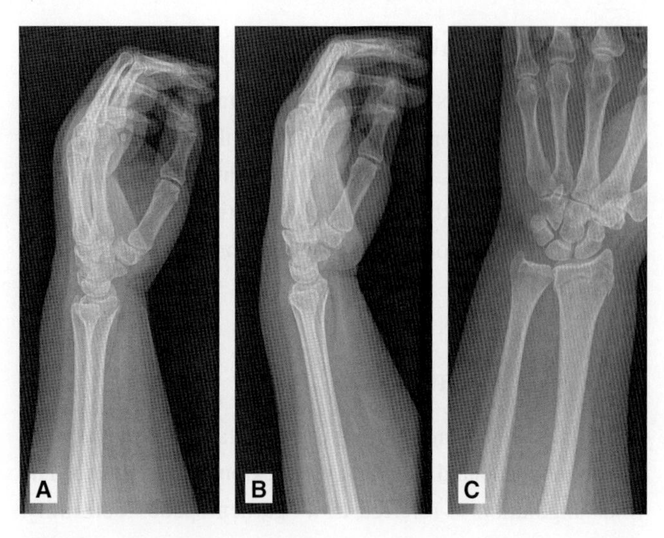

FIGURE 9.43 ■ Nondisplaced Colles' Fracture. **A-C:** PA, oblique, and lateral views of the wrist show a very subtle, nondisplaced transverse fracture through the distal radial metaphysis.

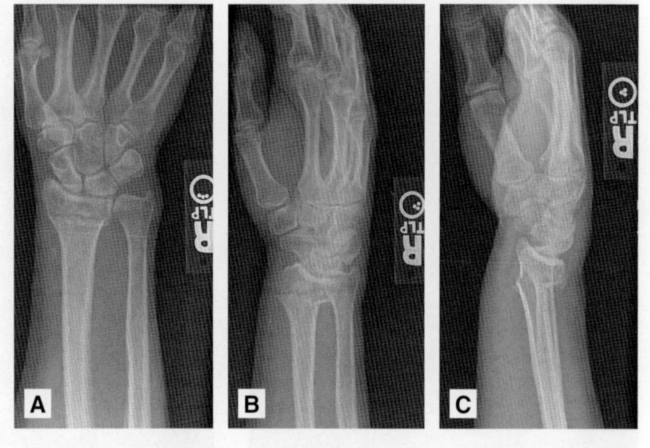

FIGURE 9.44 ■ Displaced Colles' Fracture. **A-C:** PA, oblique, and lateral views of the right wrist show a transverse distal radial metaphyseal fracture with significant dorsal tilt of the distal radial segment.

Radiographic Summary

A Smith's fracture is a fracture of the distal radius metaphysis with volar angulation. Close inspection of the DRUJ and carpal spaces is necessary to assess for additional injury. These fractures may be extra articular, intra articular, or associated with a fracture/dislocation of the radiocarpal joint (Barton's fracture).

Clinical Implications

Smith fractures occur with a backward fall onto the palm of an outstretched hand causing hyperflexion and pronation. The volar angulation is referred as a "garden spade" deformity. Smith fractures require closed reduction with hematoma block or procedural sedation and placement in a sugar-tong splint. Surgical fixation is recommended. Emergent orthopedic consultation is necessary for open fractures and median nerve injuries.

Pearls

1. Smith fractures are referred as the "garden spade deformity" because of the volar angulation.
2. The median nerve is at risk for compression due to the angulation and deformity.

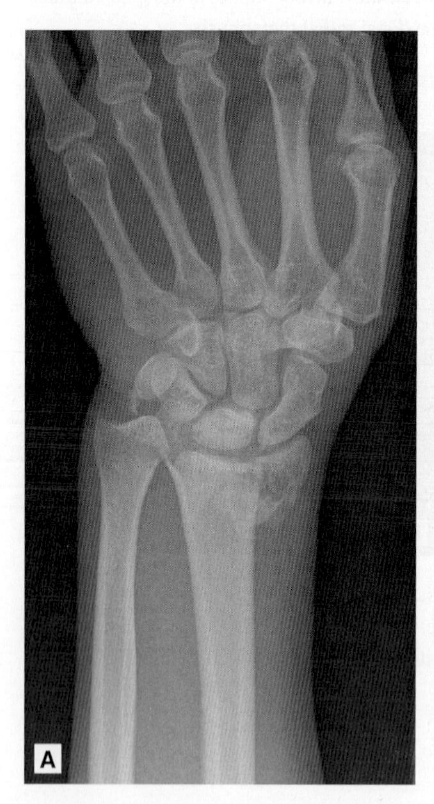

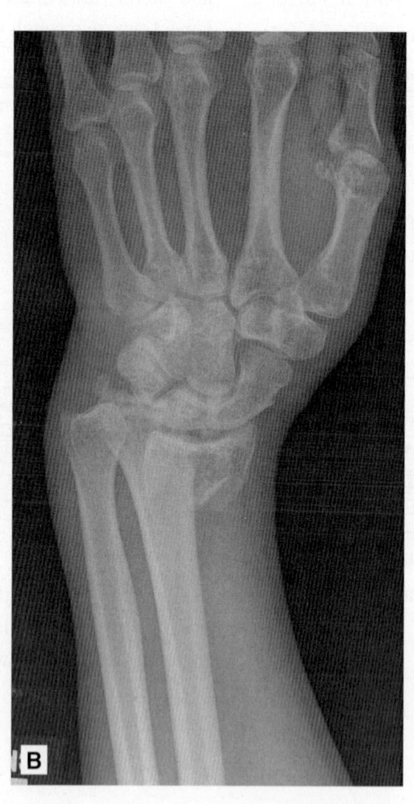

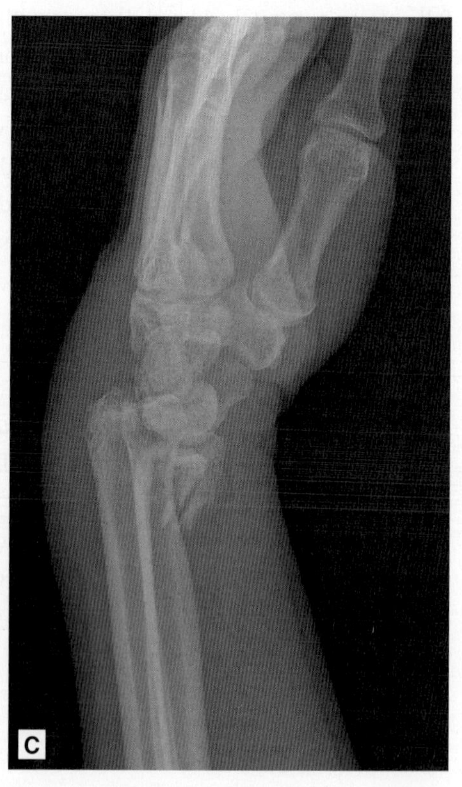

FIGURE 9.45 ■ Barton's Fracture. **A-C:** PA, oblique, and lateral views of the left wrist show a comminuted intraarticular fracture of the distal radius. A major fragment from the volar aspect of the distal radius is proximally impacted and displaced.

Radiographic Summary

Hutchinson's fracture is a fracture of the radial styloid. The mechanism of injury is typically a fall onto an outstretched hand where the force is transmitted through the scaphoid and radial styloid. It has also been referred to as the Chauffer's fracture as it used to occur when a car backfired while the chauffer was hand cranking to start the car. The crank was forced into the palm and force was transmitted from the scaphoid into the radial styloid. Associated scaphoid fractures and scapho-lunate ligament injuries may occur as well, based on the mechanism of injury.

Clinical Implications

Nondisplaced fractures with no articular depression may be treated in sugar-tong splint with thumb spica. Displaced fracture should be treated with operative fixation.

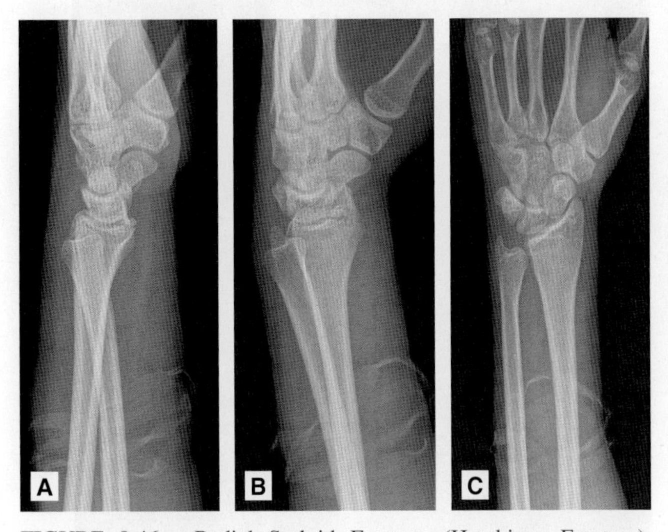

FIGURE 9.46 ■ Radial Styloid Fracture (Hutchison Fracture). **A-C:** PA, oblique, and lateral views of the left wrist show a nondisplaced fracture of the radial styloid.

Pearls

1. Associated scaphoid fractures are common with radial styloid fractures and a dedicated scaphoid view may be helpful to further assess for this injury.
2. CT scans may be helpful to determine the degree of articular involvement and assess the need for operative fixation.

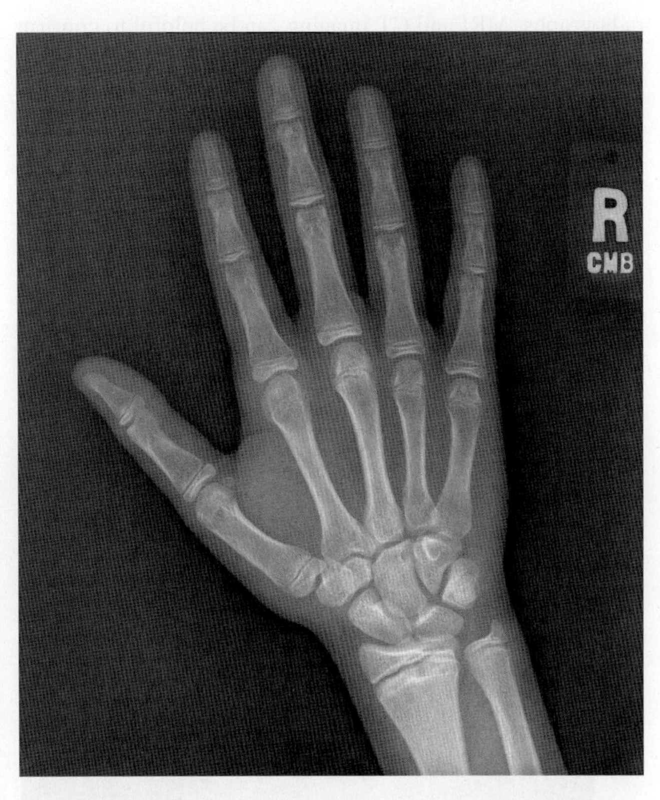

FIGURE 9.47 ■ Salter–Harris I Fracture. PA view of the right wrist shows abnormal widening and irregularity along the distal radial physis. Note that the distal radial physis is much wider than the adjacent normal distal ulnar physis. This is a Salter–Harris type 1 injury to the growth plate. The patient was a young gymnast.

Radiographic Summary

The scaphoid is the most commonly fractured carpal bone. Injury typically occurs with a fall onto an outstretched hand with dorsiflexion and radial deviation of the wrist. Standard AP, lateral, and oblique views of the wrist should be obtained to assess for the injury. A scaphoid view (AP view of the wrist obtained with ulnar deviation of the hand) can help "elongate" the scaphoid and aid in diagnosis. Up to 10% of scaphoid fractures may be incomplete and may not be seen on initial radiographs. MRI and CT imaging can be helpful to confirm or exclude the diagnosis, when necessary.

Clinical Implications

The scaphoid bone has its blood supply enter the distal pole. Nonunion and avascular necrosis are common in this fracture, particularly in fractures involving the scaphoid waist and proximal pole, because the blood supply may be limited or completely disrupted. Injuries to the scaphoid bone can cause instability of the wrist. Any displaced fractures indicate instability and should undergo operative fixation. Because of the high risk of missed diagnosis on initial radiographs and the high associated rate of nonunion and avascular necrosis, all patients with pain on palpation of the scaphoid bone (elicited

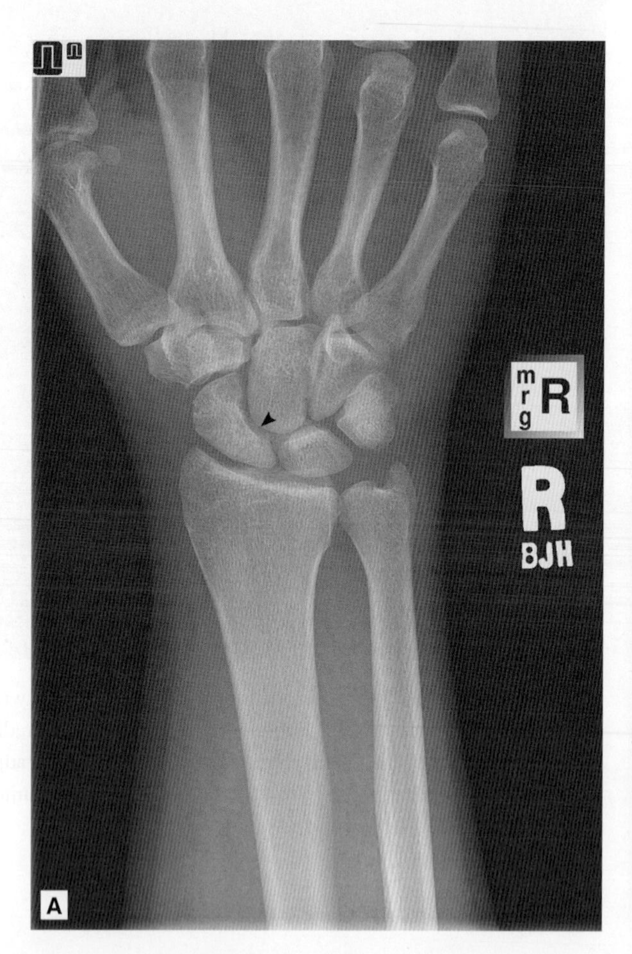

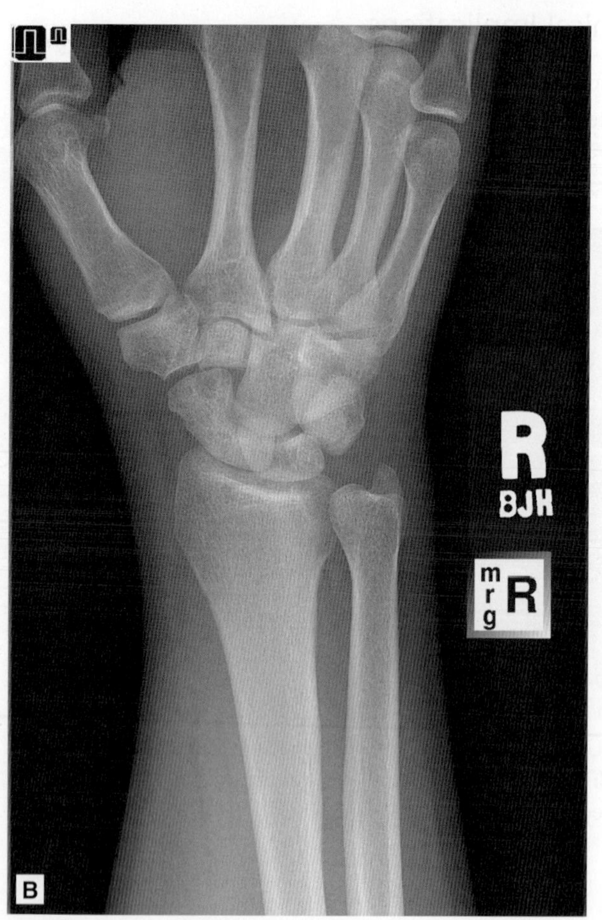

FIGURE 9.48 ■ Scaphoid Fracture. **A-D:** PA, oblique, lateral, and scaphoid views of the right wrist show a subtle fracture through the scaphoid waist. The fracture is seen best on the scaphoid and PA views (arrowhead). If a fracture of the scaphoid is suspected, it is worth obtaining an additional dedicated scaphoid view because it is often the view which best delineates the fracture.

with pressure applied to the anatomical snuff box) should be placed in a spica splint and treated for an occult fracture. Repeat physical exam and radiographs 2 weeks after the injury should be helpful in ruling in or out an initially occult fracture. When the diagnosis remains equivocal, an MRI can confirm or exclude the diagnosis.

Pearls

1. Up to 10% of fractures to the scaphoid bone are not visible on initial radiographs.
2. A scaphoid view (AP wrist with ulnar deviation) helps "elongate" the scaphoid and can be helpful to assess for a subtle fracture.
3. Because the blood supply to the scaphoid bone enters at its distal pole, the more proximal the fracture, the higher the incidence of nonunion and avascular necrosis.

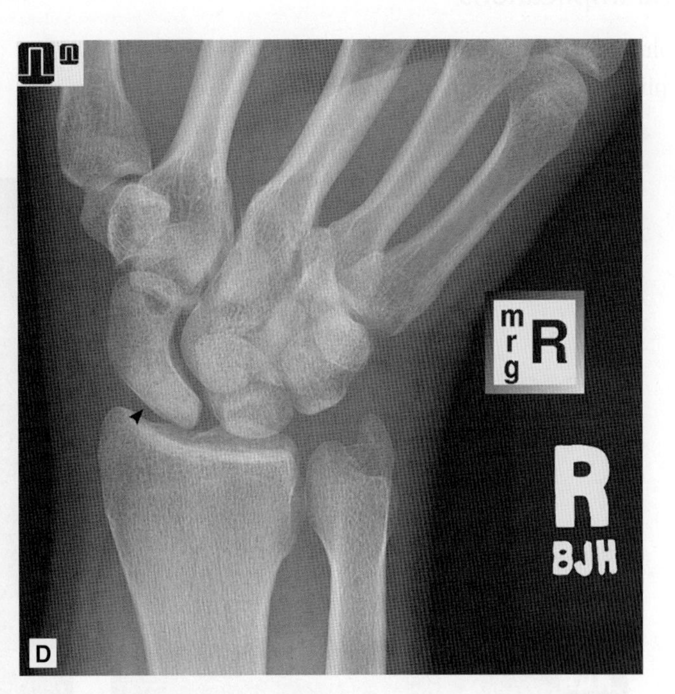

FIGURE 9.48 ■ (*Continued*) Lateral and scaphoid views of the same wrist.

Radiographic Summary

Scapholunate ligament tears are the most common and most significant ligament injury in the wrist. Injury to the ligament typically occurs with a fall onto an outstretched hand with ulnar deviation. Associated fractures of the scaphoid and radial styloid are common. AP imaging of the wrist shows increased distance between the scaphoid and lunate bones (Terry Thomas sign) as compared to the typical uniform 1-2 mm seen between all other carpal bones. A bilateral AP grip compression view of the wrist can be obtained to help identify the injury. In this view, the capitate is pushed into the space between the scaphoid and lunate during closure of the fist and will increase the space between the scaphoid and lunate when an injury to the ligament is present. MRI and wrist arthrography can also confirm the diagnosis.

Clinical Implications

Scapholunate ligament tears may be placed in a sugar-tong splint with close orthopedic follow-up. Nonoperative treatment is reserved for the elderly and those with severely arthritic joints. Most other patients will require operative fixation to prevent chronic instability and wrist pain.

Pearls

1. A bilateral grip compression view radiograph of the wrists can be obtained when the diagnosis is suspected but not evident on the conventional AP view of the wrist.
2. The scaphoid shift test can be performed to assess for ligamentous instability. The examiner holds pressure on the volar scaphoid tubercle (at the palmar crease) with the thumb and presses the index finger on the dorsal wrist behind the scaphoid. While compressing the index and thumb together, the wrist is moved from ulnar to radial deviation. Pain and a palpable clunk indicate scapholunate instability.

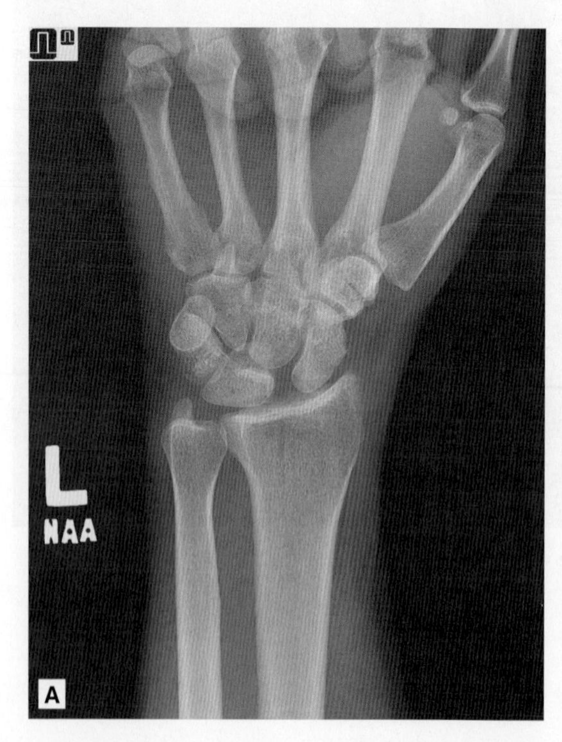

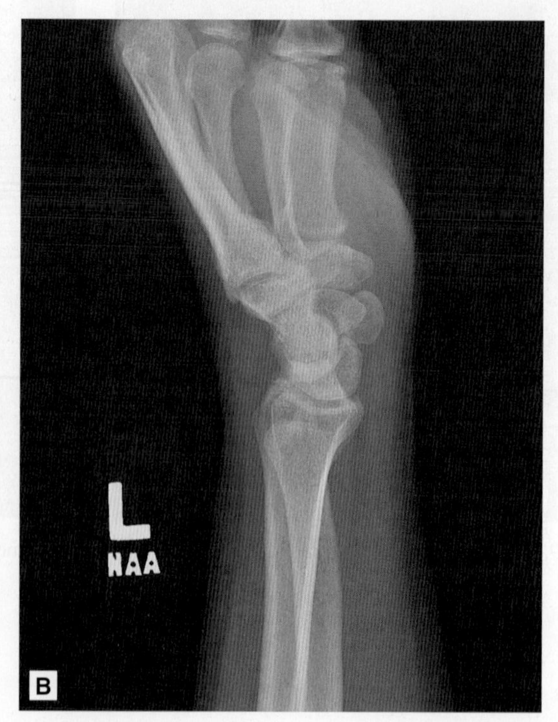

FIGURE 9.49 ■ Scapho-Lunate Ligament Tear. **A, B:** PA and lateral views of the left wrist show marked abnormal widening of the scapholunate interval consistent with insufficiency (prior tear) of the scapho-lunate ligament. One complication of this injury is the development of dorsal intercalated segmental instability (DISI). Indeed, the lateral view shows abnormal increase of the scapho-lunate angle which approaches 90° in this patient (upper normal is 60°). The findings are consistent with DISI.

Radiographic Summary

The triquetrum is the second most common carpal bone fracture. It typically occurs with a hyperextension injury to the wrist with ulnar deviation. AP radiographs are typically normal; most triquetral fractures are identified as a small dorsal avulsion fracture visible only on the lateral view of the wrist.

Clinical Features

Patients with triquetrum fractures are typically treated nonoperatively and can be splinted acutely in the emergency room with outpatient orthopedic follow-up.

Pearls

1. Triquetrum fractures are usually only seen on the lateral radiograph of the wrist.
2. CT or MRI can confirm the diagnosis when conventional radiographs are normal but clinical suspicion for the injury remains high.

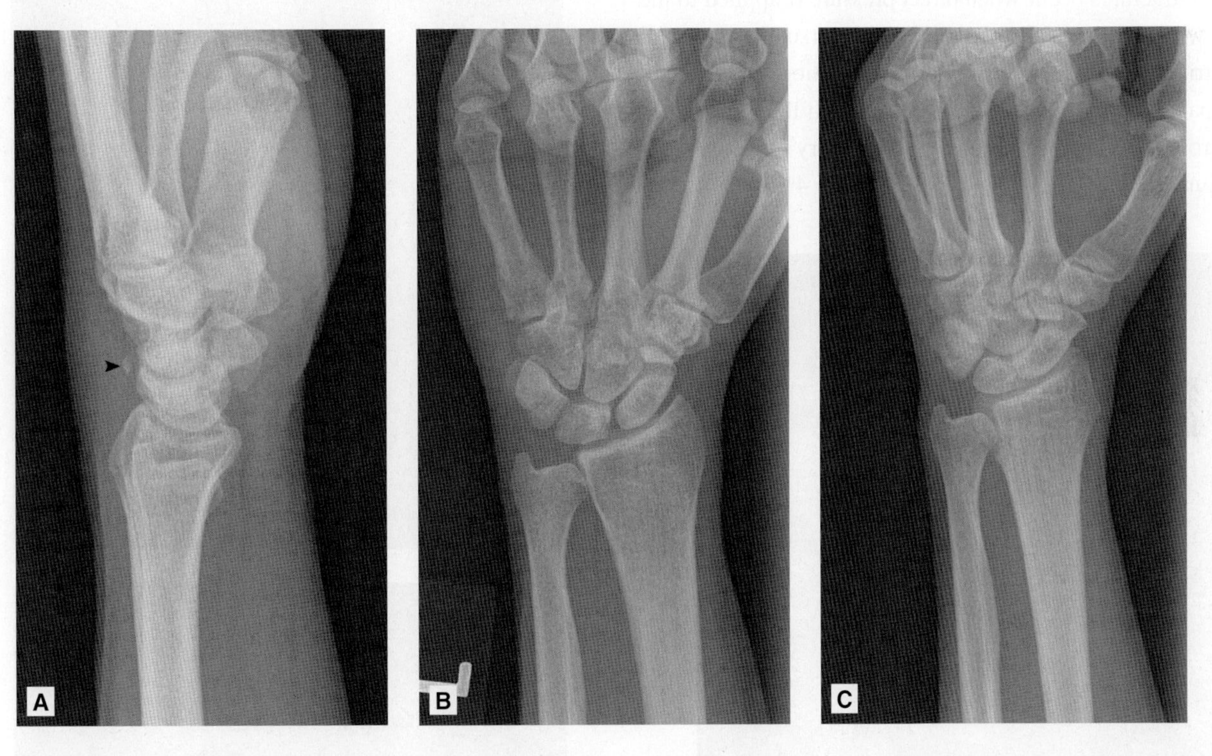

FIGURE 9.50 ■ Triquetral Fracture. **A-C:** Lateral view of the wrist shows a tiny fleck of bone just dorsal to the proximal carpal row with regional soft tissue swelling (arrowhead). This is a triquetral avulsion fracture. This fracture is usually only visible on the lateral view of the wrist. Notice that the fracture cannot be seen on the PA or oblique views (B or C).

Radiographic Summary

The hamate articulates with the 4th and 5th metacarpals. Body fractures can be seen on AP and oblique wrist radiographs as a small avulsion just proximal to the base of the 5th metacarpal. Hook of the hamate fractures are more common and are often difficult to see on standard AP, lateral, and oblique wrist radiographs. A carpal tunnel view, where the wrist is dorsi-flexed and the x-ray tube is angled 25° inferiorly to the palm, should be obtained when the diagnosis is suspected. CT imaging can be used to confirm the diagnosis.

Clinical Implications

Hamate fractures occur when direct pressure is applied to the ulnar wrist due to a fall or when an object (such as baseball bat) strikes the palm forcing it in ulnar deviation. Patients will have pain on palpation to the hamate bone. If the fracture has compromised Guyon's canal, the ulnar artery and nerve can be injured. Patients with paresthesias to the 4th and 5th digits and vascular compromise require emergent orthopedic evaluation. Definitive management varies. A trial of conservative treatment with immobilization can be attempted; however, some orthopedists recommend surgical excision in all cases.

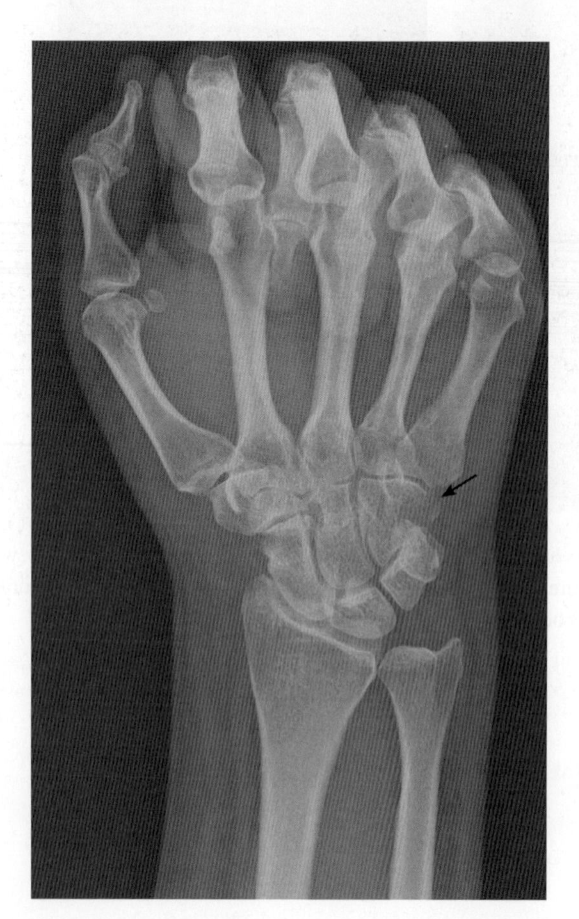

FIGURE 9.51 ■ Hamate Fracture. PA view of the wrist shows a very subtle fracture of the ulnar aspect of the hamate bone.

Pearls

1. Carpal tunnel views of the wrist or CT imaging can be used to assess for hook of the hamate fractures.
2. CT angiogram can be used to help identify the fracture and associated injury to the ulnar artery.

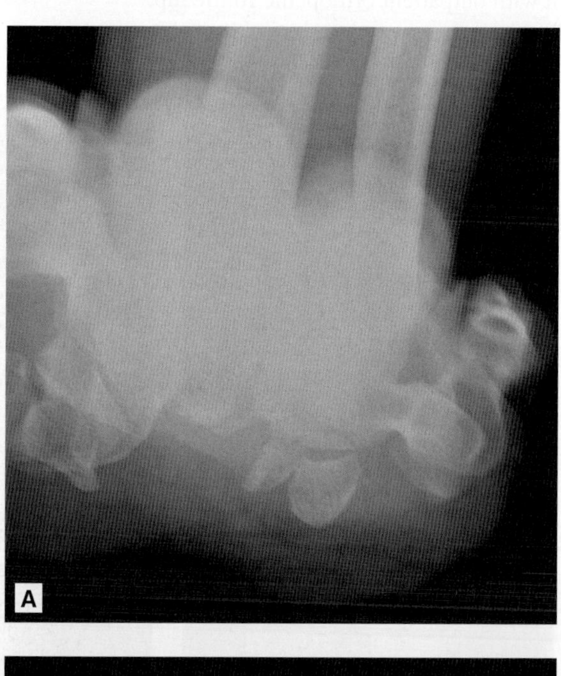

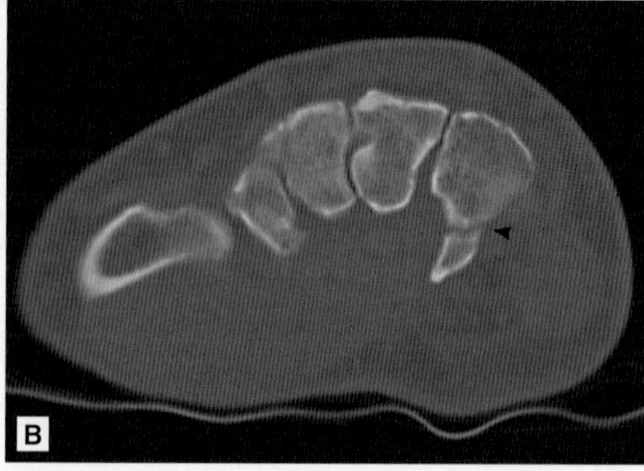

FIGURE 9.52 ■ Hamate Fracture. **A:** Carpal tunnel view shows an essentially nondisplaced fracture through the base of the hamate hook. This fracture was invisible on the conventional (AP, oblique and lateral) views of the wrist. **B:** Axial CT image done without intravenous contrast shows the fracture through the base of the hook of the hamate (arrowhead).

Radiographic Summary

Fractures to the lunate, capitate, trapezium, trapezoid, and pisiform bones are less common. These may be identified on plain radiographs of the wrist, but additional imaging including CT or MRI may be most useful in visualizing these injuries.

Clinical Implications

Frequently fractures to these bones may be associated with other fractures and ligament injuries to the wrist that may require operative management. Orthopedic consultation should be obtained to assess with definitive management.

Pearls

1. Kienbocks's disease, or avascular necrosis of the lunate, can occur when the lunate's blood supply is disrupted. It is a rare disorder that may be associated with prior wrist trauma such as a fracture of the lunate, but may also be related to injury to the arterial blood supply from a wrist sprain. Classically, Kienbock's disease is associated with ulna minus variance (the ulna is shorter than the radius).
2. CT and MRI are superior to plain radiographs in assessing bone bruising, ligament injury and occult fractures of the carpal bones. They should be obtained when radiographs are unremarkable and clinical suspicion is high.

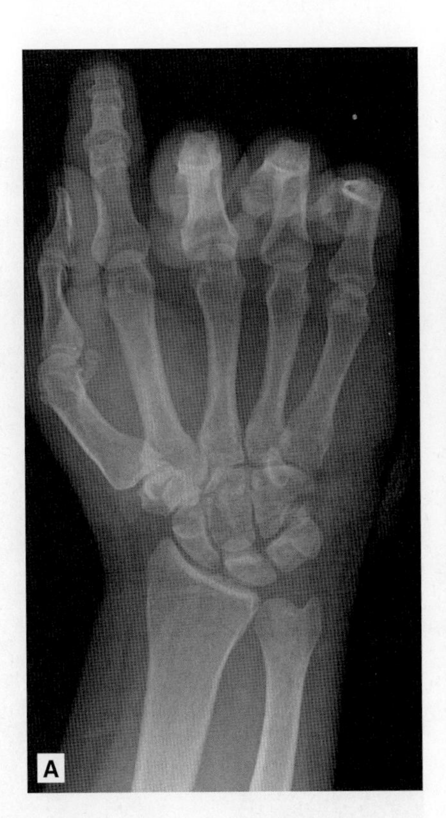

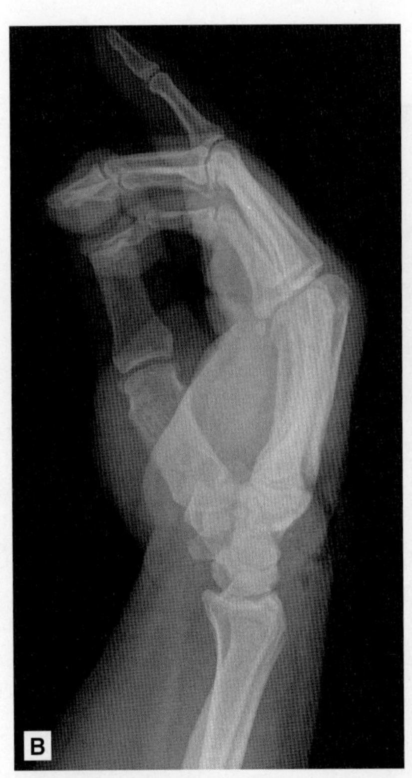

FIGURE 9.53 ■ Capitate, Hamate, and Pisiform Fractures. **A, B:** AP and lateral views of the right wrist show nondisplaced fractures of the capitate, hamate, and pisiform and a large laceration in the dorsal aspect of the wrist.

Radiographic Summary

A perilunate dislocation occurs when the lunate maintains a normal relationship with the distal radius while the capitate and other carpal bones are dislocated (typically posteriorly) in regards to the lunate. This can be seen as disruption of the "3 C sign" on both AP and lateral images. AP views will show a triangular appearance of the lunate. Lateral images show the lunate articulating with the distal radius, but the capitate and distal carpal bones are posteriorly dislocated.

Clinical Implications

Similar to lunate dislocations, perilunate dislocations are associated with significant ligamentous damage to the wrist. These are unstable and require emergent orthopedic consultation with reduction and operative stabilization.

Pearls

1. Closed reduction can be difficult and may require open reduction.
2. Median nerve injury is the most common associated injury in perilunate dislocations.
3. Volar skin can become ischemic if reduction is delayed. Prompt orthopedic assessment is necessary.

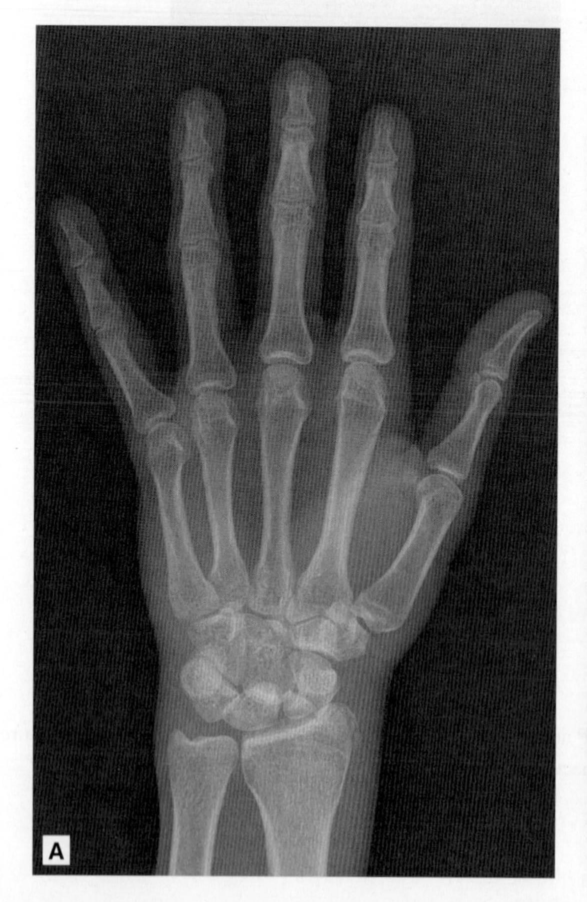

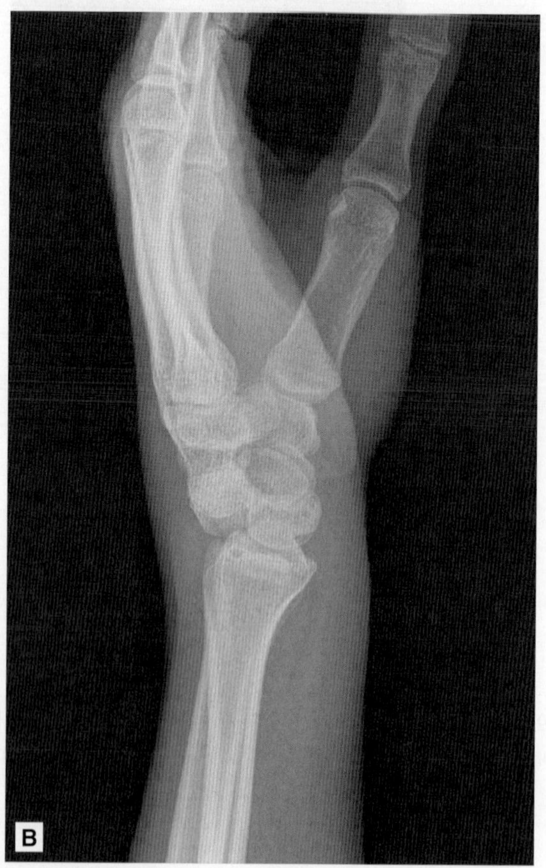

FIGURE 9.54 ■ Perilunate Dislocation. **A, B:** A PA view of the wrist shows disruption of the carpal arcs. The lateral view shows that the lunate aligns with the distal radius while the capitate and metacarpals are dislocated dorsal to the lunate.

Radiographic Summary

Lunate dislocations can be seen on AP views of the wrist with disruption of the normally 3 smooth arcs ("3 C sign"). On AP radiographs, the lunate will have a triangular or "pie shaped" appearance. On lateral radiographs, the lunate is displaced volarly and does not articulate with the capitate or radius ("spilled tea cup sign").

Clinical Features

With displacement of the lunate volarly, the median nerve and ulnar/radial arteries can be injured. Orthopedic consultation is required and often closed reductions are not successful. Lunate dislocations require surgical fixation.

Pearls

1. Lunate dislocations can be easily identified on the lateral radiographs by the presence of the "spilled tea cup sign."
2. Compression of the median nerve is common and prompt reduction followed by surgical fixation is necessary.

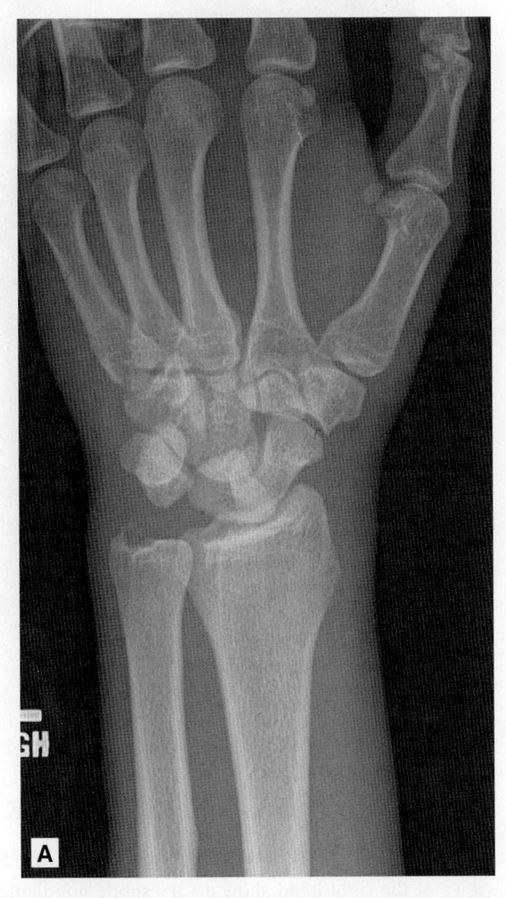

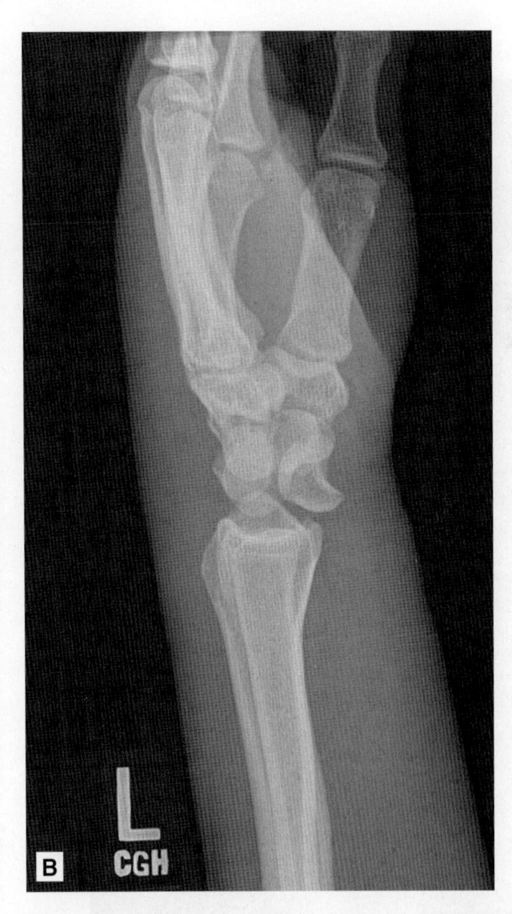

FIGURE 9.55 ■ Lunate Dislocation. **A, B:** A PA view of the wrist shows disruption of the carpal arcs. A lateral view shows volar displacement of the lunate. The radius, capitate, and third metacarpal align.

Radiographic Summary

Metacarpal fractures are common and account for a third of all hand fractures. Fractures can occur at the head, neck, shaft, or base of a metacarpal. AP, lateral, and oblique radiographs should be obtained to assess for fractures. Radiographs should be reviewed for degree of angular deformity and intra-articular involvement.

Clinical implications

Each metacarpal tolerates variable degrees of angulation with the 4th and 5th tolerating more angulation due to the increased motion of the ulnar hand. Thumb, index, and middle metacarpal fractures tolerate very little angulation and fractures with >5-10° of angulation will require surgical fixation.

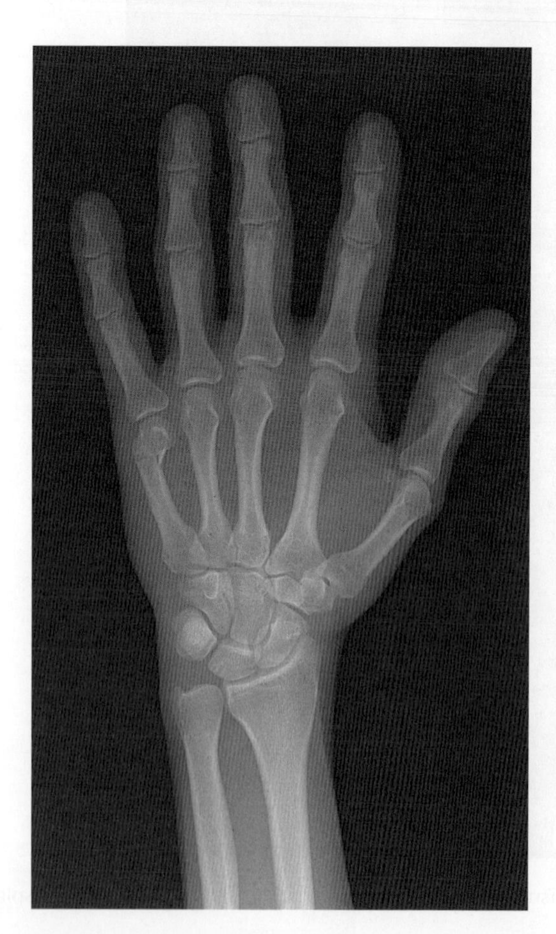

FIGURE 9.56 ■ Boxer's Fracture. A PA view of the hand shows an angulated fracture of the neck of the 5th metacarpal.

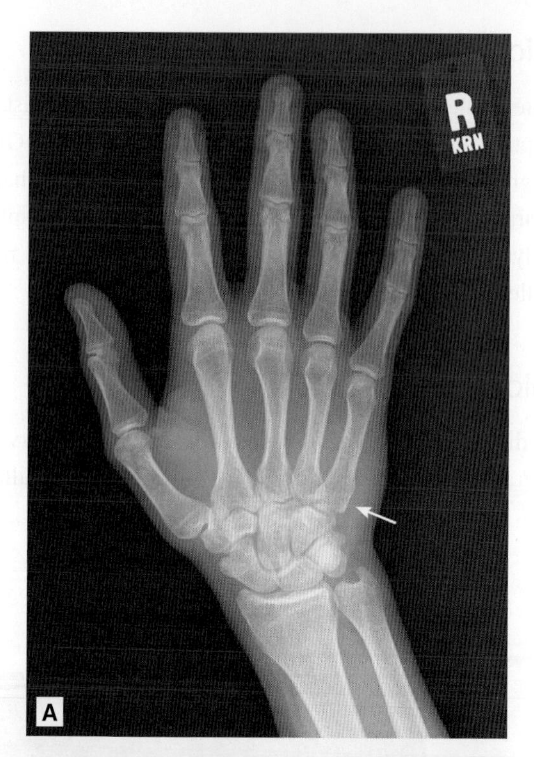

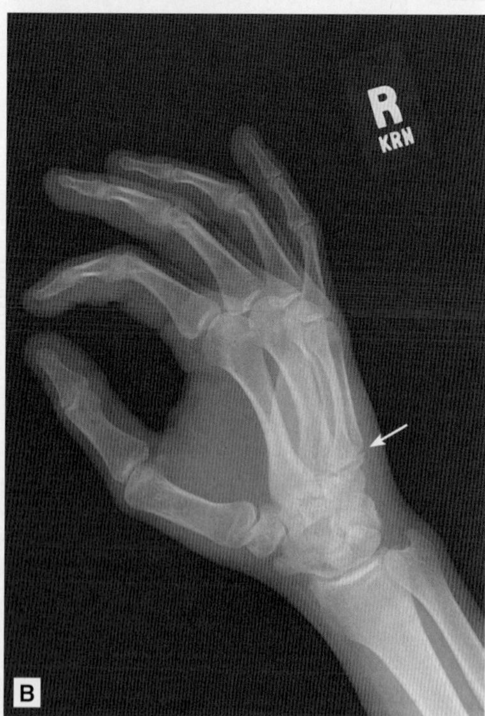

FIGURE 9.57 ■ Fifth Metacarpal Fracture. **A, B:** PA and oblique views of the right hand show a very subtle nondisplaced fracture at the base of the 5th metacarpal (arrow). The fracture is better demonstrated on the oblique view. Such fractures at the metacarpal bases can be very subtle. Look for metacarpal foreshortening and assess the alignment of the carpo-metacarpal joints on the lateral and oblique views. Dislocations without fractures can also occur at the carpo-metacarpal joints and can be very subtle radiographically.

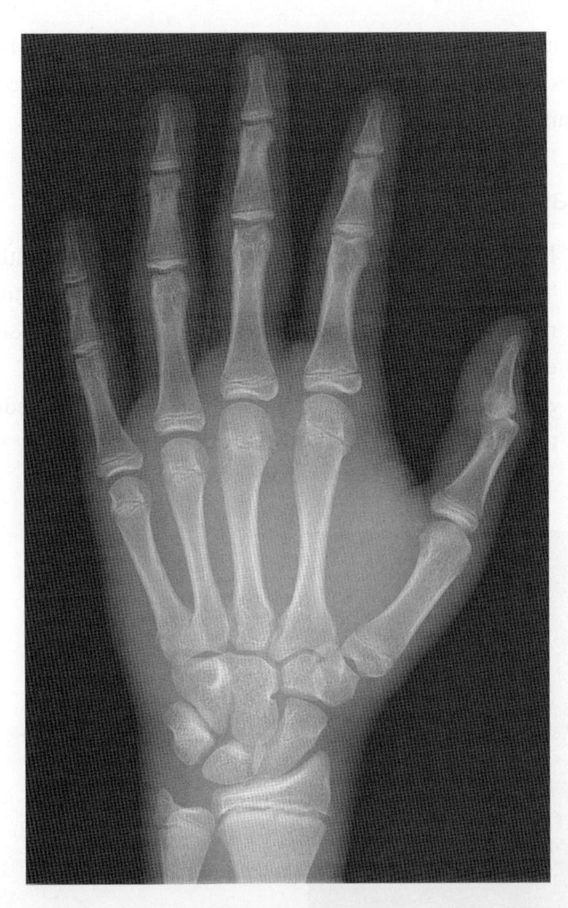

FIGURE 9.58 ■ Fifth Metacarpal Fracture. Another example of a subtle extraarticular fracture at the 5th metacarpal base.

4th metacarpal fractures may tolerate up to 30° of volar angulation and 5th metacarpal fractures up to 45°. Intra-articular fractures, fractures with foreshortening, and fractures with rotational deformity require surgical fixation. Acutely, fractures can be placed in a dorsal-volar splint to the MCP joint or ulnar gutter splint.

Pearls

1. Fractures of the 5th metacarpal base can be subtle and difficult to see. These fractures may best be seen on true lateral and/or oblique views.
2. Malrotation can be assessed by having the patient flex the fingers at the MCP joints with the tips of the fingers touching the palmar crease. Each finger should have a similar cascade. Comparison to the unaffected hand can be helpful. Malrotation can also be assessed by having the patient extend all of the digits at the MCP joints and look directly in the axial plane for differences among each extended finger.
3. Metacarpal neck and shaft fractures are unstable and repetitive reduction attempts in the emergency department are not typically beneficial.

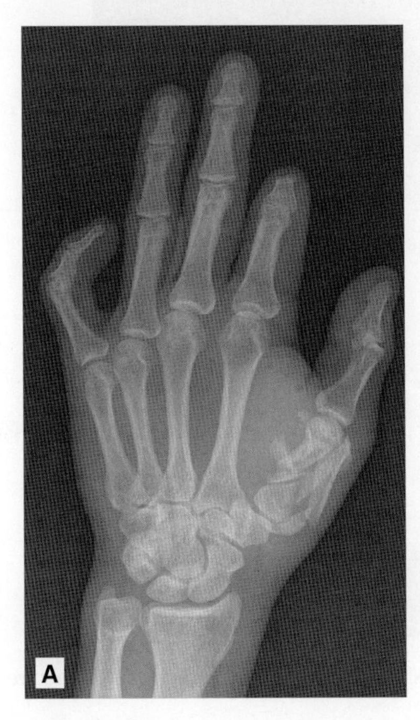

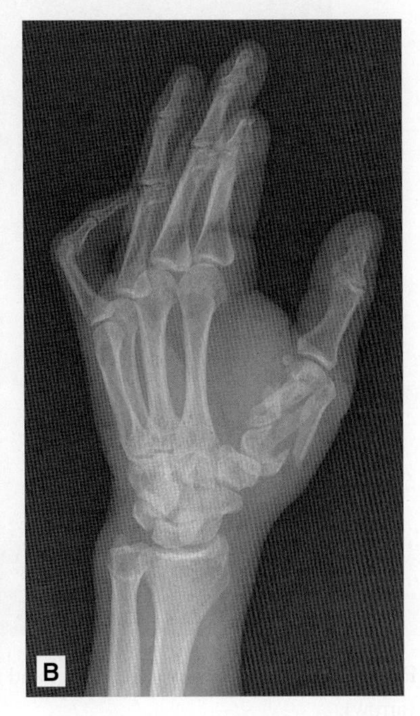

FIGURE 9.59 ■ First Metacarpal Fracture. **A, B:** Two views of the left hand show a severely comminuted fracture of the 1st metacarpal bone. The patient has had prior amputation of the distal portion of the index finger.

Radiographic Summary

Middle and proximal phalanx fractures can be assessed with AP and lateral radiographs of the injured finger.

Clinical Implications

Middle and proximal phalanx fracture have a high risk for deformity because of deforming forces of the associated tendons and ligaments. Close inspection should assess for angular and rotational deformity. Nondisplaced fractures can be treated with buddy taping or volar splint. Displaced/angulated fractures, fractures with foreshortening, intra-articular fractures, and any fracture with malrotation should be referred to a hand specialist for definitive care.

Pearls

1. Radiographs should be obtained in a patient with a "jammed finger" as subtle and not so subtle fractures may be seen on radiographs despite an unremarkable exam.
2. All PIP and DIP joint dislocations require a post reduction radiograph to assess for associated fractures.

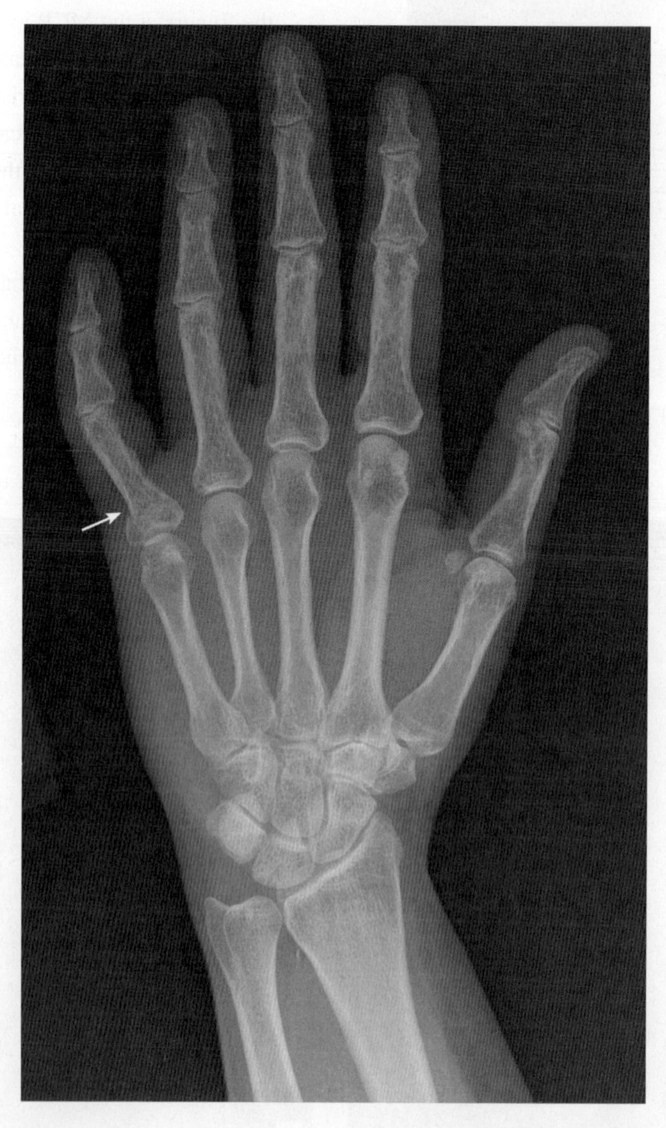

FIGURE 9.60 ■ Proximal Phalanx Fracture. PA view of the left hand shows an angulated extra-articular fracture at the base of the proximal phalanx of the pinky finger (arrow).

Radiographic Summary

Tuft fractures are fractures of the distal aspect of the distal phalanx. They can be seen on AP and lateral images of the involved finger.

Clinical implications

Closed fractures without significant comminution and displacement can be splinted and treated conservatively. Large, intra-articular, and displaced fractures may require operative fixation. Open fractures and those with associated nail bed injuries require orthopedic consultation.

Pearls

1. Subungual hematomas may be present and can often cause more pain than the fracture. Nail trephination in the setting of the fracture is controversial.
2. The extensor tendon and flexor digitorum profundus both attach on the distal phalanx. Physical exam should confirm that the tendons are intact.

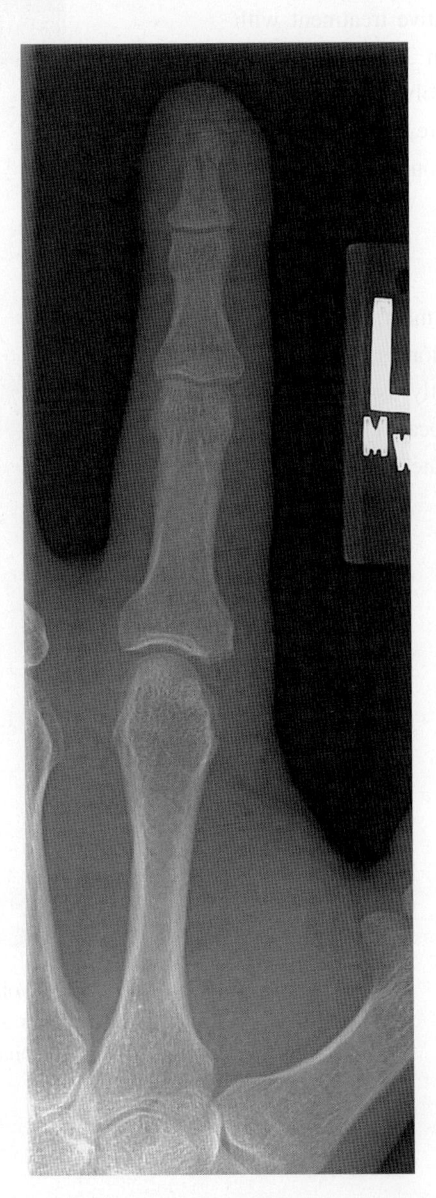

FIGURE 9.61 ■ Tuft Fracture. PA view of the left index finger shows a comminuted fracture of the tuft of its distal phalanx.

Radiographic Summary

Hyperextension or dorsal subluxation or dislocation of a finger joint can result in injury to the volar plate. The volar plate may be torn or avulsed. Lateral radiographs of the injured finger can reveal the avulsion fracture.

Clinical Implications

Patients with volar plate avulsion fractures will be tender on palpation of the affected joint. Full range of motion of the joint should be attempted and the stability of the collateral ligaments should be assessed. Nonoperative treatment with buddy taping is preferred when less than 20% of the articular surface is involved. In fractures involving greater than 20-40% of the articular surface or fractures with bony fragments that block reduction, surgical fixation is necessary.

Pearls

1. Buddy taping can effectively splint most fractures and allows for gradual early range of motion as tolerated.
2. Dorsal PIP dislocations are frequently associated with volar plate avulsion fractures. All dislocated joints require post reduction radiographs to evaluate for an avulsion fracture.

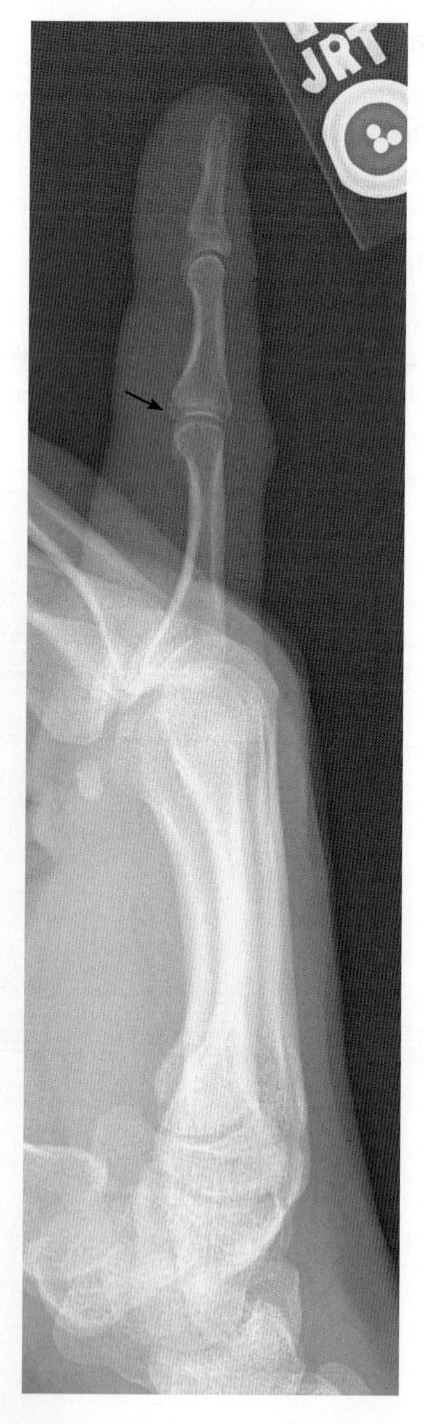

FIGURE 9.62 ■ Volar Plate Fracture. A lateral view of the right index finger shows a small volar plate avulsion fracture from the base of its middle phalanx (arrow).

Radiographic Summary

A mallet finger is a dorsal avulsion fracture from the base of the distal phalanx at the insertion of the extensor tendon. The typical mechanism of injury occurs with forced hyperflexion of the DIP joint. AP and lateral radiographs of the finger should be obtained to assess for the injury.

Clinical Implications

A mallet finger should be suspected when patients cannot actively extend the DIP joint. Bony mallet fingers involve an avulsion fracture of the extensor tendon. Minimally displaced fractures may be treated in an extension DIP splint (Stack/Stax splint) for 6 weeks. Special care should be made to protect the skin from injury during this time. Surgical fixation may be required in the presence of DIP subluxation of the distal phalanx, significant displacement of the avulsed fragment, and when significant intra-articular involvement is present.

Pearls

1. Initial conservative treatment of mallet fingers with extension splinting of the DIP joint may be attempted up to 6 weeks after the original injury.
2. Patients treated in a stack splint should always keep the DIP joint in extension, even when changing the splint. Failure to do so may create a re-tear and require 6 additional weeks of splint wear.

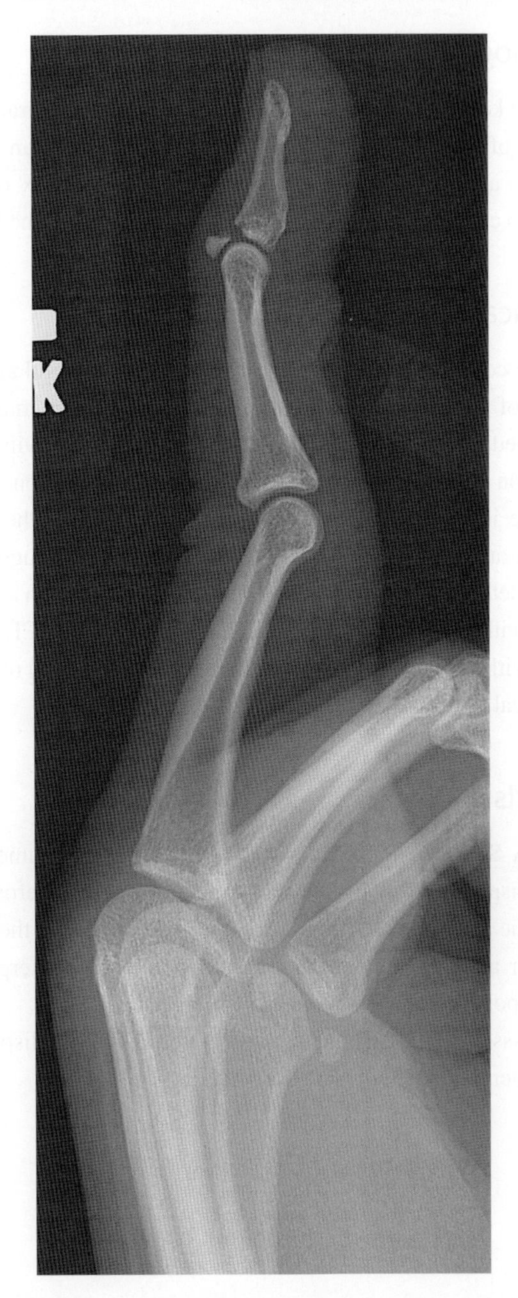

FIGURE 9.63 ■ Mallet Finger. A lateral view of the left index finger shows an avulsion fracture from the dorsal aspect of the base of its distal phalanx. There is no subluxation or dislocation. The PIP joint is hyperextended, presumably due to joint laxity.

Radiographic Summary

Game keeper's thumb is an injury to the ulnar collateral ligament of the 1st metacarpo-phalangeal joint. Often, an associated avulsion fracture along the proximal phalanx of the thumb can be seen on AP and lateral radiographs of the hand.

Clinical Implications

Ulnar collateral ligament injuries result from forceful abduction of the thumb. The ulnar collateral ligament may be strained, partially torn, or completely torn. Patients will have pain on palpation of the UCL and pain with abduction stress of the joint. Greater than 30° laxity compared to the contralateral side or absence of a definitive end point suggest a completely torn ligament. Patients should be placed in a spica cast with orthopedic referral. Complete tears and UCL injuries with displaced avulsion fractures (Stener lesions) require surgical fixation.

Pearls

1. A Stener lesion occurs when the torn UCL ligament is displaced away from the donor site with the aponerosis of the adductor pollicis muscle interposed between the torn or avulsed ligament and the donor site. The interposed aponerosis prevents the UCL from healing.
2. Associated avulsion fractures with >3 mm of displacement may require surgical fixation.

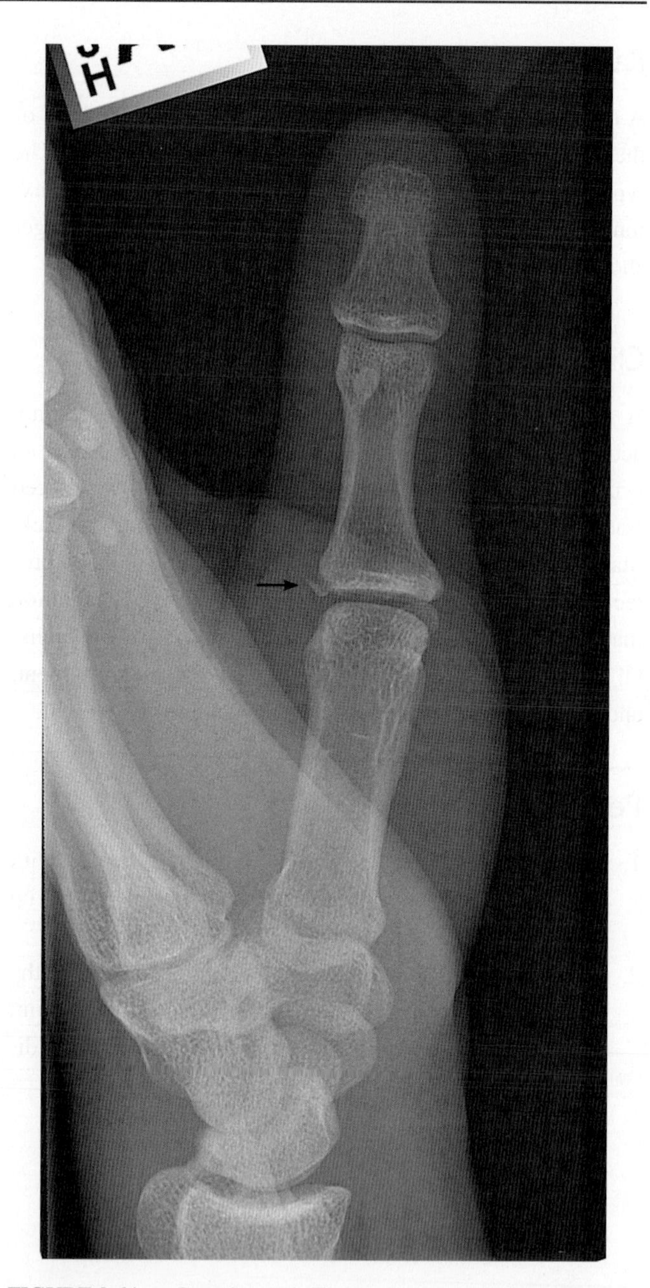

FIGURE 9.64 ■ Gamekeeper's Thumb. PA view of the right thumb demonstrates a small avulsion fracture from the ulnar base of its proximal phalanx (arrow). The alignment is normal.

Radiographic Summary

A Bennett fracture is a fracture of the base of the 1st metacarpal bone which extends into the carpometacarpal (CMC) joint. This is the most common type of fracture of the thumb and is often associated with a dislocation of the 1st carpometacarpal joint.

Clinical Implications

Bennett fractures occur with axial forces applied to a partially flexed metacarpal. Patients will have pain and swelling at the fracture site and the 1st CMC joint may be unstable. Nondisplaced fractures may be treated with spica splint and casting for 6 weeks. Fractures with greater than 1 mm of displacement should be surgically fixed.

Pearls

1. Bennett fractures require anatomic alignment to prevent osteoarthritis and chronic hand pain. Close follow-up with hand surgery is necessary.
2. CT scans can be helpful in assessing the degree of comminution and impaction of the articular surface and may aid in surgical planning.

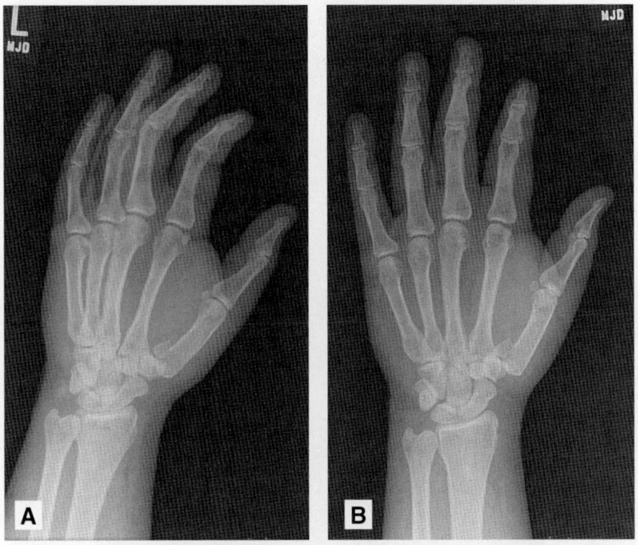

FIGURE 9.65 ■ Bennett Fracture. **A, B:** PA and oblique views of the left hand show a simple intraarticular fracture at the base of the 1st metacarpal. The fracture is mildly displaced.

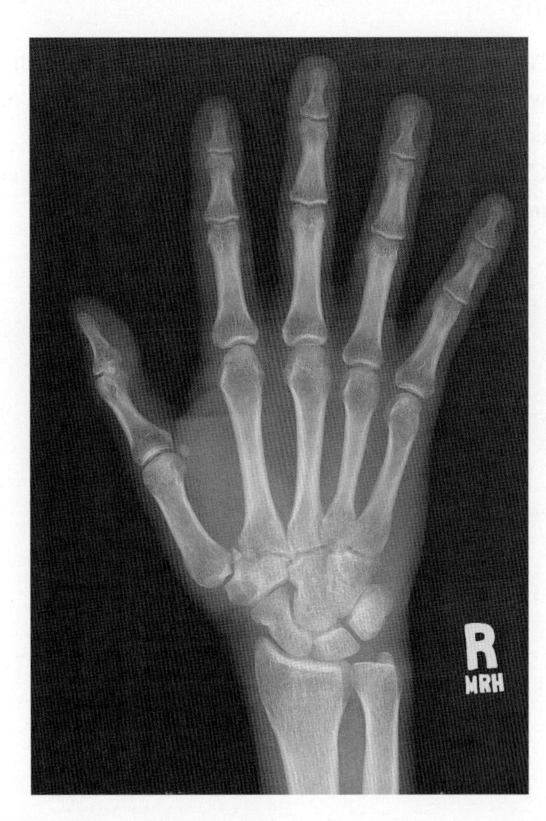

FIGURE 9.66 ■ Bennett Fracture. Companion case: a smaller Bennett fracture.

Radiographic Summary

Rolando fracture is a comminuted intra-articular fracture at the base of the 1st metacarpal bone. The injury results from an axial load, crushing the metacarpal axial surface.

Clinical Implications

Rolando fractures require operative fixation to restore the joint surface to its normal anatomical configuration. Initial management should be thumb spica for comfort and urgent orthopedic evaluation for surgical repair.

Pearls

1. Although less common, the Rolando Fracture has a worse prognosis than a Bennett Fracture because of its comminution.
2. CT scans can be useful in identifying the degree of comminution and can aid in operative planning.

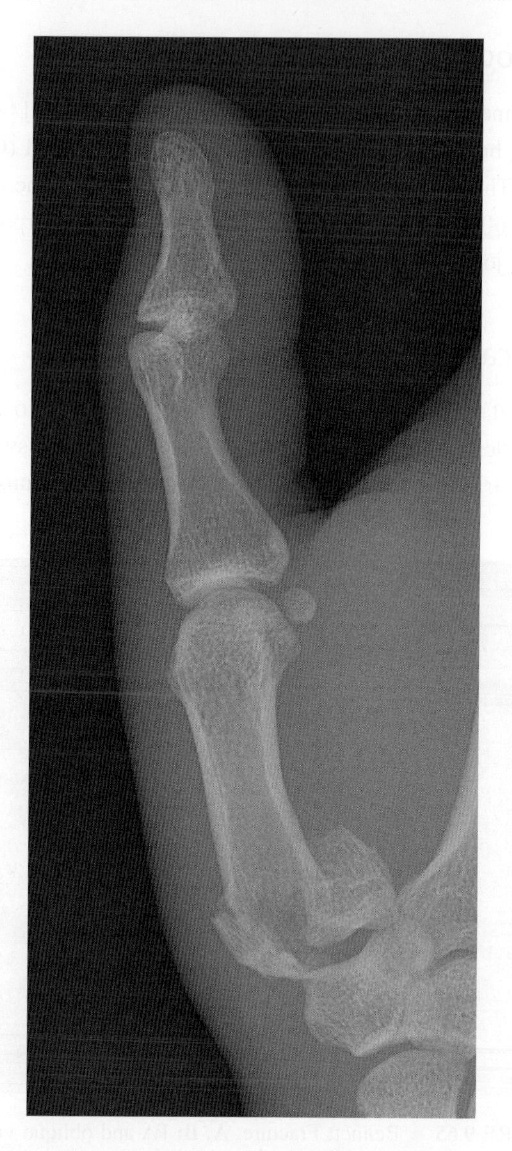

FIGURE 9.67 ■ Rolando Fracture. Oblique view of the right thumb shows a comminuted intraarticular fracture at the base of the 1st metacarpal.

Radiographic Summary

Dislocations of the 1st carpometacarpal joint can occur with axial loading of the thumb in slight adduction. This injury can be identified on AP and lateral images of the hand and may be associated with Rolando or Bennett fractures.

Clinical Implications

These dislocations can be easily reduced with axial traction and dorsal pressure applied to the carpal–metacarpal (CMC) joint, however they are very unstable. Post reduction, the thumb should be placed in a spica splint and the patient should be referred to hand surgery for evaluation. Treatment options include surgical stabilization versus prolonged cast immobilization.

Pearls

1. Dislocations of the 1st CMC joint are unstable post reduction. They should be placed in a spica splint with close orthopedic surgery follow-up.
2. Bennett and Rolando fractures are common with 1st CMC dislocations.

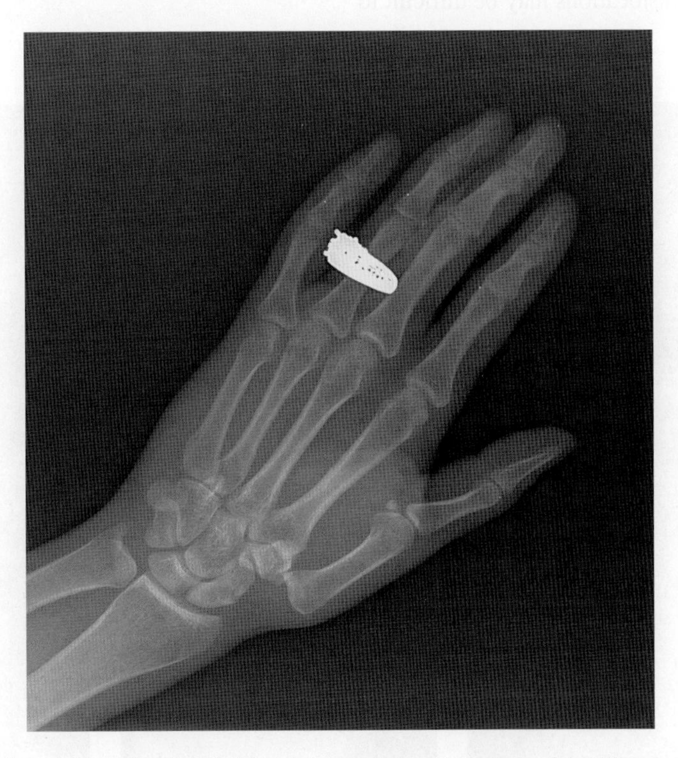

FIGURE 9.68 ■ Thumb Dislocation. A PA view of the left hand demonstrates dislocation of the 1st carpo-metacarpal joint.

Radiographic Summary

Dislocations of the DIP and PIP finger joints can be assessed radiographically with AP and lateral views of the injured finger. Both joints have similar restraints (collateral ligaments, volar plate, and extensor tendon). Dorsal PIP dislocations are most common and occur when axial and hyperextension forces are applied. Associated volar plate fractures are common. Volar PIP joint dislocations are less common.

Clinical Implications

Finger dislocations are generally easily reduced with axial traction. Occasionally, dorsal dislocations may be difficult to reduce due to entrapment of the flexor tendon or volar plate. Post reduction, dorsal dislocations can be buddy taped with an early range of motion initiation. Volar dislocations should be splinted in extension due to high associated central tendon slip injuries to prevent a boutonniere deformity.

Pearls

1. Volar PIP joint dislocations commonly cause disruption of the central tendon slip. Close orthopedic follow-up is necessary.
2. Irreducible dislocations may be due to volar plate entrapment. These may require open reduction.

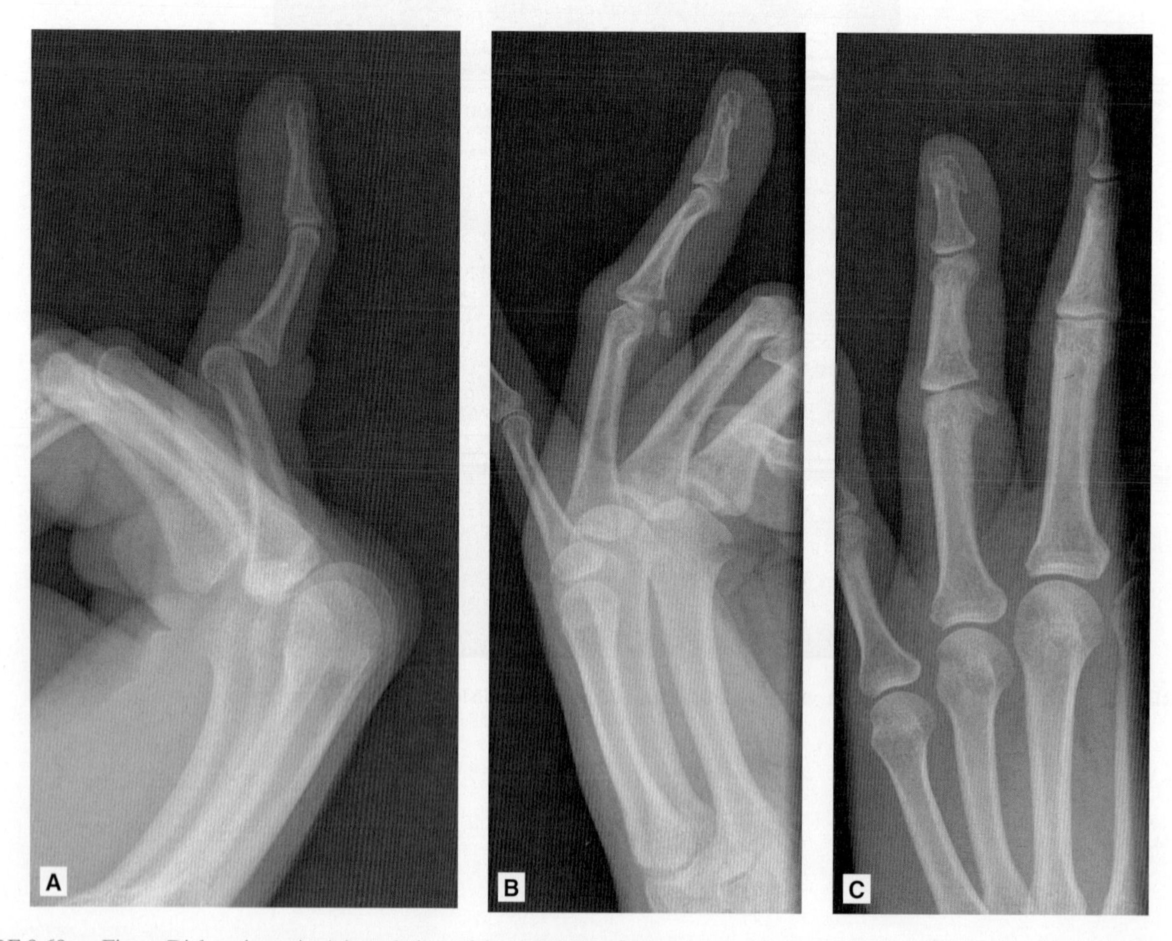

FIGURE 9.69 ■ Finger Dislocations. **A:** A lateral view of the right pinky finger demonstrates dorsal dislocation of the middle phalanx at the proximal interphalangeal joint. No fractures are evident. **B, C:** Oblique and lateral views of the left ring finger of a different patient show a large volar plate avulsion fracture from the base of its middle phalanx. These radiographs are obtained post reduction of the middle phalanx which had dislocated dorsally at the PIP joint.

Radiographic Summary

A deep vein thrombosis (DVT) is an inappropriate clot or thrombus within the deep veins of the upper extremity. They are most commonly due to central venous catheter placement and will embolize. Compressive ultrasound is the imaging modality of choice to assess for upper-extremity DVT. More proximal thrombi in the subclavian vessels may be difficult to assess under the clavicle and a CT venogram may be necessary to confirm or exclude the diagnosis.

Clinical Implications

The prevalence of upper-extremity deep venous thrombosis (DVT) has grown with the increased use of central venous catheters and pacemakers. Patients typically present with swelling and pain. Compressive ultrasound is the initial study of choice, however, CT venogram may be required for definitive diagnosis and remains the gold standard. Pulmonary embolism is less common with upper-extremity DVT, but treatment is similar to lower extremity DVT with 3 months of warfarin therapy.

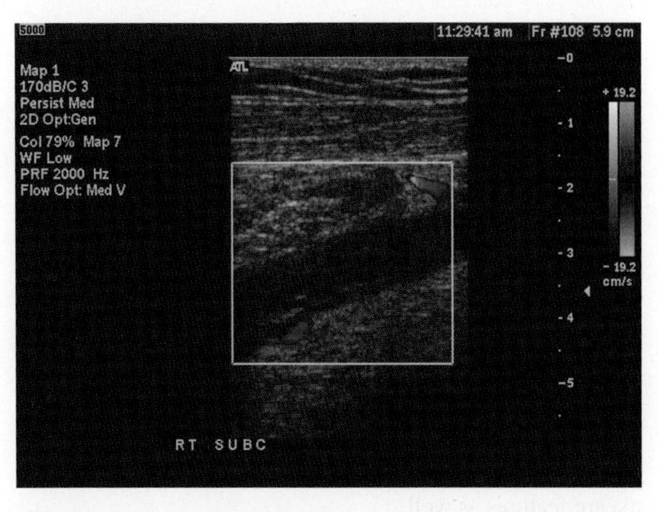

FIGURE 9.70 ■ Subclavian Vein Thrombosis. A single long axis image along the right subclavian vein with Doppler shows no flow within the vein. Echogenic material is present within the subclavian vein. The findings are consistent with subclavian vein thrombosis.

Pearls

1. Effort thrombosis should be suspected in baseball pitchers and overhead athletes who present with arm pain and swelling. The axillosubclavian vein and artery course through a tunnel formed by the first rib, clavicle, and scalene muscles. Repetitive motion can lead to arterial compression and/or DVT. Definitive treatment may require resection of the first rib and vascular surgery should be consulted.
2. In suspected cases of upper-extremity DVT, ultrasound should be performed first. If the ultrasound is negative, CT venogram should be obtained if suspicion remains high.

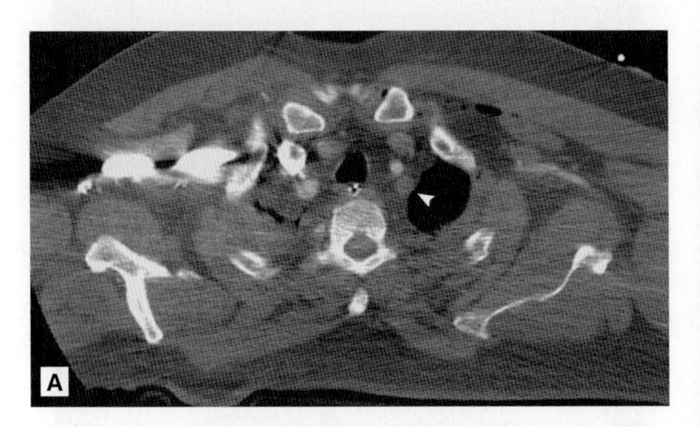

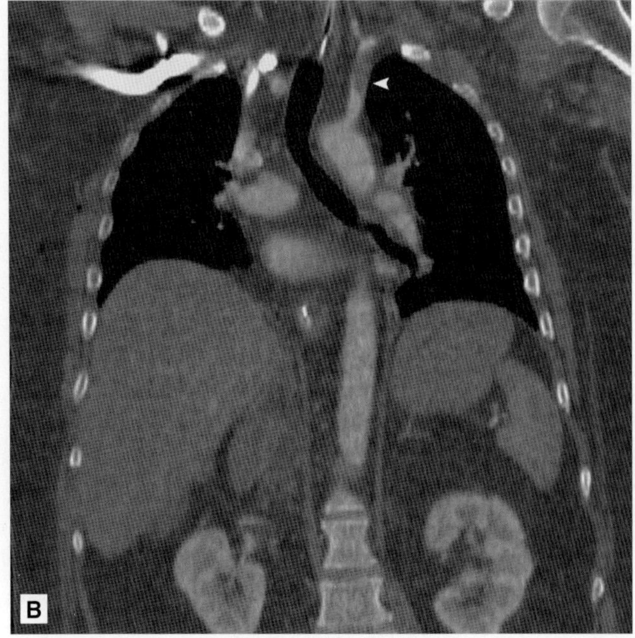

FIGURE 9.71 ■ Subclavian Artery Thrombosis. **A, B:** Axial and coronally reformatted CT images with IV contrast show a filling defect within the proximal left subclavian artery consistent with thrombosis (arrowheads).

Radiographic Summary

Arthritis, in the broadest sense, is a disease of a joint causing pain. There are two main categories of arthritis: degenerative and inflammatory. Degenerative arthritis (osteoarthritis) causes nonuniform joint space narrowing, subchondral sclerosis, subchondral cyst formation, and marginal osteophyte formation; focal cartilage defects, loose osteochondral bodies, joint effusions, and fibrocartilagenous degeneration may be present as well. Inflammatory arthritis (e.g., rheumatoid arthritis) is characterized by the uniform destruction of the hyaline cartilage and, therefore, the joint space; periarticular erosions, joint effusions, synovitis, and periarticular osteopenia are features as well.

Clinical Implications

There are over 100 different types of arthritis including osteoarthritis, rheumatoid arthritis, psoariatic arthritis, septic arthritis, and gout to name a few. Treatment varies depending on the type of arthritis and is aimed at decreasing the inflammation and providing pain relief. Osteoarthritis is the most common type of arthritis resulting from chronic "wear and tear" of joints or as a result of prior trauma. Rheumatoid arthritis is an autoimmune disorder that occurs in younger patients and symmetrically affects fingers, wrists, knees, and elbows. Septic arthritis is caused by an infection of the joint that requires prompt treatment to prevent permanent joint damage. Gout is caused by deposition of uric acid crystals in the joint causing inflammation. Pseudogout is caused by rhomboid-shaped crystals of calcium pyrophosphate dihydrate deposited within the cartilage and capsule of a joint. Certain types of arthritis can mimic each other clinically; for example, gout, pseudogout, and septic arthritis can be clinically indistinguishable at initial presentation. In such cases, arthrocentesis and analysis of synovial fluid are necessary to establish the diagnosis.

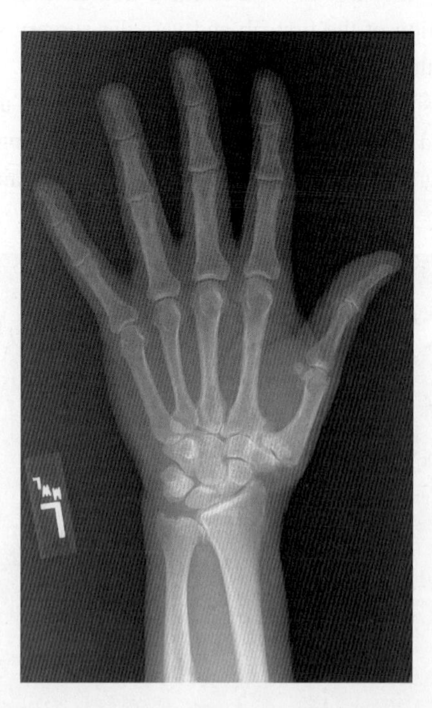

FIGURE 9.72 ■ Osteoarthritis. PA view of the hand shows severe nonuniform narrowing of the 1st carpo-metacarpal joint with subchondral sclerosis, marginal osteophyte formation, and loose osteochondral bodies. These are the features of osteoarthritis, severe in this joint. Similar but milder arthritic changes are present in the distal radio-ulnar joint and distal interphalangeal joint of the index finger.

Pearls

1. Rheumatoid arthritis affects younger patients with symmetrical involvement of multiple joints. Elevated ESR and rheumatoid factor are typically present.
2. Gouty crystals are strongly birefringent under polarized light and needle shaped.
3. Pseudogout crystals are weakly birefringent and rhomboid shaped.
4. Chondrocalcinosis (calcium pyrophosphate dihydrate) may be seen on radiographs and may aid in the diagnosis of pseudogout.

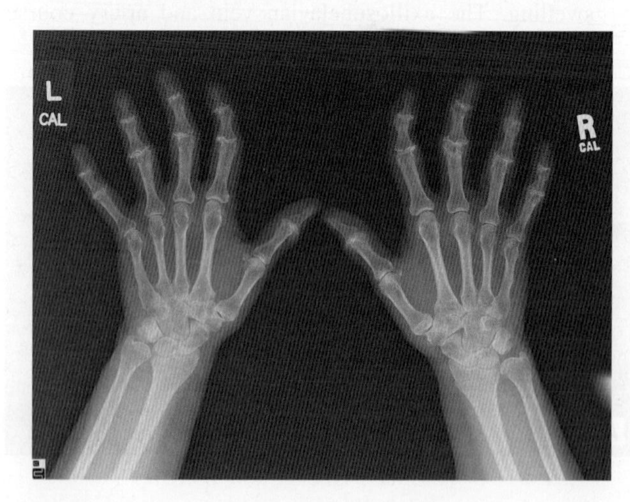

FIGURE 9.73 ■ Erosive Osteoarthritis. PA views of both hands demonstrate severe narrowing of all of the interphalangeal joints bilaterally and 1st carpo-metacarpal joints bilaterally. There is subchondral sclerosis and marginal osteophyte formation. The distribution is typical of osteoarthritis. Several of the interphalangeal joints, however, demonstrate central erosions with gull wing deformities; these are features of erosive osteoarthritis.

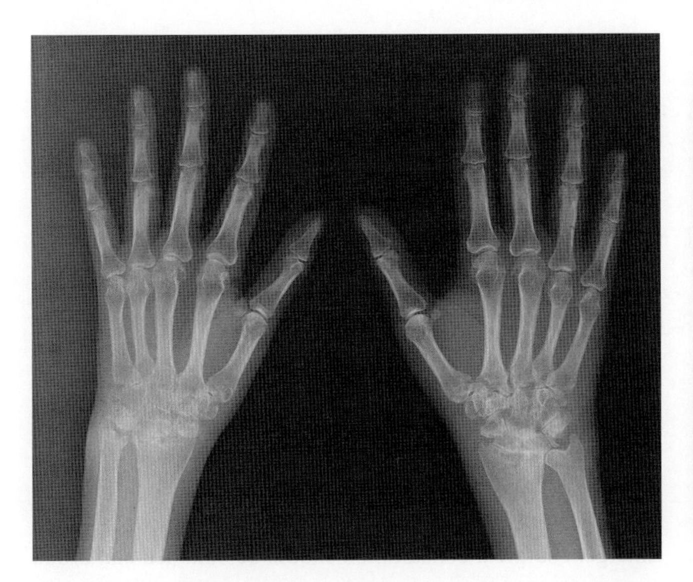

FIGURE 9.74 ■ Rheumatoid Arthritis. PA views of the hands show severe, uniform, bilateral, and symmetric narrowing of the carpal joint spaces. There are multiple large erosions in multiple carpal bones bilaterally, as well as within the second and third metacarpal heads bilaterally, distal radii bilaterally, and distal left ulna. The disease distribution, erosions, and pattern of joint destruction are consistent with rheumatoid arthritis. There is a suggestion of mild bilateral periarticular osteopenia.

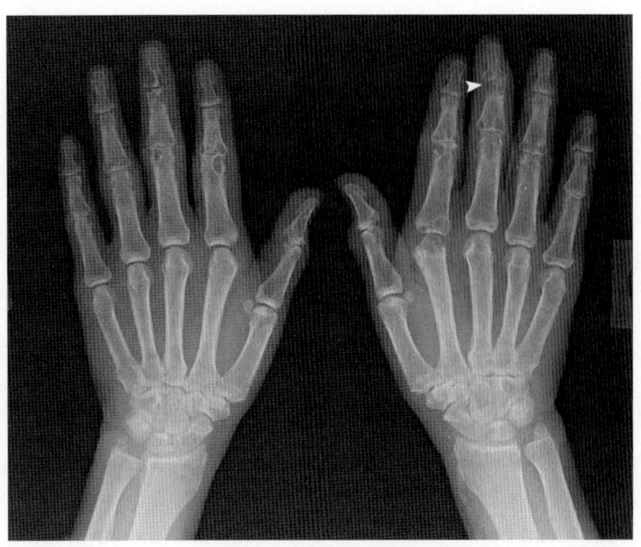

FIGURE 9.76 ■ Gout. PA views of the hands demonstrate multiple large cortical periarticular erosions about the interphalangeal joints of both hands and 2nd MCP joint of the right hand. The joint spaces are relatively preserved. Some of these erosions (arrowhead) have overhanging edges (head of the middle phalanx of the right middle finger). Soft tissue swelling is present about multiple joints. Carpal erosions are also present bilaterally but the carpal joint spaces are preserved.

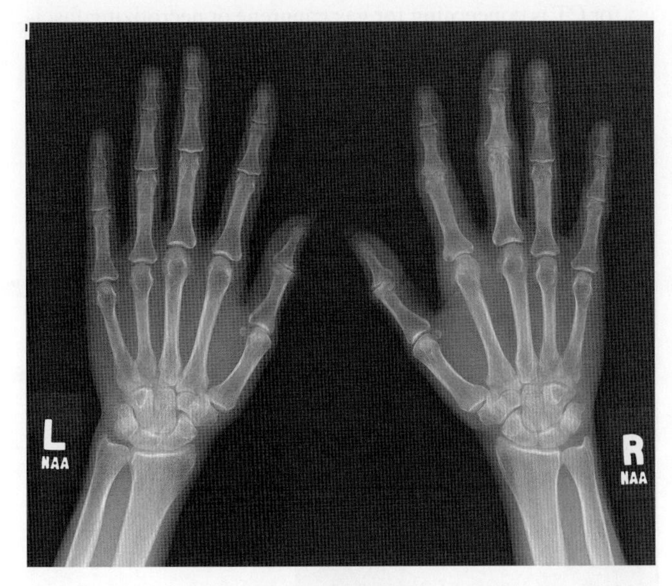

FIGURE 9.75 ■ Rheumatoid Arthritis (Companion Case). PA view of both hands. In this patient, there is a typical "bare area" erosion in the radial aspect of the base of the proximal phalanx of the right index finger. Smaller periarticular erosions are evident about the PIP joints of the right index and long fingers. There is associated mild uniform joint space narrowing and periarticular soft tissue swelling. Notice the lack of subchondral sclerosis or marginal osteophyte formation. These are the features of rheumatoid arthritis.

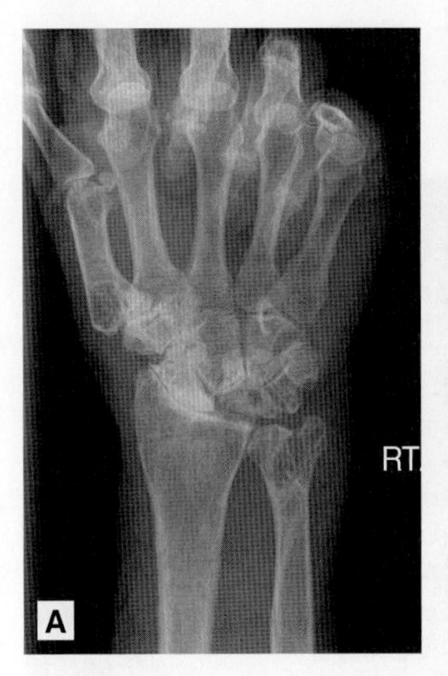

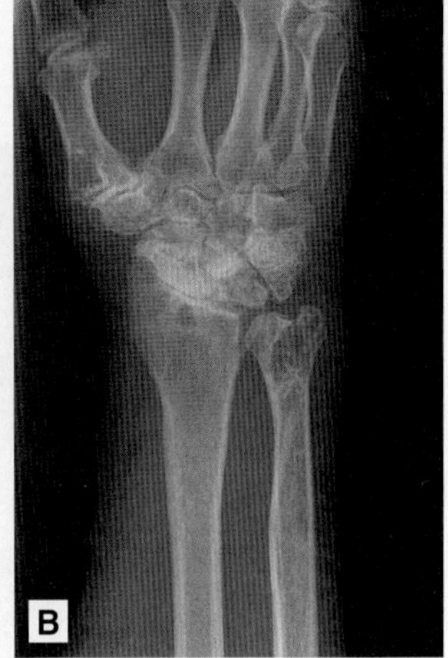

FIGURE 9.77 ■ SLAC Wrist. **A, B:** PA and oblique views of the right wrist show advanced degenerative changes in multiple carpal joint compartments but predominantly in the radio-carpal and luno-capitate articulations. Cysts or erosions are present in the distal ulna and radius and in several carpal bones. There is abnormal widening of the scapho-lunate interval attributable to scapholunate ligament tear. The capitate bone has migrated proximally. The findings represent scapho-lunate advanced collapse (SLAC wrist). SLAC wrist may be due to prior trauma, pyrophosphate arthritis, or rheumatoid arthritis.

Radiographic Summary

Imaging studies can be helpful in assessing infections of soft tissue and bone. Osteomyelitis is an infection of bone that can be due to hematogenous seeding, contiguous spread from soft tissue infections, or direct inoculation of the bone from trauma or surgery. Conventional radiographs may reveal soft tissue swelling, gas, osteolysis, cortical destruction, and periosteal new bone formation: these are features of acute or ongoing osteomyelitis. The changes are visible 7-10 days after the onset of infection. Acute osteomyelitis (the first few days after the onset of infection) are radiographically occult but may be detected with MRI. Features of chronic osteomyelitis include bony sclerosis and remodeling, a bony sequestrum (dead bone) within a bony involucrum (the enveloping bone), a sinus tract (cloaca), and a large chronic decubitus ulcer extending to the affected bone. CT with intravenous contrast can be helpful in assessing the soft tissue component of the infection, evaluate for soft tissue abscesses, as well as for the presence of gangrene. MRI is the most sensitive imaging modality and is superior to CT in evaluating the extent of infection. Tagged white blood cell scan is an option for patients who cannot undergo MRI or in cases where other processes (e.g., neuropathic arthritis) may mimic infection, limiting the specificity of MRI.

Clinical Implications

Osteomyelitis can be a difficult diagnosis to make. When radiographs are unremarkable, additional labs such as ESR, CRP, and total white blood cell count can be helpful in establishing the diagnosis. MRI can be confirmatory. Blood cultures should be obtained to assess for a blood-borne pathogen. Bone biopsies should be considered if blood cultures are unrevealing. Definitive treatment is antibiotics, and in some cases bone resection and amputation. MRI is particularly helpful in demonstrating the presence of any devitalized bone that would not respond to antibiotic therapy and would require debridement. When gas is noted within the soft tissues on radiographs or CT, necrotizing fasciitis should be considered. Emergent surgical consultation should be obtained and broad spectrum antibiotics should be administered.

Pearls

1. A high index of suspicion is necessary to diagnose osteomyelitis. Radiographs are normal in the first 7-10 days after the onset of infection. MRI is the imaging modality of choice in this early period.
2. The presence of gas within the soft tissues on radiographs or CT is concerning for gas gangrene or necrotizing fasciitis and necessitates emergent surgical consultation.

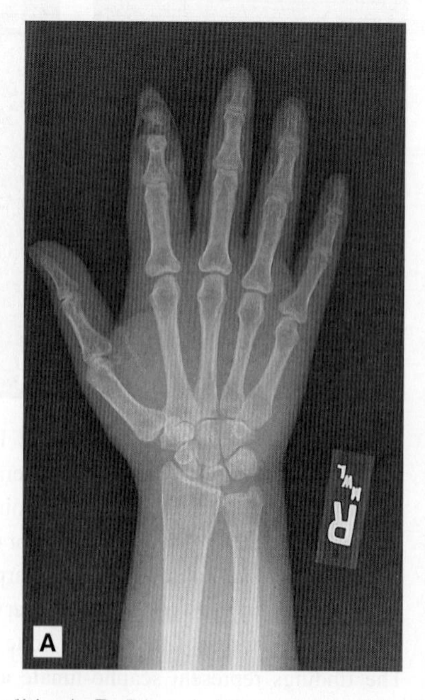

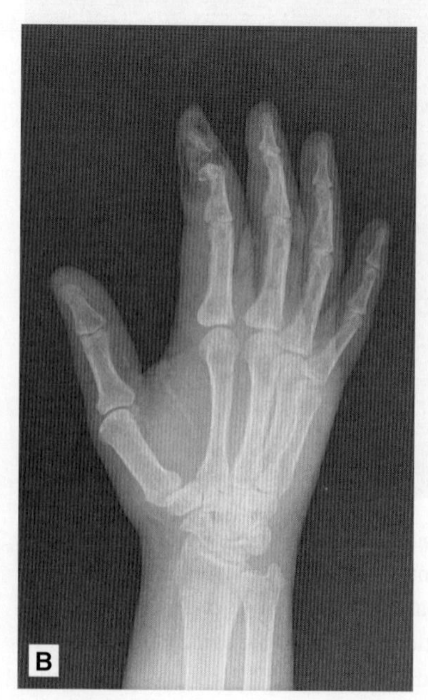

FIGURE 9.78 ■ Osteomyelitis. **A, B:** PA and oblique views of the right hand show advanced osteolysis of the distal phalanx of the index finger and extensive soft tissue swelling and gas around the destroyed phalanx. The findings represent a gangrenous digit with osteomyelitis.

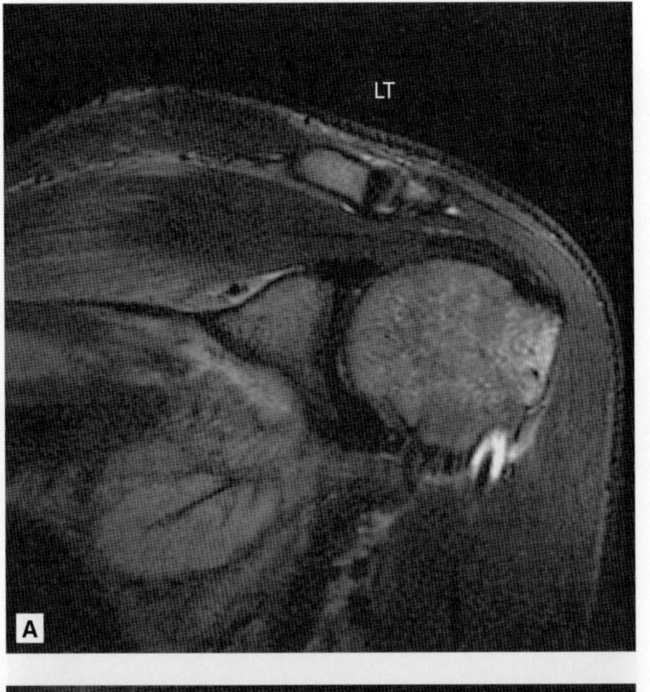

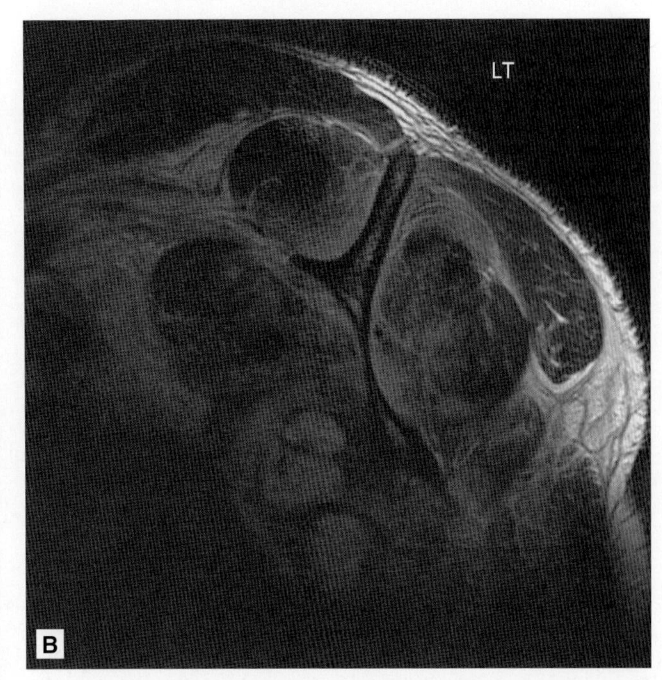

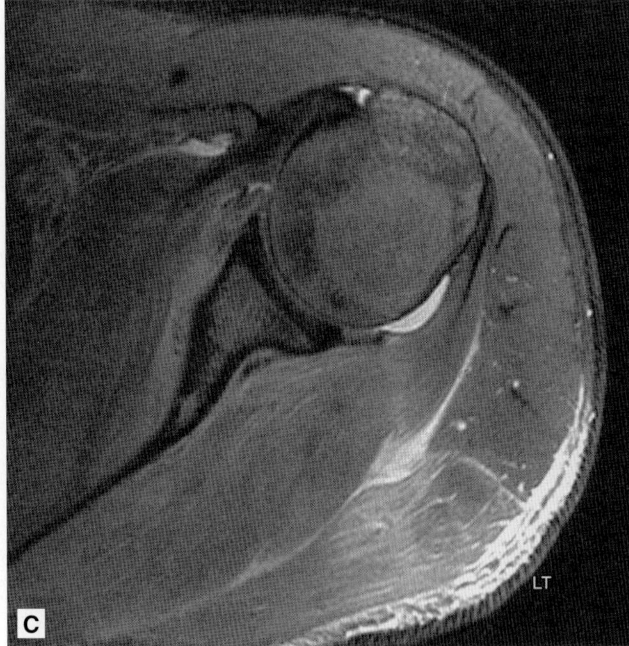

FIGURE 9.79 ■ Pyomyositis. **A-C:** Coronal T2-weighted, oblique sagittal T2-weighted, and axial FS PD-weighted images of the left shoulder show extensive edema within the muscles of the rotator cuff and large abscesses within the subscapularis muscle. This is a young adult who presented to the ER with acute MRSA pyomyositis. The patient had had a pustule on his skin approximately 3 weeks earlier which was treated with oral antibiotics.

Radiographic Summary

Vascular injuries to the upper extremity can occur from blunt and penetrating trauma as well as from repetitive compressive forces. Doppler ultrasonography can be utilized to assess for arterial injuries. While conventional angiography remains the "gold standard," CT angiography has largely replaced conventional angiography as the initial diagnostic study of choice. CT angiography is fast, sensitive, and specific. The evaluation of terminal arterial branches (e.g., the digital arteries), may be limited, if there is motion artifact or the timing of the contrast bolus is suboptimal.

Clinical Implications

Arterial injuries should be suspected in patients presenting with the following: active hemorrhage, expanding hematoma, bruits, evidence of ischemia, and absent or diminished pulses. Depending upon the injury pattern, orthopedic and vascular surgery should be emergently consulted for stabilization. Penetrating trauma is the leading cause of upper-extremity arterial injuries with brachial artery involvement being the most common. Blunt trauma resulting in fractures is also a common cause of vascular injury; all displaced fractures and fracture-dislocations should be thoroughly assessed for associated neurovascular injuries.

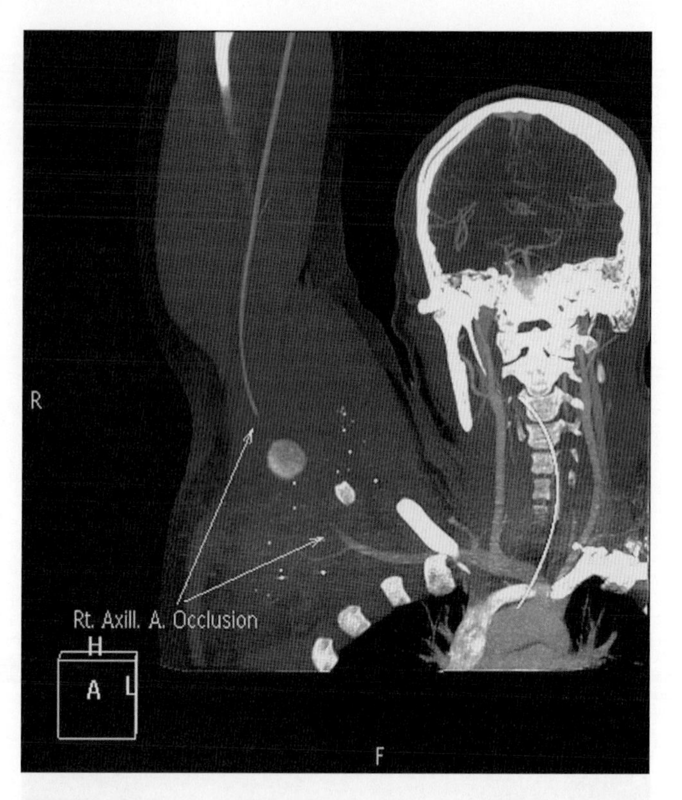

FIGURE 9.80 ■ Axillary Artery Injury. Coronally reformatted image from a contrast-enhanced CT scan shows ballistic transection of the right axillary artery. A long segment of the artery is occluded (arrows). The brachial artery reconstitutes via collaterals.

Pearls

1. Direct pressure should be the first step in management of arterial hemorrhage. Tourniquet use should be reserved for major amputations and mangled extremities and total tourniquet time should be minimized to prevent further tissue ischemia.
2. Hypothenar hammer syndrome results from repetitive palmar trauma leading to injury of the ulnar artery as it passes around the hook of the hamate bone. Patients will present with pallor and numbness of the 4th and 5th digits. CT angiography and vascular consultation are necessary for definitive management.
3. A palpable radial pulse does not exclude a proximal vascular injury.
4. The arterial pressure index (API) or arm–arm pressure index (A-A index) measured with a hand-held Doppler unit can be used to assess for vascular injury. The systolic pressure of the injured upper extremity divided by the noninjured upper extremity should be greater than 0.90. Values less than 0.90 should cause concern for occult arterial injury and additional evaluation is mandatory.

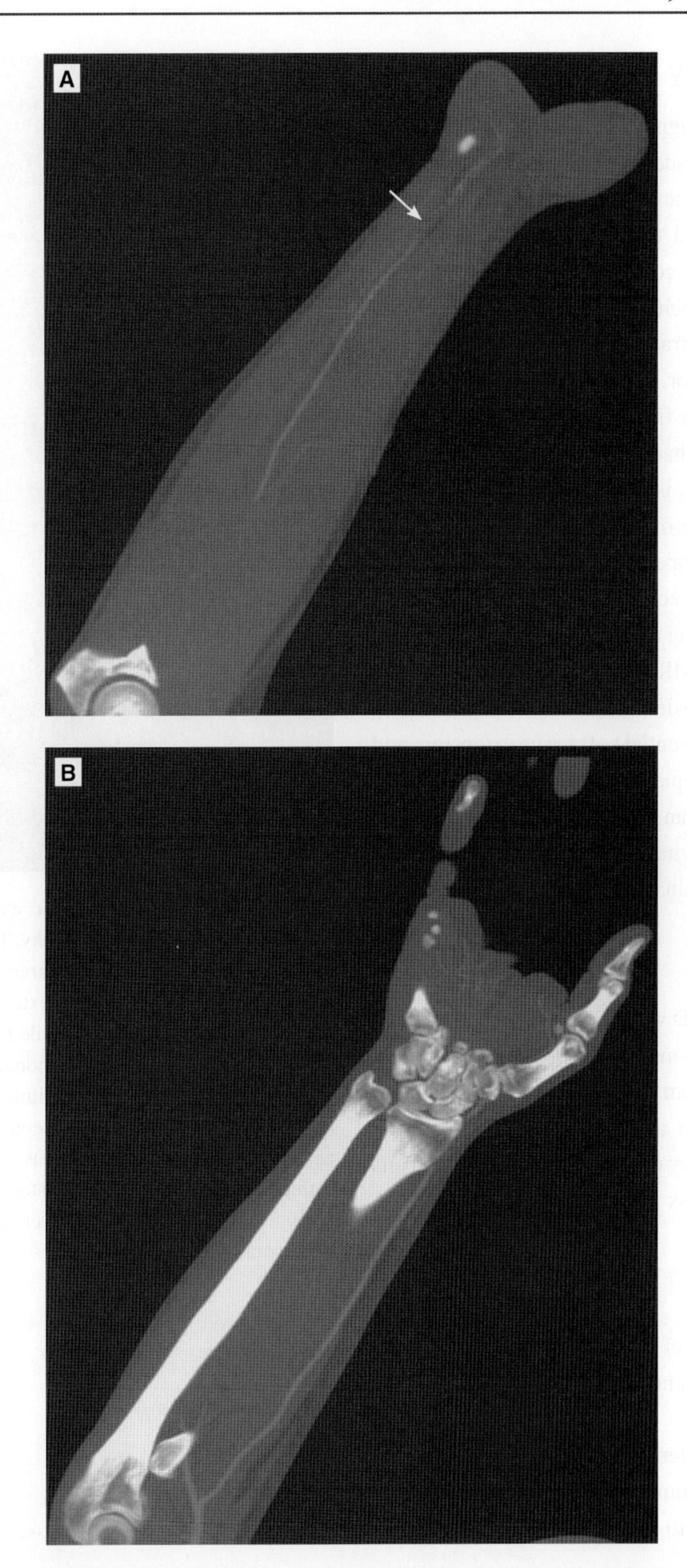

FIGURE 9.81 ■ Hypothenar Hammer Syndrome. **A, B:** Two coronally reformatted CT images from a CT angiogram of a forearm show occlusion of the distal ulnar artery at the level of the carpus (arrow). The radial artery is normal. The patient was a mechanic. These are the findings of hypothenar hammer syndrome.

Radiographic Summary

A variety of benign and malignant neoplasms may develop within the bones and soft tissues of the upper extremity. A detailed discussion and illustration of the entire spectrum of possible neoplasms is beyond the scope of this book. The Emergency physician should consider the possibility of an underlying neoplasm if the mechanism of injury does not adequately explain the resulting fracture (e.g., a long bone fracture resulting from only minor trauma). Radiographs of the injured bone would reveal the fracture and may demonstrate the underlying lesion. The characterization of the underlying bone neoplasm, if visible, is accomplished on the radiographs; the presence and type of a specific pattern of matrix calcification is critical. The appearance of most osseous neoplasms on MRI is rather nonspecific (T1 isointense to muscle, T2 hyperintense, and enhancing after intravenous Gadolinium administration). The role of MRI is to depict neoplasms that are radiographically occult, to define the exact size and extent of bone neoplasms and any potential soft tissue extension, and to characterize soft tissue neoplasms that are typically radiographically occult. MRI does an excellent job in depicting the relationship of the tumor to vital regional structures such as nerves and vessels, and is invaluable in preoperative planning.

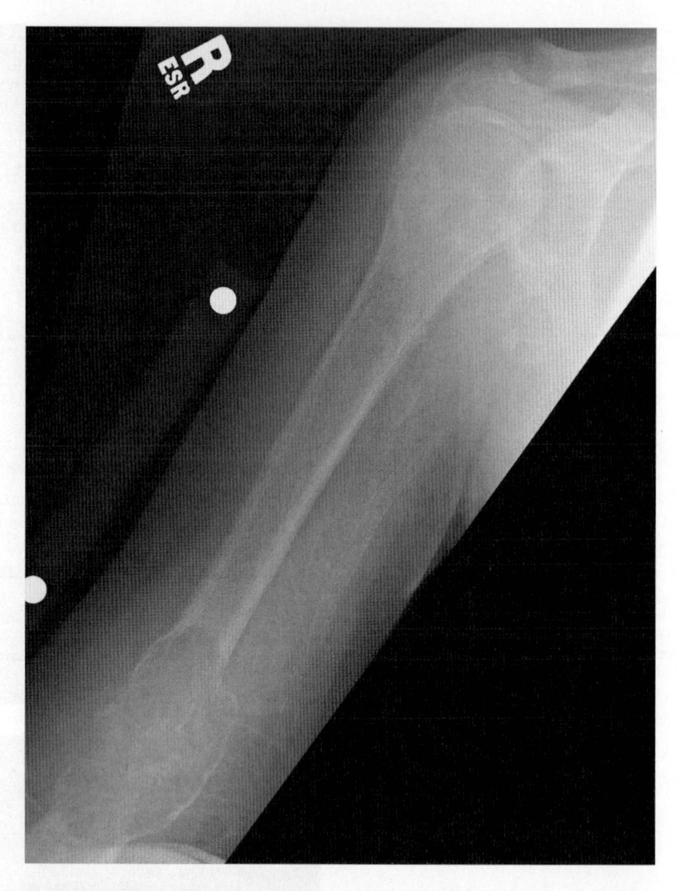

FIGURE 9.82 ■ Brown Tumor with a Pathologic Fracture in a Patient with Renal Osteodystrophy. The bones are diffusely osteopenic and have a "chalky" appearance. The distal right clavicle is partially resorbed. There are extensive vascular calcifications in the arm. There is a large expansile lytic lesion in the distal humeral shaft through which there is a nondisplaced pathologic fracture. A second lytic lesion is present within the glenoid. Although the differential diagnosis for lytic osseous lesions is broad and includes entities such as metastatic disease and multiple myeloma, in this patient with features of renal osteodystrophy, the best diagnosis is Brown tumors. Indeed, these were proven to be Brown tumors of hyperparathyroidism.

Clinical Implications

Patients may present to the ED with long bone fractures after minimal trauma. Soft tissue masses lead to regional mass effect and may cause pain from neurovascular impingement, central necrosis, erosion into a nearby bone or ulceration through the skin. Large primary or metastatic bone neoplasms place patients at significant risk for a pathologic fracture.

Pearls

1. Consider the possibility of a pathologic fracture if the mechanism of injury does not adequately account for the resulting fracture.
2. Bone tumors are characterized on conventional radiographs. MRI defines the tumor extent, soft tissue involvement, and relationship to the regional neurovascular structures.

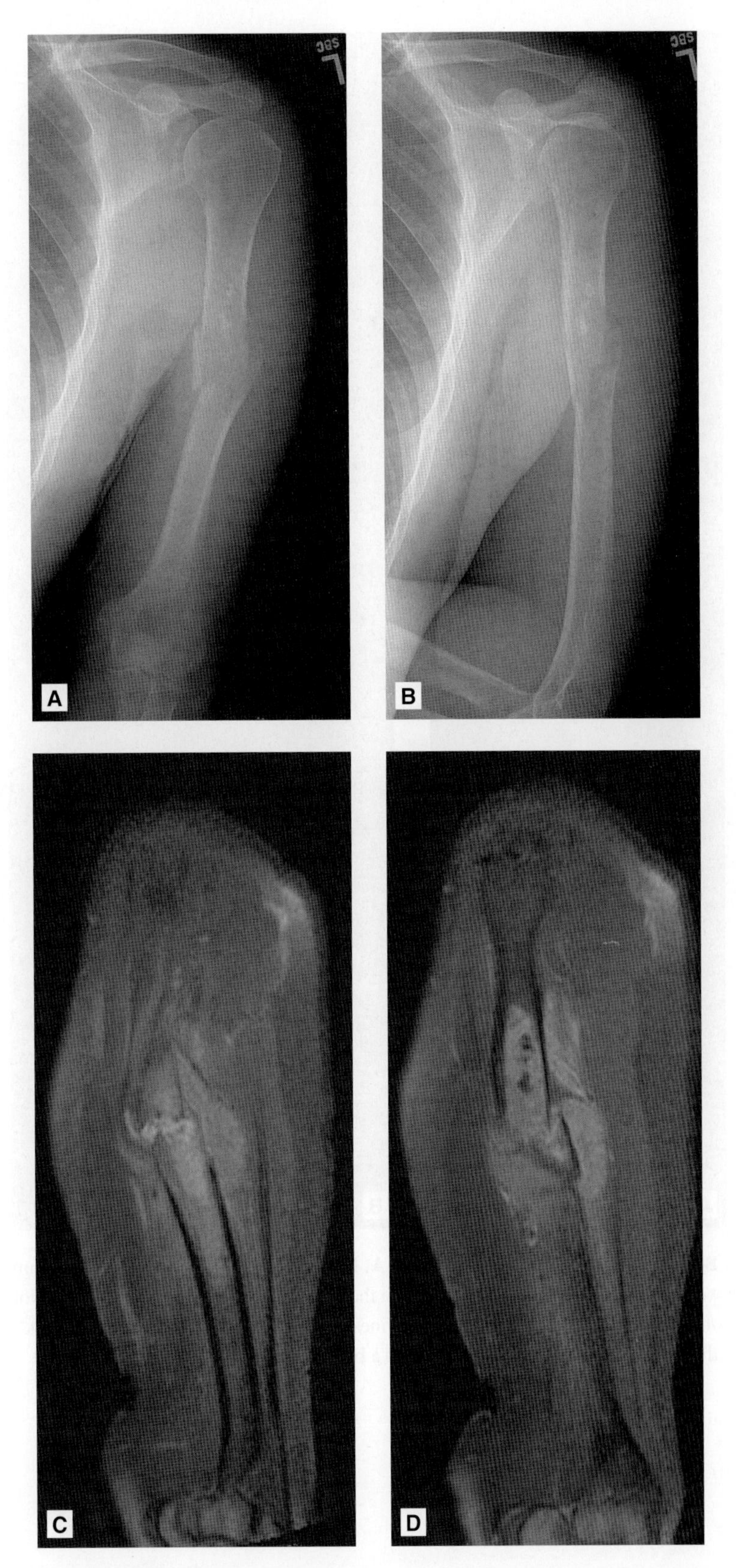

FIGURE 9.83 ■ Chondrosarcoma of the Humerus with a Pathologic Fracture. **A-D:** AP and lateral views of the left humerus show a pathologic fracture through an aggressive lytic lesion within the mid left humeral shaft. Two selected sagital MRI images (fat saturated T1 with IV Gadolinium) demonstrate a large underlying lesion, a proven chondrosarcoma.

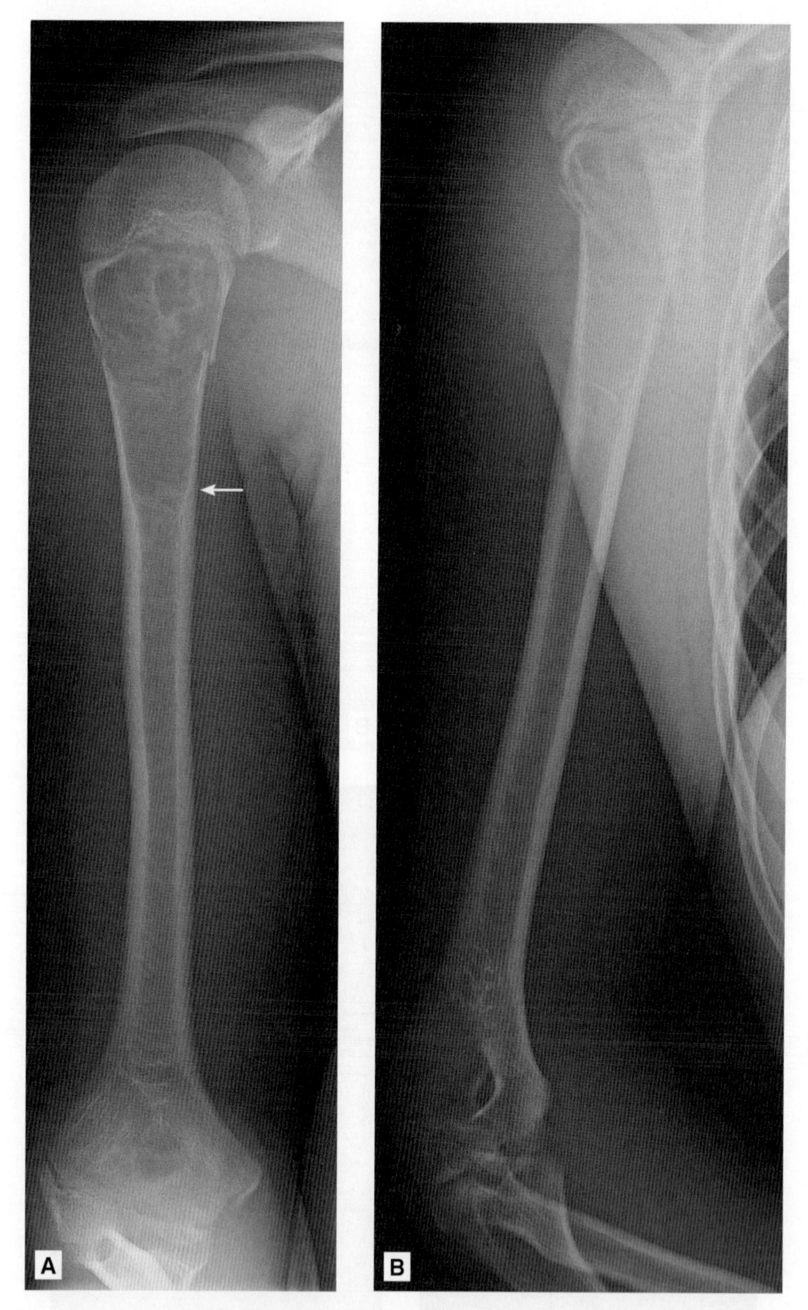

FIGURE 9.84 ■ Unicameral Bone Cyst with a Pathologic Fracture. **A, B:** AP and lateral views of the right humerus of a young child show a pathologic fracture through a well-defined, mildly expansile lesion in the proximal humeral diametaphysis. Notice the tiny "fallen fragment" within the dependent portion of the lesion (arrow); this fragment defines the lesion as a unicameral bone cyst. A unicameral bone cyst is the only truly hollow bone lesion that would allow such displacement of a bone fragment within the lesion.

Chapter 10

LOWER EXTREMITY

Martin I. Jordanov
James F. Fiechtl

Radiographic Summary

Radiographs of the pelvis are sufficient to demonstrate a hip dislocation. Hips can dislocate posteriorly, anteriorly, or inferiorly. With posterior dislocation, the femoral head migrates posteriorly and superiorly and partially projects over the acetabular roof on an AP view of the pelvis. Anterior dislocations, conversely, result in anteroinferior migration of the femoral head. Radiographs can also show associated injuries of the acetabulum and femoral head. CT scan (preferably after reduction) can better define the injury, evaluate for associated fractures, ensure the congruity of the joint, and assess for retained intra-articular fragments.

Clinical Implications

Hip dislocations require a significant amount of force to occur. These patients should be treated as trauma patients and quickly evaluated for other injuries. The most common direction of dislocation is posterior (90%), followed by anterior (approximately 10%) and inferior (much less than 1%). Visual inspection of the patient will reveal a leg that is internally rotated, shortened, and adducted with a posterior dislocation. Patients with an anterior dislocation will have more subtle changes of slight external rotation and abduction. Physical exam should also include a thorough neurovascular exam to ensure distal blood flow and sciatic nerve function. Treatment is reduction (preferably within 6 hours) to reduce the likelihood of avascular necrosis of the femoral head.

Pearls

1. Hip dislocations are caused by a significant amount of force; evaluate the patient for life-threatening concomitant injuries.
2. The most common hip dislocation is posterior.
3. Hips should be reduced within 6 hours to reduce the likelihood of avascular necrosis of the femoral head.

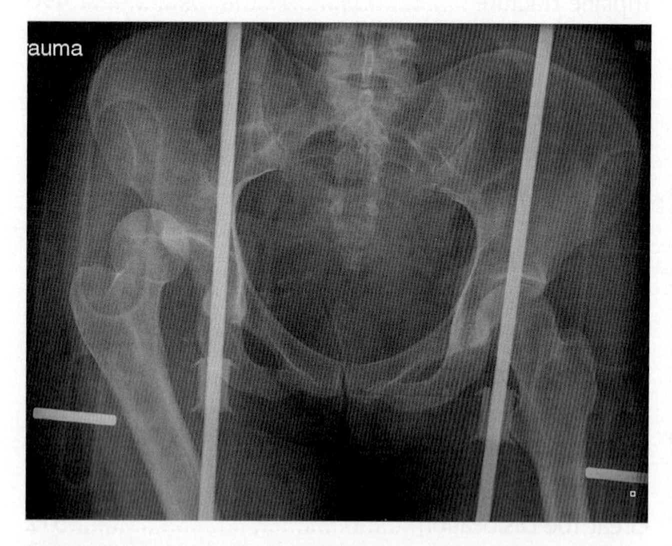

FIGURE 10.1 ■ Posterior Hip Dislocation. An AP view of the pelvis shows posterior dislocation of the right femoral head. The right lower extremity is shortened, markedly internally rotated, and adducted (the classic "shy girl" configuration seen with posterior dislocation of the hip).

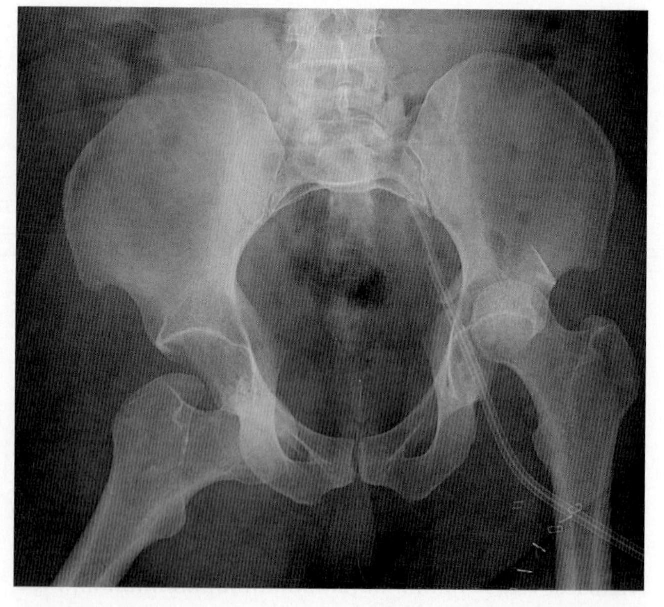

FIGURE 10.2 ■ Hip Dislocation. AP view of the pelvis demonstrates posterior dislocation of the left hip joint and anterior dislocation of the right hip joint. There is also a fracture of the left posterior acetabular wall.

Radiographic Summary

Plain radiographs can usually identify a femoral neck fracture, which is almost always associated with a hip dislocation. CT scan can be used to better define the fracture and evaluate for associated fractures. Subtle fractures may only be visible on CT.

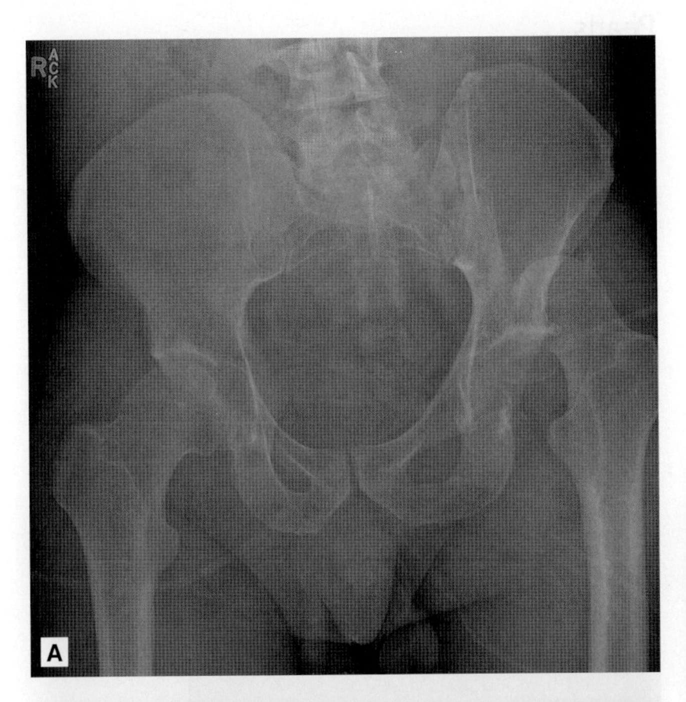

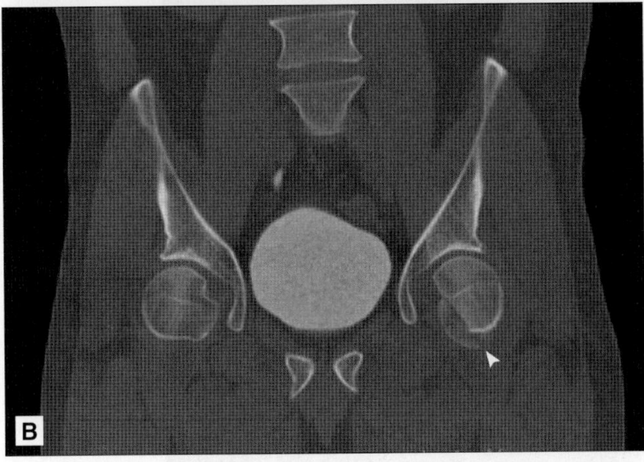

FIGURE 10.3 ■ Femoral Head Fracture—Pipkin Type I. **A, B:** AP view of the pelvis and a coronally-reformatted CT image of the pelvis of the same patient show a Pipkin type I fracture of the left femoral head (arrowhead). The fracture plane is distal to the fovea. On the radiograph (image A), the left femoral head is posteriorly dislocated while the Pipkin fracture fragment is rotated and resides within the empty acetabular fossa.

Clinical Implications

Femoral head fractures have an incidence of approximately 10% with hip dislocations. These fractures are classified based on the fracture location in relation to the fovea of the femoral head and associated injuries. The classification system is called the Pipkin system. For the emergency physician, the presence of a femoral head fracture is not a contraindication to hip reduction; however, it may make the reduction more difficult. The treatment of these fractures is predominately operative unless the fragment is nondisplaced and stable.

Pearls

1. Femoral head fractures occur with hip dislocations.
2. The presence of a Pipkin fracture is not a contraindication to hip reduction; however, it may make the reduction more difficult.

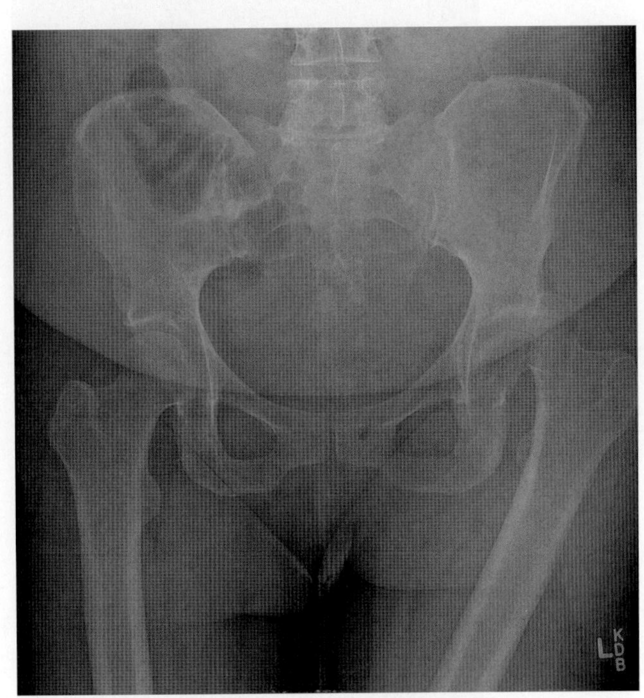

FIGURE 10.4 ■ Femoral Head Fracture—Pipkin Type II. An AP view of the pelvis shows a large Pipkin fracture on the left extending proximal to the fovea: this is a Pipkin type II fracture. The left femoral head is posteriorly dislocated while the large Pipkin fracture fragment resides within the empty acetabulum.

Radiographic Summary

A subchondral fracture of the femoral head occurs as an insufficiency or fatigue fracture. Initial radiographs are often normal, but as the disease progresses, flattening of the femoral head or a sclerotic subchondral line can be seen on radiographs. An MRI is the imaging modality of choice for initial evaluation and can demonstrate the fracture, any associated marrow edema, and the degree of subchondral collapse, if any.

Clinical Implications

A subchondral fracture of the femoral head is an infrequent cause of atraumatic hip pain. These are typically insufficiency fractures (stress fractures that occur in abnormal, demineralized bones due to physiologic, everyday stresses). These patients are generally older and do not have the common risk factors for osteonecrosis, such as smoking, alcohol abuse, trauma, or steroid use. Nondisplaced fractures heal spontaneously. Fractures that result in subchondral collapse may eventually require a total hip arthroplasty.

Pearls

1. Include in the differential diagnosis for older patients that present with sudden-onset, progressively worsening atraumatic hip pain.
2. These patients do not have the common risk factors for osteonecrosis.

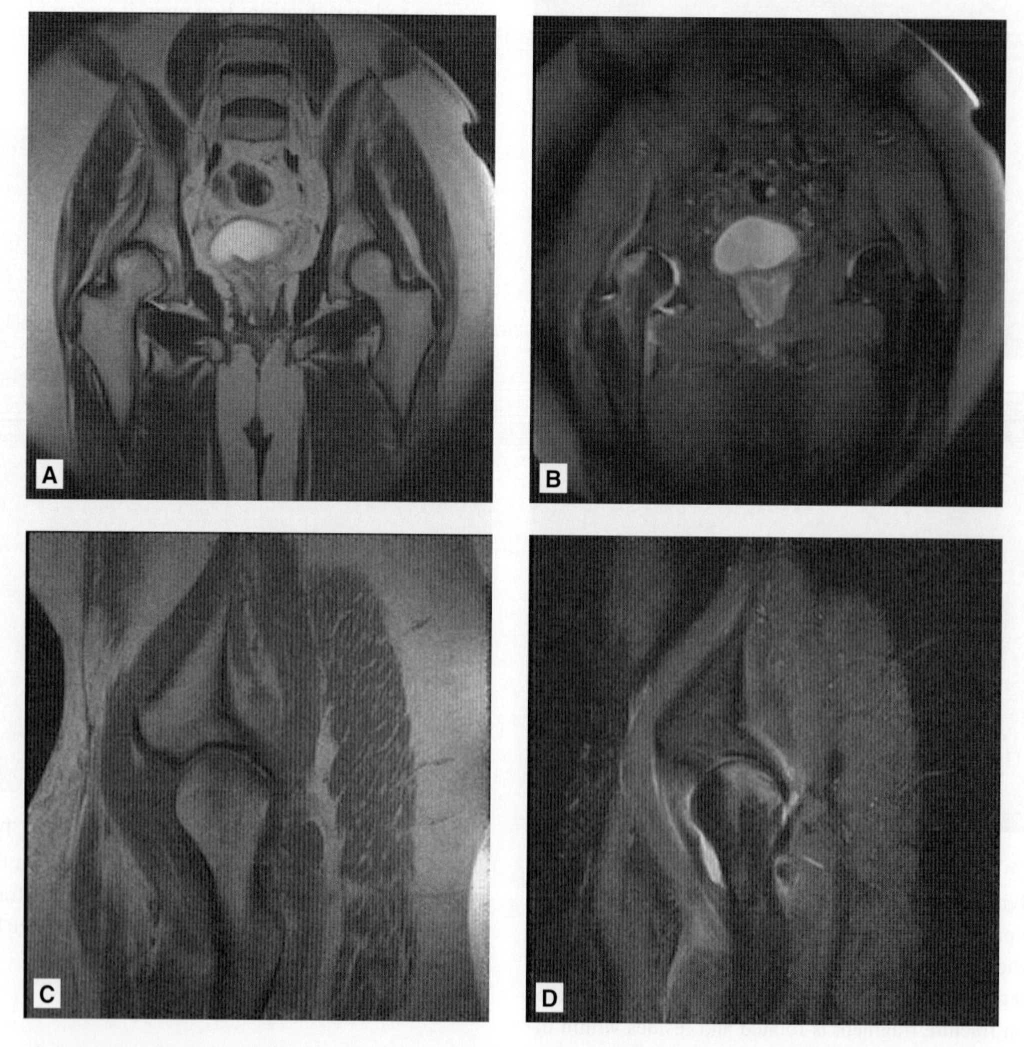

FIGURE 10.5 ■ Subchondral Fracture. **A-D:** Coronal T1 and FS T2-weighted images of the pelvis and sagital T1 and FS T2-weighted images of the right hip show marrow edema in the superior aspect of the right femoral head. A faint T1 and T2 hypointense line parallels the superoposterior articular surface. The findings are consistent with a subchondral fracture. There is no subchondral collapse.

Radiographic Summary

Radiographs are sufficient to demonstrate even minimally displaced fractures through the femoral neck. Radiographs obtained with gentle axial traction may be required to differentiate between a femoral neck fracture and a basicervical fracture.

Clinical Implications

These patients present with groin pain and an inability to ambulate. The leg may be foreshortened depending on the amount of displacement. Treatment involves pain control and subsequent surgical treatment with screws, hemiarthroplasty, or total hip arthroplasty. Traction has been shown to be ineffective with these fractures. Several classification schemes are used to describe these fractures, but no single one has been shown to be clinically relevant.

Pearls

1. If the patient is unable to perform a straight leg raise, defer range of motion testing until the radiographs are obtained (the goal is to avoid displacing a nondisplaced fracture).
2. Traction radiographs can help differentiate between a femoral neck fracture and a basicervical femoral neck fracture (the two require different treatments).

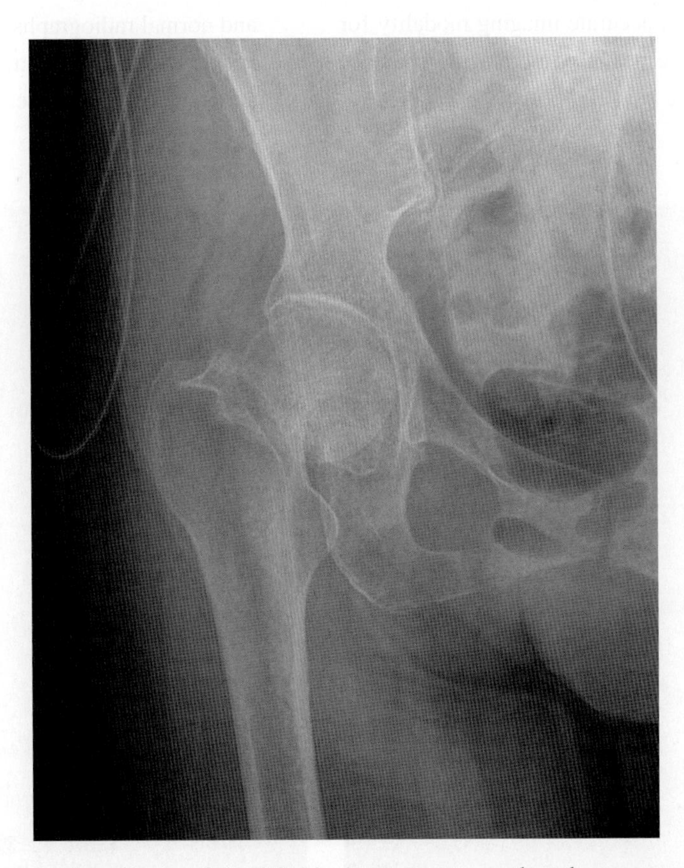

FIGURE 10.6 ■ Femoral Neck Fracture. An AP view of the right hip demonstrates a moderately varus-angulated and impacted subcapital right femoral neck fracture.

Radiographic Summary

Initial radiographs may be normal. Disease progression creates subchondral sclerosis and cysts. With further progression, radiographs may show the crescent sign, which is due to compaction of the trabecular bone deep to the subchondral plate with rebound of the subchondral plate itself; this is a brief and transient phase. Eventually, the subchondral plate loses its ability to rebound into its normal spherical shape and permanent subchondral collapse occurs. Radiographs of chronic osteonecrosis also reveal serpiginous sclerotic lines forming geographic outlines within the superior aspect of the femoral head: these are the classic radiographic features of osteonecrosis. Radiographs during the end-stage of this disease reveal joint space narrowing and a deformed femoral head. An MRI is the most accurate imaging modality for femoral head osteonecrosis, especially in the acute phase of the disease when radiographs are still normal.

Clinical Implications

Femoral head osteonecrosis presents with insidious pain, predominately in the groin, in a younger subset of patients. This process occurs most commonly in patients aged 20 to 50 years. Patients may have an antalgic gait and will have pain with hip range of motion, especially internal rotation. Risk factors for osteonecrosis include trauma, corticosteroid use, alcohol abuse, smoking, HIV, and sickle cell disease among others. Treatment is based on the stage of disease, and ranges from activity/risk factor modification to total hip arthroplasty.

Pearls

1. Consider this diagnosis in a younger patient with hip pain and normal radiographs.
2. Risk factors include trauma, HIV, sickle cell disease, smoking, alcohol abuse, and chronic steroid use.

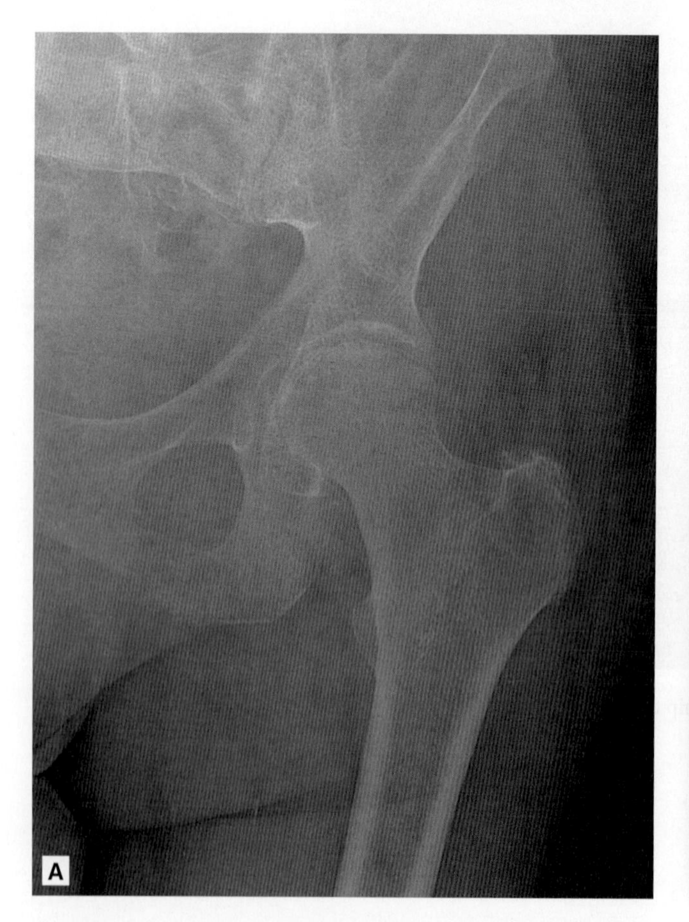

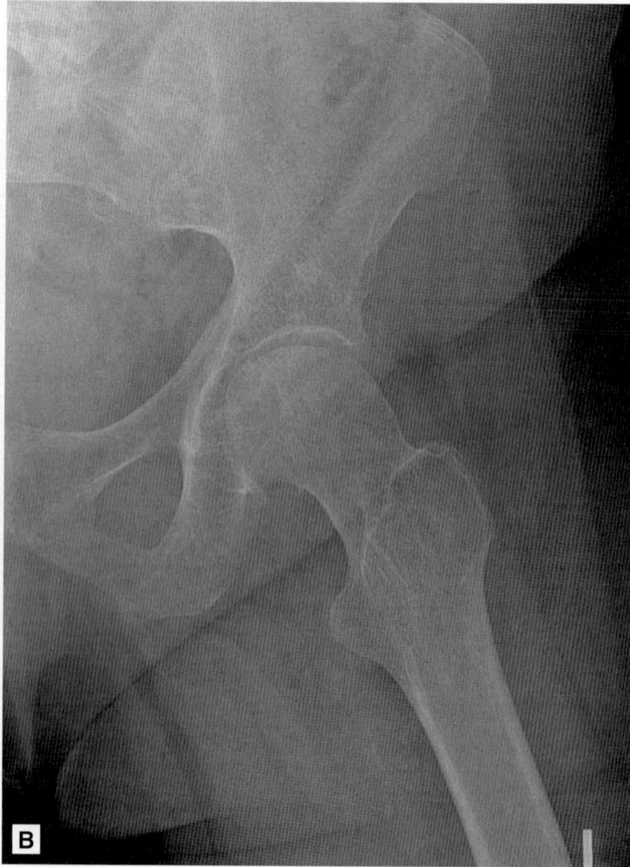

FIGURE 10.7 ■ Femoral Head Osteonecrosis. **A, B:** AP and frog leg lateral view of the left hip demonstrate a geographic area of sclerosis in the superior aspect of the left femoral head consistent with osteonecrosis. Both the AP and frog leg lateral view demonstrate some subchondral collapse of the superior aspect of the left femoral head.

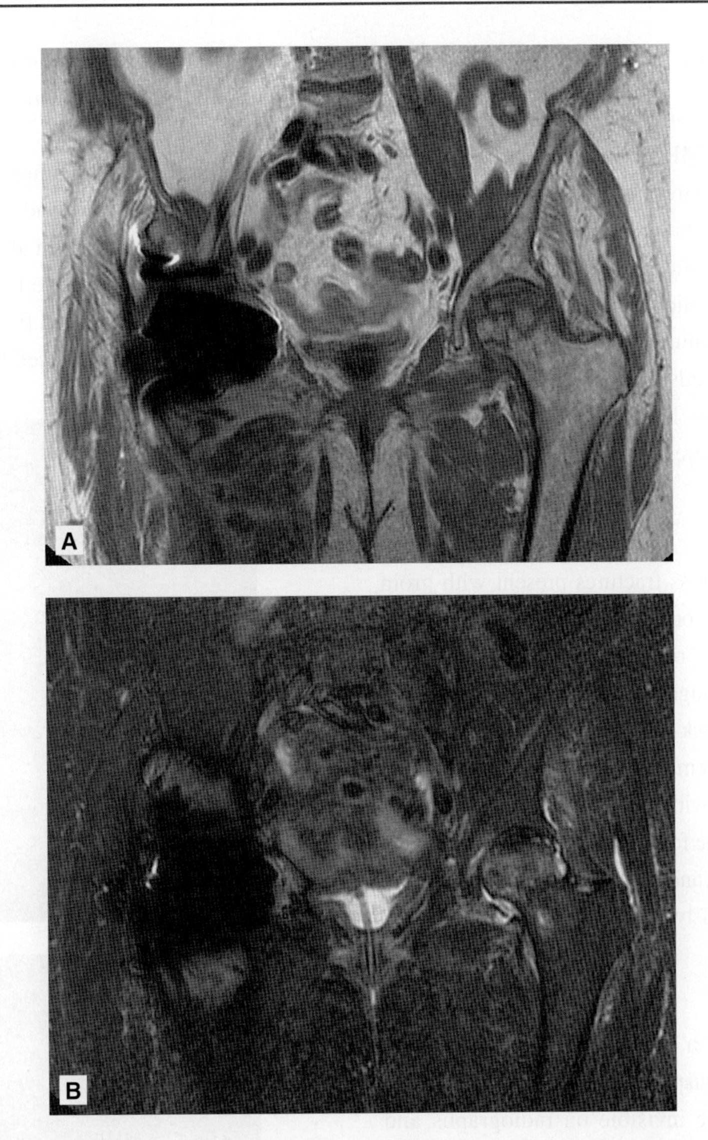

FIGURE 10.8 ■ Femoral Head Osteonecrosis. **A, B:** Coronal T1 and STIR images of the pelvis (same patient as in figure 10.7) show a serpigenous hypointense line forming a geographic area within the superior aspect of the left femoral head consistent with osteonecrosis. Minor subchondral collapse is evident on this study as well.

Radiographic Summary

Acute stress fractures are invisible on radiographs and CT; they can be detected with an MRI. In the days before MRI, a bone scan was used to detect stress fractures. Stress fractures can be detected on radiographs and CT 7-10 days after the injury as jagged, fuzzy sclerotic lines within the trabecular bone; in long tubular bones, solid periosteal new bone formation will be seen over the healing stress fracture at this later stage. The sclerosis corresponds to the fracture line demonstrable on MRI and represents healing. MRI is the study of choice when a femoral neck stress fracture is suspected.

Clinical Implications

Patients with femoral neck stress fractures present with groin pain, which can be either acute or insidious. On physical exam, they will have difficulty performing a straight leg raise. If they are able to perform a straight leg raise, testing hip range of motion will cause pain. Risk factors include osteoporosis, older/postmenopausal age, female, and corticosteroid use. Younger athletes can present with these stress fractures, especially when associated with the female athlete triad. Treatment is dependent on patient factors and includes fixation with femoral neck screws, hemiarthroplasty, or total hip arthroplasty.

Pearls

1. Making the diagnosis of a femoral neck stress fracture requires a high index of suspicion.
2. Acute stress fractures are invisible on radiographs and CT. For a fracture to be visible on these modalities, there must be cortical disruption. Therefore, CT does not add anything in the evaluation for an acute stress fracture and should not be obtained.
3. An MRI is the only imaging modality that can demonstrate an acute stress fracture and should be obtained if the index of suspicion remains high after normal radiographs.
4. An MRI can demonstrate the whole spectrum of injuries from normal to displaced fracture (normal-stress reaction-stress fracture-nondisplaced fracture, displaced fracture).

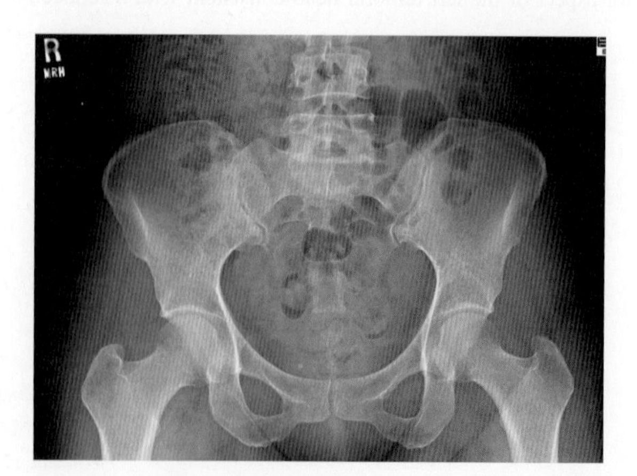

FIGURE 10.9 ■ Femoral Neck Stress Fracture. AP view of the pelvis demonstrates no osseous or articular abnormality. This patient presented with acute-onset right hip pain. There is no fracture. The joint spaces are normal.

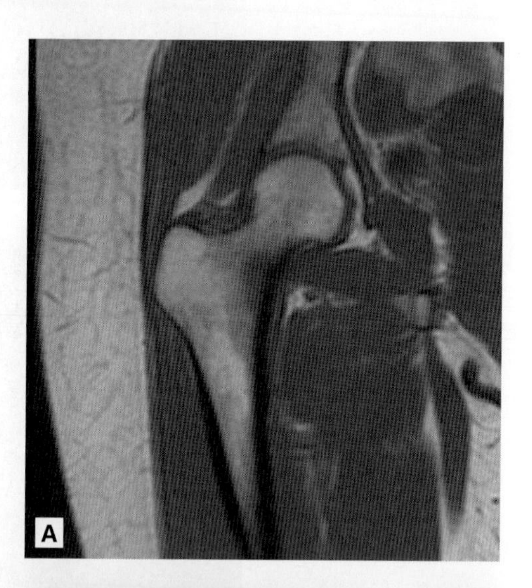

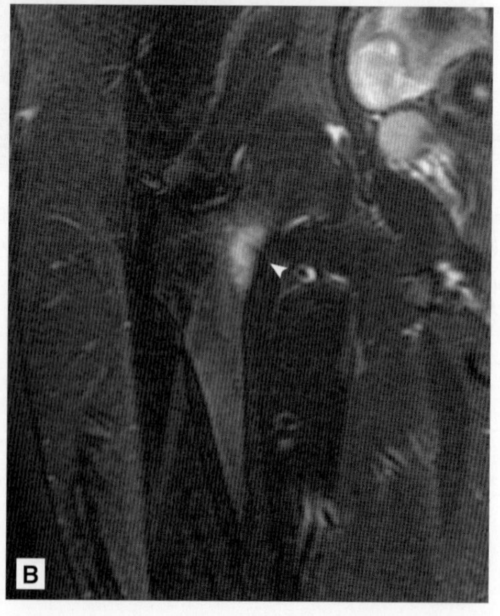

FIGURE 10.10 ■ Femoral Neck Stress Fracture. **A, B:** Coronal T1 and STIR images of the right hip (same patient as in figure 10.9) show an area of marrow edema within the medial aspect of the right femoral neck. In the middle of this area of edema and adjacent to the medial cortex, there is a thin T2 hypointense line, oriented perpendicular to the cortex of the femoral neck (arrowhead). The findings are consistent with an acute stress fracture.

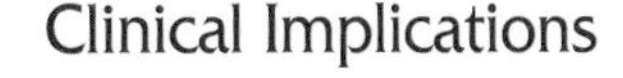

Radiographic Summary

Acute stress fractures of the pubic rami are radiographically occult. After 7-10 days, they become visible as sclerotic lines indicating healing. If these fractures become displaced, they become visible radiographically. Radiographs miss approximately 20% of subtle pubic rami fractures. An MRI is the only modality that can demonstrate acute stress fractures. Subtle, minimally displaced/nondisplaced fractures can be seen on CT.

Clinical Implications

Pubic rami stress fractures generally occur in elderly, osteoporotic patients. These patients present with pain localized to the rami. Treatment involves pain control and immobilization, but ramoplasty has been described.

Pearls

1. Though not nearly as common as femoral neck stress fractures, pubic rami stress fractures do occur.
2. An MRI should be obtained if the index of suspicion remains high after normal radiographs.

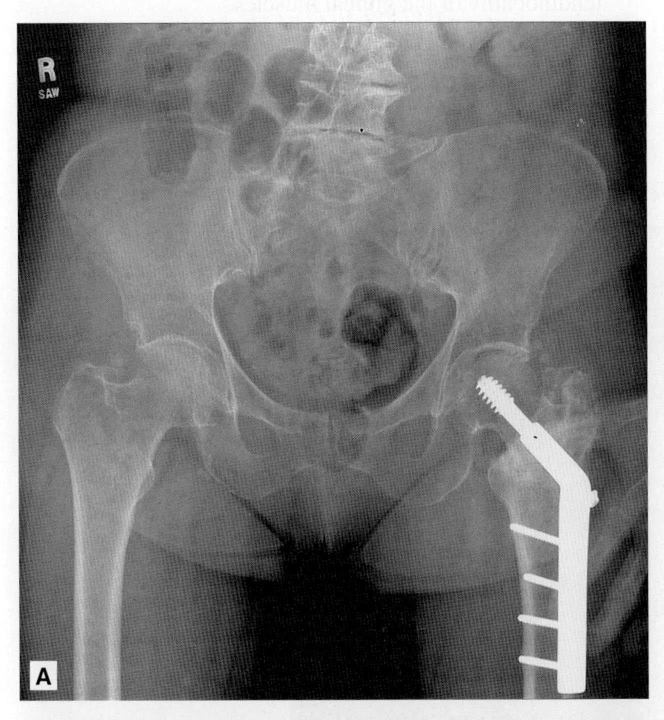

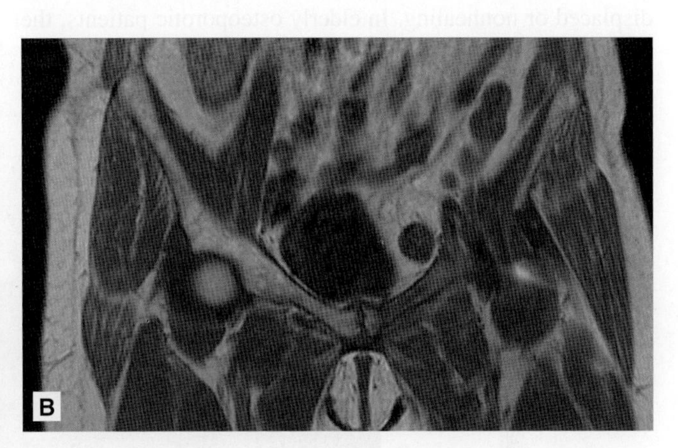

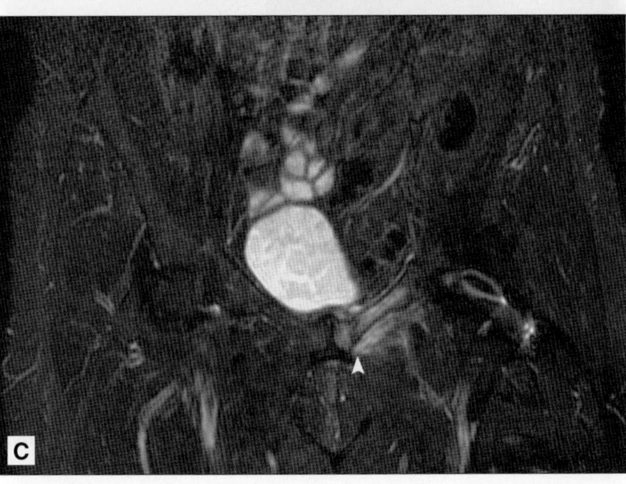

FIGURE 10.11 ■ Pubic Ramus Stress Fracture. **A:** AP view of the pelvis shows an old healed left intertrochanteric femoral fracture repaired with a dynamic hip screw. Mild osteoarthritic changes are present in the hip joints bilaterally and degenerative disk disease is evident in the lower lumbar spine. The bones are diffusely demineralized. There is no evidence of an acute fracture. There is no dislocation. **B, C:** Coronal T1 and STIR images of the pelvis through the superior pubic rami show a jagged T1 and T2 hypointense line through the left superior pubic ramus (arrowhead) surrounded by a large amount of marrow edema that fills most of the left superior pubic ramus. The findings represent a nondisplaced fracture of the left superior pubic ramus. Regional periosteal edema is present as well. Notice that while the metal of the left dynamic hip screw produces some regional susceptibility artifact, it does not preclude evaluation of the pubic rami.

Radiographic Summary

The anteroposterior pelvis radiograph is usually sufficient to demonstrate the injury. In elderly patients and those with osteoporosis, an MRI can be helpful to determine the presence of any intertrochanteric fracture extension.

Clinical Implications

These fractures predominately result from the forceful contraction of the hip abductors or a direct fall. Pain is generally localized to the greater trochanter area. Treatment of isolated greater trochanter fractures is conservative with operative intervention reserved for those fractures that are greatly displaced or nonhealing. In elderly osteoporotic patients, the possibility of intertrochanteric extension should be strongly considered because this changes the fracture category and markedly alters patient management. In these patients, the intertrochanteric extension is sometimes occult on radiographs but can be demonstrated on MRI or, sometimes, CT. In such cases, the visible, greater trochanter portion of the fracture is called "the tip of the iceberg" sign.

Pearls

1. With elderly or osteoporotic patients, consider an MRI to evaluate for intertrochanteric extension, as the treatments are vastly different.
2. It is important to differentiate this fracture from calcific tendinopathy of the gluteal muscles.

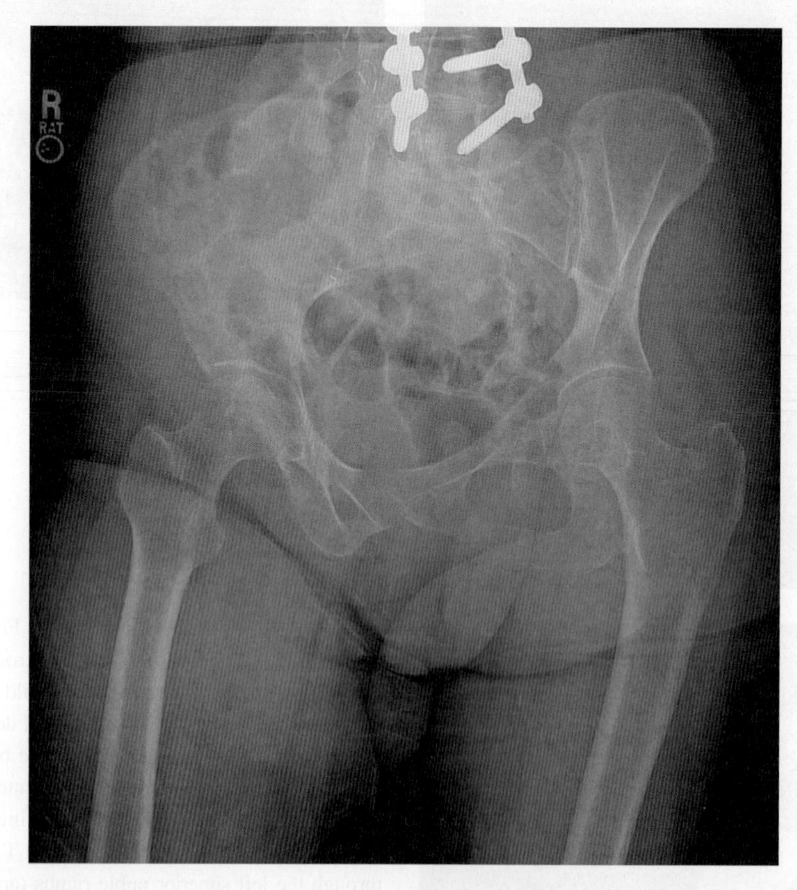

FIGURE 10.12 ■ Greater Trochanter Fracture. AP view of the pelvis shows a nondisplaced fracture of the left greater trochanter.

Radiographic Summary

The lesser trochanter can be evaluated with an anterior–posterior pelvis radiograph. Externally rotating the leg helps to evaluate the lesser trochanter. This is one of the classic pathologic avulsion fractures in adults (typically due to a metastasis at the base of the lesser trochanter). An MRI can be obtained to evaluate the extent of the fracture and to assess for an underlying lesion.

Clinical Implications

Lesser trochanter fractures are uncommon in adults and should be considered a pathological fracture until proven otherwise. These fractures cause pain either in the groin or in the posterior buttock worsened by resisted hip flexion. Treatment is usually conservative.

Pearls

1. In adults, these fractures are pathological until proven otherwise.
2. Lesser trochanter avulsion fracture is the least common avulsion fracture involving the pelvis (anterior superior iliac spine, anterior inferior iliac spine, and ischial tuberosity are all more common).

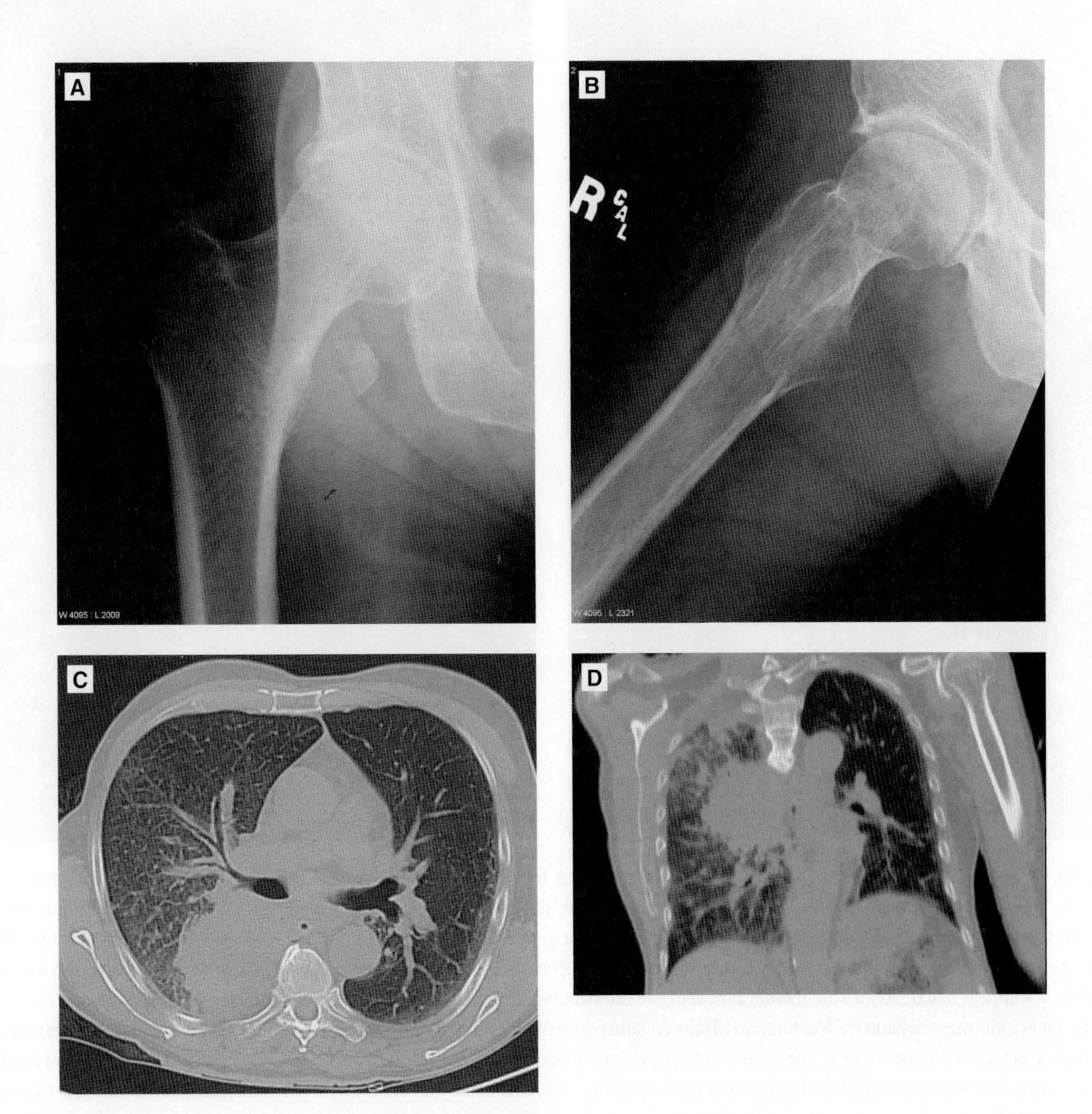

FIGURE 10.13 ■ Lesser Trochanter Avulsion Fracture. **A-D:** AP and frog leg lateral views of the right hip show an avulsion fracture of the lesser femoral trochanter. This is a classic pathologic avulsion fracture. Indeed, this patient had metastatic lung cancer. Selected axial and coronally-reformatted CT images of the chest show a very large mass in the superior segment of the right lower lobe.

Radiographic Summary

Intertrochanteric fractures by definition involve both trochanters. If there is a cortical break or any degree of displacement, the diagnosis can be established on conventional radiographs. In subtle cases, however, an MRI may be required to differentiate between an isolated trochanteric fracture and an intertrochanteric femoral fracture. Treatment options vary markedly between the two.

Clinical Implications

In younger patients, these fractures are the result of high energy impact and the patient should be evaluated for concomitant

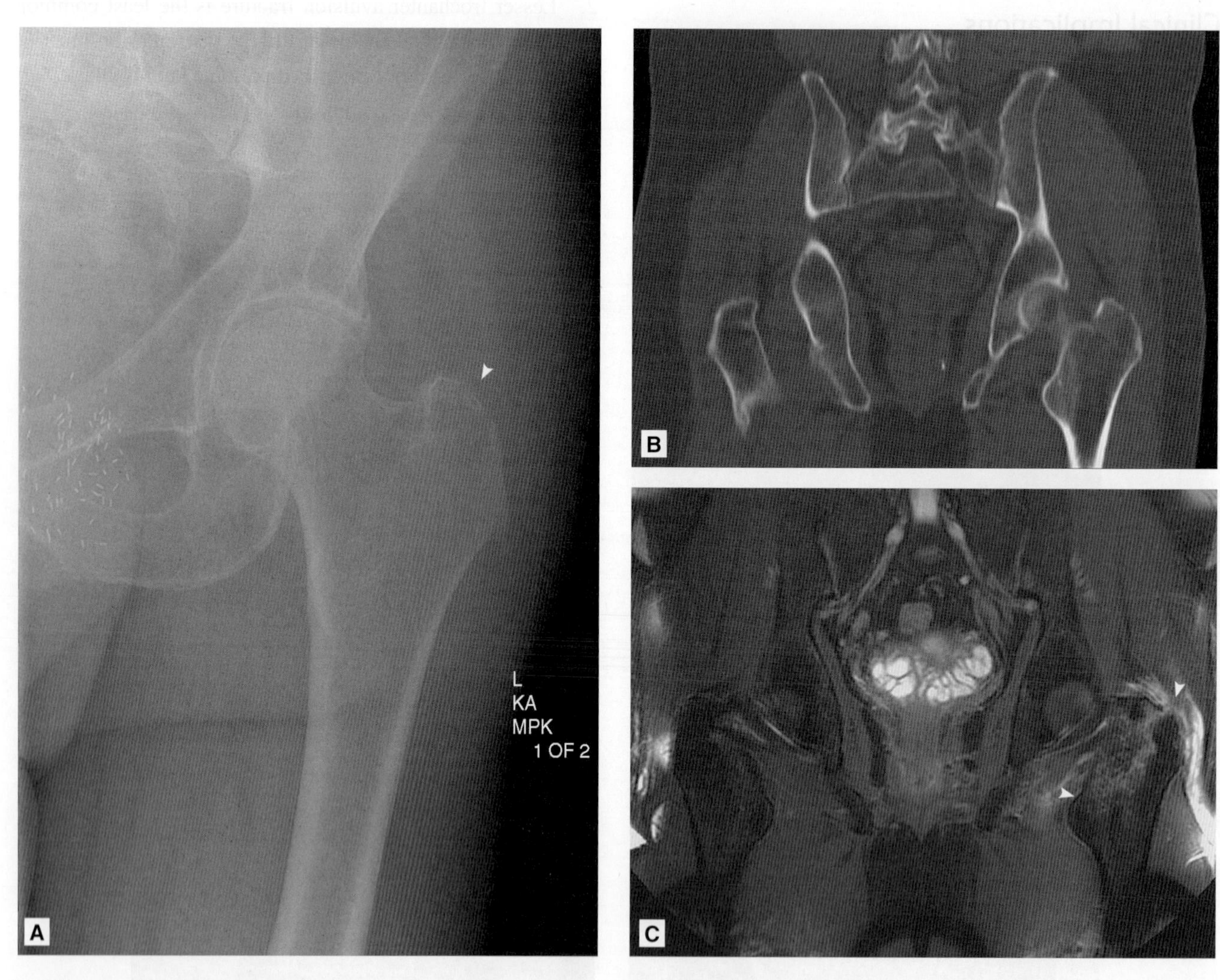

FIGURE 10.14 ■ Intertrochanteric Fracture. **A:** AP view of the left hip shows a nondisplaced fracture of the greater femoral trochanter (arrowhead). The fracture is seen extending through the lateral cortex of the femur. It is not clear, based on this conventional radiograph, how far medially the fracture extends. This could be an isolated fracture of the greater trochanter or a nondisplaced intertrochanteric fracture. **B:** A CT scan of the pelvis was obtained to evaluate the fracture further. This coronally reformatted image shows a fracture of the greater trochanter. The fracture does not appear to extend into the medial aspect of the intertrochanteric region. **C:** Because the orthopoedic surgeon was concerned that this may be an occult intertrochanteric fracture, an MRI was subsequently obtained for further evaluation. This coronal FS T2-weighted image demonstrates a jagged T2 hyperintense line extending all the way through the intertrochanteric portion of the left femur (arrowheads). The findings are consistent with a nondisplaced intertrochanteric fracture. An MRI is the best modality to demonstrate such a fracture. Conventional radiographs and CT can underestimate the extent of the fracture.

injuries. Conversely, the elderly can sustain this fracture from minor trauma. Nonetheless, elderly patients require careful evaluation for associated injuries as well. Intertrochanteric fractures require operative intervention, which should be performed within 24-48 hours of the injury.

Pearls

1. Look for additional injuries when you see this fracture.
2. An MRI can be used to determine intertrochanteric extension if the radiographs are equivocal.

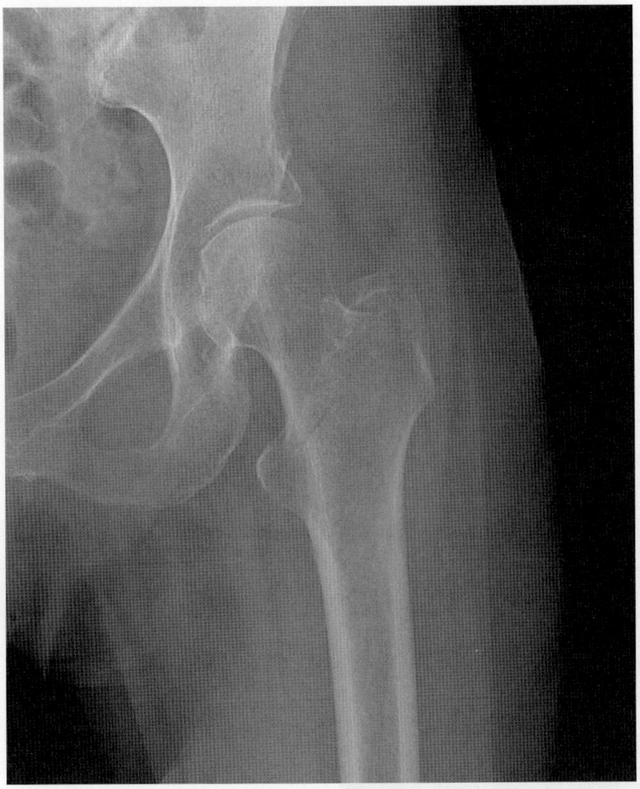

FIGURE 10.15 ■ Intertrochanteric Fracture (Companion Case). AP view of the left hip shows a nondisplaced intertrochanteric fracture.

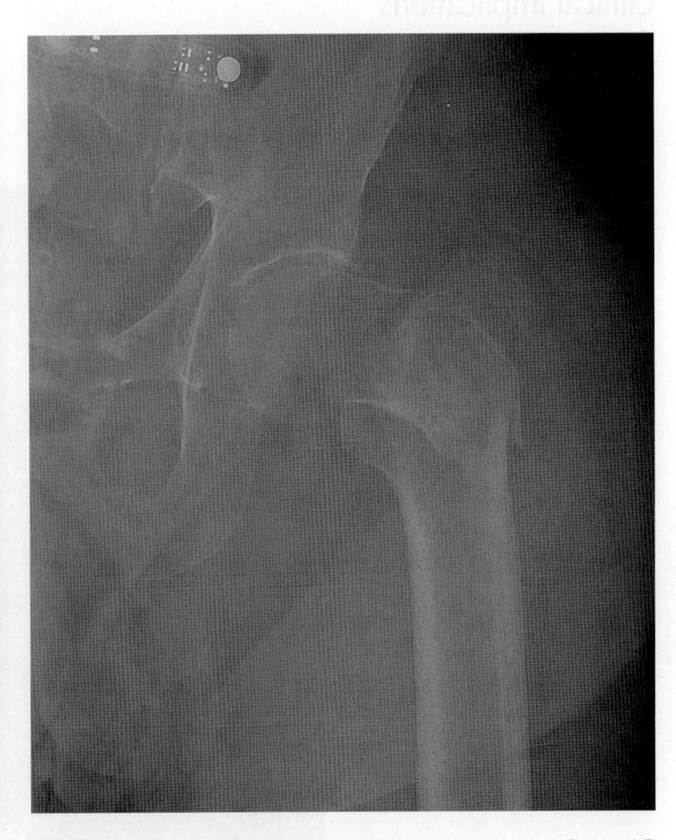

FIGURE 10.16 ■ Intertrochanteric Fracture (Companion Case). AP view of the left hip shows a markedly varus-angulated and mildly displaced intertrochanteric fracture of the left femur.

Radiographic Summary

Radiographs are usually sufficient to demonstrate this injury. This fracture is defined by being within 5 cm of the lesser trochanter, but not involving the lesser trochanter.

Clinical Implications

Similar to the intertrochanteric fracture, a subtrochanteric fracture can be the result of high-energy or, in the elderly, seemingly low-energy mechanisms. Concomitant injuries are common and should be sought. Treatment is surgical fixation.

Pearls

1. Always look for additional injuries when you see this fracture.
2. Radiographs are usually sufficient to demonstrate this injury.

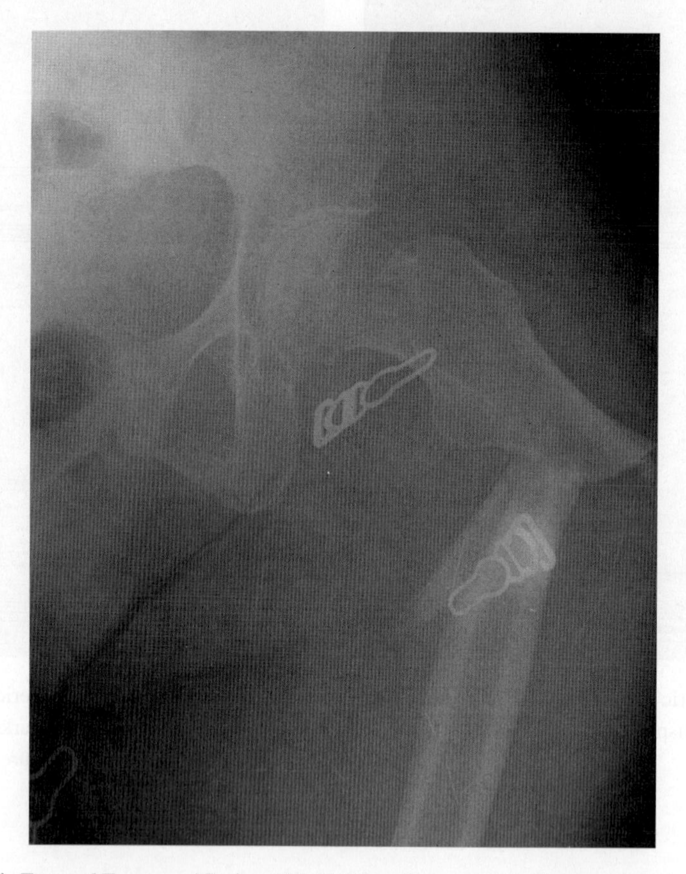

FIGURE 10.17 ■ Subtrochanteric Femoral Fracture. AP view of the left hip shows a markedly varus angulated and displaced subtrochanteric femoral fracture.

Radiographic Summary

Conventional radiographs are sufficient to demonstrate the fracture and can usually demonstrate the periprosthetic osteolysis or loosening. CT or MRI can demonstrate periprosthetic osteolysis better than conventional radiographs in complex, overlapping anatomical sites (e.g., in the pelvis or foot). At the hip, the most common site of loosening and fractures is on the femoral side.

Clinical Implications

Fortunately, periprosthetic fractures are a rare complication of total hip arthroplasty. The fractures range from nondisplaced greater trochanter fractures, which are generally stable to the fracture illustrated that will require operative fixation. Treatment is based on the stability of the implants and the type of the fracture.

Pearls

1. Femoral-sided fractures are more common. The entire implant should be included within the field of view of the radiographs and carefully evaluated for periprosthetic osteolysis, loosening, or fracture.
2. Full-length femur radiographs should be obtained to assist operative planning.

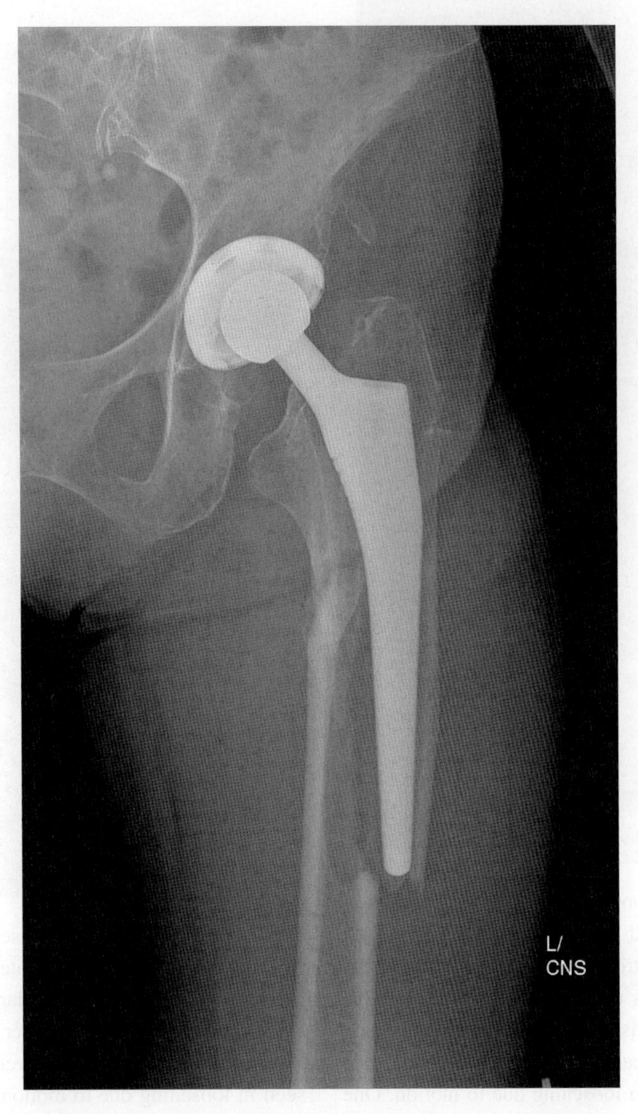

FIGURE 10.18 ■ Periprosthetic Fracture. AP view of the pelvis shows a noncemented total left hip prosthesis which is located. There is an acute periprosthetic fracture at the tip of the femoral stem which extends proximally to the lateral intertrochanteric region.

Radiographic Summary

Radiographs reveal a zone of lucency along the implants. Perfectly straight zones of lucency ("windshield wiper effect") are seen with implant motion and loosening. Lumpy and undulating zones of lucency are caused by particle disease and infection. Any type of orthopedic implant can be affected.

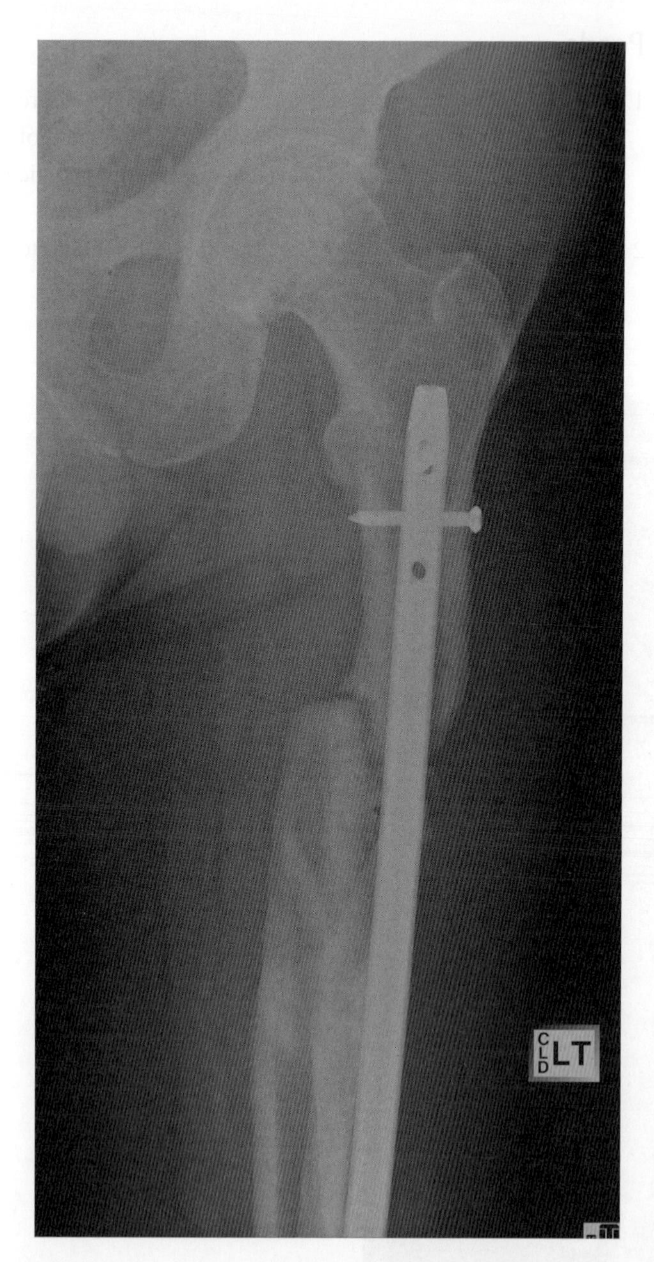

FIGURE 10.19 ■ Periprosthetic Loosening. An AP view of the left hip shows prior open reduction and internal fixation of the proximal femoral shaft fracture with a retrograde intramedullary nail and interlocking screws. The fracture is ununited: 10 months after the injury the fracture plane is clearly visible and the fracture edges are sclerotic and flared. There is a linear zone of lucency medial and lateral to the IM rod consistent with loosening due to motion. One could easily envision how a "windshield wiper" motion of the IM rod would create this zone of lucency.

Clinical Implications

The three most common causes of periprosthetic osteolysis or loosening are particle disease, implant motion, and infection. Patients present with pain and limited function. The degree of limited function is dependent on the implant location and the degree of loosening. The presence of infection should always be considered and must be differentiated from particle disease. Orthopedic referral is required.

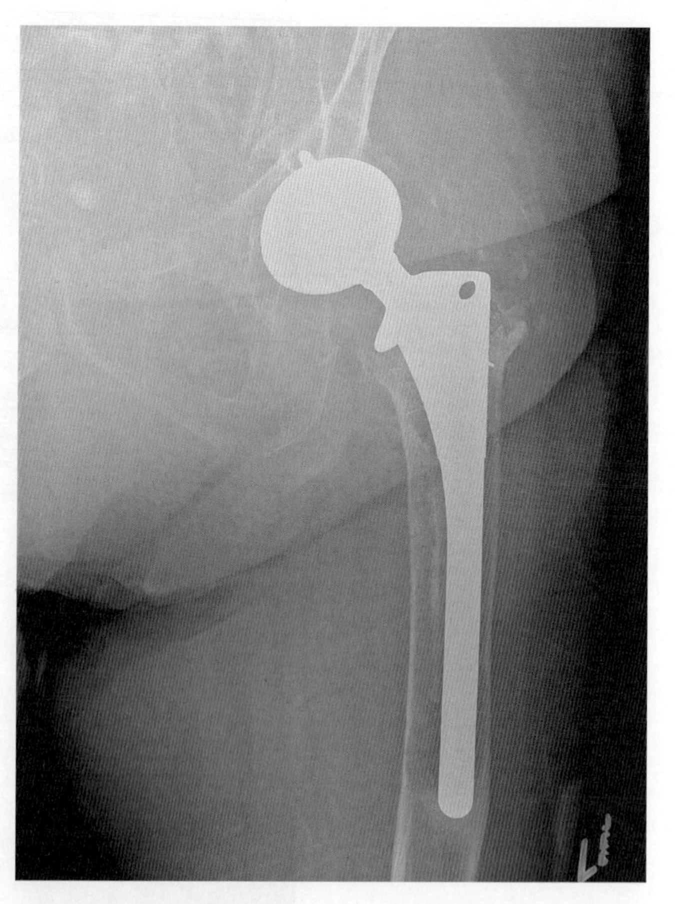

FIGURE 10.20 ■ Particle Disease Versus Infection. An AP view of the left femur shows a located total left-hip prosthesis. There is extensive "lumpy" and irregular osteolysis along the femoral endostem, in the greater trochanter, and medial to the acetabular cup. This pattern of osteolysis is very different from the linear pattern seen in loosening due to motion. There is no way in which motion could result in this pattern of osteolysis. The differential diagnosis in this case includes particle disease and infection.

Pearls

1. The three most common causes of periprosthetic osteolysis or loosening are particle disease, implant motion, and infection.
2. If left unattended, loose prostheses either dislodge or cause periprosthetic fractures.
3. Loosening is a common cause of pain.

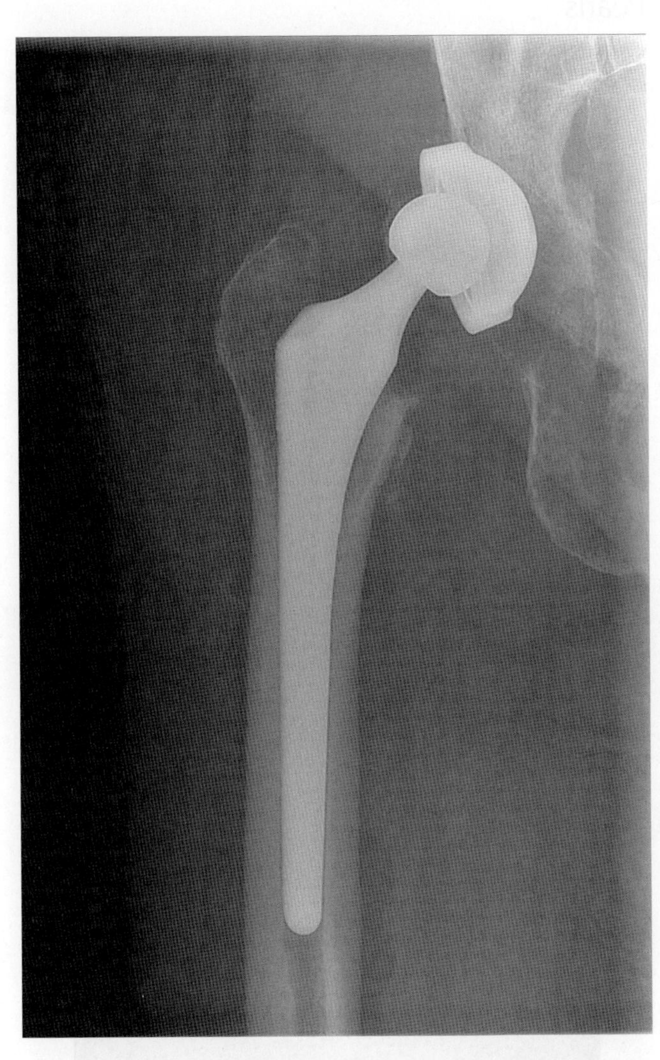

FIGURE 10.21 ■ Particle Disease Versus Infection (Companion Case). AP view of the right hip shows osteolysis within the greater trochanter and right acetabulum. The differential diagnosis again includes particle disease and infection. The acetabular cup has migrated superolaterally. There is a pathologic fracture through the significantly lysed and weakened medial right acetabular wall.

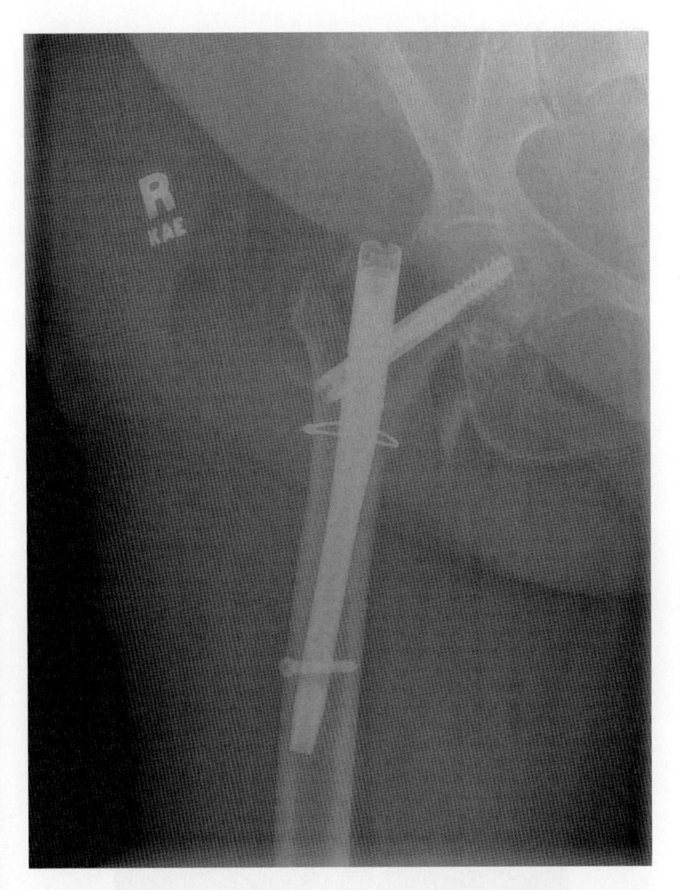

FIGURE 10.22 ■ Infection. An AP view of the right hip shows prior repair of an intertrochanteric fracture with a gamma nail device. There is extensive osteolysis within the greater femoral trochanter and superior aspect of the femoral neck. The differential diagnosis includes infection and neoplastic disease. A biopsy demonstrated osteomyelitis.

Radiographic Summary

Radiographs may reveal evidence of a healing stress fracture (periosteal new bone formation), typically in the lateral cortex of the proximal to mid femoral diaphysis; however, an MRI may be warranted if the radiographs are negative or equivocal.

Clinical Implications

Bisphosphonate fractures result from a decreased bone turnover, leading to bone fragility. Multiple case reports of patients treated with bisphosphonates have described stress fractures in the subtrochanteric region (typically laterally)—an "atypical" stress fracture. Patients will present with mid-thigh pain. Treatment includes activity modification and bisphosphonate discontinuation.

Pearls

1. Consider these atypical stress fractures in patients on bisphosphonate therapy.
2. An MRI should be considered if the clinical suspicion is high and the initial radiographs are normal or equivocal.

FIGURE 10.23 ■ Bisphosphonate Fracture. An AP view of the proximal right femur shows a healing stress fracture in the lateral cortex of the proximal right femoral diaphysis (arrowhead). This location is typical for a stress fracture occurring in a patient who has been or is currently on bisphosphonate therapy for osteopenia/osteoporosis.

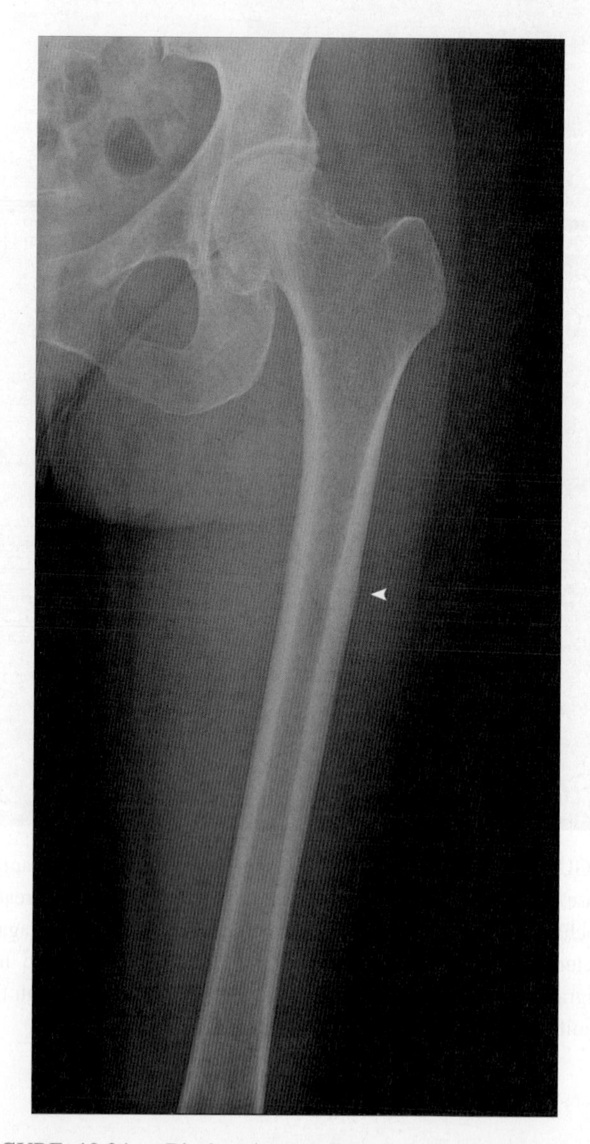

FIGURE 10.24 ■ Bisphosphonate Fracture (Companion Case). AP view of the proximal left femur of a different patient shows a very subtle stress fracture in the lateral cortex of the proximal left femoral diaphysis (arrowhead). Note how similar the location of the fracture is.

Radiographic Summary

Radiographs are sufficient to demonstrate the injury.

Clinical Implications

Femoral fractures in young patients are the result of high-energy impact. Elderly patients may suffer this injury with lower-energy mechanisms, such as a same-level fall. Femoral fractures can be associated with significant blood loss, and therefore patients should be evaluated for concomitant injuries. Profuse bleeding caused by these fractures can lead to hypotension. Treatment is surgical.

Pearls

1. Most femoral fractures are due to high-energy impact.
2. Assess all patients with femoral fractures for associated injuries.

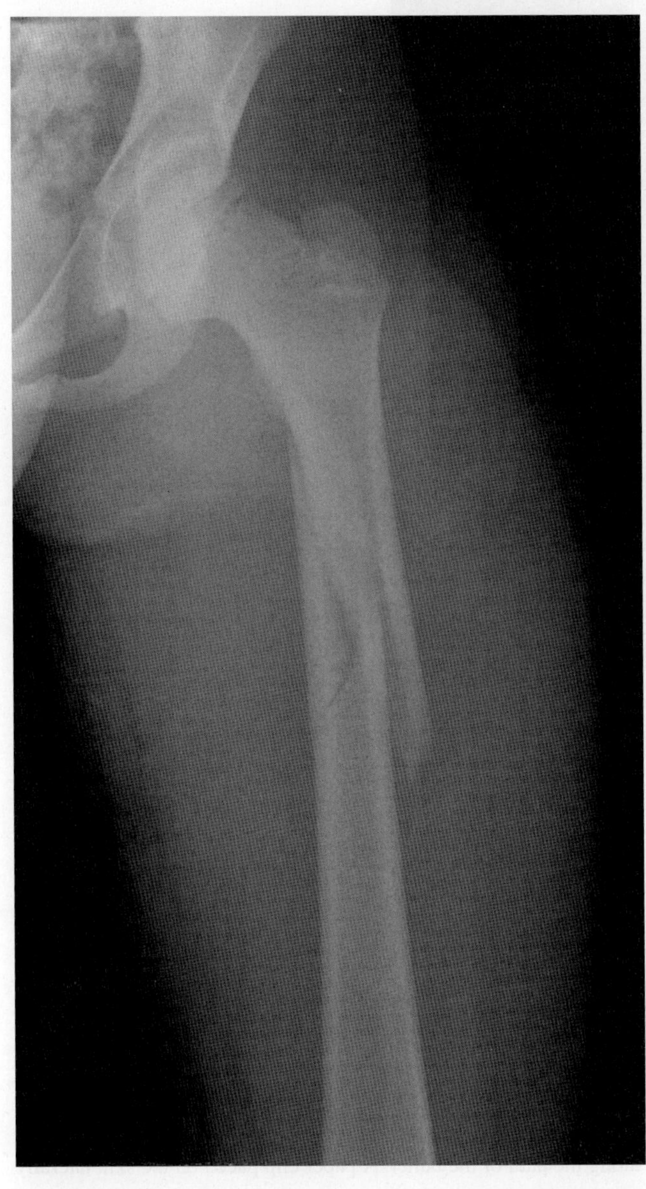

FIGURE 10.25 ■ Spiral Femur Fracture. An AP view of the proximal left femur shows a spiral fracture of the proximal left femoral diaphysis.

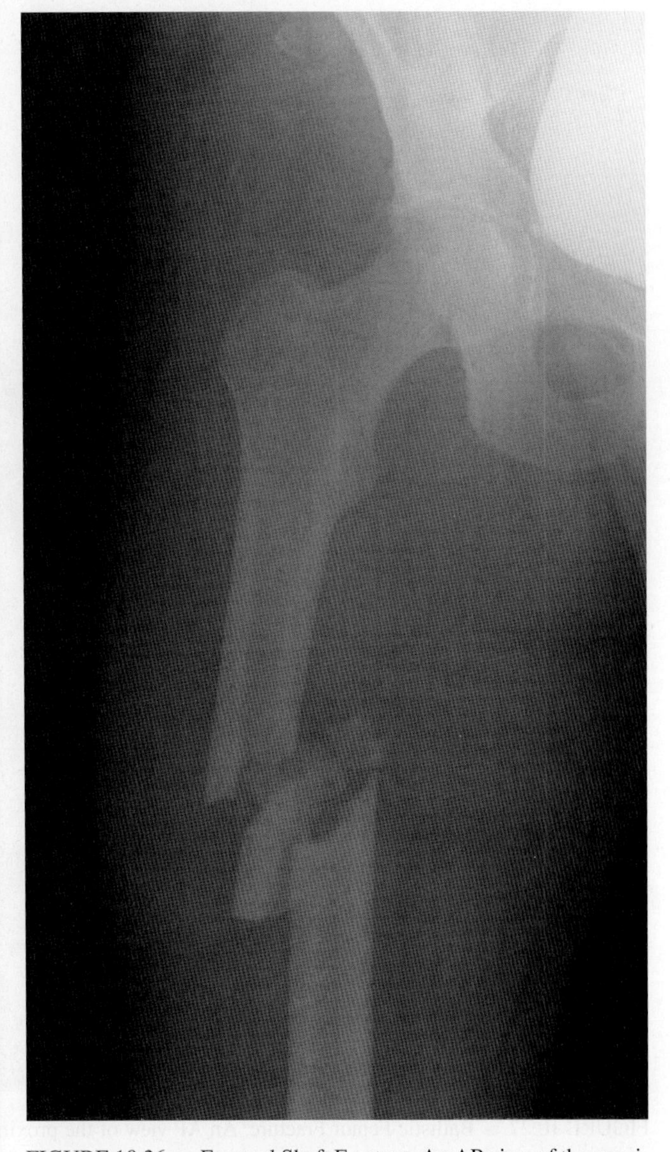

FIGURE 10.26 ■ Femoral Shaft Fracture. An AP view of the proximal right femur shows a comminuted fracture of the proximal femoral shaft. The distal femoral segment is medially displaced by one shaft width.

Radiographic Summary

Radiographs are the imaging study of choice and are sufficient to demonstrate the injury.

Clinical Implications

These injuries are usually obvious with a ballistic wound and deformity. Focus should be on resuscitation and ensuring adequate distal blood flow. Treatment is surgical.

Pearls

1. Resuscitate the patient and check for distal pulses.
2. Vascular imaging may be required based on the patient's exam. CT arteriogram and venogram are the studies of choice.

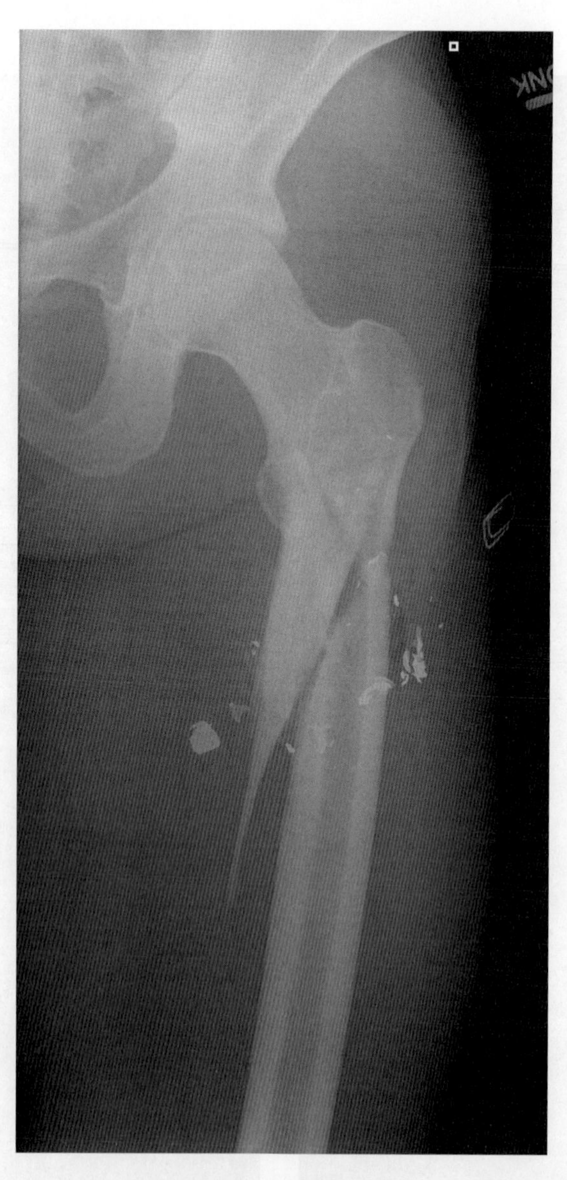

FIGURE 10.27 ■ Ballistic Femur Fracture. An AP view of the proximal left femur shows a comminuted ballistic fracture of the low intertrochanteric and subtrochanteric left femur. Bullet fragments are present along the path of the bullet. A paper clip paced on the skin laterally denotes an entry or exit wound.

Radiographic Summary

Radiographs are sufficient to demonstrate the injury.

Clinical Implications

Supracondylar fractures can result from high-energy mechanisms in younger patients, but may occur with low-energy mechanisms in the elderly. Patients present with an obvious deformity and pain proximal to the knee. Exam reveals tenderness in this area. The clinician should differentiate this injury from a knee dislocation by palpating the joint line. A thorough neurovascular exam should be performed as well. Treatment for these fractures is operative fixation.

Pearls

1. Differentiate this fracture from a knee dislocation by palpating the joint line.
2. Vascular injuries do occur due to the proximity of the femoral artery to the fracture site.

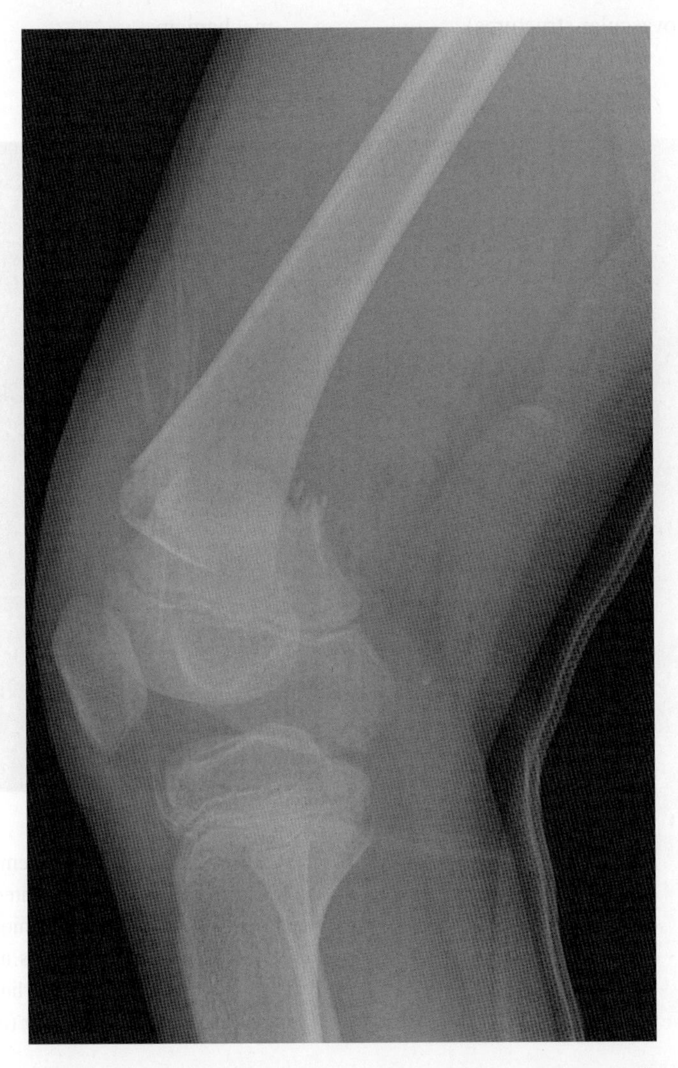

FIGURE 10.28 ■ Femoral Supracondylar Fracture. A lateral view of a child's distal femur shows a displaced distal femoral supracondylar fracture.

FEMORAL FRACTURE—PATHOLOGIC

Radiographic Summary

Radiographs can demonstrate the fracture and are very helpful in characterizing the underlying osseous lesion. It is the radiographs that reveal the matrix calcification pattern, if present, as well as define the type of underlying lesion (type of osteolysis, pattern of sclerosis, type of periosteal new bone formation). Most tumors are quite nonspecific on MRI (isointense to muscle on T1, hyperintense on T2, enhance after IV Gadolinium injection). The role of an MRI is to define the precise extent of the underlying neoplasm, the degree of osseous involvement, the soft tissue extension of the mass, and the relationship of the mass with other soft tissue structures (particularly the regional neurovascular structures).

Clinical Implications

Pathological femoral fractures are uncommon and generally result from low-energy mechanisms. The pathology can be either from metastasis (most common), primary bone tumors, or abnormal bone, such as Paget's disease. Treatment is surgical.

Pearls

1. Breast, lung, prostate, kidney, and thyroid are the common cancers that metastasize to bone.
2. Consider pathological fractures with low-energy mechanisms.

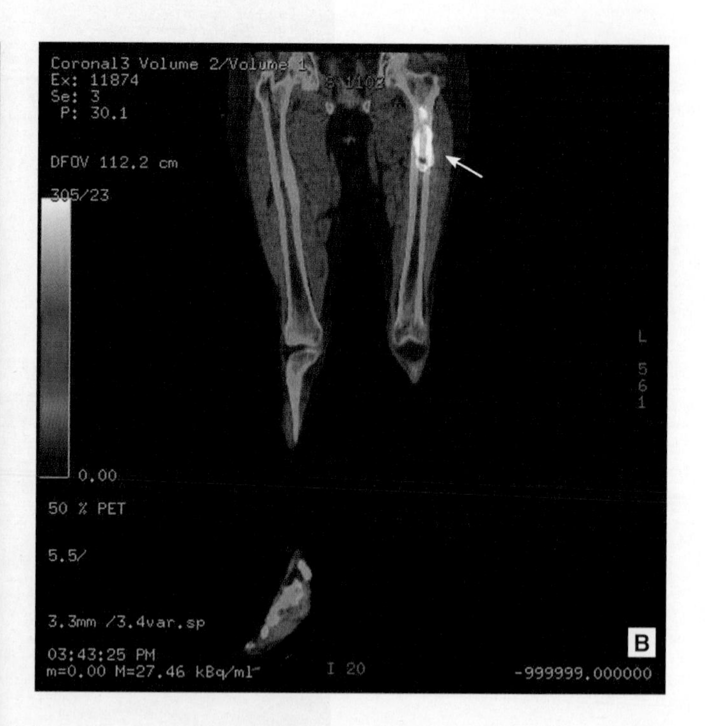

FIGURE 10.29 ■ Pathologic Femur Fracture. **A, B:** An AP view of the left hip shows a varus-angulated and mildly displaced pathologic fracture through an aggressive, moth-eaten, lytic lesion in the proximal left femoral diaphysis. This unfortunate patient had just had a PET CT examination 7 days earlier showing a large FDG-avid lytic lesion in the proximal left femur (arrow).

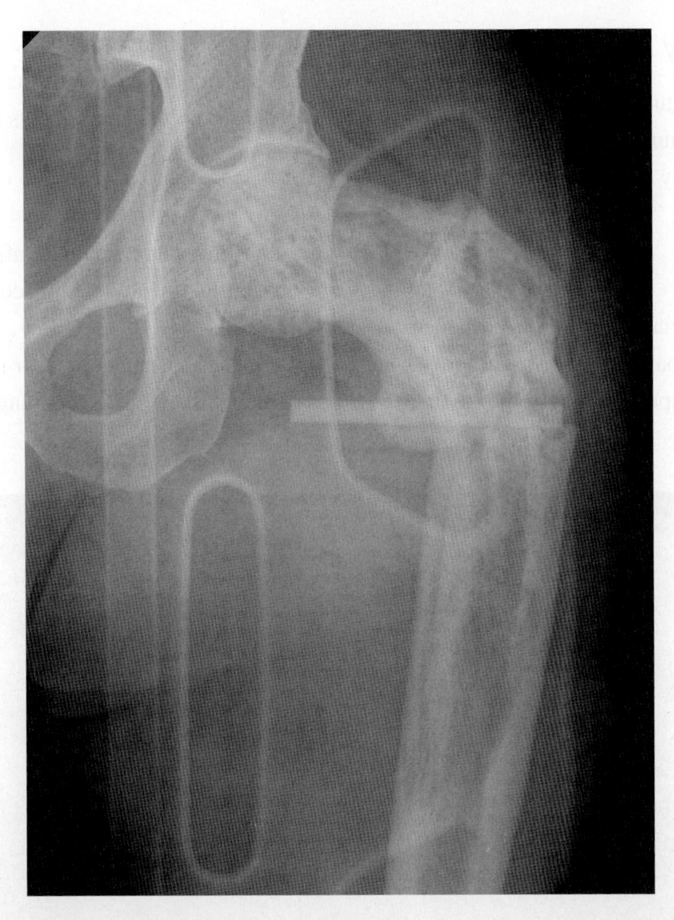

FIGURE 10.30 ■ Pathologic Intertrochanteric Fracture. An AP view of the left hip shows a pathologic low intertrochanteric fracture in a patient with Paget's disease. Notice the classic features of Paget's affecting the proximal left femur: the bone is mildly expanded and diffusely sclerotic, the cortex is thickened, and the trabeculae are coarse and disorganized.

Radiographic Summary

Radiographs are the imaging study of choice and usually sufficient in demonstrating the injury. A CT may aid in the diagnosis if the fracture is markedly comminuted.

Clinical Implications

Periprosthetic fractures associated with total knee arthroplasty are more common in patients with osteoporosis and after revision surgery. The supracondylar femoral fractures are related to notching the femur during surgery. Treatment can be nonoperative as long as the fracture is not significantly displaced and the components are stable.

Pearls

1. Periprosthetic fractures after total knee arthroplasty can occur with any of the components: femoral, tibial, or patellar.
2. Full-length tibia or femur radiographs will be required to assist in operative planning.

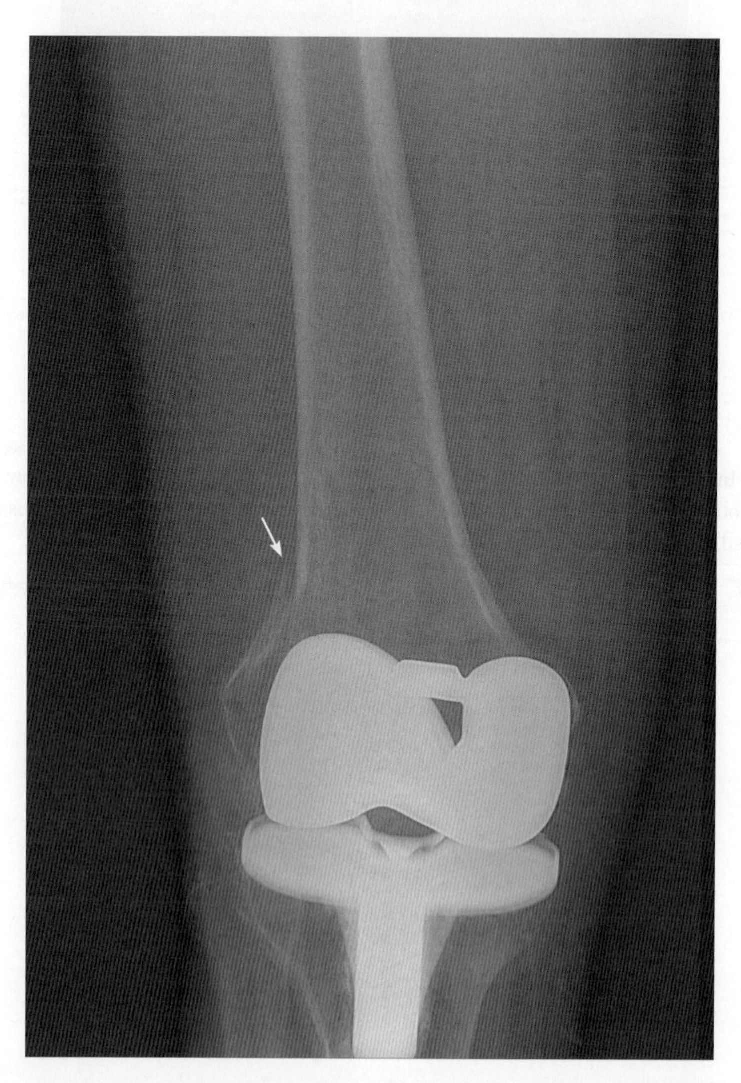

FIGURE 10.31 ■ Periprosthetic Fracture. An AP view of the distal right femur shows a minimally displaced periprosthetic fracture adjacent to the femoral component of a total knee prosthesis (arrow).

Radiographic Summary

Radiographs are sufficient to demonstrate the injury, if the joint is still dislocated. Reduced and splinted joints may appear radiographically normal, as the alignment would be restored. Look carefully for abnormal widening of joint spaces or subtle malalignment. The ligamentous injuries associated with a knee dislocation can be evaluated with an MRI.

Clinical Implications

These patients often present dramatically. The most common dislocation is anterior, but the dislocation can also be posterior, medial, lateral, or rotatory. Approximately 50% of knee dislocations spontaneously reduce in the field. These patients will not have the same dramatic physical deformity but will complain of severe pain. Spontaneously reduced dislocations still carry the same likelihood of neurovascular injury. A careful neurovascular exam should be performed to assure some degree of distal blood flow; if absent, emergent reduction should be performed. After reduction, further testing, including the ankle-brachial index (ABI), should be performed. If the ABI is less than 0.9, vascular imaging should be performed. Definitive treatment is dependent on the ligaments that are injured.

Pearls

1. Approximately 50% of knee dislocations spontaneously reduce in the field; however, they carry the same likelihood of neurovascular injuries.
2. Look carefully for abnormal widening of joint spaces or subtle malalignment.
3. The ligamentous injuries associated with a knee dislocation can be evaluated with an MRI.

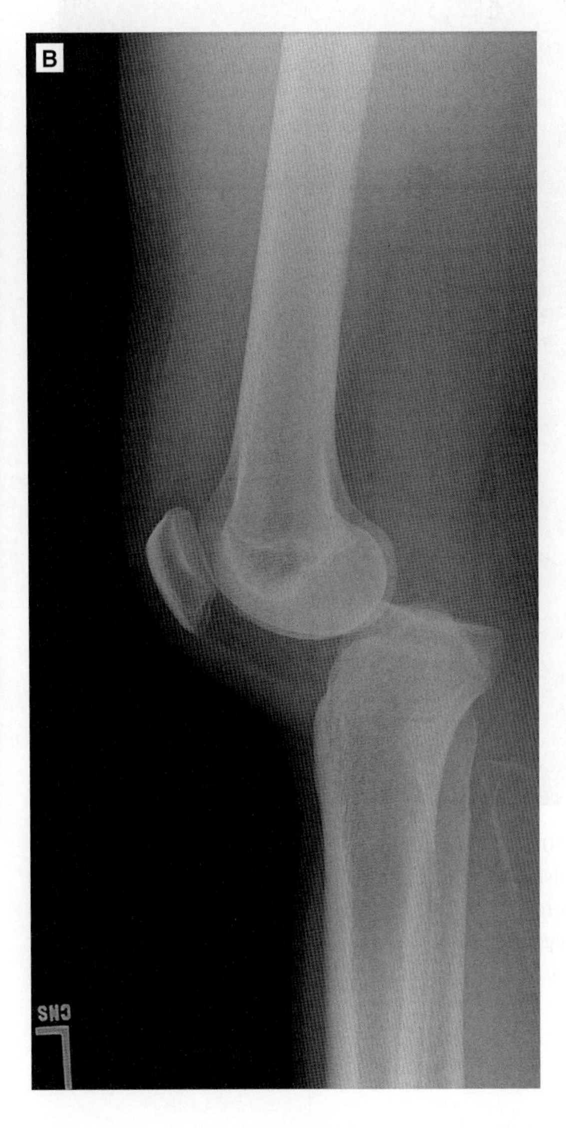

FIGURE 10.32 ■ Posterior Knee Dislocation. **A, B:** AP and lateral views of the left knee demonstrate posterior dislocation of the tibia. A joint effusion is present.

Radiographic Summary

Anterior cruciate ligament (ACL) injuries are best imaged with an MRI; however, there are certain radiographic abnormalities (the Segond fracture, deep sulcus sign, and anterior tibial spine avulsion fracture) that have an extremely high association with ACL tears. These findings are not sensitive but they are very specific for concomitant ACL tears.

Clinical Implications

Patients will prevent after an instability event with knee pain. Initial physical exam may be limited due to pain. The vast majority of patients will have a joint effusion. Specific knee-ligament injuries are difficult to discern based on a clinical exam. Initial treatment in the ER is conservative with compression (not a knee immobilizer), ice, and pain control.

Pearls

1. ACL tears are diagnosed with an MRI, but the presence of a Segond fracture, deep sulcus, or anterior tibial spine avulsion on the initial radiographs can point to the diagnosis.
2. These indicators are specific but not sensitive for ACL tear.

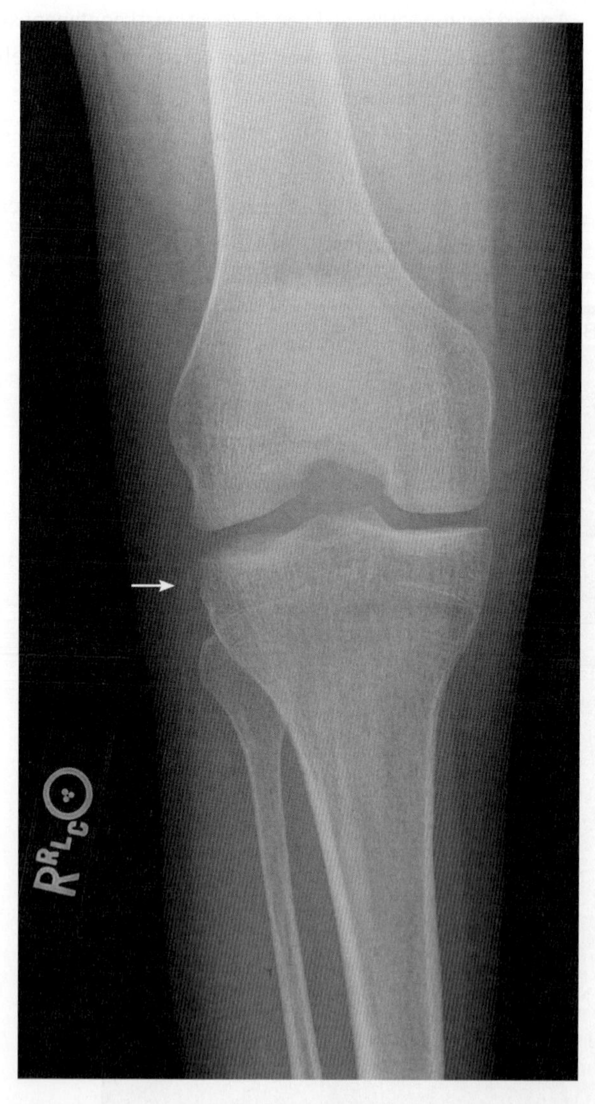

FIGURE 10.33 ■ Segond Fracture. An AP view of the knee shows a tiny avulsion fracture from the lateral aspect of the lateral tibial plateau (arrow). This is an avulsion of the lateral capsule and is called a Segond fracture. It has a very high (>90%) association with a tear of the anterior cruciate ligament.

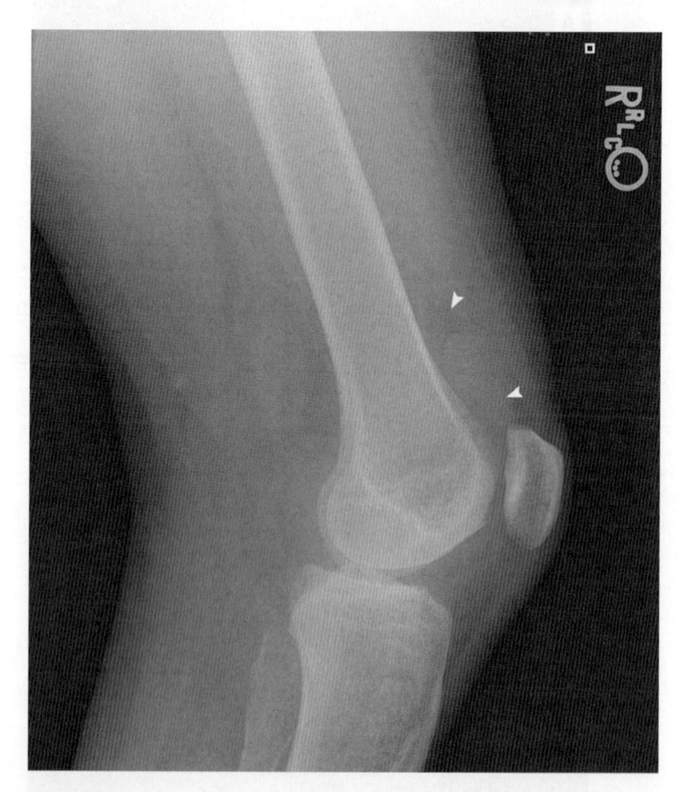

FIGURE 10.34 ■ Segond Fracture. A lateral view of the knee of the same patient shows a moderate joint effusion (arrowheads).

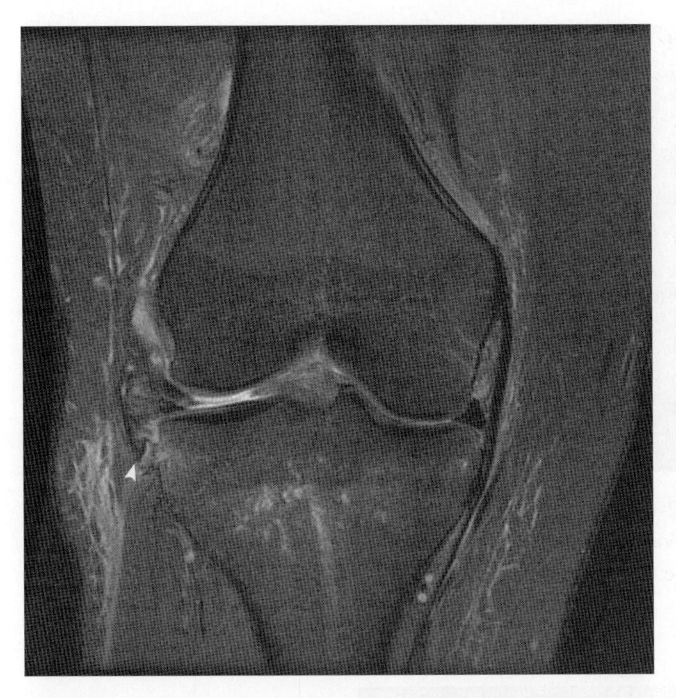

FIGURE 10.35 ■ Segond Fracture. A coronal FS PD-weighted image of the same patient's knee shows the Segond fracture (arrowhead). Notice the lateral joint capsule attached to the avulsion bony fragment.

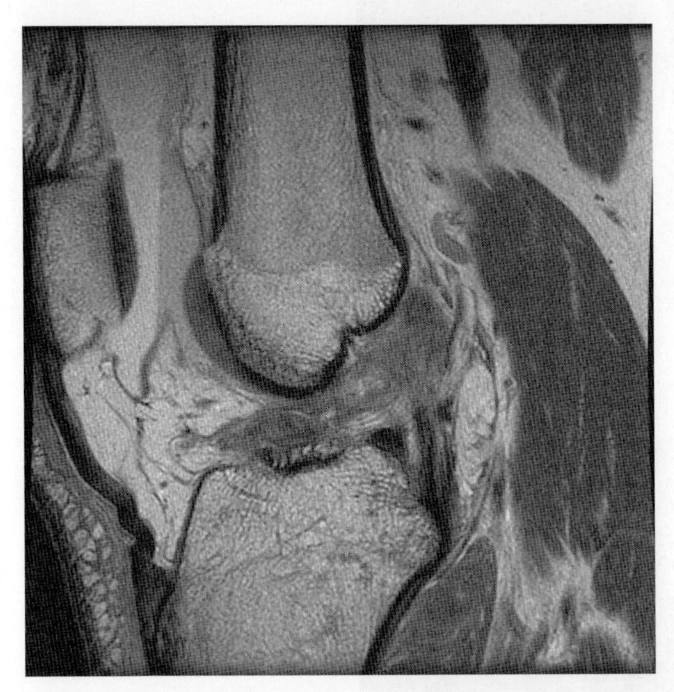

FIGURE 10.36 ■ Anterior Cruciate Ligament Injury. A sagittal PD-weighted MR image of the same patient's knee shows a tear of the proximal ACL: the ACL is indistinct and its fibers are lax, redundant, and no-longer parallel to the roof of the intercondylar femoral notch.

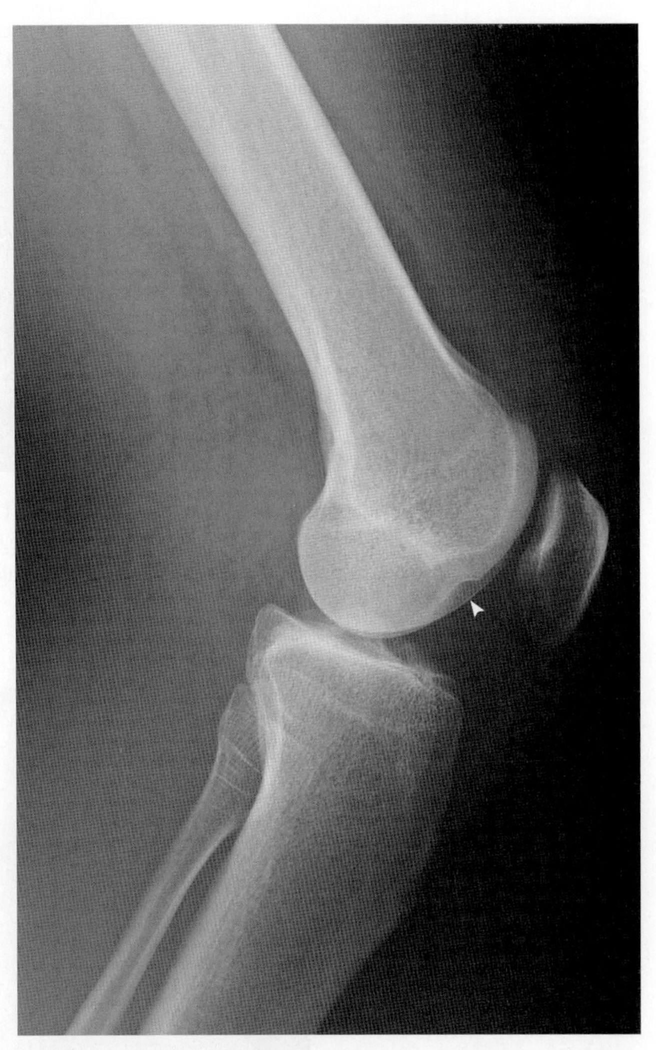

FIGURE 10.37 ■ Subchondral Fracture. A lateral view of the left knee shows a subtle subchondral fracture in the region of the sulcus terminalis of the lateral femoral condyle (arrowhead). In the setting of ACL injury, the femur rotates in such a fashion that the lateral femoral condyle often impacts against the posterior aspect of the lateral tibial plateau. This frequently results in "kissing" contusions or areas of marrow edema in the lateral femoral condyle and posterior lateral tibial plateau. If the impaction forces are greater still, then a subchondral fracture of the lateral femoral condyle can occur, as seen in this patient.

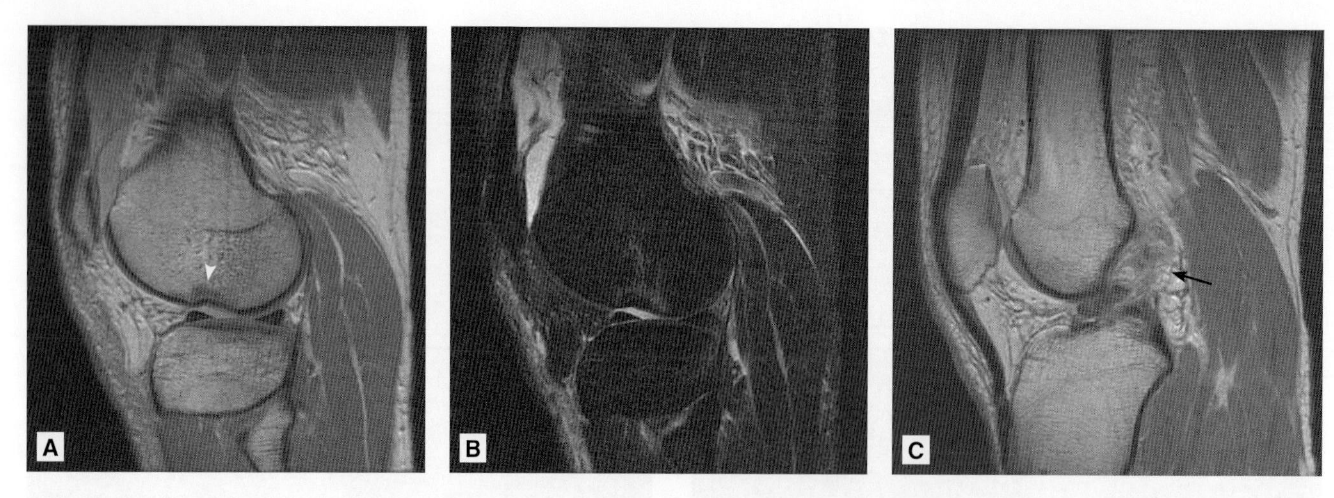

FIGURE 10.38 ■ Subchondral Fracture. **A-C:** Sagital PD and FS T2-weighted images through the lateral knee compartment of the same patient as in figure 10.37 show a subtle subchondral fracture in the region of the sulcus terminalis of the lateral femoral condyle (arrowhead). There is some associated marrow edema. A sagital PD-weighted image through the intercondylar notch shows a proximal ACL tear (arrow).

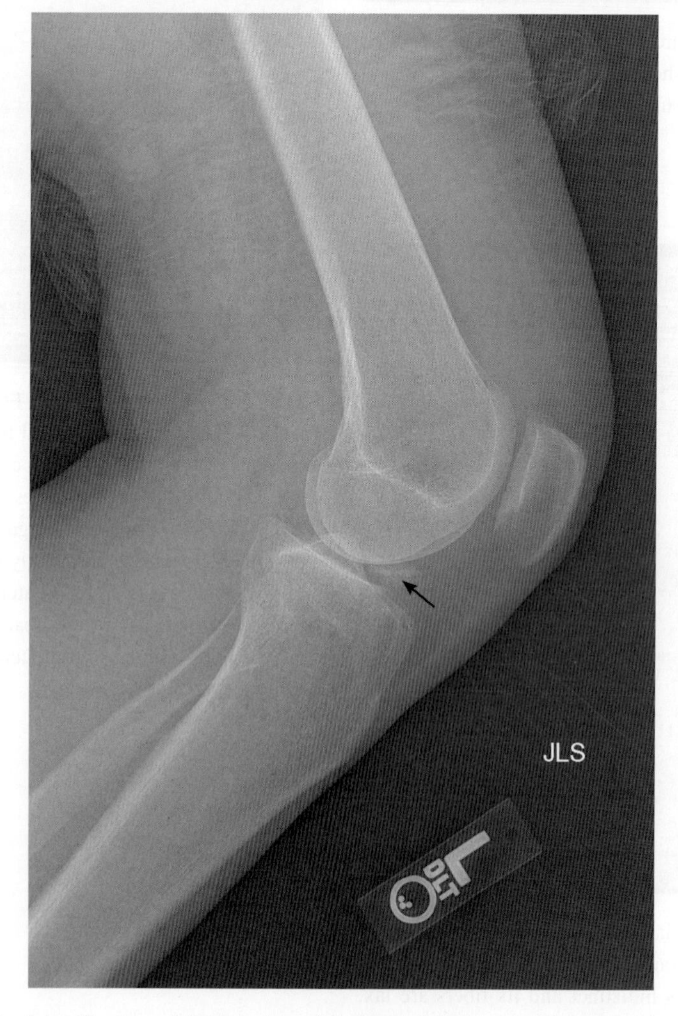

FIGURE 10.39 ■ Tibial Spine Avulsion Fracture. A lateral view of the knee shows an avulsion fracture of the anterior tibial spine (arrow). The bony fragment is distracted proximately and posteriorly. A joint effusion is present.

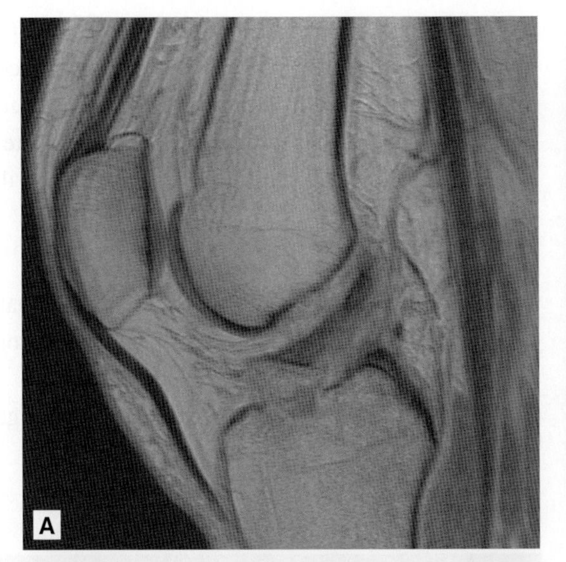

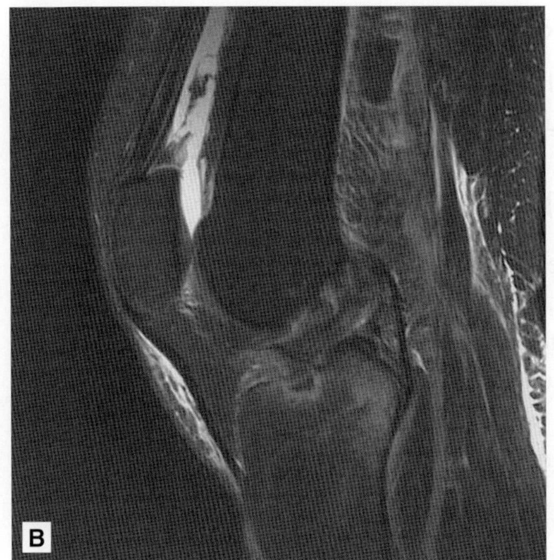

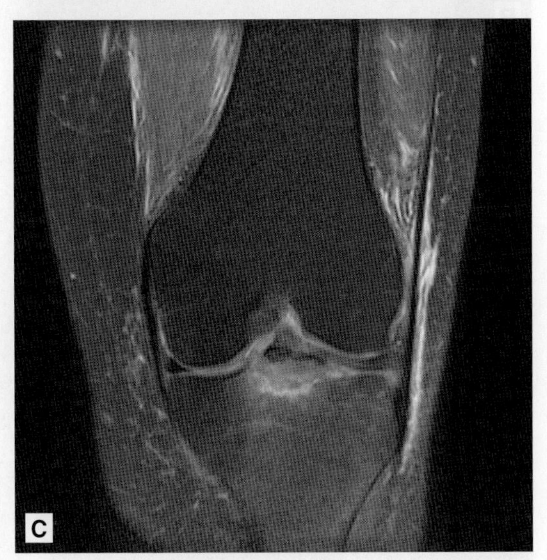

FIGURE 10.40 ■ Tibial Spine Avulsion Fracture. **A-C:** Sagital PD and FS T2-weighted and coronal FS PD-weighted images of the knee of the same patient as in figure 10.39 show an intact ACL attaching into an avulsed anterior tibial spine. Joint effusion, tibial marrow edema, and periarticular soft tissue edema and fluid are also present.

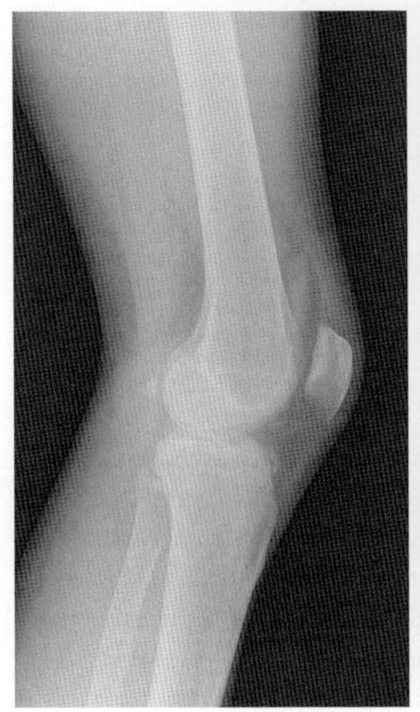

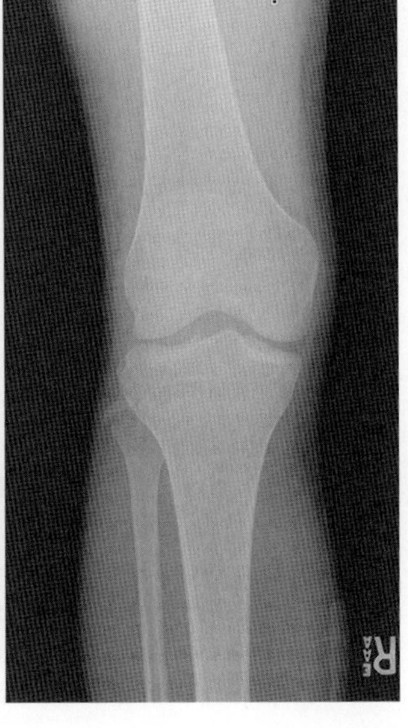

FIGURE 10.41 ■ Multiple Knee Fractures (Companion Case). Segond fracture, anterior tibial spine avulsion, and arcuate fracture. These AP and lateral views of the right knee show evidence of extensive ligamentous injury, including injury to the ACL and postero-lateral corner. The avulsed fragment of the fibular head is the site of attachment of the fibular collateral ligament and biceps femoris tendon: two of the major stabilizers of the postero-lateral corner of the knee.

Radiographic Summary

Radiographs typically reveal a joint effusion. The specific ligamentous injuries are demonstrable on MRI.

Clinical Implications

Posterolateral corner injuries may involve the biceps femoris tendon, fibular collateral ligament, popliteus tendon or muscle, lateral capsule, and a number of other less important ligaments that are not usually visible on conventional MRI sequences (arcuate ligament, popliteofibular ligament, etc). These injuries are rarely seen in isolation; ACL and/or PCL tears are usually present. Patients will present with pain, instability, and a knee effusion. Treatment depends on co-existing ligamentous injuries. It is critical that posterolateral corner injuries are identified and repaired with the cruciate ligament (usually ACL) repair; otherwise, the ACL repair will fail.

Pearls

1. Posterolateral corner injuries require a great deal of force; always keep the possibility of a knee dislocation on your mind when evaluating these injuries.
2. An MRI is the study of choice to evaluate for ligamentous injuries.

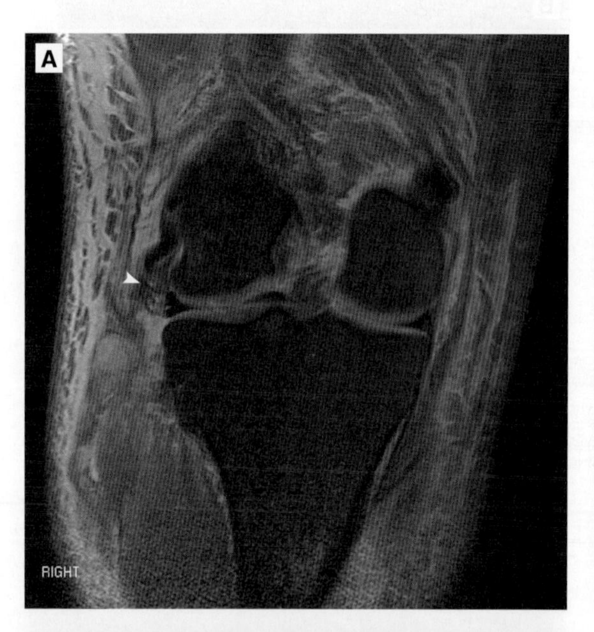

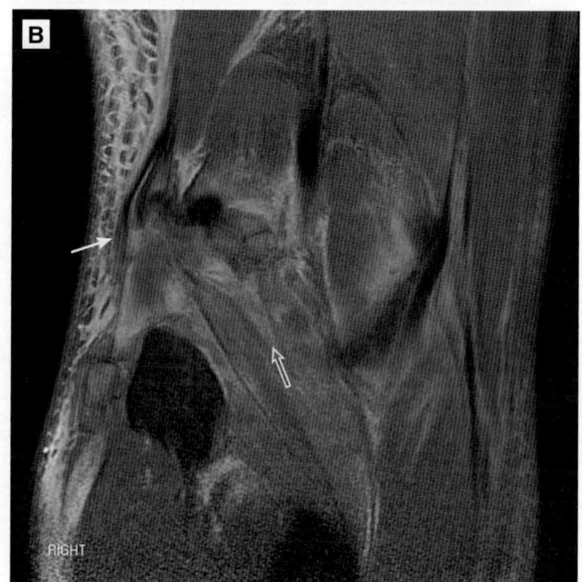

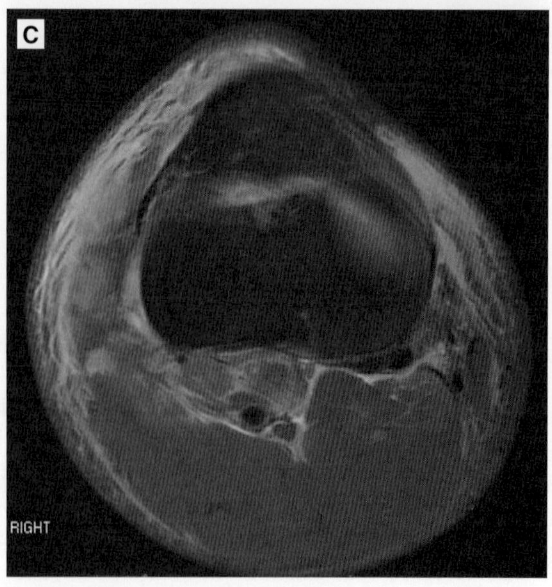

FIGURE 10.42 ■ Posteriolateral Corner Injury. **A-C:** Selected coronal FS PD and axial FS PD-weighted images of a knee show tears of the distal biceps femoris tendon (arrow), proximal lateral collateral ligament (arrowhead), and hemorrhage within the popliteus muscle (open arrow). Extensive periarticular soft tissue edema and hemorrhage is present as well. The patient had an ACL tear as well (not shown).

Radiographic Summary

Radiographs are normal, except for a possible effusion. Occasionally, a radiograph may demonstrate an extruded meniscus containing chonrocalcinosis (tiny deposits of calcium pyrophosphate dihydrate crystals). An MRI is the study of choice. Meniscal tears are hyperintense signal abnormalities within a meniscus that reach a meniscal surface (the superior surface, inferior surface, or free edge of the miniscus). Globular signal abnormalities within the substance of a meniscus that do not reach a meniscal surface are either areas of myxoid degeneration (usually in older patients) or meniscal contusion (in acute injuries, younger patients). An MRI can demonstrate the exact type and extent of the meniscal tear, as well as associated abnormalities (flipped or displaced meniscal fragments, perimeniscal cyst, intrameniscal cyst, bone contusion patterns, cartilage loss).

Clinical Implications

Meniscal tears can be either acute or chronic. Patients will present with knee pain and mechanical symptoms such as catching or locking. Physical exam can reveal joint line tenderness and possibly an effusion. It is extremely important to assess the injured joint's range of motion as a bucket-handle meniscal tear can limit extension and necessitate expedited surgical intervention. Treatment for acute meniscal tears is surgical; treatment for chronic tears varies.

Pearls

1. It is important to assess the injured joint's range of motion as a bucket-handle meniscal tear can limit extension and necessitate expedited surgical intervention.
2. An MRI is the test of choice.

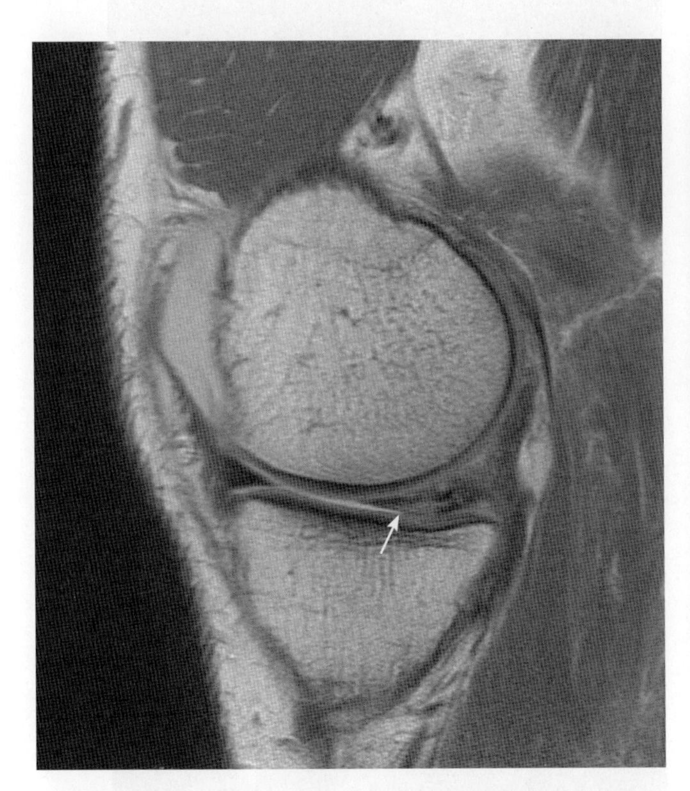

FIGURE 10.43 ■ Medial Meniscal Tear. A sagital PD-weighted image through the medial compartment of a knee joint shows a linear PD-hyperintense signal abnormality within the posterior horn of the medial meniscus (arrow). Notice that this linear signal abnormality reaches the inferior meniscal surface. This is a meniscal tear. No flipped or displaced meniscal fragment is evident on this image.

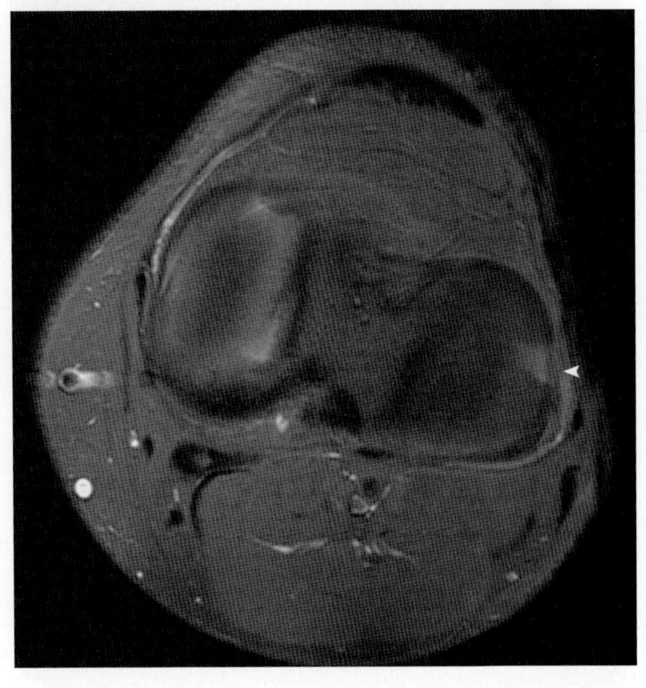

FIGURE 10.44 ■ Lateral Meniscal Tear. A selected axial FS PD-weighted image of a knee at the level of the femoro-tibial joint space shows a radial tear through the body of the lateral meniscus (arrowhead). The gap measures approximately 5 mm in width and is filled with fluid. The axial plane can be very helpful in the diagnosis of radial meniscal tears that could be indistinct or even completely undetected on the sagital and coronal images.

POSTERIOR CRUCIATE LIGAMENT (PCL) AND MEDIAL COLLATERAL LIGAMENT (MCL) TEAR

Radiographic Summary

Radiographs are generally normal, except for the presence of a joint effusion. Rarely, an avulsion of the posterior tibial spine where the PCL inserts can be discovered. An MRI is the imaging modality of choice. Old injuries to the MCL result in heterotopic new bone formation adjacent to the medial femoral condyle (Pellegrini–Steada lesion).

Clinical Implications

Patients with PCL injuries present after a blow to the knee or falling onto the knee with a plantarflexed foot. They will have knee pain, an effusion, and a positive posterior drawer test. Unlike ACL injured patients, the symptoms are mild and the patient may unwittingly return to sport. Treatment is primarily conservative.

Pearls

1. PCL injuries are not nearly as dramatic as ACL injuries. The symptoms are generally mild.
2. Treatment of these injuries is usually conservative.

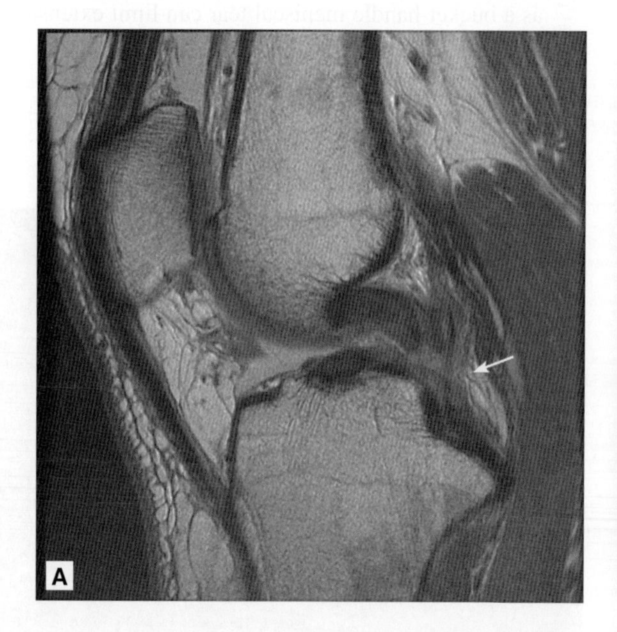

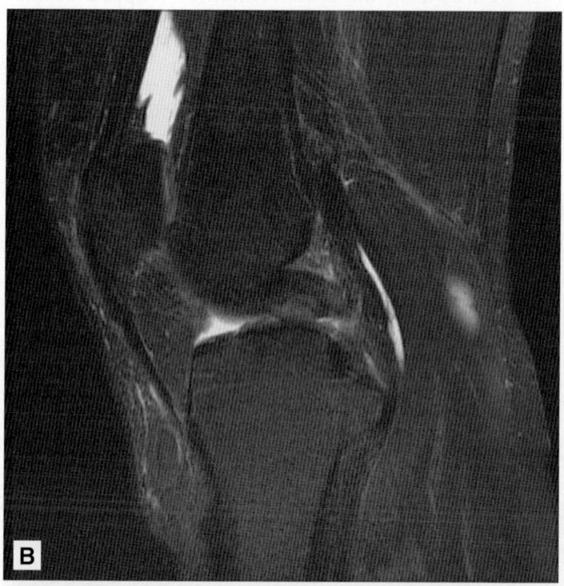

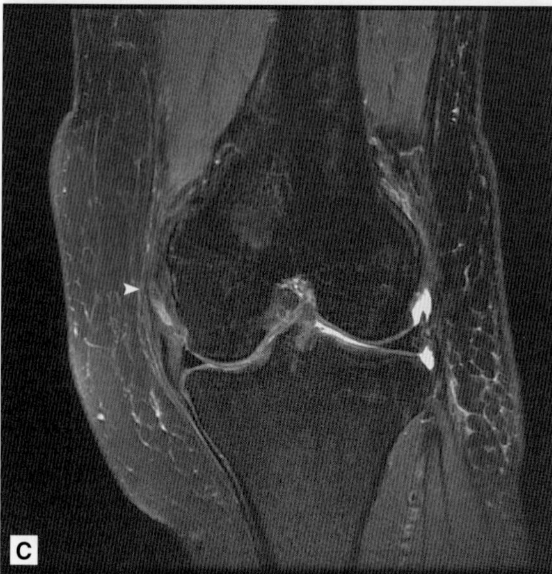

FIGURE 10.45 ■ Posterior Cruciate Ligament Tear. **A-C:** Sagittal PD and FS T2-weighted and coronal FS PD-weighted images of a knee show a tear of the distal PCL (arrow) and a complete tear at the origin of the medial collateral ligament (arrowhead).

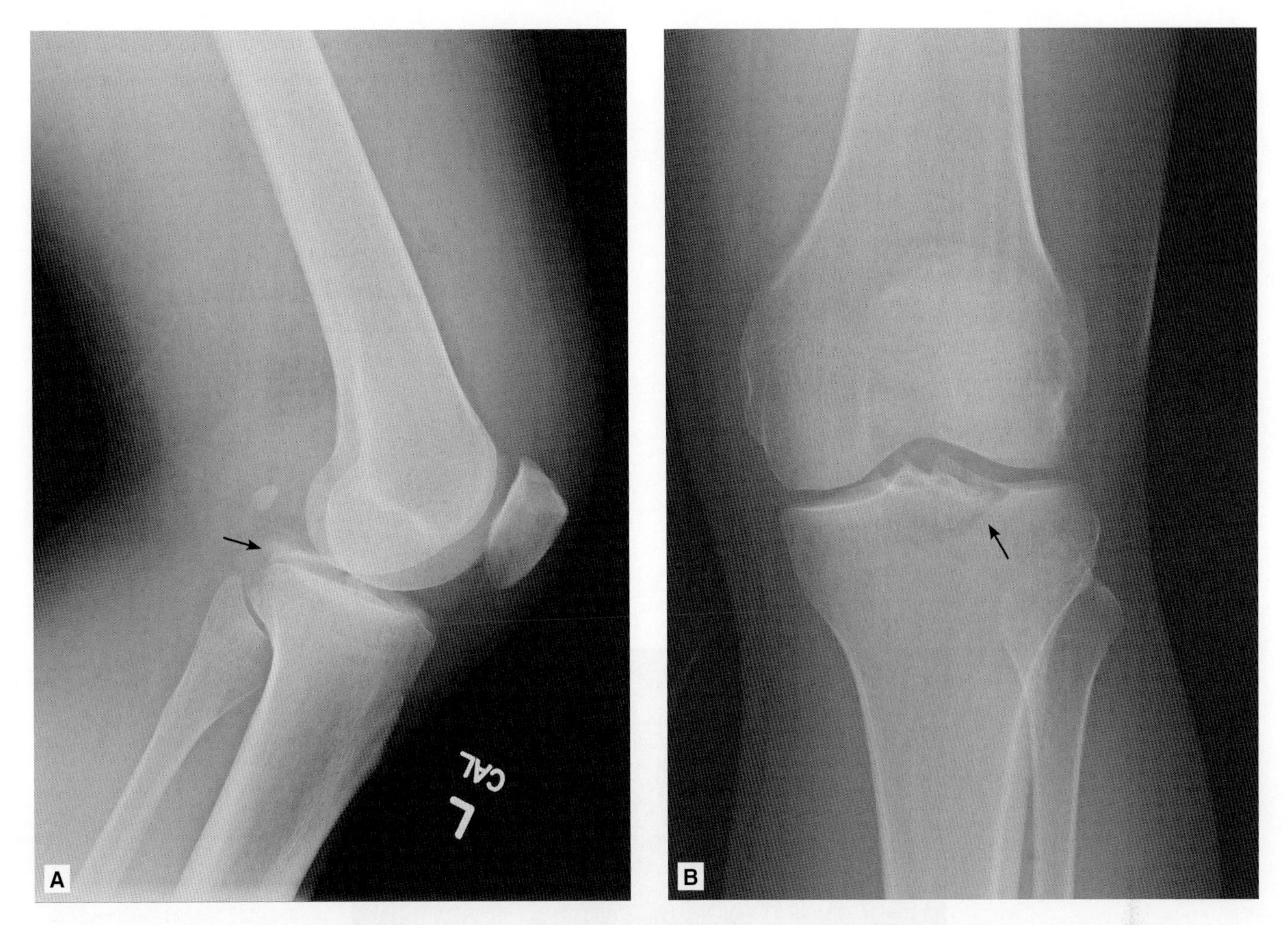

FIGURE 10.46 ■ Posterior Tibial Spine Avulsion Fracture. **A, B:** Lateral and AP views of the left knee show a nondisplaced avulsion fracture of the posterior tibial spine (arrows). This is the site of insertion of the PCL. A large joint effusion is present.

Radiographic Summary

Radiographs show subchondral collapse, most commonly on the lateral aspect of the medial femoral condyle. An MRI depicts the abnormality in much greater detail. It demonstrates the cartilage defect, if any, including delaminating injuries (an unstable cartilage fragment undermined by joint fluid resembling a door on a hinge), the exact size of the lesion, the stability of the lesion, the degree of subchondral collapse, and any associated subchondral changes such as cysts or edema.

Clinical Implications

Patients will present with knee pain and possibly mechanical symptoms (catching or locking). Physical exam reveals a knee effusion and possibly tenderness over the medial femoral condyle in a flexed-knee position. Treatment depends on the size of the lesion and age of the patient.

Pearls

1. The most common location of OCD in the knee is the lateral aspect of the medial femoral condyle.
2. An MRI can be utilized to determine size of the lesion and help determine stability.

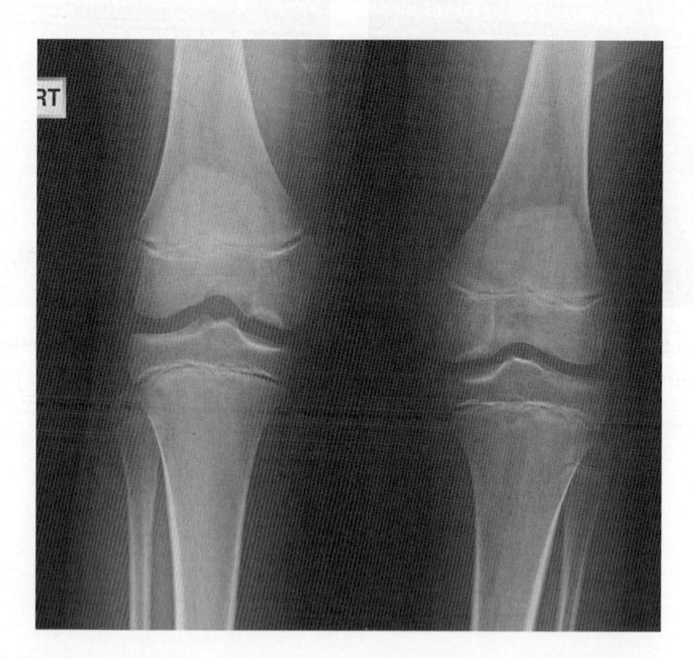

FIGURE 10.47 ■ Osteocondritis Dessicans. AP view of the knees shows bilateral subchondral collapse in the weight-bearing aspects of the medial femoral condyles. These are osteochondral lesions.

Radiographic Summary

Patella baja means a "low lying patella." A lateral radiograph of the knee is used to assess for the condition. A patella baja implies injury or tendinopathy of the quadriceps tendon or muscle.

Clinical Implications

When patella baja is discovered, injury to the quadriceps muscle or tendon should be expected. Rarely, patella baja can be congenital.

Pearls

1. A low-lying patella (patella baja) suggests quadriceps muscle or tendon tear.
2. A lateral radiograph of the knee reveals the abnormality. Patella baja may be occult on the AP view.

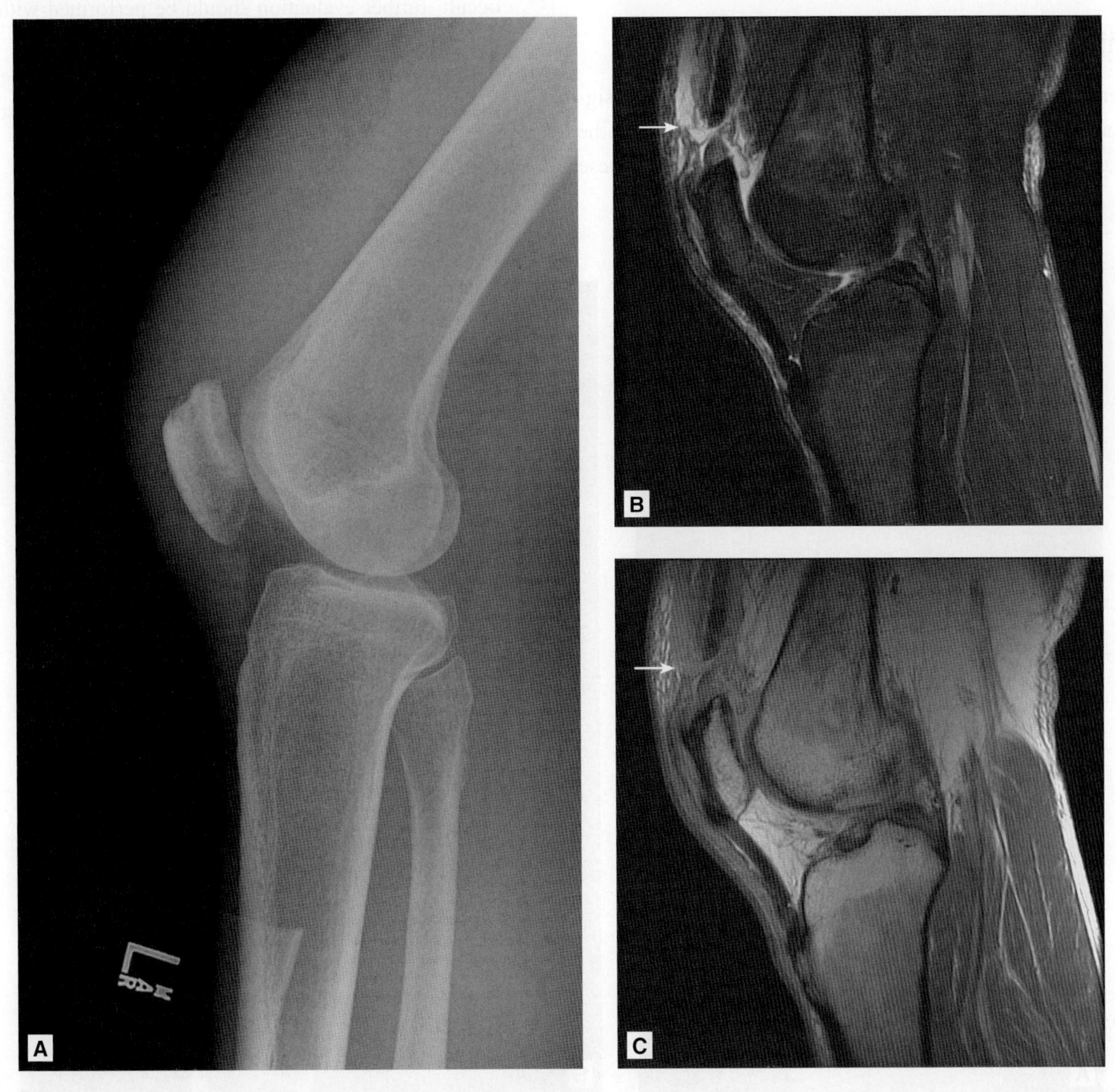

FIGURE 10.48 ■ Patella Baja. **A-C:** A lateral view of the left knee shows that the patella is too distally positioned or "low-lying." Hence, the term "patella baja." There is extensive soft tissue swelling in the anterior aspect of the distal right thigh. The findings are consistent with injury to the distal quadriceps muscle or tendon, allowing the patella to migrate distally. Sagitally oriented PD and FS T2-weighted images of the same knee show a complete tear of the distal quadriceps tendon (arrows). Fluid extends through the gap.

Radiographic Summary

Radiographs are typically sufficient to demonstrate these fractures. Very subtle fractures may be radiographically occult and can be detected with CT (if there is an actual cortical break or any degree of displacement) or MRI (if the fracture is completely nondisplaced). A knee lipohemarthrosis indicates the presence of an intra-articular fracture. If the fracture is radiographically occult, further evaluation should be performed with CT or MRI. Occult fractures of the lateral tibial plateau are particularly common.

Clinical Implications

Patients will present with knee pain, most likely due to significant trauma. Physical exam can find tenderness over the lateral and/or medial tibial plateau and a knee effusion. These fractures, though less likely than tibial shaft fractures, are associated with vascular injuries and compartment syndrome; careful and repeated assessments should be performed. These fractures require orthopedic referral. Emergent referral is warranted for open fractures, displaced fractures, compartment syndrome, and vascular injuries.

Pearls

1. A knee lipohemarthrosis indicates the presence of an intra-articular fracture. If the fracture is radiographically occult, further evaluation should be performed with CT or MRI.
2. Perform repeated soft tissue and vascular exams with these injuries because they are associated with vascular injuries and compartment syndrome.

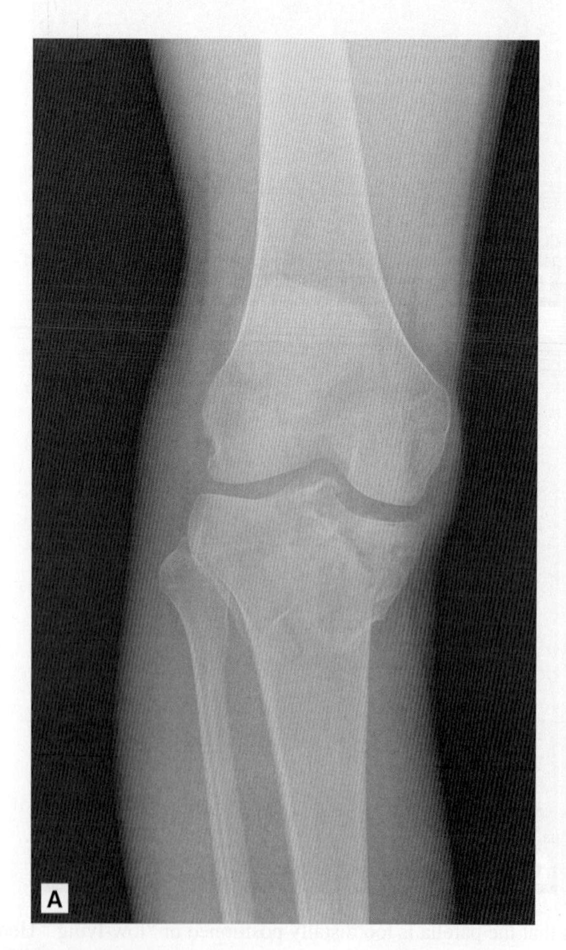

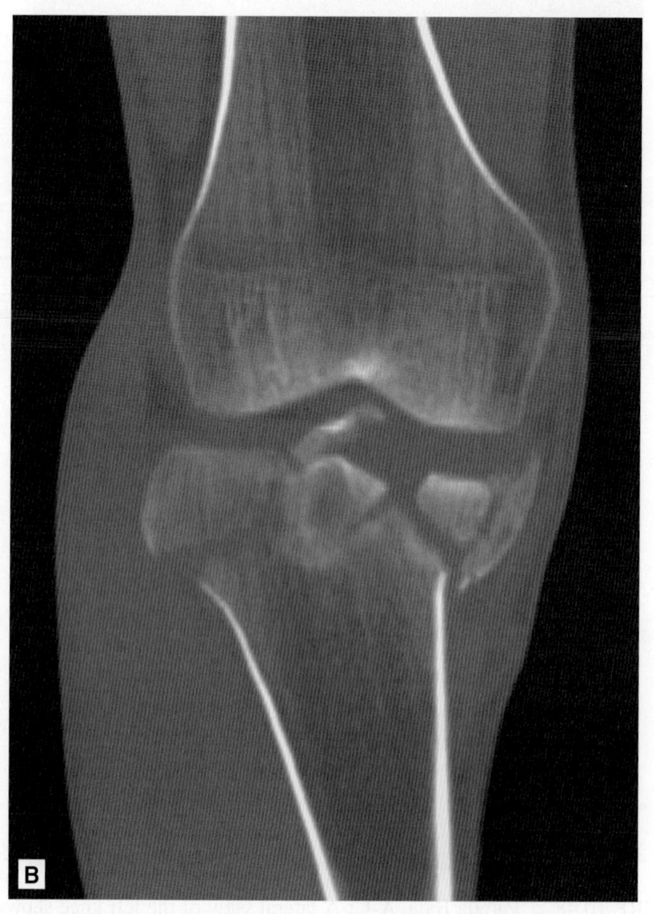

FIGURE 10.49 ■ Tibial Plateau Fracture. **A, B:** AP view of the right knee and a coronally reformatted CT image of the same knee show a comminuted and depressed fracture of the medial tibial plateau and a mildly displaced fracture of the lateral tibial plateau. Fracture planes also extend through the tibial spines; these are better delineated on the CT.

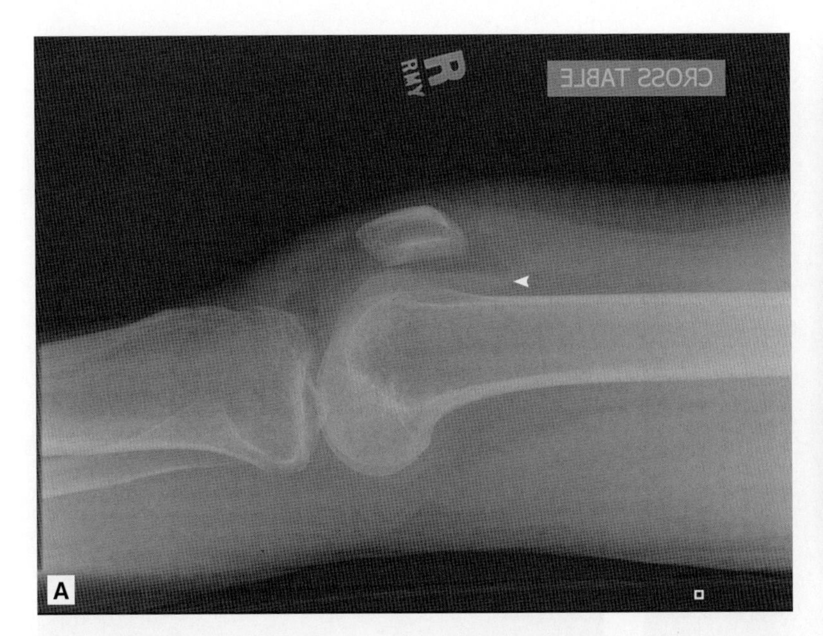

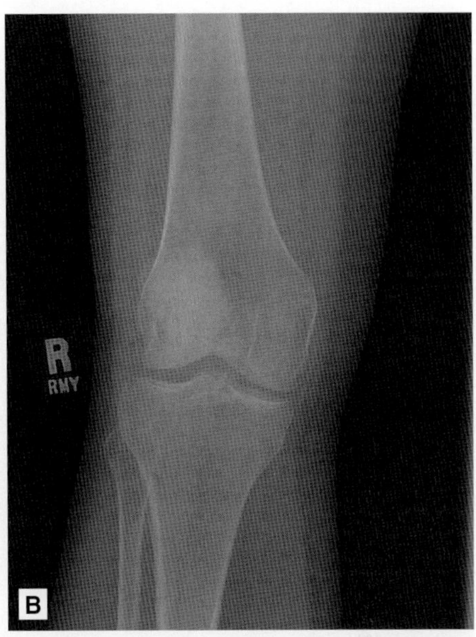

FIGURE 10.50 ■ Lateral Tibial Plateau Fracture with Liphemarthrosis. **A:** A lateral cross-table lateral view of the right knee shows lipohemarthrosis (arrowhead). This indicates the presence of an intra-articular fracture. Upon close inspection, a very subtle fracture line is evident in the lateral tibial plateau. **B:** AP view of the same knee fails to demonstrate a fracture.

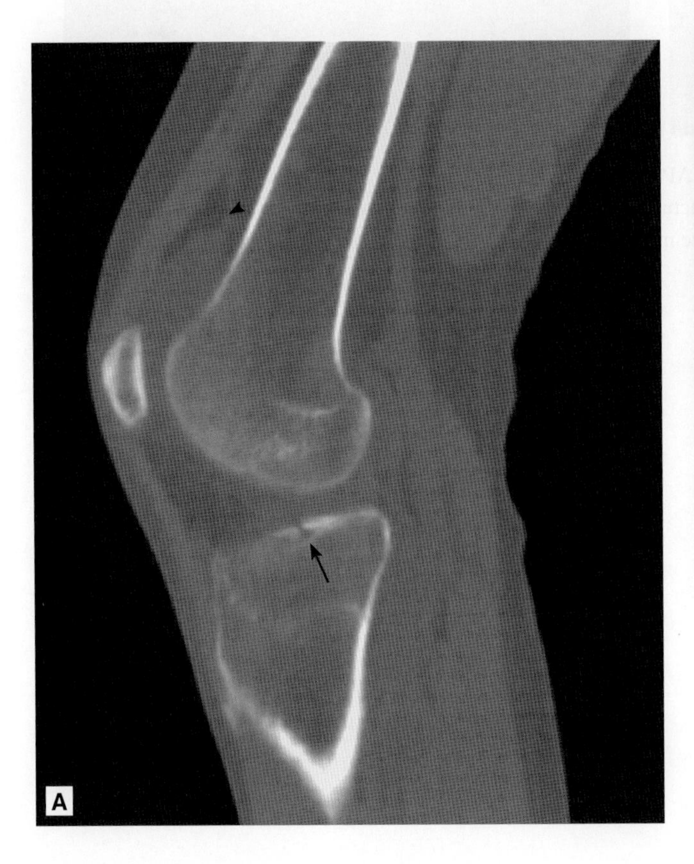

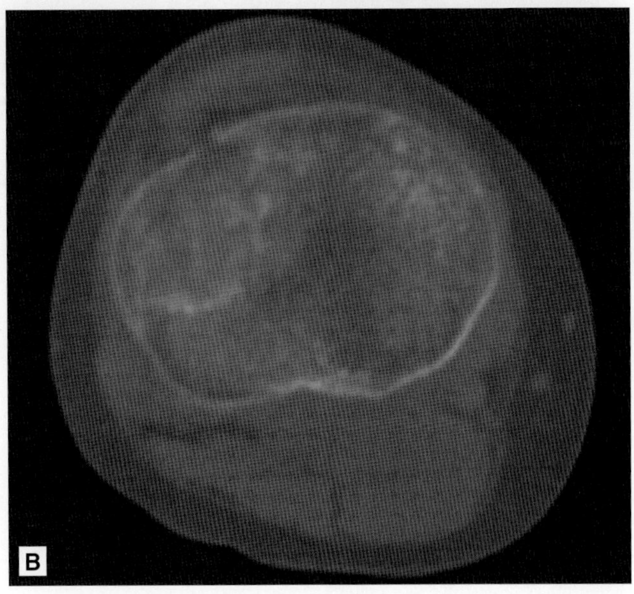

FIGURE 10.51 ■ Lateral Tibial Plateau Fracture with Liphemarthrosis. **A, B:** Axial and sagitally reformatted CT images of the same knee show a subtle, nondepressed, and nondisplaced fracture of the lateral tibial plateau (arrow) with associated lipohemarthrosis (arrowhead).

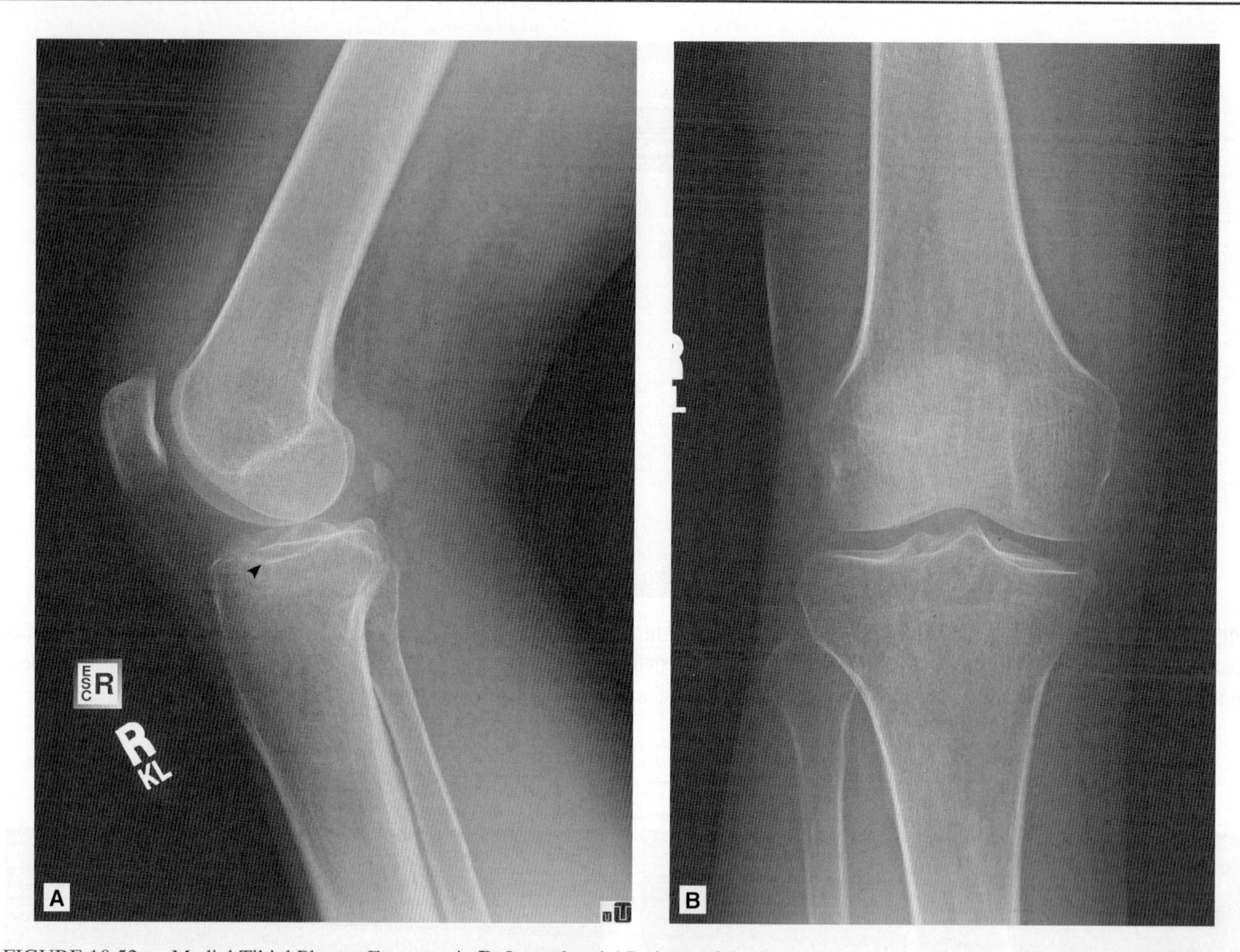

FIGURE 10.52 ■ Medial Tibial Plateau Fracture. **A, B:** Lateral and AP views of the knee show a joint effusion and a very subtle minimally depressed fracture of the medial tibial plateau (arrowhead). The fracture is best seen on the lateral view and not readily apparent on the AP view. Slight increase in bony markings can be seen underneath the medial tibial plateau resulting from trabecular compression.

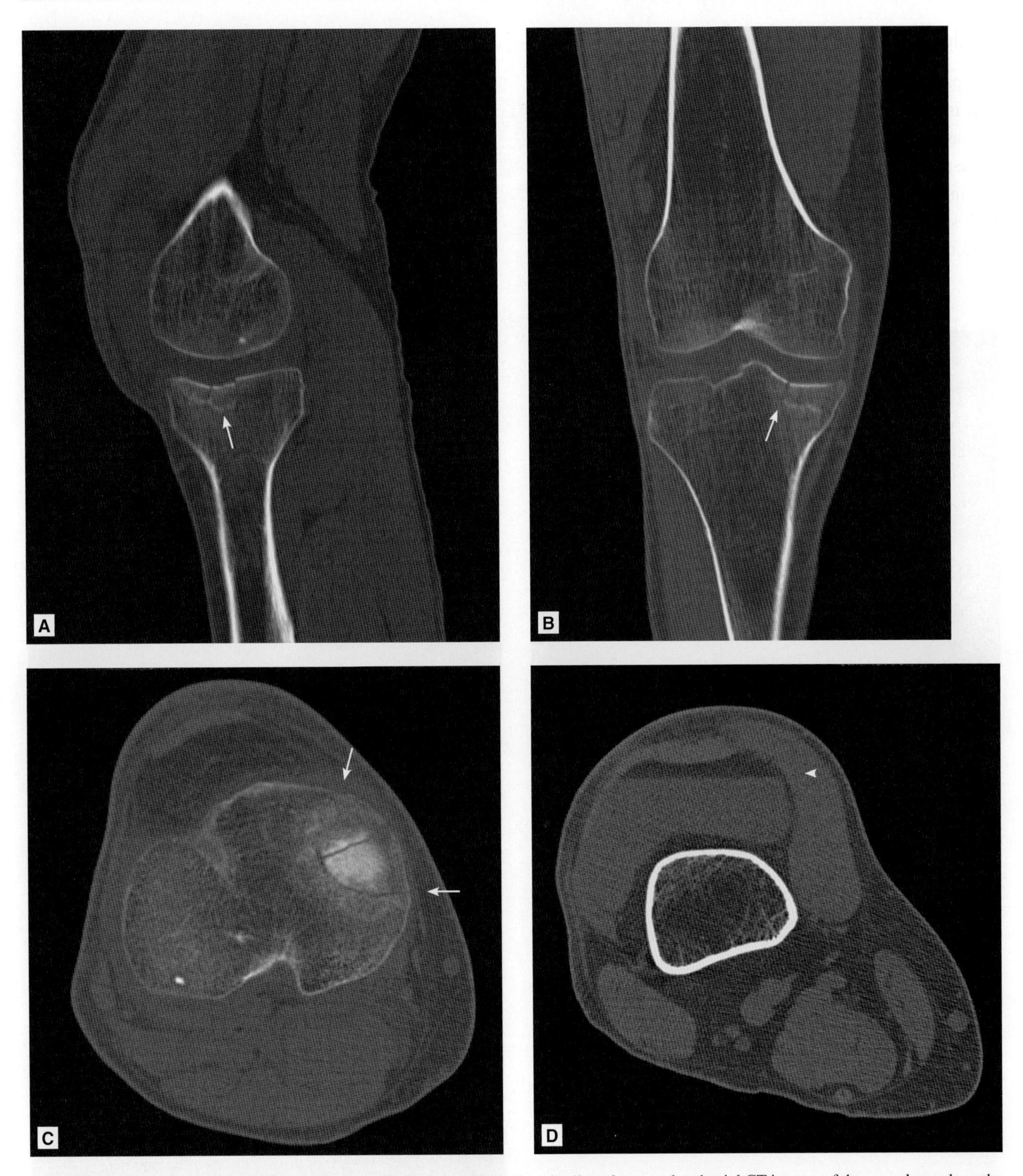

FIGURE 10.53 ▪ Medial Tibial Plateau Fracture. **A-D:** Coronally and sagittally reformatted and axial CT images of the same knee show the medial tibial plateau fracture (arrows) and lipohemarthrosis (arrowhead).

Radiographic Summary

The patella almost always dislocates laterally. If the dislocation is still present when the radiographs are obtained, AP and sunrise-patellar views of the injured knee would demonstrate the dislocation. Usually, by the time the radiographs are obtained, the patella has relocated. Sunrise-patellar views of both knees may reveal soft tissue edema in the anteromedial aspect of the injured knee due to patellar retinacular sprain or tear. A joint effusion may be present as well. An MRI is the imaging modality of choice and can reveal retinacular injuries as well as patellar cartilage injuries. "Kissing contusions" in the medial patellar facet and lateral surface of the lateral femoral condyle are almost always seen and occur due to impaction at the time of the dislocation. Rarely, an acute cartilage fracture may be seen on the sunrise-patellar view (if the subchondral plate is sheared off as well and the fragment is displaced).

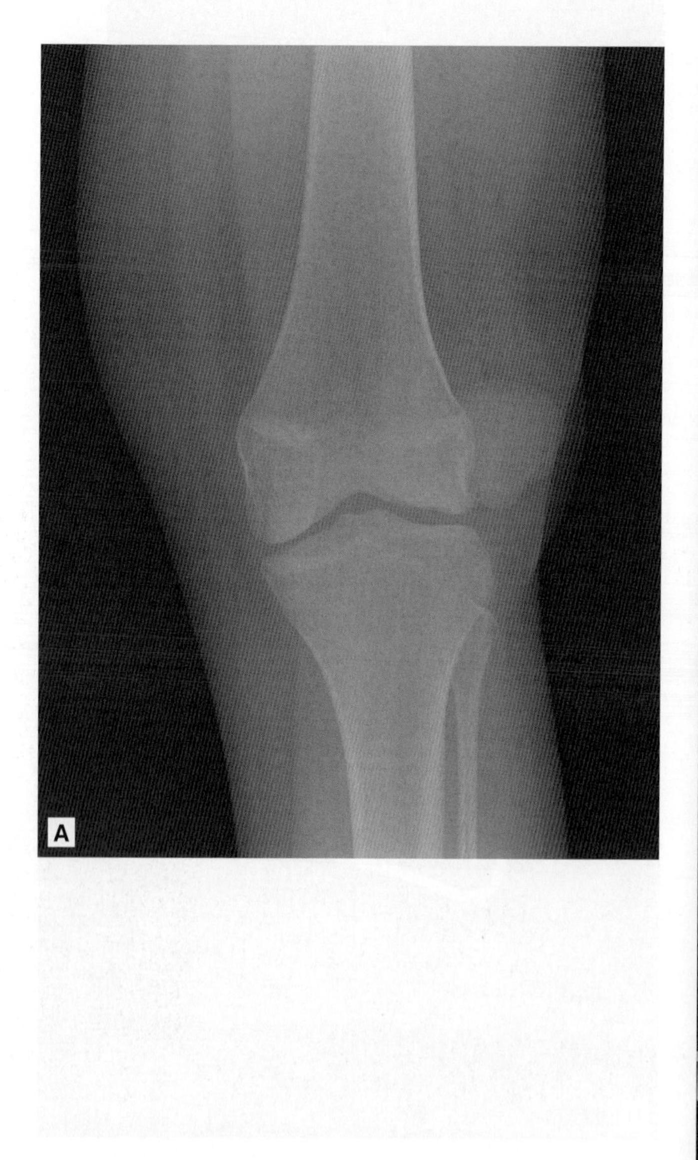

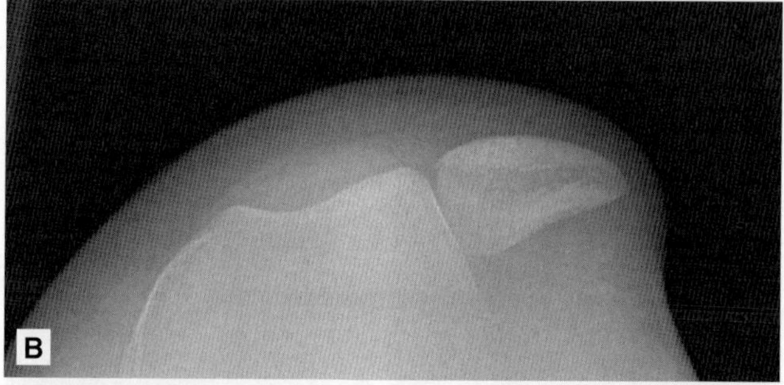

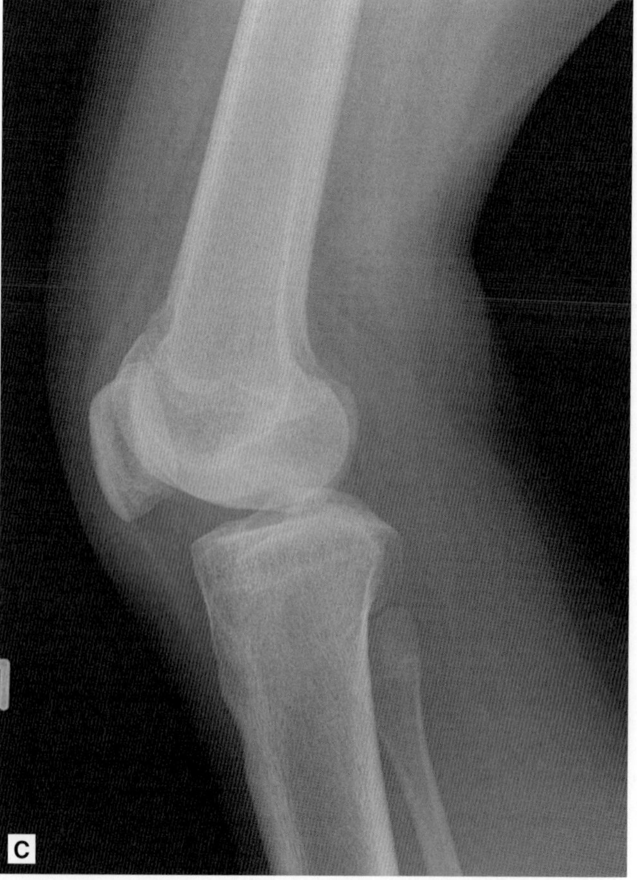

FIGURE 10.54 ■ Patellar Dislocation. **A-C:** AP, sunrise-patellar, and lateral views of the left knee show a laterally dislocated patella and extensive periarticular soft tissue edema.

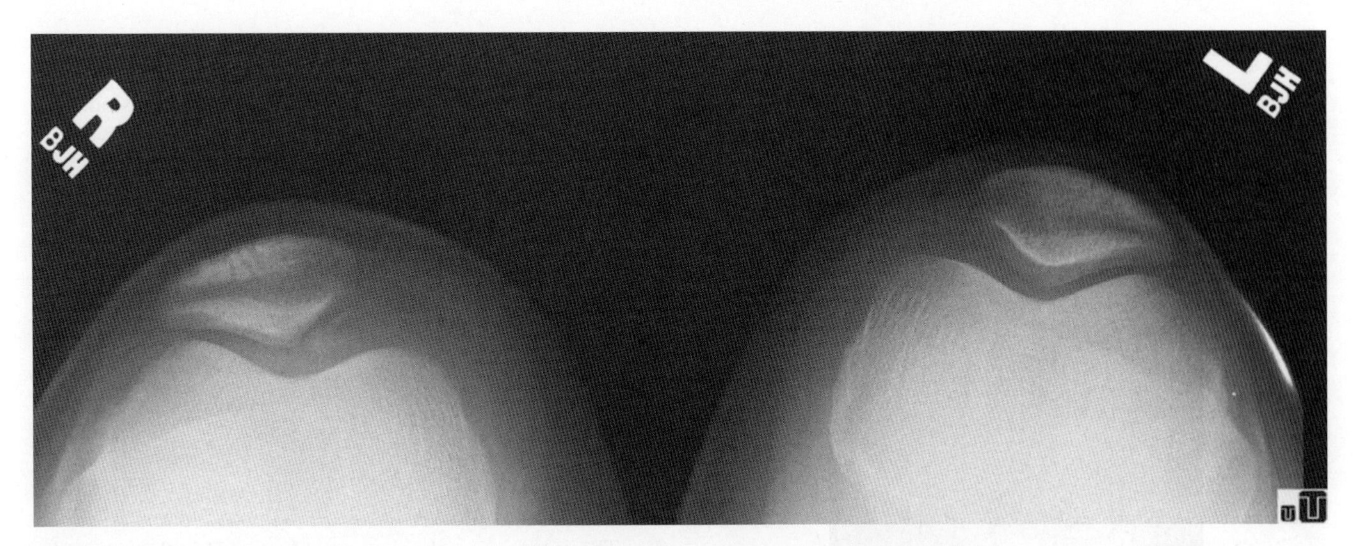

FIGURE 10.55 ■ Sheared Osteochondral Fracture Due to Patellar Dislocation. Sunrise-patellar views of the knees show mild soft tissue swelling in the medial aspect of the right knee joint. A small linear fleck of bone is present between the medial patellar facet and medial femoral condyle of the right knee. The fleck of bone is a sheared osteochondral fracture fragment that sometimes occurs during the lateral patellar dislocation or subsequent patellar reduction.

Clinical Implications

Patients will present with an obvious deformity with the knee in a flexed position and the patella displaced laterally. The patella should be reduced as soon as possible to alleviate the pain. Reduction is performed by flexing the hip slightly and extending the leg. Gentle, medial force is placed upon the patella. Difficult reductions will require hyperextending the leg. Patellar dislocations represent one of the few times a knee immobilizer is indicated.

Pearls

1. Reduction is the best pain relief for these patients.
2. The sunrise-patellar view is the most helpful radiographic view in assessing subluxations, dislocations, anteromedial soft tissue injuries and potential avulsions, and osteochondral fractures.
3. An MRI is the imaging modality of choice and can reveal the presence and type of medial retinacular injury, cartilage injuries, and bone marrow contusions.

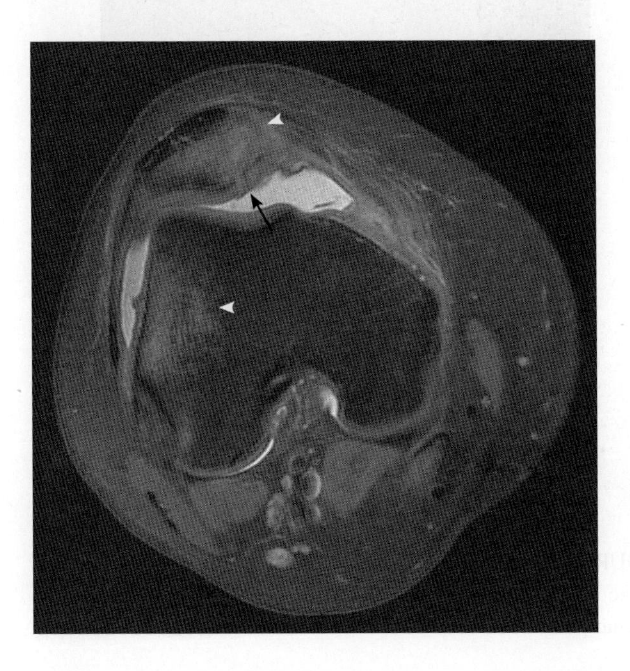

FIGURE 10.56 ■ "Kissing Contusions" of Patellar Dislocation. A selected axial FS PD-weighted image of the same knee shows the classic "kissing contusions" on the medial patellar facet and lateral aspect of the lateral femoral condyle which occur with transient lateral patellar dislocation (arrowheads). A small cartilage fissure is present in the medial patellar facet near the patellar ridge (arrow). The medial patellar retinaculum is thick and markedly edematous consistent with high-grade sprain or tear. A joint effusion is present. At this time, the patella is located.

Radiographic Summary

Radiographs are sufficient to demonstrate the vast majority of these injuries. AP, sunrise-patellar, and lateral views should be obtained. Some fractures may be invisible on a single view. Associated findings are joint effusion and soft tissue edema.

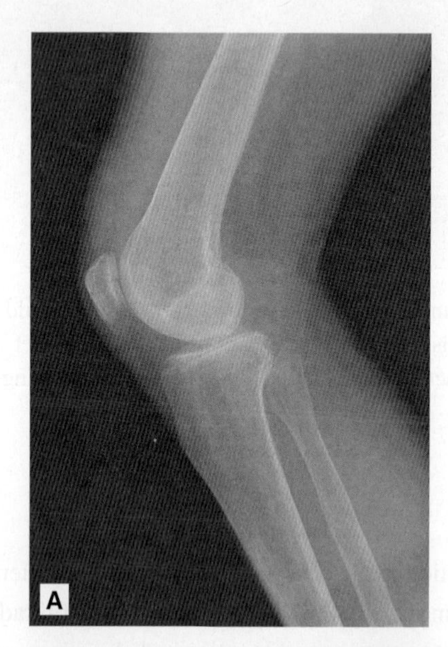

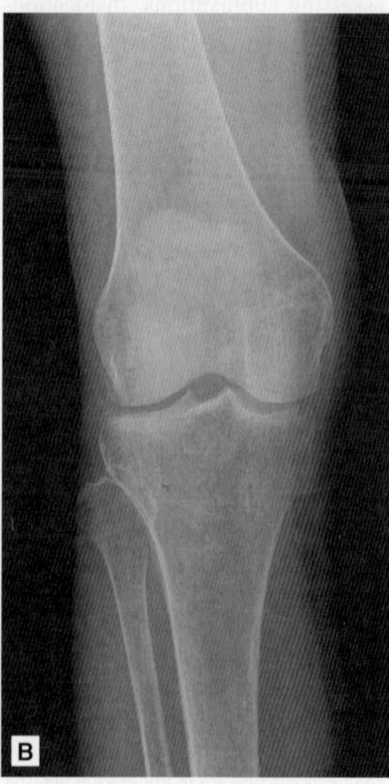

FIGURE 10.57 ■ Transverse Patellar Fracture. **A, B:** AP and lateral views of the right knee show a nondisplaced transverse fracture of the patella. A joint effusion is present.

Clinical Implications

Patients will present with knee pain and an effusion. The extensor mechanism must be evaluated, as its disruption is one of the indications for operative fixation. The patient should be asked to extend the knee from a flexed position. Inability to extend the lower leg against gravity indicates the extensor mechanism has been disrupted. Other indications for surgical intervention include displacement of fractured fragments greater than 2-3 mm or articular surface incongruity greater than 2-3 mm.

Pearls

1. The extensor mechanism must be tested in these patients by making them extend the lower leg against gravity.
2. AP, sunrise-patellar, and lateral views should be obtained to characterize the fracture type and assess the displacement and any potential articular incongruity.

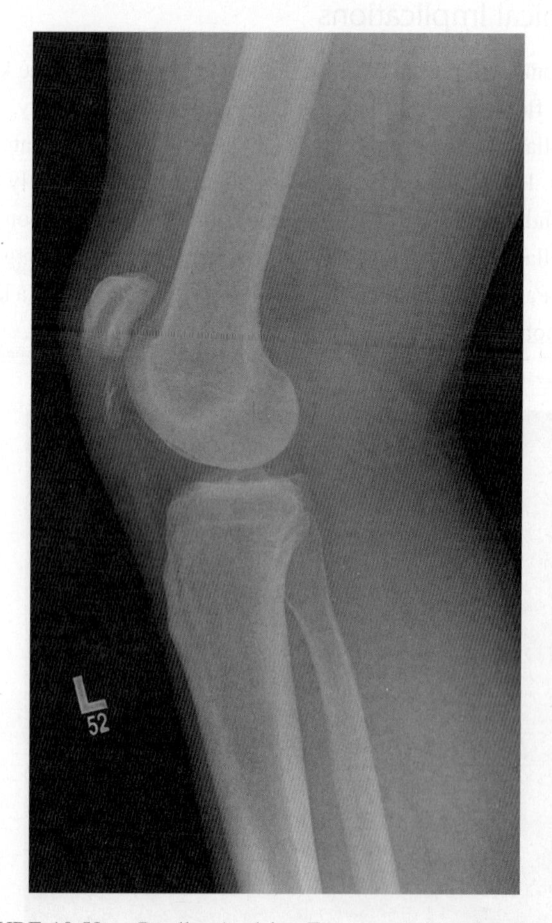

FIGURE 10.58 ■ Patellar Avulsion Fracture. A lateral radiograph of the left knee shows a distracted avulsion fracture of the inferior patellar pole.

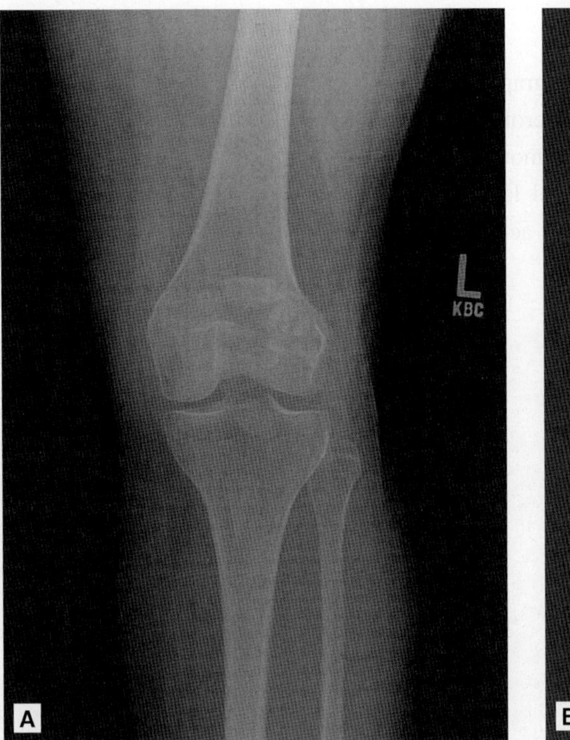

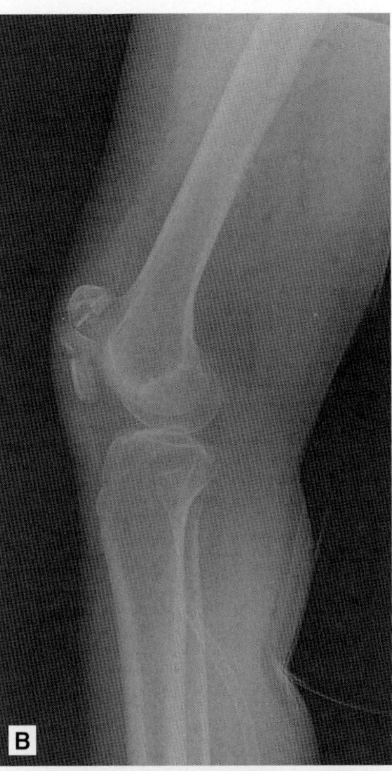

FIGURE 10.59 ■ Comminuted Patellar Fracture. **A, B:** AP and lateral views of the left knee show a severely comminuted fracture of the patella with some distraction of the proximal and distal fragments.

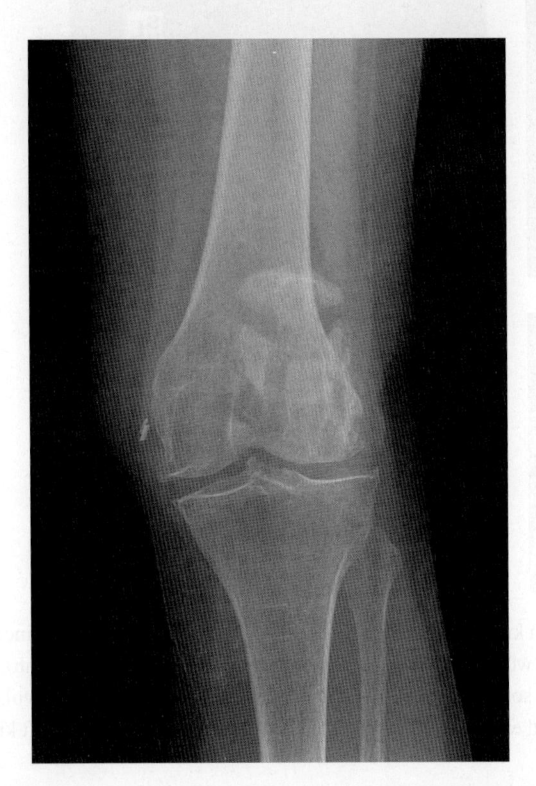

FIGURE 10.60 ■ Comminuted Patellar Fracture. An AP view of the left knee shows a stellate comminuted fracture of the left patella with mild displacement and distraction of the fractured fragments.

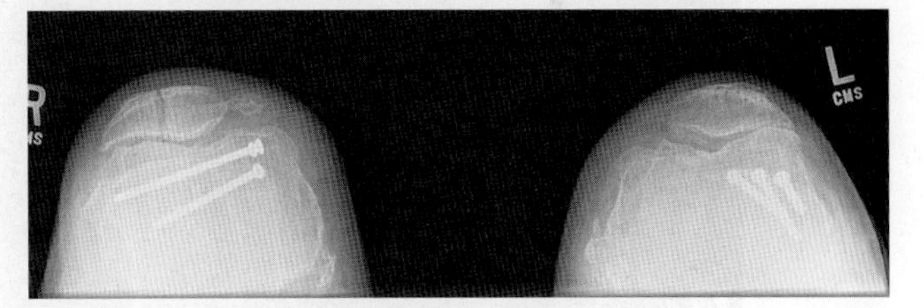

FIGURE 10.61 ■ Sagittal Patellar Fracture. A sunrise-patellar view of both patellae shows a nondisplaced sagitally oriented fracture of the right patella. Severe osteoarthritic changes are present in the patello-femoral compartments bilaterally.

Radiographic Summary

The bipartite patella can mimic a patellar fracture. Radiographs reveal a rounded ossicle, most commonly in the superolateral corner of the patella. The edges are sclerotic and smooth unlike with fractures where the edges are jagged and lack sclerosis ("naked trabeculi" are instead observed with acute fractures). Also, unlike with fractures, the components of a bipartite patella cannot be mentally reduced into a perfect patellar shape. Multipartite patellae exist as well; in those, multiple small ossicles are observed (again, typically in the superolateral patellar corner). The findings may be unilateral or bilateral.

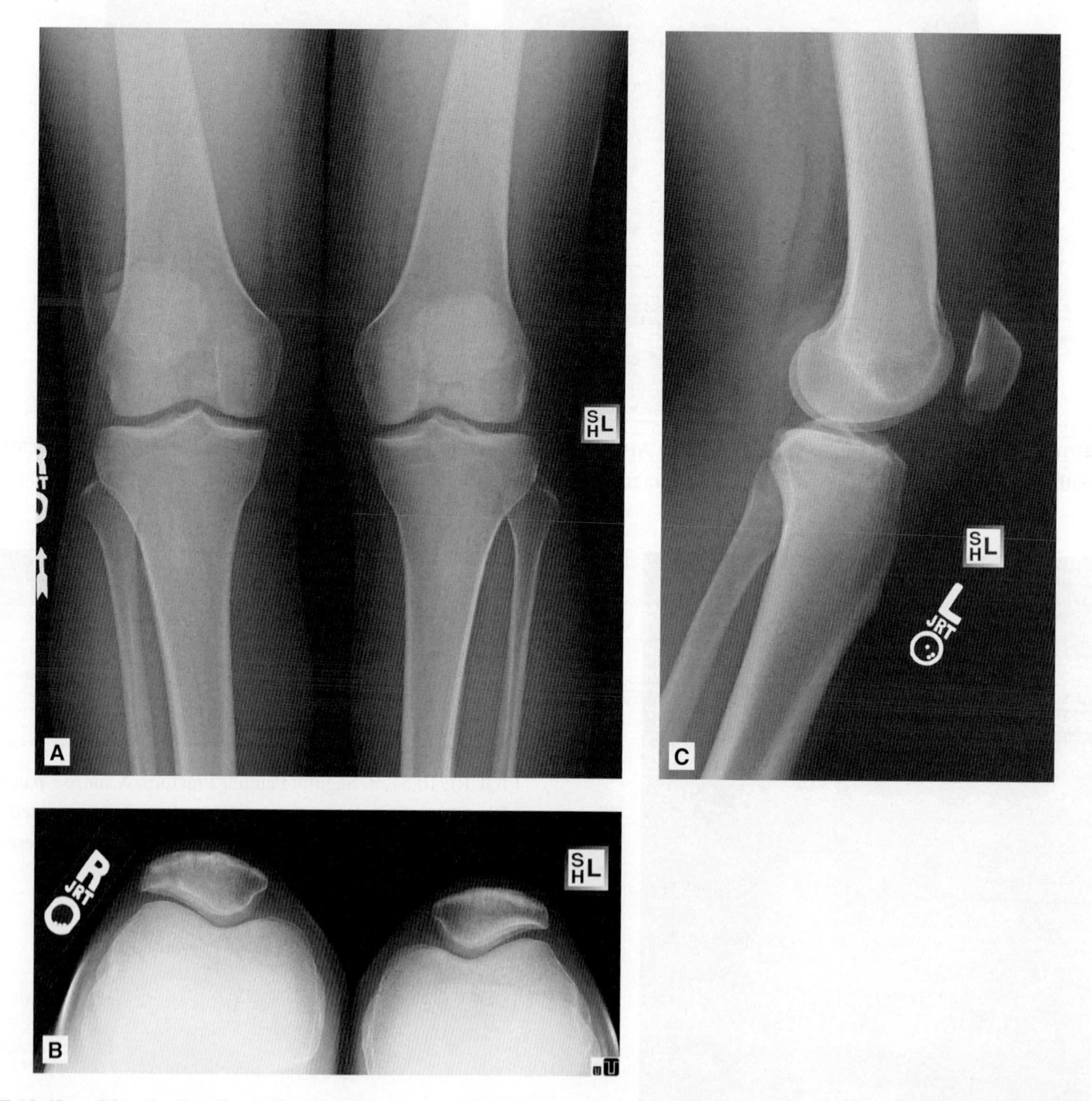

FIGURE 10.62 ■ Bipartite Patella. **A-C:** AP and sunrise-patellar views of both knees show a bipartite right patella. This is due to the incomplete fusion of an ossification center and is a normal variant. Notice how the two parts of the right patella could not be "reduced" into one perfect patella. The unfused ossification center is somewhat rounded and has a sclerotic edge. Incidentally, this patient has an acute avulsion fracture of the inferior pole of the left patella. This is visible on the AP view and even better demonstrated on the lateral view of the left knee.

Clinical Implications

Generally, the finding is asymptomatic and may be considered a normal variant. It is important to recognize it as such and not mistake it for a patellar fracture. Bipartite and multipartite patellae result from incomplete fusion of one or more of the patellar ossification centers.

Pearls

1. Rounded, smooth, and sclerotic edges characterize these normal variants. Conversely, acute fractures have jagged edges and "naked trabeculi," and can mentally be reduced into a perfect patellar shape.
2. Mimickers may be bilateral.

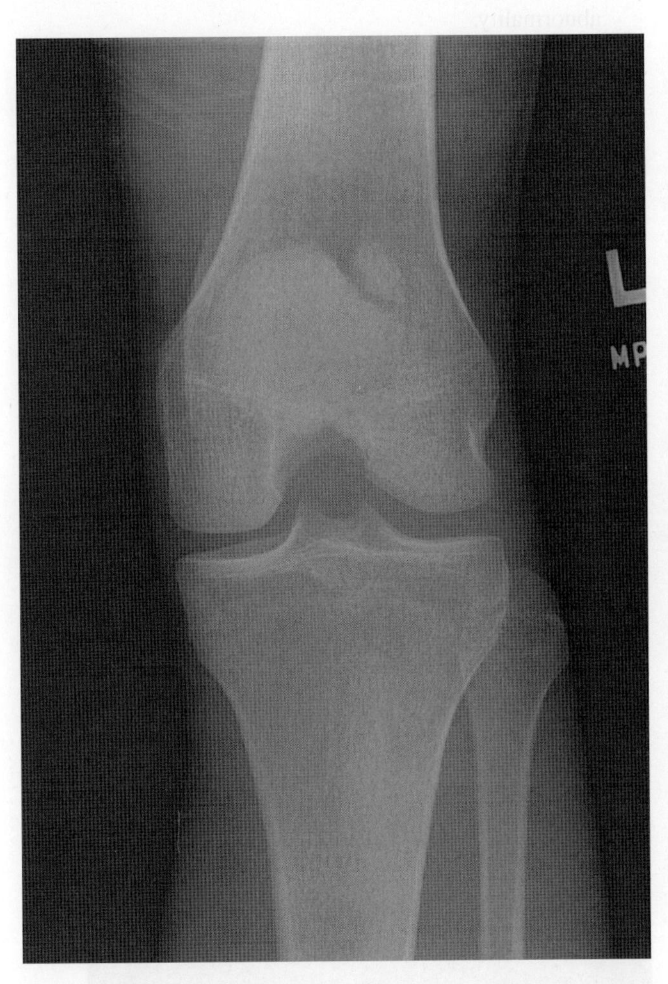

FIGURE 10.63 ■ Bipartite Patella. Another example of a bipartite patella, a normal variant. It most commonly occurs in the superolateral corner of the patella.

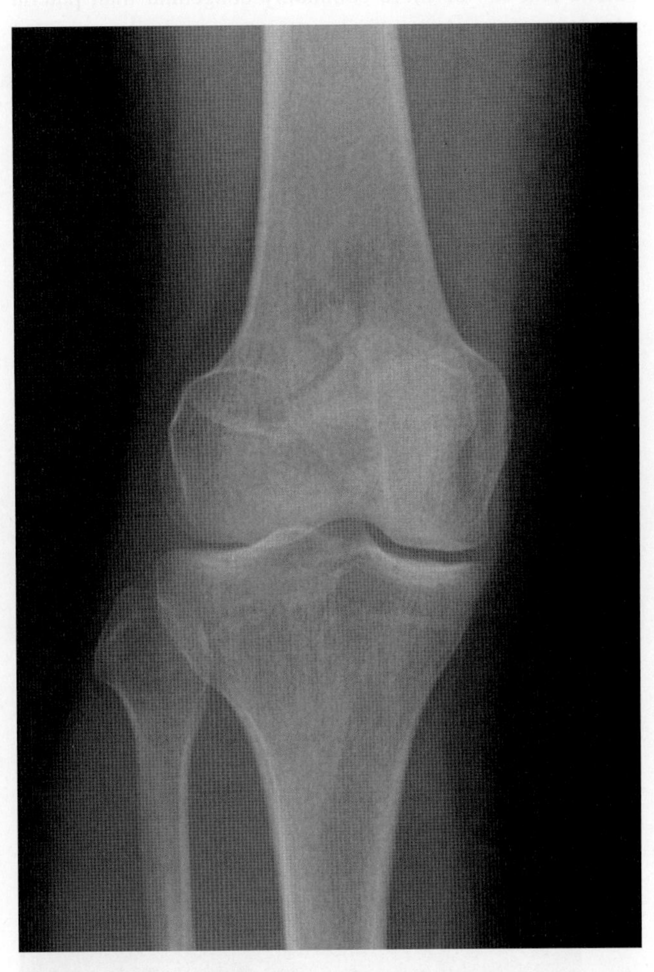

FIGURE 10.64 ■ Multipartite Patella. AP view of the right knee shows a multipartite patella: usually, the location is the same as seen in bipartite patellae but instead of just one accessory ossification center there are several. Also a normal variant. Should not be confused with a comminuted patellar fracture.

Radiographic Summary

Patella alta means a "high riding" patella and implies injury to the patellar ligament. A lateral radiograph is necessary to evaluate for the abnormality.

Clinical Implications

Patella alta can be more commonly congenital than patella baja; however, when associated with an acute injury and effusion, the patellar tendon is usually torn. An MRI can further characterize the injury.

Pearls

1. In the setting of an acute injury, patella alta indicates a tear of the patellar ligament.
2. A lateral radiograph is necessary to evaluate for the abnormality.

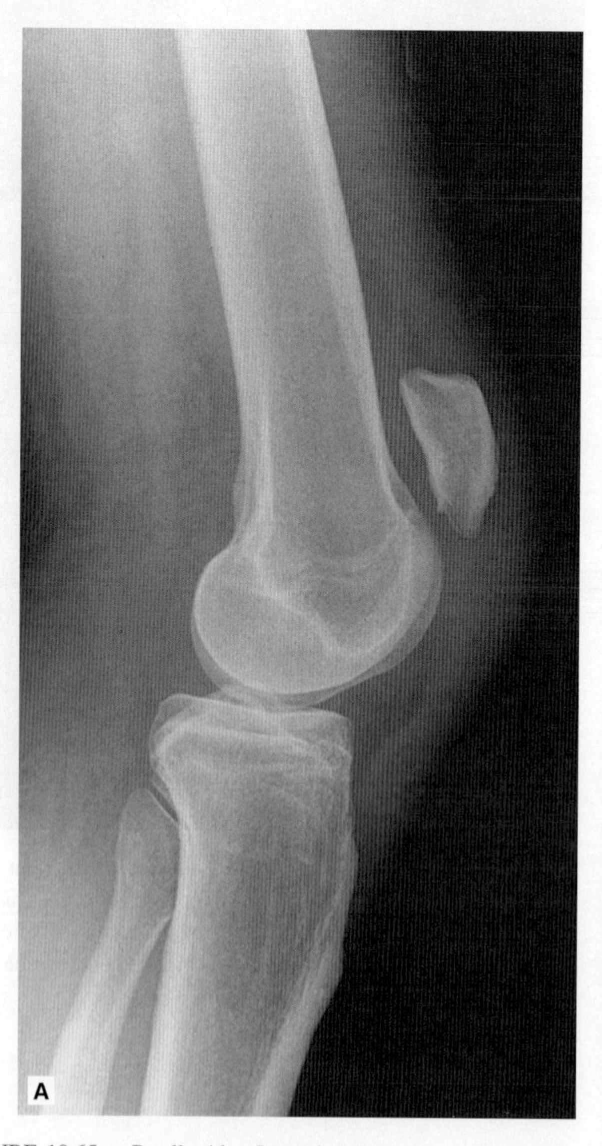

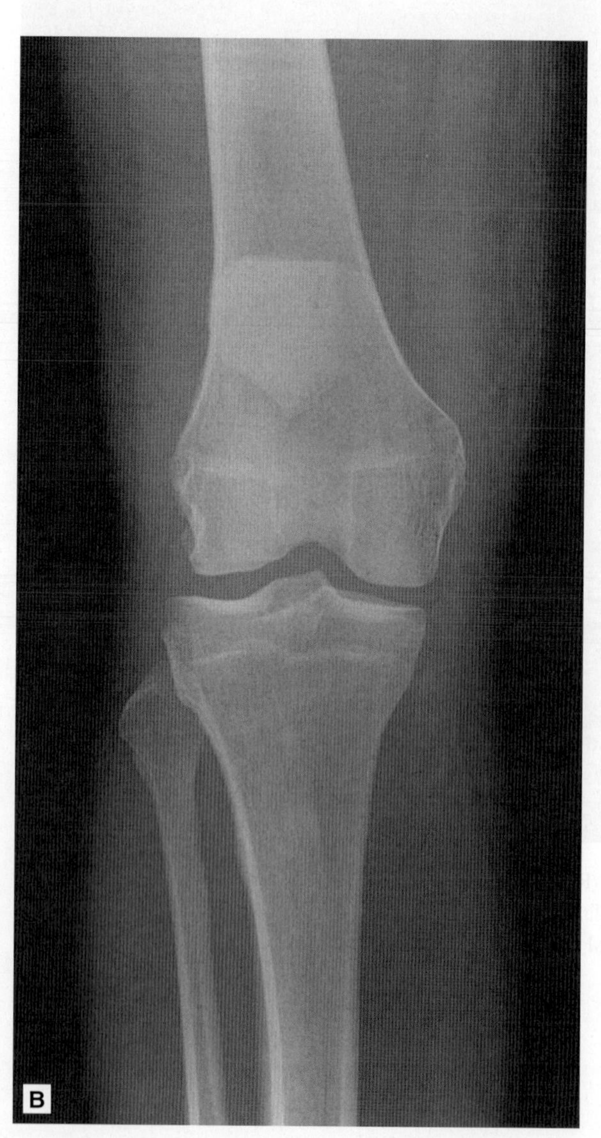

FIGURE 10.65 ■ Patella Alta. Lateral and AP views of the knee show a patella that resides too high: patella alta. There is thickening and edema around the patellar ligament both proximally and distally. The findings are consistent with injury to the patellar ligament.

Radiographic Summary

The lateral radiograph is the most important view to evaluate for the presence of Osgood–Schlatter disease. A lateral radiograph reveals fragmentation of the tibial tuberosity as well as elevation of the tubercle. Soft tissue edema may also be evident around the distal patellar ligament and in the inferior aspect of Hoffa's fat pad.

Clinical Implications

Patients present with anterior knee pain, localizing to the tibial tubercle. On exam, direct pressure over the tibial tuberosity elicits pain. Erythema can be seen at this site as well. Otherwise, the knee exam should be normal.

Pearls

1. Osgood–Schlatter disease is a clinical diagnosis. Radiographs are performed to rule out other conditions such as tumor or acute fracture.
2. A lateral radiograph of the knee reveals fragmentation of the tibial tuberosity.

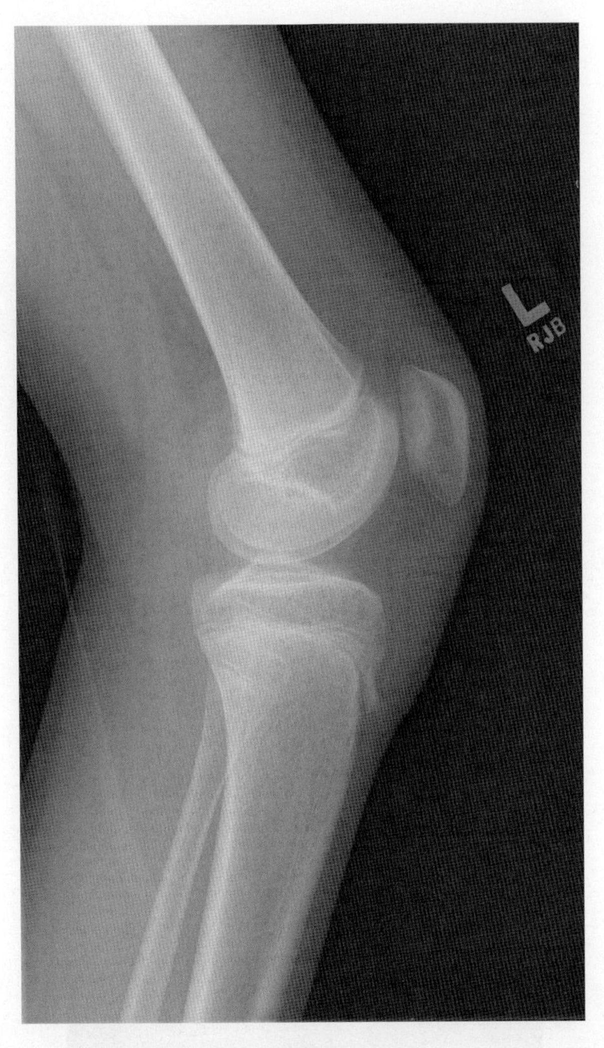

FIGURE 10.66 ■ Osgood–Schlatter Disease. A lateral view of the left knee of a child shows some fragmentation of the tibial tuberosity and extensive edema around the distal patellar ligament. The findings are consistent with Osgood–Schlatter disease.

Radiographic Summary

Radiographs are usually sufficient to demonstrate these injuries, especially in adults. Children can have subtle nondisplaced or minimally displaced oblique or spiral fractures that can be more difficult to discern.

Clinical Implications

Patients will present with leg pain, occasionally with an obvious deformity depending on the degree of angulation and displacement. The physical exam should include a careful neurovascular, soft tissue, and skin assessment. Leg fractures are associated with vascular injuries and compartment syndrome; careful and repeated assessments should be performed. Treatment is based on the type of fracture. Closed, nondisplaced fractures may be treated with a long-leg cast; otherwise, most orthopedic surgeons would recommend operative fixation.

Pearls

1. Pay close attention to the vascular system and soft tissues; monitor for compartment syndrome.
2. Be aware that children can have subtle nondisplaced or minimally displaced oblique or spiral fractures that can be more difficult to discern.

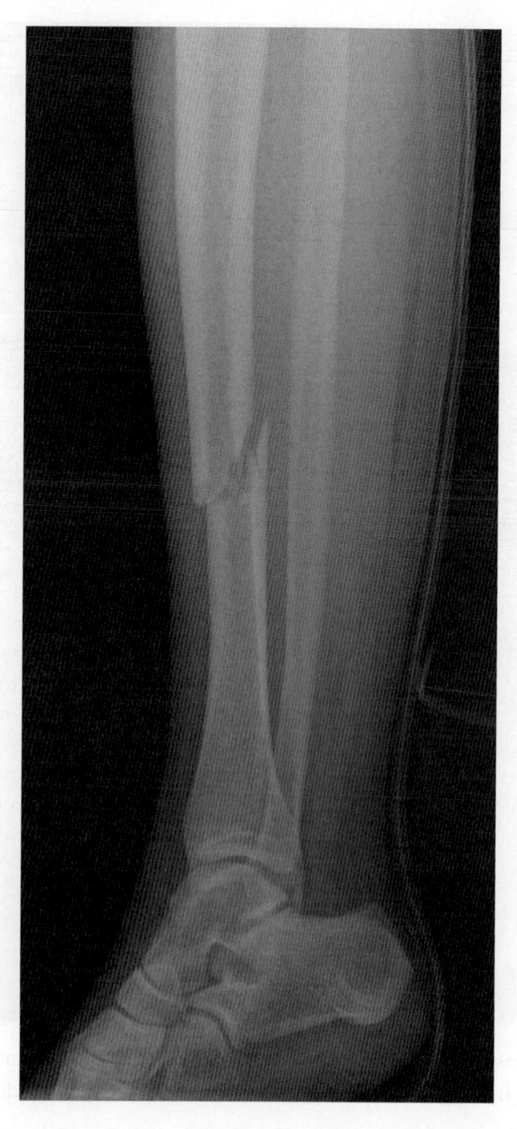

FIGURE 10.67 ■ Tibial Diaphysis Fracture. A lateral view of the distal leg shows a transverse fracture through the distal tibial diaphysis. The fracture is essentially nondisplaced.

Radiographic Summary

A Maisonneuve injury consists of injury to the medial ankle (medial malleolar fracture or deltoid ligament complex injury), distal tibio-fibular syndesmotic injury, injury to the interosseous membrane, and a proximal fibular fracture. An AP or mortise view of the ankle shows a medial malleolar fracture or abnormal widening of the medial joint space. If the distal tibio-fibular syndesmotic space is abnormally wide but there is no "exit" distal fibular fracture, a proximal fibular fracture and, therefore, a Maisonneuve injury should be suspected. An AP radiograph of the leg will demonstrate the proximal fibular shaft fracture.

Clinical Implications

A Maisonneuve injury is a proximal fibular fracture associated with an external rotation injury to the ankle. The energy enters the ankle medially and travels proximally along the syndesmosis membrane, subsequently exiting through the proximal fibula. Patients present with an ankle injury and tenderness over the proximal fibula. Other physical exam findings included tenderness over the anterior tibio-fibular ligament, positive squeeze test, and pain with external rotation. This injury requires a high index suspicion and radiographs of the leg, in addition to the AP, mortise, and lateral radiographs of the injured ankle. The treatment for this injury depends upon the stability of the ankle and the syndesmosis. This stability can be assessed with gravity stress views of the ankle.

Pearls

1. The ankle exam always starts at the knee.
2. If a patient sustains a medial ankle injury and the distal tibio-fibular syndesmotic space is abnormally wide but there is no "exit" distal fibular fracture, a proximal fibular fracture and, therefore, a Maisonneuve injury should be suspected. An additional AP radiograph of the leg should be obtained and will demonstrate the proximal fibular shaft fracture.

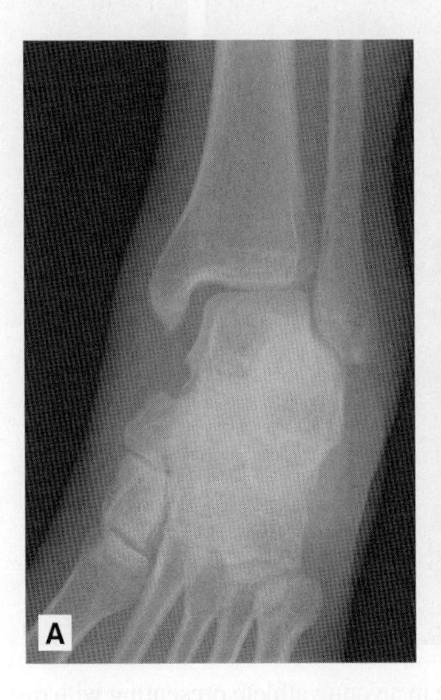

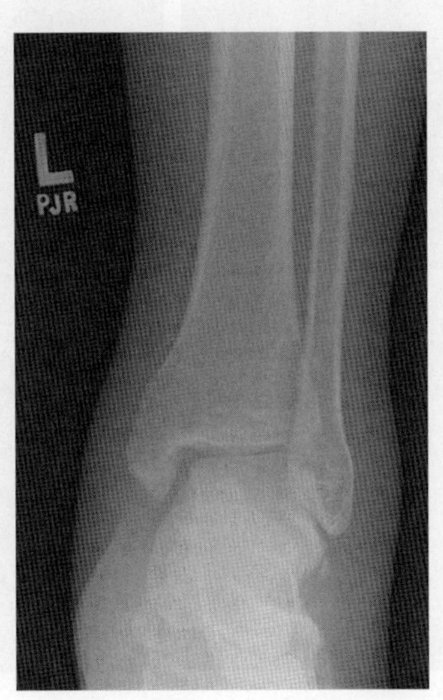

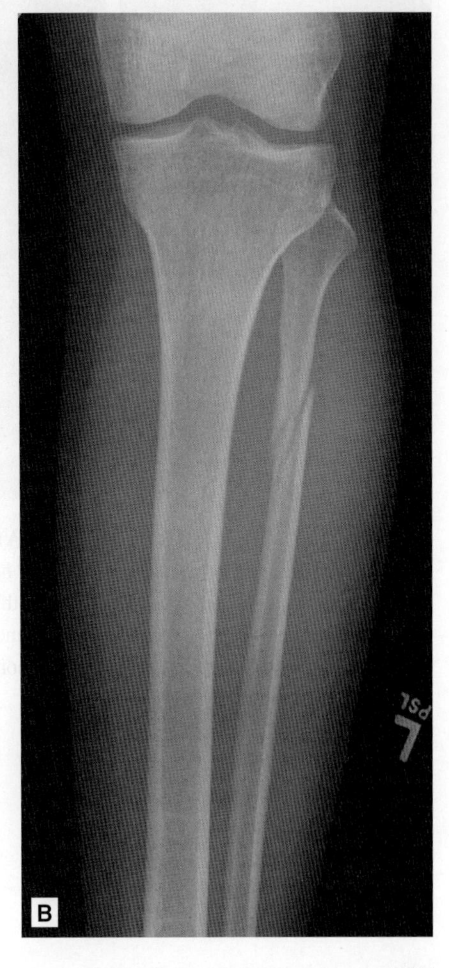

FIGURE 10.68 ■ Maisonneuve Fracture. **A, B:** AP view of the left ankle shows abnormal widening of the medial aspect of the ankle mortise, abnormal widening of the distal tibio-fibular syndesmosis, and slight lateral subluxation of the talar dome. No avulsion fracture is evident from the medial malleolus. The findings are consistent with injury to the deltoid ligament complex and distal tibio-fibular syndesmotic injury. Because no fracture is present on the distal fibula, a fracture of the proximal fibula was suspected by the radiologist. The clinician was called and an AP view of the leg was recommended. An AP view of the upper left leg shows a nondisplaced oblique fracture of the proximal fibular shaft. These are the findings of Maisonneuve injury. Most of the time, the clinician suspects this type of injury because of tenderness to palpation over the proximal fibula. In this case, the clinicians were unaware of the injury.

Radiographic Summary

Acute stress fractures are radiographically occult. Seven to ten days after a stress fracture develops, radiographs can detect periosteal new bone formation at the level of the fracture or a sclerotic band within the medullary bone corresponding to the healing fracture. Acute stress fractures can be detected only with an MRI.

Clinical Implications

Tibial stress fractures can be either low risk (posterior–medial) or high risk (anterior–lateral). Patients present with localized pain exacerbated with impact and occasionally swelling at the site. For tibial stress fractures, consider presumptive treatment with radiographic follow-up in 7-10 days. If immediate imaging confirmation is required, this can be accomplished with an MRI.

Pearls

1. Consider this diagnosis in patients who have recently started or increased their training regimens and present with tibial pain.
2. Acute stress fractures are radiographically occult; stress fractures become visible on radiographs in 7-10 days.
3. Acute stress fractures can be diagnosed only with an MRI. CT cannot detect acute stress fractures.

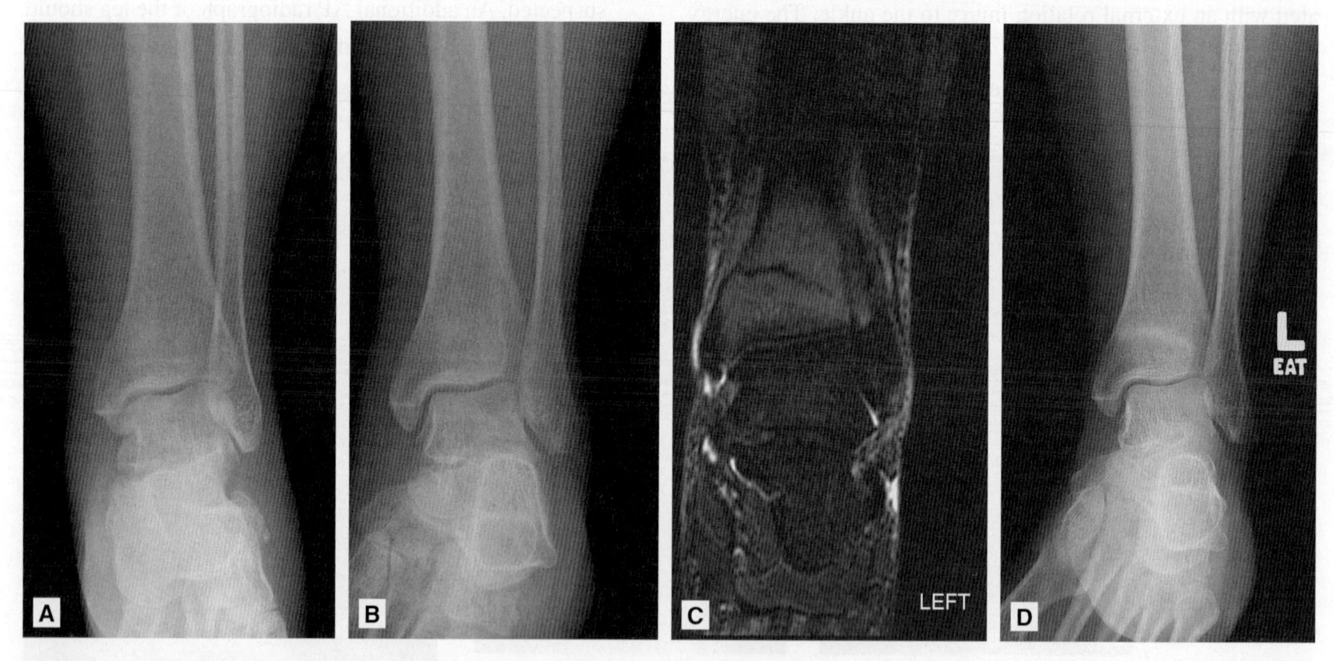

FIGURE 10.69 ■ Tibial Stress Fracture. AP (**A**) and oblique (**B**) views of the left ankle in a young athlete presenting with distal tibial/ankle pain show no fracture. The bones and joints appear normal. **C:** An MRI was obtained to evaluate for a stress fracture. This coronal FS T2-weighted image shows a jagged T2 hypointense line within the medial aspect of the distal tibial metaphysic extending perpendicular to the long axis of the bone. This is a stress fracture that is surrounded by extensive marrow edema. **D:** Healing tibial stress fracture. One month later, an AP view of the ankle shows a band of sclerosis corresponding perfectly to the stress fracture seen on the prior MRI. This is the typical appearance of a healing stress fracture.

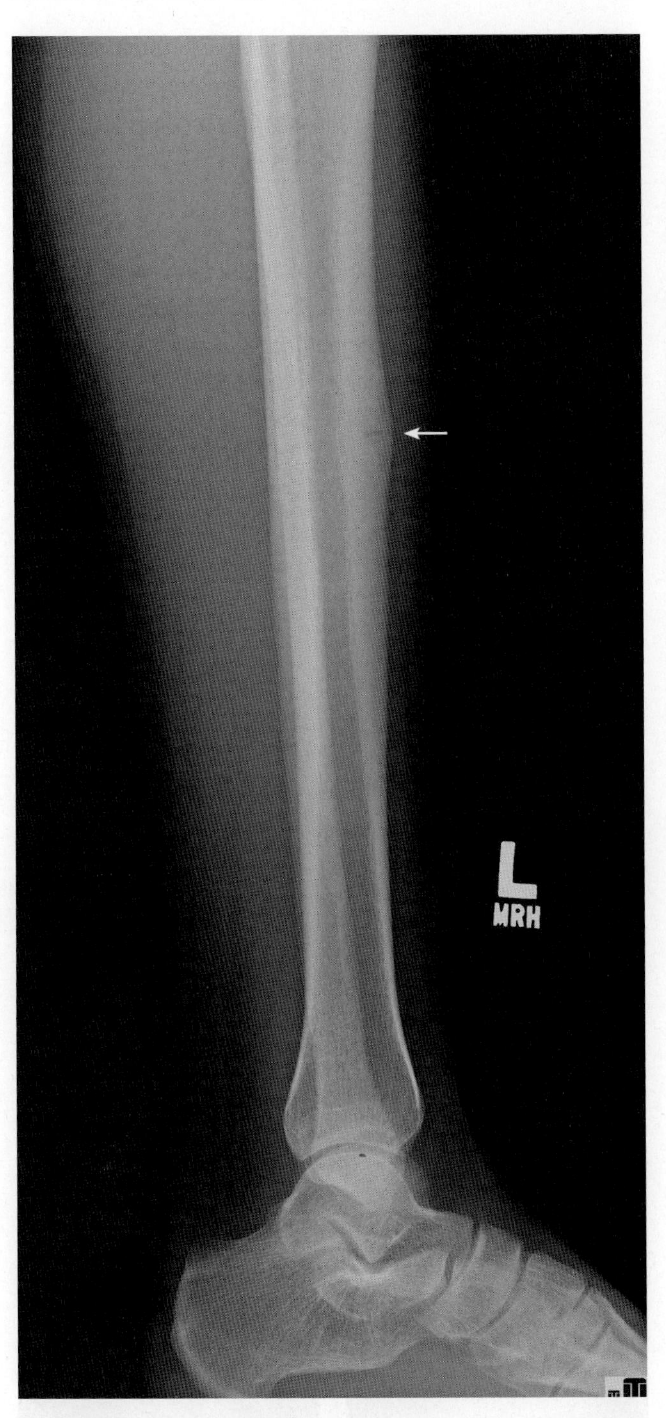

FIGURE 10.70 ■ Healing Tibial Stress Fracture. A lateral view of the distal left leg shows a small linear lucency within the anterior cortex of the mid tibia (arrow). This is covered by a small amount of solid periosteal new bone formation. The findings represent a healing cortical stress fracture in a young runner.

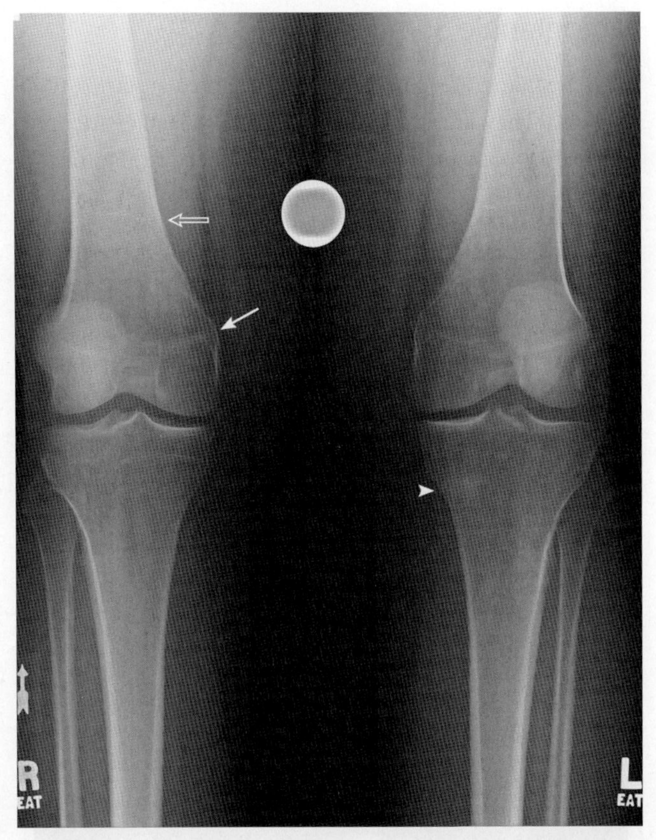

FIGURE 10.71 ■ Healing Tibial Stress Fracture. An AP view of the knees shows a fuzzy thick band of sclerosis in the medial aspect of the proximal left tibial metaphysis (arrowhead). This is a healing stress fracture. Notice the fused growth plates (arrow) and growth arrest lines (open arrow): these are much thinner white lines and should not be confused for stress fractures.

PILON FRACTURE

Radiographic Summary

Pilon fractures are comminuted intra-articular distal tibial fractures. They are inherently extremely unstable. AP, mortise, and lateral views of the ankle can delineate the fracture planes in most instances. A CT of the ankle is often necessary for complete characterization of the fracture planes, intra-articular fracture extension, and articular surface congruity.

FIGURE 10.72 ■ Pilon Fracture. AP view of the left ankle shows a severely comminuted intra-articular distal tibial fracture and a fracture of the distal fibular shaft.

Clinical Implications

Pilon fractures, the combination of an ankle fracture and distal tibial metaphyseal fracture usually with intra-articular extension, result from the talus being driven into the tibia. Patients will present with an obvious deformity and pain. Associated injuries include compression fractures, tibial plateau fractures, and neurovascular injuries. The soft tissues can be compromised with these injuries and compartment syndrome can occur. Treatment for these injuries is operative.

Pearls

1. Monitor the patient closely for compartment syndrome and soft tissue necrosis.
2. A CT scan may be required to accurately and completely characterize these fractures.

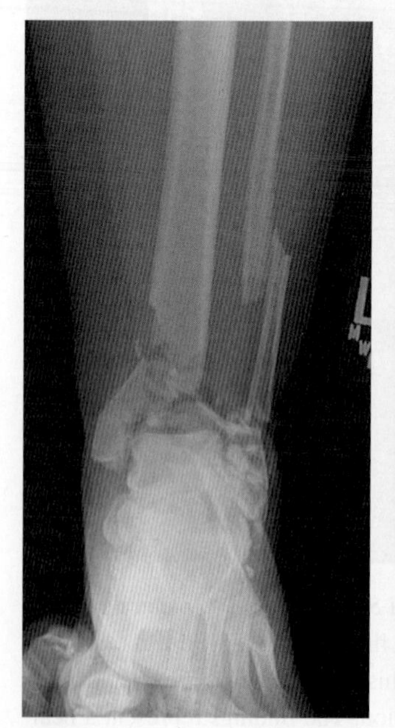

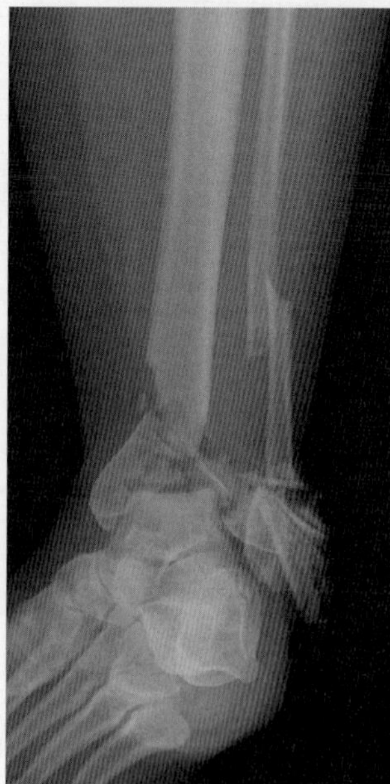

FIGURE 10.73 ■ Pilon Fracture (Companion Case). AP and oblique views of the left ankle show a severely comminuted intra-articular distal tibial and a comminuted distal fibular fractures.

Radiographic Summary

Eversion ankle injuries result in a transverse medial malleolar fracture (or injury to the deltoid ligament complex) and an oblique fracture of the distal fibula. AP, lateral, and mortise views of the ankle are sufficient to characterize the fractures. Look carefully for signs of distal tibiofibular syndesmotic injury if the distal fibular fracture is above the level of the syndesmosis. Stress views can help in this regard.

Clinical Implications

Treatment of these fractures depends upon ankle stability. If the stress views are positive, operative fixation is indicated. Patients with negative stress views can be treated with a posterior sugar tong splint and kept non-weight-bearing.

Pearls

1. The ankle exam starts with the knee.
2. Stress views can help to assess for stability.
3. Don't forget to evaluate the posterior malleolus with these injuries.

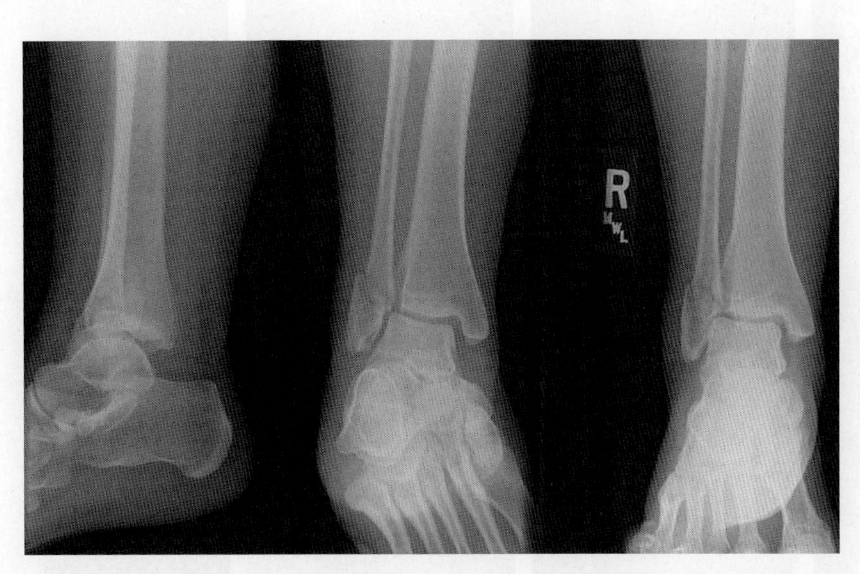

FIGURE 10.74 ■ Ankle Eversion Injury. AP, mortise, and lateral views of the right ankle show slight widening of the medial aspect of the ankle mortise and an oblique fracture of the lateral malleolus extending medially to the level of the tibio-talar joint. There is some soft tissue swelling about the right ankle joint.

Radiographic Summary

Radiographs are usually sufficient to reveal the fracture. It is important to obtain the entire ankle series consisting of anterior–posterior, lateral, and mortise views. Stress views may be necessary to evaluate ankle stability.

Clinical Implications

The ankle consists of three malleoli: lateral, medial, and posterior. Any combination of fractures and/or ligamentous injuries can occur. A stress view is often helpful in evaluating ankle stability. Treatment is based on fracture location and ankle stability.

Pearls

1. If there is concern for ligamentous injury, stress views can be helpful.
2. Stress views also help in assessing the distal tibio-fibular syndesmosis.
3. Don't forget to evaluate the posterior malleolus.

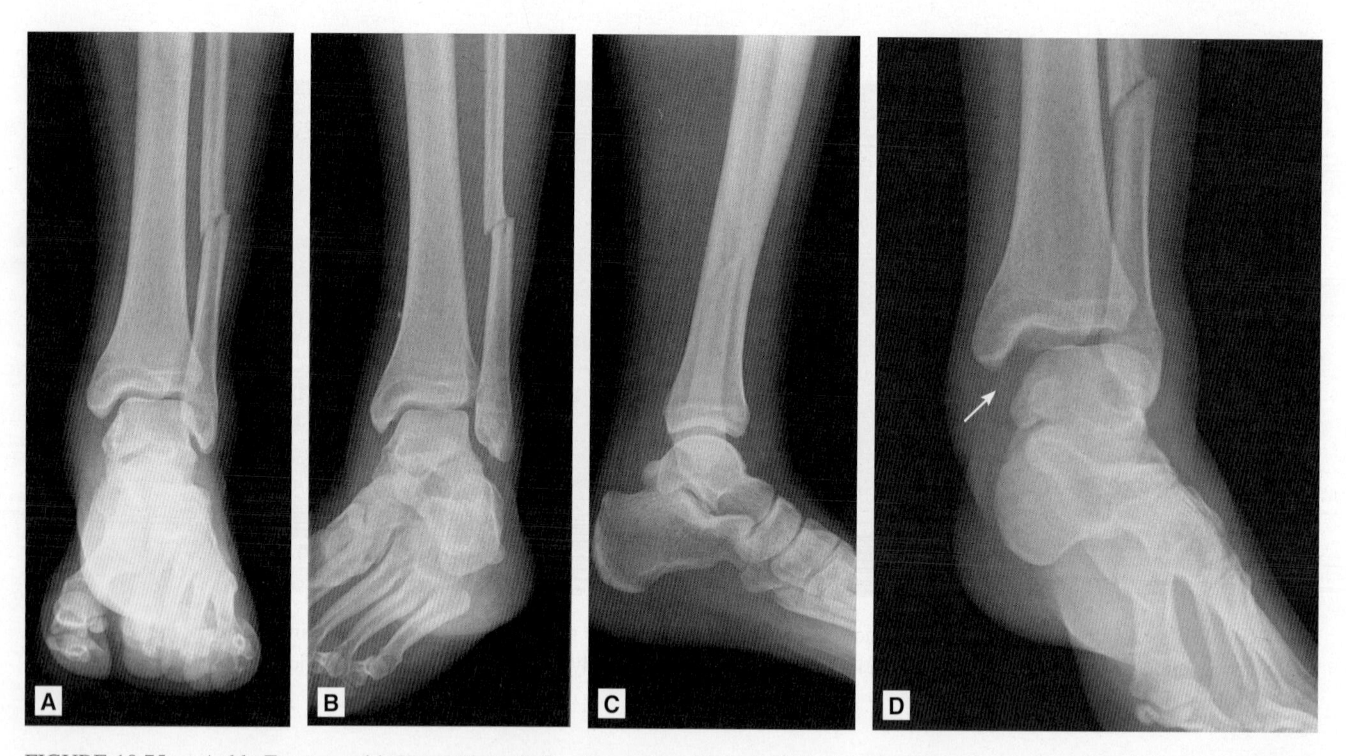

FIGURE 10.75 ■ Ankle Fracture with Stress View. **A-C:** AP mortise and lateral views of the ankle show an oblique fracture of the distal fibular shaft. The alignment of the ankle mortise is normal on these views. The pattern of the distal fibular fracture suggests an eversion injury. A stress view (**D**) was performed to evaluate the stability of the deltoid ligament complex. This additional view shows marked abnormal widening of the medial aspect of the ankle mortise (arrow) consistent with the rupture of the deltoid ligament complex due to an eversion injury.

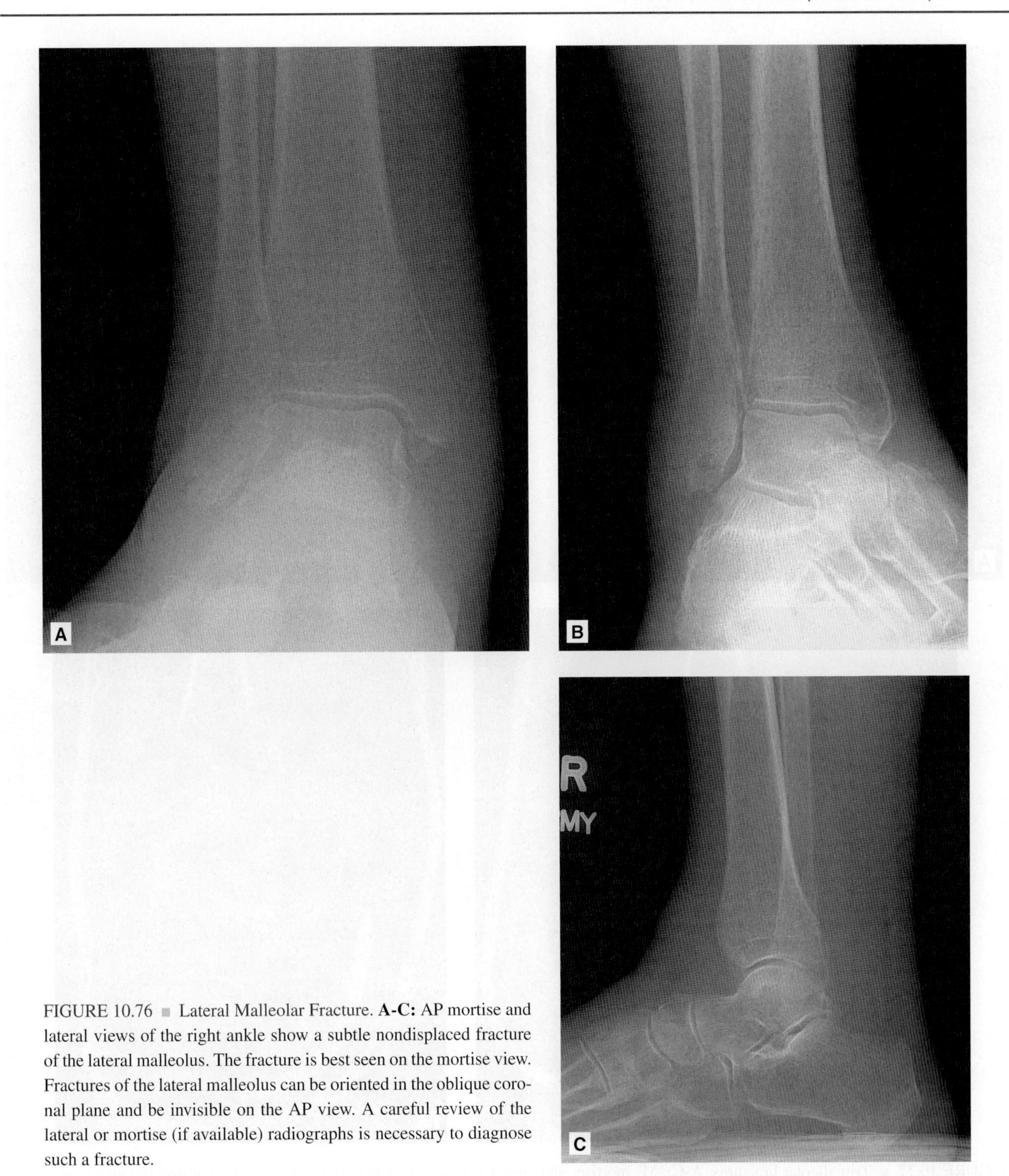

FIGURE 10.76 ■ Lateral Malleolar Fracture. **A-C:** AP mortise and lateral views of the right ankle show a subtle nondisplaced fracture of the lateral malleolus. The fracture is best seen on the mortise view. Fractures of the lateral malleolus can be oriented in the oblique coronal plane and be invisible on the AP view. A careful review of the lateral or mortise (if available) radiographs is necessary to diagnose such a fracture.

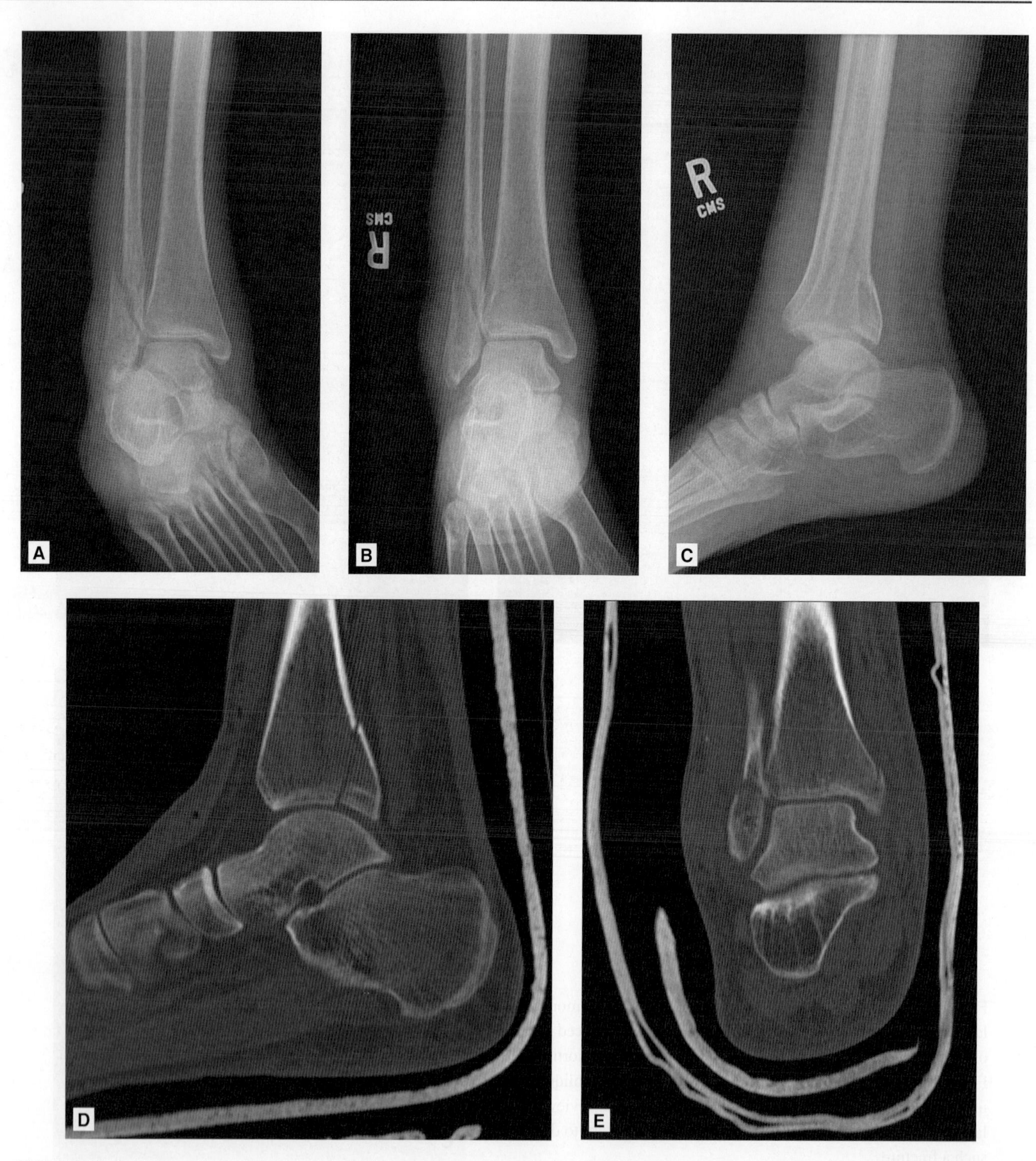

FIGURE 10.77 ■ Trimalleolar Fractures. **A-C:** AP, mortise, and lateral views of the right ankle show a tiny avulsion fracture from the tip of the medial malleolus, an oblique fracture of the lateral malleolus, and an oblique fracture of the posterior lip of the distal tibia (posterior malleolus). There is extensive soft tissue edema. **D, E:** Coronally and sagitally reformatted CT images nicely demonstrate the same fractures.

Radiographic Summary

This injury involves a transverse fracture of the lateral malleolus (or rupture of the lateral collateral ligaments) and an oblique fracture of the medial malleolus. Radiographs are sufficient to demonstrate the fractures. It is important to obtain the entire ankle series consisting of anterior–posterior, lateral, and mortise views.

Clinical Implications

These fractures require operative fixation.

Pearls

1. These fractures are usually treated surgically due to the medial malleolus fracture.
2. Don't forget to evaluate the posterior malleolus with these injuries.

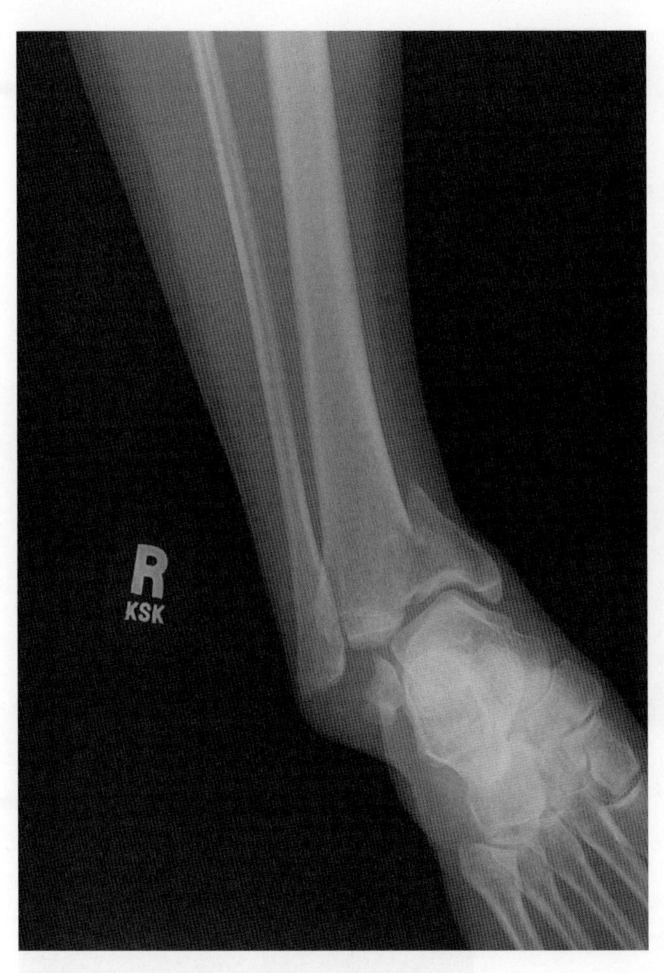

FIGURE 10.78 ■ Ankle Inversion Injury. AP view of the right ankle shows a transversely oriented avulsion fracture of the lateral malleolus, medial subluxation of the talar dome, and an obliquely oriented fracture of the medial malleolus. Notice that the lateral malleolar fracture is transverse (it got pulled off) and the medial malleolar fracture is oblique (it got pushed aside).

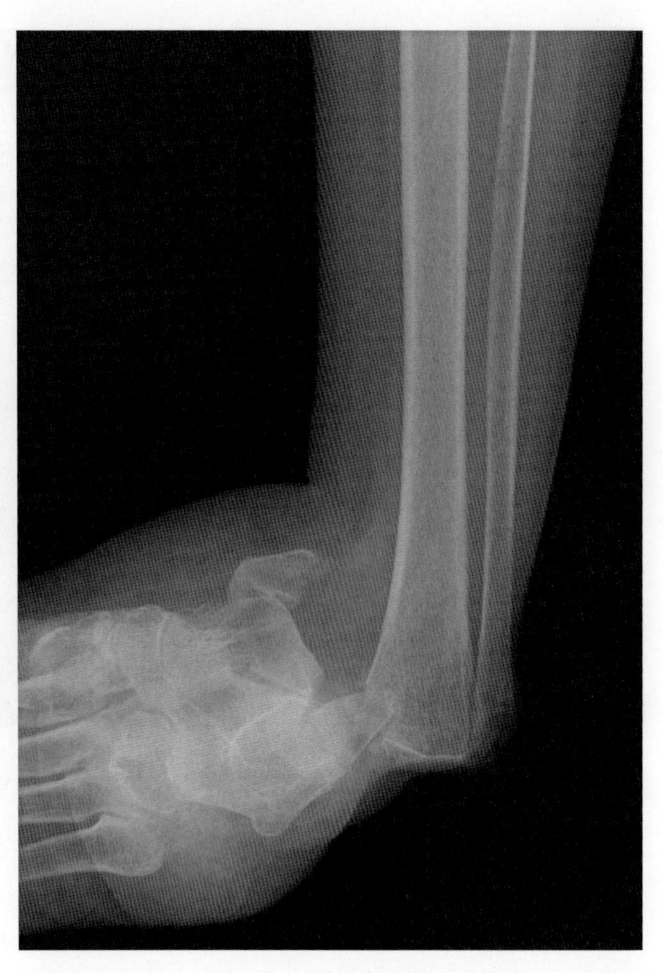

FIGURE 10.79 ■ Ankle Inversion Injury (Companion Case). Severe injury with medial dislocation of the talar dome and medial and lateral malleolar fractures.

TRIPLANE FRACTURE

Radiographic Summary

Radiographs are usually sufficient to demonstrate the injury. A CT scan can be utilized to better delineate the fracture planes.

Clinical Implications

Triplane fractures occur in adolescents and require open growth plates. This fracture derives its name from the three fracture planes that it creates: a coronal fracture through the distal tibial metaphysis, a transverse fracture through a portion of the distal tibial physis, and a sagital fracture through the distal tibial epiphysis. These patients present with pain and swelling. Treatment is surgical.

Pearls

1. Triplane fractures are associated with a high risk of premature physeal closure.
2. Although radiographs are usually sufficient to demonstrate the injury, CT may be utilized to better delineate the fracture planes and assist in operative planning.

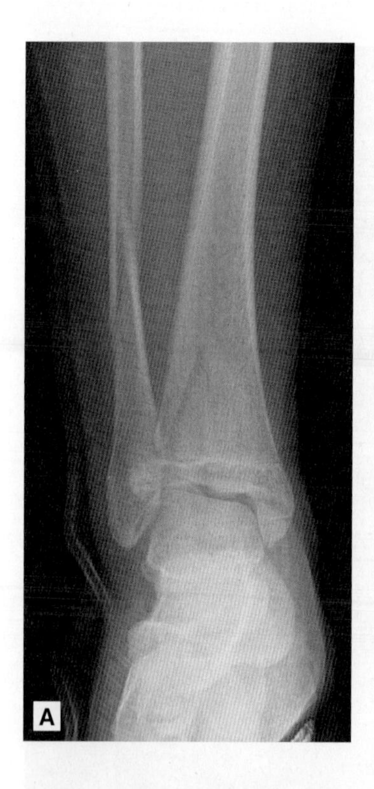

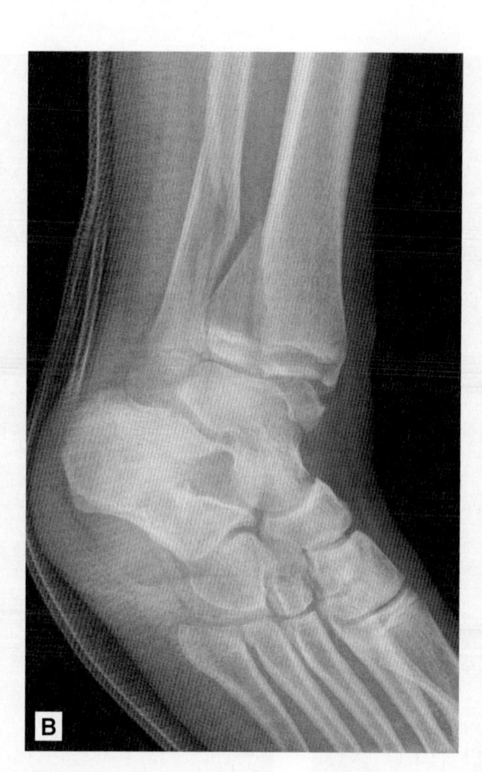

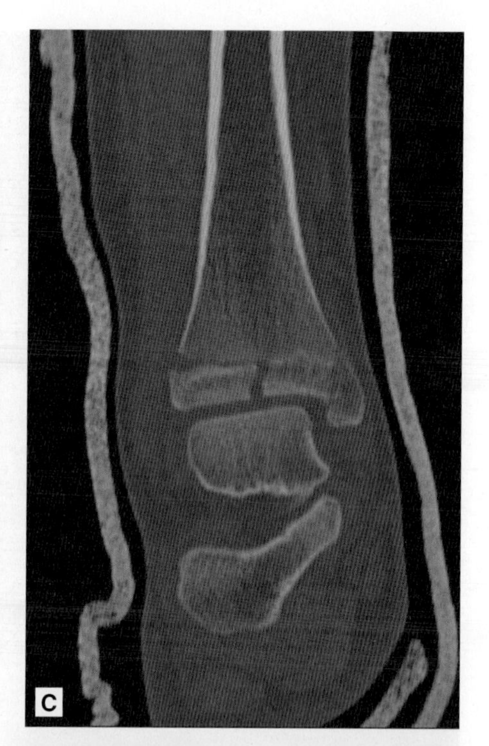

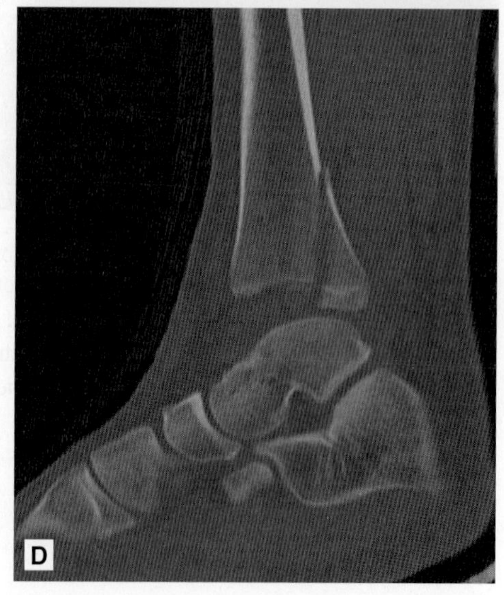

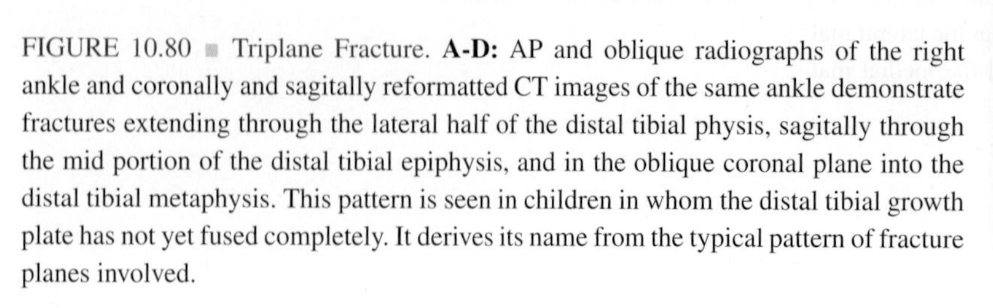

FIGURE 10.80 ■ Triplane Fracture. **A-D:** AP and oblique radiographs of the right ankle and coronally and sagitally reformatted CT images of the same ankle demonstrate fractures extending through the lateral half of the distal tibial physis, sagitally through the mid portion of the distal tibial epiphysis, and in the oblique coronal plane into the distal tibial metaphysis. This pattern is seen in children in whom the distal tibial growth plate has not yet fused completely. It derives its name from the typical pattern of fracture planes involved.

Radiographic Summary

Radiographs are usually sufficient to demonstrate these uncommon injuries. A CT may be utilized to better delineate the fracture plane.

Clinical Implications

The talar dome is an unusual fracture site. Fractures of the talar dome can occur with direct axial load or with ankle twisting. Treatment depends on the degree of displacement.

Pearls

1. Talar fractures may be very subtle on conventional radiographs. Carefully assess the talar dome on the AP and mortise views. Coronally-oriented fractures may only be visible on the lateral view.
2. CT scan can be used to better delineate the fracture and assist in operative planning.

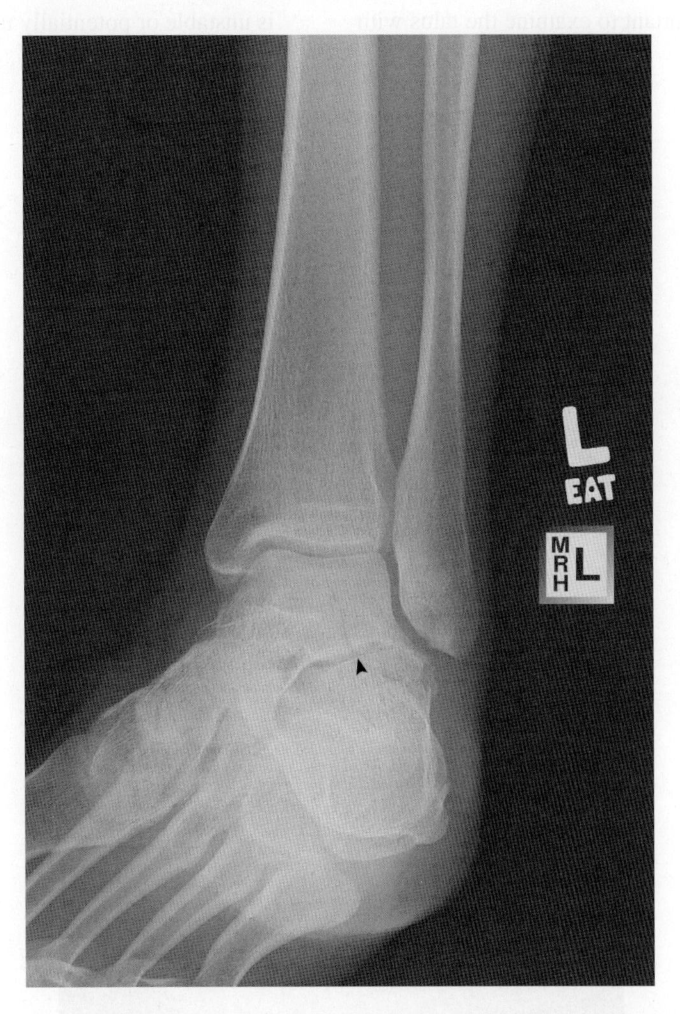

FIGURE 10.81 ■ Talar Dome Fracture. A mortise view of the left ankle shows a very subtle nondisplaced fracture extending in a sagital fashion through the talar dome (arrowhead).

Radiographic Summary

Initial radiographs can be normal in 1/3 of cases. Lesions can be either medial or lateral and are similar in appearance to knee OCD lesions (sclerotic, rounded edges).

Clinical Implications

Talar OCD lesions generally result from trauma disrupting blood flow to the talar dome or a subchondral bone fracture. Patients will present with pain, reduced range of motion, and possibly with mechanical symptoms. They may be tender on exam over the talus. It is important to examine the talus with the foot in plantarflexion to assess the anterolateral dome and in dorsiflexion to assess the posteromedial dome. If the radiographs are normal but clinical suspicion remains high, an MRI should be obtained for further evaluation.

Pearls

1. Palpate the talus with the foot in various positions to assess for the presence of a talar osteochondral lesion.
2. An MRI is the study of choice to evaluate for talar OCD lesions. It can identify lesions that are invisible on conventional radiographs. It can also determine if the lesion is unstable or potentially unstable.

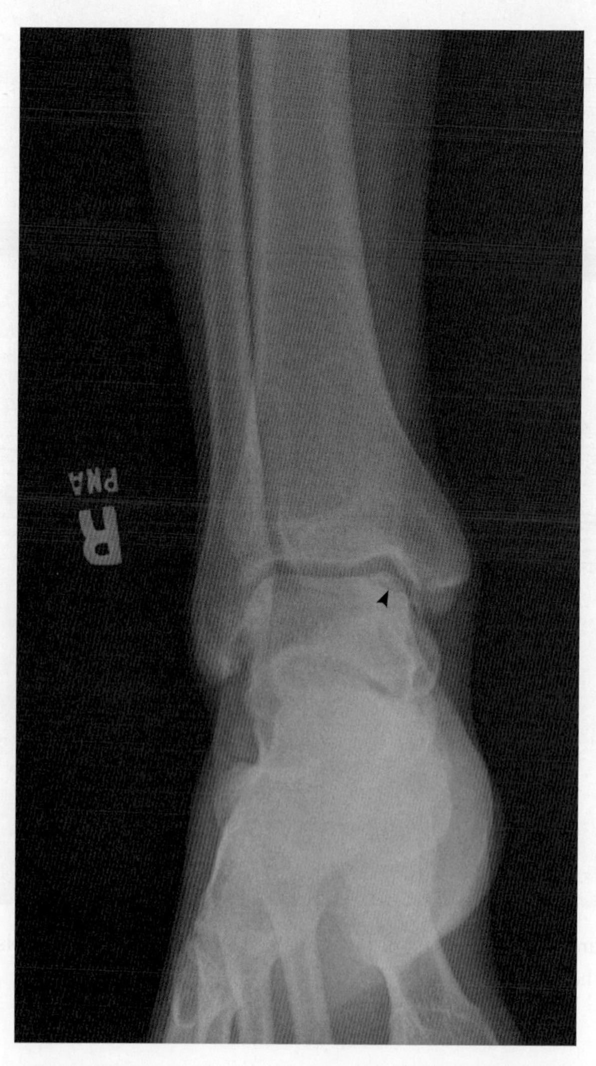

FIGURE 10.82 ■ Subchondral Fracture or Osteochondral Lesion. This AP view of the right ankle shows a subtle subchondral lucency in the most medial aspect of the talar dome (arrowhead). This is consistent with a subchondral fracture or an osteochondral lesion, depending on the clinical scenario (acute injury vs. more chronic pain). There is no evidence of subchondral collapse at this time.

Radiographic Summary

Radiographs are usually sufficient to demonstrate the fracture. CT can better delineate the location and extent of the fracture.

Clinical Implications

Talar neck fractures are due to high energy imparted to the foot while in a dorsiflexed position. The talar neck is driven into the anterior tibia. A classification system devised by Hawkins is frequently used to describe these fractures. This classification system portends more to the likelihood of ostenecrosis as a complication of the fracture type than acute treatment. Patients will present with pain, swelling, and ecchymosis over the anterior ankle. Closed reduction should be performed as soon as possible because these fractures are associated with high rates of talar dome osteonecrosis. Treatment involves operative fixation.

Pearls

1. Displaced fractures of the talar neck require emergent reduction.
2. CT scan should be utilized to better delineate the fracture and assist in operative planning.

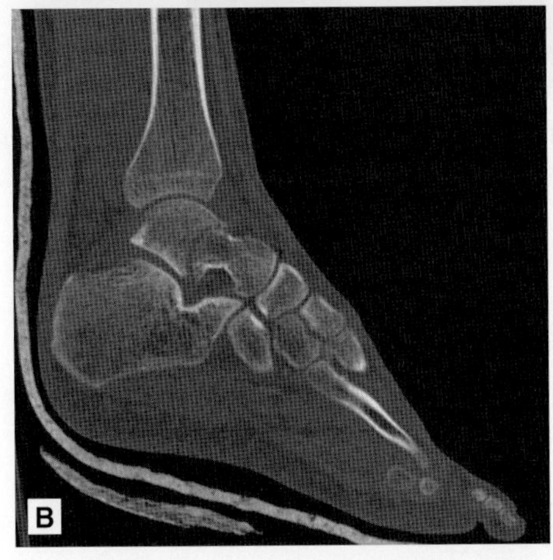

FIGURE 10.83 ■ Talar Neck Fracture. **A:** A lateral view of the left foot shows a very subtle nondisplaced fracture of the talar neck. There is some soft tissue edema about the ankle. **B:** A CT was performed as well. This sagitally reformatted CT image nicely demonstrates the nondisplaced fracture of the talar neck and precisely delineates the extent and directionality of the fracture. This can be invaluable to the orthopoedic surgeon for surgical planning.

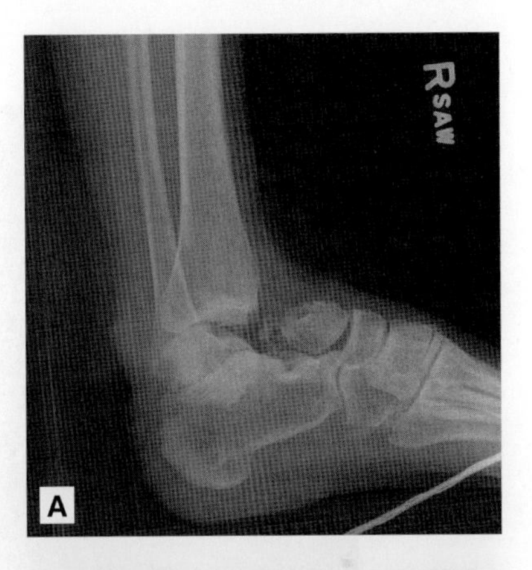

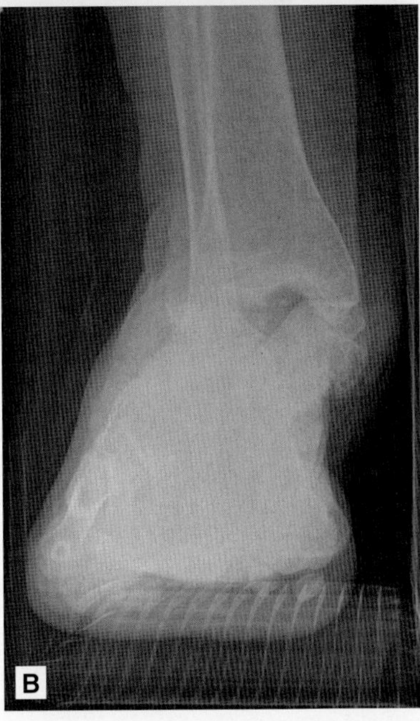

FIGURE 10.84 ■ Talar Neck Fracture (Companion Case). **A, B:** Lateral and AP views of the right ankle show a severely displaced talar neck fracture with subtalar dislocation and medial ejection of the talar dome. Such severely displaced talar neck fractures (Hawkins 4) have a very high association with the subsequent development of talar dome osteonecrosis.

Radiographic Summary

AP and mortise views of the ankle are optimal to evaluate for this fracture. A CT may be obtained if the radiographs are negative but clinical suspicion remains high.

Clinical Implications

The lateral process of the talus is commonly injured during snowboarding. Patients present with anterolateral ankle pain and are often misdiagnosed with anterolateral ankle sprain. Nondisplaced fractures can be treated with a short leg cast, while displaced or comminuted fractures require operative fixation.

Pearls

1. Classically described as "the snowboarder's fracture".
2. Consider this injury in patients with pain in the anterolateral ankle. Mimics lateral ankle sprain.

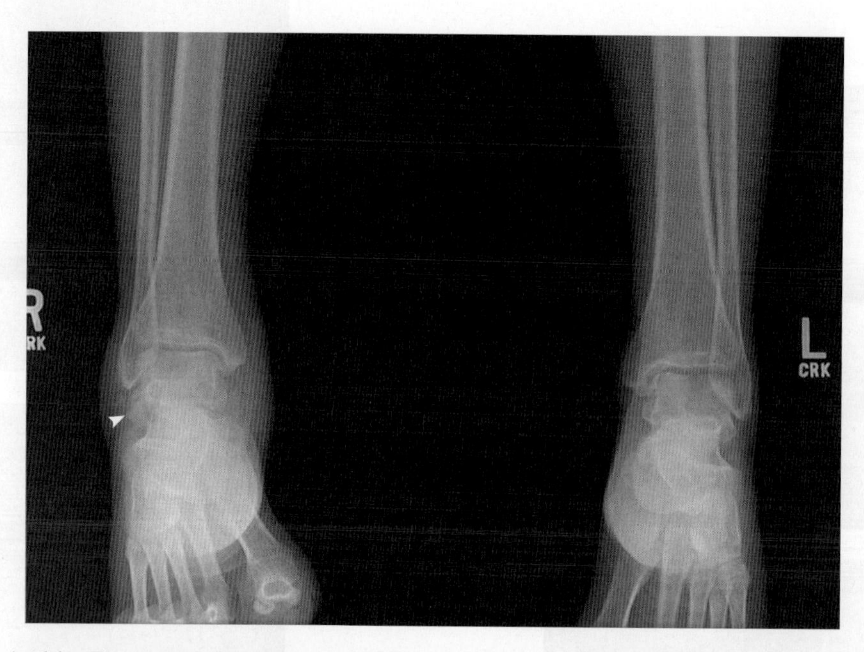

FIGURE 10.85 ■ Talar Avulsion Fracture. AP view of the ankles shows an avulsion fracture from the lateral process of the right talus (arrowhead) associated with extensive soft tissue swelling. The alignment is normal.

Radiographic Summary

AP, mortise, and lateral views of the ankle may all reveal this injury. The lateral view is usually the most helpful. Look for associated fractures. As usual, CT can provide further detail, if clinically necessary.

Clinical Implications

Patients present with an obvious posterior foot deformity and pain. Often, the skin is under extreme tension, necessitating emergent reduction. Neurovascular injuries are associated with subtalar dislocations. Treatment is based upon the presence of any associated fractures.

Pearls

1. Closely evaluate the soft tissues and neurovascular structures; emergent reduction may be required.
2. CT scan may be required to assess for associated fractures.

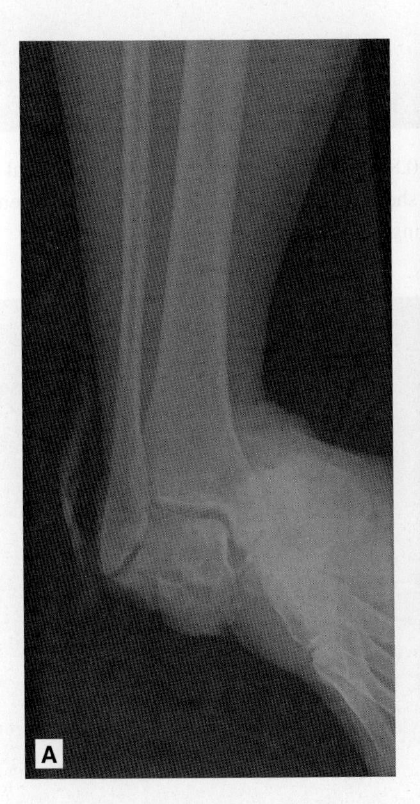

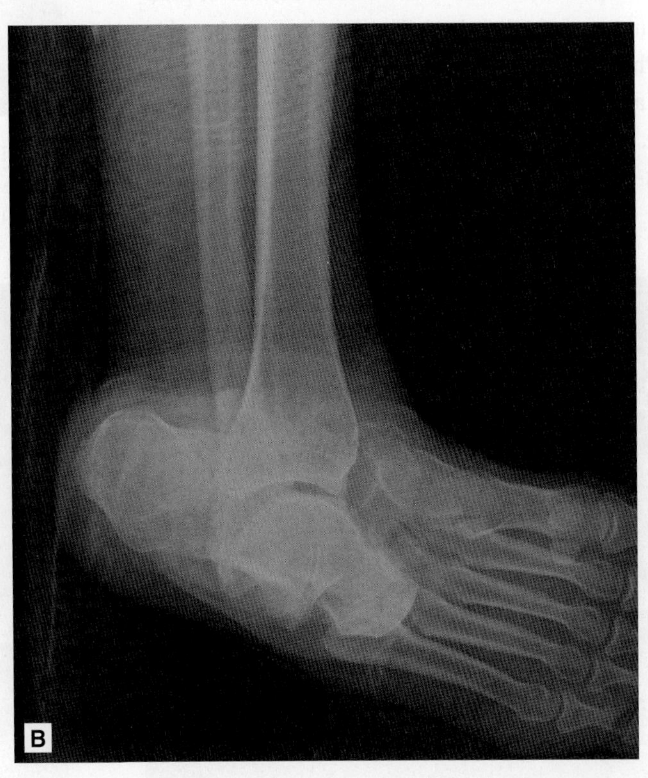

FIGURE 10.86 ■ Subtalar Dislocation. **A, B:** AP and lateral views of the right ankle show complete medial dislocation of the hindfoot at the subtalar joints.

CALCANEAL STRESS FRACTURES

Radiographic Summary

Acute stress fractures are radiographically occult. 7-10 days after the stress fracture occurs, faint sclerosis may be appreciated within the bone and corresponds to the healing stress fracture; periosteal new bone formation may be evident as well at this time. Acute stress fractures may be detected with an MRI.

Clinical Implications

Calcaneal stress fractures occur in runners, military recruits, and as insufficiency fractures in the elderly. Patients with stress fractures present with several weeks to months of gradually worsening pain in their heel. The pain is exacerbated by activities. Physical exam will reveal tenderness over the calcaneus and a positive squeeze test (compression from medial and lateral). Treatment includes a walking boot for 6 weeks with weight-bearing allowed.

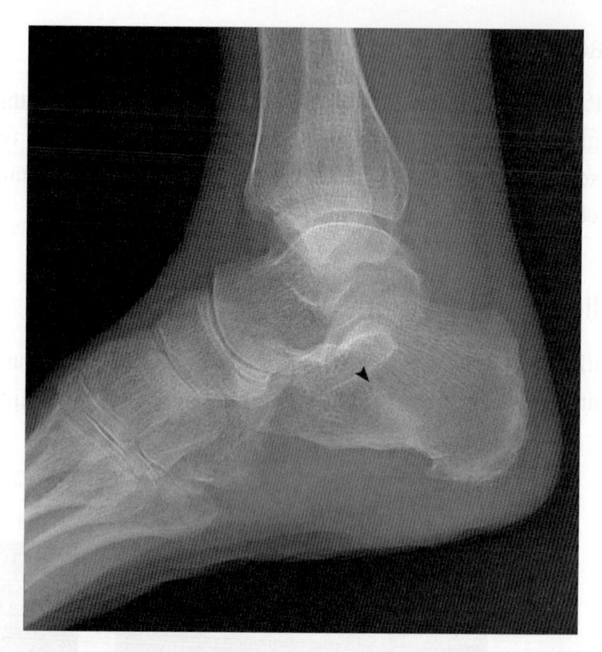

FIGURE 10.88 ■ Calcaneal Stress Fracture. A lateral view of the right ankle shows a band of sclerosis in the mid calcaneus consistent with a healing stress fracture (arrowhead).

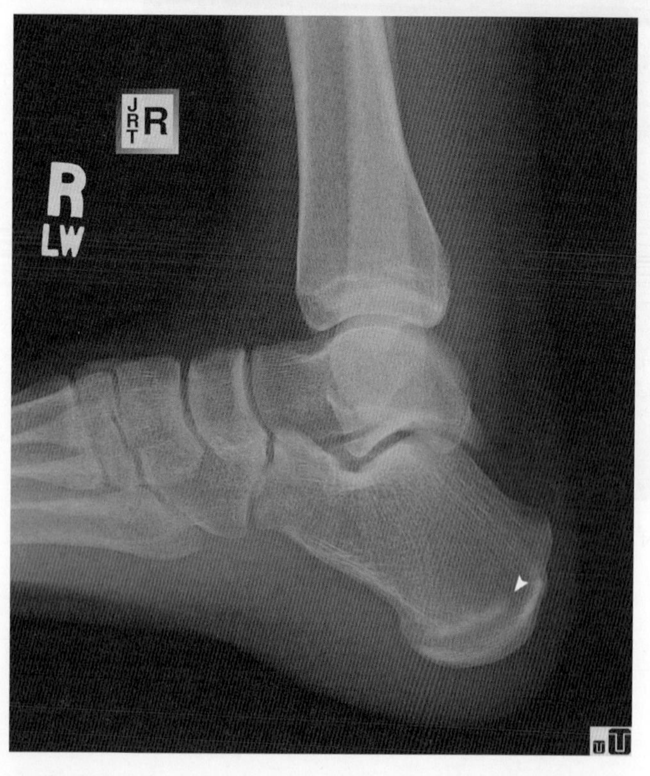

FIGURE 10.87 ■ Calcaneal Stress Fracture. Lateral view of the right ankle shows a fuzzy broad band of sclerosis extending transversely to the major compressive trabecular lines in the posterior calcaneus (arrowhead). This is the typical appearance of a healing stress fracture in one of the common locations of a stress fracture in the calcaneus.

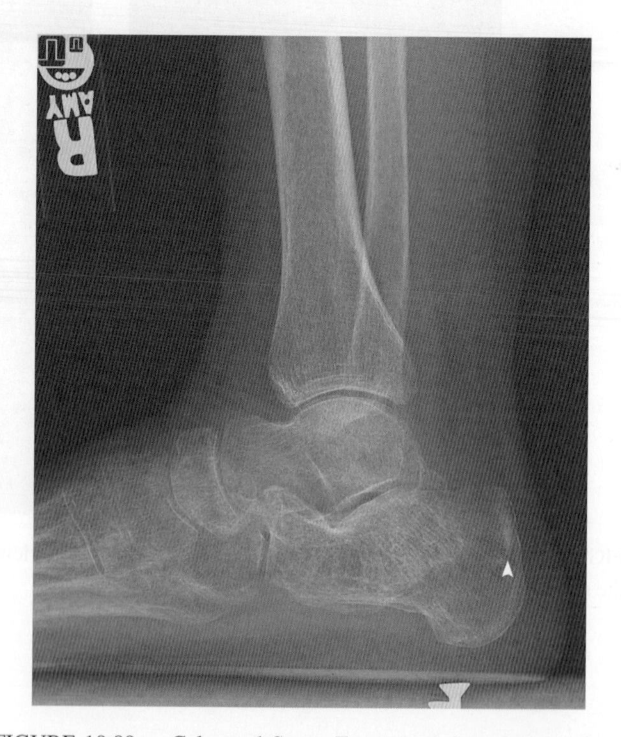

FIGURE 10.89 ■ Calcaneal Stress Fracture. A lateral view of the right ankle shows a healing comminuted fracture of the right calcaneus with flattening of Bohler's angle. There is generalized bony demineralization, likely related to disuse or altered weight-bearing related to the healing calcaneal fracture. In the supero-posterior calcaneus there is a fuzzy sclerotic band extending parallel to the posterior calcaneal cortex (arrowhead). This is a subacute healing calcaneal stress fracture.

Pearls

1. Consider this diagnosis in runners and military recruits with heel pain.
2. If the initial radiographs are negative but clinical suspicion remains high, obtain an MRI. An MRI can demonstrate acute stress fractures that are radiographically occult.

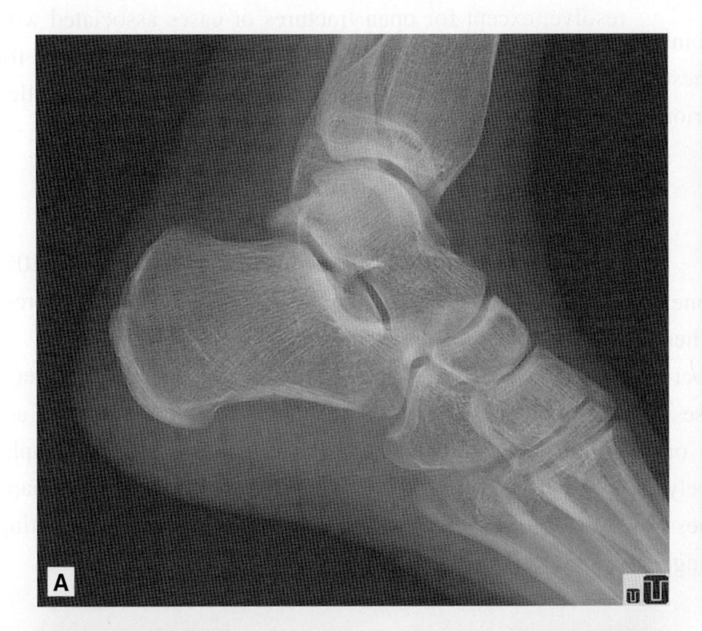

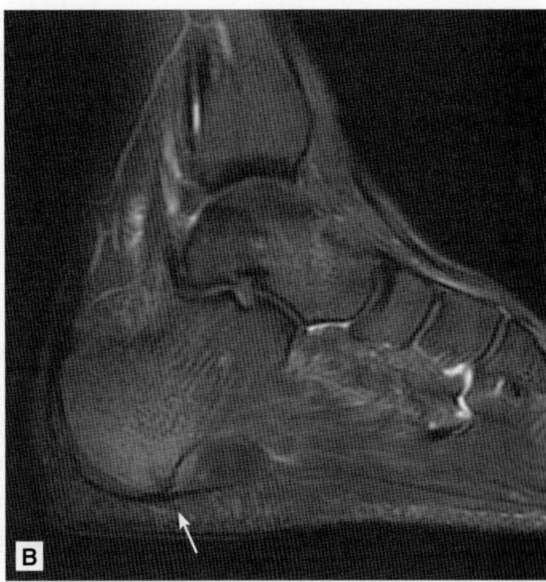

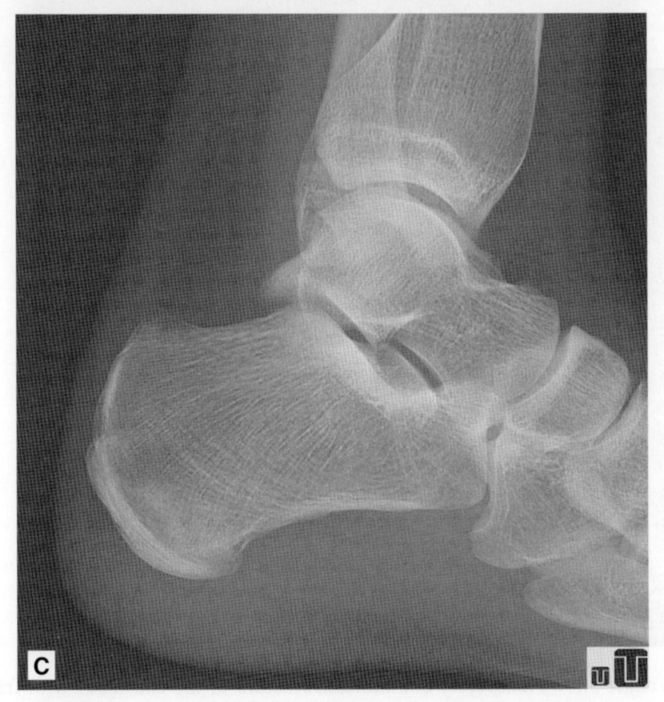

FIGURE 10.90 ■ Calcaneal Stress Fracture. **A:** Lateral view of the left ankle shows no fracture or malalignment. This is a young athlete. The clinicians suspected a stress fracture and an MRI was performed for further evaluation. **B:** A sagital FS PD-weighted image of the left foot shows a PD-hypointense line in the posterior calcaneus extending inferiorly to the plantar fascia origin (arrow). This is a stress fracture. It is surrounded by extensive marrow edema. **C:** A lateral view of the ankle in the same patient obtained 3 weeks later shows a fuzzy band of sclerosis in the posterior calcaneus consistent with a healing stress fracture. The orientation of the fracture corresponds to the fracture seen on the MRI.

Radiographic Summary

A lateral view of the ankle or foot is best to evaluate for this fracture. Bohler's angle can be measured to evaluate for more subtle injuries resulting in subtle calcaneal flattening but with no obvious fracture. The angle is measured at the intersection of the following two lines: one is drawn from the highest point of the anterior calcaneal tuberosity to the highest point of the posterior facet; the second is drawn from the highest point of the posterior facet to the highest point of the posterior tuberosity. The angle should be between 20 and 40°.

Clinical Implications

The calcaneus is the most commonly fractured tarsal bone. Patients present after a fall, motor vehicle collision, or other high-energy mechanism. Calcaneal fractures are associated with spine compression fractures in 10% of the cases. Calcaneal fractures can either be extraarticular (30%) or intra-articular (70%) and are bilateral in approximately 10% of the cases. Physical exam will reveal tenderness to palpation over the calcaneus and soft tissue swelling. Compartment syndrome can occur with these injuries. Treatment is usually conservative for extraarticular fractures (except for Achilles avulsion fractures). Operative fixation is the treatment mainstay for most intra-articular fractures, unless they are nondisplaced. The timing of surgery is usually delayed 10 to 14 days to allow the soft tissue edema to resolve, except for open fractures or cases associated with compartment syndrome. If patients are being discharged for home, they should be placed in a big, bulky dressing called a Jones dressing.

Pearls

1. Remember the rule of 10's for calcaneal fractures: 10% are bilateral and 10% are associated with spine compression fractures.
2. CT scan can be utilized to further delineate the fracture(s) and assist in operative planning. Calcaneal fractures are difficult to completely characterize with radiographs alone because of the complex, three-dimensional shape of the calcaneus and multiple overlying and articulating bones.

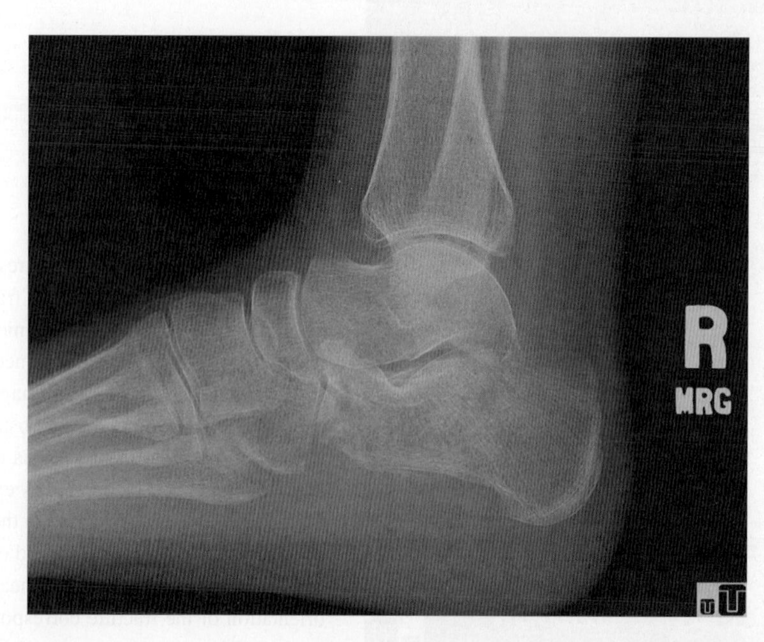

FIGURE 10.91 ■ Calcaneal Fracture. A lateral view of the right ankle shows a severely comminuted fracture of the calcaneus with fracture planes extending thorough the middle and posterior subtalar joints and undermining the sustentaculum tali. The calcaneus has partially collapsed with resultant flattening of Bohler's angle.

Radiographic Summary

A lateral view of the ankle or foot is best for visualizing this injury. A lateral view shows the avulsion fracture from the superior–posterior calcaneus, at the site of insertion of the Achilles tendon.

Clinical Implications

Calcaneal insufficiency avulsion fractures result from two main mechanisms: either a direct blow or, in the elderly, a forceful contraction of the gastrocnemius–soleus complex. These fractures are classically seen in diabetic patients. Patients present with pain directly at the site and will have variable residual Achilles function. These patients can develop skin necrosis due to the lack of soft tissue in the posterior ankle and the displacement of the fracture. Treatment is operative fixation in the majority of cases unless the patient is older, nonmobile, or the fracture is nondisplaced.

Pearls

1. Pay close attention to the soft tissues as skin necrosis can occur quickly.
2. Lateral radiographs of the ankle or foot are sufficient in demonstrating this injury.
3. These injuries are classically seen in diabetic patients.

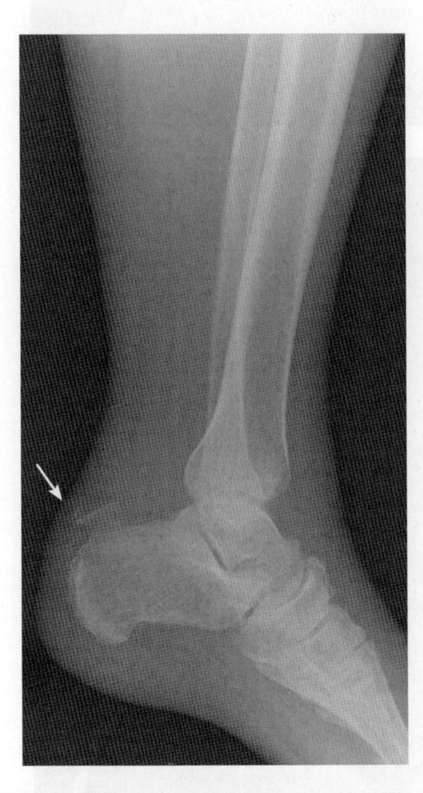

FIGURE 10.92 ■ Calcaneal Insufficiency Avulsion Fracture. A lateral view of the ankle shows an avulsion fracture of the supero-posterior calcaneus at the site of insertion of the Achilles tendon (arrow). There is extensive soft tissue edema.

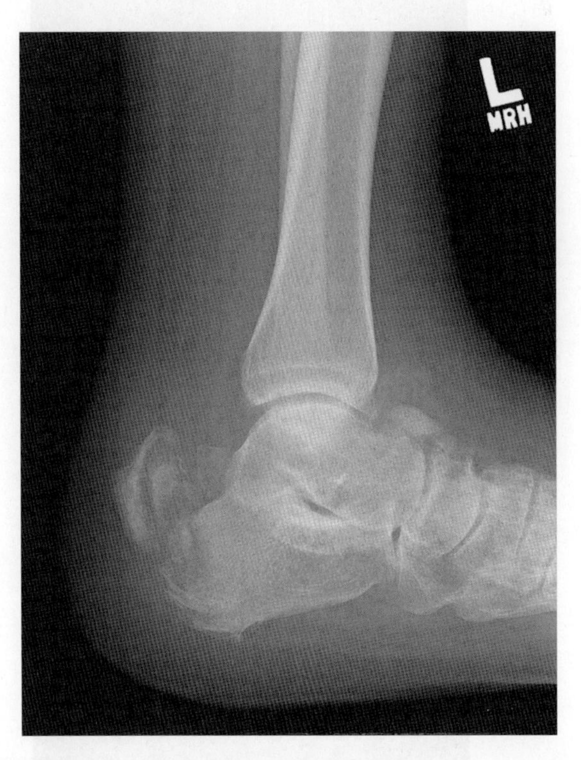

FIGURE 10.93 ■ Calcaneal Insufficiency Avulsion Fracture (Companion Case). A lateral view of the left ankle shows a large avulsion fracture of the supero-posterior calcaneus at the site of insertion of the Achilles tendon.

Radiographic Summary

Dorsoplantar and oblique radiographs of the foot can demonstrate most midfoot fractures; however, CT is usually required to better delineate the fractures and typically reveals additional fractures that were not visible on the initial radiographs. Acute stress fractures are radiographically occult. If there is a strong clinical suspicion for a stress fracture, an MRI should be obtained. An MRI can demonstrate subtle injuries such as stress reaction, stress fracture, or nondisplaced fracture.

Clinical Implications

Isolated tarsal fractures are rare. Usually, multiple tarsal fractures occur simultaneously. Navicular fractures, especially navicular stress fractures, may occur in isolation. Patients with navicular stress fractures will present with insidious arch pain. These stress fractures are in the high-risk category and it is critical that they are discovered in a timely manner, preferably before they complete and displace. Physical exam should help discern which

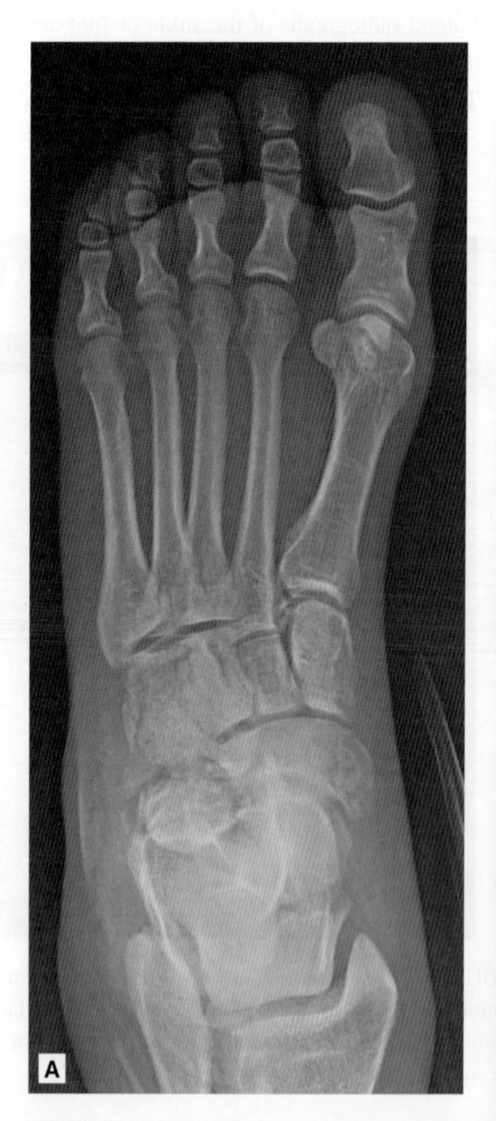

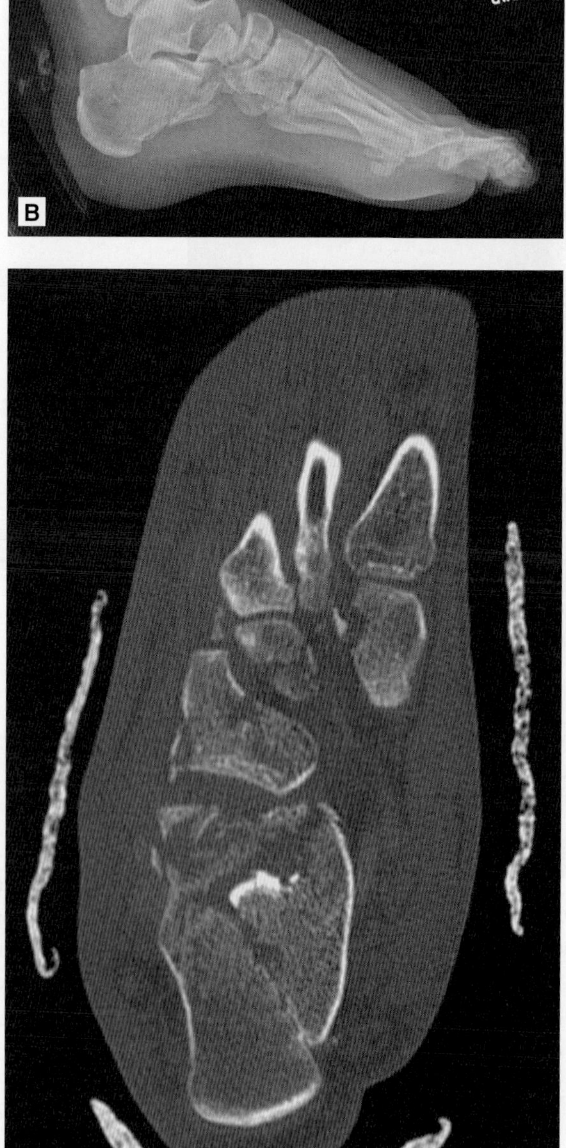

FIGURE 10.94 ■ Midfoot Fractures. **A-C:** Dorsoplantar and lateral views of the left foot and a selected axial CT image of the same foot show multiple fractures of the calcaneus, cuboid, medial, middle, and lateral cuneiforms and navicular bone. The alignment of the midfoot is normal on these non-weight-bearing views.

of the tarsal bones is injured. Midfoot fracture treatment involves splinting and non-weight-bearing, unless the fractures are displaced. Displaced fractures require operative fixation.

Pearls

1. Midfoot fractures typically occur in combination; navicular fractures may occur in isolation.
2. Consider obtaining a CT to better characterize midfoot fractures. A CT frequently reveals additional fractures that were not visible on the initially obtained radiographs.
3. An MRI is the imaging modality of choice to evaluate for an acute stress fracture. Acute stress fractures are radiographically occult. After 7-10 days, a sclerotic line corresponding to the healing fracture and periosteal new bone develop and can be identified on radiographs.

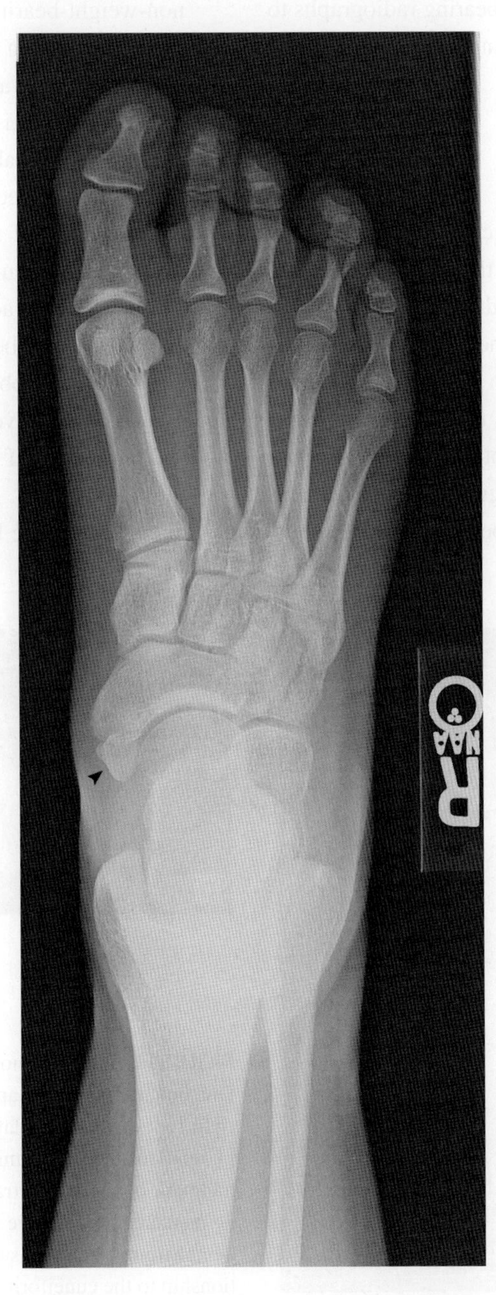

FIGURE 10.95 ■ Accessory Tarsal Navicular. Dorsoplantar view of the right foot reveals an accessory navicular bone (arrowhead).

Radiographic Summary

Dorsoplantar, oblique, and lateral radiographs of the foot are initially obtained to evaluate a Lisfranc injury. The alignment of the midfoot should be evaluated by ensuring that the medial cortex of the 2nd metatarsal aligns perfectly with medial cortex of the middle cuneiform on the standard dorsoplantar view. The medial aspect of the 4th metatarsal should align with the medial aspect of the cuboid on the oblique view. The cuneiforms should align with the respective metatarsal bases on the lateral view. Significant injuries are readily seen. Subtle injuries, however, may require weight-bearing radiographs to stress the Lisfranc ligament and make any potential malalignment more obvious.

Clinical Implications

These injuries can be the result of a direct blow to the midfoot or a force creating dorsiflexion while the plantarflexors are firing. These mechanisms stress the midfoot and the Lisfranc ligament that runs from the medial cuneiform to the base of the 2nd metatarsal. Patients present with pain and swelling in this area. Physical examination reveals tenderness and exacerbated pain with stressing the midfoot. Treatment depends on the type of fracture, but if the radiographs are normal and suspicion remains, the patient should be treated with a short leg splint and made non-weight-bearing. An MRI can be utilized to confirm the injury; an MRI can directly evaluate the ligament itself and demonstrate whether it is intact or torn.

Pearls

1. These injuries can be extremely subtle and it is absolutely critical that they are not missed. A missed Lisfranc ligament injury can progress to gross dislocation of the midfoot with significant morbidity.
2. If even a minor malalignment is perceived on the initial non-weight-bearing radiographs or if there is a strong clinical suspicion for the injury but the initial radiographs are negative, always obtain stress views to further evaluate for a subtle Lisfranc injury.
3. The most valuable view is the dorsoplantar view. Demand a perfect view that adequately demonstrates the alignment of the medial cortices of the 2nd metatarsal and middle cuneiform. Suboptimal (slightly oblique) DP views do not adequately demonstrate this relationship and should not be accepted as diagnostic; a repeat DP view should be obtained.
4. Treat conservatively with a short leg splint and non-weight-bearing if suspicion remains high, despite negative radiographs. Consider obtaining an MRI that can directly visualize Lisfranc's ligament.

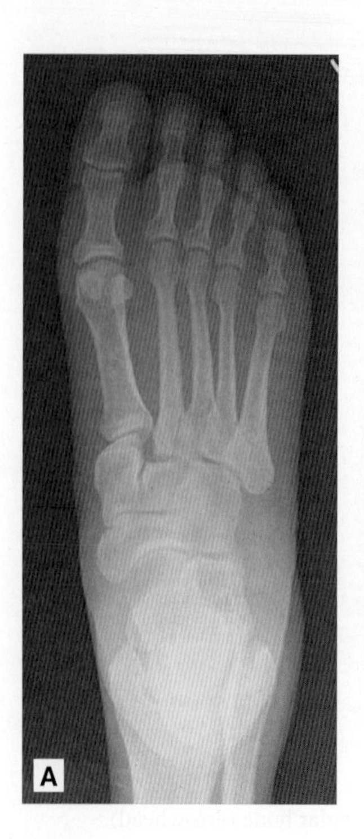

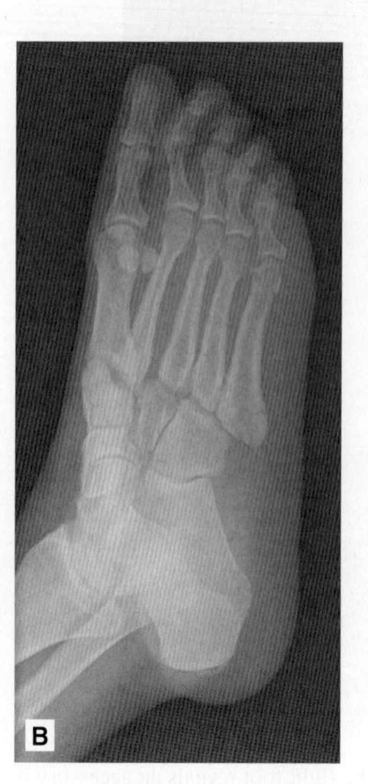

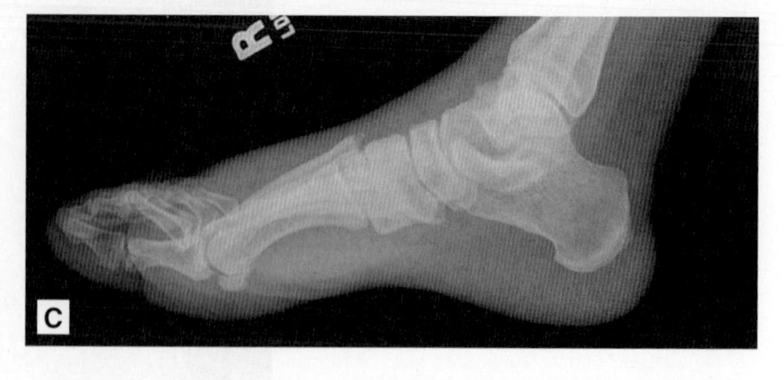

FIGURE 10.96 ■ Homolateral Lisfranc Fracture-Dislocation. **A-C:** Dorsoplantar, oblique, and lateral non-weight-bearing views of the right foot demonstrate lateral subluxation of the 2nd metatarsal base in relationship to the middle cuneiform. This is the radiographic hallmark of a Lisfranc fracture-dislocation. Notice that the first and 3rd metatarsal bases have migrated laterally as well. The lateral view demonstrates superior subluxation of the metatarsal bases in relationship to the cuneiform bones.

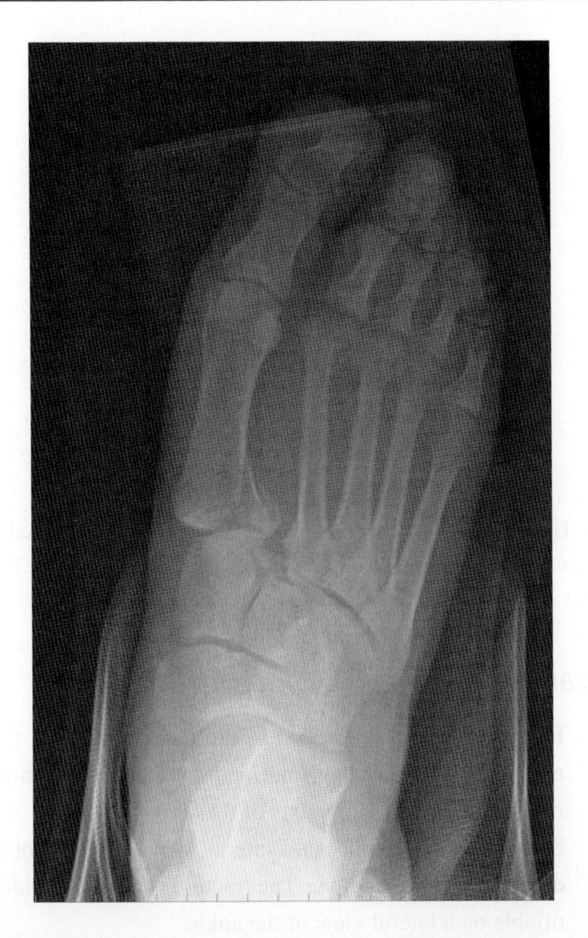

FIGURE 10.97 ■ Divergent Lisfranc Fracture-Dislocation. A dorsoplantar view of the right foot shows lateral subluxation of the 2nd metatarsal base and medial subluxation of the first metatarsal base with a fracture of the lateral aspect of the fifth metatarsal base. This is an example of a divergent Lisfranc fracture-dislocation.

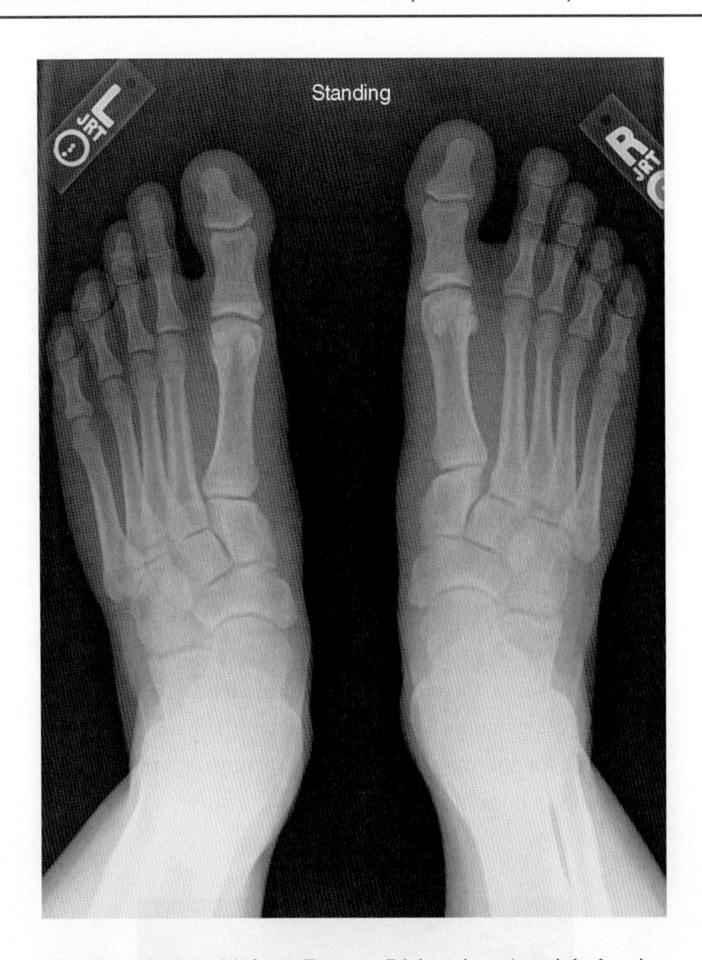

FIGURE 10.98 ■ Lisfranc Fracture-Dislocation. A weight-bearing dorsoplantar view of both feet shows a very subtle malalignment of the right midfoot with very subtle lateral subluxation of the 2nd metatarsal base. The alignment was normal on the non-weight-bearing view. Notice the normal alignment of the medial cortices of the 2nd cuneiform and 2nd metatarsal on the left.

Radiographic Summary

Dorsoplantar, oblique, and lateral views of the foot are sufficient to demonstrate this fracture. The fracture can be seen on any of the above views. Avulsion fractures of the 5th metatarsal base involve its tuberosity: the distal attachment site of the peroneus brevis tendon and lateral cord of the plantar fascia. Avulsion fractures of the 5th metatarsal base can be distinguished from the normal apophysis seen at this location in children by the direction of the observed lucency: fractures are perpendicular to the long axis of the 5th metatarsal while the normal synchondrosis runs parallel to the long axis of the 5th metatarsal.

Clinical Implications

Patients present after a forced inversion injury with the foot in the plantarflexed position. Patients will have pain and swelling over this area. Physical exam will find tenderness over the proximal 5th metatarsal, exacerbated with resisted eversion. Treatment for the majority of these fractures is conservative with walking boot immobilization.

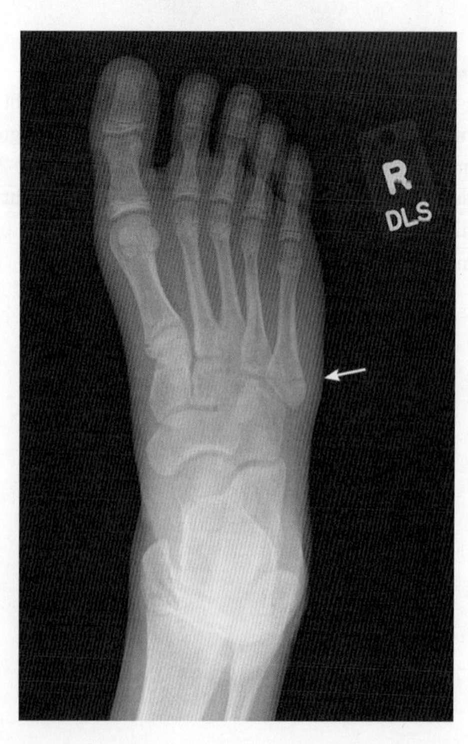

FIGURE 10.99 ■ Avulsion Fracture Proximal 5th Metatarsal. A dorso-plantar view of the right foot shows a nondisplaced avulsion fracture at the base of the 5th metatarsal bone (arrow).

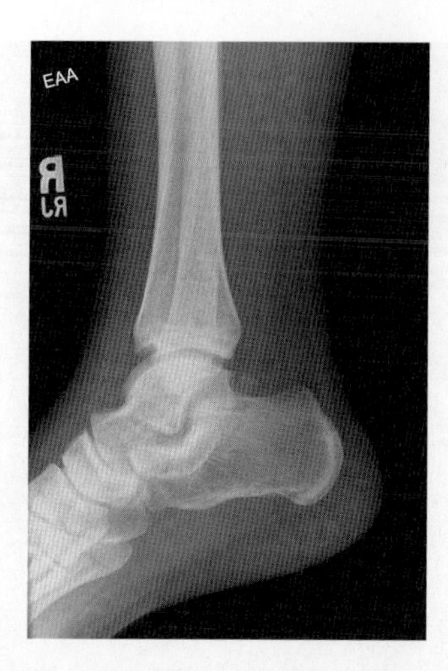

FIGURE 10.100 ■ Avulsion Fracture Proximal 5th Metatarsal. A lateral view of the right ankle shows the same fracture. These fractures are clearly seen on a lateral view of the ankle.

Pearls

1. Fractures are perpendicular to the long axis of the fifth metatarsal while the normal apophyseal synchondrosis runs parallel to the long axis of the 5th metatarsal.
2. Dorsoplantar, oblique, and lateral views of the foot all demonstrate this fracture. The fracture is also easily identifiable on a lateral view of the ankle.

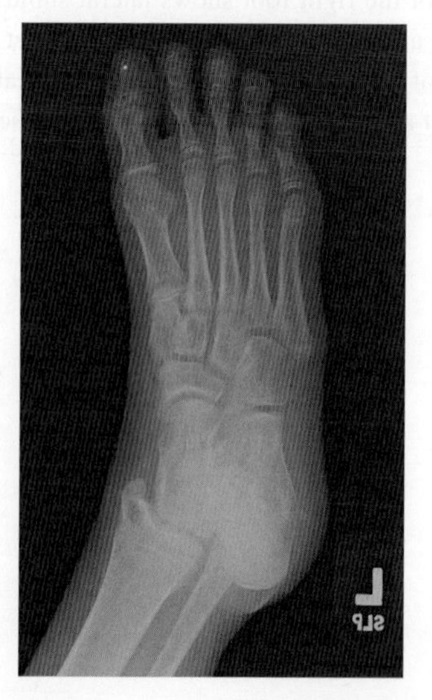

FIGURE 10.101 ■ Companion Case: Normal Apophysis. Oblique view of the left foot in a 12-year-old child shows a linear lucency at the base of the 5th metatarsal bone which extends parallel to the long axis of the 5th metatarsal bone. This is the classic appearance of an unfused apophysis at the base of the 5th metatarsal. This is a normal finding in a child of this age and should be distinguished from a fracture. Fractures extend transversely through the 5th metatarsal base.

Radiographic Summary

A Jones fracture is a fracture of the 5th metatarsal diaphysis. Dorsoplantar, oblique, and lateral views of the foot are sufficient to identify this injury.

Clinical Implications

The classic Jones fracture results from an acute injury to the 5th metatarsal. The site of the fracture can be identical to the site of a stress fracture of the proximal diaphysis, but the history from patients presenting with a stress fracture will be vastly different. Patients with stress fractures in this area generally have pain for months, especially with activity, unlike patients presenting with a Jones fracture who develop pain acutely as a result of a memorable injury. Physical examination elicits tenderness over the 5th metatarsal with associated swelling and ecchymosis. ED treatment for these fractures (Jones and stress fractures) is similar t posterior splinting. Definitive treatment is controversial. Patients with both types of fractures should be evaluated by an orthopoedic surgeon as outpatients.

Pearls

1. Jones fractures are typically acute and occur in the diaphysis of the 5th metatarsal bone.
2. 5th metatarsal stress fractures occur in the same location but the presenting clinical history is vastly different: weeks or months of insidious pain exacerbated with activity.
3. Consider an MRI to evaluate for a stress fracture in patients presenting with persistent pain in the 5th metatarsal with negative or equivocal radiographs.

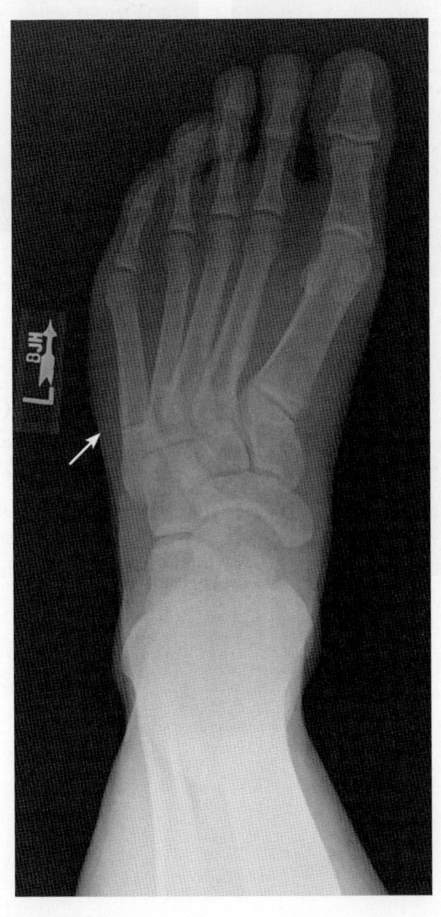

FIGURE 10.102 ■ Jones Fracture. A dorso-plantar view of the left foot demonstrates a transverse fracture of the proximal shaft of the 5th metatarsal bone (arrow). There is no displacement.

Radiographic Summary

Dorsoplantar, oblique, and lateral views of the foot or affected toe are sufficient to demonstrate this injury. Associated avulsion fractures are common and are usually easier to see on the post-reduction radiographs. Therefore, post-reduction radiographs should always be obtained.

Clinical Implications

The great toe is extremely important for ambulation and jumping. Dislocations should be reduced and immobilized. Indications for orthopedic referral include fracture-dislocations, unstable dislocations, and displaced fractures. Treatment is conservative with a walking boot, with or without a toe plate.

Pearls

1. Treat great toe fractures much more conservatively than lesser toe fractures.
2. Advanced imaging is generally not required.

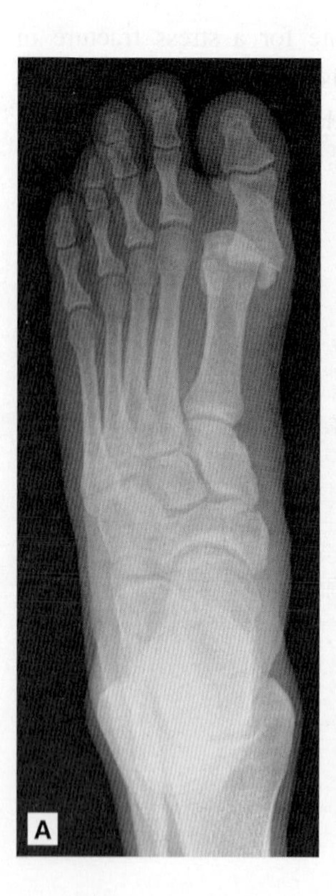

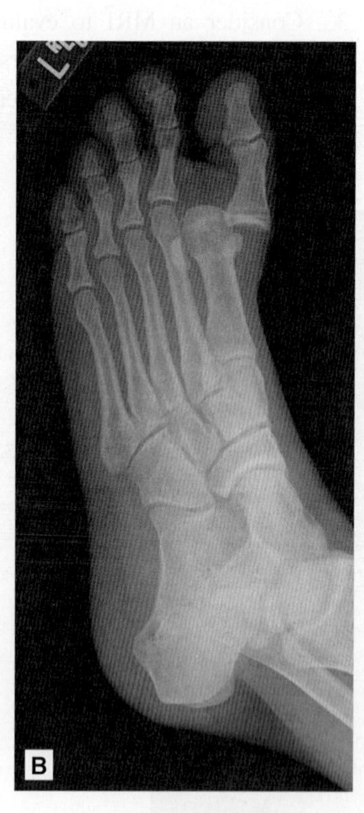

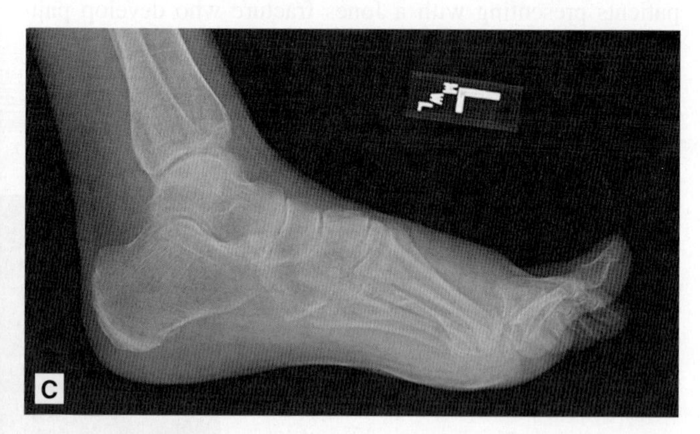

FIGURE 10.103 ■ Great Toe Dislocation. **A-C:** DP, oblique, and lateral views of the left foot show a dorsal dislocation of the base of the proximal phalanx of the great toe. There is also a small avulsion fracture of the distal aspect of the lateral great toe sesamoid. Notice how the great toe sesamoids are splayed apart. This is consistent with injury to the volar plate.

Radiographic Summary

Dorsoplantar, oblique, and lateral views of the foot or great toe are usually sufficient to demonstrate the fracture. A dedicated sesamoid view may be helpful, if the standard views are insufficient. An MRI can be used to diagnose nondisplaced fractures, if the radiographs are negative but clinical suspicion remains high.

Clinical Implications

Patients with sesamoid fractures present with pain that localizes to the plantar surface of the first metatarsophalangeal joint. Physical exam reveals tenderness over the respective sesamoid, exacerbated by resisted toe plantarflexion. Radiographs are required to differentiate a displaced fracture from sesamoiditis or stress fracture. Treatment ranges from a pad (to unload the sesamoid) to a short leg cast. Initial emergency department treatment can start with a postoperative shoe and cut-out padding.

Pearls

1. Patients with sesamoid fractures present with pain that localizes to the plantar surface of the first metatarsophalangeal joint.
2. An MRI may be required for definitive diagnosis and treatment planning.

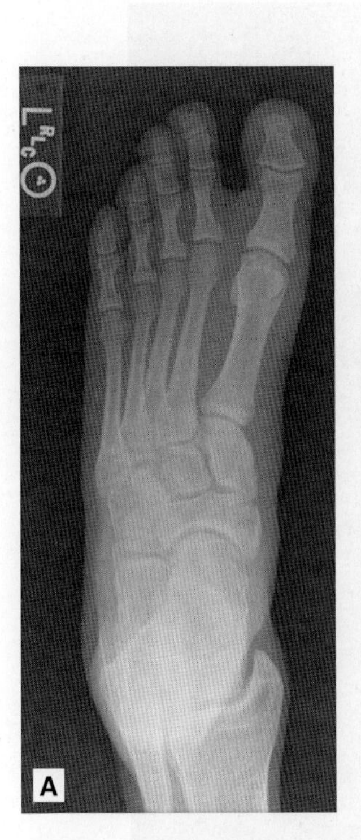

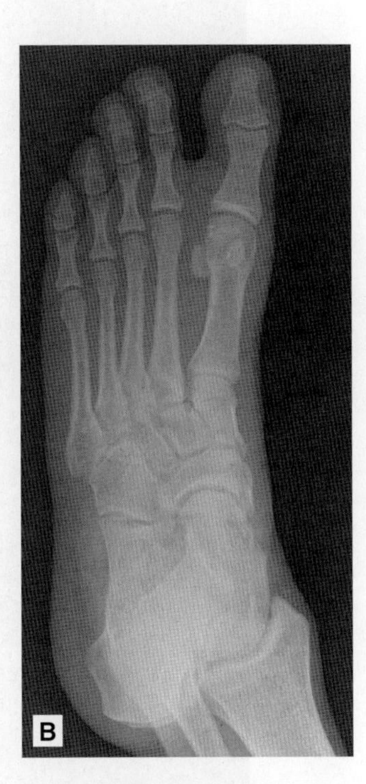

FIGURE 10.104 ■ Sesamoid Fracture. **A, B:** DP and oblique views of the left foot show splaying of the great toe sesamoids consistent with an injury to the volar plate. There is a tiny avulsion fracture from the distal aspect of the lateral great toe sesamoid as well.

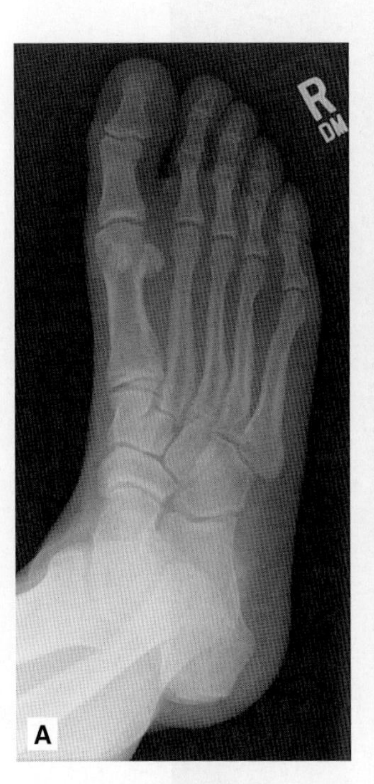

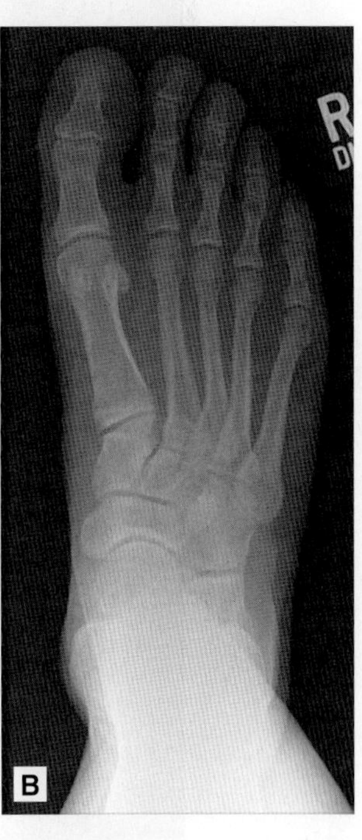

FIGURE 10.105 ■ Sesamoid Fracture. **A, B:** DP and oblique views of the right foot show a nondisplaced oblique fracture of the lateral great toe sesamoid.

Radiographic Summary

Similar to the bipartite patella, a bipartite sesamoid consists of two halves; it has the appearance of two round pebbles, stacked upon one-another. The edges of the two halves are rounded and smooth. They could not be mentally reduced into one complete shape. Conversely, sesamoid fractures are thin and jagged; the resulting fragments have sharp, angular edges, and could be mentally reduced into one whole ossicle.

Clinical Implications

A bipartite sesamoid is a common normal variant. The vast majority are asymptomatic. It is important to be aware of their existence and distinguish them from sesamoid fractures. Some authors believe that bipartite sesamoids may be more prone to the development of sesamoiditis.

Pearls

1. Not all lines are fracture lines; don't forget to consider bipartite sesamoids if the edges are rounded and well-corticated.
2. An MRI can be utilized to assess for sesamoiditis.

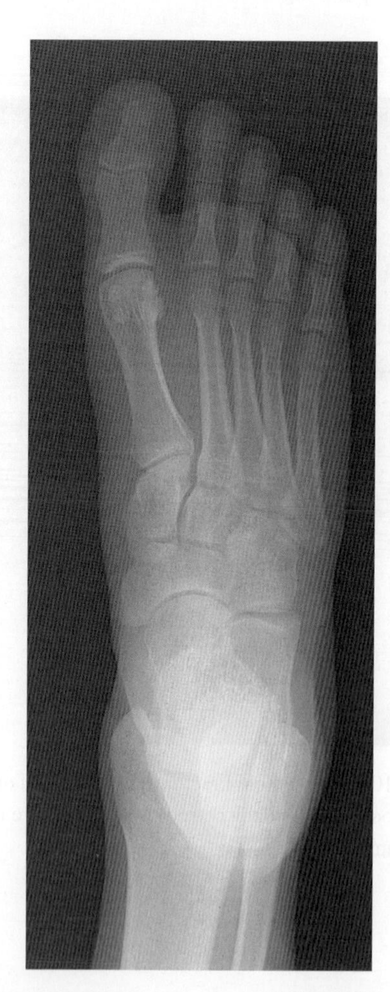

FIGURE 10.106 ■ Bipartite Sesamoids. A DP view of the right foot shows that both the medial and lateral great toe sesamoids are bipartite. Notice the rounded and well-corticated appearance of the two halves of each sesamoid. The two halves could not be mentally "reduced" into one perfect round sesamoid. In the case of a fractured sesamoid, the fractured fragments could be reduced into one perfect sesamoid.

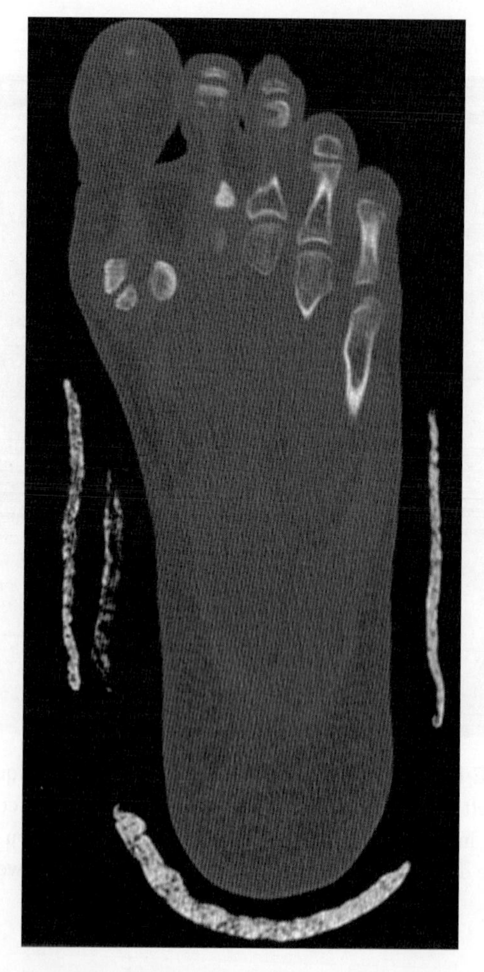

FIGURE 10.107 ■ Bipartite Sesamoid. A selected coronal CT image of a foot shows a bipartite medial great toe sesamoid.

Radiographic Summary

Dorsoplantar, oblique, and lateral views of the injured foot or toe are usually sufficient to demonstrate these fractures.

Clinical Implications

Patients will present with pain localizing to the injured toe. Important aspects of the physical exam include nail evaluation and assessment for open wounds. The lesser toes (2-5) generally do better than great toe fractures, and rarely require orthopedic referral. Indications for referral include open injuries, displaced intra-articular fractures, and irreducible fractures. Treatment involves reduction when needed and buddy-taping. Some patients may require further immobilization with a post-operative shoe and/or a toe plate.

Pearls

1. Normal alignment should be restored or, at least, approximated prior to buddy-taping.
2. Advanced imaging is generally not required with these injuries.

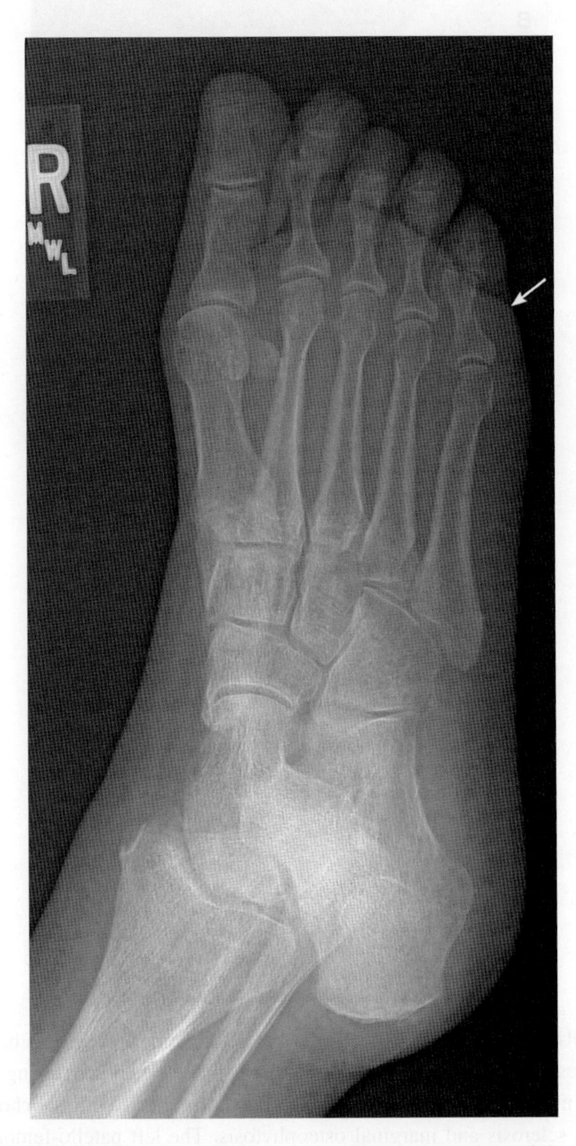

FIGURE 10.108 ■ Toe Fracture. An oblique view of the right foot shows an oblique, nondisplaced, and extraarticular fracture of the shaft of the proximal phalanx of the 5th toe (arrow).

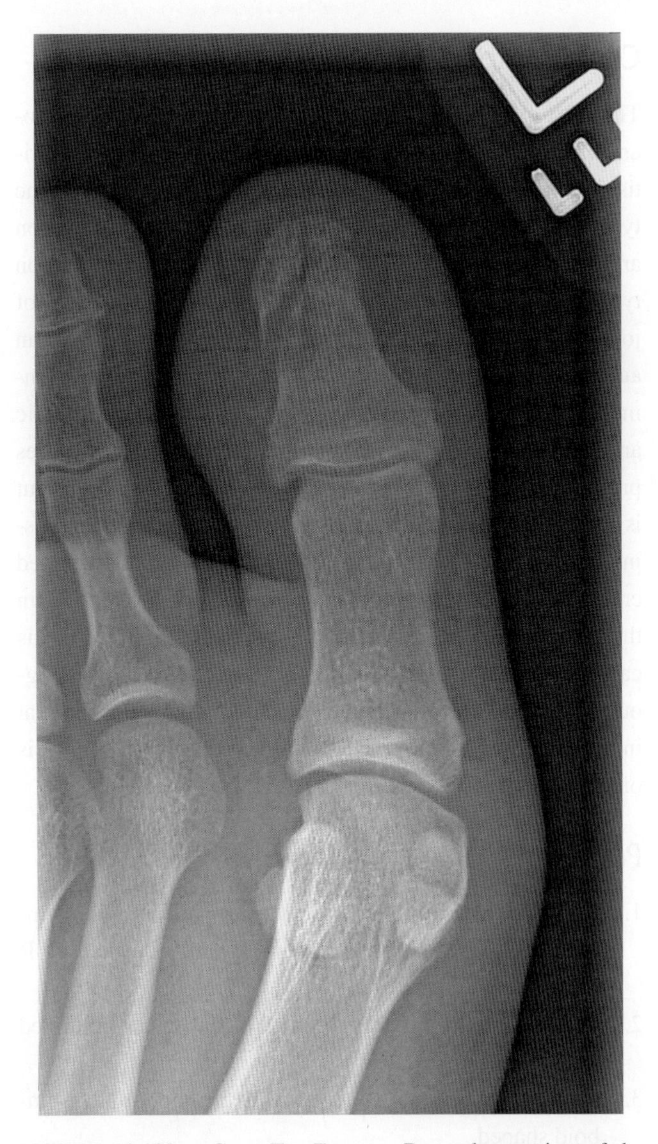

FIGURE 10.109 ■ Great Toe Fracture. Dorsoplantar view of the left great toe shows a comminuted fracture of the tuft of the distal phalanx of the great toe.

Radiographic Summary

Arthritis, in the broadest sense, is a disease of a joint causing pain. There are two main categories of arthritis: degenerative and inflammatory. Degenerative arthritis (osteoarthritis) causes non-uniform joint space narrowing, subchondral sclerosis, subchondral cyst formation, and marginal osteophyte formation; focal cartilage defects, loose osteochondral bodies, joint effusions, and fibrocartilagenous degeneration may be present as well. Inflammatory arthritis (e.g., rheumatoid arthritis) is characterized by uniform destruction of the hyaline cartilage and, therefore, the joint space; periarticular erosions, joint effusions, synovitis, and periarticular osteopenia are features as well.

Clinical Implications

There are over 100 different types of arthritis including osteoarthritis, rheumatoid arthritis, psoariatic arthritis, septic arthritis, and gout to name a few. Treatment varies depending on the type of arthritis and is aimed at decreasing the inflammation and providing pain relief. Osteoarthritis is the most common type of arthritis resulting from chronic "wear and tear" of joints or as a result of prior trauma. Rheumatoid arthritis is an autoimmune disorder that occurs in younger patients and symmetrically affects fingers, wrists, knees, and elbows. Septic arthritis is caused by an infection of the joint that requires prompt treatment to prevent permanent joint damage. Gout is caused by deposition of uric acid crystals in the joint causing inflammation. Pseudogout is caused by rhomboid-shaped crystals of calcium pyrophosphate dihydrate deposited within the cartilage and capsule of a joint. Certain types of arthritis can mimic each other clinically; for example, gout, pseudogout, and septic arthritis can be clinically indistinguishable at initial presentation. In such cases, arthrocentesis and analysis of synovial fluid are necessary to establish the diagnosis.

Pearls

1. Rheumatoid arthritis affects younger patients with symmetrical involvement of multiple joints. Elevated ESR and rheumatoid factor are typically present.
2. Gouty crystals are strongly birefringent under polarized light and needle shaped.
3. Pseudogout crystals are weakly birefringent and rhomboid shaped.
4. Chondrocalcinosis (calcium pyrophosphate dihydrate) may be seen on radiographs and may aid in the diagnosis of pseudogout.

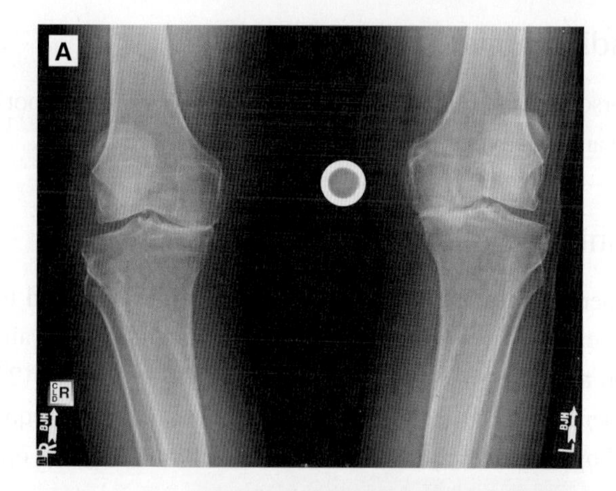

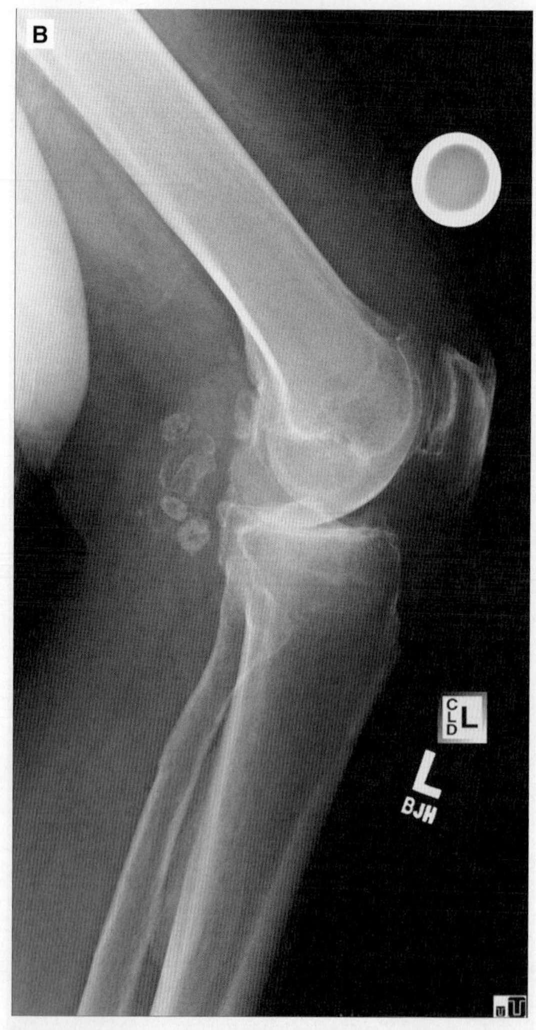

FIGURE 10.110 ■ Osteoarthritis. **A, B:** Standing AP view of both knees and a lateral view of the left knee show severe narrowing of the medial knee joint spaces bilaterally associated with subchondral sclerosis and marginal osteophytosis. The left patello-femoral compartment is moderately narrowed as well. Multiple loose osteochondral bodies of various sizes are present posterior to the left knee joint; these are trapped within a Baker's cyst.

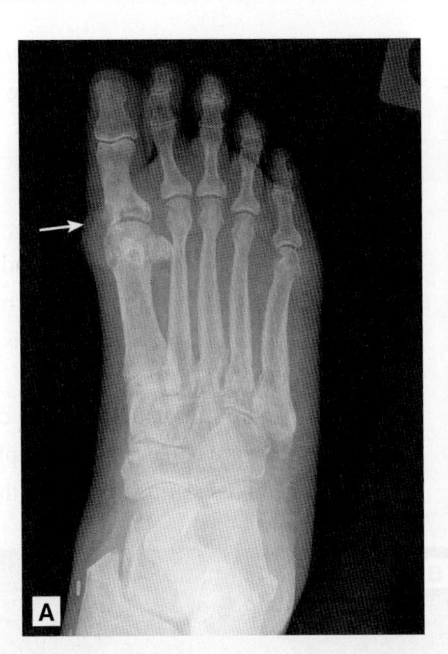

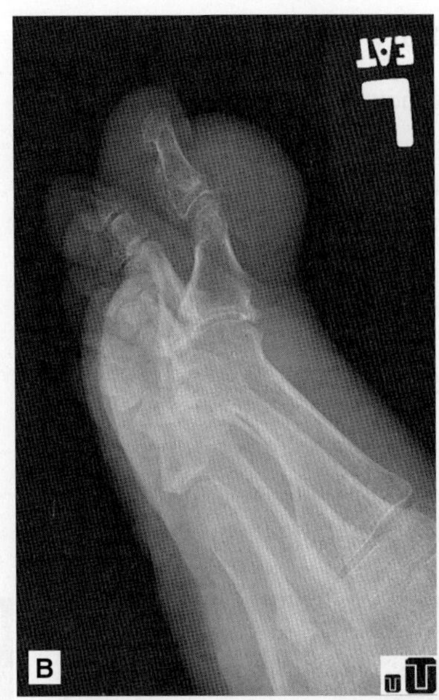

FIGURE 10.111 ■ Gout. **A:** An oblique view of the right foot shows multiple large corticated periarticular erosions about the first metatarso-phalangeal joint. The erosion at the medial base of the proximal phalanx of the great toe has an "overhanging edge (arrow)." Notice the relative preservation of the 1st MTP joint space, despite the numerous large periarticular erosions. There is periarticular soft tissue swelling. The findings are classic for gout. Multiple similar erosions are also present about the 2nd through 5th tarso-metatarsal joints. This distribution is also frequently seen in gout. **B:** A lateral view of the left great toe shows large corticated periarticular erosions with overhanging edges about the first metatarso-phalangeal and interphalangeal joints. Marked soft tissue swelling with central density is present on the dorsal aspect of the first interphalangeal joint. The findings are classic of tophaceous gout.

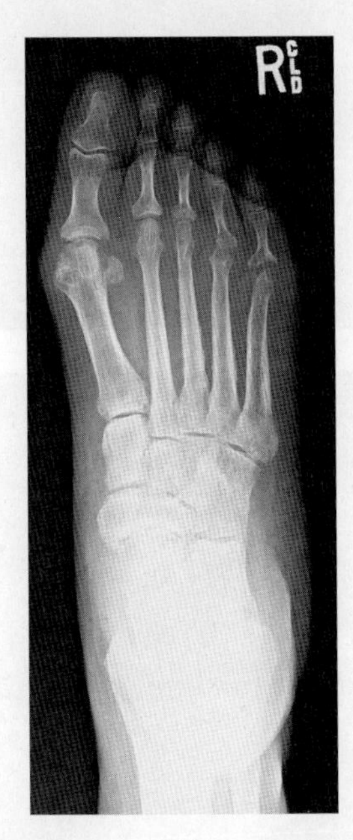

FIGURE 10.112 ■ Rheumatoid Arthritis. A DP view of the right foot shows uniform narrowing of the 1st, 3rd, 4th, and 5th metatarso-phalangeal joints with prominent periarticular erosions. The "bare areas" erosions in the base of the proximal phalanx of the great toe are classic for inflammatory arthritis. The involvement of the MTP joints is also typical of inflammatory arthritis. There is extensive periarticular soft tissue edema.

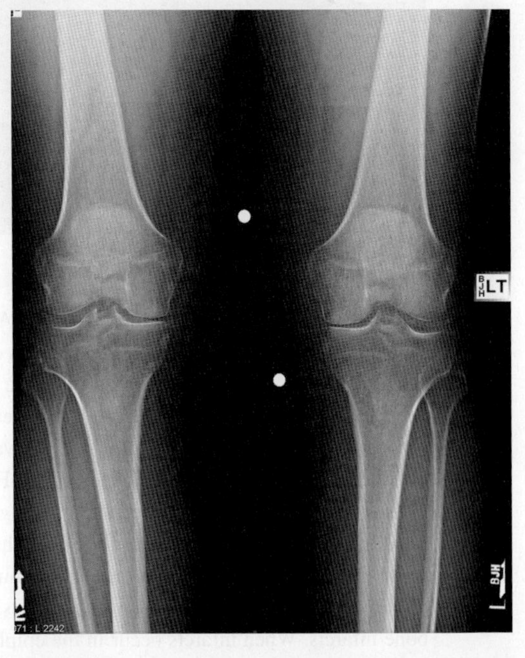

FIGURE 10.113 ■ Pyrophosphate Arthritis. Standing AP view of both knees shows chondrocalcinosis within the medial and lateral menisci bilaterally. The differential diagnosis for this includes calcium pyrophosphate dihydrate deposition disease, hyperparathyroidism, and hemochromatosis. There is moderate narrowing of the medial knee joint space bilaterally.

Radiographic Summary

Radiographs reveal serpigenous sclerotic lines forming geographic outlines or ill-defined areas of sclerosis within the medullary space of a bone. An MRI is the imaging modality of choice and can be used to differentiate between acute and chronic infarcts based upon the amount of edema present.

Clinical Implications

Bone infarcts are due to an interrupted blood supply to a certain area of the bone. Infarction within the epiphysis is called osteonecrosis; diaphyseal lesions are called bone infarcts. Common risk factors for bone infarcts/osteonecrosis include chronic steroid use, hemoglobinopathies (sickle cell disease), and alcoholism.

Pearls

1. Radiographically, bone infarcts, and osteonecrosis appear as serpigenous sclerotic lines forming geographic outlines or ill-defined areas of sclerosis within the medullary space of a bone.
2. An MRI is the study of choice and can reveal many more infarcts than are apparent radiographically.
3. An MRI can determine the age of the infarct.

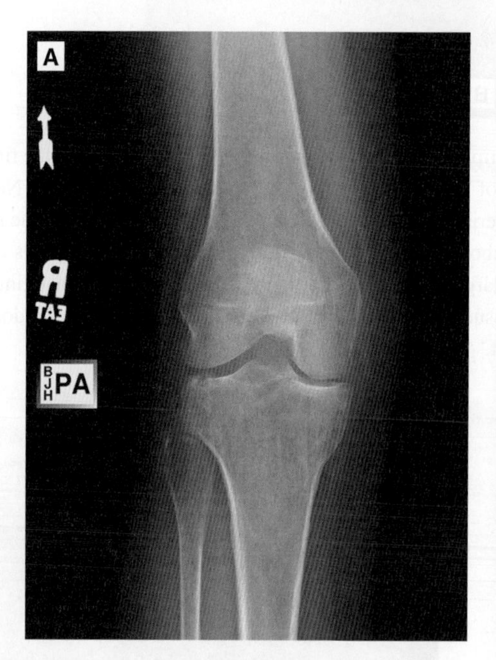

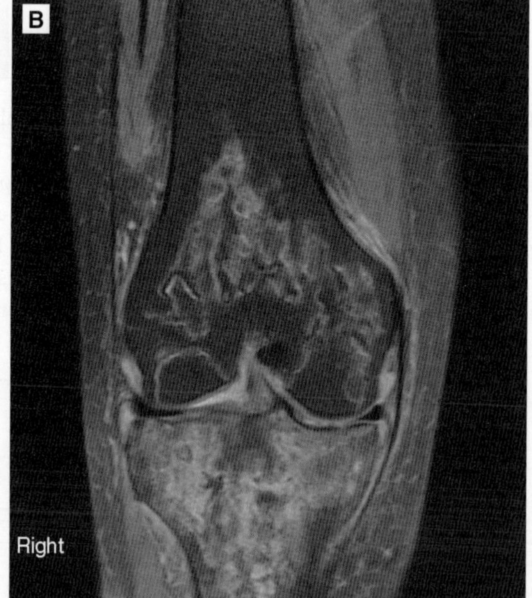

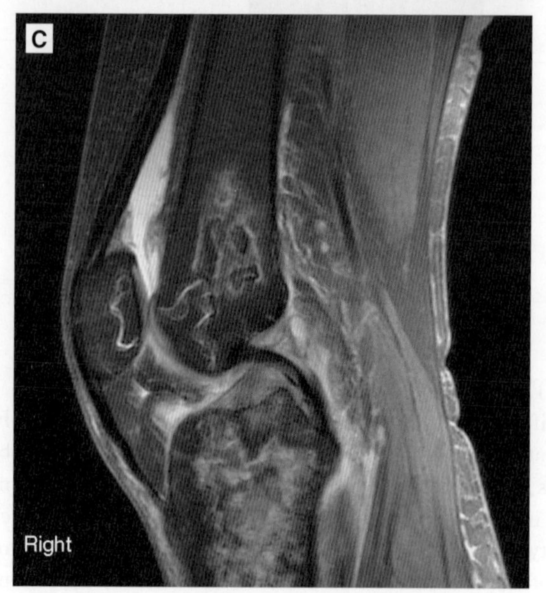

FIGURE 10.114 ■ Bone Infarction. **A:** An AP view of the right knee shows ill-defined areas of sclerosis within the proximal right tibia. There is no fracture or malalignment. Bone infarcts were suspected. **B, C:** An MRI of the right knee was obtained. These coronal FS PD and sagital FS T2-weighted images of the knee show serpiginous hypo- and hyperintense parallel lines that form geographic outlines in the distal femur, proximal tibia, and patella. These are classic bone infarcts. When infarcts occur in the epiphyses they are called osteonecrosis and when they occur in the diaphysis they are called bone infarcts. There is a lot of edema in the proximal tibia indicating that this infarct is acute. The infarcts of the distal femur and patella are not surrounded by edema and are indolent.

Radiographic Summary

There are two types of neuropathic arthritis: hypertrophic and atrophic. In the shoulder (a non-weight-bearing joint), one typically encounters the atrophic type characterized by a "gillotined" appearance; differential considerations for this form of neuropathic arthritis include prior infection, surgical resection, and advanced inflammatory arthritis. In weight-bearing joints (hip, knee, ankle, and the joints of the foot), the hypertrophic form is typically observed and is characterized by severe joint space destruction, subluxations or dislocations, marked periarticular sclerosis and fragmentation, joint effusions and intra-articular debris. Hypertrophic neuropathic arthritis is characterized by multiple Ds (dislocation, destruction, density, debris).

Clinical Implications

The etiology of neuropathic (Charcot) arthritis is likely multifactorial: loss of sensation, dysautonomia, and vascular compromise all likely playing a role. Diabetes is the most common cause of a Charcot arthropathy. Patients present with pain, reduced function, swelling, and erythema. The differential for this arthropathy includes osteomyelitis, septic joint, gout, and complex regional pain syndrome. Patients generally have good distal pulses, as blood flow is required for bone resorption. The presence of good distal pulses makes vascular insufficiency less likely.

Pearls

1. Diabetes is the most common cause of a Charcot arthropathy.
2. Infection must be ruled out.
3. An MRI may be of some help. However, be aware that infection and early neuropathic arthritis may look alike. A radiolabeled WBC scan is the most specific imaging modality for ruling in osteomyelitis.

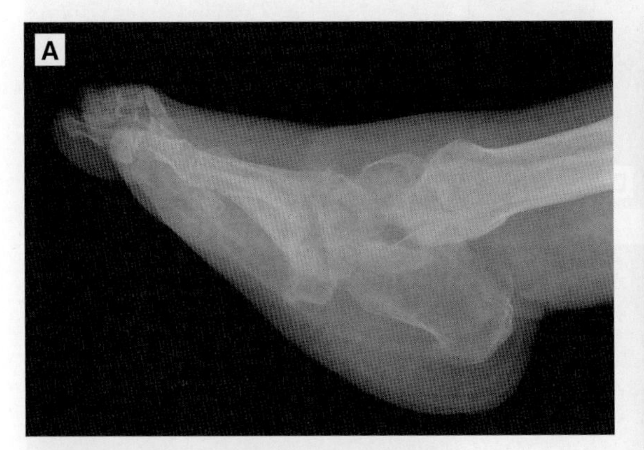

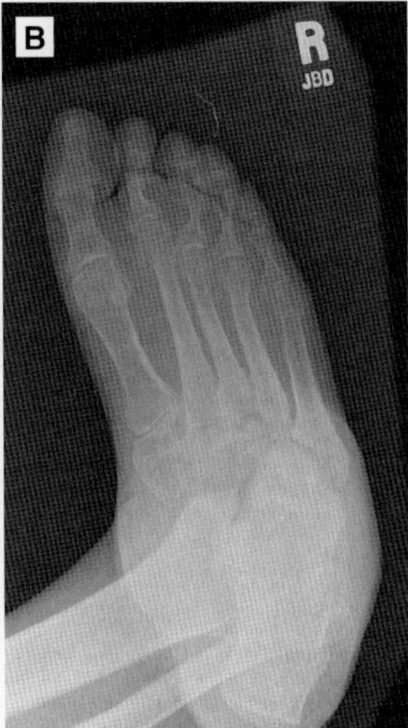

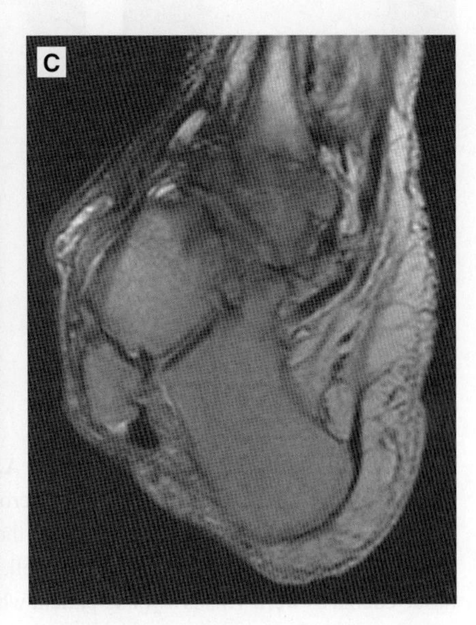

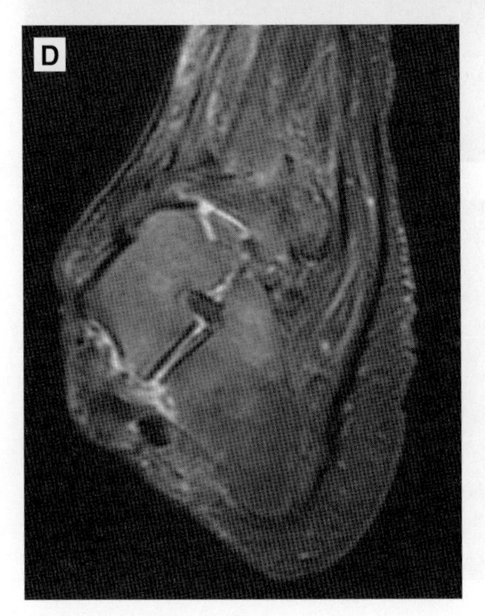

FIGURE 10.115 ■ Neuropathic Arthrits. **A-D:** DP and lateral views of the right foot show markedly increased sclerosis of the bones of the hindfoot and midfoot. The tarso-metatarsal joints are severely narrowed, the midfoot has collapsed, and the cuboid is extruded distally. There is extensive soft tissue edema. These are classic findings of neuropathic arthritis. The clinical presentation and, sometimes, the radiographic presentation mimic chronic osteomyelitis. The utility of MRI in the assessment of these patients is very limited. Joint destruction with subluxations and bone fragmentation, extensive periarticular marrow edema, and soft tissue edema are the usual findings on MRI, as seen on these axial FS T2 and T1-weighted images. The MRI findings can be seen in the setting of infection as well. Findings on radiographs or MRI, which would favor a superimposed osteomyelitis would be new osteolysis and new ulcer or soft tissue abscess extending to an actively lysed bone cortex.

Radiographic Summary

Initial radiographs may be normal. 7 to 10 days after the onset of osteomyelitis, radiographs reveal cortical osteolysis or erosions, periosteal new bone formation, or subtle permeation of the trabecular bone, as well as soft tissue swelling. Chronic osteomyelitis results in sclerotic, deficient, or "whitled" bones. Dead bone (the "sequestrum") becomes enveloped by normal bone (the "involucrum"). Sometimes, a sinus tract ("the cloaca") may be appreciated. Acute osteomyelitis may be diagnosed with an MRI.

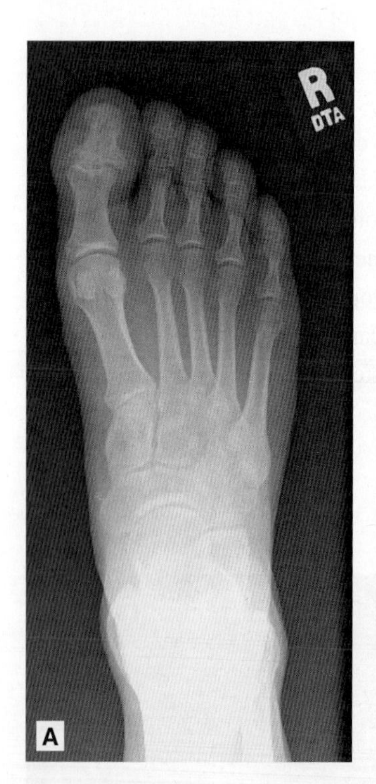

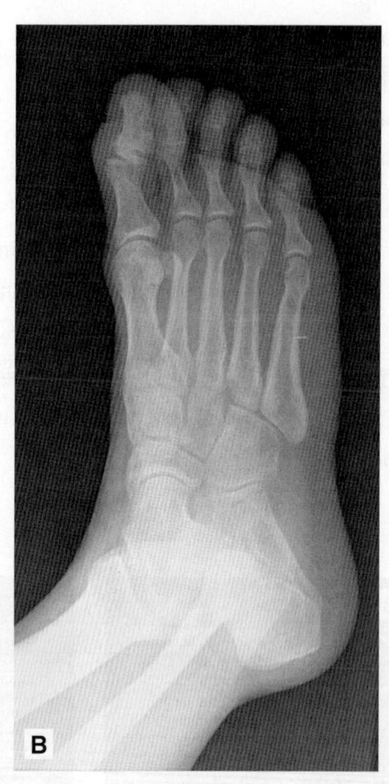

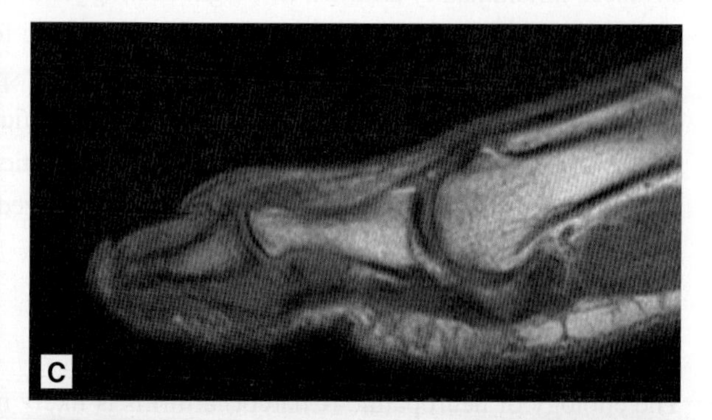

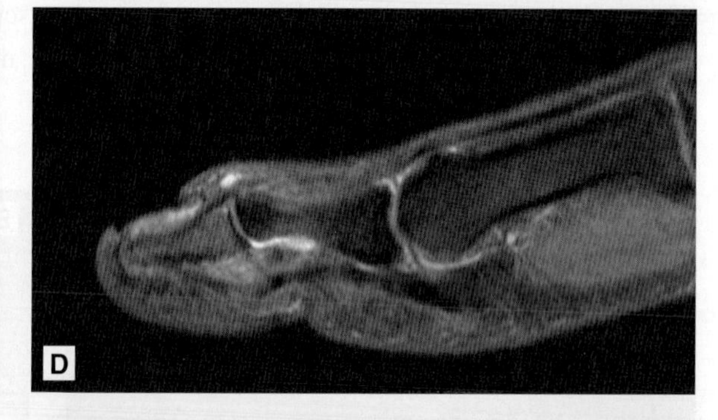

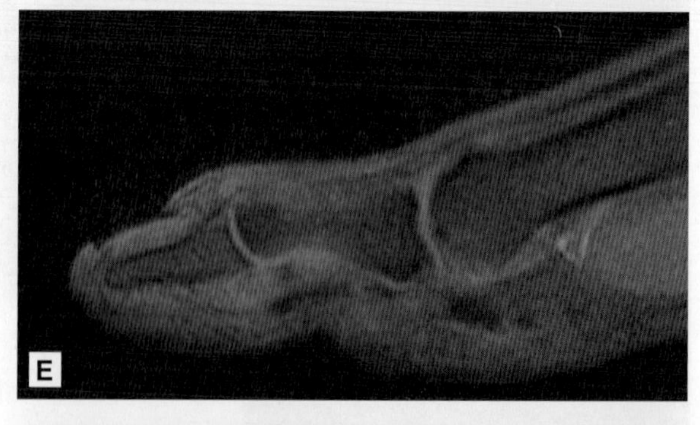

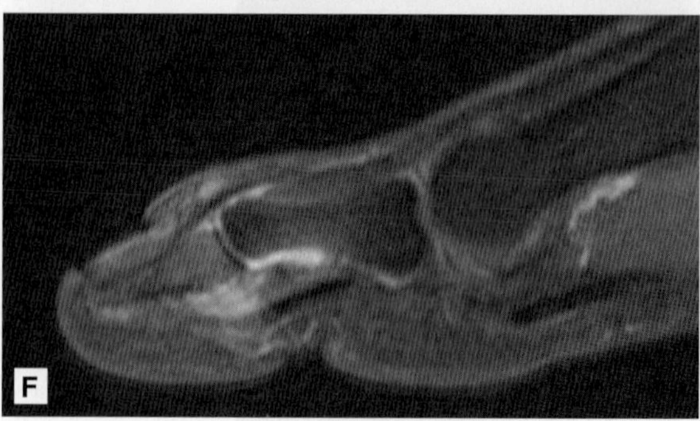

FIGURE 10.116 ■ Chronic Osteomyelitis. **A, B:** DP and oblique radiographs of the right foot show increased sclerosis of the distal phalanx of the great toe. Small erosions are present at the base of the distal phalanx and there is some hypertrophic change as well. There is some regional soft tissue edema as well. This is a young patient who fell off a tree a few weeks earlier, broke his great toe nail, and presented to the ED with a red, swollen, and painful toe. The radiographic findings are consistent with chronic osteomyelitis. Reactive arthritis and psoriatic arthritis are in the differential and can produce an identical radiographic appearance of the distal phalanx of the great toe but the clinical information fits chronic osteomyelitis better. **C-F:** Sagital T1, FS T2, Fs T1, and Gd-enhanced FS T1-weighted images of the great toe show subtle replacement of the normal T1 hyperintense marrow signal with T1 isointense signal, as well as marrow edema and mild enhancement. There is mild surrounding soft tissue edema and enhancement. There is no joint effusion. There are no abscesses. There is no unenhancing (devitalized) bone.

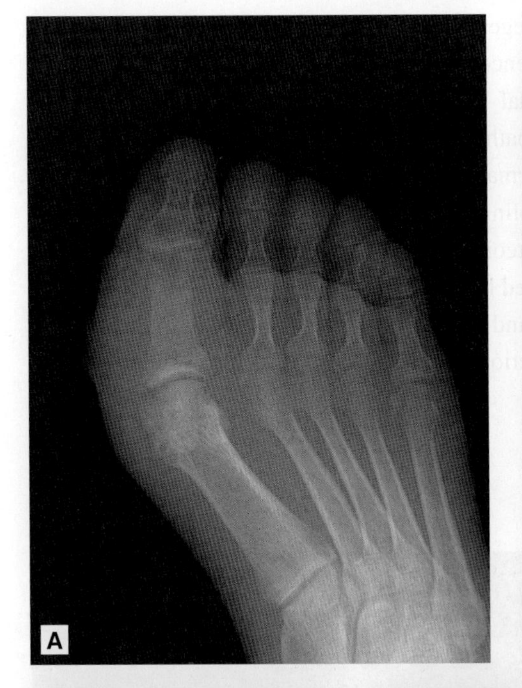

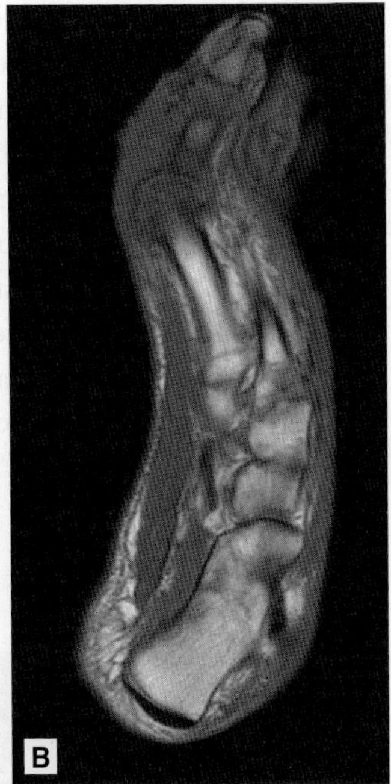

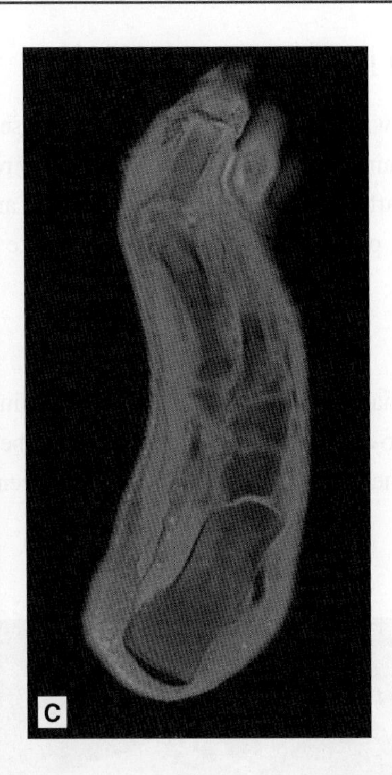

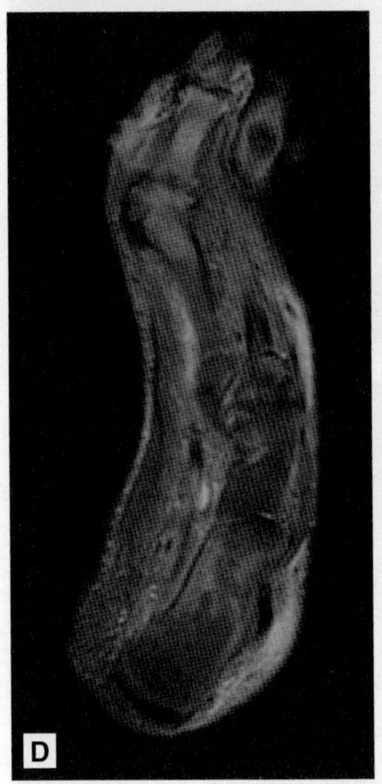

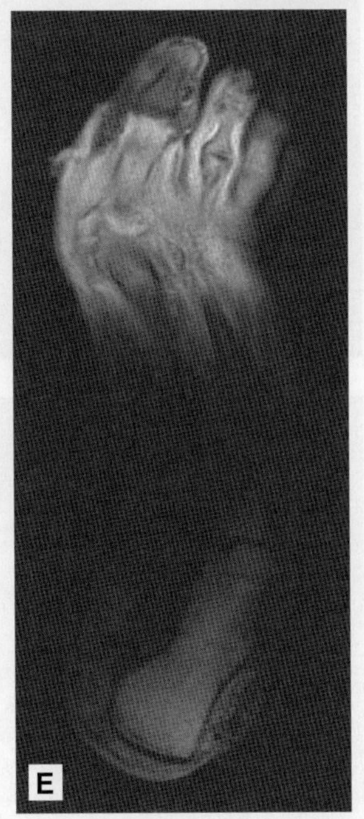

FIGURE 10.117 ■ Septic Arthritis with Gangrene. **A:** A DP view of the toes shows marked soft tissue edema in the foot and particularly in the great toe, as well as a very large amount of soft tissue gas within the great toe. The findings represent cellulitis and soft tissue gangrene. There is significant osteolysis of the head of the proximal phalanx of the great toe with destruction of the medial cortex. There is some apparent osteolysis of the distal phalanx as well. The interphalangeal joint of the great toe is severely narrowed; is the setting of infection, septic arthritis is suspected. **B-E:** Coronal T1, FS T1, Fs T2, and Gd-enhanced Fs T1-weighted images of the same foot show replacement of the normal T1 hyperintense marrow signal within the proximal and distal phalanges of the great toe as well as the first metatarsal head. There is extensive marrow edema and corresponding enhancement within the same bones. Prominent erosions are evident in the first metatarsal head, not visible on the conventional radiographs, even in retrospect. There are no areas within the affected bones which fail to enhance; therefore, there is no evidence of devitalized bone. There is extensive edema and enhancement within the surrounding soft tissues consistent with cellulitis. The small foci of signal dropout are due to the soft tissue gas. There are no fluid collections.

Clinical Implications

Patients with osteomyelitis generally present with several days of pain with fevers. Physical exam may reveal tenderness over the affected bone, as well as erythema and swelling. For diabetics, probing an ulcer to bone can make the diagnosis.

Pearls

1. Edema on MRI is a very nonspecific finding. It may be due to early osteomyelitis but may also be due to a myriad of other causes: reactive edema to adjacent inflammation, injury, degenerative change. More specific findings for the presence of osteomyelitis include: replacement of the normal T1-hyperintense signal, cortical destruction, abscess bathing the abnormal bone or ulcer extending to the abnormal bone.
2. IV Gadolinium is not necessary to make the diagnosis of osteomyelitis. It is, however, necessary to detect devitalized bone (which would not respond to antibiotic therapy and must, therefore, be resected) and can make the detection of soft tissue abscesses easier and more reliable.

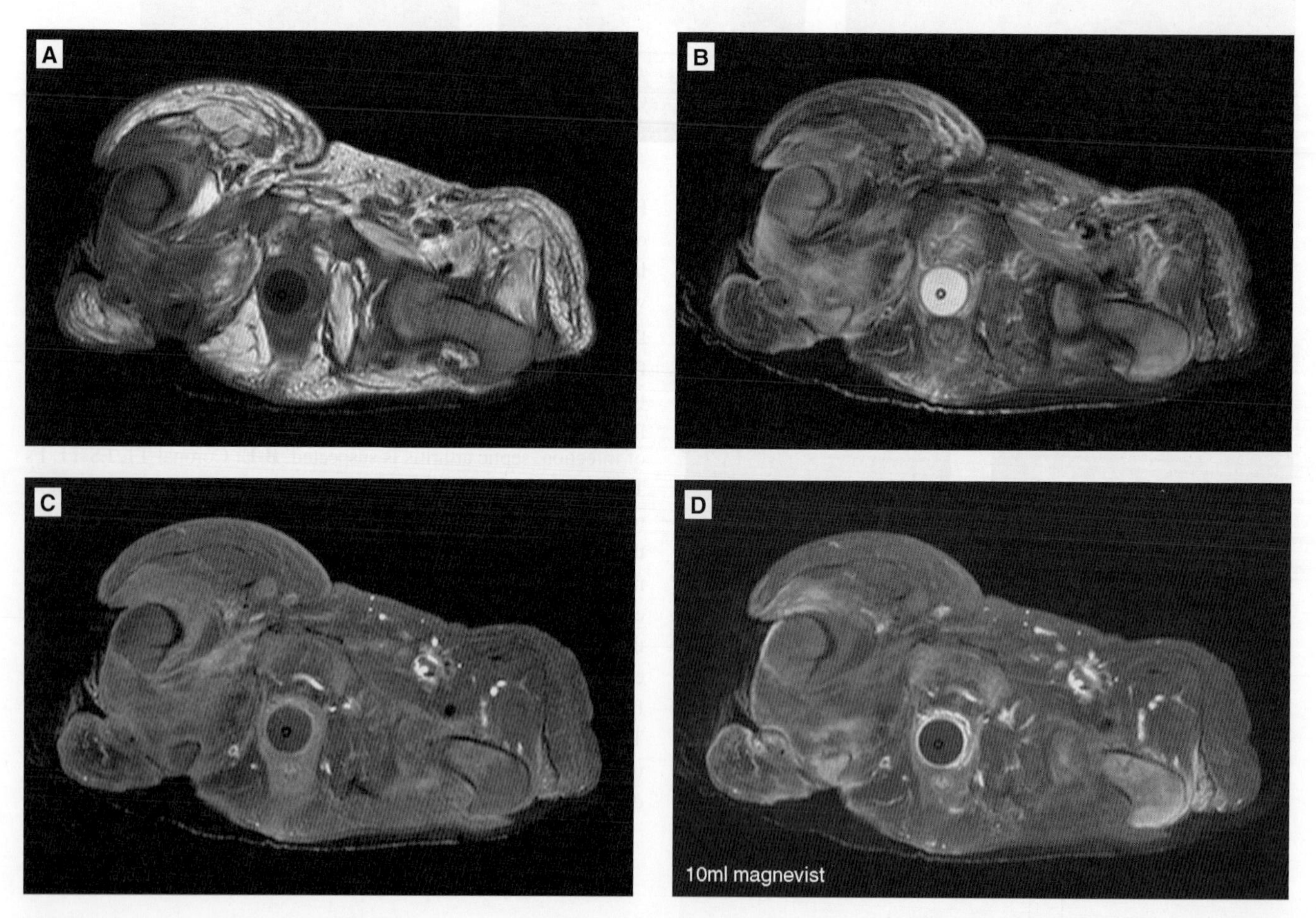

FIGURE 10.118 ■ Dead Bone. **A-D:** Axial T1, Fs T2, Fs T1, and Gd-enhanced FS T1-weighted images of the pelvis show features of osteomyelitis (T1 marrow signal replacement, marrow edema, large decubitus ulcers extending to the bone cortices) of the proximal femurs bilaterally. This patient with large decubitus ulcers has had recurrent and chronic osteomyelitis bilaterally. The Gd-enhanced T1-weighted images show marked abnormal enhancement of the affected proximal left femur indicating this bone is still vital. Conversely, the proximal right femur shows no enhancement after intravenous Gd administration. This indicates that it is devitalized or dead. The ability to detect devitalized bone is one of the main reasons to give intravenous Gd when evaluating for osteomyelitis. The other main advantage is improved sensitivity and specificity in the detection and characterization of soft tissue (and intraosseous) abscesses.

Radiographic Summary

Radiographs are initially normal. If the condition is unrecognized and untreated, the cartilage of the joint is rapidly and uniformly destroyed. In a matter of days to weeks, radiographs would demonstrate gradual and rapid uniform loss of joint space. An MRI is the study of choice: in addition to the joint effusion that is typically present but rather non-specific, an MRI can demonstrate periarticular edema, bone edema, and, sometimes, bone erosions. Ultrasound may identify an effusion and assist the aspiration. If septic arthritis is suspected, arthrocentesis should be performed promptly.

Clinical Implications

Patients with a septic hip will present with hip pain, limited and irritable range of motion, and fever. The knee is the most common joint involved, but the wrist, ankle, and hips are other common joints affected. If septic arthritis is clinically suspected, arthrocentesis must be performed to make or exclude the diagnosis. While an MRI can be strongly suggestive of septic arthritis, it cannot definitively rule in or out the diagnosis; arthrocentesis would still be necessary.

Pearls

1. Septic hip arthritis requires a high index of suspicion.
2. Ultrasound can be used to assess for a joint effusion and to assist the aspiration.
3. If septic arthritis is clinically suspected, an arthrocentesis should be performed promptly. Delays in establishing the diagnosis can lead to irreversible cartilage damage and increase the patient's risk for sepsis and death.

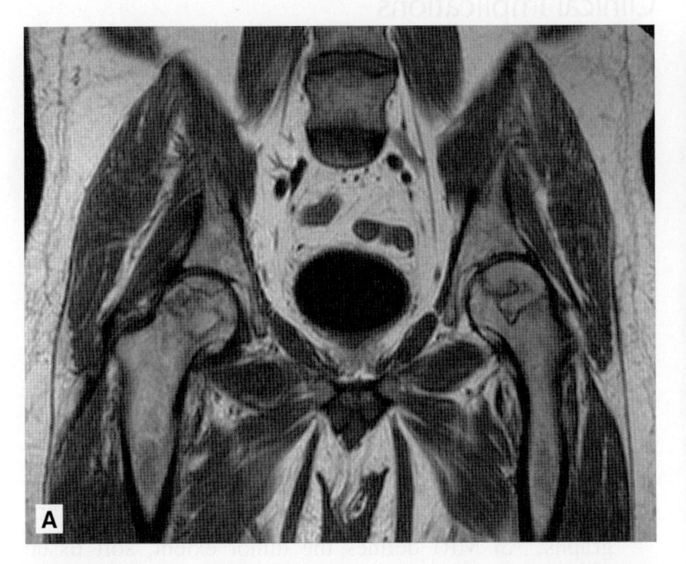

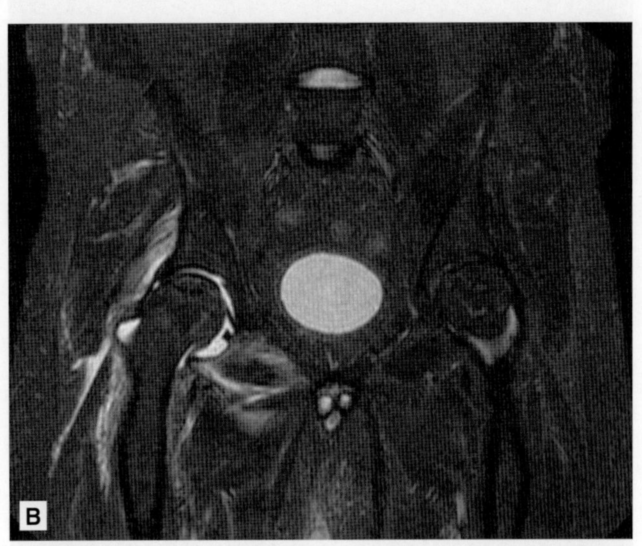

FIGURE 10.119 ■ Septic Arthritis. **A, B:** Coronal T1-weighted and STIR images of the pelvis demonstrate a large right hip joint effusion with significant periarticular soft tissue edema. These findings are very suspicious for septic arthritis. Arthrocentesis of the right hip was performed under fluoroscopic guidance shortly after the MRI examination and ~ 10 cc of pus were aspirated. Note the bilateral femoral head osteonecrosis which appears indolent (no associated marrow edema is present).

Radiographic Summary

A variety of benign and malignant neoplasms may develop within the bones and soft tissues of the lower extremity. A detailed discussion and illustration of the entire spectrum of possible neoplasms is beyond the scope of this book. The Emergency physician should consider the possibility of an underlying neoplasm if the mechanism of injury does not adequately explain the resulting fracture (e.g., a long bone fracture resulting from only minor trauma). Radiographs of the injured bone would reveal the fracture and may demonstrate the underlying lesion. The characterization of the underlying bone neoplasm, if visible, is accomplished on the radiographs; the presence and type of a specific pattern of matrix calcification is critical. The appearance of most osseous neoplasms on MRI is rather nonspecific (T1 isointense to muscle, T2 hyperintense, and enhancing after intravenous Gadolinium administration). The role of an MRI is to depict neoplasms that are radiographically occult, to define the exact size and extent of bone neoplasms and any potential soft tissue extension, and to characterize soft tissue neoplasms that are typically radiographically occult. An MRI does an excellent job in depicting the relationship of the tumor to vital regional structures such as nerves and vessels, and is invaluable in preoperative planning.

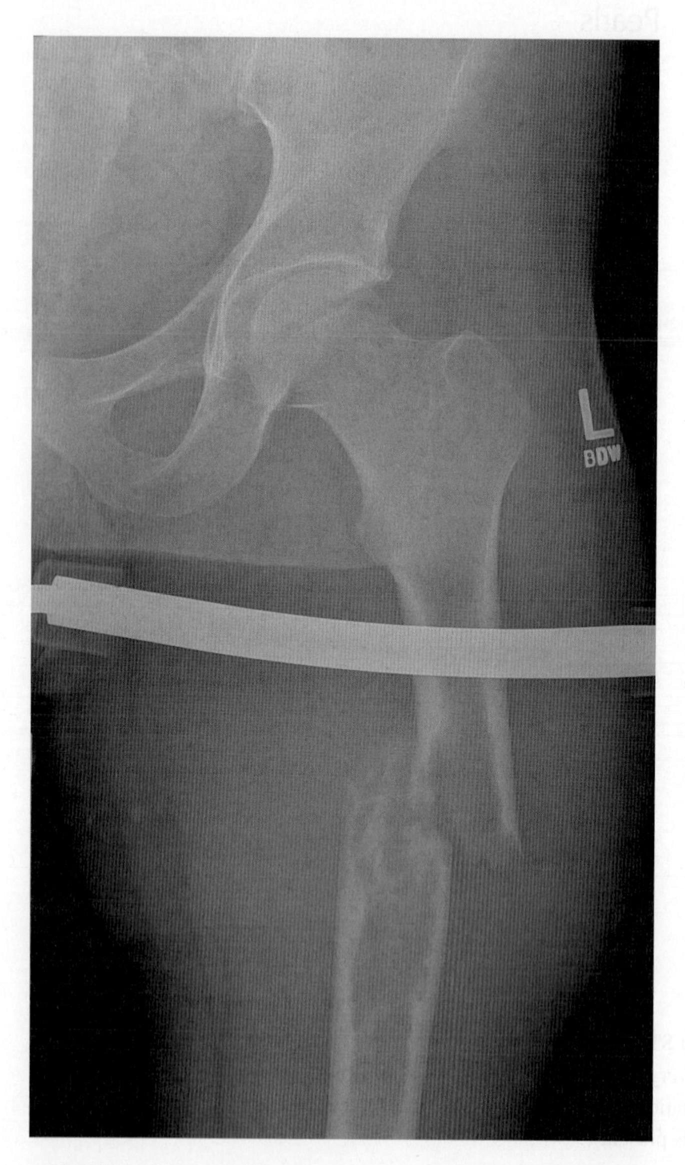

FIGURE 10.120 ■ Pathologic Fracture due to Ewing's Sarcoma. An AP view of the left hip shows a displaced pathologic fracture through an aggressive lytic lesion in the proximal left femoral diaphysis. This proved to be a Ewing's sarcoma.

Clinical Implications

Patients may present to the ED with long bone fractures after minimal trauma. Soft tissue masses lead to regional mass effect and may cause pain from neurovascular impingement, central necrosis, erosion into a nearby bone, or ulceration through the skin. Large primary or metastatic bone neoplasms place patients at significant risk for a pathologic fracture.

Pearls

1. Consider the possibility of a pathologic fracture if the mechanism of injury does not adequately account for the resulting fracture.
2. Bone tumors are characterized on conventional radiographs. An MRI defines the tumor extent, soft tissue involvement, and relationship to the regional neurovascular structures.

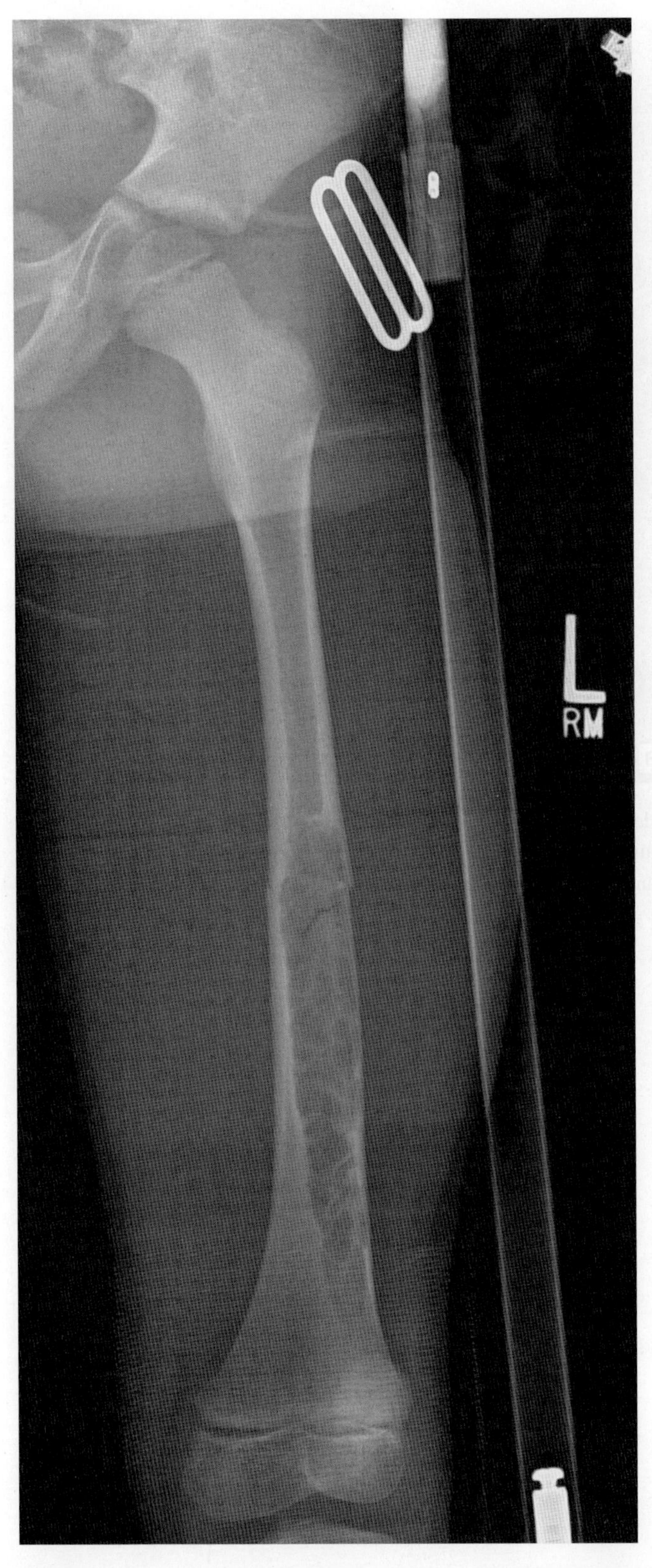

FIGURE 10.121 ■ Pathologic Fracture. AP view of a young child's left femur shows a pathologic fracture through a large lytic lesion in the distal femoral diaphysis. The lesion is well circumscribed, has a lobulated appearance, and a well-defined thin sclerotic margin. This is a large nonossifying fibroma.

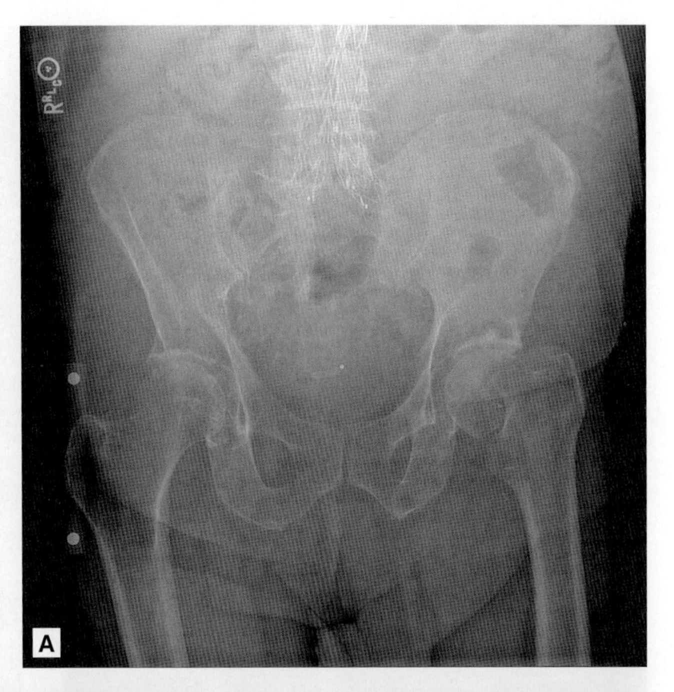

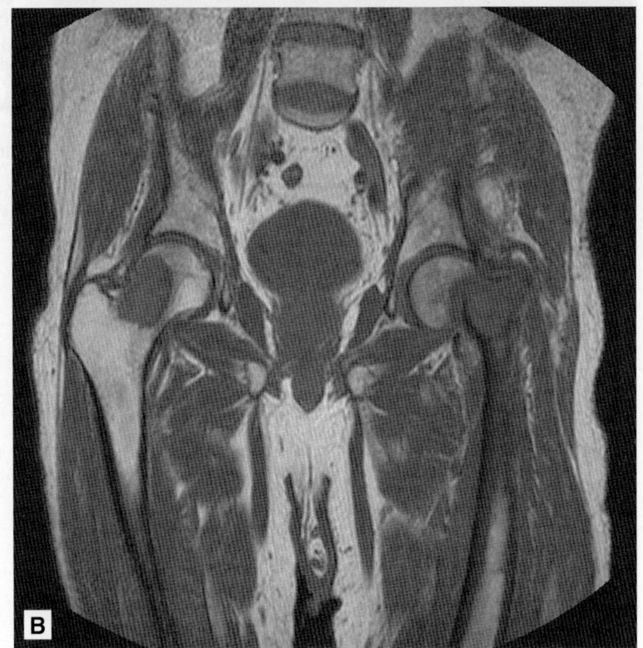

FIGURE 10.122 ■ Lung Metastases. **A, B:** An AP view of the pelvis demonstrates diffuse bony demineralization and an acute angulated and impacted fracture of the left femoral neck. A coronal T1-weighted MRI image at the level of the femoral necks shows a large underlying marrow-replacing lesion, in this case a lung cancer metastasis. Note the very large metastasis within the right femoral neck which is radiographically occult; this metastasis is also at significant risk for a future pathologic fracture.

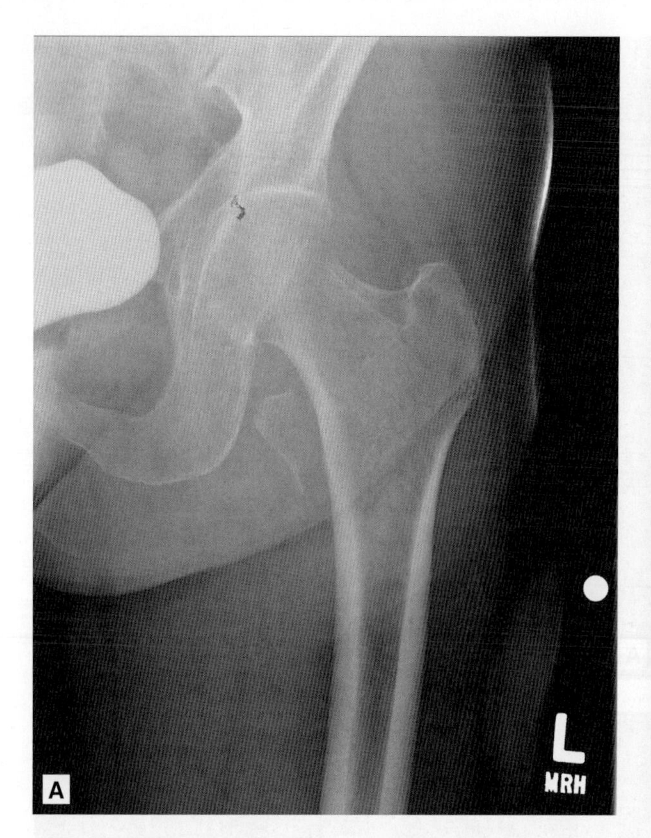

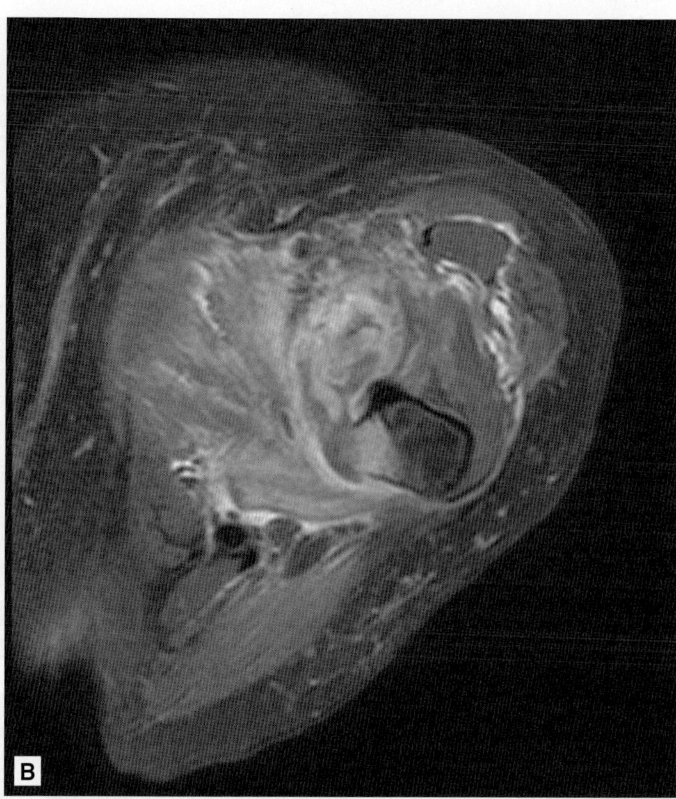

FIGURE 10.123 ■ Lesser Trochanter Fracture. **A, B:** AP view of the left proximal femur shows an acute avulsion fracture of the left lesser trochanter. In adults, this is a classic pathologic fracture and strongly suggests an underlying metastatic lesion. A selected axial fat-saturated T1-weighted image after IV Gadolinium administration shows an enhancing marrow-replacing metastasis in the region of the avulsed lesser femoral trochanter.

Radiographic Summary

Radiographs may reveal gas in the soft tissues. This radiographic finding, however, is not very sensitive as soft tissue gas is not always present. An MRI is the study of choice and can demonstrate fluid and abnormal thickening, gas, or lack of enhancement of the involved fascial planes. A CT may be of some value as well as it may demonstrate small quantities of gas in the tissues, fluid in the fascial planes, or abnormal thickening of the deep fascia.

Clinical Implications

Imaging should not delay surgical intervention in obvious cases of necrotizing fasciitis. Patients can present with rapidly progressing pain, with or without skin findings. Rapidly progressing pain without skin findings of erythema or warmth suggests a deep space infection. Diabetics may not have the same degree of pain due to neuropathy. Immediate actions are required including stabilization, broad-spectrum antibiotics, and surgical consultation.

Pearls

1. Gas in the soft tissues is very specific, but not very sensitive in diagnosing necrotizing fasciitis.
2. Be aggressive in the care of these patients and do not delay surgical consultation to obtain imaging studies.
3. An MRI is the study of choice (preferably with IV Gadolinium) but a noncontrasted, emergent CT scan may be of value as well and may be obtained rapidly in the ER.

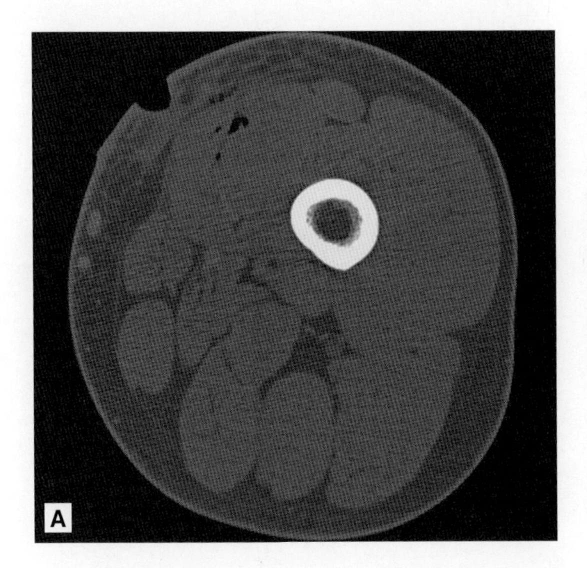

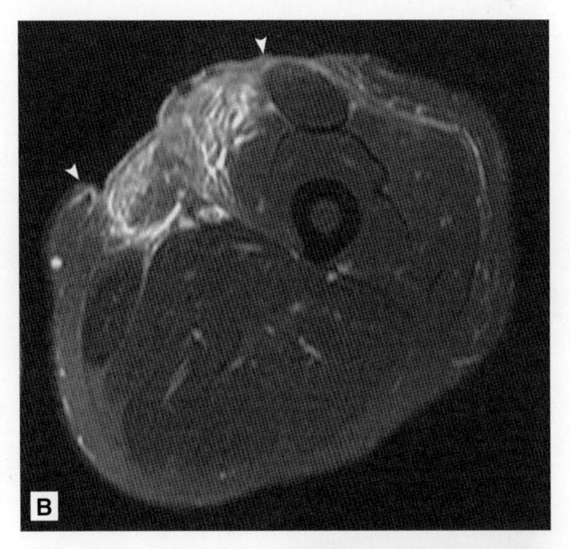

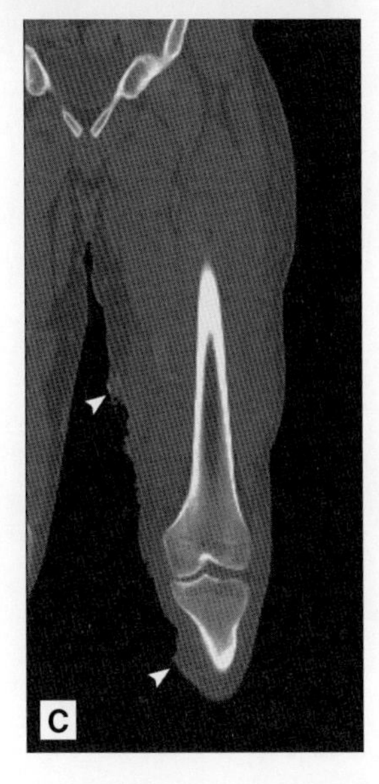

FIGURE 10.124 ■ Necrotizing Fasciitis. **A:** Selected axial CT image shows a large skin defect with adjacent subcutaneous stranding. Gas is present within the subjacent vastus medialis muscle. The superficial fascia over the vastus medialis muscle is markedly thickened. This is necrotizing fasciitis from a brown recluse spider bite. **B, C:** An axial FS T2-weighted image at the level of the original spider bite and a reformatted coronally oriented CT image from a subsequent CT show the extensive debridement of necrotic tissue that the patient required, spanning more than 20 cm in the cranio-caudal dimension (between the arrowheads). The MRI image shows extensive regional fascial edema and thickening as well as regional subcutaneous and muscular edema.

Chapter 11

PATHOLOGIC CONDITIONS OF THE SPINE

Katherine G. Hartley
Jason Dowling
Allison D. Bollinger

Radiographic Summary

A true flexion teardrop fracture appears as a small fractured bony fragment at the anteroinferior border of the vertebral body. Generally, these occur at mid-cervical levels, and are three-column injuries with anterior column fractures, disruption of the posterior longitudinal ligament, and facet disruption. On plain radiographs, this injury is best seen on lateral view, with kyphosis and anterolisthesis at the affected level. The most common radiographic features also include prevertebral soft tissue swelling, a triangular anterior vertebral body avulsion fracture (teardrop fragment), posterior vertebral body subluxation, possible vertebral body displacement into the spinal canal, and spinous process fracture.

Clinical Implications

Flexion teardrop fractures are the most severe injuries to the cervical spine. They are caused by hyperflexion of the neck with additional compressive forces that result in disruption of the posterior ligaments. Flexion teardrop fractures are highly unstable fractures and may be associated with spinal cord injury in up to 50% of cases. Treatment may include rigid c-collar in certain patient populations that have minimal fracture displacement, minimal kyphosis, no neurologic symptoms, and no posterior longitudinal ligament injury. Otherwise, treatments include a halo or operative intervention.

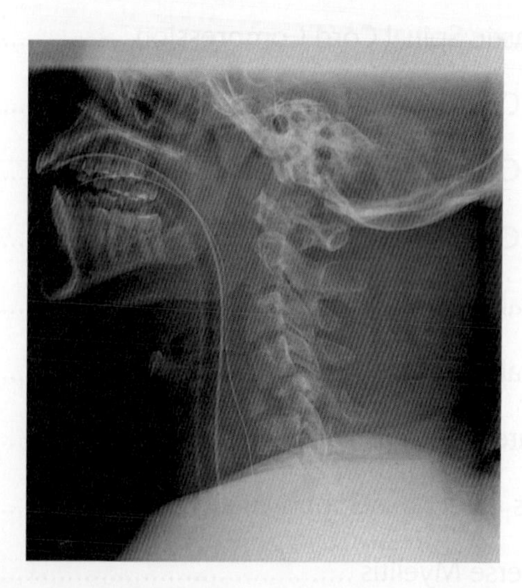

FIGURE 11.1 ■ Flexion Teardrop Fracture. Cross-table lateral radiograph of the cervical spine shows a flexion teardrop injury at the C5 level. In addition to the fracture of the anterior, inferior aspect of the C5 vertebral body, there is disruption of the facet joints, with widening and malalignment of the posterior elements between C4 and C5.

Pearls

1. Flexion teardrop fractures are most common at the C5 level.
2. This particular fracture may be associated with anterior cord syndrome with loss of motor, pain, and temperature sensation, with preservation of proprioception and fine touch.

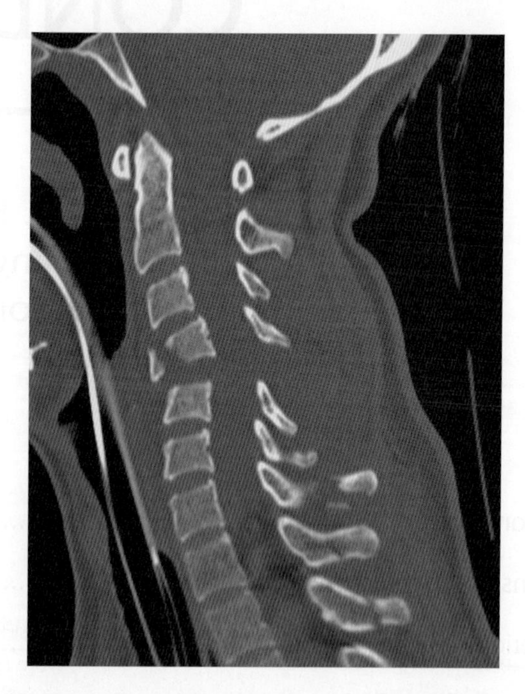

FIGURE 11.2 ■ Flexion Teardrop Fracture. Sagittal CT image in a different patient shows a flexion teardrop fracture at C4. Note widening between the C4 and C5 spinous processes and distraction of the C4–C5 disk space.

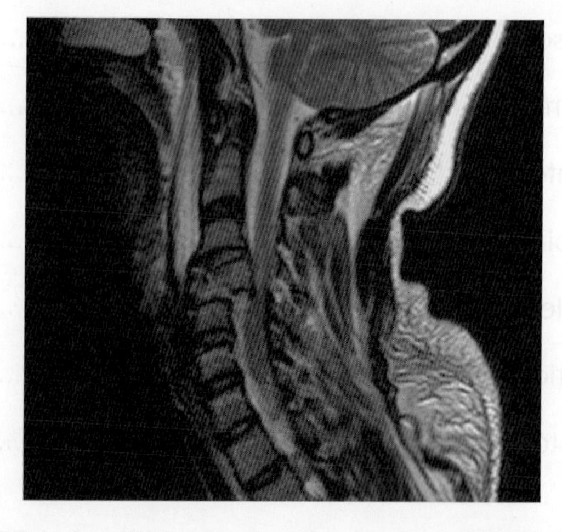

FIGURE 11.3 ■ Flexion Teardrop Fracture. Sagittal T2 MR image shows disruption of the C4–C5 disk space and posterior subluxation of the C4 vertebral body. Increased signal within the spinal cord at the level of injury indicates a cord contusion.

Radiographic Summary

Extension corner avulsion fractures result from avulsion of the anterior longitudinal ligament from the inferior margin of C2, and are a result of extreme hyperextension. These fractures are sometimes referred to as "extension teardrop" injuries, due to the triangular fracture fragment produced, but should be distinguished from the flexion teardrop fracture pattern. In extension corner avulsion fractures, the alignment of the posterior aspect of the vertebral bodies and the posterior elements remain normal, and thus it is a single-column fracture. On plain radiographs, this fracture is best seen on lateral views and is frequently associated with prevertebral soft tissue swelling.

Clinical Implications

Extension corner avulsion fractures are the result of severe hyperextension of the neck. This injury most commonly occurs during MVCs or diving accidents. Extension corner avulsion fractures may be unstable in extension. Treatment is usually conservative with a rigid cervical collar. Surgical treatment is rarely needed, but may be necessary if there are more complex injury patterns involving the posterior longitudinal ligament.

Pearls

1. Extension corner avulsion or "extension teardrop" fractures are most common at C2.
2. Distinguish extension corner avulsion fractures from the more ominous flexion teardrop fractures by the lack of posterior element involvement in extension corner injuries.

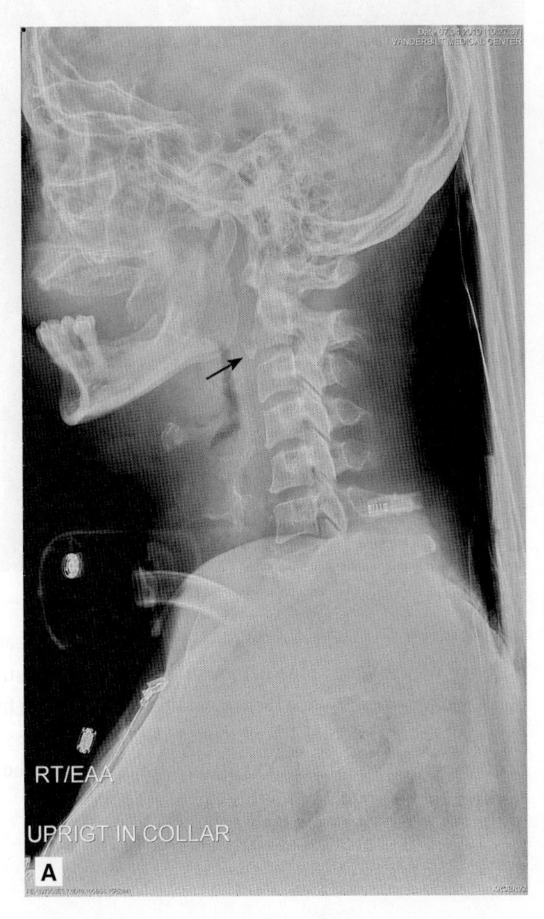

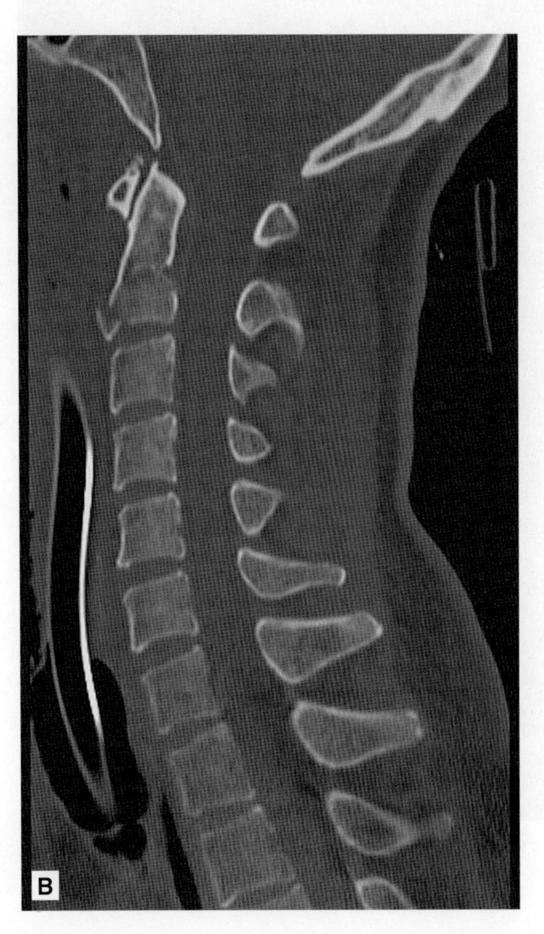

FIGURE 11.4 ■ Extension Corner Avulsion Fractures. **A:** Lateral cervical spine radiograph demonstrates a triangular fracture fragment arising from the anterior inferior endplate of C2 (arrow) and prevertebral soft tissue swelling. Notice that the alignment of the posterior vertebral body cortex remains normal in this single-column injury. **B:** The reformatted sagittal CT images in the same patient redemonstrate the extension injury fracture and normal middle and posterior column alignment.

Radiographic Summary

Anterior subluxation injuries occur when the posterior ligaments are torn and disrupted as a result of hyperflexion. This injury is most common at lower cervical levels and can result in kyphosis at the level of injury, anterior displacement of the involved vertebra (<25% the diameter of the vertebral body), displacement of the articulating facets, anterior narrowing and posterior widening of the disk space, and increased interlaminar/interspinous distances. As the injury progresses from less to more severe, ligamentous disruption can be accompanied by unilateral or bilateral perched and then jumped facets. Anterior subluxation is best appreciated radiographically on lateral radiographs, however, MRI is a far more sensitive modality for detecting ligamentous injury not accompanied by significant bony displacement. Some anterior subluxation injuries are radiographically occult.

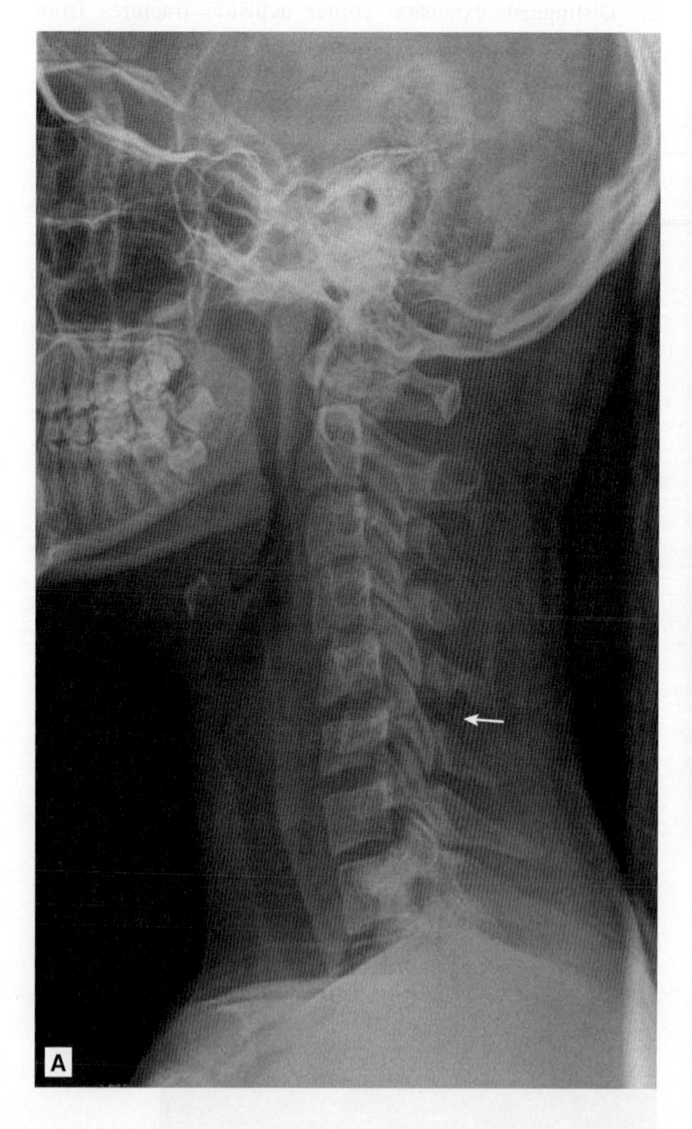

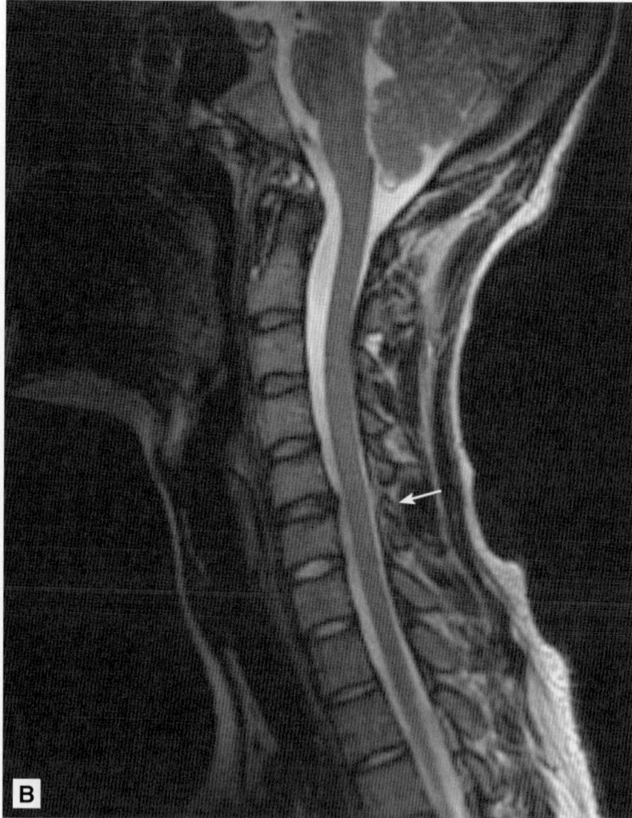

FIGURE 11.5 ■ Anterior Subluxation Injury. **A:** Lateral radiograph of the cervical spine demonstrates subtle interlaminar widening at the C5–6 interspace (arrow) in this patient with a hyperflexion strain injury. **B:** Sagittal T2-weighted MR image in the same patient demonstrates disruption of the ligamentum flavum at the C5–6 level (arrow), with a small post-traumatic disk bulge.

Clinical Implications

Anterior subluxation injury occurs after forceful hyperflexion of the spine. It is rarely associated with neurologic injury. This injury is generally regarded as stable since the anterior column ligaments remain intact. However, there is a risk of delayed instability with significant displacement when the neck is flexed and therefore, these injuries should be regarded as potentially unstable. Surgical intervention may be required to prevent delayed neck instability.

Pearls

1. Nontraumatic anterior subluxation can occur in rheumatoid arthritis and is most common at C5/6.
2. In children, there is a physiologic anterior subluxation of C2 on C3 due to ligamentous laxity (pseudosubluxation). Pseduosubluxation exists if the spinolaminar line drawn between C1 and C3 intersects or is within 2 mm anterior to the C2 spinolaminar line.

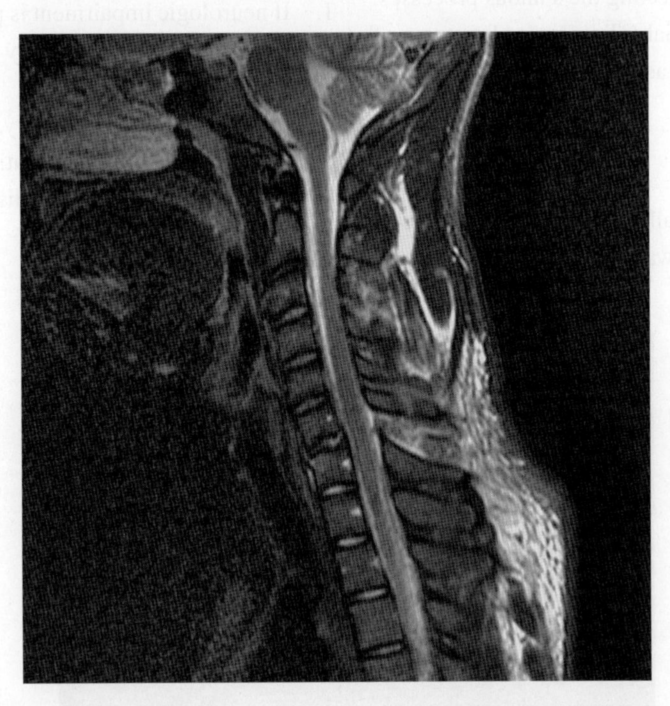

FIGURE 11.6 ■ Anterior Subluxation Injury. MRI of the cervical spine in a different patient shows marrow edema in the C6 spinous process, as well as increased T2 signal in multiple interspinous spaces. Ligamentum flavum disruption is visible at C6–7. The interspinous signal denotes a hyperflexion sprain injury (whiplash).

Radiographic Summary

In a unilateral facet dislocation injury (unilateral "locked" or "jumped" facet), the posterior ligaments are disrupted due to flexion and rotation. One of the inferior articular facets of the upper vertebra moves superior and anterior to the superior articular facet of the lower vertebra, coming to rest in the intervertebral foramen. On lateral views, the involved vertebra will be displaced anteriorly 25-50% the diameter of the vertebral body, and rotational deformity may be visible. Oblique radiographs may help further assess facet malalignment. AP view will show offset of the line connecting the spinous processes. Look for a "naked" facet on axial CT imaging. Fractures of involved facet tips may occur in association with this injury.

Clinical Implications

Unilateral facet dislocation usually occurs following a rotational injury combined with forward or lateral flexion of the neck. This injury is also referred to as a unilateral "locked facet." Neurologic impairment is uncommon. Unilateral facet dislocations are generally stable injuries since the vertebrae are "locked" into place, however, more complex facet fracture patterns may be present, increasing the potential for instability and delayed neurologic injury. These patients are usually treated with halo traction to reduce the facet dislocation and restore alignment.

Pearls

1. If neurologic impairment is present, it is usually a peripheral nerve injury secondary to impingement at the intervertebral foramen.
2. Anterior subluxation injury, unilateral facet dislocation, and bilateral facet dislocation are on a spectrum from mild to more severe anterolisthesis on lateral radiographs.

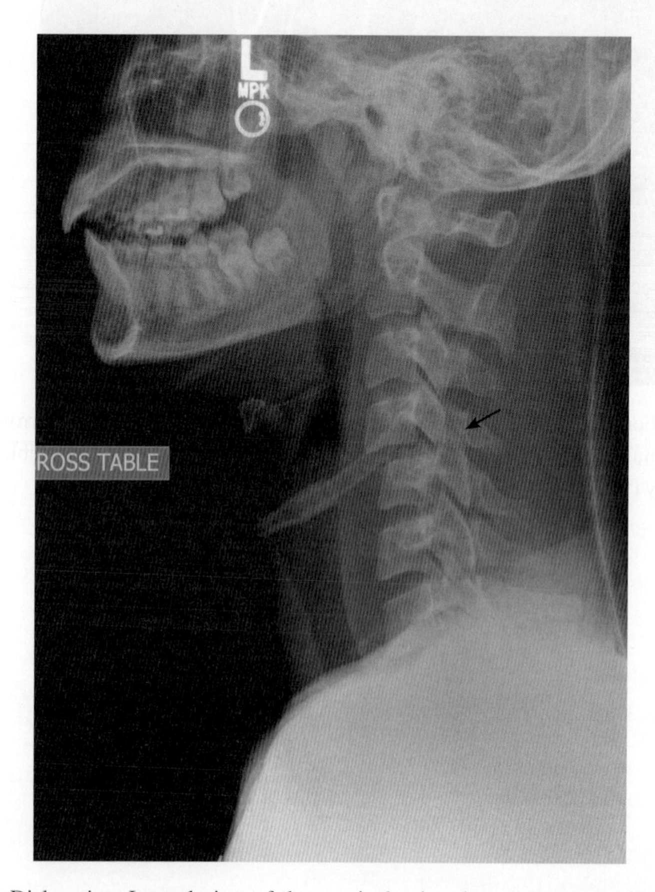

FIGURE 11.7 ■ Unilateral Facet Dislocation. Lateral view of the cervical spine demonstrates a unilateral facet dislocation at the C4–5 level. Note the malalignment of the facet articulation (arrow), and 25% anterolisthesis at C4–5. A rotational deformity is present at the site of injury, typical of unilateral facet dislocations. Vertebrae above the level of injury appear in true lateral projection, while more inferior levels demonstrate rotation. (Image contributor: Jake Block, MD.)

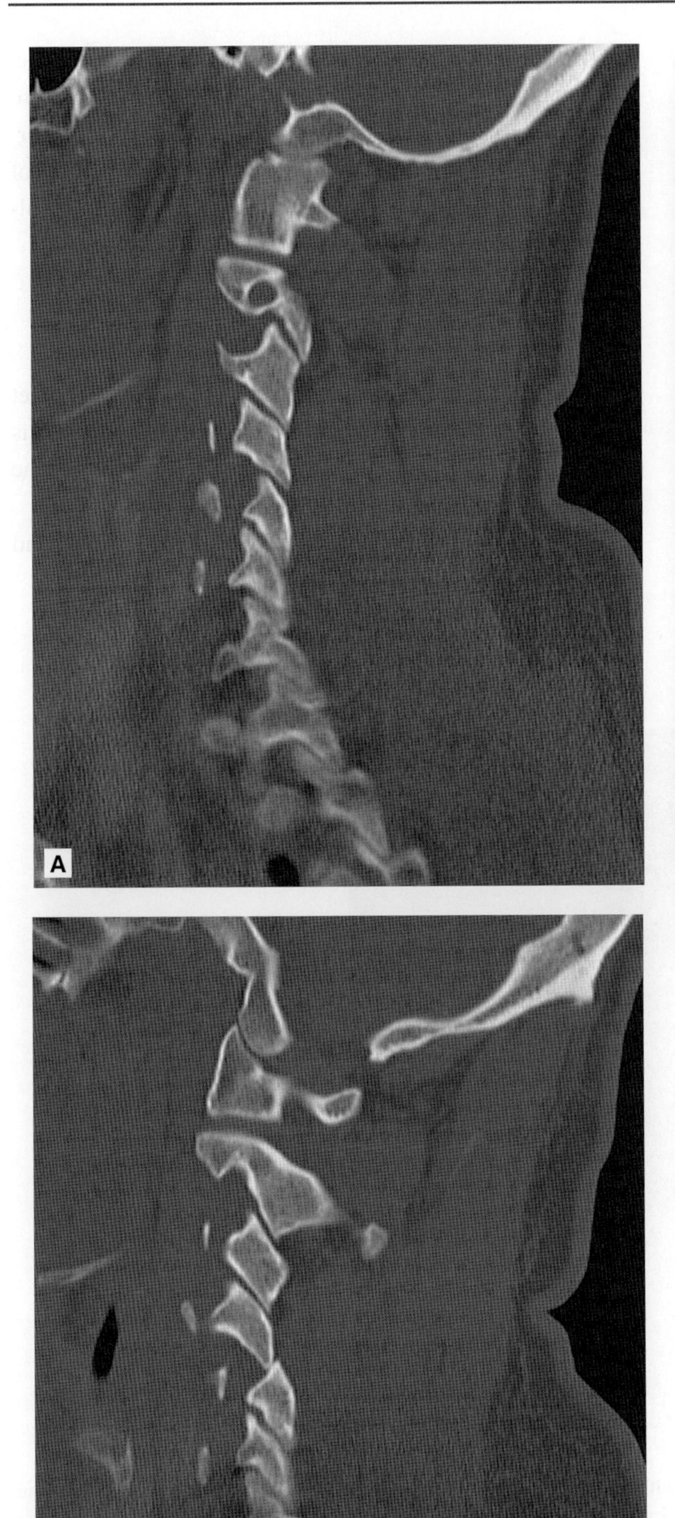

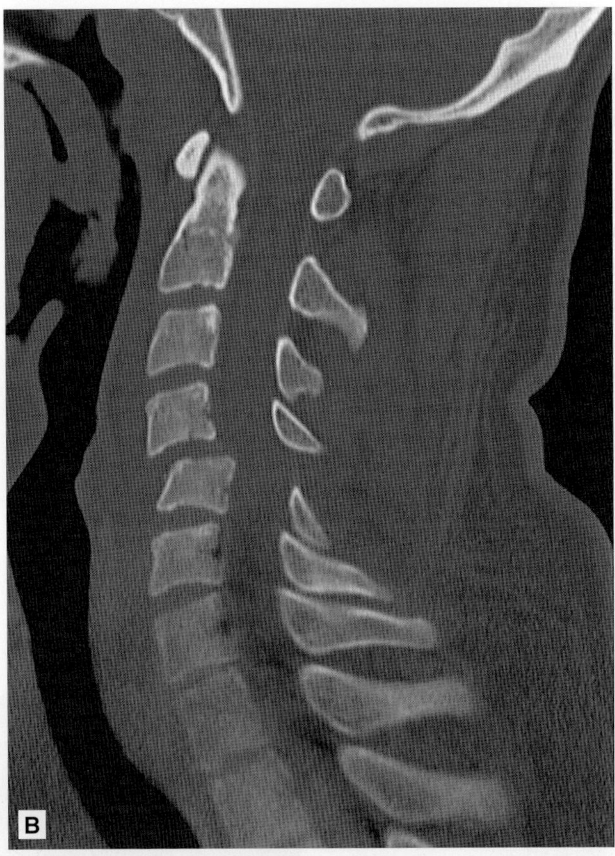

FIGURE 11.8 ■ Unilateral Facet Dislocation. **A-C:** Sagittal reconstructed CT images from a trauma series show normally reduced facet articulations on one side (A). The midline CT image (B) demonstrates the involved C4 vertebral body displaced 25% with respect to C5 inferiorly, typical of unilateral facet dislocation. (C) CT reconstructed sagittal images through the contralateral facet joints show the inferior articular facet of C5 displaced anterior to the superior articular facet of C5, thus a unilateral jumped facet (given the reduced contralateral articulation).

Radiographic Summary

In a bilateral facet dislocation (bilateral "locked" or "jumped" facets), the anterior longitudinal ligaments, annulus fibrosus, and posterior ligamentous complex are injured. This allows both of the inferior articular facets of the superior vertebra to move anterior to the superior articular facets of the inferior vertebra. On lateral view, there is a displacement of greater than 50% of the AP diameter of the vertebral body, and abrupt kyphosis at the affected level. On AP view, there is widening of the interspinous distance at the injury level. On CT scan, the "naked facet" sign shows the uncovered articulating processes.

Clinical Implications

Bilateral facet dislocations occur after extreme neck flexion and anterior subluxation. This is an unstable injury since the integrity of all the stabilizing ligaments and articular facet joints is lost. Disk herniation can occur and contribute to spinal-cord impingement. Careful neurologic exam is imperative as neurologic deficits occur in approximately 75% of patients. Initial management includes closed reduction followed by surgical stabilization.

Pearls

1. Unlike unilateral facet dislocations, bilateral facet dislocation injuries are distinguished by anterolisthesis of 50% or greater, and lack of rotational deformity at the level of injury.
2. CT is important to evaluate for associated facet and posterior arch fractures.

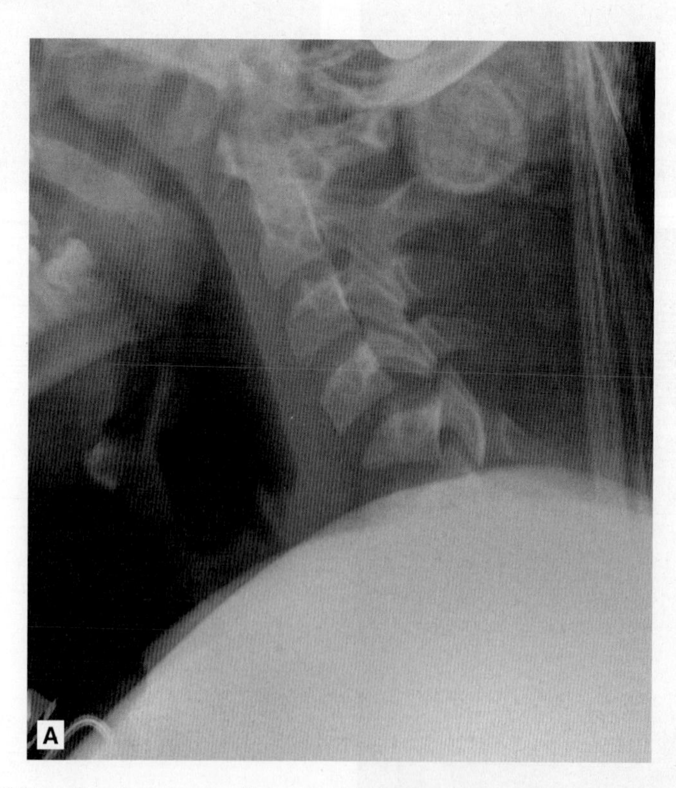

FIGURE 11.9 ■ Bilateral Facet Dislocation. **A:** Lateral radiograph with displacement of both inferior articular facets of C4 anterior to the superior articular facets of C5. Note 50% anterior displacement of C4 on C5, and the lack of rotational deformity typical of bilateral facet dislocation injuries.

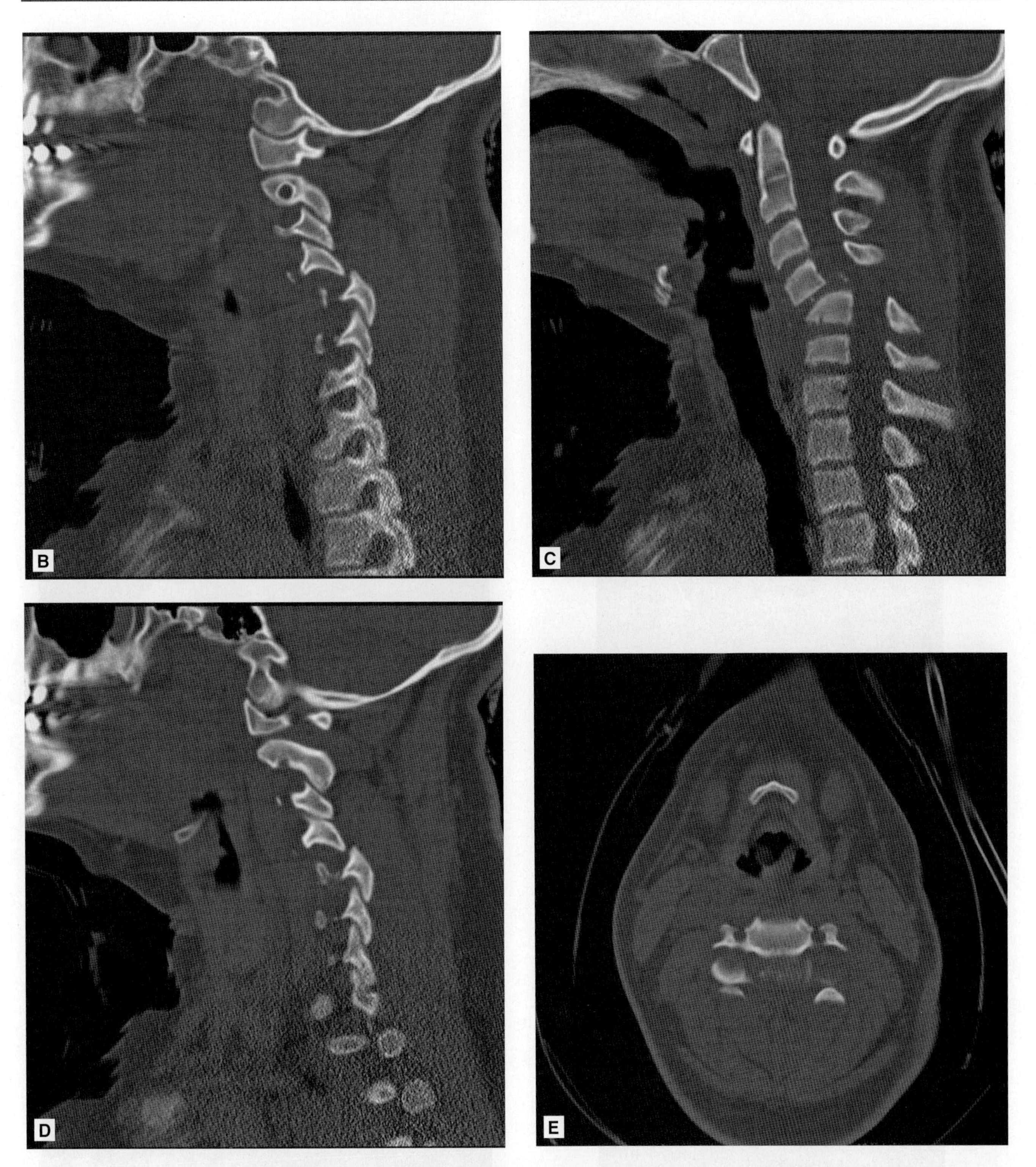

FIGURE 11.9 ■ (*Continued*) **B-D:** Sagittal reconstructed CT images through the cervical spine redemonstrate the severe hyperflexion related bilateral facet dislocation. Notice greater than 50% anterolisthesis of C4 on C5. **E:** An axial CT image through the bilateral dislocation shows four discrete round structures, the articular facets of C4 and C5, without normally anticipated anatomic overlap ("naked facet" sign).

Radiographic Summary

The clay shoveler fracture is an avulsion fracture of the spinous process of any of the lower cervical or upper thoracic vertebra. The spinous process tip is displaced inferiorly. In a simple clay shoveler fracture, the vertebral bodies are normally aligned and the lamina is not affected. More extensive fracture patterns may extend to involve the lamina and spinal canal. This injury is best seen on lateral radiograph.

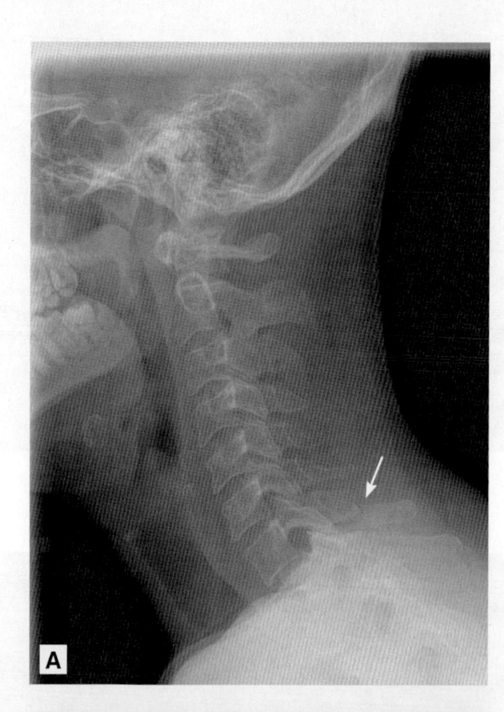

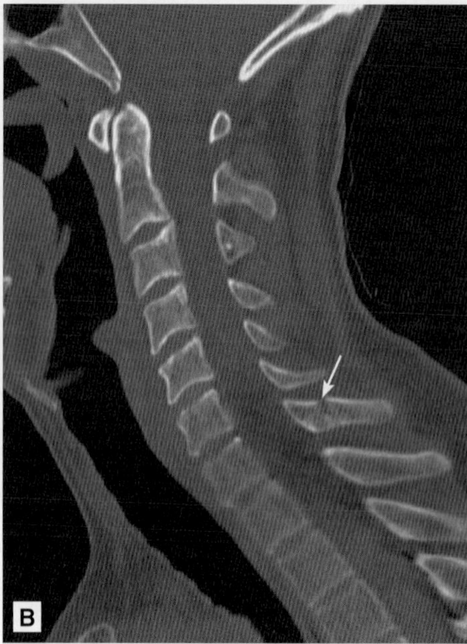

FIGURE 11.10 ■ Clay Shoveler Fracture. **A, B:** Lateral radiograph and sagittal CT image of the cervical spine show a mildly displaced fracture of the spinous process of C7 (arrows).

Clinical Implications

Patients with this type of fracture often present following a hyperflexion injury during contraction of the paraspinous muscles. This injury is classically seen after shoveling clay or snow, but may also occur during an MVC or forceful blow to the back. Pain is usually located between the shoulder blades. This is considered a stable fracture (unless the avulsion extends into the lamina) and the usual treatment is with a cervical collar.

Pearl

1. The clay shoveler fracture is most common at C6 and C7.2. It is almost always a stable fracture that can be treated with a cervical collar.

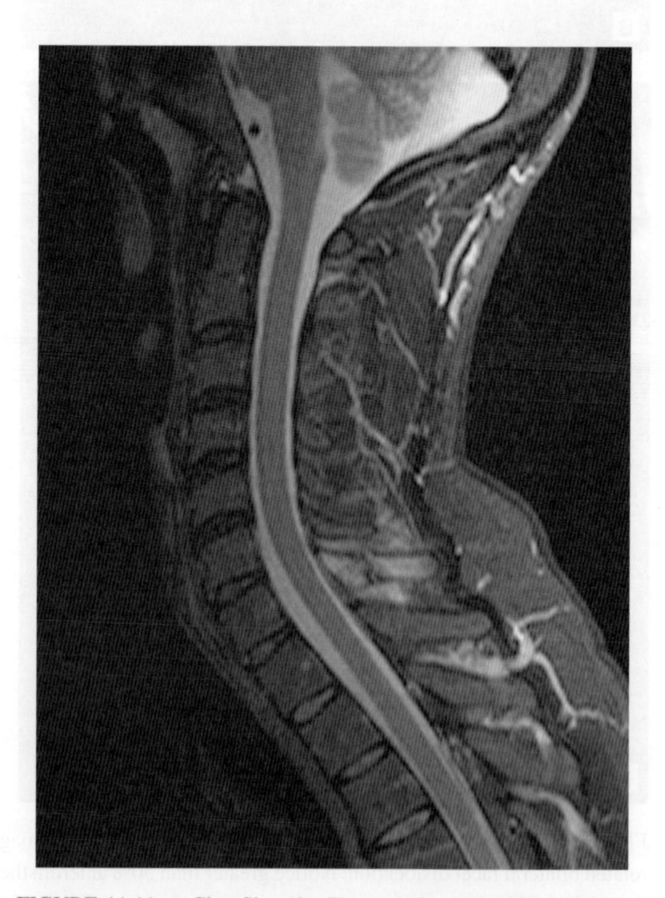

FIGURE 11.11 ■ Clay Shoveler Fracture. Sagittal STIR MR image illustrates not only hyperintense marrow edema around the hypointense avulsion fracture line, but also edema in the intraspinous ligament. Note the lack of spinal canal compromise in this typical clay shoveler's fracture.

Radiographic Summary

Jefferson's fracture is classically considered a four-part fracture of the C1 ring (atlas) with combined anterior and posterior arch fractures, although two and three-part fractures also occur. On plain radiographs, this fracture is best seen on an open-mouth odontoid view. On this view, the distance between the C1 ring lateral masses and odontoid process will be increased either unilaterally or bilaterally. In addition, there will be lateral displacement of the articular portion of the ring of C1 in relation to the lateral margin of C2. However, CT is still the most sensitive way to detect this fracture. Avulsion fractures of the transverse ligament from the inner ring of C1 indicates further instability.

Clinical Implications

Jefferson's fracture occurs secondary to an axial load injury while the neck is in a neutral position. The most common mechanisms for this fracture are from a dive into shallow water, an impact against the roof of a vehicle in an MVC, or from a fall. These fractures are unstable. Treatment depends on the severity of fracture of the anterior arch and whether or not the transverse ligament is functionally intact. Treatment can include a rigid cervical collar, traction, a halo, or surgery.

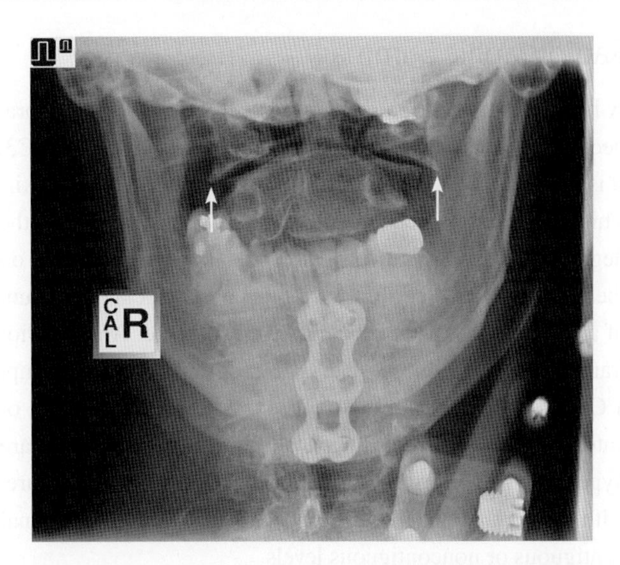

FIGURE 11.13 ■ Jefferson's Fracture. In this patient with Jefferson fracture, the odontoid view of the cervical spine shows lateral displacement of the lateral masses of C1 in relation to the lateral masses of C2 (arrows).

Pearls

1. Associated C2 fractures occur in approximately one half of patients.
2. This fracture rarely leads to spinal cord injury since the fractured fragments have a tendency to fall outward away from the canal and brainstem.

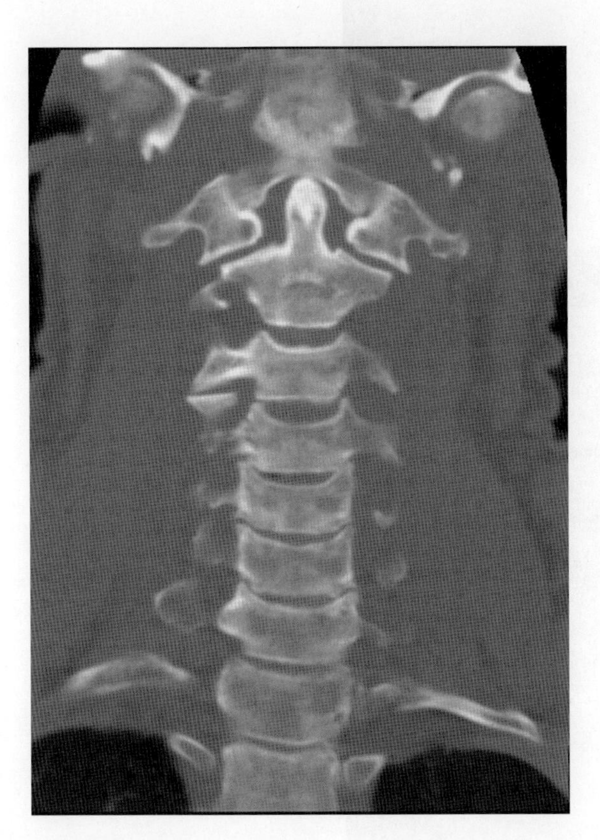

FIGURE 11.12 ■ Jefferson's Fracture. Coronal reformatted image of the cervical spine confirms the widening of the C1 arch with lateral subluxation of the lateral masses of C1.

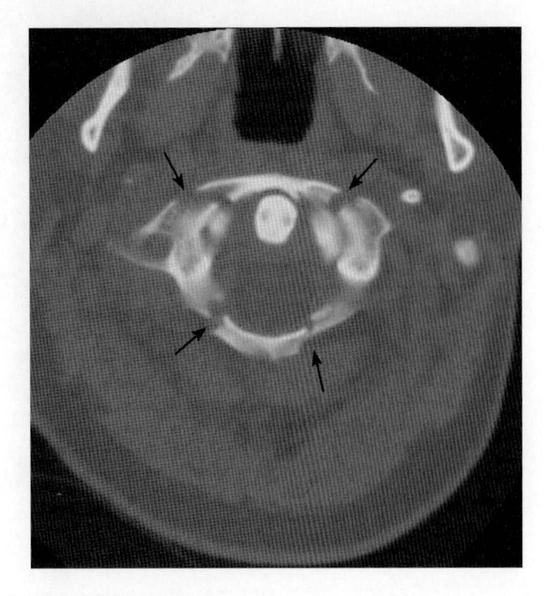

FIGURE 11.14 ■ Jefferson's Fracture. Axial image through the C1 arch shows a classic four-part fracture of the C1 ring (arrows).

Radiographic Summary

A hangman's fracture involves the fracture of both vertebral pedicles at C2 (axis) with or without translation of C2 on C3. It is also referred to as traumatic spondylolisthesis of the axis. This injury is classified into three types, which help stratify the degree of injury and guide treatment. The types are based on the degree of translation of C2 on C3 and associated amount of angulation with type 3 being the most severe. Any anterior translation of C2 on C3 seen on radiographs should prompt a CT even if no fracture is seen. Despite the appearance of anterior displacement and kyphosis at C2-3, these injuries are hyperextension injuries. This is often not an isolated fracture, with many patients having cervical spine injury at additional contiguous or noncontiguous levels.

Clinical Implications

This injury results from forceful hyperextension of the head with neck distraction. MVCs and falls are responsible for the majority of these injuries. Type 1 Hangman's fractures are stable, types 2 and 3 are unstable. These fractures are unlikely to cause neurologic injury, except in type 3 fractures, where the likelihood of spinal cord injury is higher. Type 1 fractures are usually treated with a c-collar, type 2 fractures are usually treated with a halo vest, and type 3 fractures may require operative management.

Pearls

1. Up to 30% of patients with a hangman's fracture will also have other cervical spine pathology.
2. The term "hangman's fracture" is often misleading, as this injury pattern is uncommon following a judicial hanging, and more likely the result of an MVC or fall.

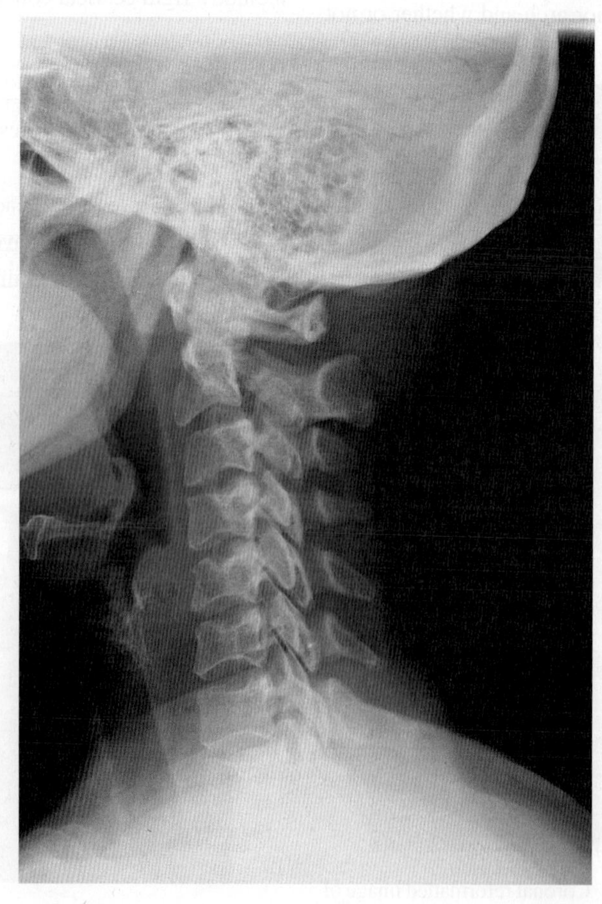

FIGURE 11.15 ■ Hangman's Fracture. Lateral radiograph of the cervical spine shows a fracture through the posterior elements of C2 with mild anterior subluxation of C2. (Image contributor: Jake Block, MD.)

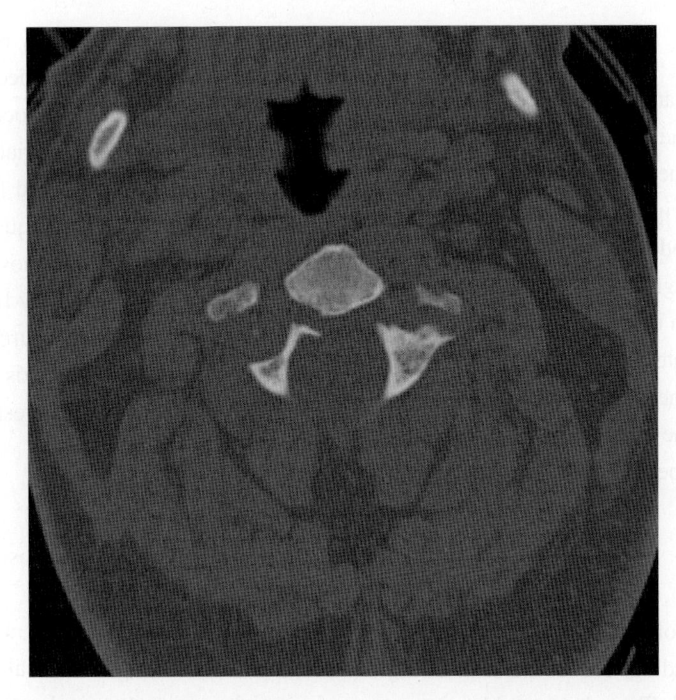

FIGURE 11.16 ■ Hangman's Fracture. Axial CT image through the upper cervical spine shows the fracture extends through both C2 pedicles.

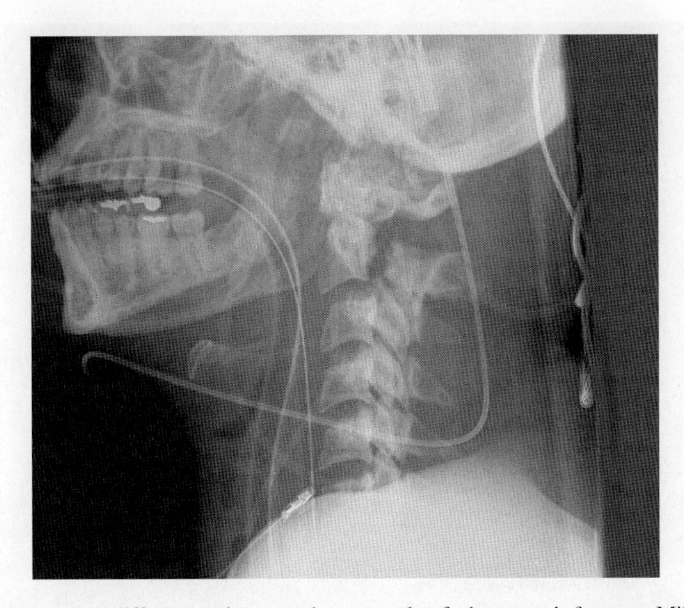

FIGURE 11.17 ■ Hangman's Fracture. In a different patient, another example of a hangman's fracture. Mild anterior displacement of the C2 vertebral body indicates a type 2 injury. Despite the appearance of anterior displacement, hangman's fractures are extension injuries.

Radiographic Summary

Odontoid (axis) fractures occur at C2 and are classified into three types. Type 1 odontoid fractures occur at the tip of the odontoid process (dens) above the level of the alar ligaments (that connect the dens to the occiput). Type 2 odontoid fractures occur at the base of the odontoid process and type 3 odontoid fractures occur through the C2 vertebral body. These injuries may be evident on both the open-mouth odontoid radiograph, as well as the lateral projection of the cervical spine. Careful evaluation of the bone cortex of the anterior portion of the C2 vertebra on the lateral x-ray is critical for detecting subtle nondisplaced type 2 or type 3 fractures.

Clinical Implications

Flexion loading is the usual cause of injury; however, this injury can also occur from extension loading. These fractures usually occur following an MVC or fall. Type 1 odontoid fractures are stable and neurologic injury is uncommon since the alignment of C1 on C2 is maintained. Type 1 fractures are very rare, with many abnormalities occurring at the tip of the dens indicative of developmental variations (osodontoideum) rather than fractures. Type 2 odontoid fractures are unstable, prone to nonunion, and are more frequently associated with neurologic deficits. These are the most common type of odontoid fractures. Type 3 fractures may be comminuted and unstable and may be associated with neurologic injury if fragments are displaced. Management depends on the type of fracture and may include a c-collar, a halo vest, or operative intervention.

Pearls

1. Type 2 fractures are the most common and most unstable fracture of the odontoid.
2. The rare type 1 fractures are usually managed with a c-collar, but occipitocervical instability must be ruled out since it requires surgical management.

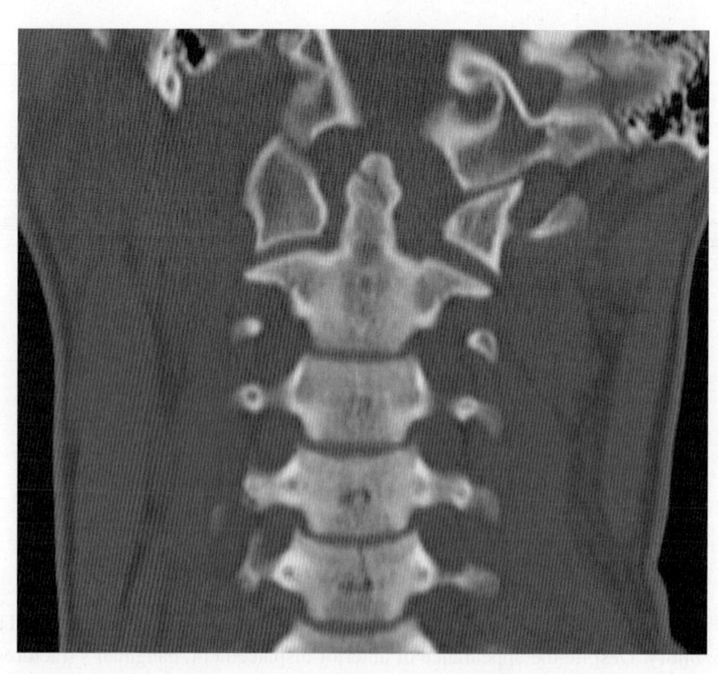

FIGURE 11.18 ■ Type 1 Odontoid Fractures. Type 1 odontoid fracture: coronally reformatted CT image of the cervical spine shows a fracture line extending through the tip of the odontoid process. These fractures are quite rare and difficult to see on radiographs.

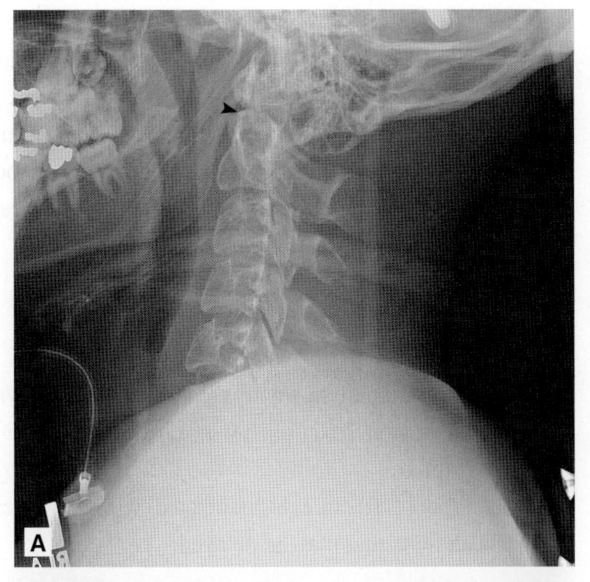

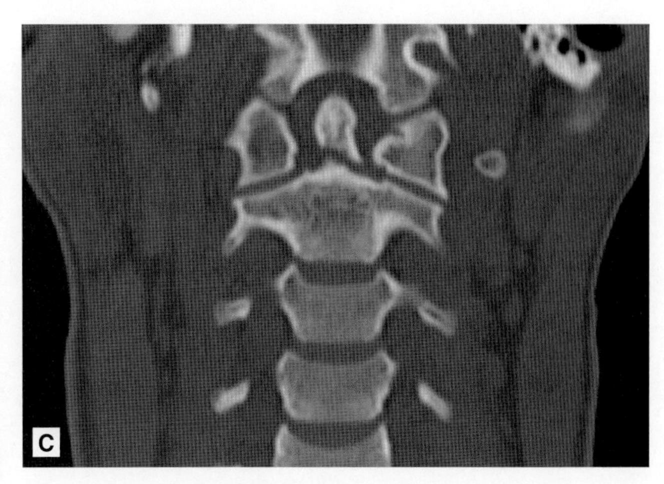

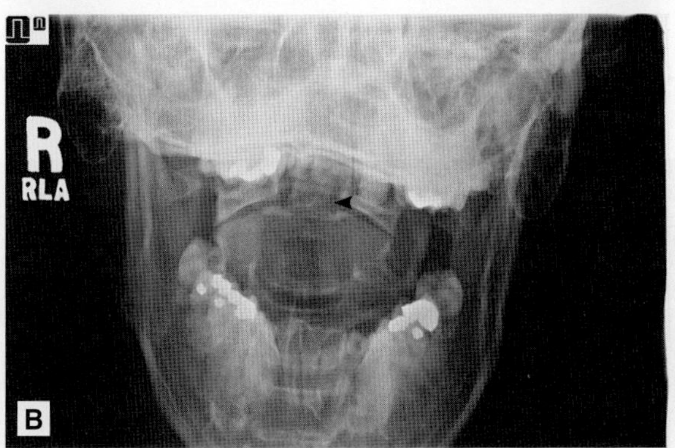

FIGURE 11.19 ■ Type 2 Odontoid Fractures. **A, B:** Lateral and open mouth odontoid views of the cervical spine show subtle disruption and step off at the base of the odontoid process (arrowheads) and a fracture plane through the base of the dens. **C:** Reformatted CT image in the coronal plane better illustrate the fracture line and show that the vertebral body is not involved.

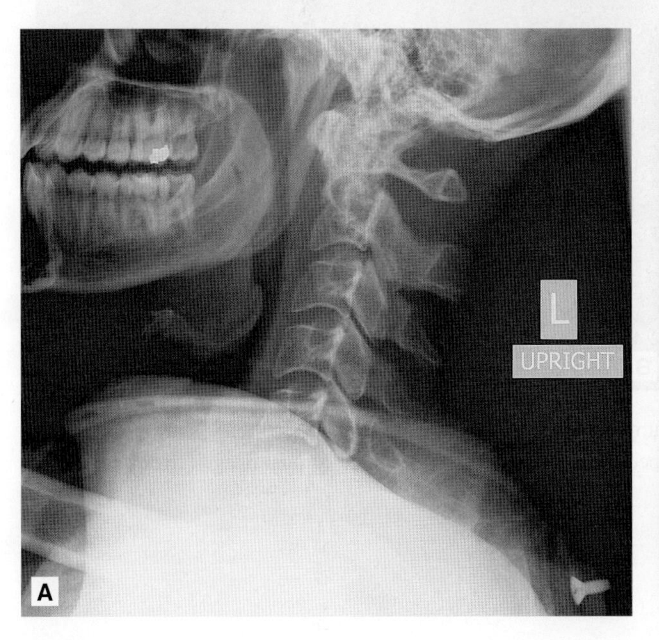

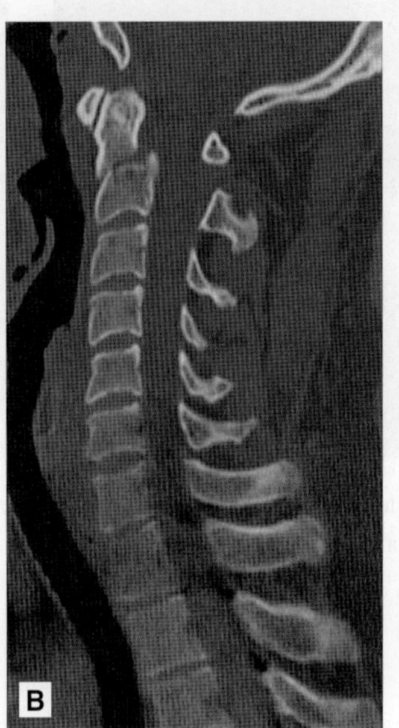

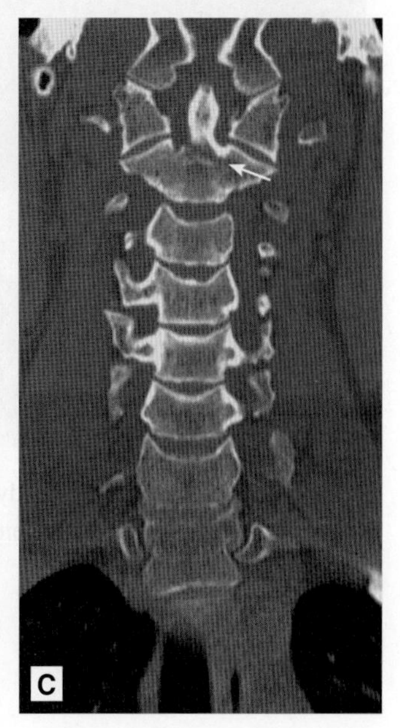

FIGURE 11.20 ■ Type 3 Odontoid Fractures. **A-C:** Lateral cervical spine radiograph shows anterior angulation of the dens, with cortical disruption of the anterior C3 vertebral body. The CT reformatted images confirm that the fracture line extends into the C2 vertebral body (arrow) with mild comminution, differentiating this type 3 fracture from a type 2.

Radiographic Summary

There are three types of occipital condyle fractures. Type 1 fractures are comminuted but not displaced. Type 2 fractures are extensions of basilar skull fractures. In type 3 fractures, the condyle is avulsed and there is disruption of the contralateral alar ligament and tectorial membrane. While the occipital condyles are poorly visualized on x-ray and fractures are rarely visible, the plain radiographs may demonstrate prevertebral soft tissue swelling, and should increase the suspicion that an upper cervical spine injury may have occurred. Ultimately, CT is necessary for fully characterizing these injuries.

Clinical Implications

Occipital condyle fractures are usually the result of either an axial load injury or significant rotational force. Patients who are conscious and neurologically intact may describe pain at the base of the skull and may present with a slight head tilt or poor mobility at the occipito-cervical joint. Type 1 and type 2 fractures are stable and may be treated with a rigid cervical collar. Type 3 fractures are associated with extensive ligamentous injury and often require halo immobilization.

Pearls

1. An occipital condyle fracture can be either an avulsion or compression fracture, but is rarely visible on plain radiographs.
2. This type of fracture is associated with lower cranial nerve deficits that may be delayed.

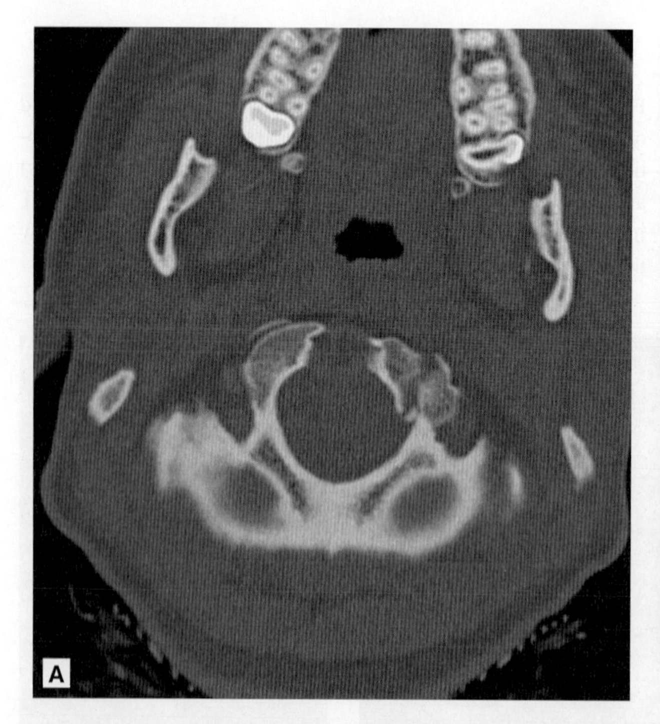

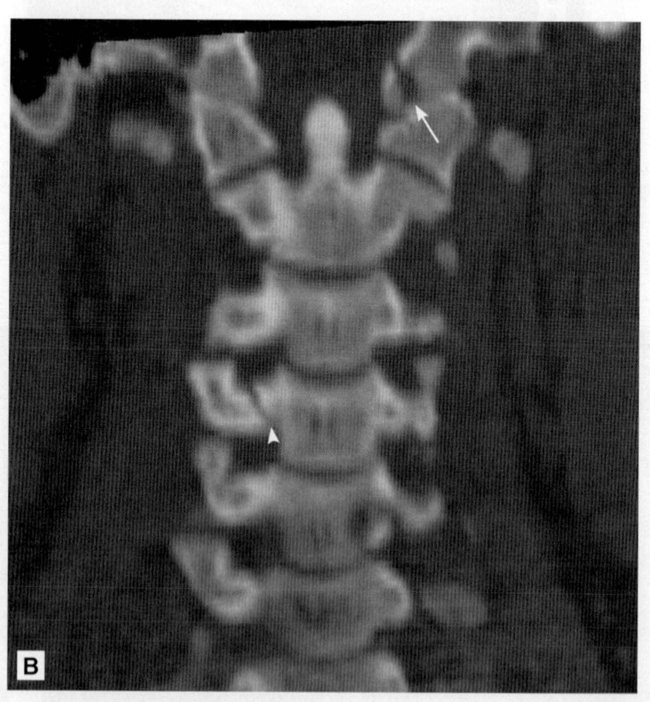

FIGURE 11.21 ■ Occipital Condyle Fracture. **A, B:** Axial and coronal reformatted CT images through the skull base show a moderately displaced fracture of the left occipital condyle (arrow). Note a right C4 pedicle fracture also visible on the coronal image (arrowhead).

Radiographic Summary

A simple wedge compression fracture results in a wedge-shaped deformity with loss of height exclusively along the anterior aspect of the vertebral body, and with preservation of the posterior vertebral body height. The anterior column is involved, but the middle and posterior columns remain intact, including the posterior cortex of the vertebral body, the pedicles, lamina, and spinous processes. Posterior ligamentous structures are unaffected. Simple wedge compression fractures demonstrate less than 50% loss of height. Unlike burst fractures, retropulsion of bone into the spinal canal does not occur with simple wedge compression injuries.

Clinical Implications

Simple wedge compression fractures result from axial loading of the spine in flexion and can present following both trauma or as insufficiency injury. The most significant risk factor for this type of fracture is osteoporosis, which may predispose the patient to fractures even after trivial trauma. These fractures are generally stable without neurologic involvement; however, as with all spinal injuries, a careful neurologic assessment is imperative. Assessment for more complex injury patterns is important, and may include neurologic involvement when the adjacent vertebrae are affected, when anterior wedging is greater than 50%, if there is severe hyperkyphosis (greater than 20°), if there is a rotational component to the injury, or if bone fragments are suspected in the spinal canal. Treatment is usually conservative with bracing of the affected area, pain control, and physical therapy. Surgery is rarely necessary.

Pearls

1. CT scanning is often necessary in patients with wedge compression fractures found on plain radiographs since it is often difficult to differentiate simple wedge compression fractures from burst fractures with plain radiographs alone.
2. These fractures can occur with even trivial trauma in patients with severe osteoporosis or metastatic cancer.
3. Compression fractures should be considered in any patient presenting with calcaneal fractures following a fall.

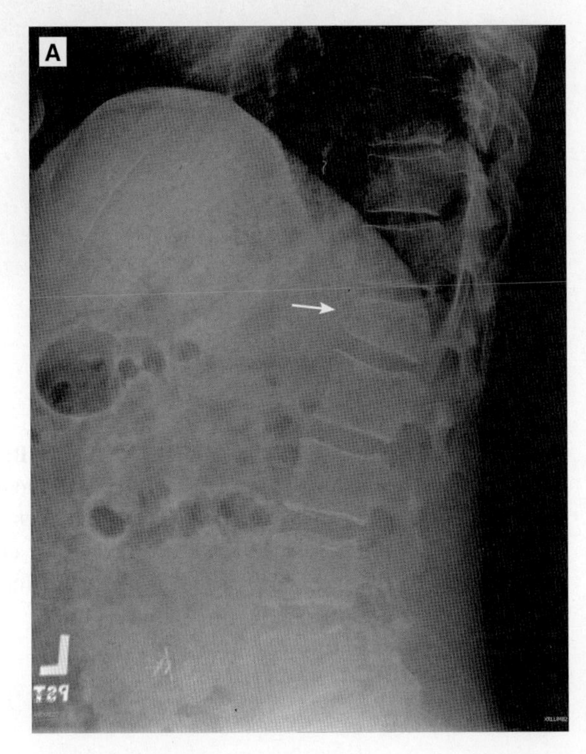

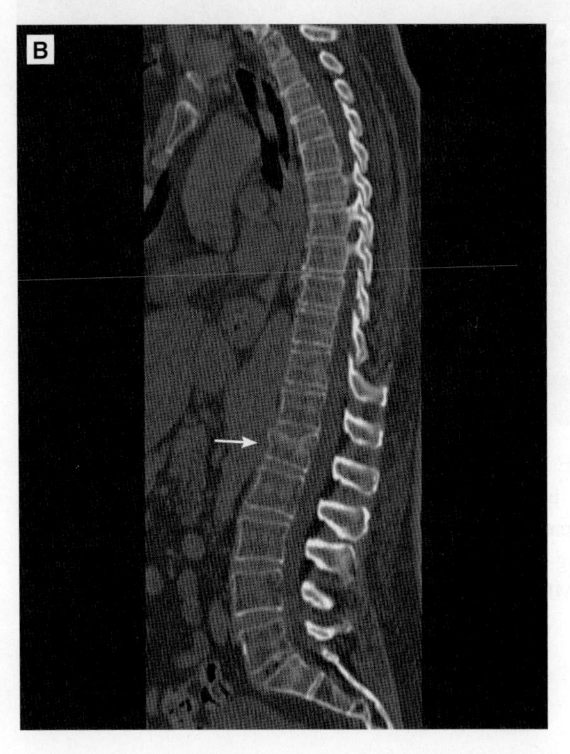

FIGURE 11.22 ■ Simple Wedge Compression Fracture. **A:** Lateral lumbar spine radiograph shows a simple wedge compression fracture of L1 (arrow). The anterior column shows 20-30% height loss but the middle and posterior columns are intact. **B:** CT reformatted image (in the sagittal plane) redemonstrates this patient's L1 compression fracture (arrow) and confirms no middle or posterior column involvement. Note preservation of posterior vertebral body height and no retropulsion of fragments into the spinal canal.

Radiographic Summary

In an anterior atlanto-axial dislocation, the transverse ligament that stabilizes the articulation between C1 and C2 is disrupted and the atlanto-dental interval (ADI) is increased. The ADI is the distance between the odontoid process and the posterior border of the anterior arch of the atlas on lateral view. An ADI of greater than 2 mm (or 5 mm in children less than 8 years) is abnormal and suggests instability. Acute atlanto-axial injuries are often associated with prevertebral soft tissue swelling. Of note, the ADI can increase by as much as 2 mm with neck flexion and may be pathological but not traumatically increased in certain conditions such Down's syndrome and rheumatoid arthritis.

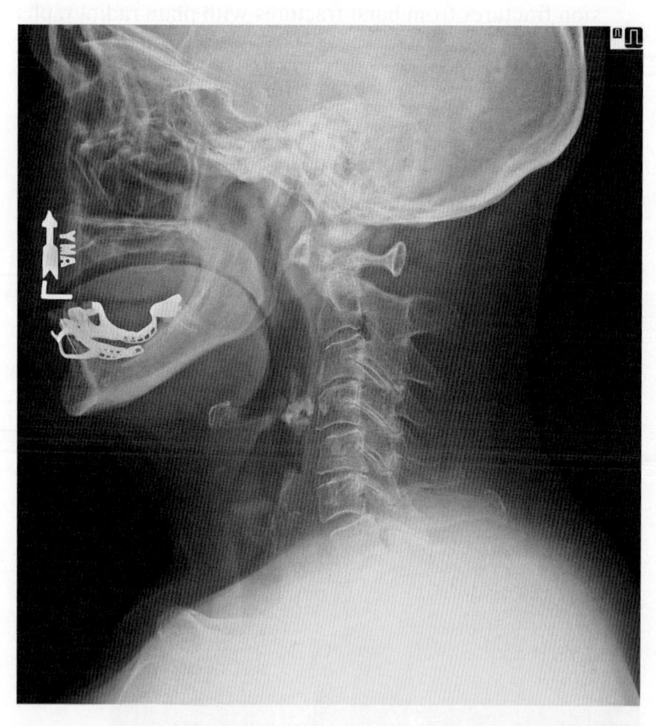

FIGURE 11.23 ■ Anterior Atlanto-Axial Dislocation. Notice that the predental space is considerably wider than 2 mm in this elderly patient involved in a motor vehicle collision. This pathologic widening indicates ligamentous injury. (Image contributor: Jake Block, MD.)

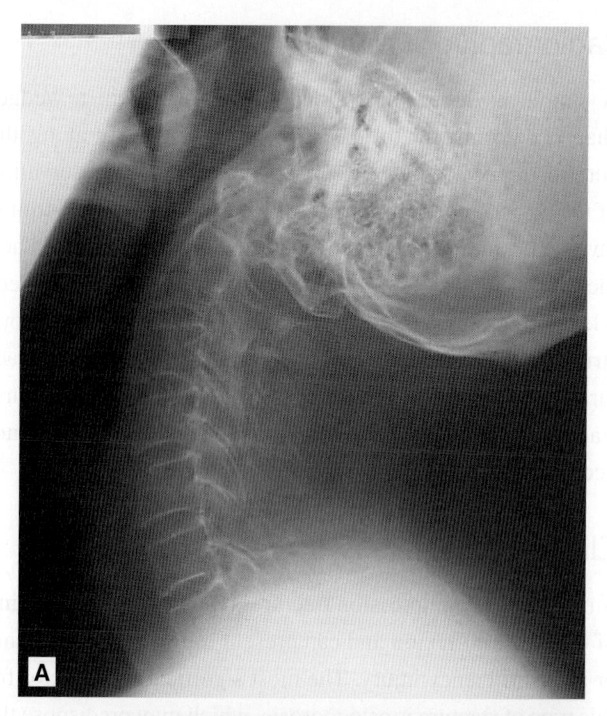

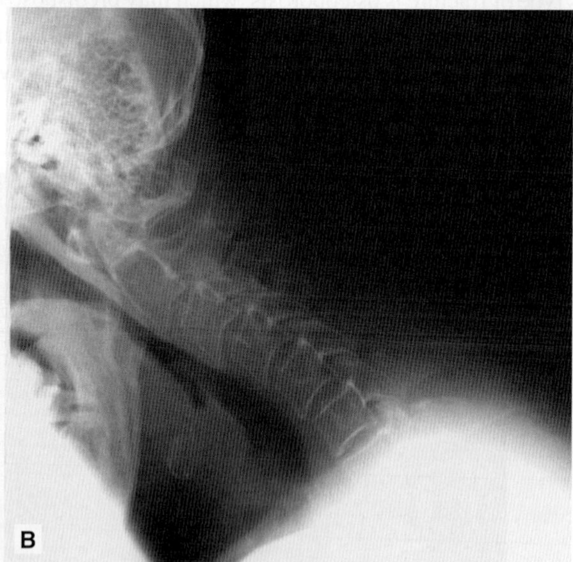

FIGURE 11.24 ■ Anterior Atlanto-Axial Dislocation. **A, B:** Lateral flexion and extension radiographs in a patient with rheumatoid arthritis show widening of the predental space on flexion which reduces when the patient extends. Note the generalized osteopenia and small dens erosions related to her underlying inflammatory arthropathy.

Clinical Implications

Traumatic anterior atlanto-axial dislocation occurs with hyperflexion of the neck. The most common causes of traumatic anterior atlanto-axial dislocations are MVCs and sports-related injuries. This is an unstable injury. Spinal cord injury can occur, but is less common due to the wide spinal canal at this level. Treatment is with a hard collar and sometimes halo placement. These injuries will often eventually require internal fixation.

Pearls

1. Nontraumatic atlanoto-axial dislocation can occur in conditions such as Down's syndrome and rheumatoid arthritis, and may be evaluated with flexion and extension views.
2. Grisel's syndrome is a rare pharyngeal tissue infection that can cause nontraumatic atlanto-axial dislocation.
3. This injury is rare in adults and more common in children due to the laxity of the surrounding ligaments.

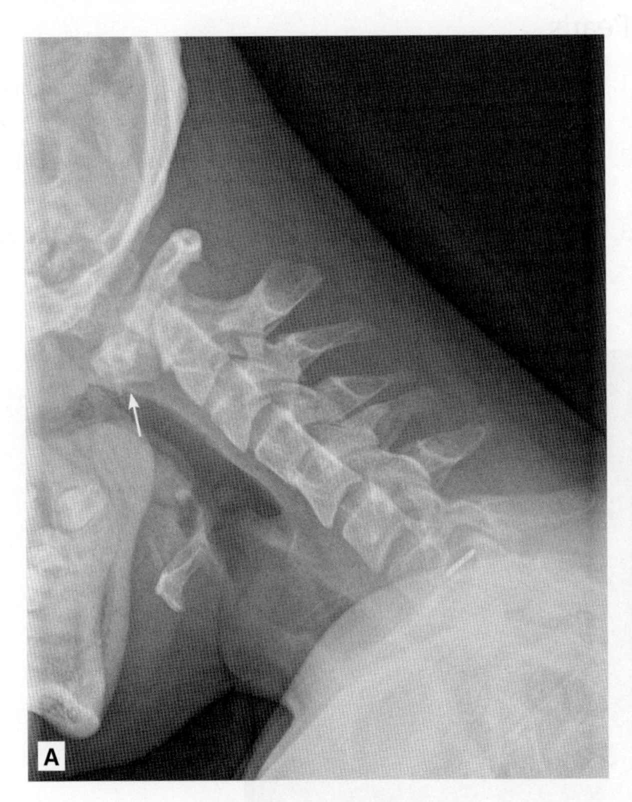

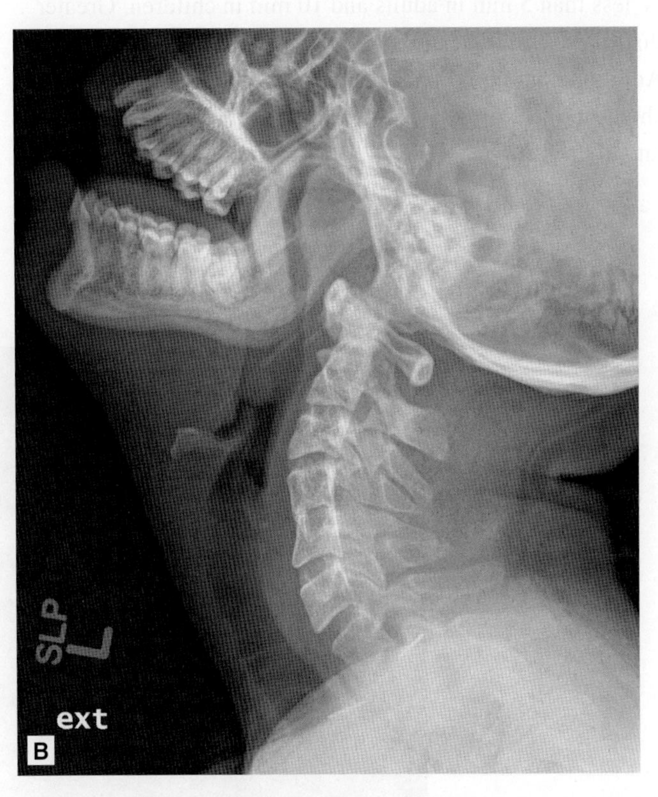

FIGURE 11.25 ■ Anterior Atlanto-Axial Dislocation. **A, B:** This patient with Down's syndrome also shows features of atlantoaxial instability with an osodontoidium present (arrow). In flexion, the ring of C1 and the os translate anteriorly but reduce in extension.

Radiographic Summary

Atlanto-occipital dislocation is often referred to as "internal decapitation" as it results in the complete dissociation of C1 from the occiput with disruption of the ligaments that join C1 to the skull. This injury can easily be missed on plain radiographs and CT scan since the joints may reapproximate between the incident and time of imaging. Many methods have been developed to determine the presence of this injury but, if the injury has reapproximated, it may only be evident on MRI. On radiographs and CT, the distance from the basion (tip of the clivus) to the odontoid should be less than 5 mm in adults and 10 mm in children. Greater distances are indicative of atlanto-occipital dislocation. Additionally, in normal patients, the mastoid processes should project posteriorly to the dens in a well-positioned lateral projection.

Clinical Implications

Atlanto-occipital dislocations are frequently fatal secondary to brainstem injury and respiratory arrest. They result from hyperextension, distraction, and rotary forces. If survived, these injuries are highly unstable and require internal fixation with fusion. Rigid cervical collar alone is inadequate at stabilizing this injury. Mandibular fractures, chin lacerations, and injury to the posterior pharyngeal wall could be clues to an underlying atlanto-occipital dislocation and should cause the emergency physician to consider the possibility.

Pearls

1. Stretching on the brainstem during this particular injury can lead to respiratory arrest and death.
2. Atlanto-occipital dislocation is twice as common in children due to their immature atlanto-occipital joint.
3. Nontraumatic atlanto-occipital dislocation can occur in Down's syndrome or rheumatoid arthritis.

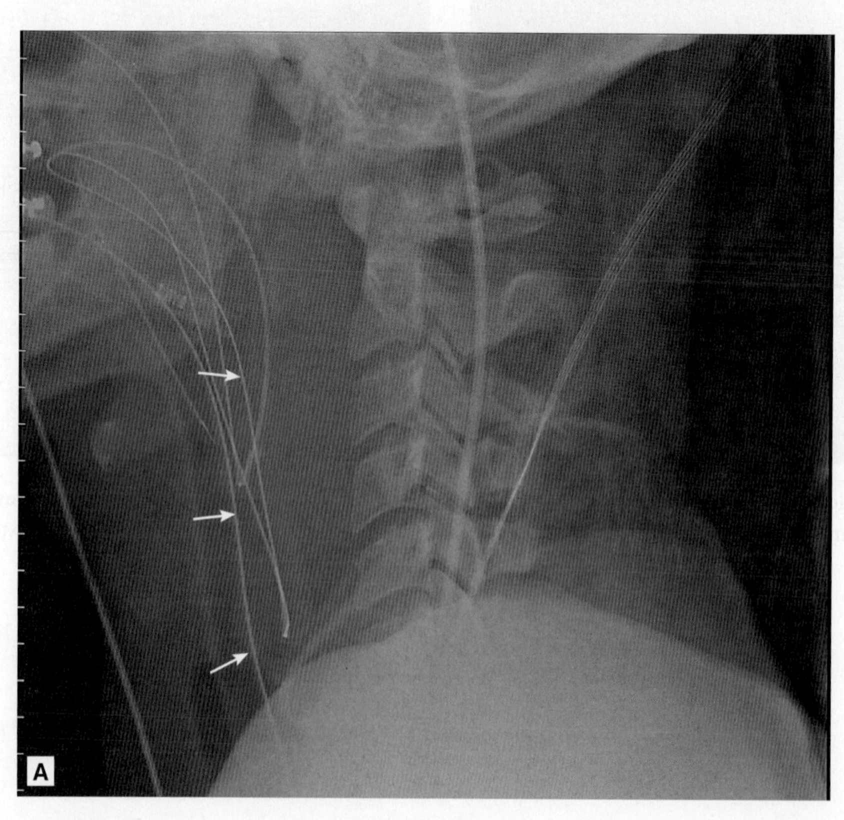

FIGURE 11.26 ■ Atlanto-Occipital Dislocation. **A:** Lateral radiograph of the cervical spine shows massive prevertebral soft tissue swelling (arrows). The tip of the dens projects posterior to the mastoid air cells, indicating distraction and anterior translation of the skull base.

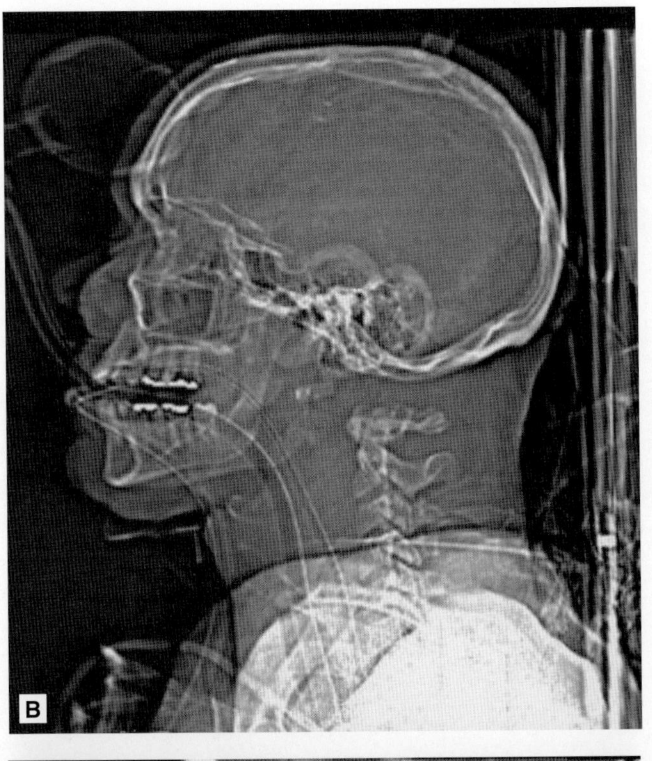

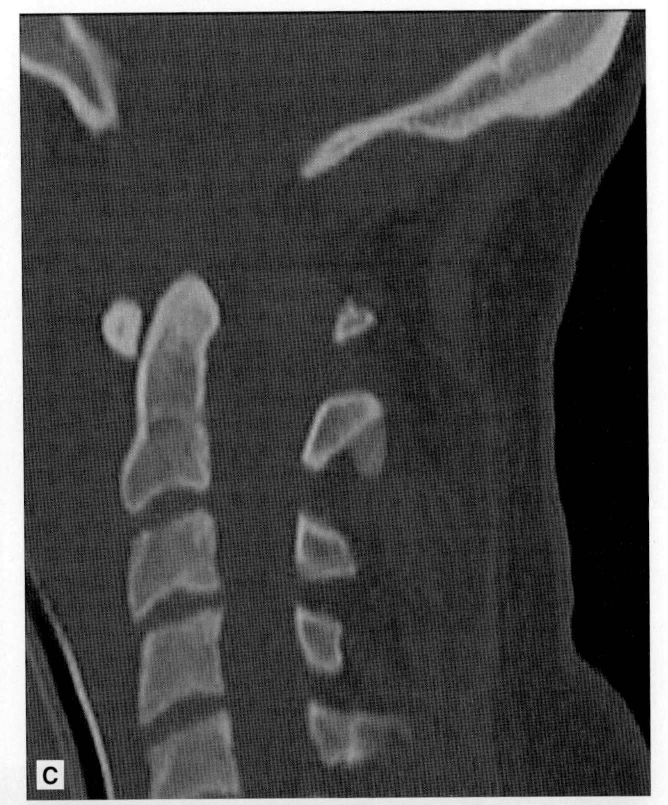

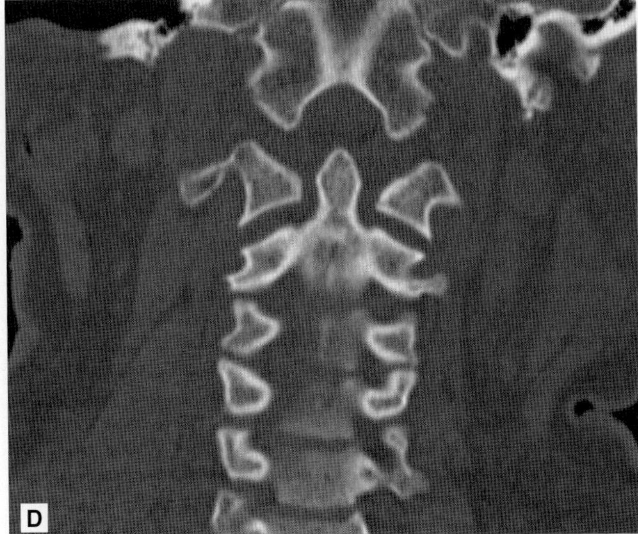

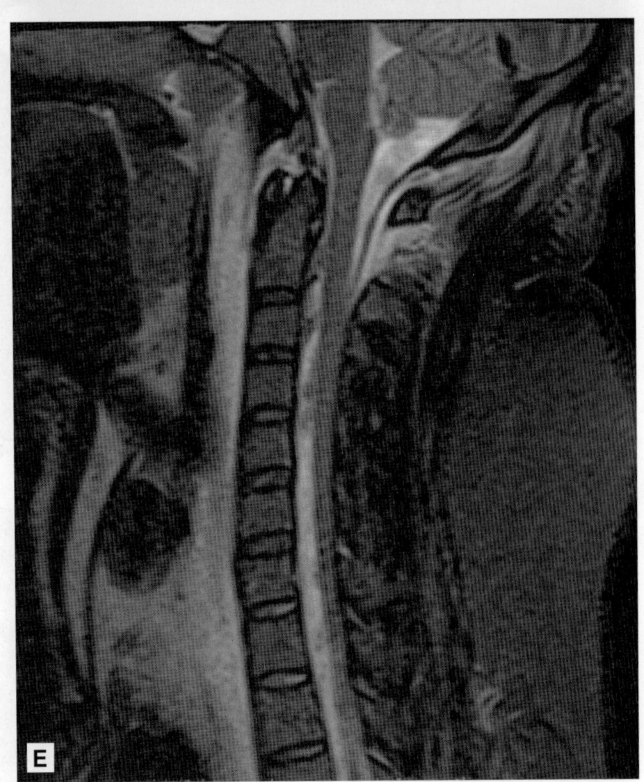

FIGURE 11.26 ■ (*Continued*) **B-D:** Scout image from CT scan shows to better advantage the anterior and cranial distraction of the skull base in relation to the C1 arch. Sagittal CT image through the midline confirms the atlantooccipital dissociation and the coronally reformatted images show marked widening of the interval between the lateral masses of C1 and the occipital condyles seen only with massive ligament disruption. **E:** Sagittal STIR MR image obtained at the time of injury shows hyperintense signal replacing the alar ligaments, indicating disruption. Note the massive amount of prevertebral edema.

Radiographic Summary

A chance fracture results from a flexion–distraction injury and is a transverse fracture through the vertebral body extending posteriorly through the pedicles, lamina, and spinous process. It involves all three columns of the spine, classically with horizontal fracture lines through the posterior elements. The interspinous and posterior longitudinal ligaments are disrupted but the anterior longitudinal ligament is usually intact. Some injury patterns may be purely ligamentous, involving the intervertebral disk space and facet ligaments without bony fracture. Chance fractures are most commonly seen at the thoracolumbar junction in adults, and in the mid lumbar region in pediatric patients.

Clinical Implications

Chance fractures are most frequently seen in patients following a head-on MVA in which only a lap belt is worn, causing violent forward flexion across a fulcrum. These fractures are rarely associated with neurologic findings. However, there is a high incidence of associated intra-abdominal injuries with Chance fractures. Chance fractures are considered unstable, but may be managed by closed reduction and immobilization in a thoracolumbosacral orthosis (TLSO) brace in appropriate patients. Internal fixation may be indicated for polytrauma patients or in patients whose size makes closed treatment difficult.

Pearls

1. Chance fractures may be associated with retroperitoneal and abdominal visceral injuries.
2. The most common long-term complications following this injury include residual kyphosis and chronic back pain.

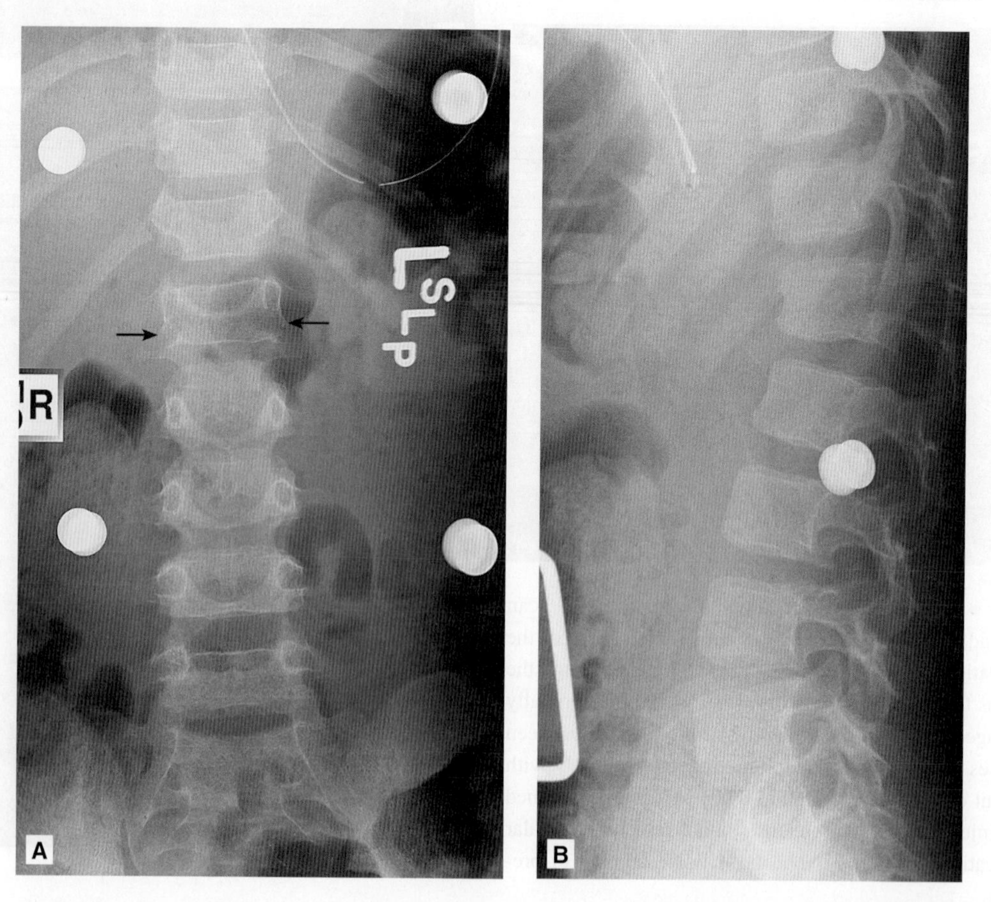

FIGURE 11.27 ■ Chance Fracture. **A, B:** Frontal and lateral radiographs of an L1 chance fracture. This three-column hyperflexion injury resulted in a transverse fracture and splaying of the posterior element fracture fragments. Note the horizontal splitting injury of the pedicles at L1, typical of this injury (arrows).

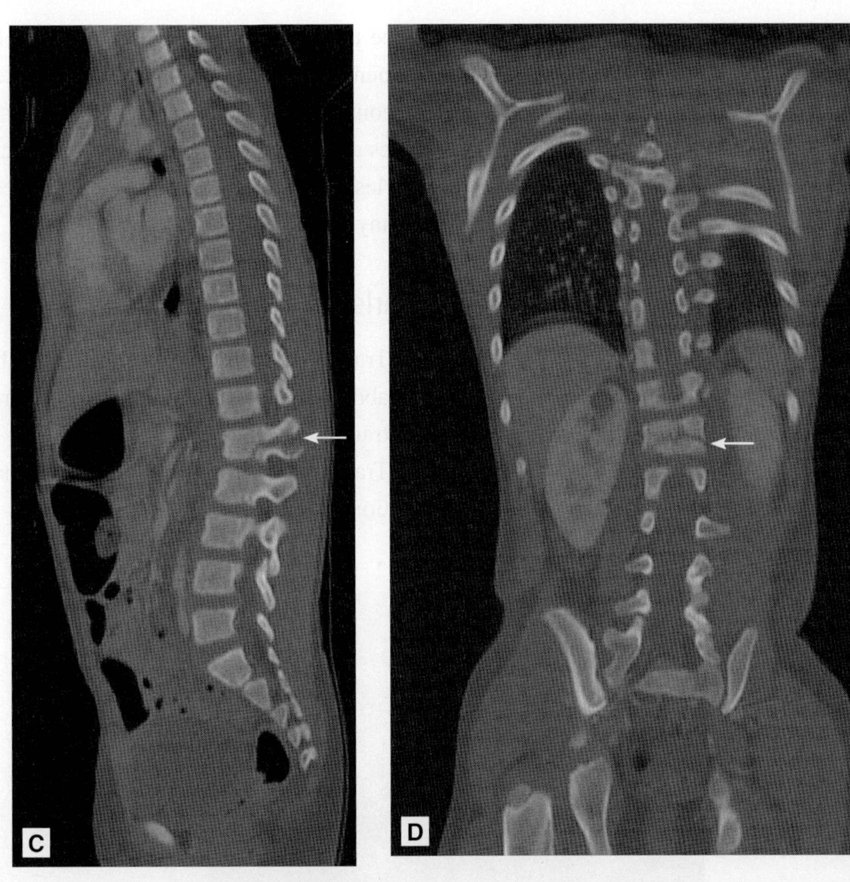

FIGURE 11.27 ■ (*Continued*) **C, D:** Sagittal and coronal CT reformatted images of the L1 chance fracture (arrows).

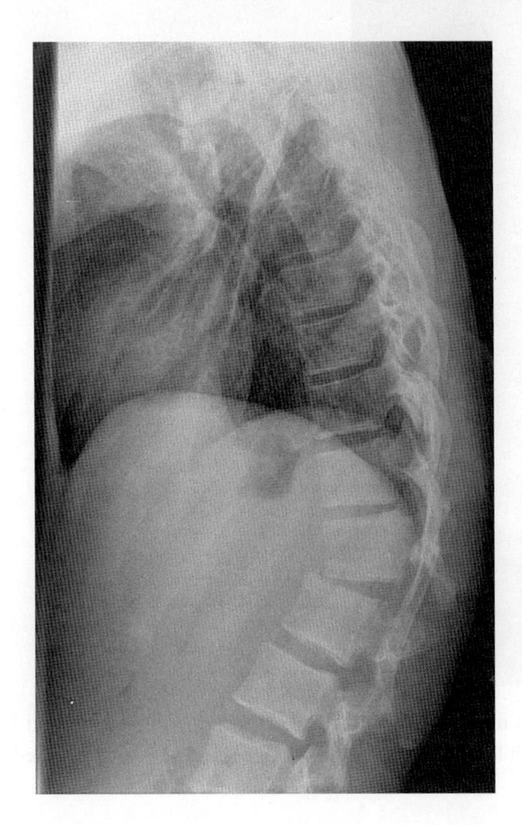

FIGURE 11.28 ■ Ligamentous Chance Injury. Lateral view of the thoracic spine demonstrates a purely ligamentous Chance injury. In this example, the disruption occurs through the disk space and posterior ligaments, without bony fractures. (Image contributor: Jake Block, MD.)

TRANSVERSE PROCESS FRACTURES

Radiographic Summary

Transverse process fractures are fractures of the bony projections that extend from the side of the vertebral body and pedicles. Most fractures are minimally displaced, and faintly visible on AP views of the spine. They may be difficult to visualize on plain radiographs and require CT scan for full visualization. These fractures are most common in the lumbar spine.

Clinical Implications

Transverse process fractures are usually a result of direct blunt trauma or extreme lateral extension–flexion forces. Sudden contraction of the psoas muscle can also cause an avulsion of the transverse process. These are stable fractures and are frequently multiple. Although transverse process fractures are considered a minor injury, they occur as a result of major forces and often co-exist with additional clinically significant injuries in trauma patients. These fractures usually heal without any treatment intervention.

Pearls

1. Transverse process fractures may be associated with abdominal visceral injuries in approximately 20% of trauma patients.
2. Transverse process fractures of L2 have a high association with renal artery thrombosis.

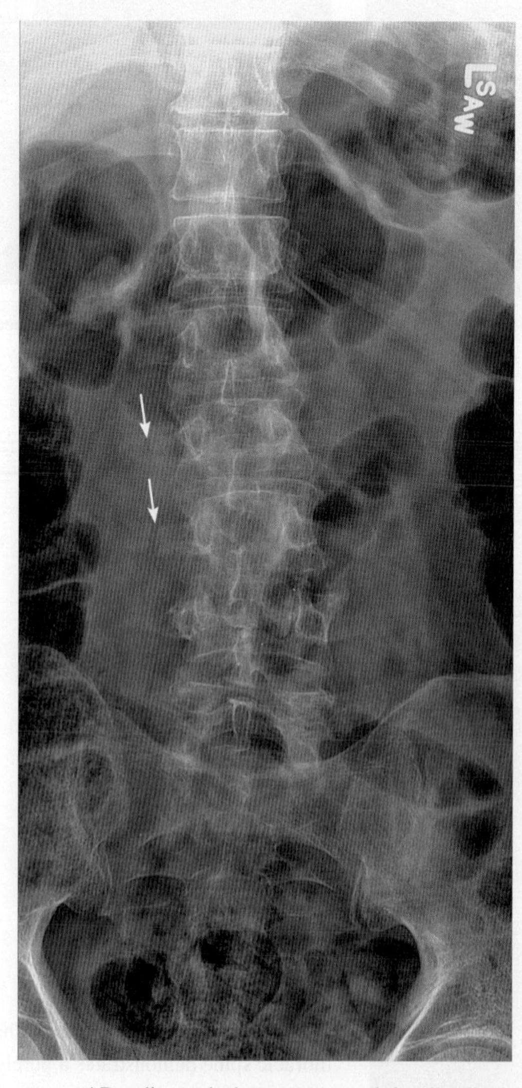

FIGURE 11.29 ■ Transverse Process Fractures. AP radiograph demonstrates minimally displaced transverse process fractures at L2 and L3 on the right (arrows). Note, this patient also had a burst fracture at L4, with loss of vertebral body height, and increased interpediculate distance.

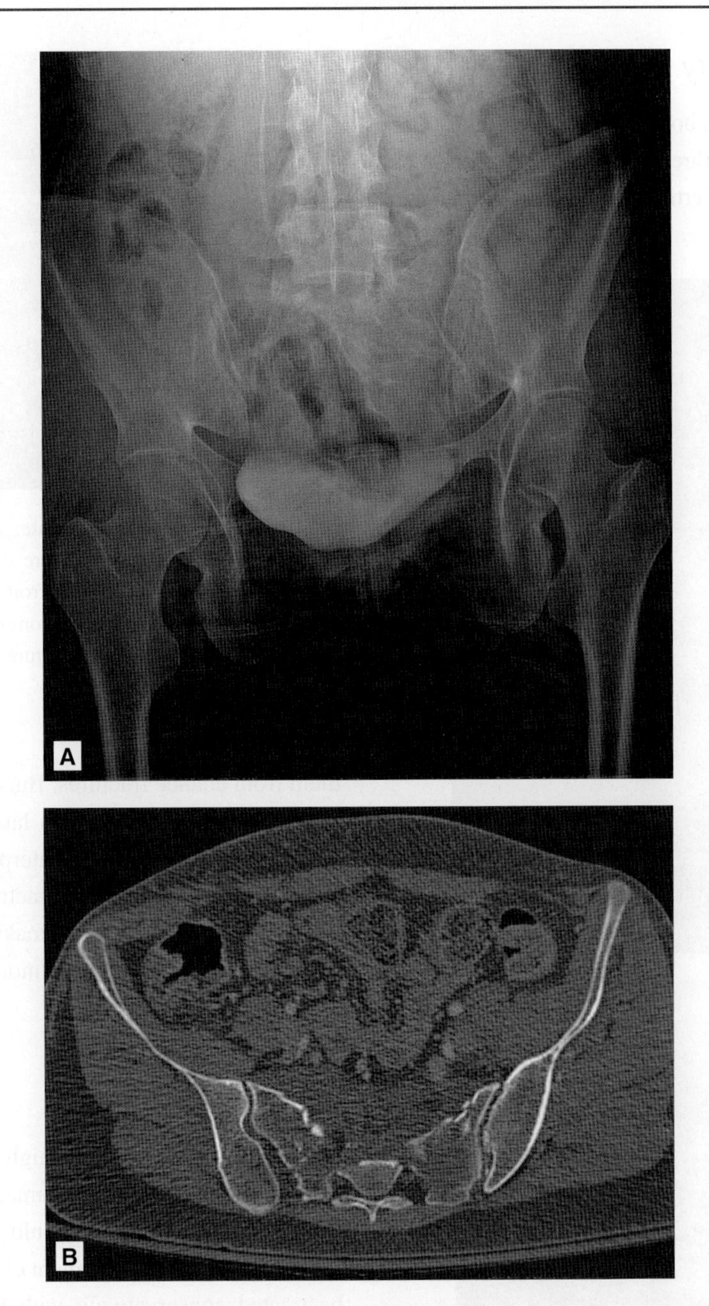

FIGURE 11.30 ■ Transverse Process Fractures. **A:** Portable pelvis obtained at initial trauma survey reveals a displaced transverse process fracture of L5 on the left. The fracture should prompt investigation for coexisting sacral injury. **B:** Axial CT image confirms bilateral sacral ala fractures in the same patient.

Radiographic Summary

A burst fracture is a vertebral body fracture resulting from an axial load which involves all three columns. The posterior element fractures are typically vertically oriented distinguishing them from chance fractures. Burst fractures have variable retropulsion of bone visible on lateral views of the spine, and may have widening of the interpedicular distance on the AP view. The posterior column fracture component may be radiographically occult however, making CT useful for diagnosis. These fractures are most commonly seen in the lower thoracic and upper lumbar spine.

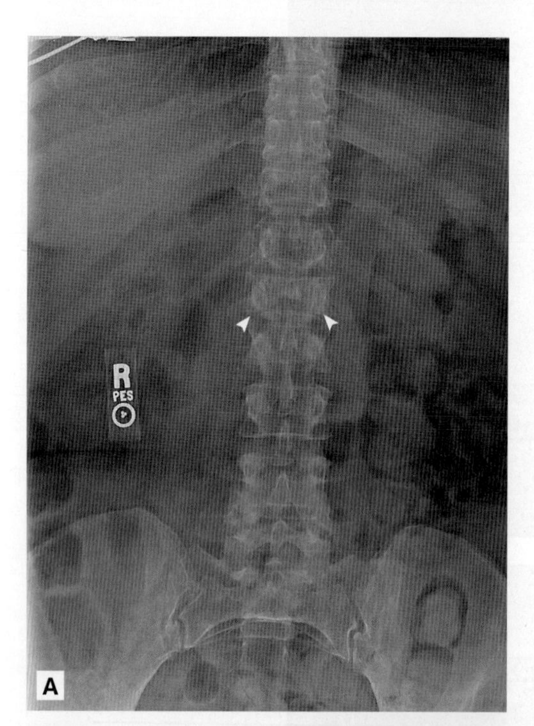

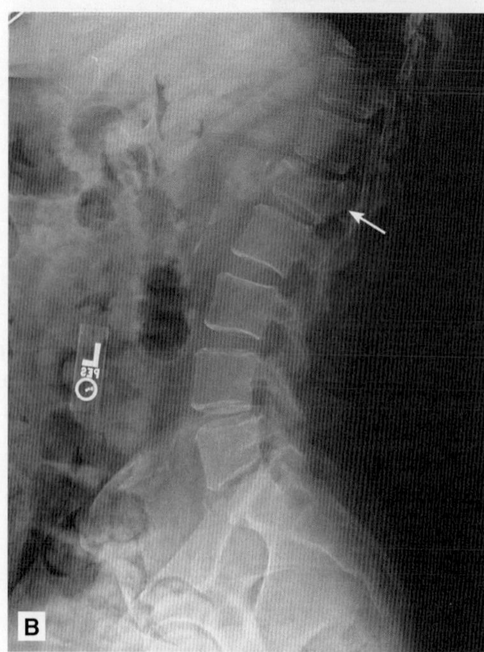

FIGURE 11.31 ■ Burst Fracture. **A:** AP radiograph shows widening of the L1 interpediculate distance (arrowheads) in this patient with a burst fracture. **B:** Posterior displacement of posterior vertebral body cortex is evident on the lateral radiograph (arrow).

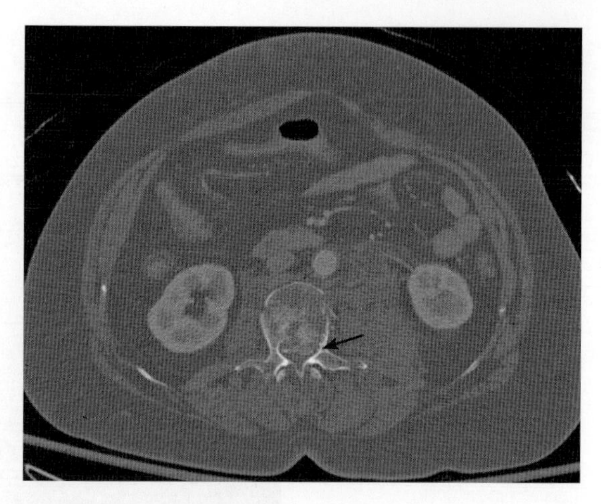

FIGURE 11.32 ■ Burst Fracture. Axial CT image in a different patient with an L2 burst fracture demonstrates involvement of all three vertebral body columns from an axial load. Notice the retropulsed bony fragments that compromise the central spinal canal (arrow). Transverse process fractures are also present.

Clinical Implications

Burst fractures result from high energy axial loading of the spine during significant trauma. They can result in severe neurologic sequelae and should be considered unstable during the emergency department evaluation. Burst fractures can be treated conservatively with bracing alone, or they may require surgical intervention if there is significant loss of height, kyphosis, extension of bone into the spinal canal, or neurologic symptoms.

Pearls

1. Subtle burst fractures can be misdiagnosed on plain radiographs. Therefore, CT scan is the modality of choice in diagnosing these fractures in the appropriate clinical setting.
2. The frequency of neurologic sequelae in burst fractures may be as high as 50%.

Radiographic Summary

MRI is the imaging modality of choice for the diagnosis of spinal cord neoplasms. Signal characteristics of these neoplasms vary depending on their etiology and the presence or absence of hemorrhage within the lesion. Both benign and malignant neoplasms and non-neoplastic intramedullary lesions may enhance following gadolinium administration. Tumors tend to expand the cord in a mass-like fashion and may have infiltrative margins.

Clinical Implications

Primary spinal cord neoplasms may be intramedullary or extramedullary. Additionally, tumors may metastasize to the spine. Metastatic disease of the spine is much more common than primary spinal cord neopslasms and is usually epidural. Primary spinal cord neoplasms are usually astrocytomas, ependymomas, and hemangioblastomas. The most common initial complaint in a patient with a spinal cord neoplasm is pain, followed by the insidious onset of neurologic deficits. Emergent radiation therapy is appropriate in certain situations in which cord compression results in neurologic dysfunction. In addition, steroids may be considered in patients with cord compression secondary to neoplasm. Surgical excision is controversial, but is another option in certain patient populations.

Pearls

1. Metastatic neoplasms are most commonly found in the thoracic spine.
2. Spinal cord neoplasms are far more likely to be from metastatic disease than a primary neoplastic process.

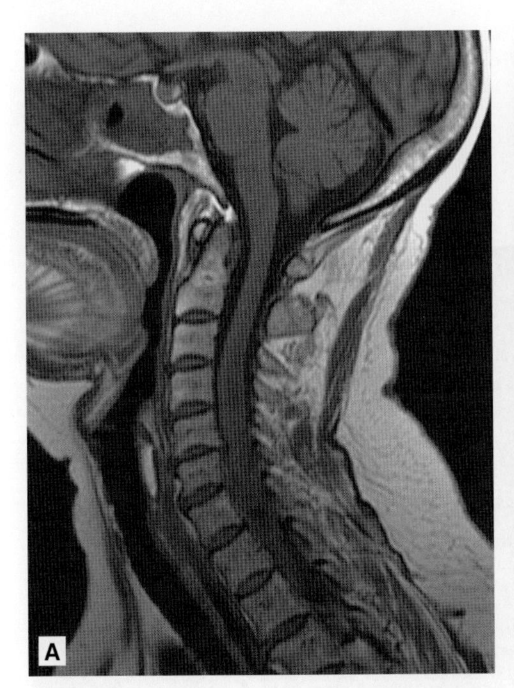

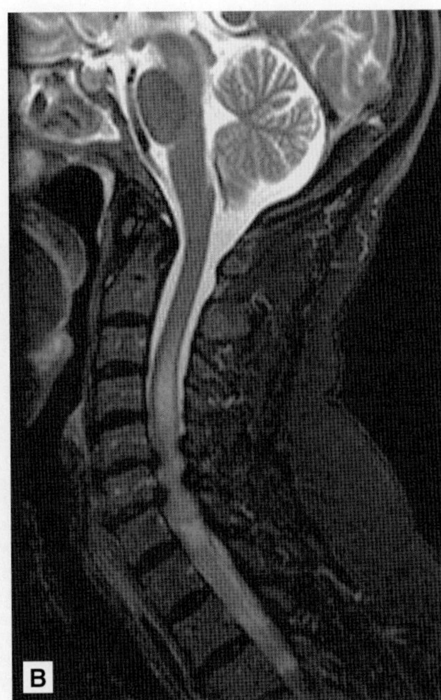

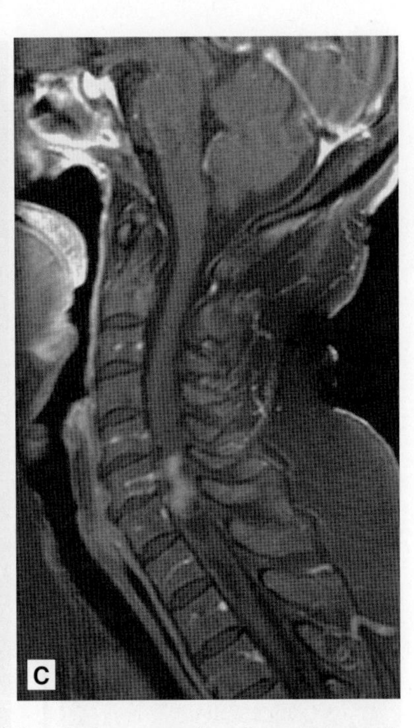

FIGURE 11.33 ■ Spinal Cord Neoplasm. **A, B:** Sagittal T1 and STIR images show an intramedullary lesion, expanding the cord, extending from C3 through C7, slightly hypointense to the cord on T1-weighted images and hyperintense on STIR. **C:** After gadolinium is given, nodular enhancement is evident. In this case, the tumor was a hemanigblastoma.

Radiographic Summary

MRI is the imaging modality of choice for the diagnosis of spinal cord compression due to neoplasm. Lesions existing within the vertebral body, posterior elements, surrounding soft tissues, or the cord itself may result in compression. These neoplasms are most commonly hyperintense on T2-weighted images, isointense or hypointense on T1-weighted images, and will typically enhance following IV administration of gadolinium contrast. Although plain radiographs may reveal vertebral collapse, bony destruction, or malalignment, the cord itself is not assessed.

Clinical Implications

Neoplastic compression of the spinal cord occurs when a primary tumor metastasizes to the spine or from a primary neoplasm of the spinal cord. Primary spinal cord tumors are usually intramedullary, while metastatic lesions are usually epidural or osseous. The most common primary cancers that metastasize to the spine are lung, breast, prostate, and renal. Neoplastic compression of the spinal cord is a true oncologic emergency. Most patients initially present with back pain, followed by the insidious onset of neurologic deficits. Emergent radiation therapy is appropriate in certain situations in which cord compression results in neurologic dysfunction. In addition, steroids may be considered. Surgical excision is controversial, but is another option in certain patient populations.

Pearls

1. Metastatic lesions cause 85% of the cases of neoplastic spinal cord compression.
2. The intervertebral disk space is usually not involved in spinal neoplasms. Therefore, if the disk space is involved on radiographs, infection is more likely.

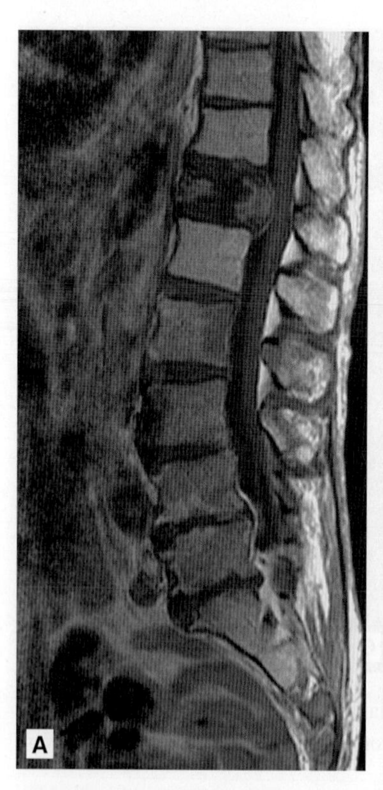

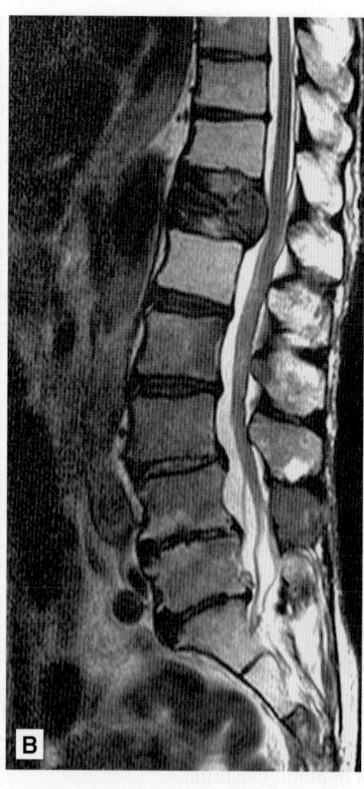

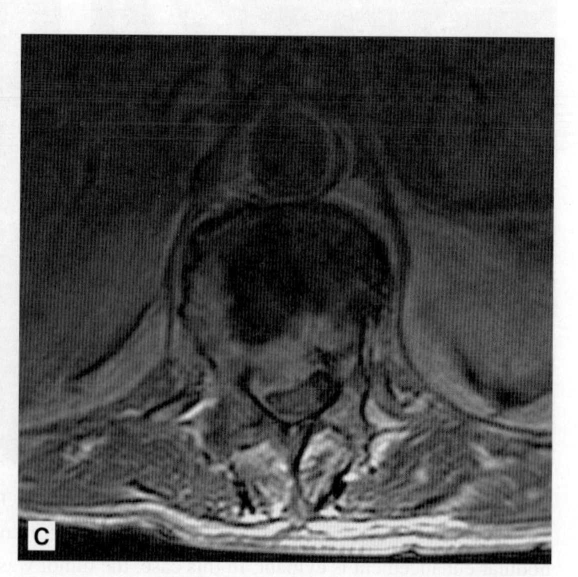

FIGURE 11.34 ■ Neoplastic Spinal Cord Compression. **A:** In this patient at T12, there is a pathologic fracture through a large metastatic lesion. The sagittal T1-weighted sequence shows replacement of normal bright fatty marrow by hypointense tumor. Notice the convex bowing of the affected vertebral body. Though not well seen at T12 due to slice selection, there is visible tumor in the posterior elements of several lumbar vertebral bodies, a feature that helps differentiate pathologic fractures from osteoporotic ones. **B:** Sagittal T2-weighted sequence show subtle cord edema at T12–L1 secondary to cord compression by the tumor related pathologic T12 fracture. **C:** Axial post contrast T1 sequence illustrates enhancing tumor deforming the thoracic cord and displacing it dorsally and to the left.

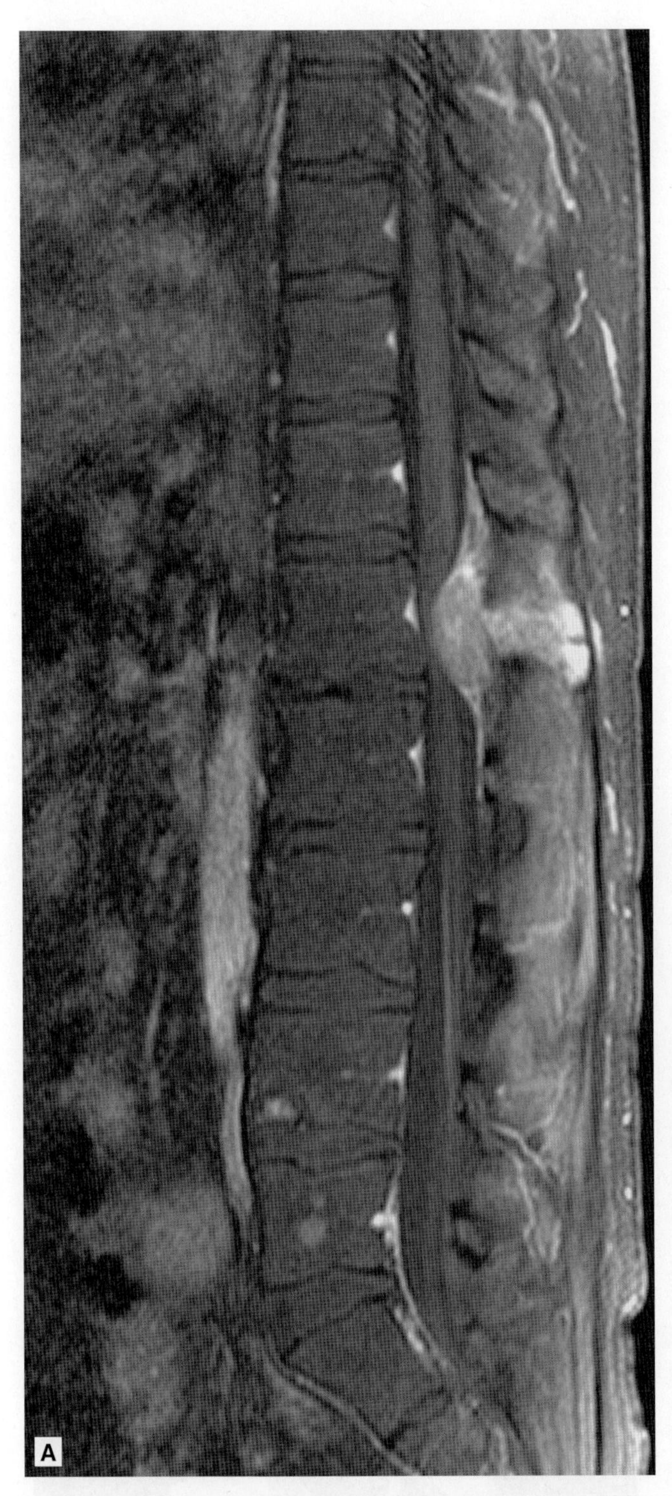

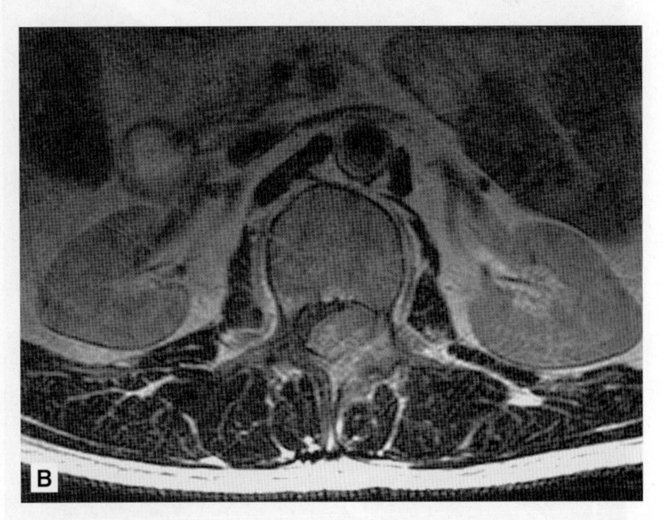

FIGURE 11.35 ■ Neoplastic Spinal Cord Compression (Different Patient). **A:** Sagittal post contrast fat saturated T1 image from a different patient with an extramedullary, extradural metastatic lesion in the left posterior elements which results in compression and displacement of the conus. **B:** Axial post contrast T1-weighted sequences help to characterize the degree of canal compromise and cord impingement that results from enhancing metastatic disease in the left posterior elements.

Radiographic Summary

Spinal cord transection is the most severe form of spinal cord injury in which the cord itself is effectively severed. It can be partial or complete. Spinal cord transection is typically noted at the level of vertebral fractures and/or dislocations on imaging studies, where the spinal canal is compromised. On MRI, there will be loss of the uniform margins defining the normal spinal cord.

Clinical Implications

Spinal cord transection usually occurs secondary to vertebral fractures or dislocations after trauma. This injury can also occur following penetrating injuries such as gunshot wounds or stab wounds. "Physiologic cord transection" refers to complete loss of motor and sensory responses below the level of injury without true external trauma to the spinal cord. This most commonly occurs in patients with multiple sclerosis. Symptoms are related to the level of injury and degree of transection (whether partial or complete). Transections above the level of C2 to C4 are usually incompatible with life, since innervation of the diaphragm is likely to be destroyed. Patients with spinal cord transection typically present with flaccid paralysis below the level of injury with loss of reflexes and sensation. Approximately 1 to 4 weeks after injury, patients will develop hyperreflexia. Treatment is the same as with spinal cord contusions and includes stabilization of the spine, reduction of cord compression, and steroid therapy. Additionally, patients with high cord lesions may require mechanical ventilatory support, since innervation to the diaphragm may be impaired.

Pearls

1. Spinal cord transection is far less common than spinal cord contusion and compression.
2. Nontraumatic vertebral dislocation can occur in patients with rheumatoid arthritis.

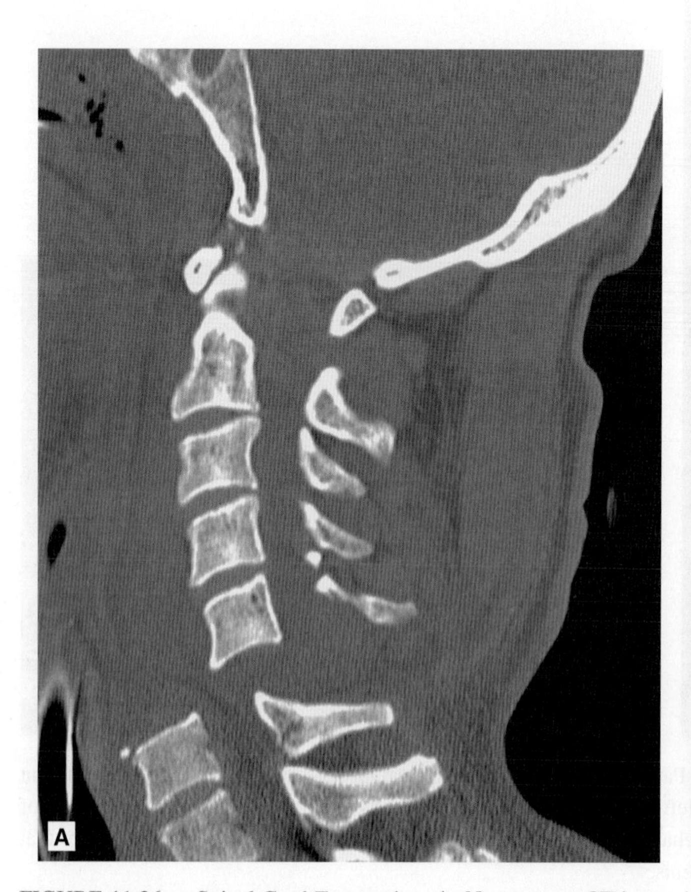

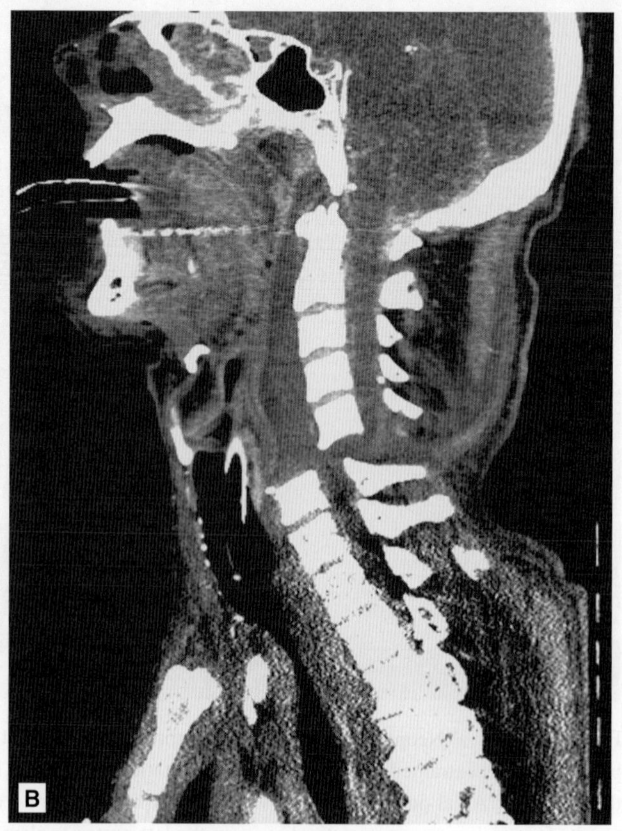

FIGURE 11.36 ■ Spinal Cord Transection. **A:** Noncontrast CT image in bone windows shows a fracture dislocation of the cervical spine at the C5–C6 level with greater than one vertebral body width displacement. **B:** Enhanced image windowed to accentuate the soft tissues demonstrates a disrupted, low-attenuation (edematous) cord with massive prevertebral and posterior edema. This patient expired before MR could be performed, succumbing to extreme spinal shock.

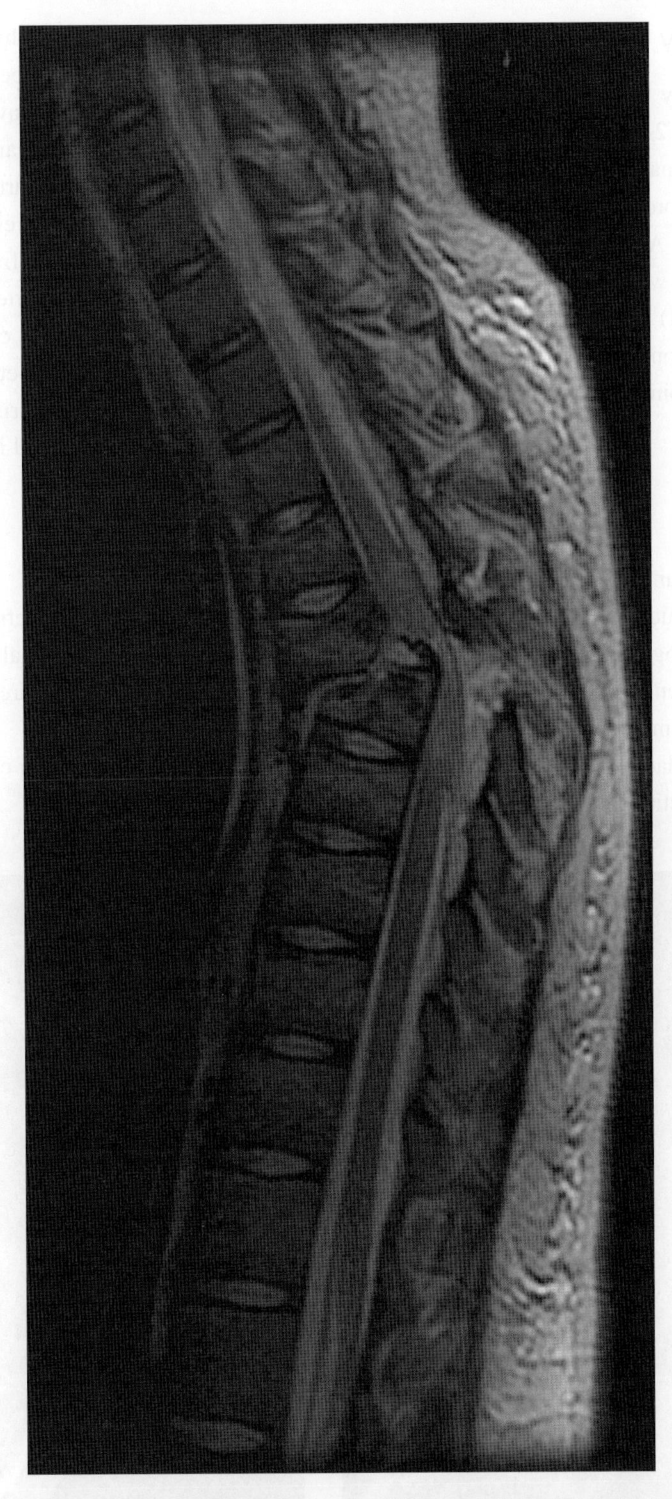

FIGURE 11.37 ■ Spinal Cord Transection. Sagittal T2W MR image in a different patient with a mid thoracic fracture dislocation and cord transection. There is hyperintense cord edema and hemorrhage on either side of the cord disruption. Note disruptions of the anterior longitudinal ligament, posterior longitudinal ligament, and intraspinous ligaments.

Radiographic Summary

MRI is the imaging modality of choice for the diagnosis of a spinal cord infarction. T2-weighted images will show a hyperintensity in the grey matter or throughout the entire cross-sectional area of the cord. T1-weighted images may show slight cord expansion. As in the brain, the area of infracted cord should restrict water diffusion making diffusion-weighted imaging (DWI) highly sensitive. DWI also helps distinguish this entity from transverse myelitis. If there is concern for a potential spinal AVM, then spinal MRA should also be performed.

Clinical Implications

Spinal cord infarctions are far less common than cerebral infarcts. Symptoms may include sudden, severe back pain and the acute onset of neurologic deficits over several minutes. Neurologic deficits depend on the level of spinal cord involvement and can include motor weakness, sensory disturbances, and bowel and bladder dysfunction. The vast majority of spinal cord infarctions occur in the territory of the anterior spinal artery, which supplies blood flow to the areas controlling pain, temperature, and touch. The posterior spinal artery is rarely involved, and supplies the areas that control proprioception and vibration sensation. A few causes of anterior spinal artery occlusion include aortic dissection, atherosclerotic embolization, trauma, AVMs, and external compression from a herniated disk, tumor, or fracture. Additionally, arteritis caused by lupus, syphilis, or other conditions may compromise blood flow to the anterior spinal artery. Diabetes, hypertension, and hyperlipidemia all increase the risk of spinal cord infarction. The treatment of spinal cord infarctions will depend on the underlying cause.

Pearls

1. Although neurologic deficits can occur without pain, greater than 80% of spinal cord infarctions are painful.
2. Spinal cord infarctions are most common in the thoracic spine.
3. Spinal venous infarction can occur as well, but is much more rare.

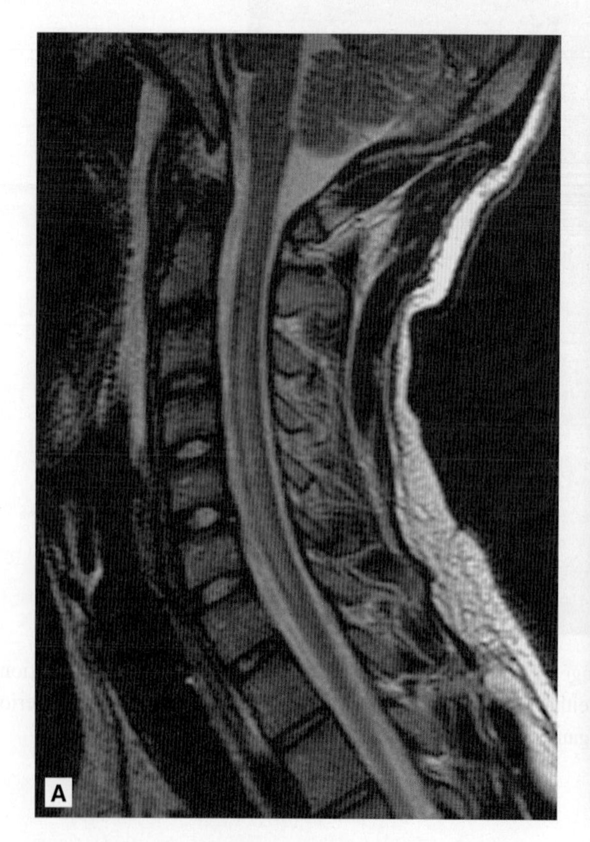

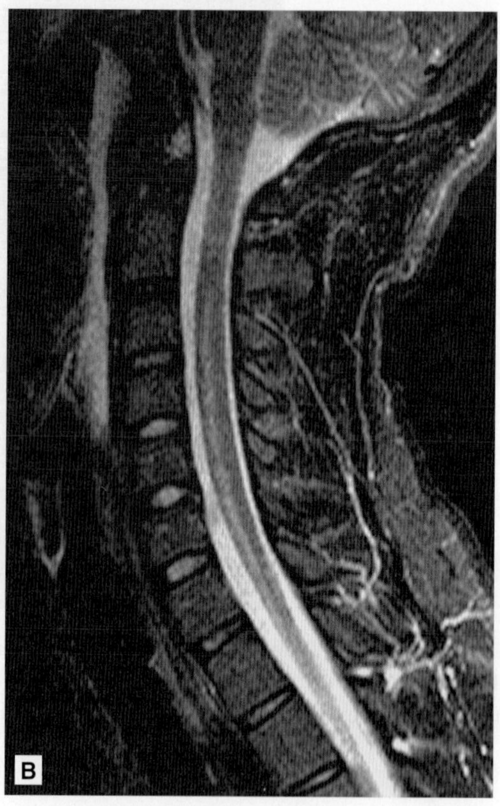

FIGURE 11.38 ■ Spinal Cord Infarction. In this patient with spinal cord infarction, Sagittal T2 and STIR sequences show central hyperintensitiy in the cord spanning multiple segments (C3–T1).

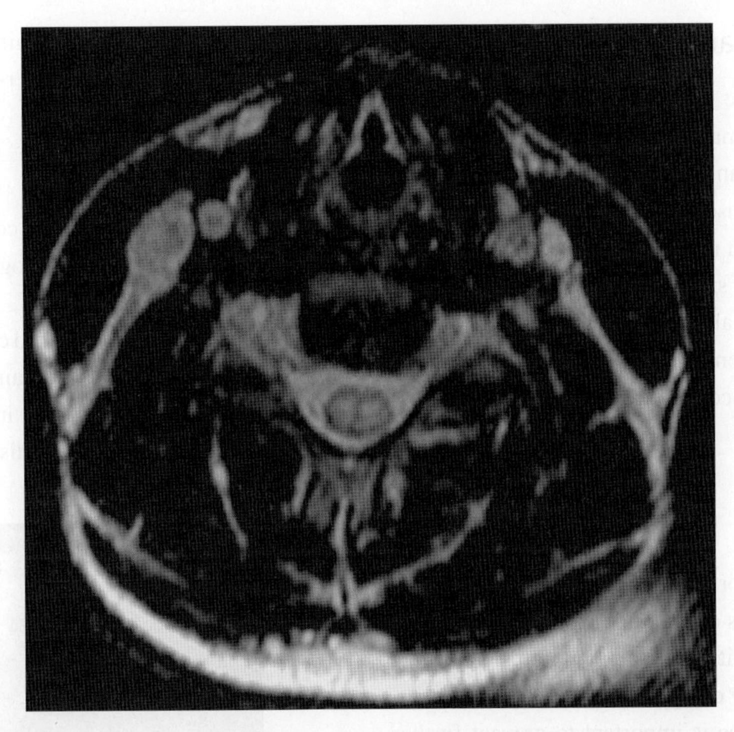

FIGURE 11.39 ■ Spinal Cord Infarction. Axial T2 3D sequence confirms increased signal in the central gray matter indicating early myelomalacia in this case of spinal cord infarction.

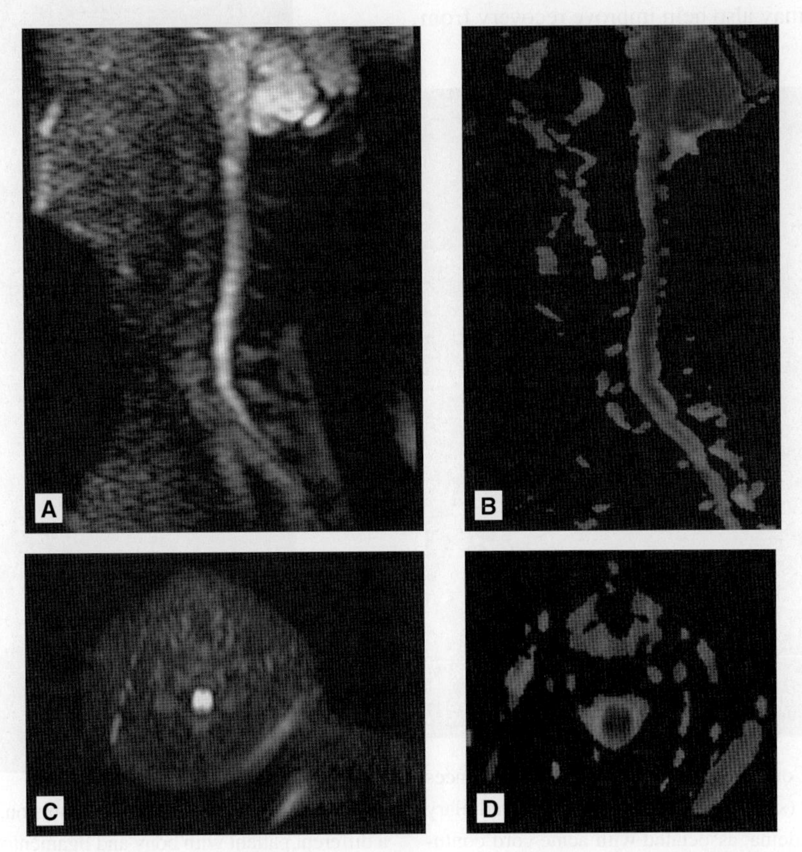

FIGURE 11.40 ■ Spinal Cord Infarction. **A-D:** Sagittal and axial DWI and ADC maps show increased and decreased signal, respectively, representing restricted diffusion in this patient with a cervical cord infarct.

Radiographic Summary

Spinal cord contusions are diagnosed by MRI. In simple contusions, T2-weighted images will show increased signal within the cord, which is an indication of contusion-related edema. They appear isointense or hypointense on T1-weighted images and usually result in mild cord swelling/enlargement. If hemorrhage is present, signal characteristics may vary. Spinal cord contusions usually occur at the site of fractures secondary to bony impingement. However, cord contusions can also occur in the absence of fractures after hyperflexion or hyperextension injuries.

Clinical Implications

Spinal cord contusion may or may not be associated with neurologic sequelae. Symptoms can include motor, sensory, and/or proprioceptive abnormalities. These symptoms can range from mild to severe. If bony or ligamentous injury exists, stabilization of the injured area is important to prevent further cord damage. In addition, if areas of cord compression exist, they may need traction or surgical stabilization. Treatment with methylprednisone may also help improve recovery from spinal cord injury if given within 8 hours of injury but this therapy remains highly controversial.

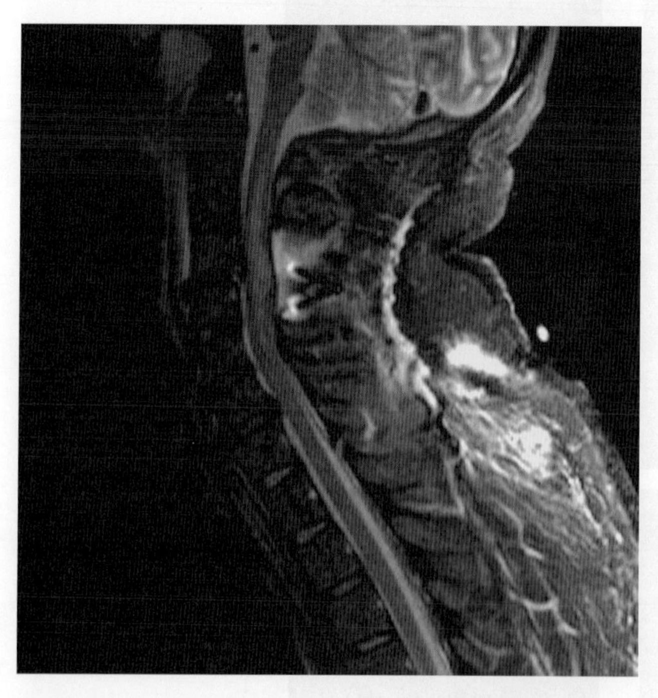

FIGURE 11.41 ■ Spinal Cord Contusion. Sagittal STIR sequences show mild cord expansion (swelling) and increased intramedullary fluid signal, representing edema, associated with acute cord contusion. The most commonly injured levels in acute spinal cord injury are C4–C6.

Pearls

1. Patients with cord lesions containing a hematoma will generally have a poorer prognosis than those with only cord edema.
2. Most people with spinal cord contusions that result in neurologic impairment will regain some functions between a week and six months after injury, but the likelihood of spontaneous recovery diminishes after six months.

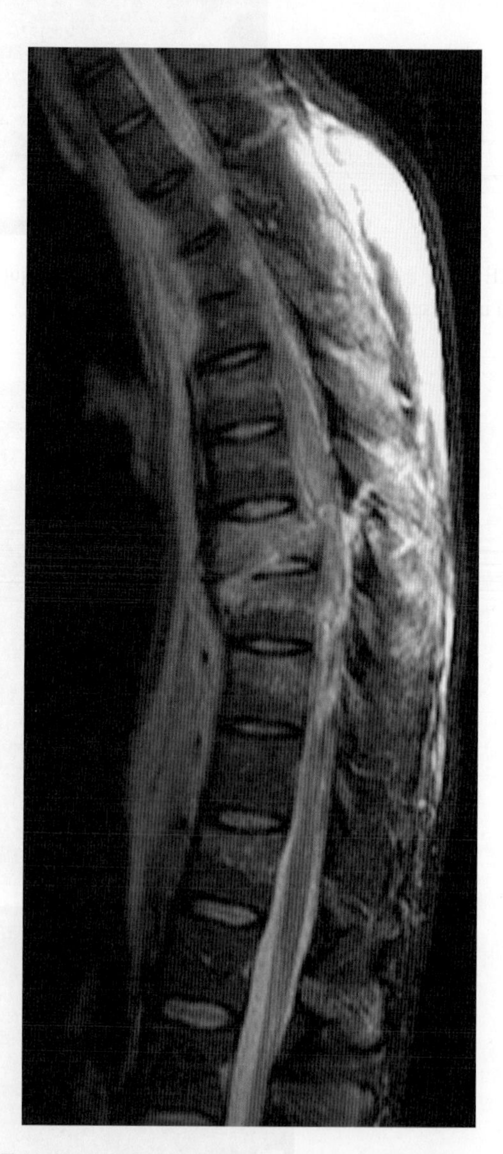

FIGURE 11.42 ■ Spinal Cord Contusion. Sagittal STIR sequence in a different patient with bony and ligamentous injuries of the lower thoracic spine in a patient with a hemorrhagic cord contusion. The increased signal in the involved thoracic cord segment is inhomogeneous.

Radiographic Summary

A spinal epidural hematoma is an accumulation of blood in the potential space between the dura and the bone of the spinal canal. MRI is the imaging modality of choice for the diagnosis of a spinal epidural hematoma. T1-weighted images usually show a hyperintense extraxial fluid collection. The collections are typically hypointense on T2-weigheted images, although the signal characteristics will vary with the age of hematoma. CT may diagnose a spinal epidural hematoma, but can give false negative results.

Clinical Implications

Spinal epidural hematoma is a rare condition that may be traumatic or spontaneous. Minor trauma from a lumbar puncture or epidural anesthesia can also cause a spinal epidural hematoma. Spontaneous hematomas may occur as a result of anticoagulation therapy, coagulopathies, vascular malformations, or neoplasms. The peridural venous plexus is the usual site of bleeding. The most common symptom is back pain with possible associated radiculopathy, weakness, and/or sensory changes. The typical treatment for spinal epidural hematomas with neurologic changes is surgical decompression. If the hematoma is secondary to trauma, then stabilization of the injured area is important to prevent further injury. If bleeding is secondary to anticoagulation therapy or a coagulopathy, then vitamin K, protamine sulfate, fresh frozen plasma, platelet transfusions, or clotting factor concentrates may be necessary.

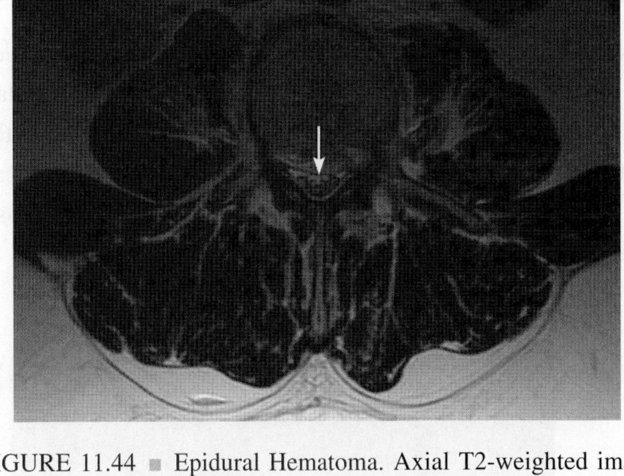

FIGURE 11.44 ■ Epidural Hematoma. Axial T2-weighted imaging shows mild dorsal displacement of the thecal sac secondary to the extradural collection (arrow).

Pearls

1. No underlying cause can be found for spontaneous spinal epidural hematoma in approximately 40 to 50% of cases.
2. Neurologic outcome in patients with spinal epidural hematoma is linked to early diagnosis and intervention.

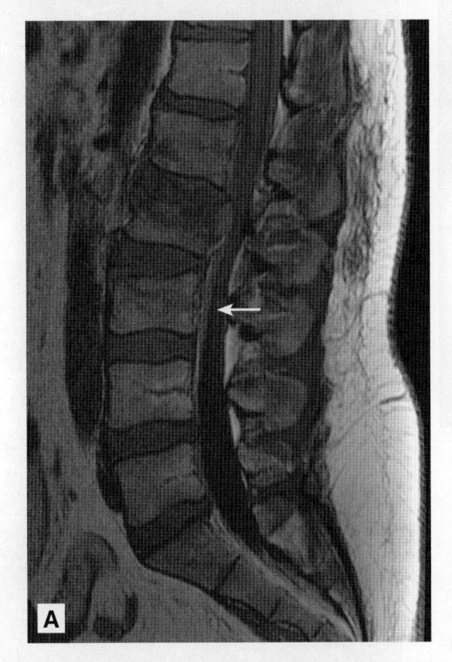

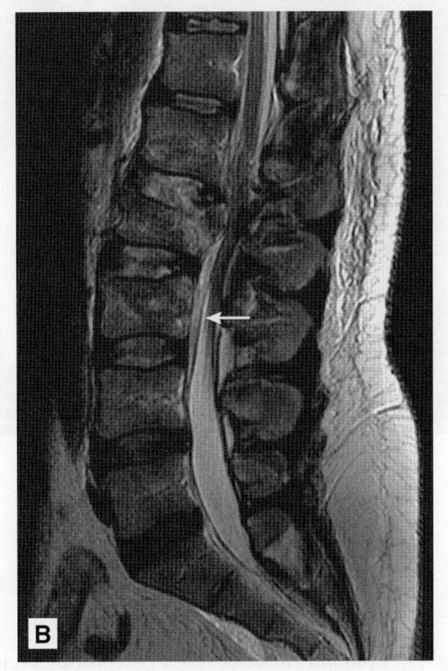

FIGURE 11.43 ■ Epidural Hematoma. L2 burst fracture with epidural hematoma. T1 and T2-weighted sequences show an extradural multisegment collection, hyperintense on T1 and hypointense on T2-weighted sequences relative to CSF, spanning the L1–L4 levels, consistent with early subacute blood (arrows). The MR signal characteristics of hemorrhage varies as intracellular oxyhemaglobin evolves into extracellular deoxyhemoglobin, methemaglobin and ferritin.

Radiographic Summary

A spinal epidural abscess is a focal collection of pus between the dura and bony spinal canal. MRI is the imaging modality of choice for diagnoses. Gadolinium contrast increases the sensitivity for the detection of an abscess. Contrasted CT scan may also demonstrate a spinal epidural abscess, but the sensitivity is greater with MRI.

MRI may reveal two basic patterns. In the first pattern, the phlegmon will result in homogeneous enhancement in the epidural space. In the second pattern, a true fluid collection exists with surrounding inflammatory tissue that has heterogeneous or peripheral rim enhancement with gadolinium.

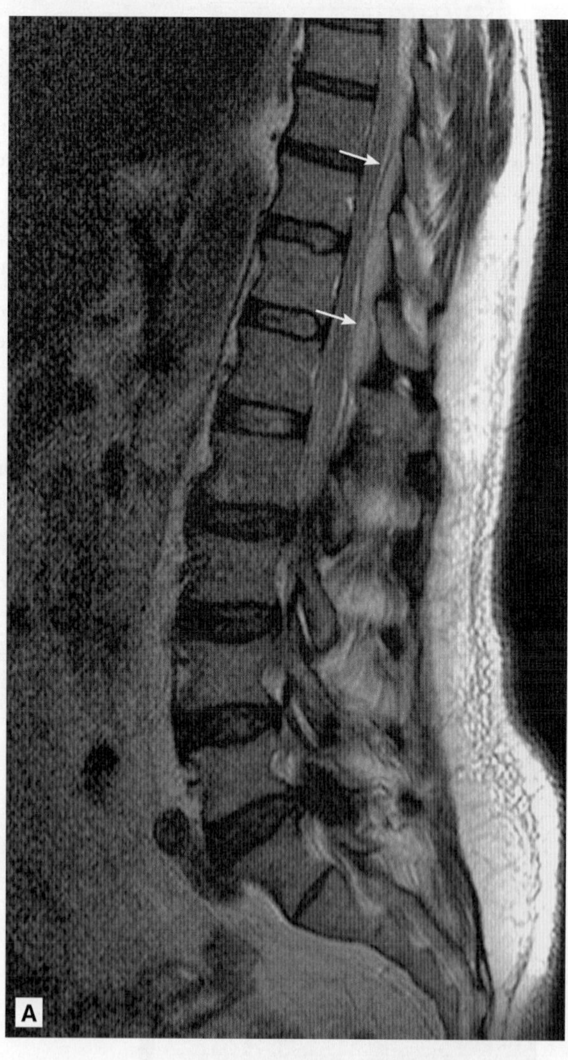
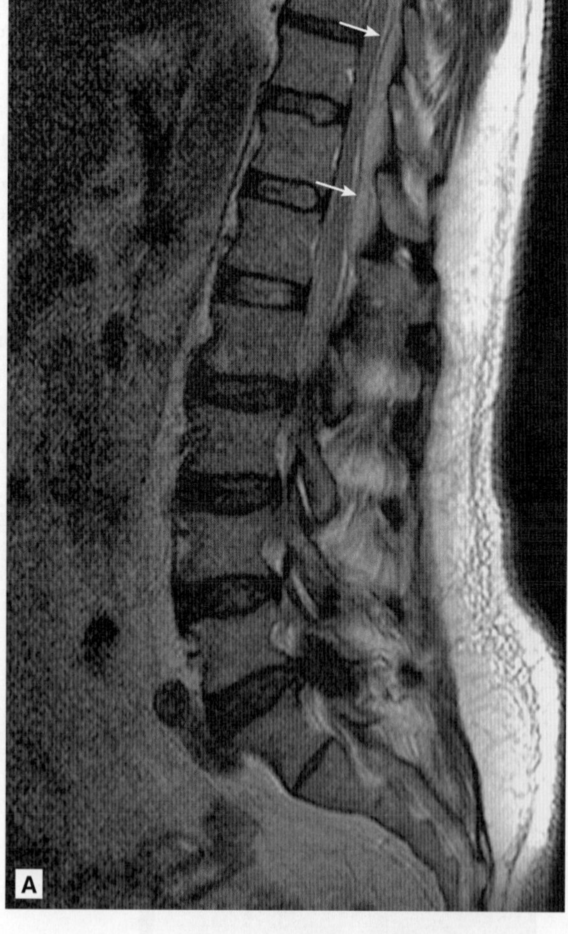

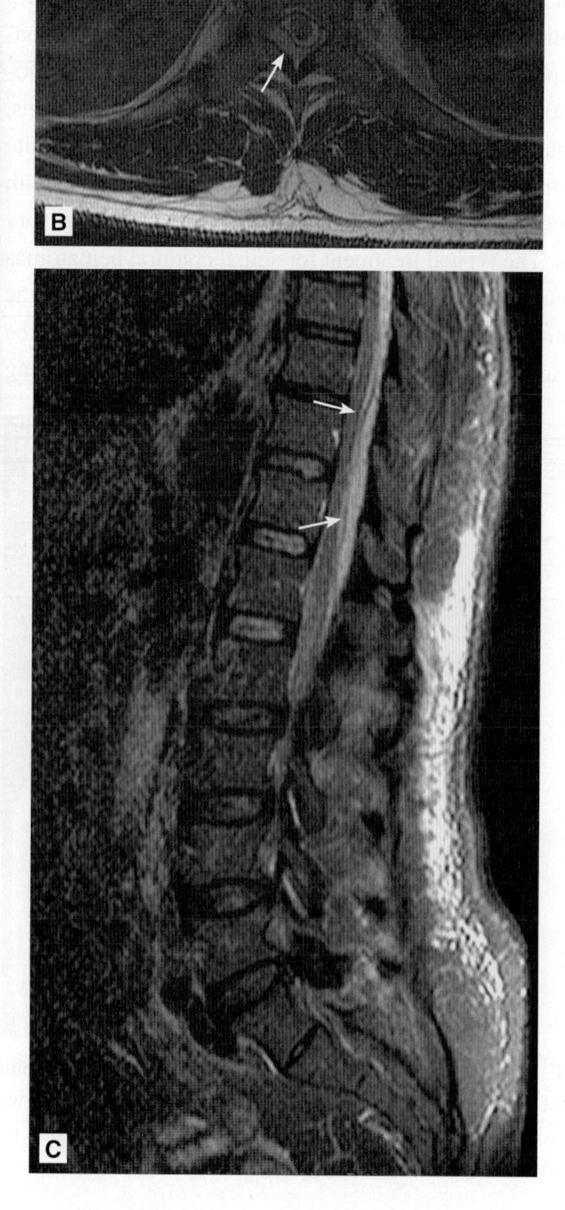

FIGURE 11.45 ■ Epidural Abscess. **A-C:** Precontrast sagittal and axial T1 and sagittal STIR sequences show a large, somewhat lobulated dorsal epidural collection that is slightly hyperintense to the cord on T1 and hyperintense on STIR (arrows). This abscess extended from C2 to the sacrum!

Clinical Implications

Epidural abscesses typically result from direct inoculation during a surgical procedure, hematogenous spread, or direct extension from an overlying soft tissue infection or osteomyelitis. Typical symptoms include back pain, fever, and possible neurologic impairment. Neurologic symptoms may include radiculopathy, weakness, sensory changes, or bowel or bladder dysfunction. Treatment includes IV antibiotics and surgical drainage.

Pearls

1. IV drug abusers, alcoholics, diabetic patients, and immunosuppressed patients are at increased risk for epidural abscesses.
2. *Staphylococcus aureus* is the most common organism found in epidural abscesses.
3. It is important to obtain blood cultures, since they are positive in approximately 60% of these patients.

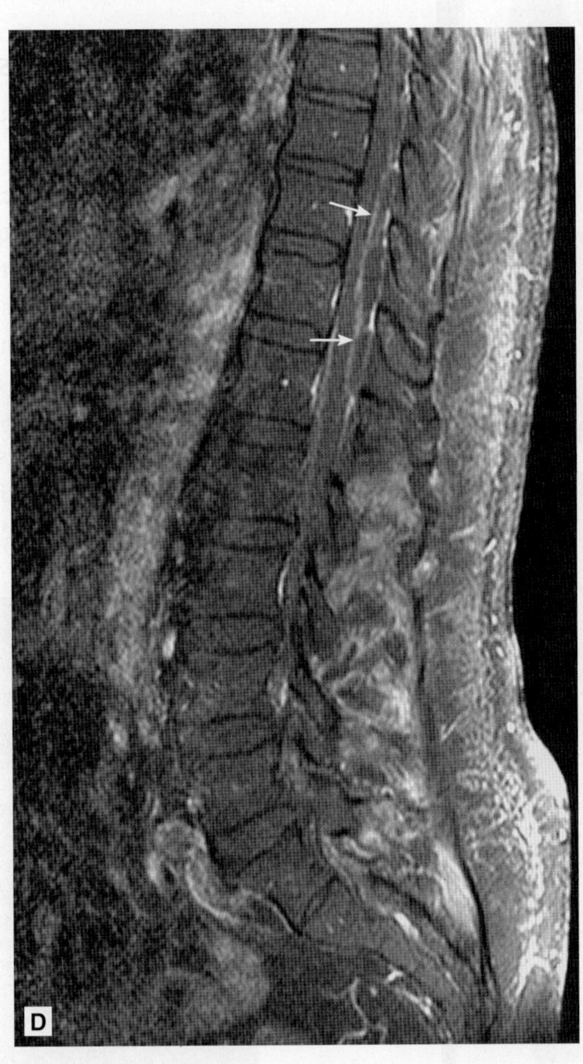

FIGURE 11.45 ■ (*Continued*) **D:** After contrast is given, the large epidural abscess shows characteristic rim enhancement (arrows). Epidural abscesses are often associated with infectious spondylodiskitis, though in this instance, there was no such evidence.

Radiographic Summary

A herniated nucleus pulposus is also referred to as a "herniated disk." It occurs when there is a disruption in the outer ring (annulus fibrosus) that surrounds the intervertebral disk and the nucleus pulposus, (the central portion of the disk), bulges out. The disk contents may or may not press against the surrounding nerves or spinal cord. Plain radiographs may increase suspicion of a herniated nucleus pulposus by showing narrowing of the disk space, but MRI provides the definitive evidence for diagnosis. T2-weighted images are best for visualization of protruded disk material into the spinal canal. Disk herniations may also occur posterolaterally into the neuroforamina, or laterally along the edge of the vertebra. IV contrast is only indicated in the postoperative patient distinguished for recurrent disk herniation from postoperative scar.

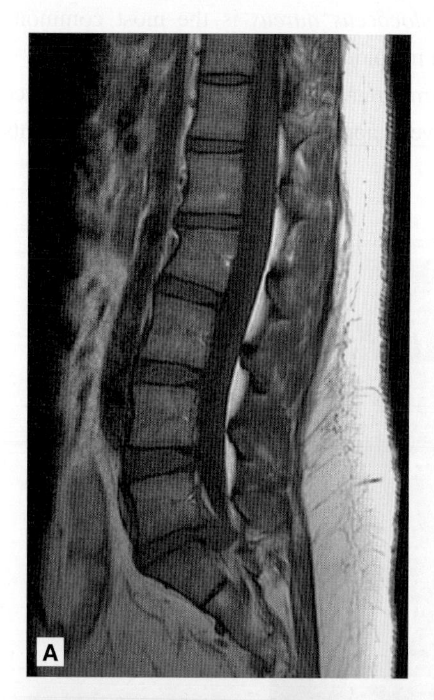

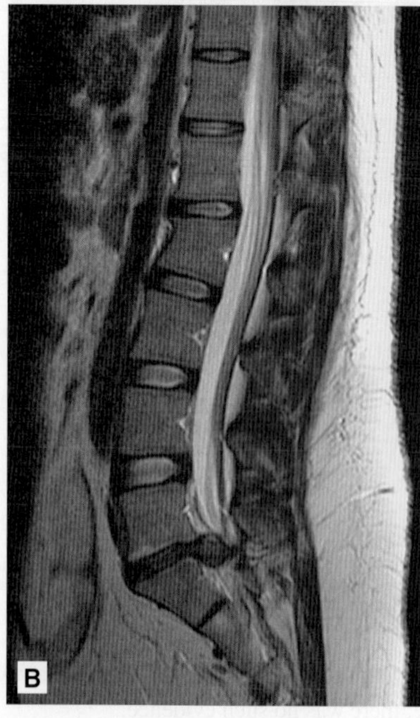

FIGURE 11.46 ■ Herniated Nucleus Pulposus. **A, B:** Sagittal T1 and T2 images of the lumbar spine show a disk extrusion at L5–S1. Notice that the extruded material is isointense to other disks on T1. The degree of disk hydration dictates T2 signal characteristics. The neck of the extrusion is narrower than any diameter of the extruded material itself making this a disk extrusion, not a herniation.

Clinical Implications

A herniated nucleus pulposus usually occurs secondary to mechanical injury. It can occur during acute trauma, or it can occur secondary to chronic mechanical forces. People who perform jobs that require heavy lifting are more prone to this type of injury. Symptoms are related to the amount of disk protrusion and impingement on surrounding nerves as well as the level of injury. Patients may have minimal to no pain if there is limited nerve compression. However, pain may become severe and symptoms may include numbness, weakness, or even paralysis if nerve compression worsens. Sciatica can occur when the disk pathology is in the lumbar spine. Lower extremity weakness and pain, urinary retention,

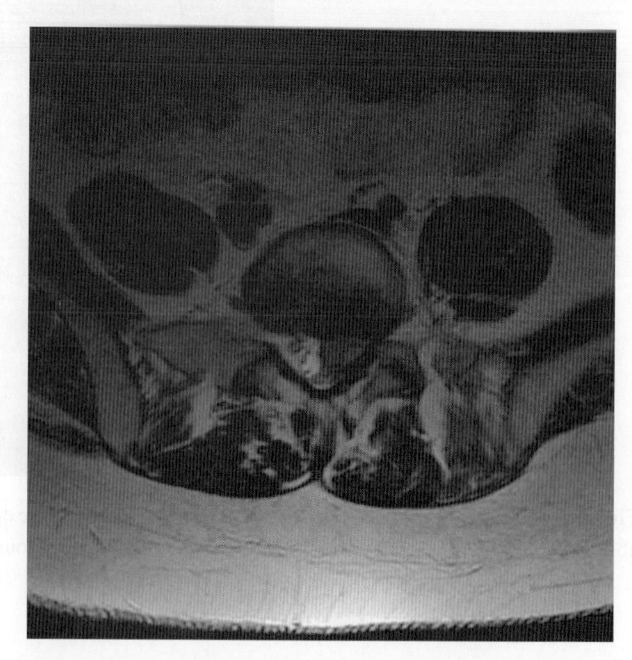

FIGURE 11.47 ■ Herniated Nucleus Pulposus. Axial T2 imaging shows obliteration of the left lateral recess by the large extruded disk and displacement of the left S1 nerve root.

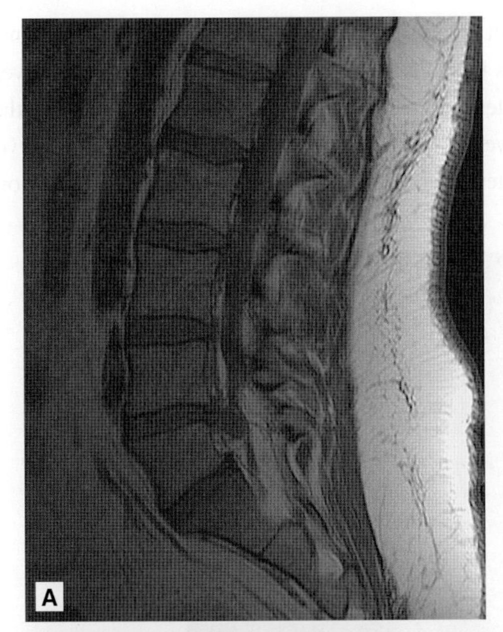

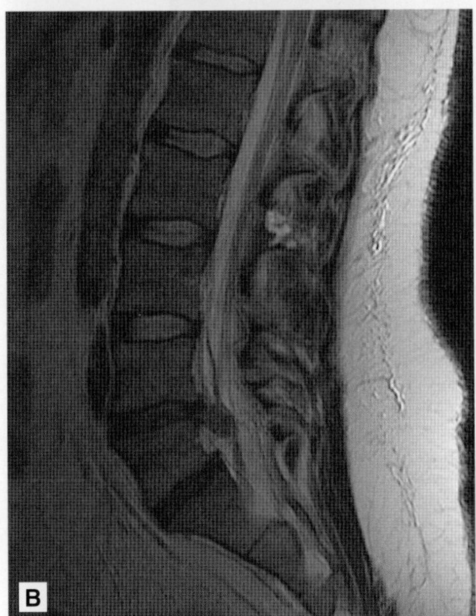

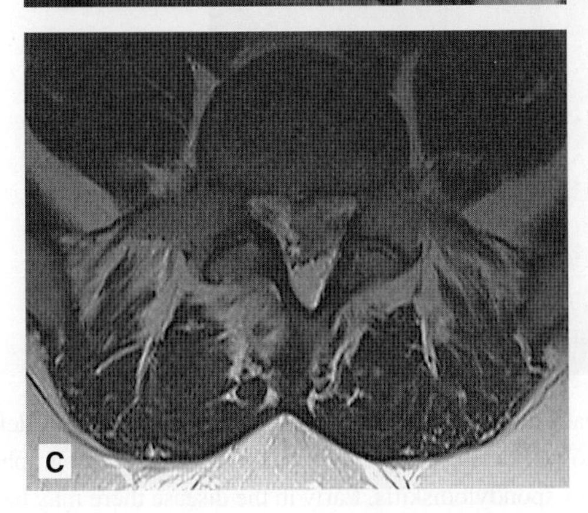

FIGURE 11.48 ■ Herniated Nucleus Pulposus. **A-C:** Sagittal T1 and T2-weighted images in another patient show a central disk extrusion.

fecal incontinence, sexual dysfunction, and saddle anesthesia (cauda equina syndrome) can occur when the nerve roots below the conus are compressed. Treatment is usually conservative, with surgical intervention reserved for those patients with significant neurologic deficits or cauda equina syndrome. Rest, pain relief, gentle stretching and massage, and physical therapy are the most common initial therapies.

Pearls

1. Herniated nucleus pulposus is most common in the lumbar spine.
2. With age, the composition of the nucleus pulposus changes and the risk of herniation reduces. It is most common when a person is in their 30s and 40s and decreases in frequency thereafter.

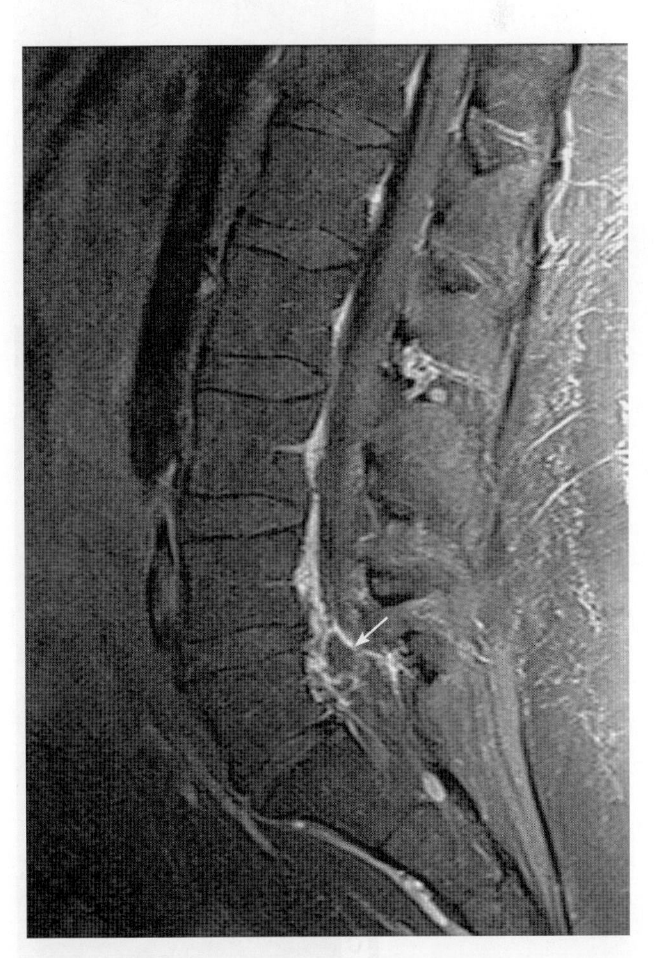

FIGURE 11.49 ■ Herniated Nucleus Pulposus. Post contrast T1-weighted sagittal image nicely demonstrates thin peripheral enhancement of the disk (arrow). Note that the disk itself does not enhance, a feature that makes pre and post contrast imaging useful in the evaluation of the postoperative patient, as scar tissue will enhance. A recurrent disk herniation will not.

Radiographic Summary

Plain radiographs are often obtained in patients presenting with symptoms of disk space infection. The most common finding on plain radiographs is intervertebral disk space narrowing with adjacent endplate osteolysis. In more chronic presentations, there is typically sclerotic irregularity of the adjacent vertebral endplates with persistent disk space narrowing. MRI is the most sensitive and specific way to diagnose infection of the vertebra and intervertebral disks. T1-weighted images will show disk

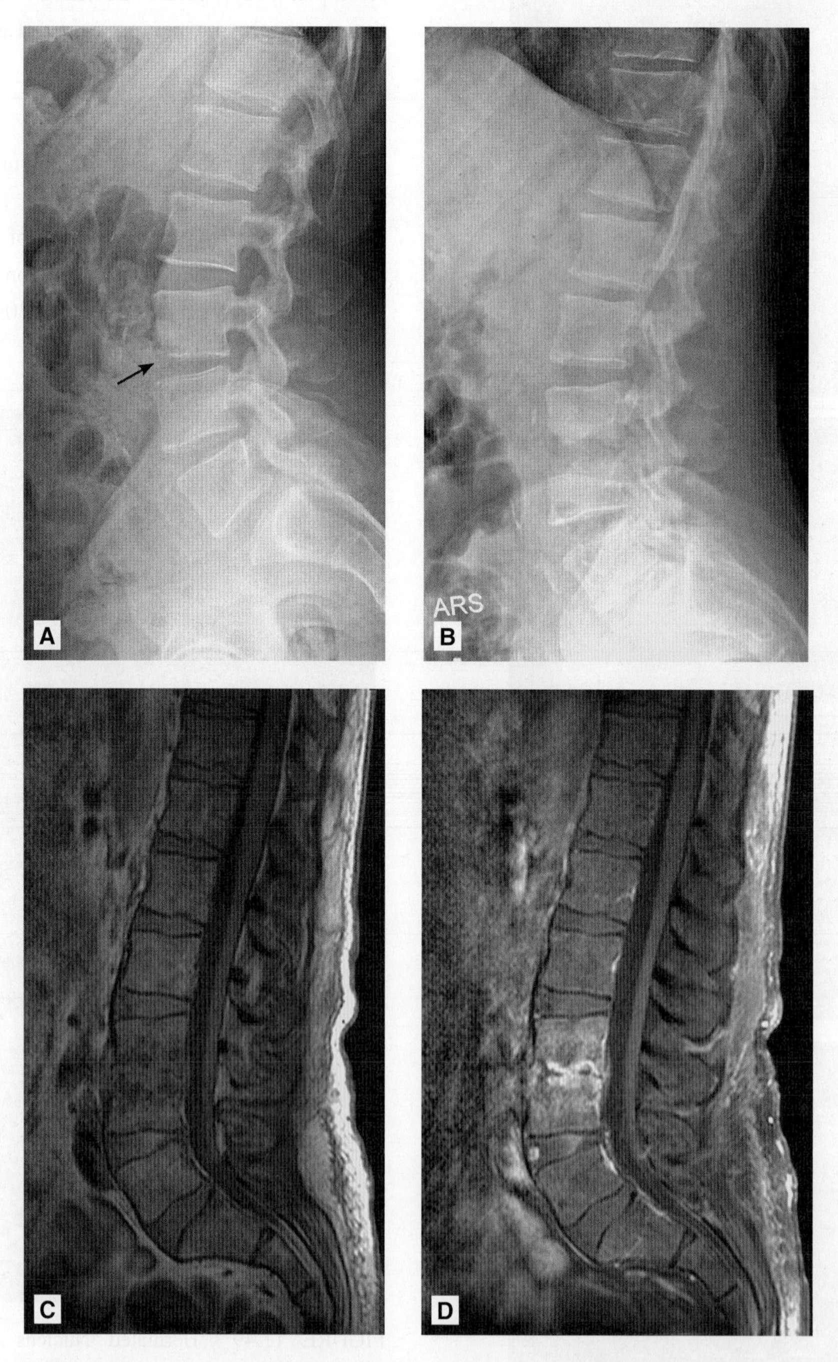

FIGURE 11.50 ■ Diskitis. **A:** This patient presented with low-grade fever and back pain. Note the subtle loss of disk height and ill-definition of the anterior portion of the adjacent L3 and L4 vertebral endplates (arrow). **B:** 6 weeks later, the patient returned. Lateral radiograph shows further endplate destruction on both sides of the affected disk, typical of infectious spondylodiskitis. Early in the disease there may be apparent disk space widening. **C, D:** An MR was obtained. Lateral T1W and post-contrast T1W MR images show characteristic cortical destruction at the involved endplates and enhancement in the involved disk space and adjacent endplates. A small epidural abscess is also present.

space narrowing and hypointense signal in the disk. T2-weighted images will show increased fluid signal in the disk and edema in the adjacent vertebral bodies. Following IV gadolinium contrast, there is enhancement of the disk space and adjacent endplates.

Clinical Implications

Diskitis is an infection of the intervertebral disk space and adjacent vertebral bodies. It may occur from hematogenous spread from a systemic infection or it may occur postoperatively. Postoperative patients usually present a few days to weeks following surgery; however, patients with spontaneous diskitis have a much more insidious onset of symptoms over weeks to months. The most common symptom is back pain with localized tenderness that is worse with movement. Less frequently, patients may have a fever. *Staphylococcus aureus* is the most common causative organism. ESR and CRP will generally be elevated, but the WBC may be normal. Treatment is usually with IV antibiotics.

Pearls

1. Diskitis is most common in the lumbar spine
2. IV drug users are at higher risk for diskitis.
3. Endplate destruction with relative preservation of the intervening disk space may be seen in cases of tuberculous diskitis.

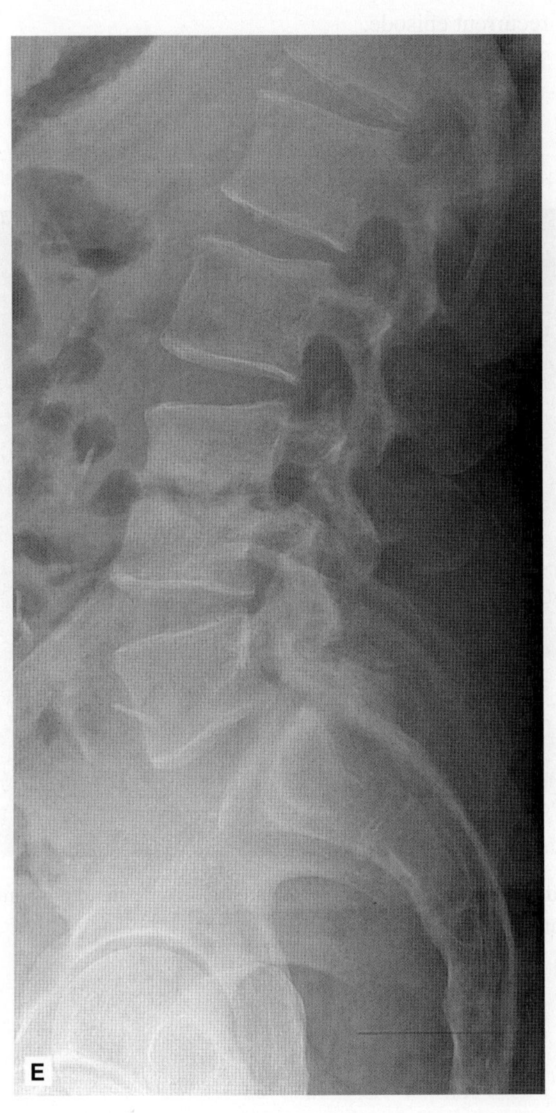

FIGURE 11.50 ■ (*Continued*) **E:** Months later, after appropriate treatment, endplate sclerosis indicates healing.

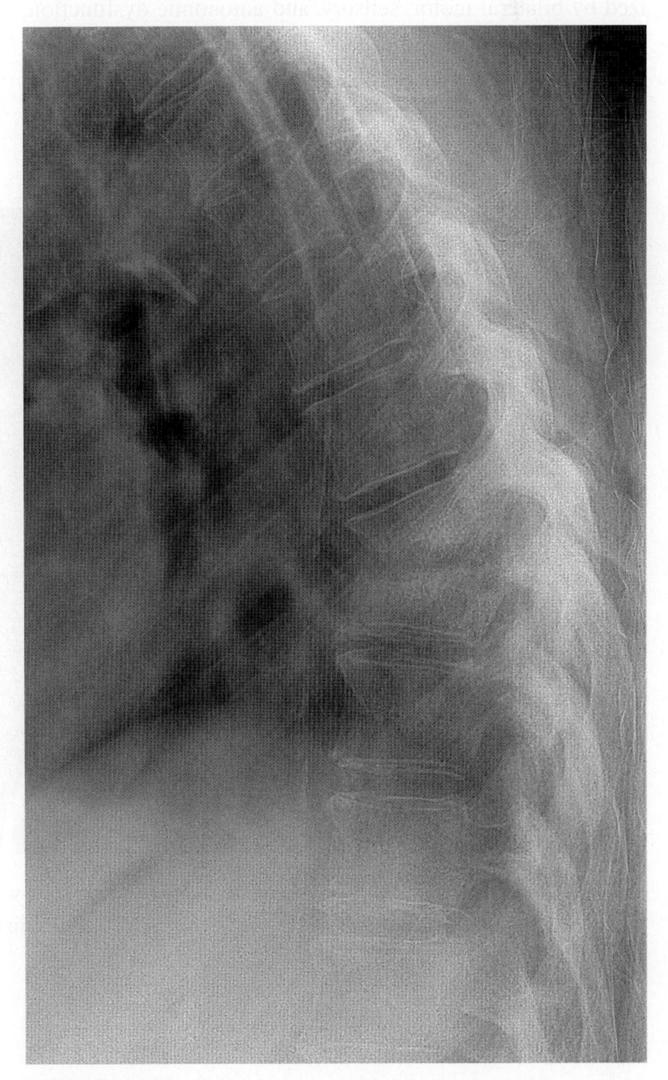

FIGURE 11.51 ■ Diskitis. Chronic thoracic spine diskitis in a different patient. Hallmark features of bone loss, endplate sclerosis, and angular kyphotic deformity are present in this case.

Radiographic Summary

Acute transverse myelitis usually presents on MRI as a central cord lesion occupying two-thirds or more of the cord and extending at least two but usually more vertebral segments in length. Lesions are usually hyperintense on T2 with variable enhancement following IV gadolinium. Smooth cord expansion may occur. Lesions may exist in any part of the spinal cord. This lesion can mimic neoplasm and can be confused with demyelinating lesions of multiple sclerosis.

Clinical Implications

Transverse myelitis is a relatively rare inflammatory process of the spinal cord that causes demyelination. It is characterized by bilateral motor, sensory, and autonomic dysfunction. The most common initial symptoms are back pain and/or radiculopathy. Symptoms may progress over several hours to days. Most cases are idiopathic. However, other cases may be related to viral or bacterial illnesses, or due to conditions like multiple sclerosis, lupus, or sarcoidosis. CSF may be normal or show a lymphocytic pleocytosis and elevated protein levels. Treatment is usually supportive. High-dose steroids are also given, although their efficacy has not been proven. Patients may make a full recovery over several weeks to months; however, some patients may never recover neurologic functions.

Pearls

1. Approximately 1/3 of patients make a full recovery, 1/3 make a partial recovery, and 1/3 have little to no recovery from neurologic deficits.
2. 5-10% of patients with transverse myelitis may have a recurrent episode.
3. The thoracic area is most commonly affected.

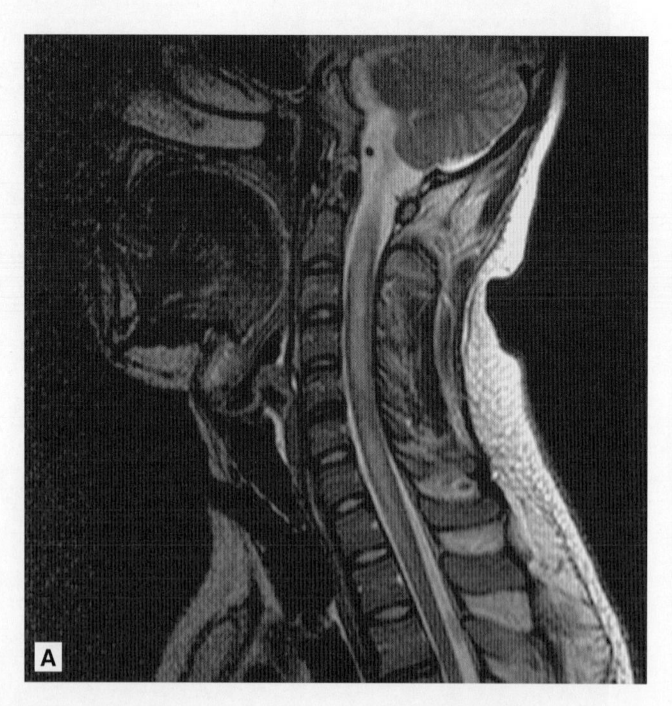

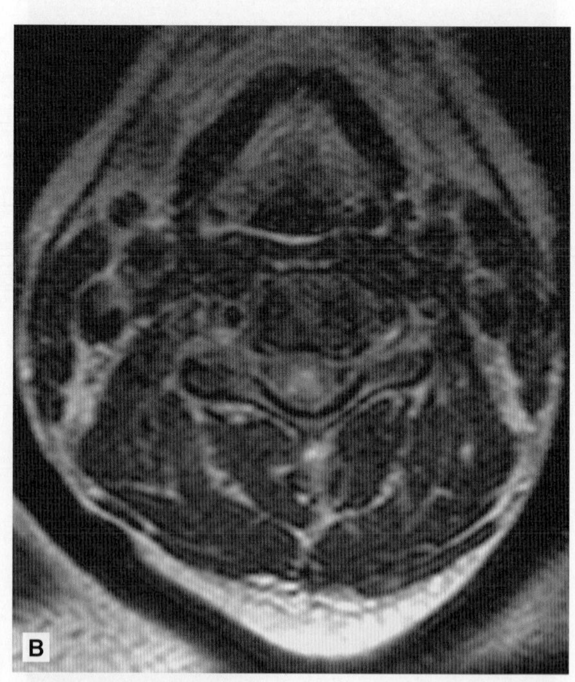

FIGURE 11.52 ■ Transverse Myelitis. **A, B:** Sagittal and axial T2-weighted images show a central hyperintense lesion extending from C2 through T2 and involving 60-70% of the cord's cross sectional area in this patient with transverse myelitis.

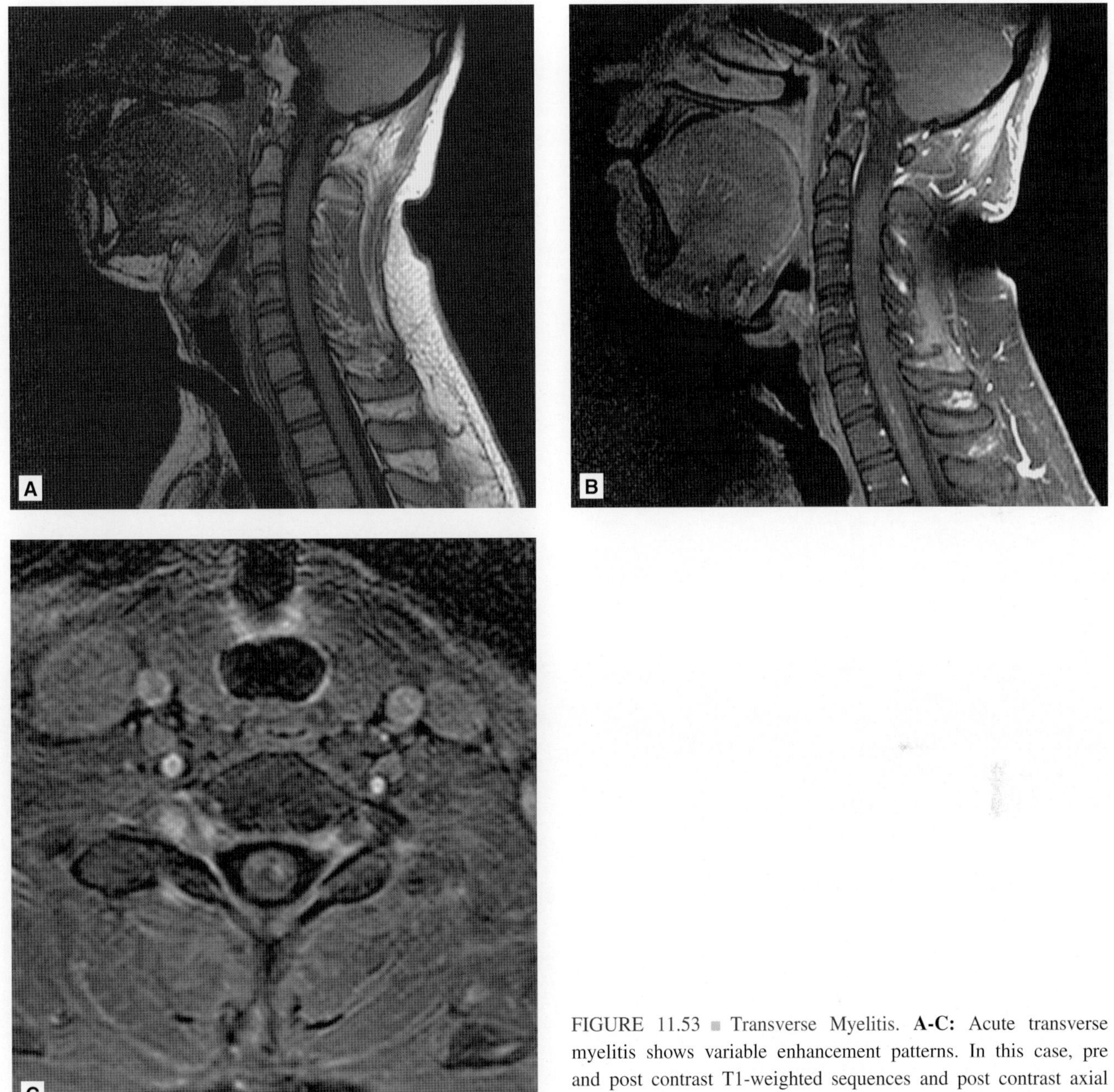

FIGURE 11.53 ■ Transverse Myelitis. **A-C:** Acute transverse myelitis shows variable enhancement patterns. In this case, pre and post contrast T1-weighted sequences and post contrast axial T1-weighted image show peripheral enhancement, a typical pattern.

Chapter 12

PEDIATRIC CONDITIONS

J. Herman Kan
Mark Meredith

Radiographic Summary

Bronchiolitis is an inflammation of the bronchioles, often seen in young children with viral respiratory infections. Although the most common radiographic finding of bronchiolitis is a normal chest radiograph, patients may also present with pulmonary hyperinflation, peribronchial thickening, and discoid atelectasis. Care should be made not to mistake an underinflation artifact with peribronchial thickening related to bronchiolitis. Alternatively, when the heart is enlarged, care should be made not to confuse pulmonary vascular congestion related to congenital heart disease with peribronchial thickening related to bronchiolitis. The utility of the chest radiograph in the evaluation of bronchiolitis is to rule out related complicating features, including superimposed pneumonia, atelectasis, and pneumothorax/pneumomediastinum. Chest x-ray may also help to rule out other causes of wheezing such as a foreign body aspiration.

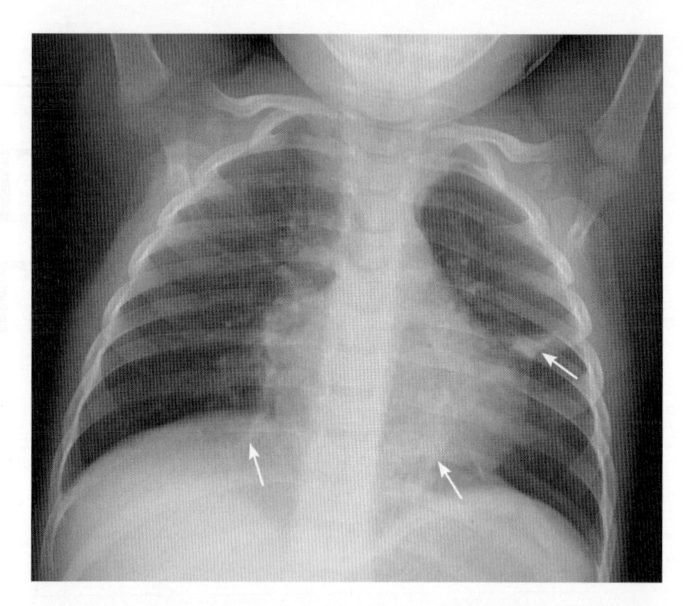

FIGURE 12.2 ■ Discoid Atelectasis. AP chest radiograph of bronchiolitis in a 2-year-old boy demonstrates bilateral multifocal discoid atelectasis (arrows).

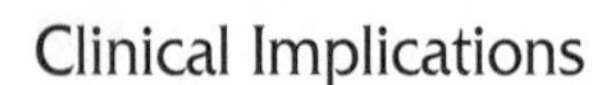

Clinical Implications

Bronchiolitis patients are often neonates to 2-year-olds and present with tachypnea, wheezing, hypoxia, copious rhinorrhea, and in more severe cases respiratory distress. Common pathogens of bronchiolitis include respiratory syncitial virus (RSV), influenza, parainfluenza, human metapneumovirus, and many other viruses. Patients who are less than one month old, born prematurely and are less than 48 weeks post-conceptual age, and those with co-morbid conditions are at

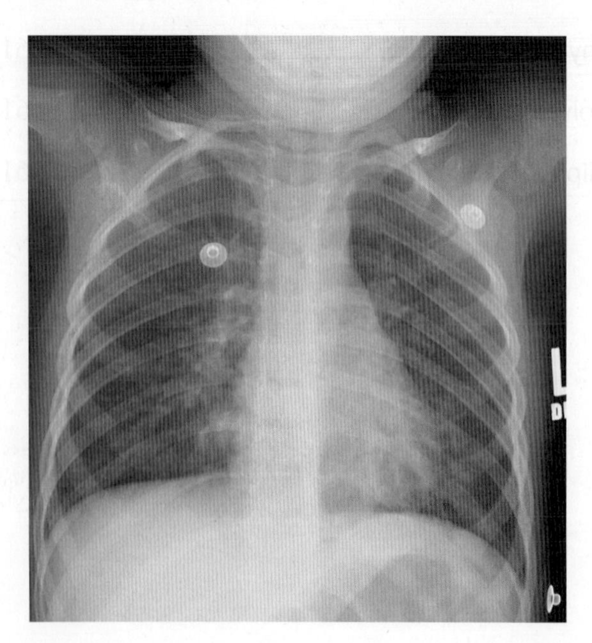

FIGURE 12.1 ■ Peribronchial Thickening. AP chest radiograph of bronchiolitis in a 3-year-old girl demonstrates diffuse bilateral peribronchial thickening and patchy and discoid atelectasis. Hyperinflation is present.

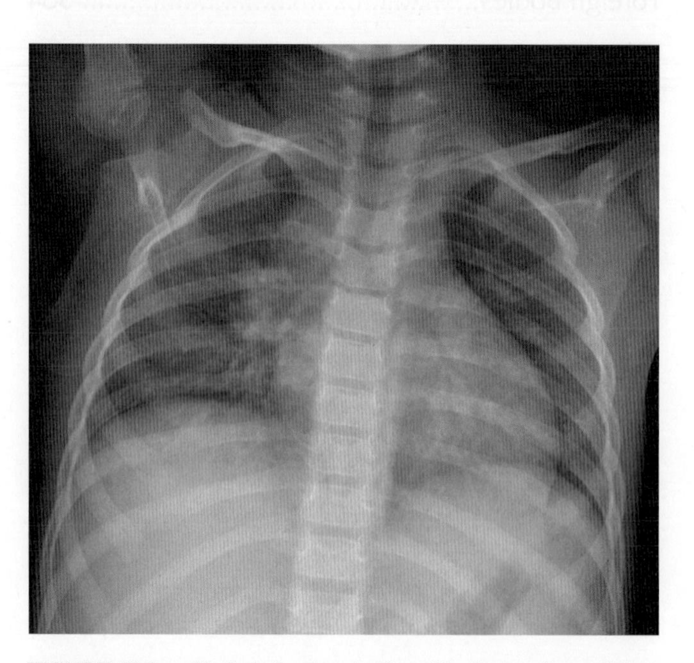

FIGURE 12.3 ■ Underinflaction Artifact. PA chest radiograph in a 6-year-old girl with a normal chest radiograph with underinflation artifact. Care should be taken not to confuse underinflation artifact for peribronchial thickening related to bronchiolitis.

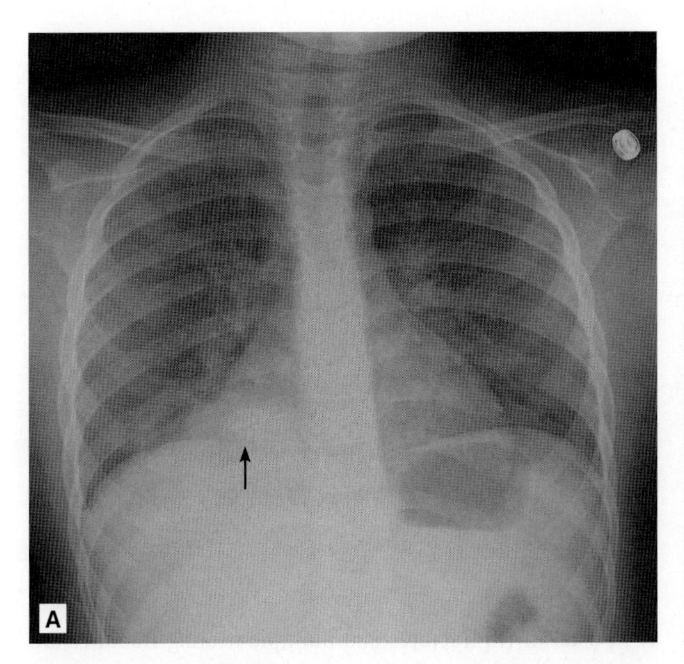

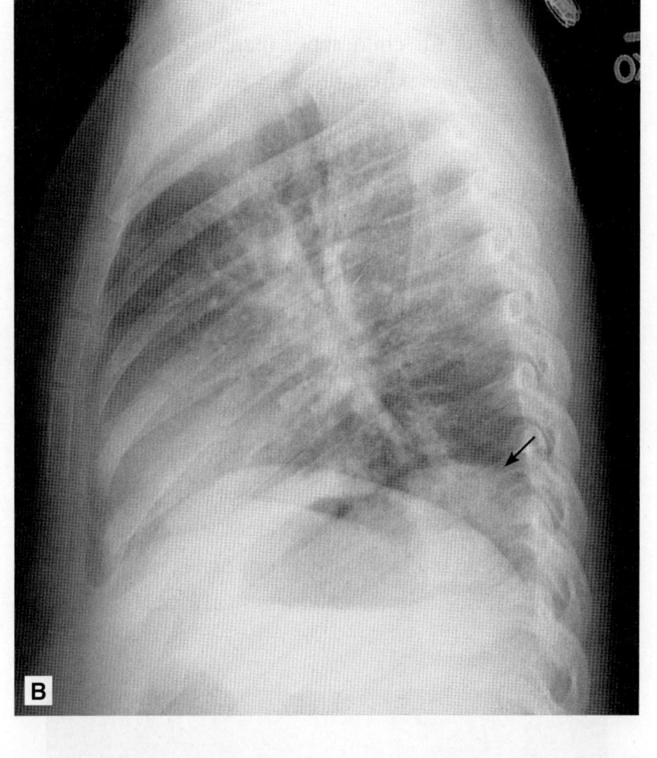

FIGURE 12.4 ■ Right Lower Lobe Pneumonia. **A, B:** PA and lateral chest radiograph demonstrate right lower lobe pneumonia (arrows) in a 5-year-old boy with clinical symptoms of bronchiolitis. Note silhouetting of portions of the right heart border and right diaphragm shadow.

risk of developing apnea. Days 3-5 are usually the most severe of the illness in regards to respiratory distress. Dehydration is a common finding in this time period as younger patients have difficulty swallowing when their respiratory rates get above 60. Treatment of bronchiolitis is ever changing but beta agonist and steroids have generally not been shown to be helpful. Criteria for discharge should include adequate hydration status, oxygenation saturations above 90%, and close follow-up within 24 hours.

Pearls

1. The chest radiograph is primarily used in bronchiolitis to rule out complicating factors such as foreign body aspiration and pneumonia.
2. Consideration should be given to whether the patient could have congenital heart disease when there is an enlarged cardiac silhouette on chest radiograph.

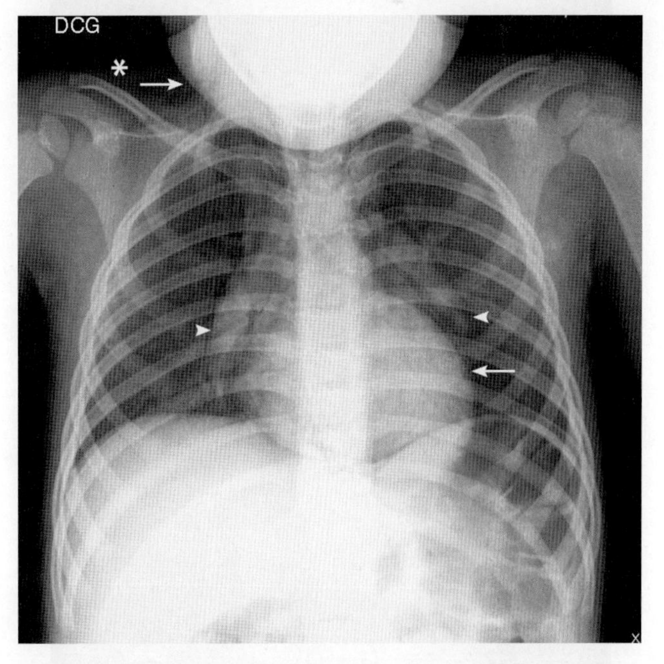

FIGURE 12.5 ■ Pneumomediastinum. AP radiograph of the chest demonstrates complications of bronchiolitis with pneumomediastinum. Note elevation of the thymus (arrowheads) and pneumopericardium (arrow). The presence of subcutaneous air in the soft tissues of the neck (arrow,*) is related to pneumomediastinum.

Radiographic Summary

Fractures specific for child abuse include classic metaphyseal fractures in the extremities and posterior rib fractures. Alternative names for the classic metaphyseal fracture of child abuse include corner fracture and metaphyseal bucket handle fracture. Without a history of major accidental trauma such as an auto accident, child abuse should also be suspected if there are fractures of the sternum, scapula, posterior element fractures of the spine, and fractures of the femur in a child not walking. However, any fracture may be a result of abuse and must be correlated with the history provided.

Clinical Implications

Where there is a possibility of child abuse, the age of the child and physical exam findings can help drive what radiologic tests should be performed. In the child less than a year of age with any fracture and an unclear or concerning history, a full skeletal survey and head CT should be performed. This allows not only an opportunity to identify acute fractures but also old healing fractures indicative of abuse. Healing fractures can further concerns for child abuse or suggest medical problems simulating abuse. For the younger patient, particular attention should be paid to radiographs of the chest looking for rib fractures and to the long bone metaphyses looking for classic metaphyseal lesions. In addition to radiographic examinations, an ophthalmologist should perform fundoscopic examination looking for retinal hemorrhages. In any case where there is suspected abuse, the local child protection services agency must be notified by law for an investigation to be completed.

Pearls

1. Posterior rib fractures and multiple healing fractures are highly concerning for child abuse.
2. When there is concern for abuse in the young child, a full skeletal survey and noncontrasted head CT should be performed.

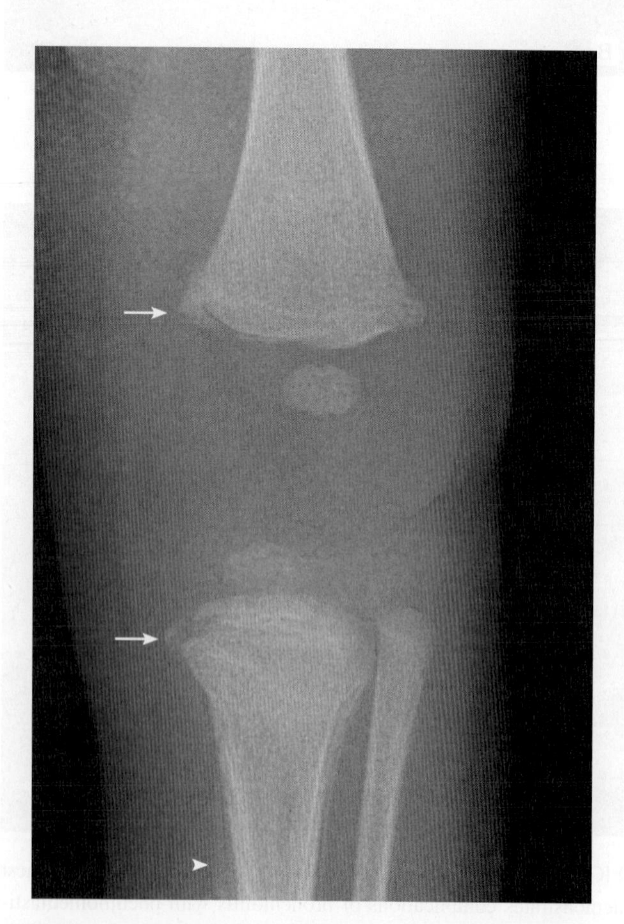

FIGURE 12.6 ■ Corner Fractures. A 2-month-old boy with classic metaphyseal "corner" fractures of child abuse affecting the distal femur and proximal tibia (arrows). Note periosteal reaction seen along the shaft of the tibia (arrowhead), indicative of healing fracture.

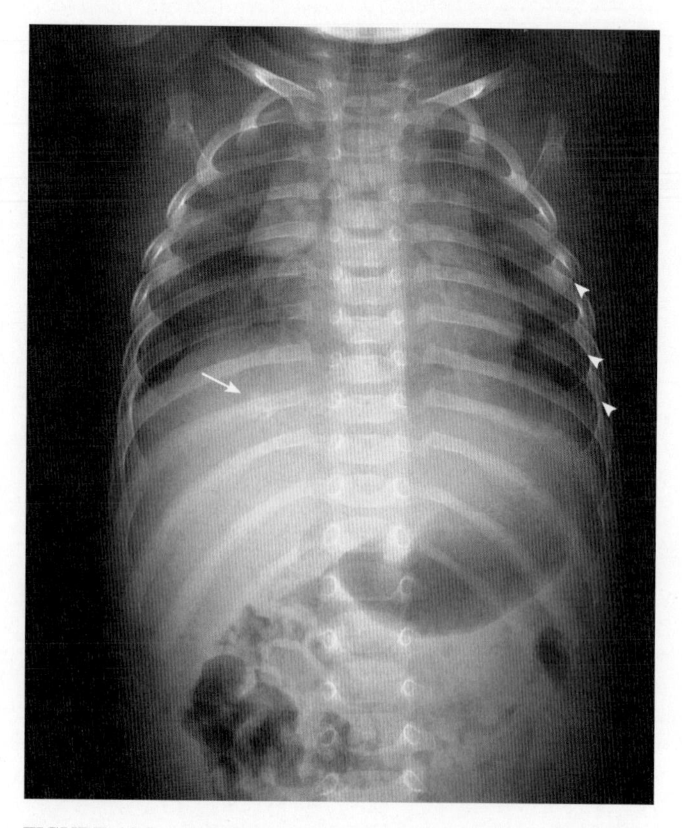

FIGURE 12.7 ■ Rib Fractures. A 3-month-old boy with multiple bilateral rib fractures of child abuse of differing ages, some of which are healing (arrow) and others that are acute (arrowheads).

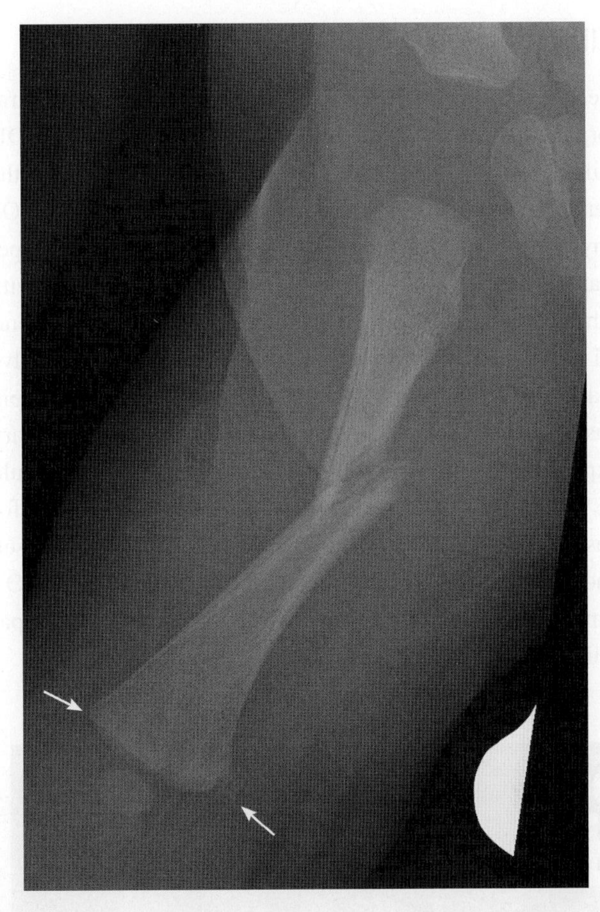

FIGURE 12.8 ■ Corner Fractures. A 7-month-old boy with femoral midshaft fracture and distal femoral metaphyseal corner fractures (arrows) indicative of child abuse.

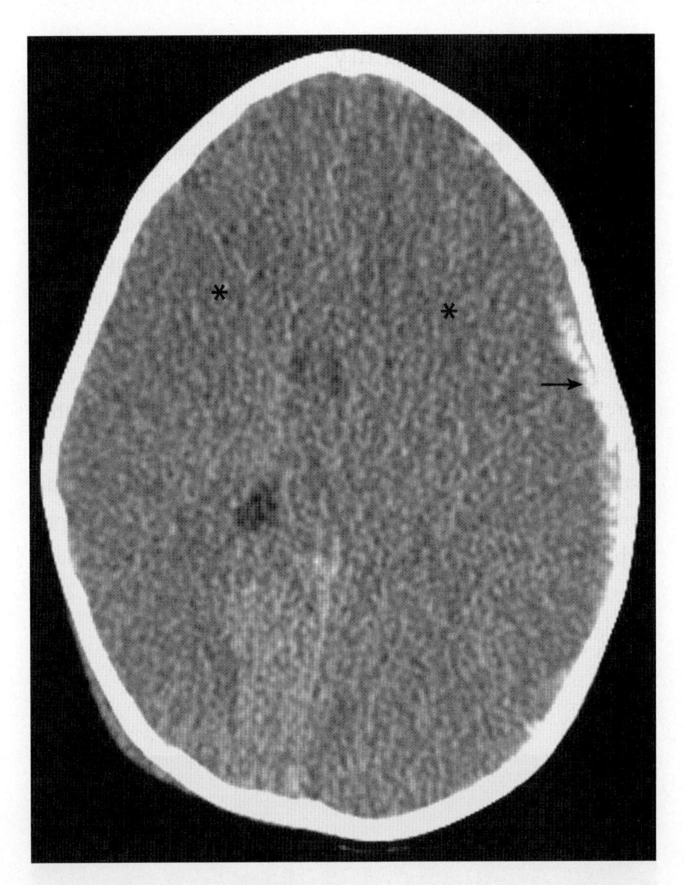

FIGURE 12.10 ■ Subdural Hematoma. An infant with nonaccidental trauma. Axial computed tomographic image at presentation show left-side frontoparietal-convexity high-density small subdural hemorrhage (arrow). There is mass effect on underlying brain parenchyma with associated midline shift to the right. Also seen is bilateral cerebral low density (*) with loss of gray–white matter differentiation indicating diffuse ischemic injury.

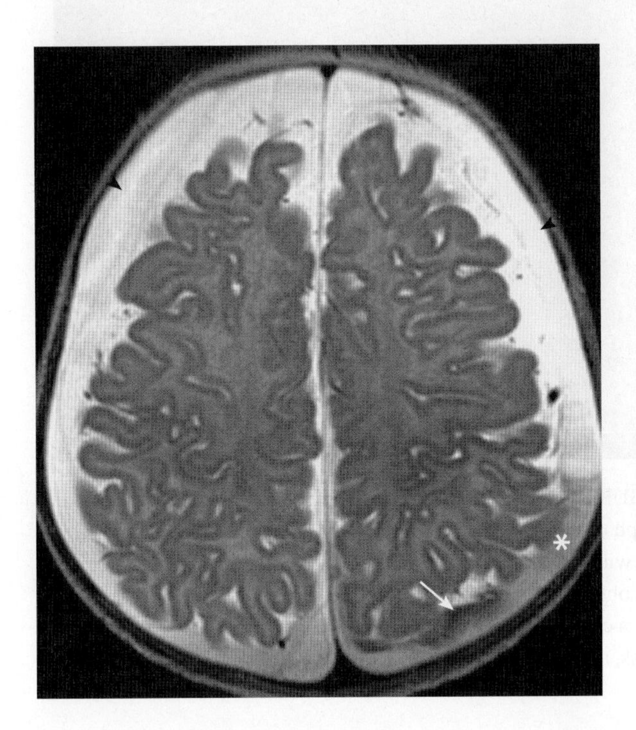

FIGURE 12.9 ■ Bilateral Subdural Hematomas. Axial T2-weighted MRI in another patient demonstrates bilateral subdural hematomas. The image shows blood products of differing ages being hyperintense (arrowheads), isointense (*), and hypointense relative to brain tissue with a blood-fluid level seen (arrow), a finding highly suggestive of child abuse. The hyperintense component indicates chronic subdural, with areas of iso and hypointensity indicating acute and subacute hemorrhage into the chronic collections.

Radiographic Summary

Congenital diaphragmatic hernia (CDH) is due to failure of a foramen in the fetal diaphragm to close, causing abdominal viscera to protrude into the thoracic cavity. CDH more commonly occurs in the left hemithorax compared with the right. When imaging is obtained early, CDH may appear as a mass, without gas delineated bowel loops. The diagnosis of CDH is usually obvious based on clinical presentation and the presence of bowel loops located in the lower chest. However, there is a differential when there is a bubbly appearing intrathoracic mass. This includes congenital cystic adenomatoid malformation (CCAM) and congenital lobar emphysema. However, both of these entities tend to occur in the upper, right middle, and lingular lobes, rarely affecting the lower chest with involvement of the diaphragm as would be seen with a CDH.

Clinical Implications

Neonates with a CDH often present with significant respiratory distress. This is due to the fact that patients with CDH will have hypoplastic lung development on the side of the hernia and therefore oxygenation may be compromised. On physician exam, one might see a scaphoid abdomen, especially if the CDH is left sided. CDHs are also associated with other congenital abnormalities, including renal and congenital heart anomalies. When these patients present, bag valve mask ventilation is contraindicated as this may cause rapid gastric insufflation and possibly further inhibit pulmonary expansion. As soon as a CDH is identified, the patient should be immediately intubated and an orogastric tube inserted for gastric decompression. Many of these patients quickly worsen and require extracorporeal membrane oxygenation (ECMO). Emergent transfer to a tertiary institution with surgical capabilities should occur.

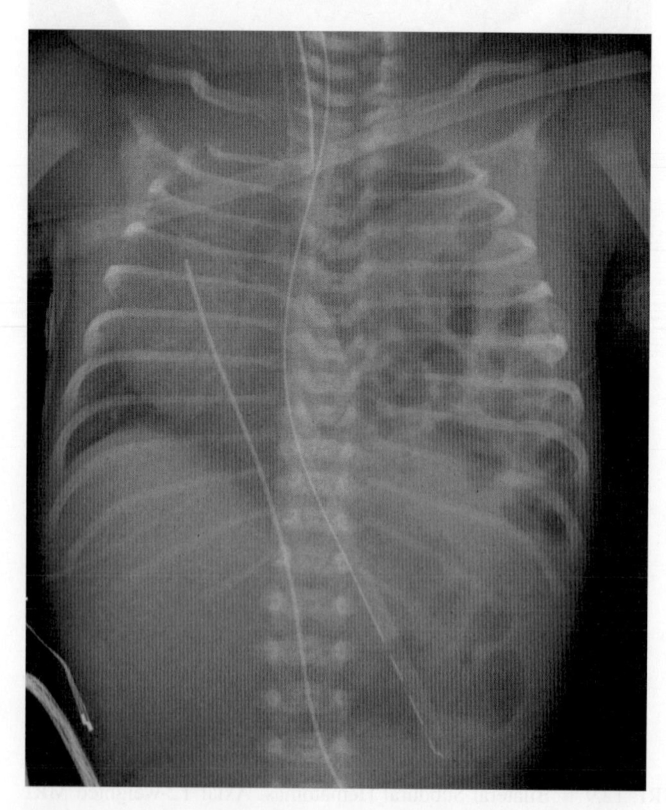

FIGURE 12.11 ■ Congenital Diaphragmatic Hernia. AP radiograph of the chest shows multiple gas delineated bowel loops occupying the left hemithorax with rightward deviation of the mediastinum consistent with congenital diaphragmatic hernia. Note that the enteric tube tip is present in the stomach located in the left hemiabdomen.

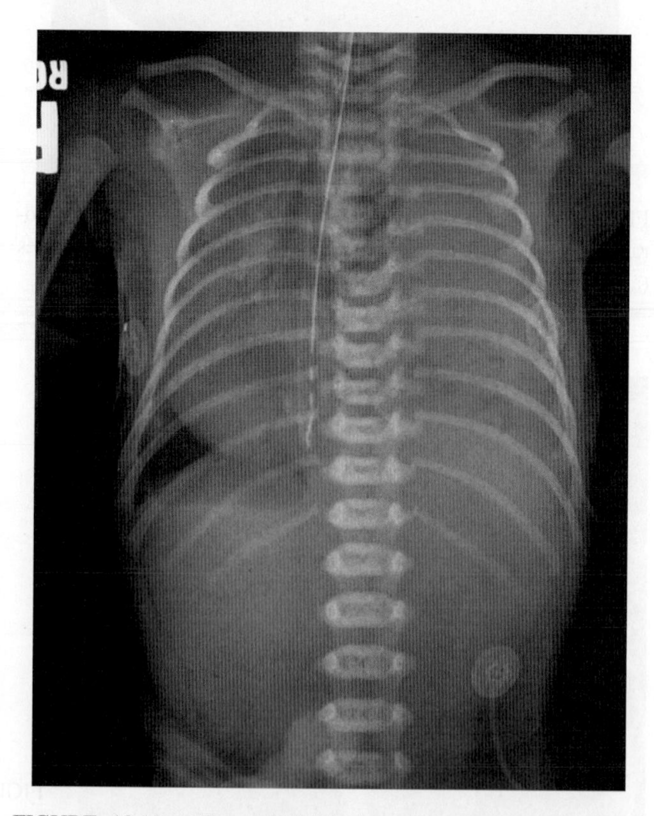

FIGURE 12.12 ■ Congenital Diaphragmatic Hernia. AP radiograph of the chest shows complete opacification of the left hemithorax with rightward deviation of the mediastinum. When radiographs are obtained early in life, bowel loops may not be gas delineated and a congenital diaphragmatic hernia can mimic a space-occupying mass, as in this example.

Pearls

1. The chest radiograph of a neonate with CDH will show a hypoplastic lung and bowel protruding into the thoracic cavity.
2. CDH should be treated with immediate intubation and orogastric tube placement. Bag valve mask ventilation should be avoided to prevent worsening respiratory compromise by gastric insufflation.

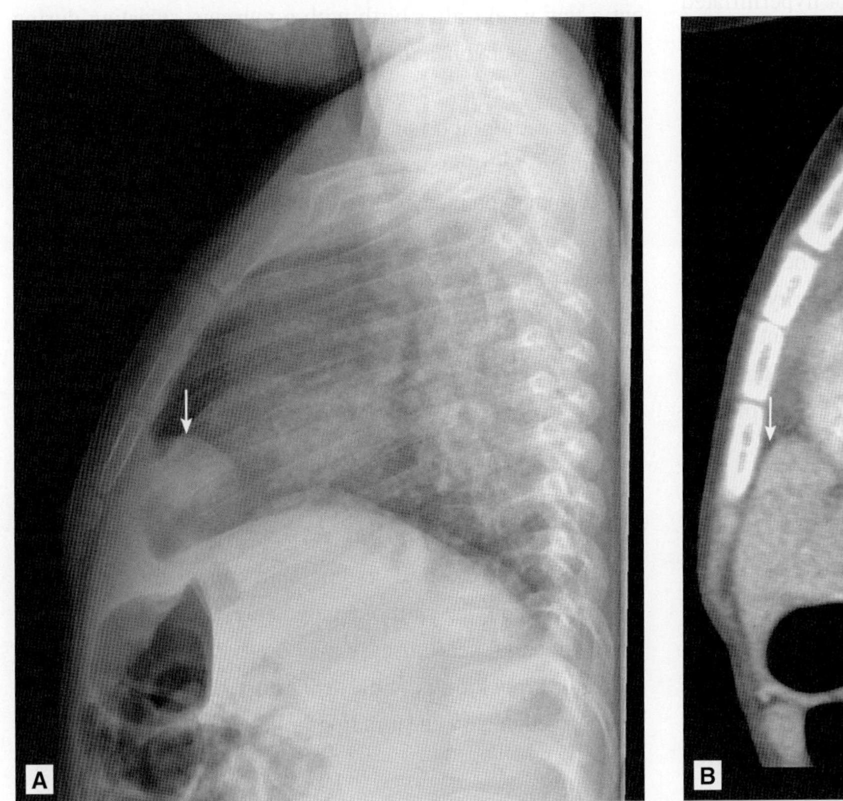

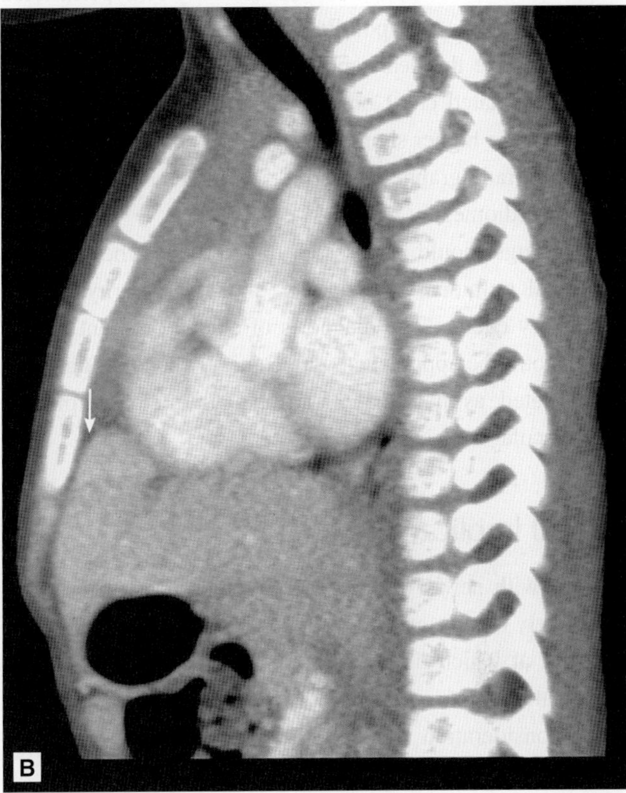

FIGURE 12.13 ■ Congenital Diaphragmatic Hernia. **A, B:** Lateral radiograph of a 15-month-old boy shows a retrosternal mass (arrow). CT with sagittal reconstruction shows an intrathoracic herniated liver (arrow) related to a congenital Morgagni hernia.

Radiographic Summary

Congenital heart disease refers to a problem with the heart's structure and function due to abnormal heart development. The chest radiograph can be helpful to assess for cardiomegaly and pulmonary edema. Care should be made to only diagnose an enlarged cardiac silhouette in a normally or hyperinflated chest radiograph. A hypoinflated chest radiograph may artifactually make the heart appear larger than normal. With a normally inflated chest on AP radiograph, a cardiothoracic ratio of 0.6 or higher should be considered cardiomegaly. On a PA chest radiograph, a ratio of 0.5 or higher should be considered cardiomegaly.

The lungs should be assessed to determine whether there is normal pulmonary vascularity, shunt vascularity, and/or pulmonary edema. The diagnosis of edema or shunt vascularity should be approached with caution when the lungs are hypoinflated, as there may be artifactually increased pulmonary vascular markings.

Clinical Implications

Patients with newly discovered congenital heart disease are most likely to present with respiratory distress or feeding difficulties, at which time a murmur may be auscultated. For those patients presenting in the first week of life with cyanosis, consideration should be given to whether or not this is due to cyanotic congenital heart disease such as truncus arteriosus, transposition of the great vessels, tricuspid atresia, Tetralogy of Fallot, or total anomalous pulmonary venous return. For these patients, prostaglandins should be initiated immediately to open and maintain the patency of the ductus arteriosus. Patients with a ventricular septal defect may present a few weeks after birth with a murmur, sweating during feeds, and tachypnea and a chest radiograph consistent with pulmonary edema.

Chest radiographs should be obtained in pediatric patients presenting with the new onset of wheezing, chest pain, syncope, or unexplained tachycardia. In these patients, a chest radiograph may show cardiomegaly or pulmonary edema. Consideration should then be given to whether this could be myocarditis, anomalous left coronary artery arising from the left pulmonary artery, or whether an intracardiac shunt is present. These patients require an expedited workup with labs and an echocardiogram.

Pearls

1. Hypoinflated chest radiographs may give the false impression that cardiomegaly is present.
2. Congenital heart disease may present similar to a patient with bronchiolitis, with respiratory distress, and pulmonary edema on chest radiograph.

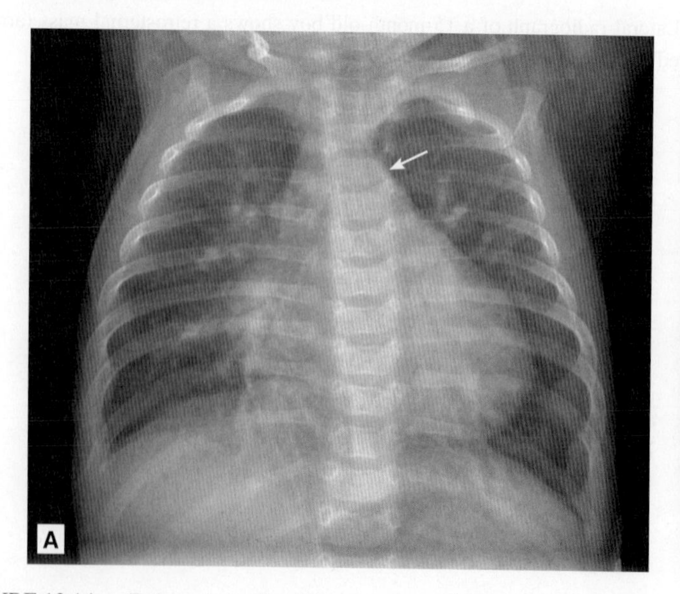

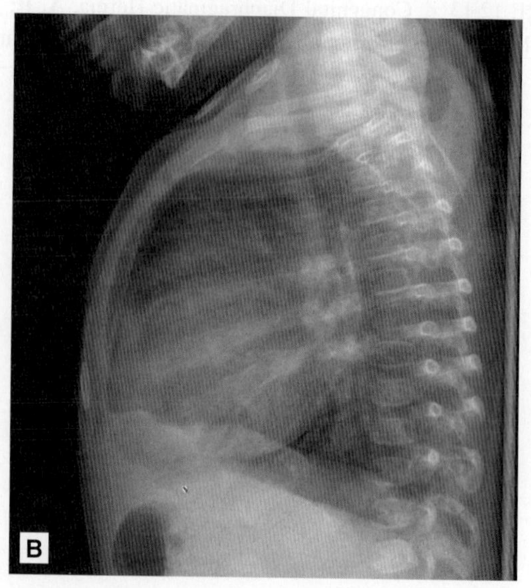

FIGURE 12.14 ■ Enlarged Cardiac Silhouette from VSD. **A, B:** AP and lateral radiograph in a 3-month-old female with a VSD shows mild cardiomegaly and prominent bilateral pulmonary vascularity consistent with shunt vascularity without frank pulmonary edema. Note pulmonary hyperinflation with flattened diaphragms, best appreciated on the lateral projection. Note left aortic arch (arrow).

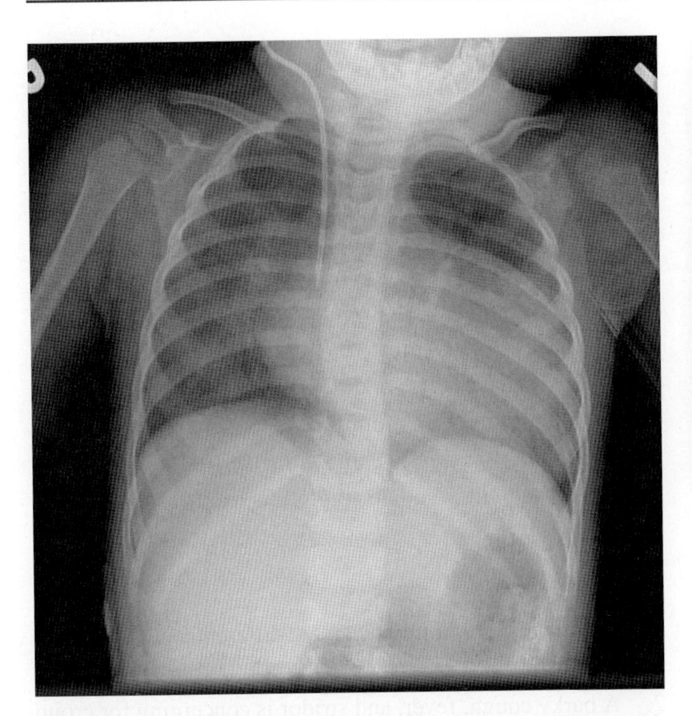

FIGURE 12.15 ■ Dilated Cardiomyopathy. A 1-year-old boy with dilated cardiomyopathy with endocardial fibroelastosis. There is marked cardiomegaly but without pulmonary edema.

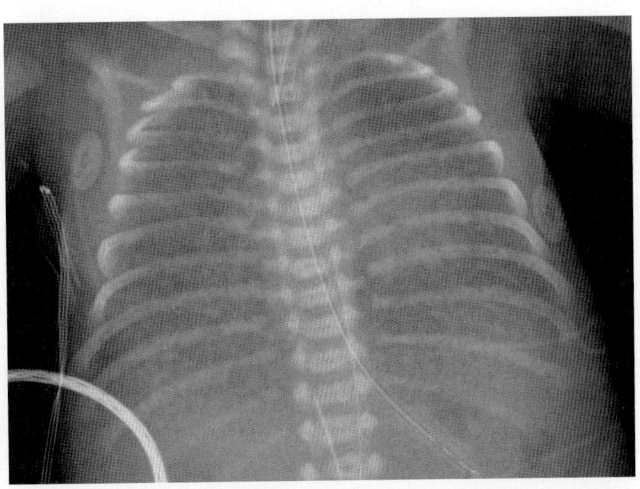

FIGURE 12.17 ■ Hypoplastic Left Heart Syndrome. Newborn child with hypoplastic left heart syndrome. Note diffuse interstitial edema bilaterally with obscuration of the heart border.

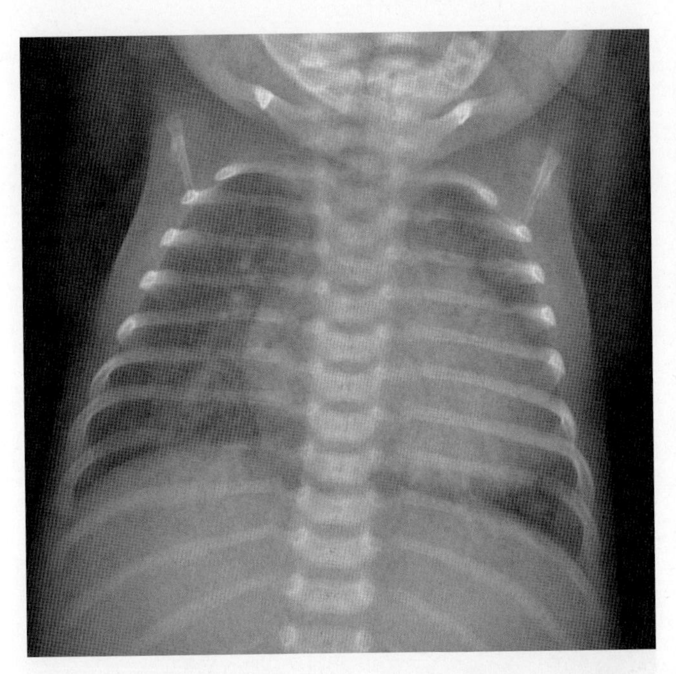

FIGURE 12.16 ■ Ventricular Septal Defect. AP radiograph in a 2-week-old female with a VSD shows mild cardiomegaly with no evidence of shunt vascularity or pulmonary edema.

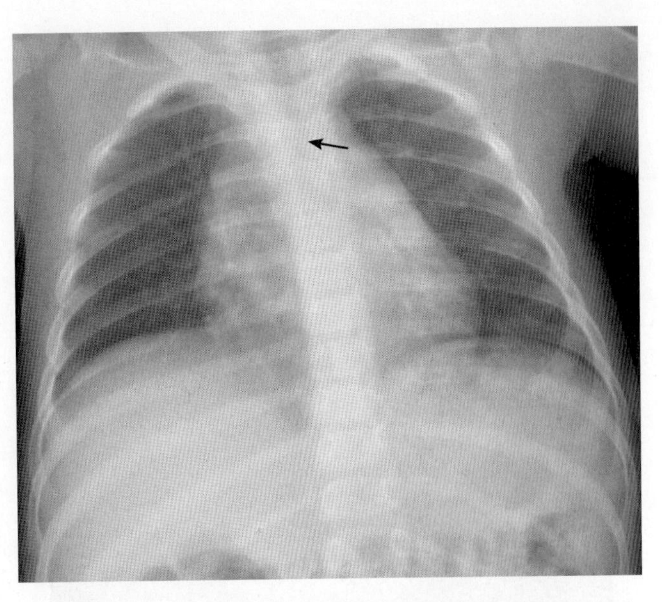

FIGURE 12.18 ■ Right Aortic Arch. AP radiograph in a 19-month-old boy demonstrates a right aortic arch. Note deviation of the trachea (arrow) to the left related to right aortic arch. The heart size and pulmonary vasculature appear normal.

Radiographic Summary

Croup is an infection and inflammation of the larynx and trachea in children. It is a clinical diagnosis based on the age of the child and characteristic presentation. The role of imaging is to exclude other entities that may mimic croup. The classic imaging finding of croup is the "steeple sign". The steeple sign is seen on the AP view and is a reverse V-shaped tapered appearance to the subglottic trachea. The normal trachea on AP view should have a normal lateral convexity. The lateral view will show diffuse subglottic tracheal narrowing in the setting of croup. The radiologic differential for croup includes subglottic stenosis (from prior intubation, trauma, or infection), subglottic hemangioma (the steeple sign has an asymmetric shape), epiglottitis, tracheitis, and foreign body.

Clinical Implications

Croup is a clinical diagnosis described as a sudden onset of a barky cough, fever, and upper airway obstruction. Stridor is a common finding but is not necessary for the diagnosis. Stridor is often found when the patient is agitated and crying. If the patient has stridor at rest, nebulized racemic epinephrine aerosol should be considered. All patients with a history of stridor either at home or in the emergency department should be given corticosteroids, with dexamethasone 0.6 mg/kg either po, IV, or IM preferred. Sometimes croup may present in a clinically similar fashion to epiglottitis. Epiglottitis was more common twenty years ago as the most common pathogen was *Haemophilus influenza* B. Since the advent of the HiB vaccine, this condition is rarely seen; however, it should be considered in an unvaccinated child or in patients not responding to racemic epinephrine aerosols. Neck radiographs can help differentiate epiglottitis from croup.

Pearls

1. Croup and epiglottitis can be differentiated on radiographs of the neck.
2. A barky cough, fever, and stridor is concerning for croup but should respond to corticosteroids and aerosolized racemic epinephrine.

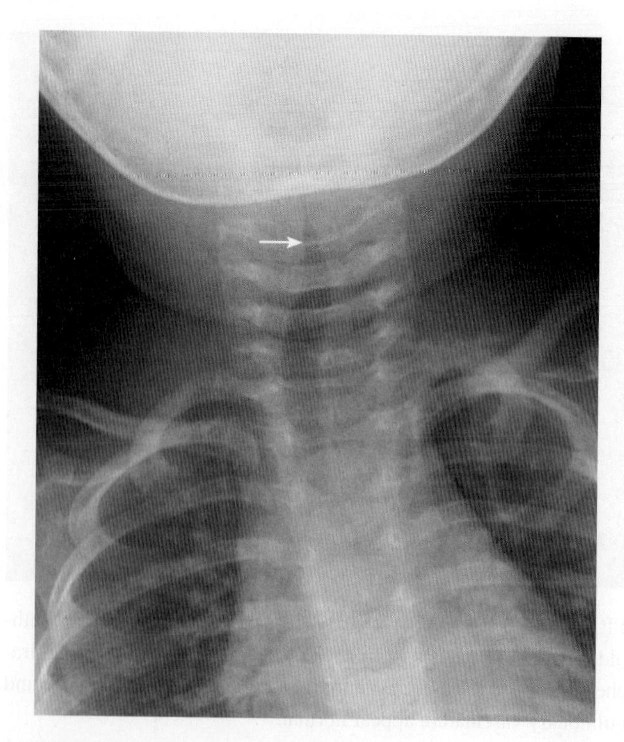

FIGURE 12.19 ■ Steeple Sign. AP soft-tissue neck radiograph shows abnormal tapering of the subglottic trachea consistent with the steeple sign (arrow) in a patient with croup.

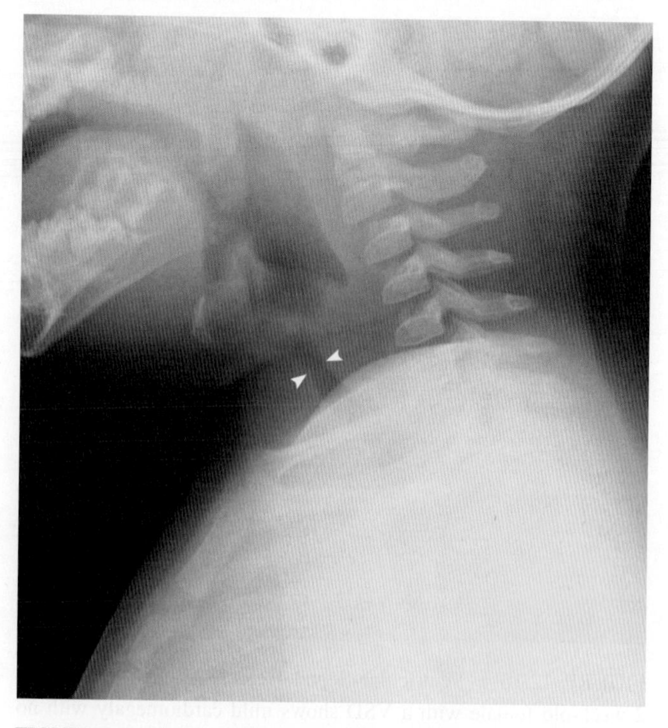

FIGURE 12.20 ■ Subglottic Tracheal Narrowing. Lateral soft-tissue neck radiograph in a different patient with croup shows diffuse subglottic tracheal narrowing (arrowheads).

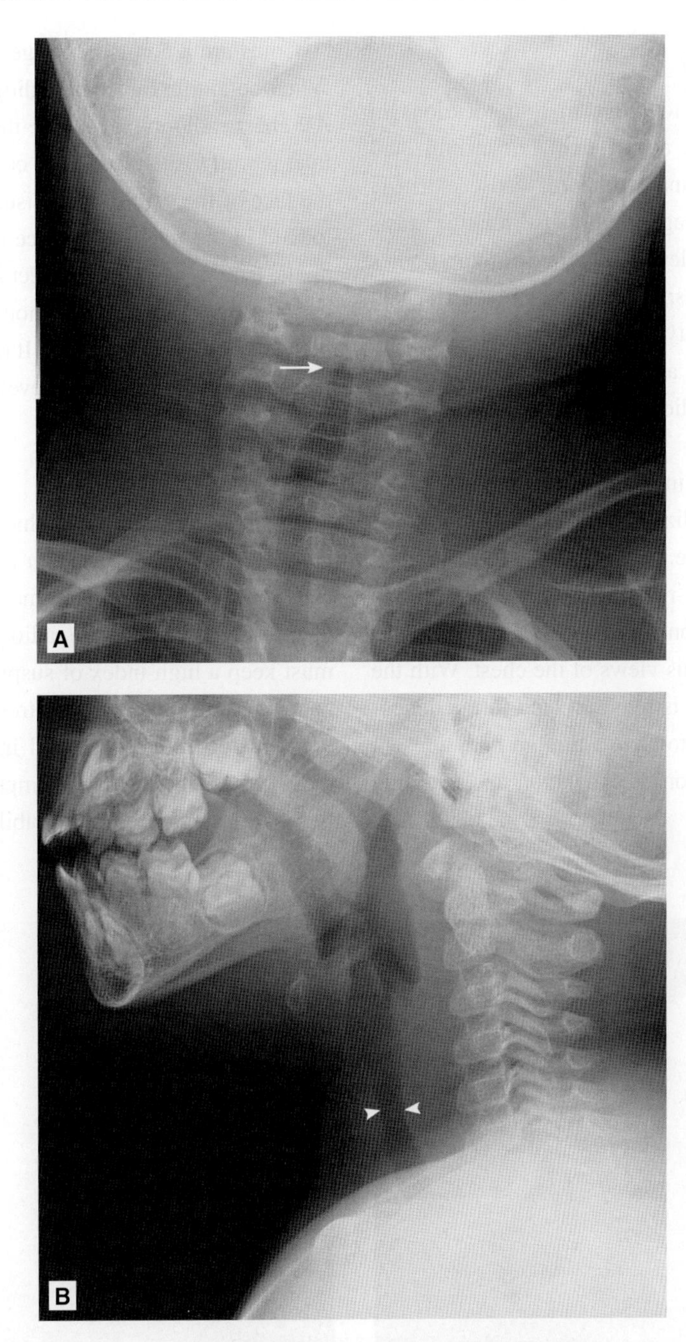

FIGURE 12.21 ■ Normal Soft Tissue Neck Radiographs. **A, B:** Normal AP and lateral soft tissue of the neck radiographs show the normal lateral convexity of the subglottic trachea (arrow). The lateral view demonstrates the normal luminal caliber of the subglottic trachea (arrowheads).

Radiographic Summary

Ingested foreign bodies tend to lodge in four locations in the esophagus: thoracic inlet, aortic arch, left atrium, and GE junctions. These mediastinal structures cause extrinsic compressions upon the esophagus and cause relative stasis of ingested materials at these levels. Ingested foreign bodies should be distinguished from aspirated foreign bodies located within the airway. The majority of food products are radiolucent. Therefore, radiolucent aspirated foreign bodies may demonstrate a normal chest radiograph or may show evidence of airway obstruction.

The AP radiograph should include the lower neck so that the thoracic inlet is well visualized as this is a common location for larger objects to lodge. If there is hyperinflation or asymmetry present on chest x-ray or if an aspirated foreign body is suspected clinically, consideration should be given to obtaining bilateral AP decubitus views of the chest. With the decubitus views, the lung that is hyperinflated in the dependent (down) position is likely to have a foreign body present due to the obstructive limitation of exhalation and resulting hyperexpansion.

Coins are a commonly ingested foreign body in children. When obtaining the chest radiograph, it is important that the AP chest radiograph include the lower neck so the thoracic inlet is well visualized. If the coin is lodged in the esophagus, the face of the coin will be visualized on the AP view. If it is lodged in the trachea, the face of the coin will be visualized on the lateral view. If the object looks wider than a coin on the lateral view, consideration should be made to ensure that the object is not a button battery. If a button battery is ingested, its radiographic hallmark is a beveled appearance.

Clinical Implications

Foreign body ingestions can happen with children of all ages, but most commonly occur in those younger than 5 years of age. Food is the most commonly aspirated object and will therefore generally not be radiopaque. Clinically, the provider must keep a high index of suspicion for any toddler with the acute onset of respiratory distress or choking as there is often not a history of a witnessed ingestion. Even with negative radiographs, if a child is symptomatic with respiratory distress, persistent cough, or inability to handle secretions then

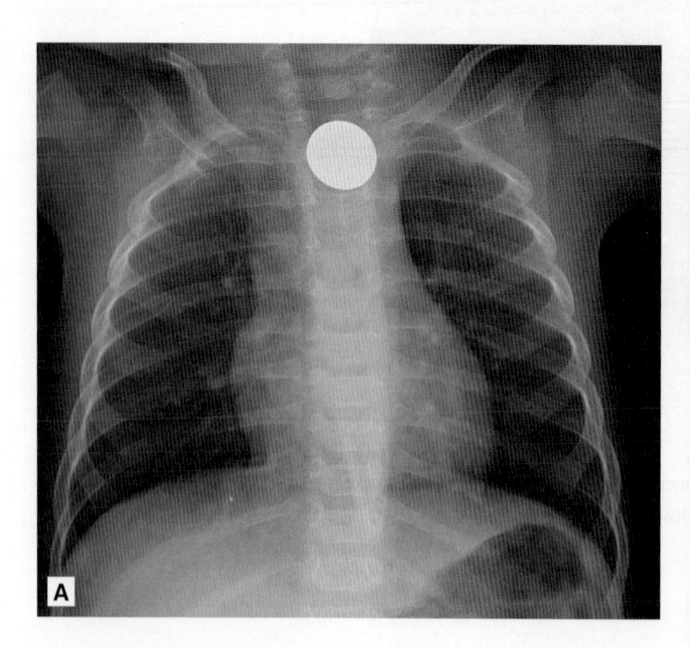

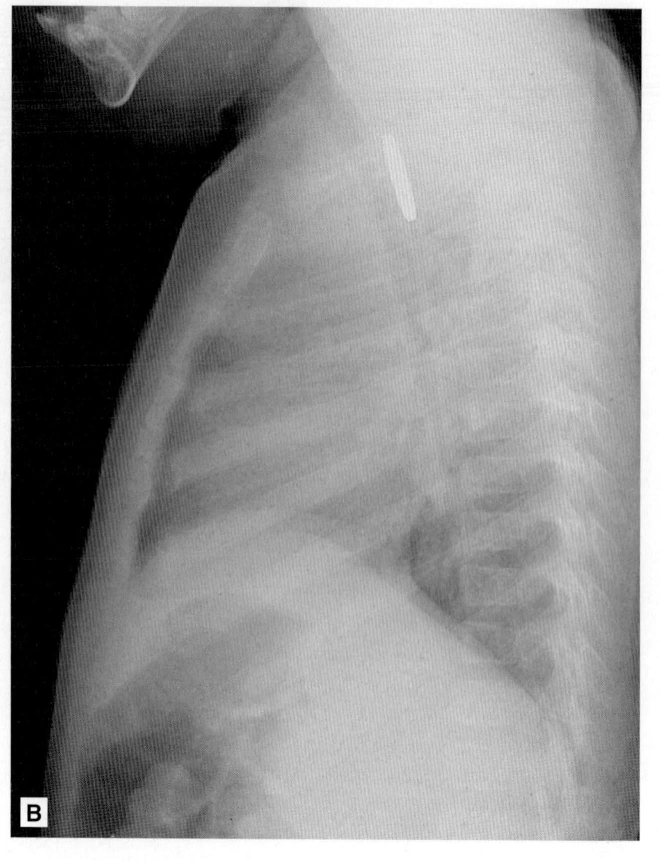

FIGURE 12.22 ■ Esophageal Foreign Body. **A, B:** Frontal and lateral chest radiographs demonstrate a coin in the upper mediastinum above the aortic arch. The coin is seen en face on the AP view, and on edge on the lateral view, typical for the esophageal location. Note the tracheal air column anterior to the coin.

they should be taken to the OR for direct laryngoscopy and bronchoscopy for removal of the foreign body.

Button batteries that are lodged in the esophagus should be considered a surgical emergency and taken out expeditiously because of the risk of erosion of the esophagus. For button batteries that make it past the esophagus in the asymptomatic patient, x-rays should be repeated weekly to ensure the battery passes. Any symptomatic patient should have the foreign body removed by endoscopy.

For other objects that pass out of the esophagus, expectant management is the norm as objects have a 90% chance of successful passage. There are a few special considerations to help guide when surgical removal should be considered. The ingestion of more than one magnet carries the risk of attachment between two parts of the small bowel, potentially leading to ischemia. The ingestion of objects longer than 5 cm or wider than 2 cm can also be problematic because of the inability to pass the duodenal sweep or through the pylorus. For most foreign bodies, the caregivers can monitor the child's bowel movements for the object. If it is not visualized, weekly x-rays are appropriate until the object passes.

Pearls

1. Patients with a high likelihood of aspiration but negative x-rays and who are symptomatic should go to the OR for direct laryngoscopy and bronchoscopy.
2. Foreign bodies that pass out of the esophagus have a 90% chance of successful passage.
3. The majority of aspirated food foreign bodies are radiolucent. Only indirect signs of aspirated foreign body may be seen, such as air trapping.
4. If a circular foreign body has a beveled appearance on the radiograph, a button battery is presumed until proven otherwise.

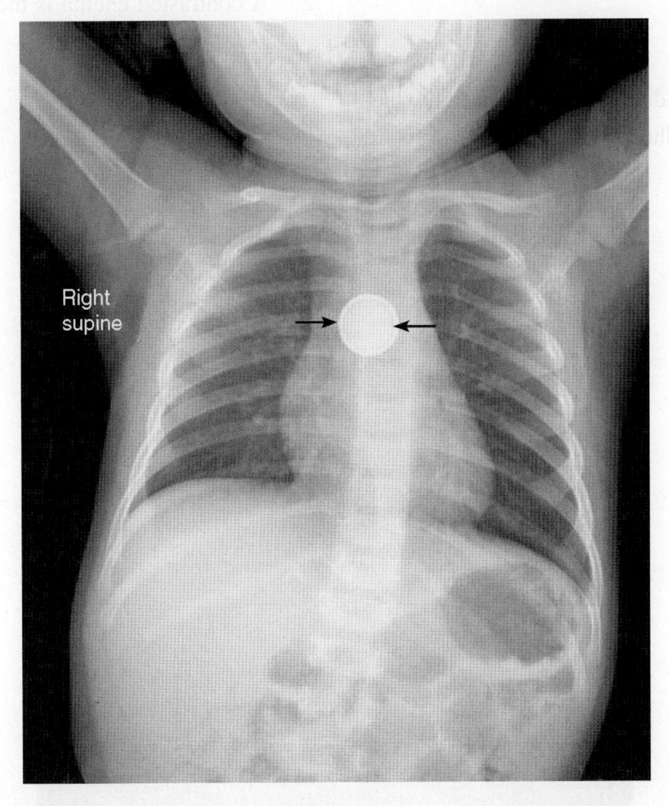

FIGURE 12.23 ■ Esophageal Button Battery. AP chest radiograph in a 15-month-old boy demonstrates a beleveled appearance to the esophageal foreign body (arrows), consistent with an ingested button battery.

Radiographic Summary

Hirschsprung's disease is a congenital abnormality of the bowel in which there is absence of parasympathetic ganglion cells in the wall of the colon. The radiologic differential for a low-lying obstruction on x-ray includes imperforate anus, Hirschsprung's disease, colonic atresia, ileal atresia, small left colon syndrome, and meconium ileus. Contrast enema is the next step in the work-up of Hirschsprung's disease. Prior to contrast enema, there should be no rectal stimulation for at least 24 hours. Rectal stimulation may alter the rectal caliber, leading to a false negative exam. The classic radiologic finding on contrast enema is reversal of the rectosigmoid ratio with the rectal caliber smaller than the sigmoid caliber. In the normal child, the rectal:sigmoid ratio should be approximately 1:1 or larger. If small left colon syndrome is encountered, repeat enema in the future may be performed since a small percentage of Hirschsprung's disease may present radiologically as small left colon syndrome.

Clinical Implications

Patients with Hirschsprung's disease can present anywhere from early in life to late childhood with difficulty in having normal bowel movements. A history of a lack of a meconium stool in the first 24 hours of life or for the need to give either a suppository or enema for the patient to have a bowel movement may often be elicited. Because the rectosigmoid colon is devoid of intramural ganglion cells, it is not able to relax and facilitate the movement of stool. This is more commonly seen in males than females (4:1) and older patients may present with failure to thrive, decreased appetite, and intermittent bouts of diarrhea. Patients with Hirschsprung's disease are at an increased risk for rectal prolapse and enterocolitis. In severe cases of enterocolitis, the patient is at risk for perforation and peritonitis. Diagnosis can be achieved through radiographic tests in addition to rectal manometry and biopsy of the affected tissue.

Pearls

1. In the infant presenting with chronic constipation and a significant stool burden but without stool in the rectal vault, Hirschsprung's disease should be considered.
2. A contrasted enema is the radiographic test of choice to assist in the diagnosis.

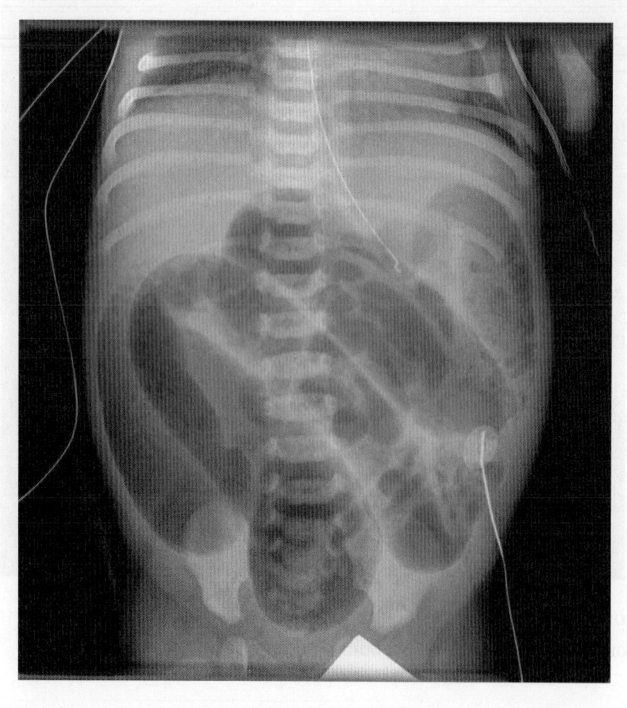

FIGURE 12.24 ■ Dilated Bowel Loops. Frontal radiograph of the abdomen demonstrates multiple dilated loops of bowel throughout the abdomen extending to the rectal vault in this patient with Hirschsprung's Disease.

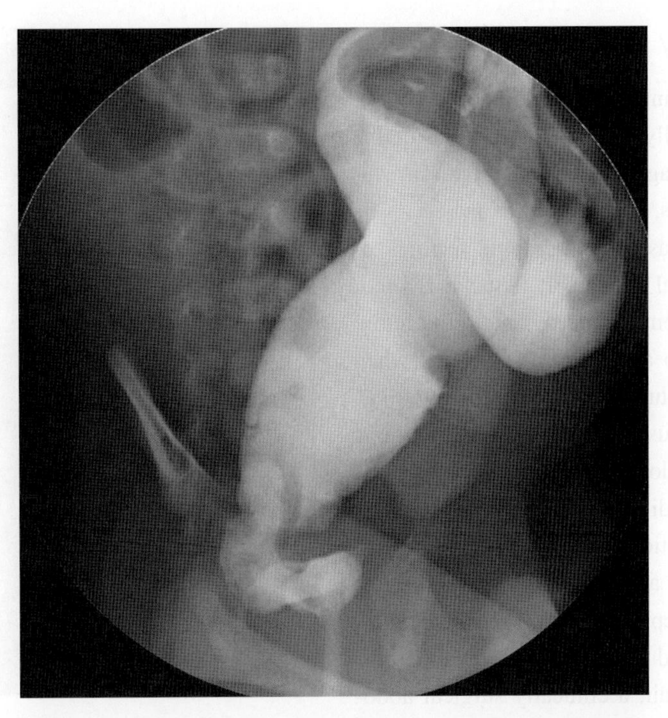

FIGURE 12.25 ■ Rectosigmoid Ratio Reversal. Water-soluble contrast enema demonstrates reversal of the rectosigmoid ratio, typical of Hirschsprung's Disease. The rectal caliber is smaller compared with the sigmoid colon caliber.

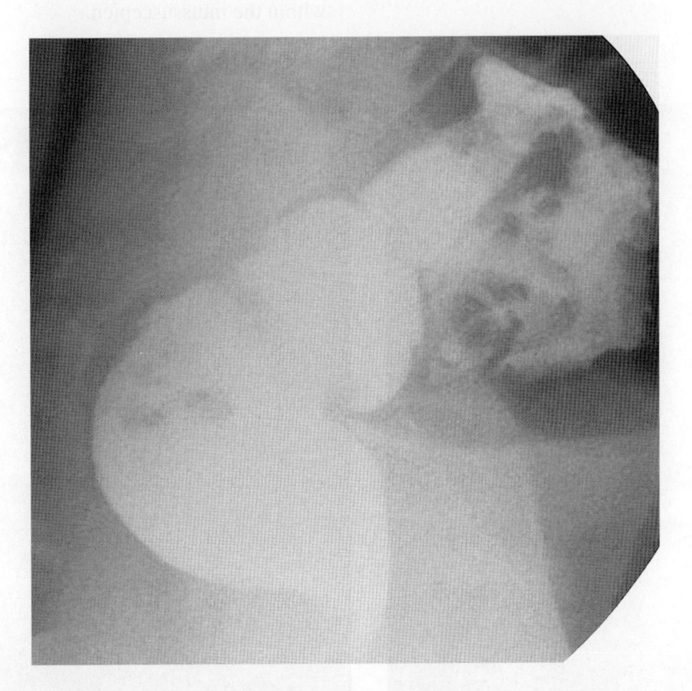

FIGURE 12.26 ■ Normal Rectosigmoid Ratio. Lateral radiograph from contrast enema demonstrates a normal rectosigmoid ratio in a 6-year-old boy. The rectal caliber is larger compared with the sigmoid colon caliber.

Radiographic Summary

Intussusception is the telescoping of one portion of the bowel into another portion, potentially leading to ischemia of the affected bowel. The initial imaging work-up of intussusception is abdominal radiographs, including AP and left side down decubitus view. The classic radiographic features of intussusception include a focal dense soft tissue mass and/ or nonspecific gasless right hemiabdomen. Often, the initial radiographs can be normal so a sonogram is needed when there is clinical concern for intussusception or when the initial radiographs suggest intussusception. Ultrasound findings for intussusception include a "donut sign" or a "pseudokidney sign." Care should be taken to differentiate ileocolic intussusceptions, which require reduction, from small bowel–small bowel intussusceptions, which are transient. The majority of idiopathic ileocolic intussusceptions can be reduced radiologically with a pneumatic reduction. Contraindications for pneumatic reduction are free air, a clinically surgical abdomen, or hemodynamic instability.

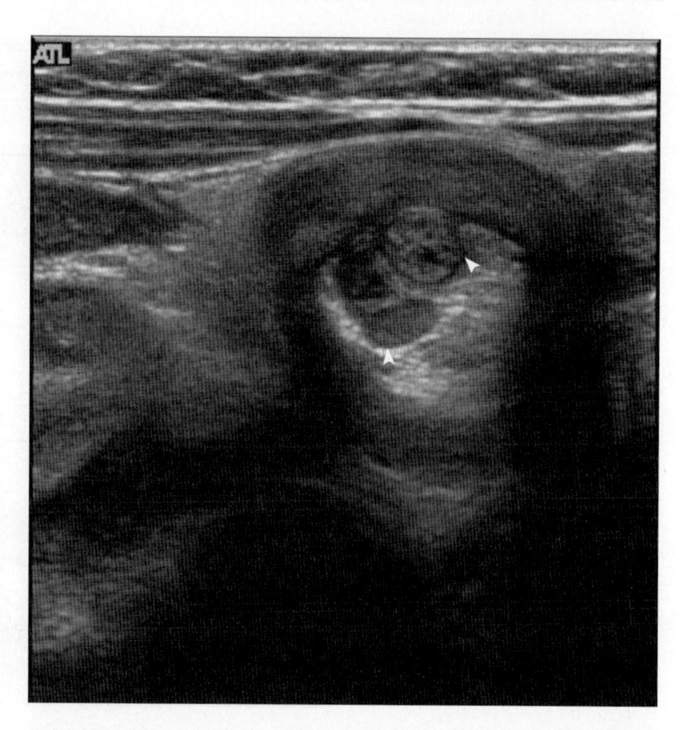

FIGURE 12.28 ■ Donut Appearance of Intussusception. Transverse sonogram of the right hemiabdomen demonstrates the "donut" appearance of intussusception, with multiple lymph nodes (arrowheads) within the intussuscepien.

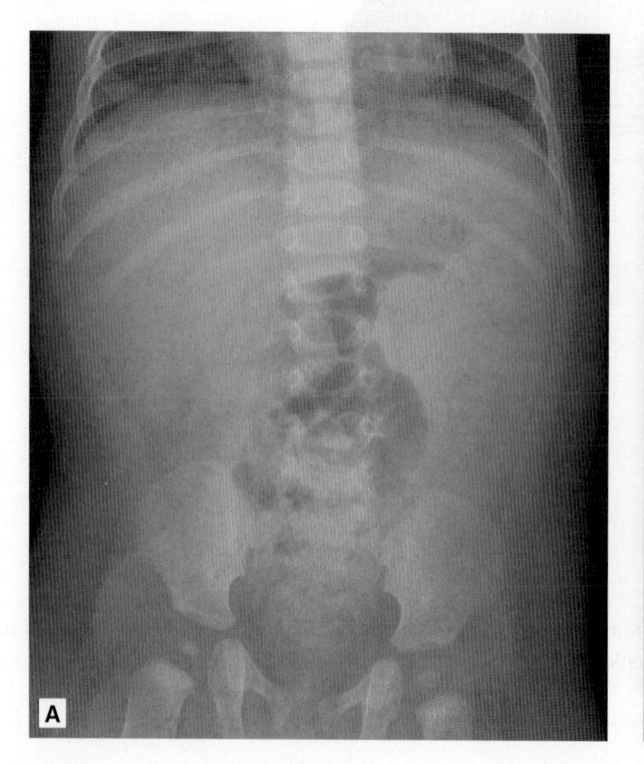

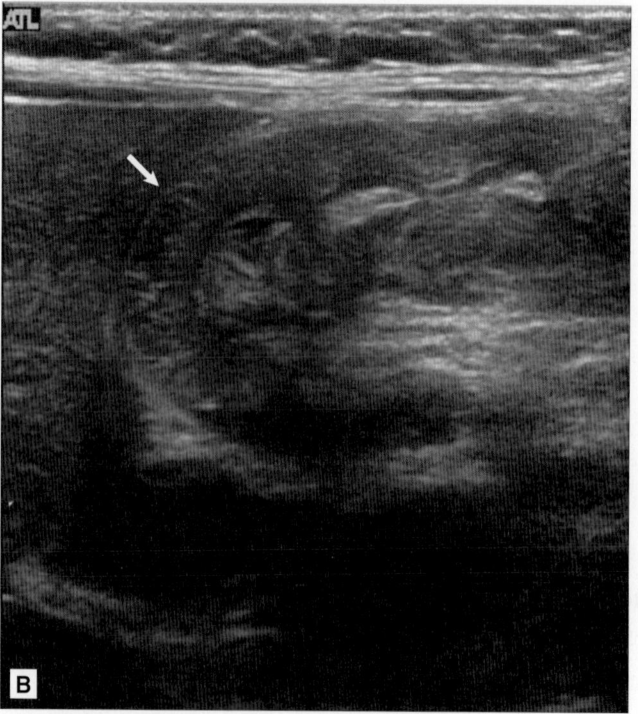

FIGURE 12.27 ■ Paucity of RLQ Bowel Gas and Pseudokidney Sign. **A, B:** AP radiograph (A) demonstrates a nonobstructive bowel gas pattern. There is a paucity of bowel gas in the right hemiabdomen. Longitudinal sonogram of the right hemiabdomen demonstrates an ileocolic intussusception with intussusceptum telescoping into the intussuscepien, producing the "pseudokidney sign" (arrow).

Clinical Implications

Intussusception is the most common cause of intestinal obstruction between the ages of 3 months and 5 years, most commonly occurring around 1 year of age. The triad of colicky abdominal pain, vomiting, and currant jelly stools is classically taught but is seen in less than one third of patients. Treatment should be focused on fluid resuscitation and making the correct diagnosis. Prior to performing, attempts at air reduction enemas should be discussed with a surgeon because if the reduction is unsuccessful or there is a perforation, the patient should be taken promptly to the operating room. For patients with intussusception that is successfully reduced, overnight observation is often warranted as the intussusception can recur.

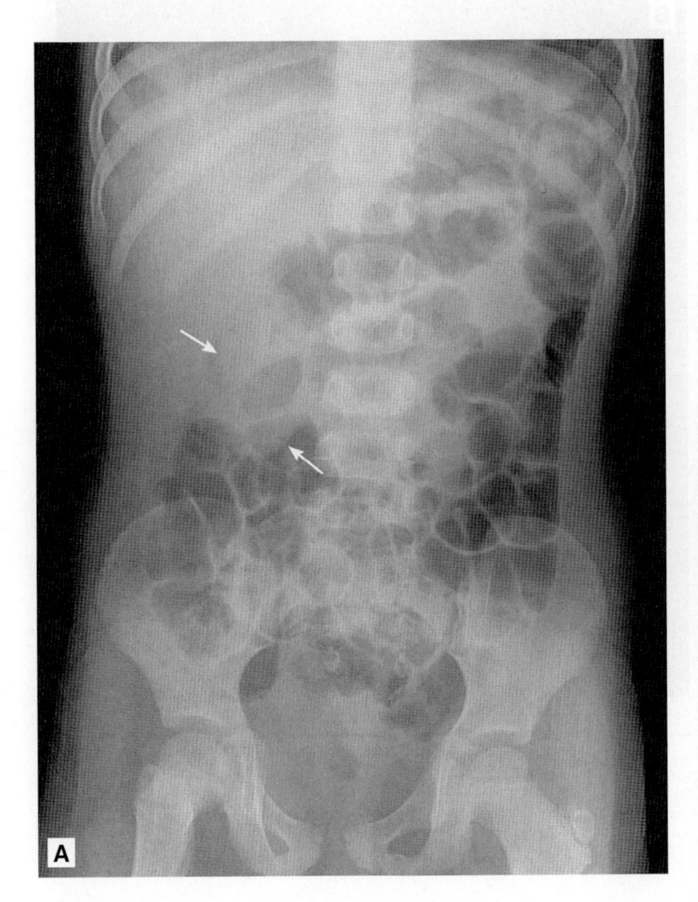

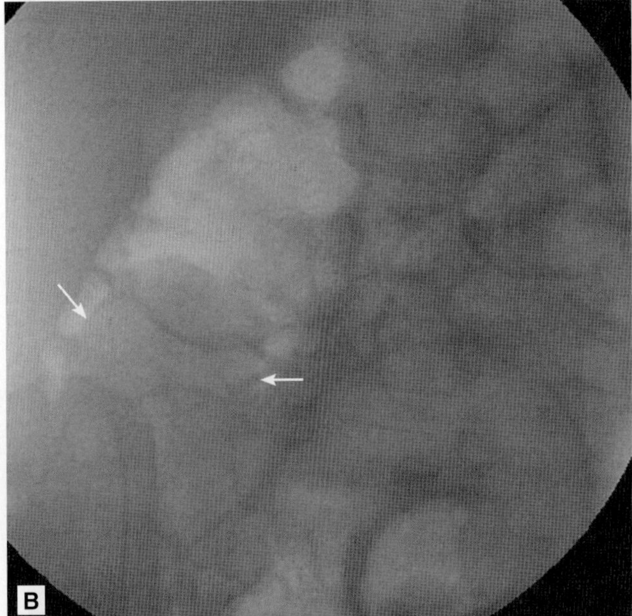

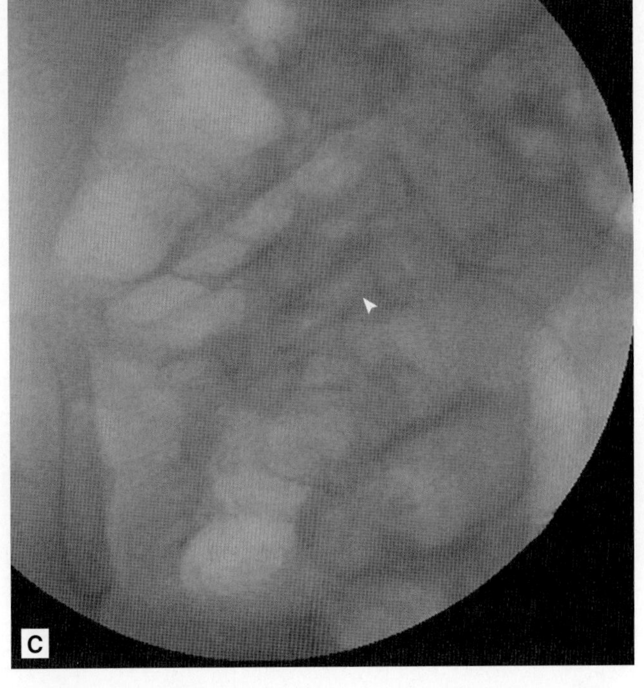

FIGURE 12.29 ■ Ileocolic Intussusception. **A-C:** AP radiograph in a 3-year-old girl shows a discrete soft-tissue mass in the right hemiabdomen consistent with ileocolic intussusceptions (arrows). AP fluoroscopic image during air reduction enema shows ileocolic intussusception in the right lower quadrant, likely near the ileocecal junction (arrows). A subsequent fluoroscopic image after success in air reduction enema shows air delineated small bowel loops (arrowhead) and the right lower quadrant ileocolic intussusception density is no longer present.

Another cause of intussusception can be a pathologic lead point such as a tumor, Meckel's diverticulum, or a duplication cyst. A pathologic lead point should be considered when the patient is outside the age range for typical ileocolic intussusception.

Pearls

1. In toddlers who have colicky abdominal pain and a lack of air in the ascending colon, the diagnosis of intussusception should be considered.
2. Consider pathologic lead points when ileocolic intussusceptions occur outside of the normal age ranges.

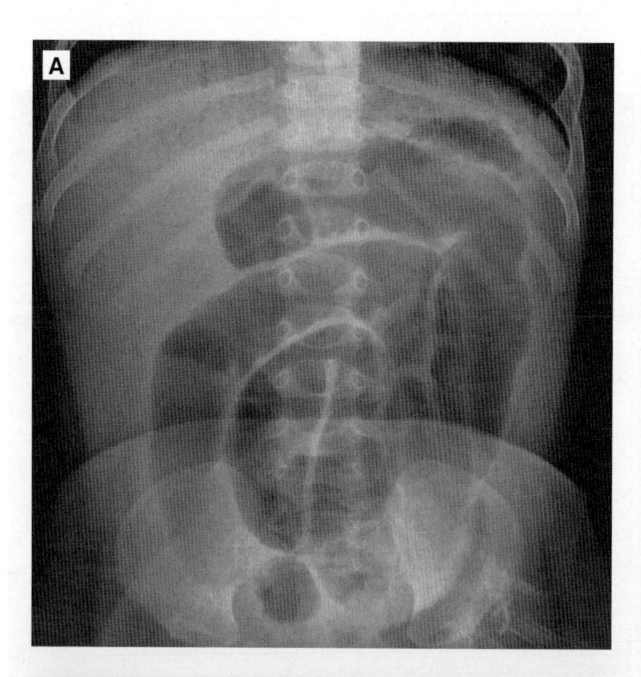

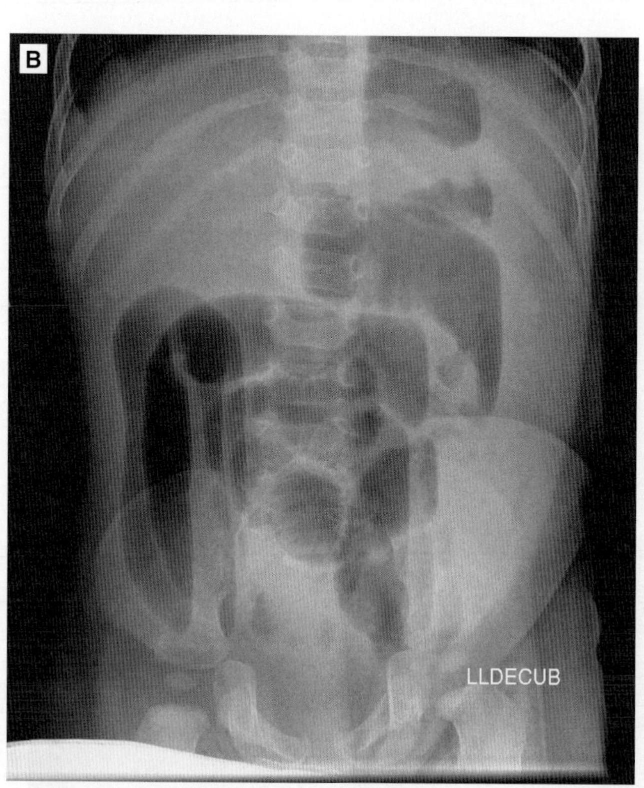

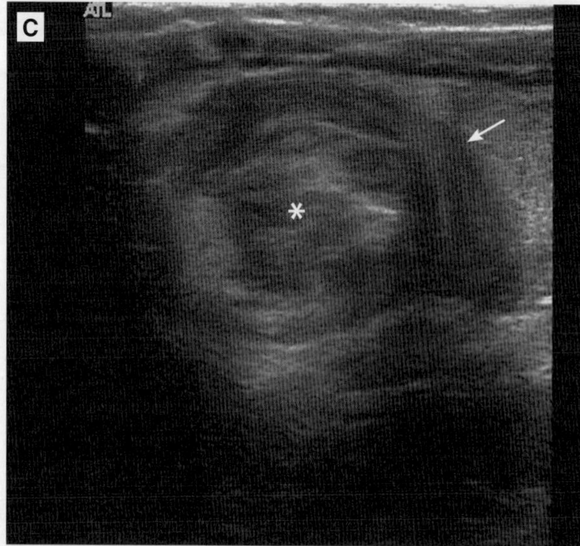

FIGURE 12.30 ■ Ileocolic Intussusception. **A-C:** AP and left side down decubitus radiographs on a 6-month-old boy demonstrates a distal obstruction with air-fluid level. No free air is seen. An ultrasound subsequently was performed demonstrating an ileocolic intussusception with intussusceptum (*) telescoping into the intussusceptum (arrow).

Radiographic Summary

Meckel's diverticulum is a congenital diverticulum in the ileum resulting from incomplete closure of the yolk sac. These children often will undergo CT or ultrasound, which are usually negative prior to referral to nuclear medicine. The optimal study to diagnose a Meckel's diverticulum is a Tc-99m pertechnetate study, but the study is dependent on whether or not the diverticulum contains functioning gastric mucosa. This is found in approximately 25% of Meckel's diverticulum patients but if present, pertechnetate uptake occurs within the functioning gastric mucosa. The diagnosis of Meckel's diverticulum can be made if there is focal, extra-gastric localization of Tc-99m pertechnetate, usually found in the right lower quadrant localized to distal ileum.

Clinical Implication

Meckel's diverticulum can be a cause of massive, painless rectal bleeding in the toddler population. The Meckel's diverticulum is the result of incomplete resolution of the omphalomesenteric duct. Rectal bleeding occurs when acid secreted by ectopic gastric tissue causes ulceration and erosion of the tissue. Patients are usually less than 2 years old when the bleeding occurs. The Meckel's diverticulum can be found within 2 feet of the ileocecal valve and is usually 2 inches in length. Boys are usually two times more affected than girls. Surgical excision is the definitive treatment.

Pearls

1. Meckel's diverticulum is usually a diagnosis of exclusion. Alternative causes for abdominal pain or gastrointestinal bleeding should be considered first.
2. Meckel's diverticulum can act as a lead point leading to ileo–ileo intussusception or ileocolic intussusception. Therefore, in a child presenting at an atypical age for idiopathic intussusception, consider Meckel's diverticulum.
3. Rectal bleeding in a child is much more commonly due to anal fissures compared with a symptomatic Meckel's diverticulum.

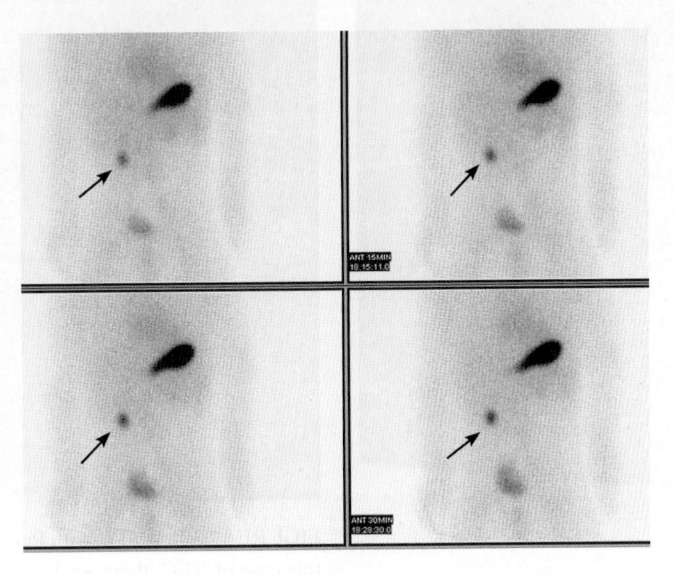

FIGURE 12.31 ■ Meckel's Diverticulum. Tc-99m pertechnetate multiple sequential images were obtained of the abdomen demonstrating increasing radiopharmaceutical uptake in the right lower quadrant, consistent with a Meckel's diverticulum (arrows). (Image used with permission from Stephanie Spottswood, MD.)

Radiographic Summary

Necrotizing enterocolitis (NEC) is most often a disease of premature infants where a serious bacterial infection causes necrosis of the bowel. Radiographic findings may include pneumatosis, portal venous gas, or free air. Pneumatosis intestinalis represents air within the mucosal wall and may appear radiographically as bubbly lucencies or linear lucencies. More severe disease will present with portal venous gas. When air migrates from the bowel wall to the mesenteric vein, it will subsequently trap within the portal vein radicals located in the liver. When there is frank perforation, free intraperitoneal air may be found. Free air may be challenging to see when the radiographs are obtained in the supine position. In the supine position, air collects along the nondependent portions of the intra-peritoneal cavity and may present with a "football sign" as an ovoid free gas collection outlines the linear hepatic falciform ligament (appearing as the seam on the football). If there is a high clinical concern for free air, cross-table lateral or a left side down decubitus view may be obtained.

Clinical Implications

Though NEC is mainly a problem of premature infants, it should be considered in full-term infants as well, particularly if there is a history of maternal drug use, prolonged delivery, midgut volvulus, or congenital heart disease. Patients can present a variety of ways and may exhibit a variety of symptoms. Universally, feeding intolerance and abdominal

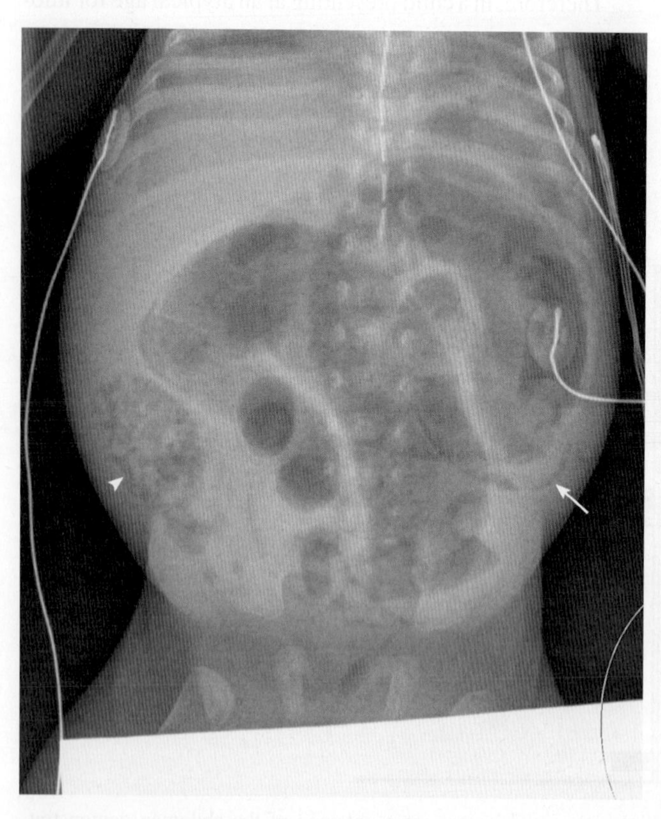

FIGURE 12.32 ■ NEC and Pneumatosis Intestinalis. Child with NEC and pneumatosis. Note linear (arrow) and bubbly (arrowhead) lucencies throughout the abdomen indicating gas within the bowel wall.

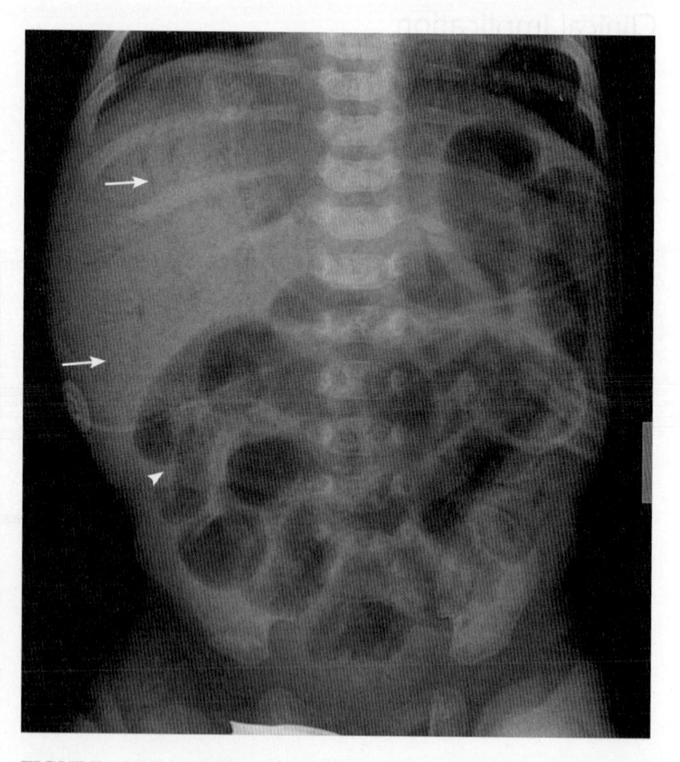

FIGURE 12.33 ■ NEC with Pneumatosis and Portal Venous Air. In this case of NEC, there are branching lucencies overlying the liver, representing portal venous gas (arrows). Note the presence of pneumatosis as well throughout the abdomen (arrowhead).

distention are present. When there is concern for NEC, the patient should be made NPO and an orogastric tube placed to low wall suction. Because of the concern for sepsis, a full sepsis evaluation should also be obtained with CBC, blood culture, catheterized urinalysis and culture, and consideration for cerebrospinal fluid studies. The patient should also be started on broad spectrum antibiotics and early surgical consultation should be obtained.

Pearls

1. Necrotizing enterocolitis is not just a disease of prematurity, and may also occur in full term infants who have midgut volvulus or congenital heart disease.
2. Pneumatosis intestinalis may be seen in children on chronic steroids and as such is not pathognomonic for NEC.

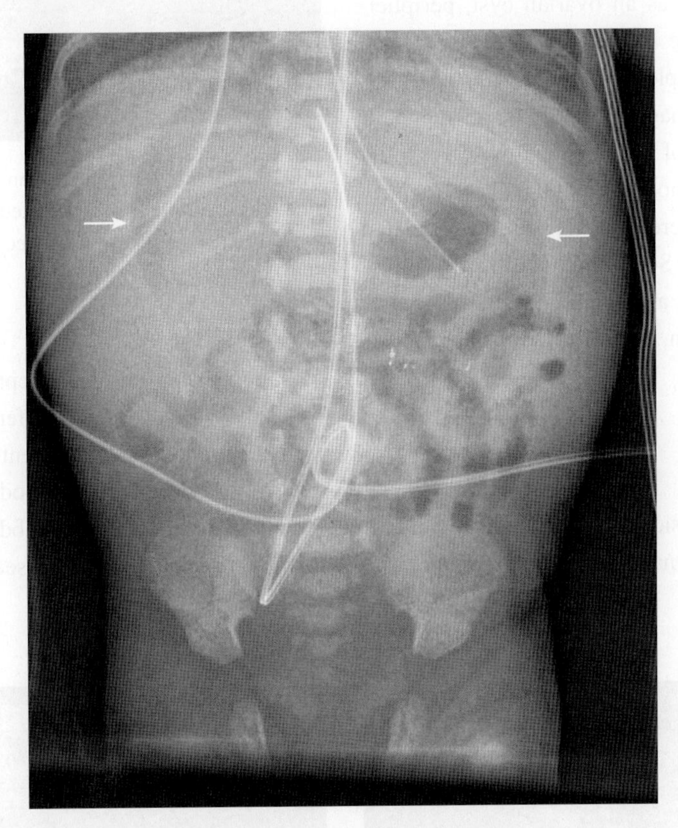

FIGURE 12.34 ■ "Football Sign" of NEC. There is a central lucency overlying the abdomen (arrows) representing the "football sign," which represents free intraperitoneal free air delineated on a supine radiograph.

Radiographic Summary

Ovarian torsion is seen when the ovary rotates to such a degree as to occlude the blood flow to the ovary. This usually occurs in the setting of a lead point, most commonly an ovarian cyst but may also be caused by teratoma. Classic imaging features of ovarian torsion include asymmetric size of the affected ovary compared with the nonaffected ovary (usually 3-4 times larger than the normal ovary), identification of a lead point such as an ovarian cyst, peripherally located follicles, midline located enlarged ovary, and absent color and spectral Doppler flow to the affected ovary. Sonography is the first-line imaging modality to evaluate for ovarian pathology. The use of abdominopelvic CT should be limited to cases where sonography is unable to identify a cause for pain or when there is a high clinical concern for undiagnosed appendicitis. Sonography is also very helpful for identifying alternative and more common causes of adnexal pelvic pain in children, including hemorrhagic cysts and ruptured ovarian cysts.

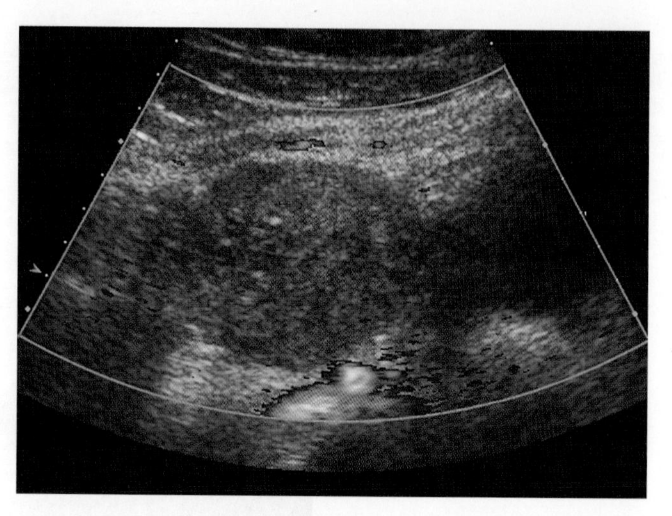

FIGURE 12.35 ■ Right Ovarian Torsion. A 10-year-old girl with right-sided ovarian torsion related to a large exophytic cyst. Right ovary is enlarged and heterogeneous with absent color flow.

Clinical Implications

Ovarian torsion should be considered in any female with unilateral lower quadrant abdominal pain. Though the majority of patients affected are of reproductive age, there are cases of premenstrual females suffering from this as well. In the teenager population, the patient is most likely to be two weeks out from her menstrual period and have the acute onset of unilateral lower quadrant abdominal pain. Approximately 70% are associated with nausea and vomiting. In any female

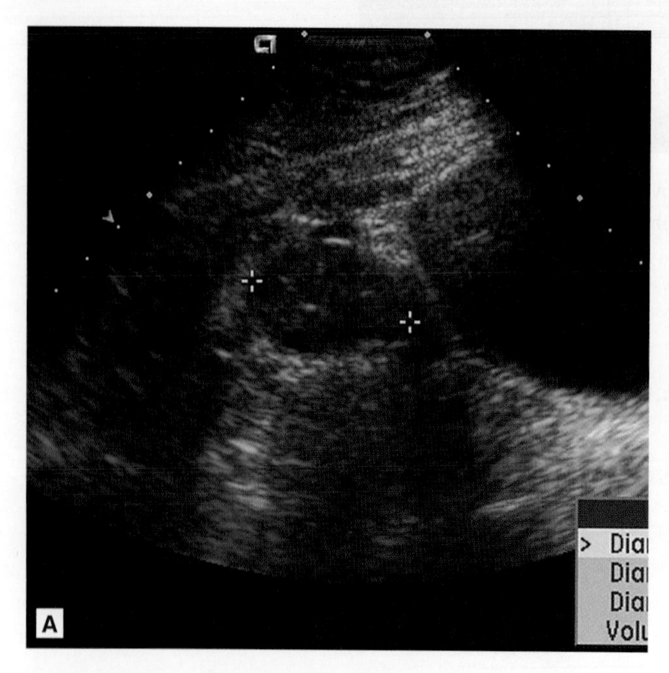

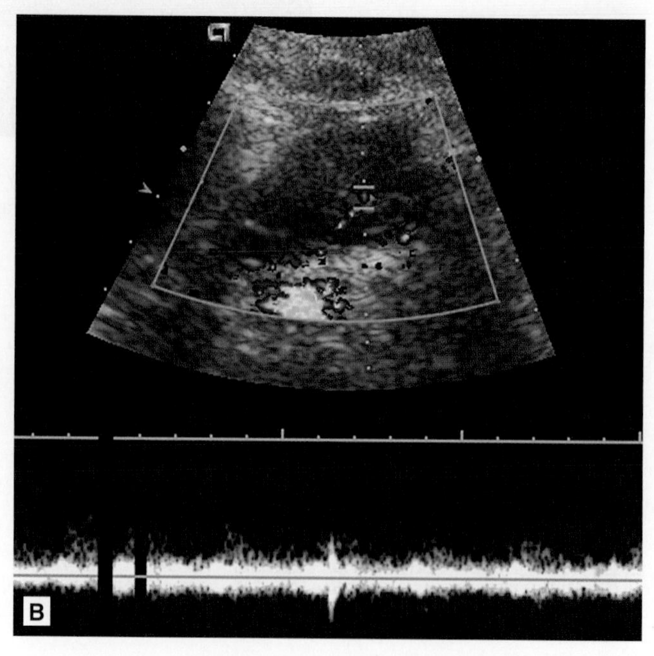

FIGURE 12.36 ■ Normal Left Ovary. **A, B:** In the same patient, the normal left ovary is identified with normal color and spectral Doppler flow. Note the size discrepancy between the left ovary and abnormal right ovary.

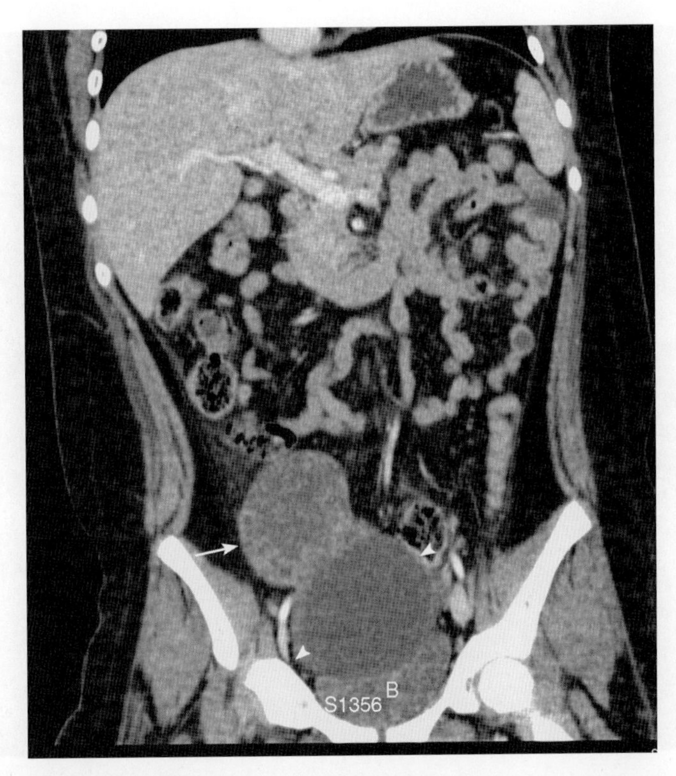

FIGURE 12.37 ■ Ovarian Torsion from Cyst. Abdominopelvic CT with contrast with coronal reformations demonstrates the enlarged right ovary and peripheral follicles (arrow). There is an exophytic cyst arising from the right ovary (arrowheads), displacing the urinary bladder (B).

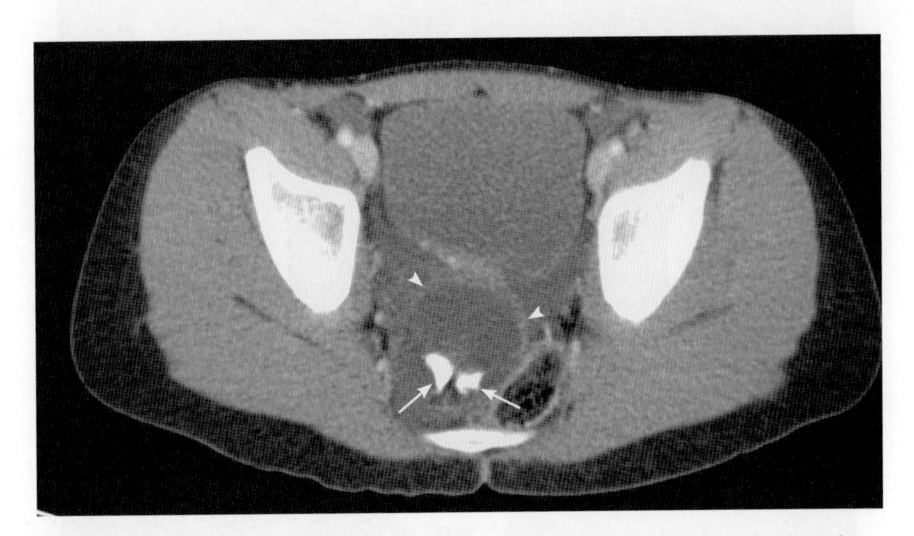

FIGURE 12.38 ■ Ovarian Torsion from Teratoma. Abdominopelvic CT with contrast in a different patient shows a midline ovary that is enlarged and replaced by a cystic (arrowheads) mass with calcifications (arrows). There is also free fluid present in the pelvic space. Surgical findings were consistent with ovarian torsion related to a teratoma lead point.

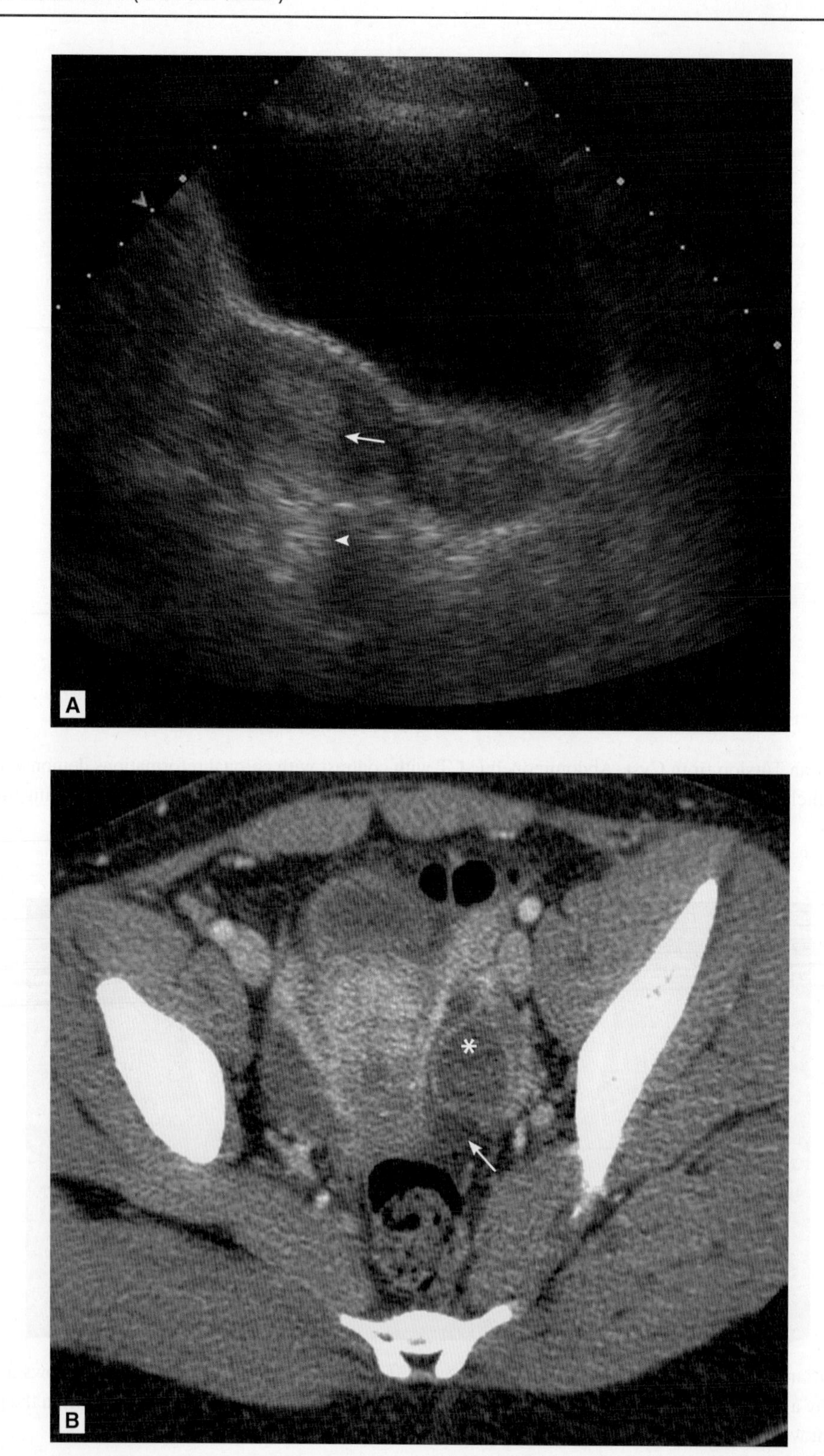

FIGURE 12.39 ■ Hemorrhagic Ovarian Cyst. **A, B:** Pelvic sonogram in an asypmtomatic 13-year-old girl demonstrates a focal echogenic lesion in the left ovary (arrow) with posterior increased through transmission (arrowhead) consistent with a hemorrhagic cyst. CT performed on the same day confirms left ovarian hemorrhagic cyst (*). Note that the hemorrhagic cyst has increased density (*) compared with free pelvic fluid (arrow). There was preserved Doppler flow with no torsion present.

presenting with these complaints, a pregnancy test should be obtained. In the sexually active patient, a pelvic exam is warranted to look for pelvic inflammatory disease (PID). If ovarian torsion is found on ultrasound, immediate surgical consultation or transfer to a facility for operative intervention should occur expeditiously.

Pearls

1. The affected ovary is usually 3-4 times larger than the unaffected ovary if ovarian torsion is present.
2. In any female patient presenting with unilateral lower quadrant abdominal pain, ovarian torsion should be considered.

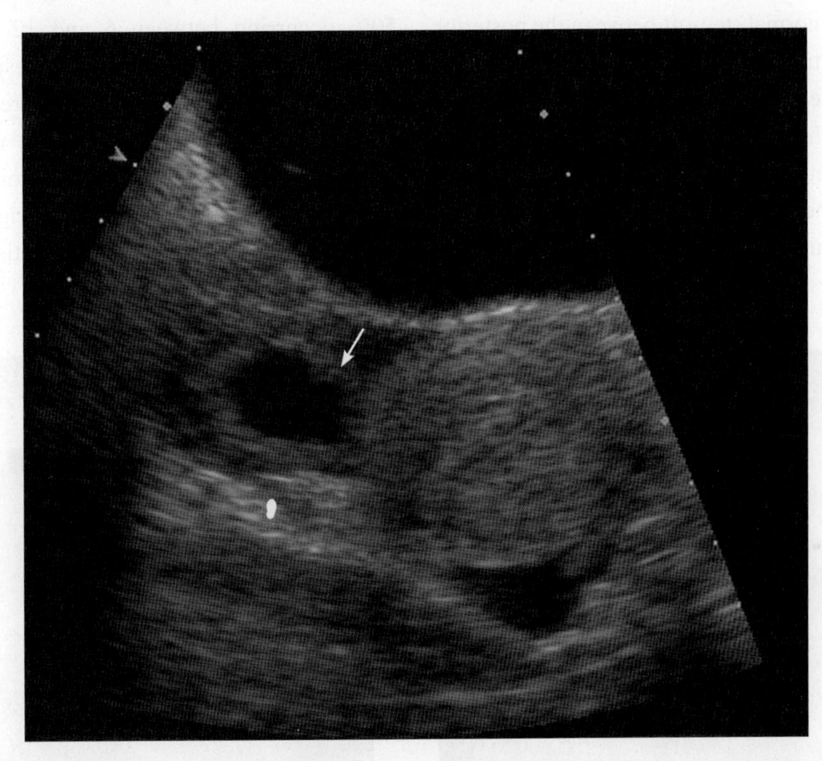

FIGURE 12.40 ■ Ruptured Ovarian Cyst. Pelvic sonogram in a 16-year-old girl demonstrates a simple cyst with a crenulated margin (arrow). Note pelvic free fluid that is present. Given its crenulated appearance, findings are consistent with a recent ruptured ovarian cyst.

Radiographic Summary

A retropharyngeal abscess (RPA) is an accumulation of pus in the prevertebral soft-tissue space of the upper airway. Imaging work-up for a retropharyngeal abscess includes soft tissue neck radiographs (AP and lateral). If there is a high clinical suspicion for abscess, neck ultrasound and/or CT should be performed irrespective of the findings on soft-tissue neck radiographs. For the normal lateral radiograph of the neck, there should be a normal step-off between the posterior wall of the larynx and trachea. In an appropriately obtained lateral radiograph, if the posterior step-off is not seen, a retropharyngeal process should be considered. Care should be made not to mistake pseudothickening of the retropharyngeal space due to the neck held in a neutral or flexed position or radiographs obtained during end-expiration. As a guideline, the normal prevertebral soft tissues should measure less than half of the vertebral body width in the upper cervical spine, and measure less than one vertebral body width in the lower cervical spine.

Clinical Implications

Most RPAs occur in patients less than 6 years of age, with 50% occurring between 6 and 12 months of age. This infection can be due to an upper respiratory infection, otitis media, or more rarely from direct penetrating trauma of the space. Patients will present with fever, dysphagia, hyperextension of the head, and noisy respirations. Some patients also present with nuchal rigidity and may mimic the presentation of acute meningitis. Airway obstruction

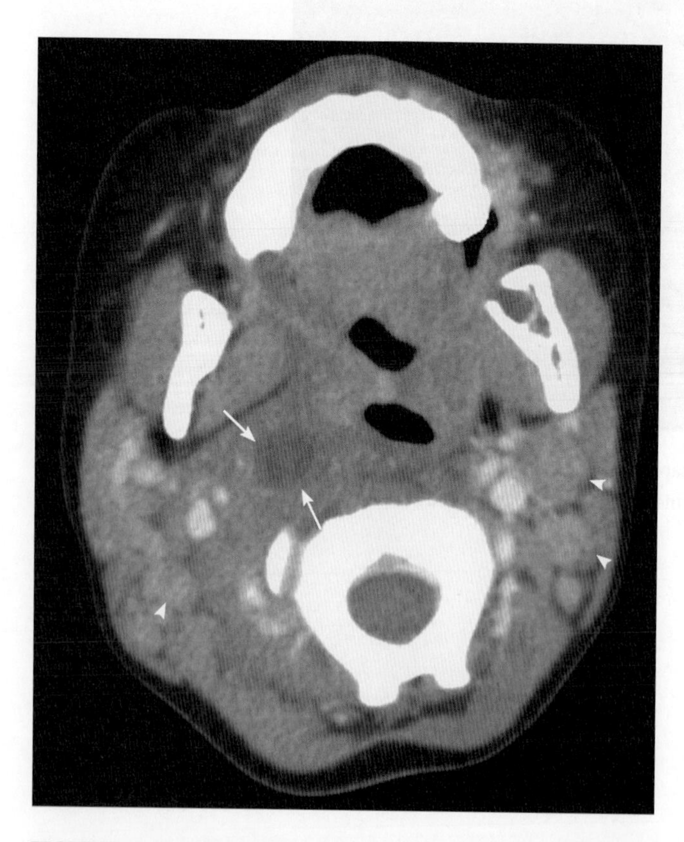

FIGURE 12.41 ■ Retropharyngeal Abscess. Contrasted CT of the neck in a 3-year-old boy demonstrates a well-defined ovoid right retropharyngeal collection (arrows) with rim enhancement consistent with a retropharyngeal abscess. Multiple bilateral lymph nodes are seen deep into the sternocleidomastoid muscle (arrowheads).

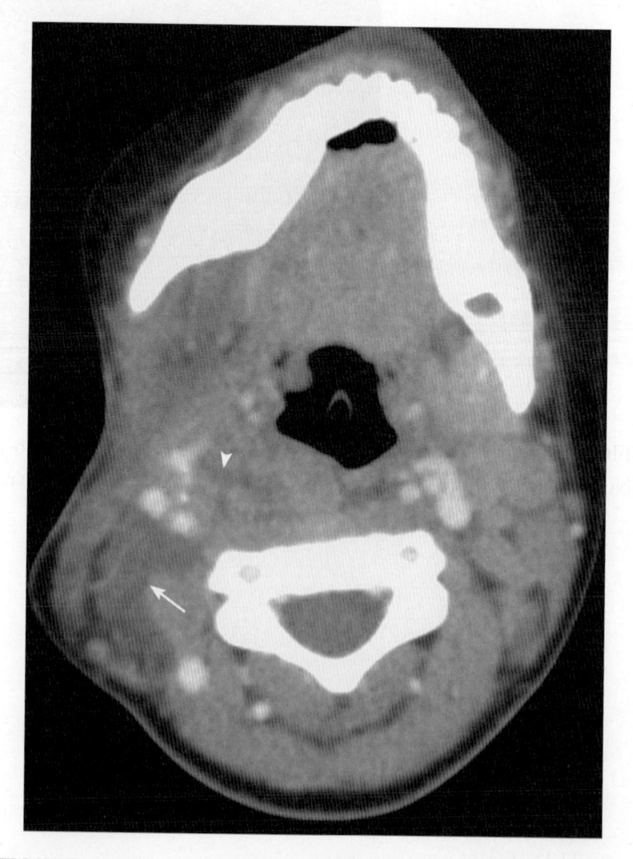

FIGURE 12.42 ■ Retropharyngeal Phlegmon. Contrasted CT of the neck in a 3-year-old girl. There is infiltrative edema in the right retropharyngeal region (arrowhead) and deep to the right sternocleidomastoid muscle (arrow) consistent with phlegmon.

and aspiration from a retropharyngeal abscess can occur. Because of the close proximity to the major vessels of the neck, hemorrhage, thrombus, and extension of the abscess into the blood vessels can occur. Treatment of the abscess is with formal incision and drainage in the operating room coupled with intravenous antibiotics. Antibiotics should cover the common pharyngeal organisms including group A streptococci, *Staphylococcus aureus*, *Haemophilus influenzae,* and anaerobes.

Pearls

1. The prevertebral soft tissues may be abnormally thickened due to neck flexion and underinflation. Consider repeating radiographs if there is a high clinical suspicion for a retropharyngeal abscess.
2. Retropharyngeal abscess should be considered in kids under 6 years old with fever, hyperextension of the neck, nuchal rigidity, and dysphagia.

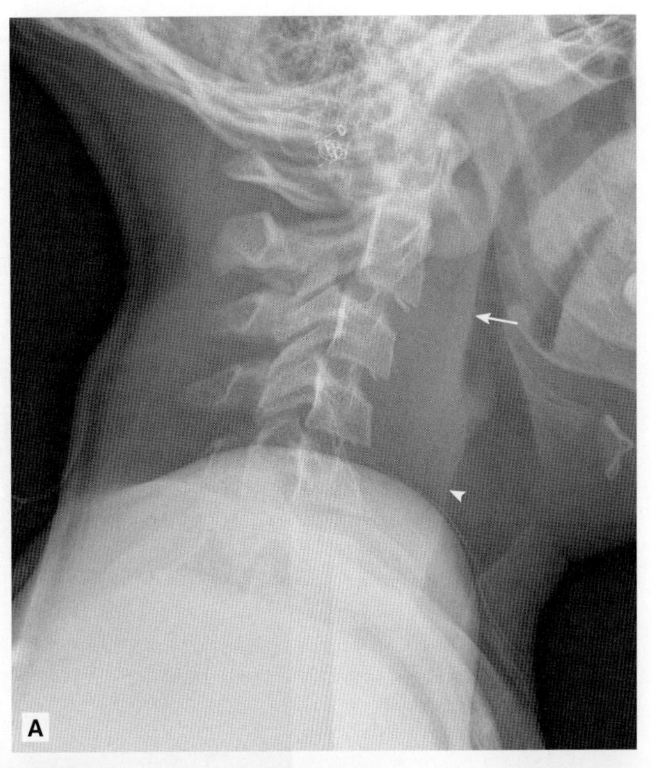

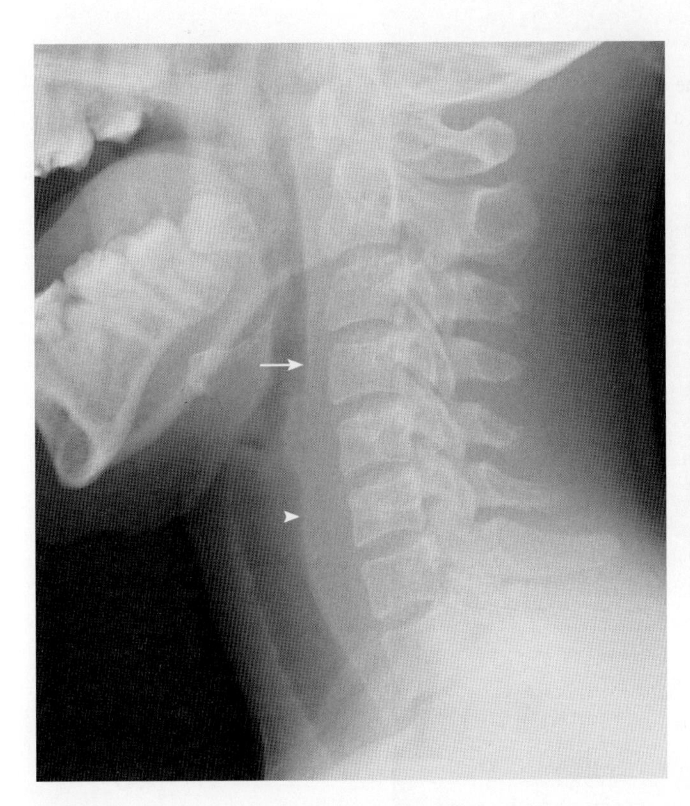

FIGURE 12.43 ■ Normal Soft Tissue Lateral Neck. Note that there is a normal step-off between the posterior wall of the larynx (arrow) and trachea (arrowhead) on a view where the child is properly in mild neck extension and in deep inspiration.

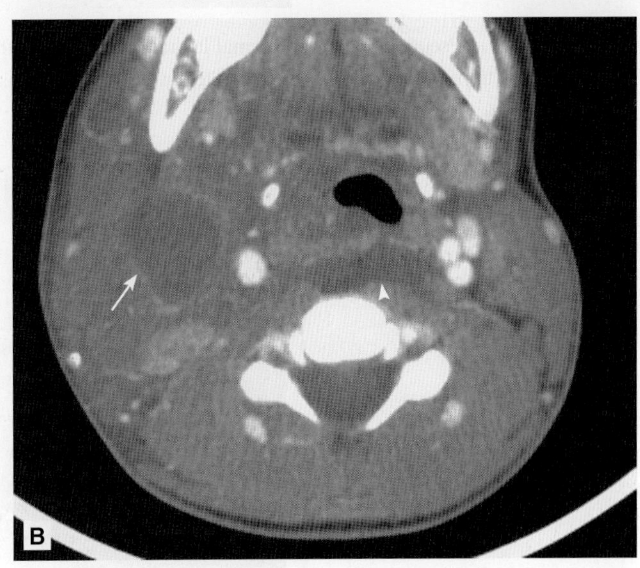

FIGURE 12.44 ■ Submandibular Abscess/Retropharyngeal Phlegmon. **A, B:** Abnormal lateral radiograph of the neck of a 12-year-old boy shows loss of the normal step-off between the posterior wall of the larynx (arrow) and trachea (arrowhead). Subsequent CT shows a right submandibular abscess (arrow) and retropharyngeal phlegmon (arrowhead).

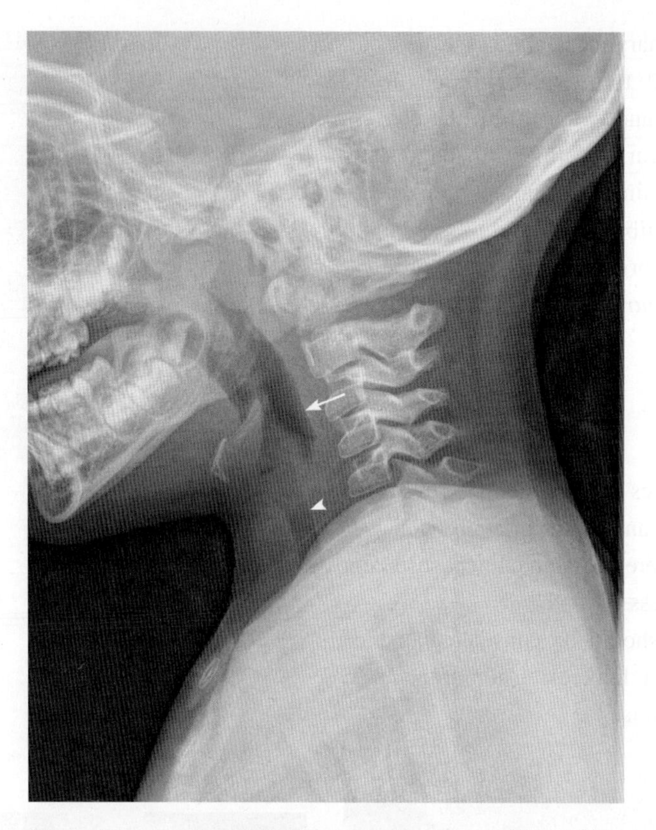

FIGURE 12.45 ■ Pseudothickening. Normal lateral radiograph of the neck in a 4-year-old boy. Note pseudothickening of the prevertebral soft tissues due to mild flexion of the neck. Note however that there is a normal step-off between the larynx (arrow) and trachea (arrowhead).

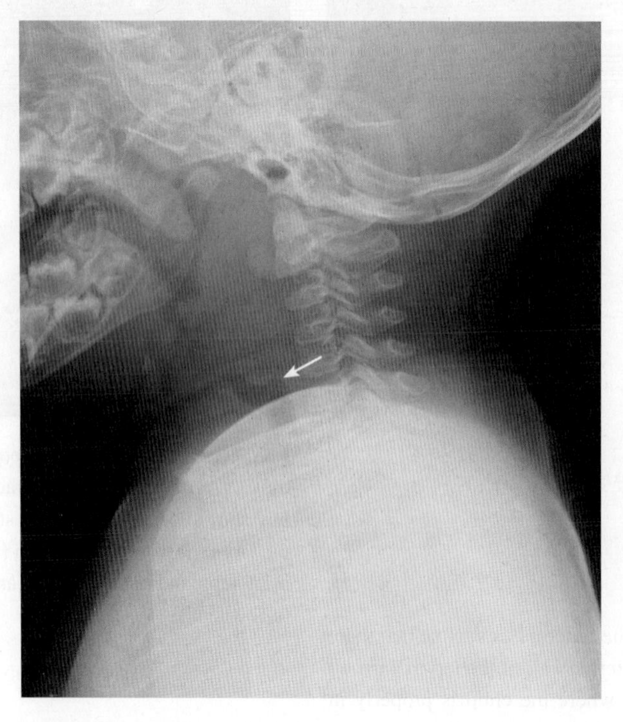

FIGURE 12.46 ■ Pseudothickening. Normal lateral radiograph of the neck in a 1-year-old boy during end-expiration. Note pseudothickening of the prevertebral soft tissues with a loss of the normal step-off between the larynx and trachea. The key to identifying underinflation artifact is to see tracheal buckling (arrow).

Radiographic Summary

Hypertrophic pyloric stenosis (HPS) is a muscular hypertrophy of the pyloric sphincter causing gastric outlet obstruction. Abdominal radiographs often reveal a normal nonobstructive bowel gas pattern but may show a gas-distended stomach. Ultrasound is the gold standard in the imaging work-up. The abnormal pyloric channel is often easily identified due to its sheer size. Sonogram criteria for HPS are a single wall thickness greater than 4 mm and longitudinal length of 1.6 cm. The normal pyloric channel can be challenging to identify compared with HPS. If the pyloric channel cannot be readily identified, giving the child something to drink may be helpful in decreasing the amount of intraluminal gas in the stomach and duodenum. As a routine component of sonographic evaluation of the pylorus, the SMA and SMV orientation is usually assessed. The SMV is to the right with respect to the SMA. If the orientation is abnormal, a diagnosis of malrotation may be suggested, and the child should undergo an upper GI contrast study. However, the converse is untrue. If the SMA and SMV are normally oriented, malrotation cannot be excluded since a 360° turn of the mesentery related to volvulus may give the SMA and SMV a normal orientation. If the diagnosis of HPS has been excluded and there remains a high clinical concern for a proximal obstruction in the infant, an upper gastrointenstinal series to rule out malrotation with midgut volvulus should be performed.

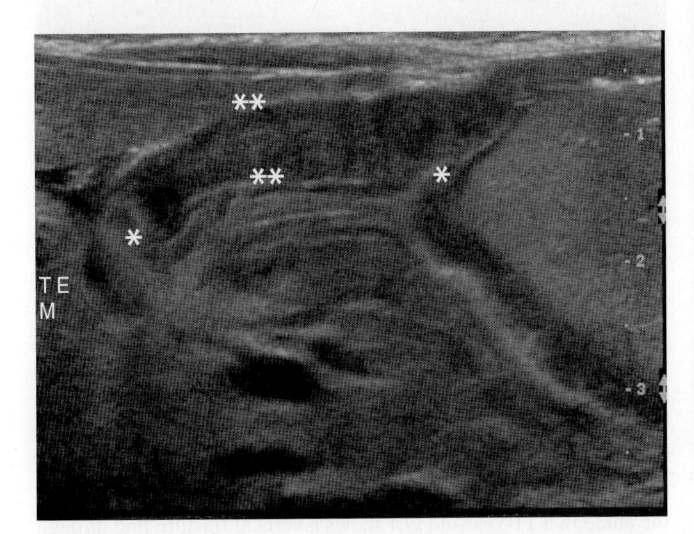

FIGURE 12.47 ■ Hypertrophic Pyloric Stenosis. Transverse sonogram of the upper abdomen demonstrates an abnormally thickened (6 mm-**) and elongated (2 cm-*) pyloric channel, typical of pyloric stenosis. There is also mucosal hypertrophy noted.

Clinical Implications

HPS is most often found in infants from three to five weeks old, though most present by 12 weeks of life. These patients present with a soft, nondistended abdomen and vomiting that progresses to projectile, nonbloody, nonbilious emesis. An olive-like mass may be palpated in the epigastrium after an episode of vomiting. The classic metabolic abnormality is a hypokalemic, hypochloremic, metabolic alkalosis. Fluid and electrolyte replacement should be promptly initiated. Once the alkalosis is corrected, the patient can be taken for operative repair.

Pearls

1. If the ultrasound is negative for HPS in an infant with progressive vomiting, an upper GI should be obtained to look for malrotation.
2. The classic metabolic abnormality is a hypokalemic, hypochloremic, metabolic alkalosis.
3. If the sonographic orientation of the SMV with respect to the SMA is abnormal, a diagnosis of malrotation may be suggested and further workup with upper GI contrast study is indicated.

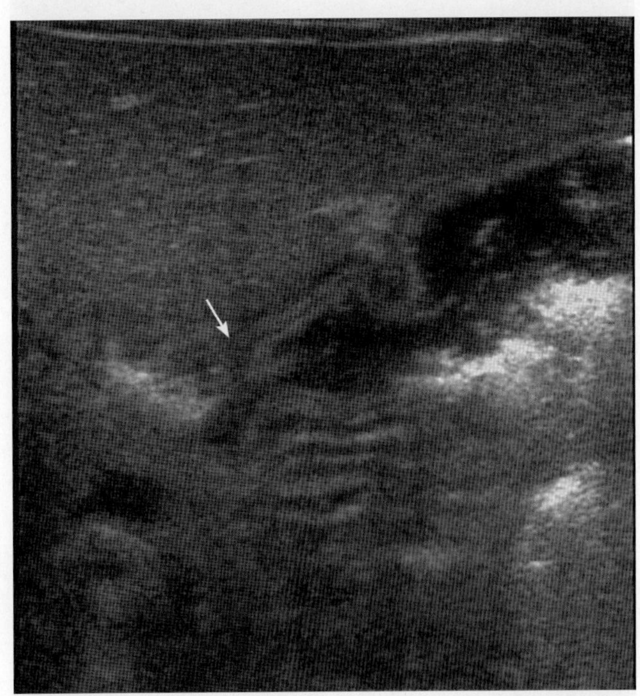

FIGURE 12.48 ■ Normal Pylorus. Transverse sonogram of the upper abdomen in a normal child demonstrates fluid distention of stomach with fluid traversing the normal pyloric channel (arrow) and emptying readily into the proximal duodenum.

Radiographic Summary

The Salter–Harris classification is useful for describing pediatric physeal fractures because it allows precise and succinct delineation of fractures in a scheme that is widely accepted amongst practitioners of differing specialties. Second, the Salter–Harris classification is also useful for delineating the severity of the fracture: the higher numeral classification of a fracture, the more severe the fracture with co-existing higher incidence for subsequent post-traumatic physeal growth disturbance and post-traumatic deformity and degeneration. The classification is as follows:

Salter–Harris:

- I: Physeal fracture only
- II: Physis and metaphysis
- III: Physis and epiphysis
- IV: Metaphysis, physis, and epiphysis
- V: Physeal crush injury

On AP view, the epiphyseal component is usually best seen. On lateral views, the metaphyseal component is best seen. For describing fractures, it is important to describe relative displacement of the distal fracture fragment, as well as describe any angulation that is present. In addition, it is important to describe if the fracture plane involves a physis, epiphysis, and whether the fracture extends to the articular margin.

Clinical Implications

Epiphyseal and metaphyseal fractures of the long bones, in particular the radius and ulna, are some of the most common pediatric fractures. A Salter Harris II fracture is the most common type of Salter Harris fracture. As with any fracture, proper radiographs are the key to diagnosis. In pediatric patients, this can sometimes be difficult secondary to pain, thus it may be helpful to treat the patient's pain with either oral, intranasal, or intravenous pain medications prior to obtaining radiographs. Once radiographs are obtained, decisions can be made as to the proper management of the fracture. Conservative or operative management of the

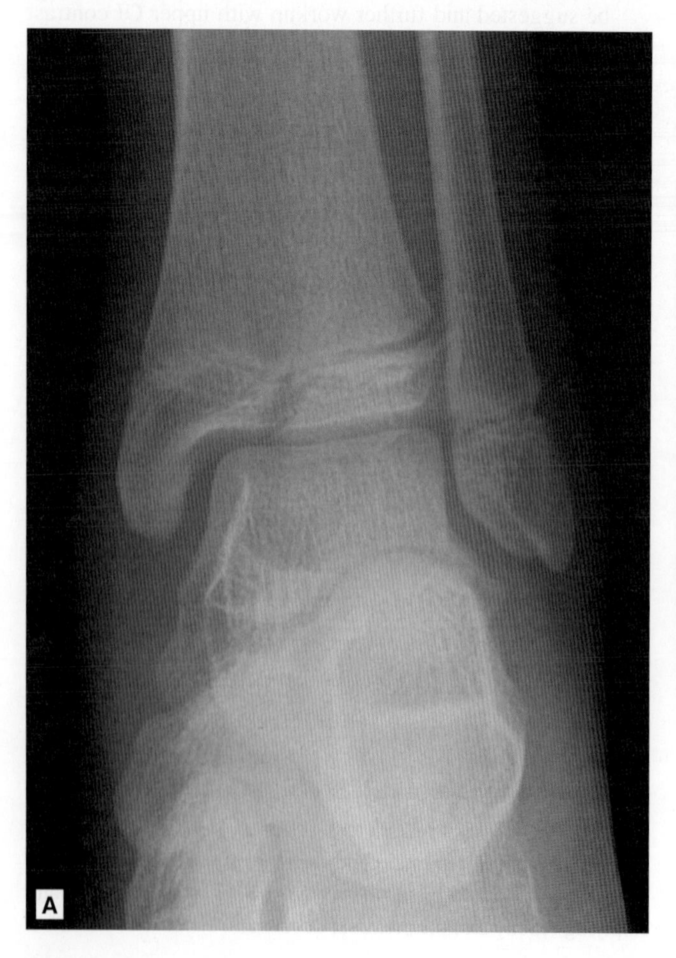

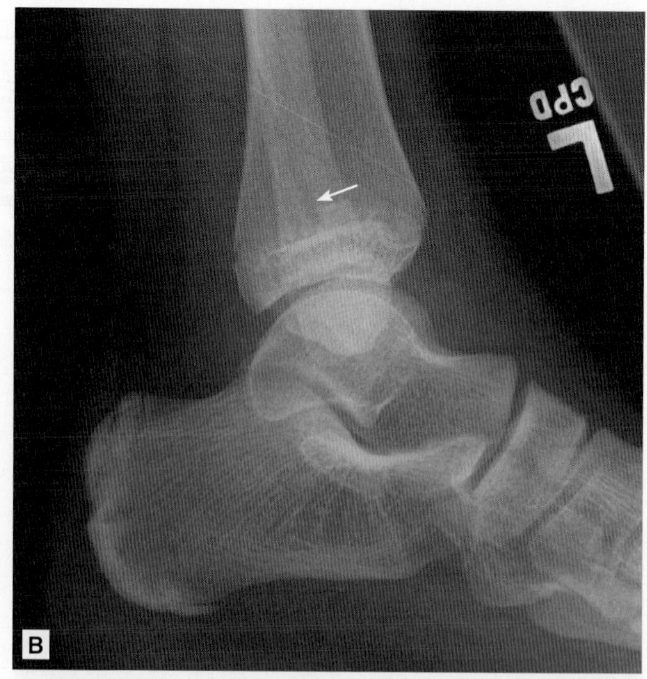

FIGURE 12.49 ■ Salter-Harris IV Fracture. **A:** AP radiograph of the ankle in a 11-year-old girl shows a vertical fracture line through the tibial epiphysis. **B:** Lateral radiograph of the ankle shows metaphyseal component of the fracture (arrow). The constellation of findings are consistent with a triplane fracture (Salter–Harris IV fracture).

fracture will depend on the location and severity of the fracture. In the presence of significant pain and bony tenderness with normal radiograph, patients should be treated for Salter Harris-I fracture with splinting and orthopaedic follow-up.

FIGURE 12.50 ■ Salter-Harris II Fracture. Lateral radiograph of the wrist in a 14-year-old boy shows a posteriorly displaced and anterior fracture apex angulation of a metaphyseal fracture of the distal radius extending to the physis, consistent with a Salter–Harris II fracture.

Pearls

1. A minimum of two planes should be used when describing a fracture to characterize relative displacement and angulation when present.
2. Apophyseal avulsion fractures in a skeletally immature child are Salter–Harris I equivalent fractures.

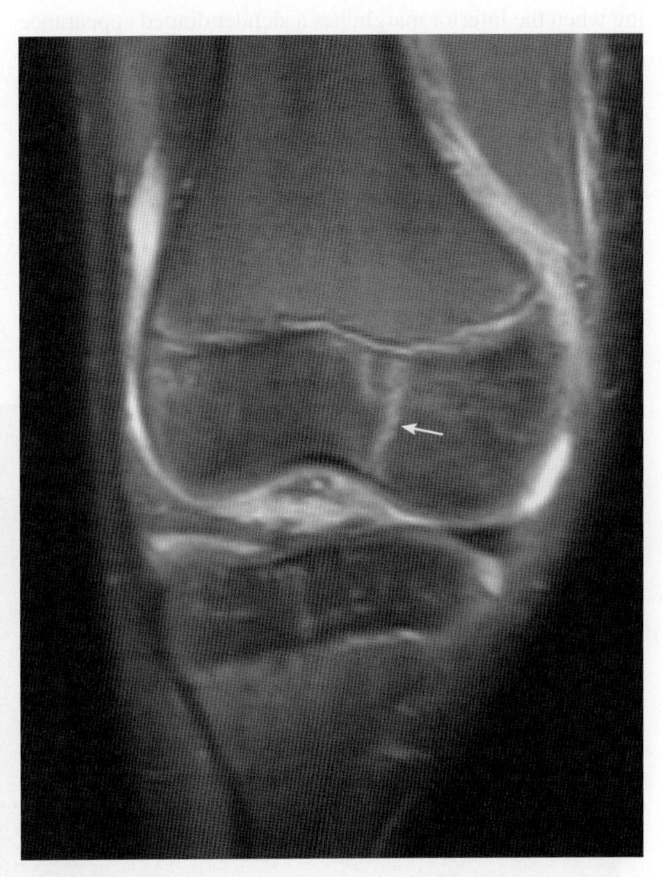

FIGURE 12.51 ■ Slater-Harris III Fracture. Coronal proton density fat saturated MRI of the knee in a 13-year-old boy shows a nondisplaced vertical fracture line through the femoral condylar epiphysis extending to the physis, consistent with a Salter–Harris III fracture (arrow).

Radiographic Summary

Standard views include AP (full extension) and lateral (90° bending) radiographs of the elbow. When a fracture line is not visible but a joint effusion is present, there is an approximately 50% incidence of occult fracture. A joint effusion may be suggested when the anterior sail sign has an inferior concave margin. The anterior fat triangle is a normal finding when the inferior margin has a slender draped appearance over the anterior humeral line. A posterior fat pad sign should always be considered abnormal, irrespective of the shape of the inferior aspect of the triangle.

Additional landmarks to consider during the review of an elbow radiograph when an obvious fracture is not present include the anterior humeral line and the radiocapitellar line. The anterior humeral line should bisect the middle third of the capitellum on the lateral view. If the anterior humeral line does not bisect the middle third of the capitellum, a displaced occult supracondylar fracture should be suspected. The radiocapitellar line is a line drawn along the radial shaft to the capitellum. The radiocapitellar line should line up with the capitellum on all views, including AP, oblique, and lateral projections. If the radiocapitellar line is not maintained, a radial head dislocation should be considered.

The most common pediatric elbow fracture is a supracondylar fracture. The majority of pediatric supracondylar fractures are extra-articular. The Gartland classification separates these fractures into three types: type 1 nondisplaced, type 2 displaced with intact posterior cortex, and type 3 displaced with no cortical contact.

The second most common pediatric elbow fracture is a lateral condylar fracture. These fractures should be considered Salter–Harris IV fractures until proven otherwise.

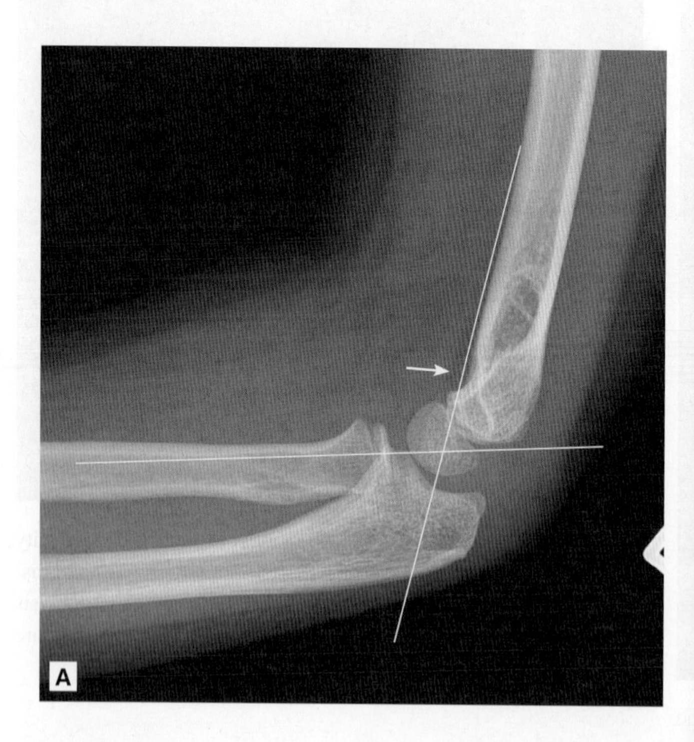

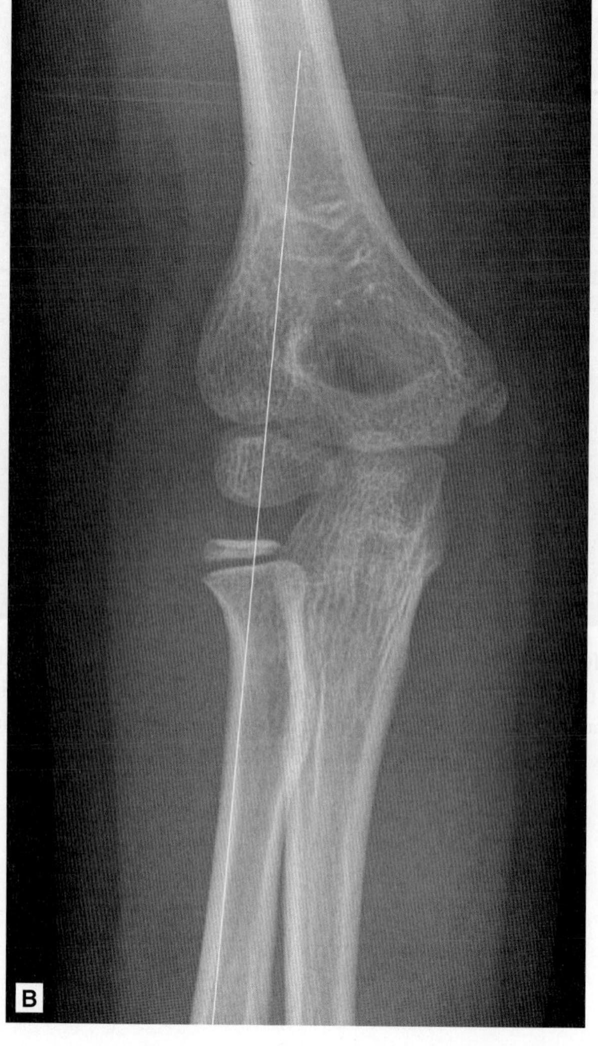

FIGURE 12.52 ■ Normal Elbow. Normal lateral (**A**) and AP (**B**) radiographs of the elbow. Note the anterior humeral line bisects the middle third of the capitellum (white line, A). Note on both lateral and AP the radiocapitellar line is maintained (white line). Note the normal appearance of the anterior fat triangle, with an inferior margin that is slender and drapes over the anterior humerus (arrow).

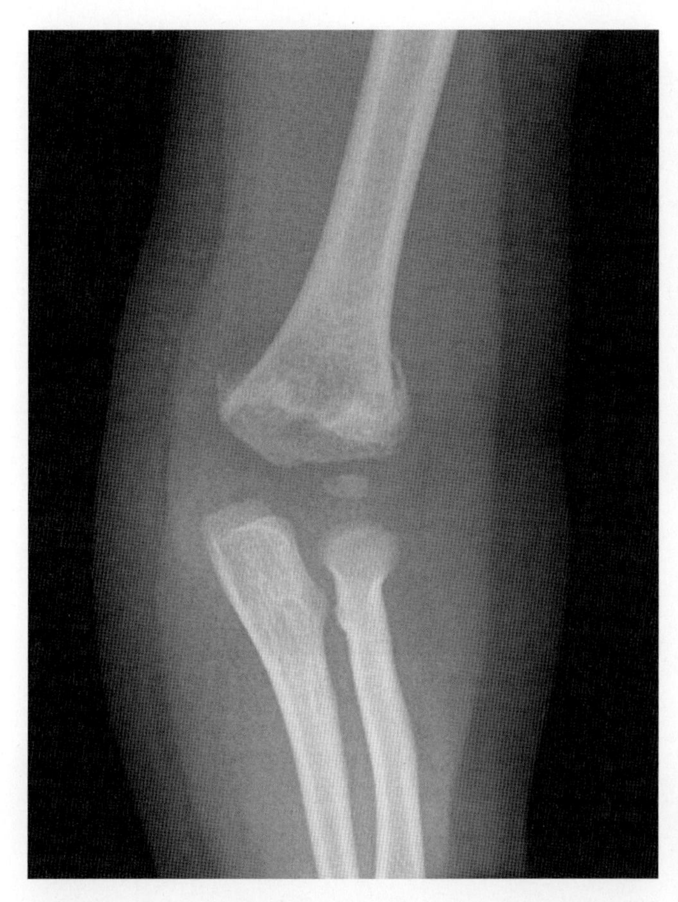

FIGURE 12.53 ■ Supracondylar Fracture. AP radiograph demonstrates a supracondylar fracture.

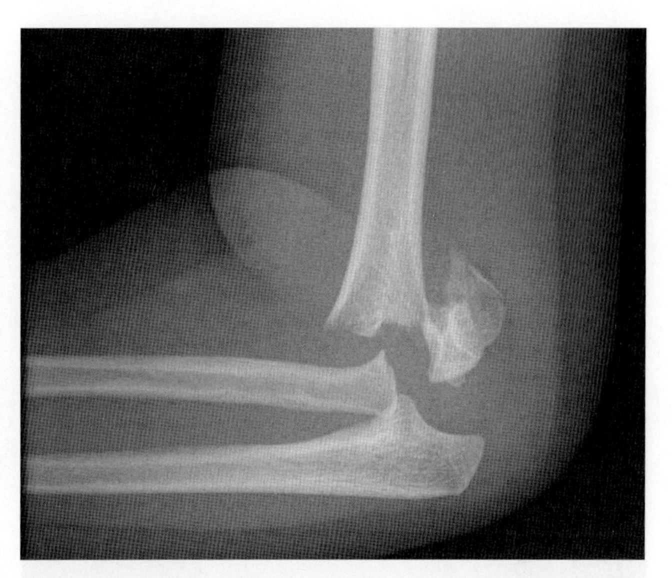

FIGURE 12.54 ■ Supraocondylar Fracture. Lateral radiograph demonstrates significant posterior displacement and angulation of a supracondylar fracture.

The third most common pediatric elbow fracture is the medial epicondylar avulsion fracture. These by definition are Salter–Harris I fractures. These fractures occur due to an avulsion injury related to the common flexor muscle origin from the medial epicondyle. A final point to remember is that the medial epicondyle ossification appears before the trochlear ossification. Therefore, if a trochlear ossification appears to be present but the medial epicondylar ossification center has not yet appeared, a displaced medial epicondylar avulsion fracture should be considered.

Clinical Implications

In pediatric patients with pain or swelling to the elbow, it should be assumed that a fracture is present. Prior to splinting, one should ensure that the patient is neurovascularly intact. The brachial artery can be injured when the fracture is displaced posteriorly. Injury to the anterior interosseous branch of the median nerve may also occur and would lead

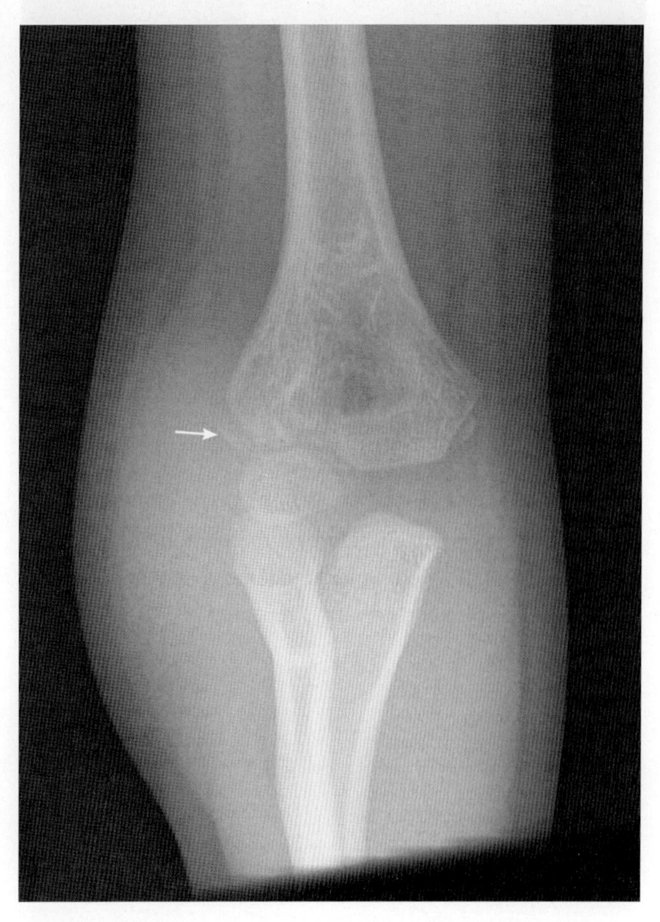

FIGURE 12.55 ■ Lateral Condylar Fracture. AP radiograph in a different child with a lateral condylar fracture (arrow).

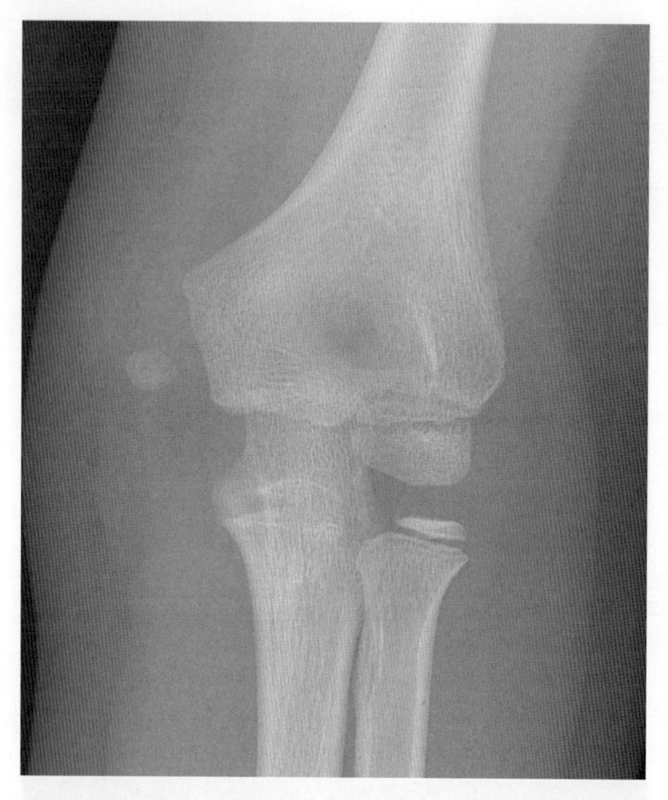

FIGURE 12.56 ■ Medial Epicondylar Fracture. AP radiograph in a different child with a displaced medial epicondylar fracture.

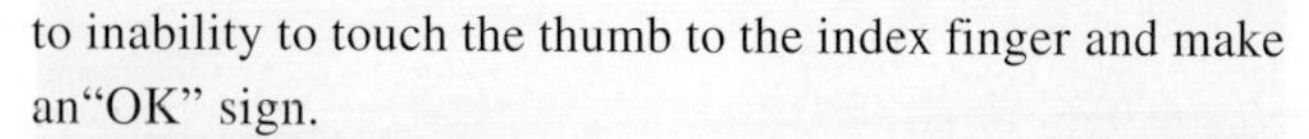

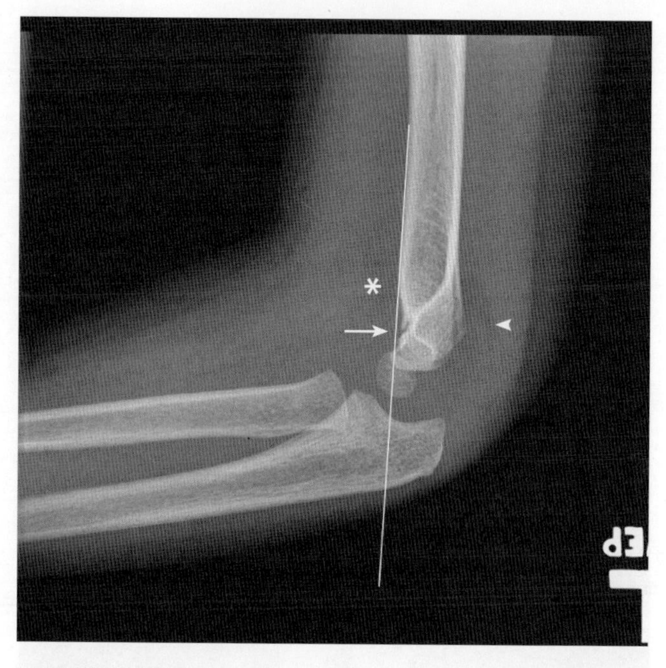

FIGURE 12.57 ■ Supracondylar Fracture. Lateral radiograph of nondisplaced supracondylar fracture (arrow). Note the presence of an abnormal anterior fat pad sign with a concave inferior margin (*) and posterior fat pad sign (arrowhead). On the lateral projection, the fracture is nondisplaced because the anterior humeral line properly bisects the middle third of the capitellum (white line).

to inability to touch the thumb to the index finger and make an"OK" sign.

For supracondylar fractures with no displacement, patients can be splinted with a posterior splint with an A-frame. Fractures with displacement and condyle fractures often require orthopaedic consultation and surgical fixation.

Pearls

1. Even with no visible fracture on radiograph, if the pediatric patient has swelling and tenderness on palpation they should be splinted and x-rays repeated in 7-10 days.
2. The chronologic age of appearance of the elbow ossification centers follows the eponym CRITOE (capitellum, radial head, internal [medial] epicondyle, trochlea, olecranon, external [lateral] epicondyle).
3. A posterior fat pad sign on lateral elbow radiographs is always pathologic. This generally indicates a supracondylar fracture in children and a radial head fracture in adults.

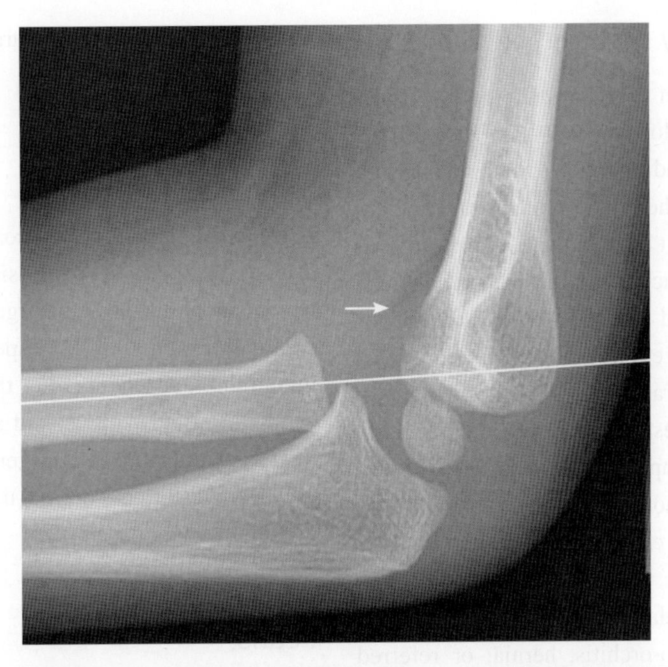

FIGURE 12.58 ■ Radial Head Dislocation. Note that the radiocapitellar line is not maintained (white line). The radial shaft line bisects superiorly to the capitellum, indicative of an anterior radial head dislocation. Note the abnormal anterior fat pad with a concave inferior margin (arrow).

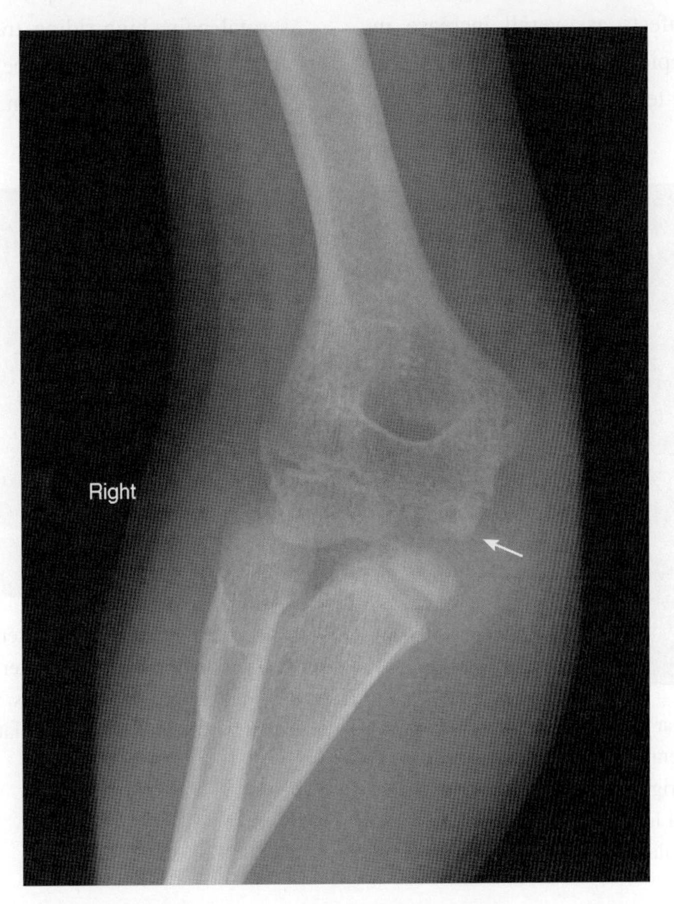

FIGURE 12.59 ■ Medial Epicondylar Avulsion Fracture. Fracture is interposed between the humerus and ulna. Note the medial epicondyle has avulsed and lies between the humerus and ulna (arrow), superficially mimicking a trochlear ossification center.

Radiographic Summary

Testicular torsion occurs when the spermatic cord becomes twisted and impedes blood flow to and from the testicle, resulting in ischemic injury and infarction. Sonography with color and spectral Doppler is helpful for diagnosing testicular torsion and differentiating it from clinical mimics such as epididymitis. In the setting of acute testicular torsion, there is absence of flow to the affected testes and the affected testes will have relatively normal size and echogenicity compared with the unaffected contralateral testes. When testicular torsion is subacute, the affected testes will show more heterogeneity and may be enlarged compared to the unaffected testes. When testicular torsion is remote, the testes volume will be small, heterogeneous, and the capsule may become thick or even calcified.

The differential for testicular pain includes epididymal appendage torsion, epididymo-orchitis, hernia, or referred pain such as seen with nephrolithiasis. Epididymal appendage torsion most commonly presents sonographically as a discrete focal extra-testicular mass associated with the epididymis. Epididymitis manifests as overall increase in size and heterogeneity of the epididymal head and tail and increased hyperemia. When the testis becomes involved, the testis may also become enlarged, heterogeneous, and show increased hyperemia.

Clinical Implications

If testicular torsion is not treated expeditiously, loss of the testicle can occur. In the classic case of testicular torsion, the patient should be taken emergently to the operating room for exploration and fixation, especially if the patient presents within the first 6 hours after the onset of pain. In nonclassic cases, a testicular ultrasound should be obtained. Testicular torsion can also be intermittent in nature and in the patient with a good story but normal ultrasound, consultation with an urologist should occur.

Pearls

1. In the acute setting of testicular torsion, the testicle can be of normal size on ultrasound.
2. The male patient who presents with the sudden onset of scrotal pain, high-riding transverse testicle, and absent cremasteric reflex should be taken immediately to the OR for exploration and fixation.

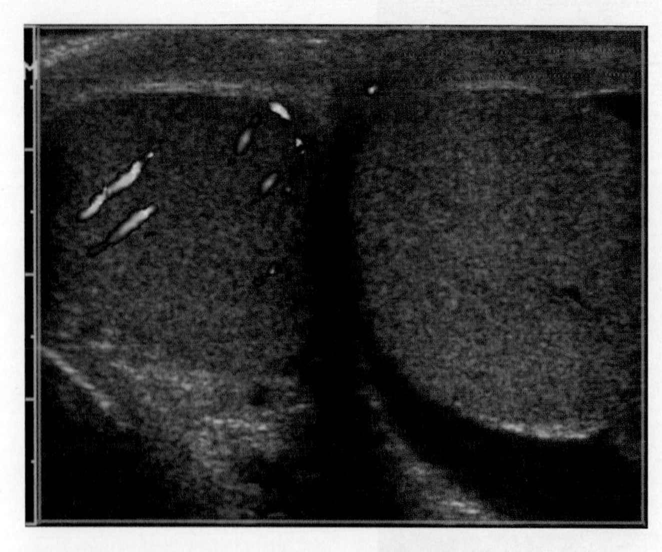

FIGURE 12.60 ■ Normal Testicular Doppler and Left Hydrocele. Transverse color Doppler of bilateral testes in a 14-year-old boy shows normal testicular flow to the right testis and absent flow to the left testis. There is also a left-sided hydrocele present. These findings are consistent with acute testicular torsion of the left testis.

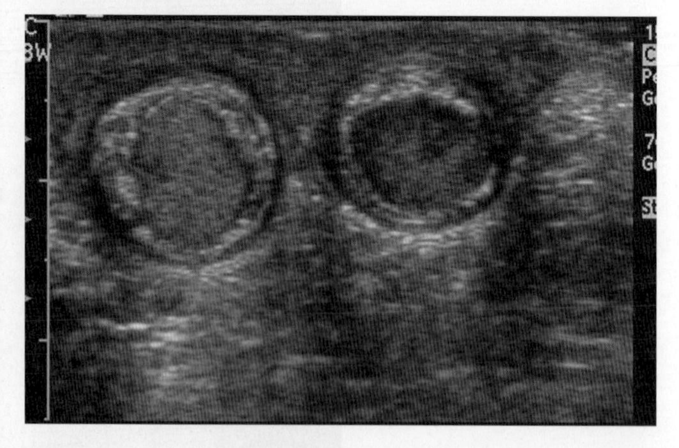

FIGURE 12.61 ■ Remote in Utero Bilateral Testicular Torsion. Transverse sonogram of the bilateral testes in an 8-week-old boy shows small heterogeneous testes with eccentric echogenic rims, consistent with remote, in utero bilateral testicular torsion.

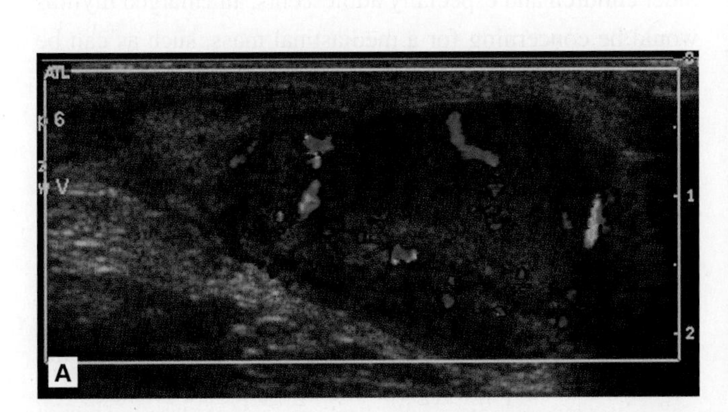

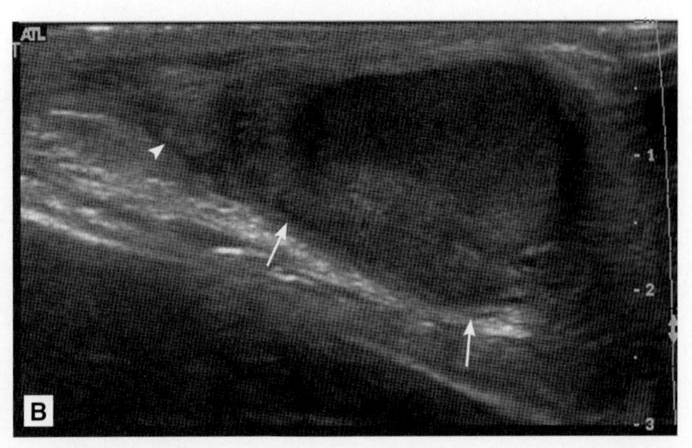

FIGURE 12.62 ■ Epididymitis. **A, B:** Color and spectral Doppler of a 12-year-old boy's right testes shows increased flow to an enlarged and heterogeneous epididymal head (arrowhead) and body (arrows), consistent with epididymitis.

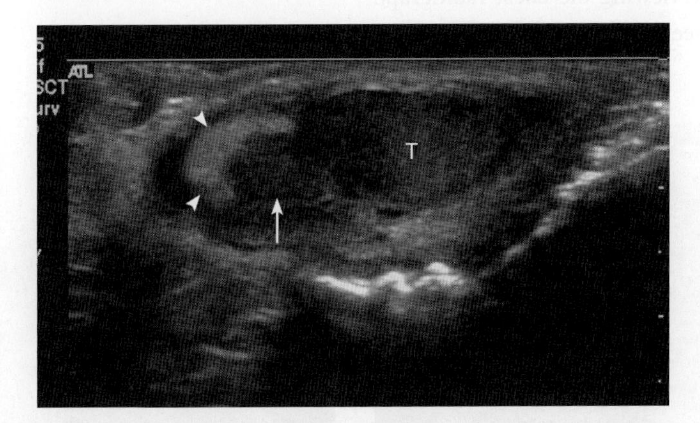

FIGURE 12.63 ■ Epididymal Appendage Torsion. A longitudinal sonogram of the testes in a 9-year-old boy shows an epididymal head mass (arrow) displacing the normal epididymis (arrowheads), consistent with epididymal appendage torsion. Normal testes (T).

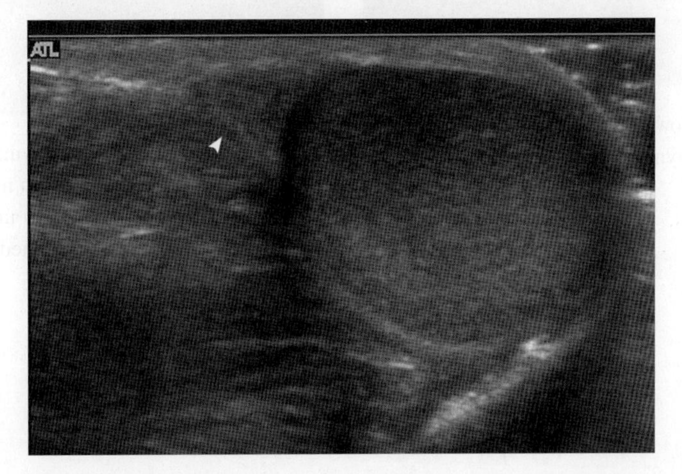

FIGURE 12.64 ■ Normal Epididmal Head. Longitudinal sonogram of the 12-year-old boy's left testes shows a normal appearance to the left epididymal head (arrowhead) for comparison.

Radiographic Summary

The normal thymic shadow in the infant may mimic cardiomegaly, a mediastinal mass, or pneumonia. The normal thymic shadow may demonstrate a "sail sign" and have normal wavy undulations along its margins related to extrinsic impression by adjacent ribs. Sometimes, the thymic shadow may be left or right side dominant, and this should not be mistaken for a mediastinal mass. The thymic shadow is usually most prominent during infancy and will become smaller over time as the child gets older.

Clinical Implications

Care should be taken when reviewing the chest radiograph to ensure that what you are seeing fits the clinic picture. In older children and especially adolescents, an enlarged thymus would be concerning for a mediastinal mass, such as can be seen in non-Hodgkin's lymphoma.

Pearls

1. The thymus is often confused for pneumonia in infants.
2. In infants, the thymus can demonstrate a "sail sign."
3. As always, placing radiographic findings in the context of the clinical picture is key and helps avoid confusing the thymus with pathological findings and vice versa.

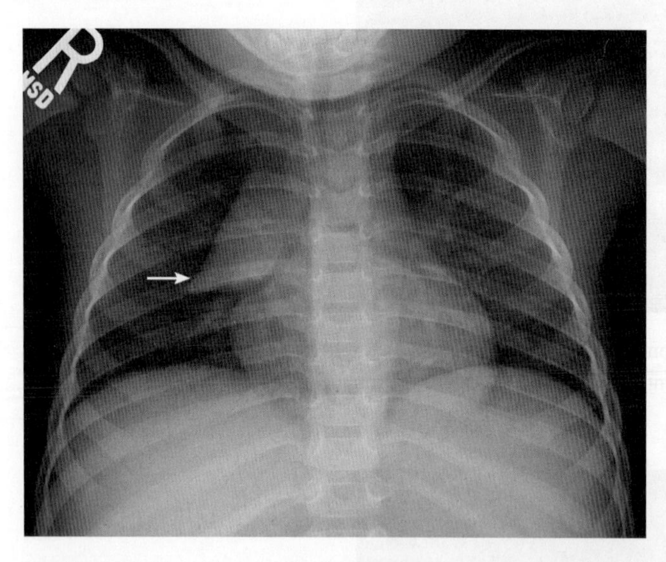

FIGURE 12.65 ■ Thymic Shadow "Sail Sign." AP radiograph in a 3-year-old boy with normal thymus demonstrating the sail sign (arrow).

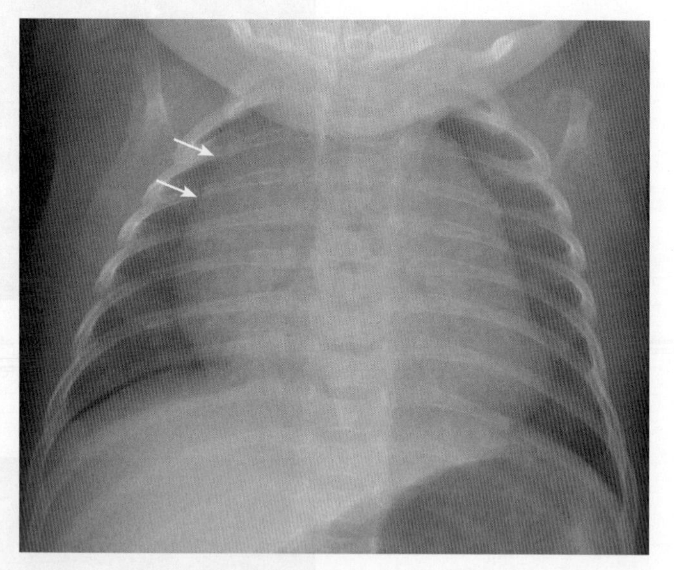

FIGURE 12.66 ■ Normal Thymic Shadow. AP radiograph in a 6-week-old boy demonstrating a normal thymus mimicking cardiomegaly with characteristic wavy undulations (arrows) characteristic of the extrinsic impressions related to the ribs.

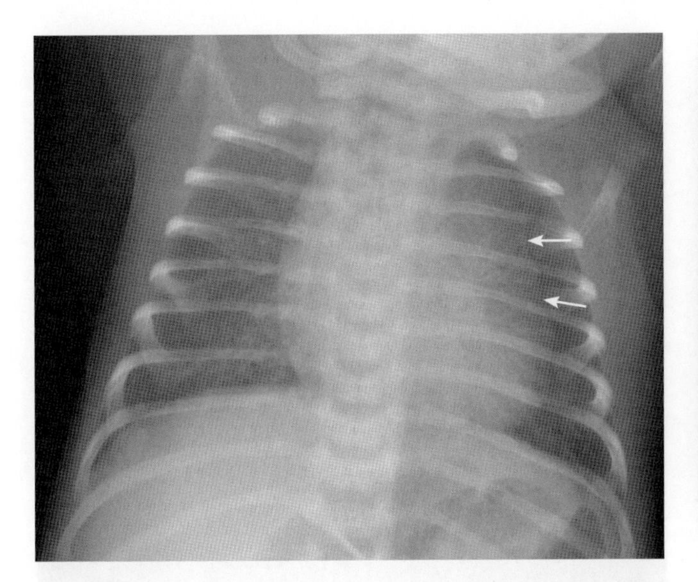

FIGURE 12.67 ■ Wavy Undulations of Thymic Shadow. AP radiograph in a 2-week-old boy demonstrating a normal thymus that is predominantly left-side dominant with characteristic wavy undulations (arrows) characteristic of the extrinsic impressions related to the ribs.

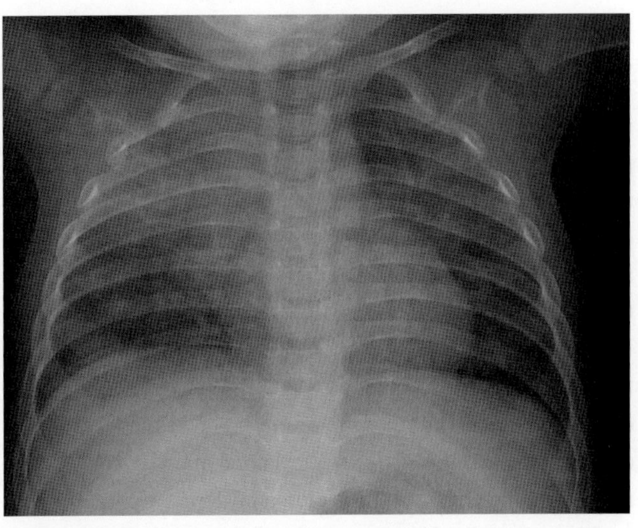

FIGURE 12.68 ■ Right Upper Lobe Pneumonia. AP radiograph in a 13-month-old girl demonstrating lobar pneumonia of the right upper lobe obscuring the right mediastinal border.

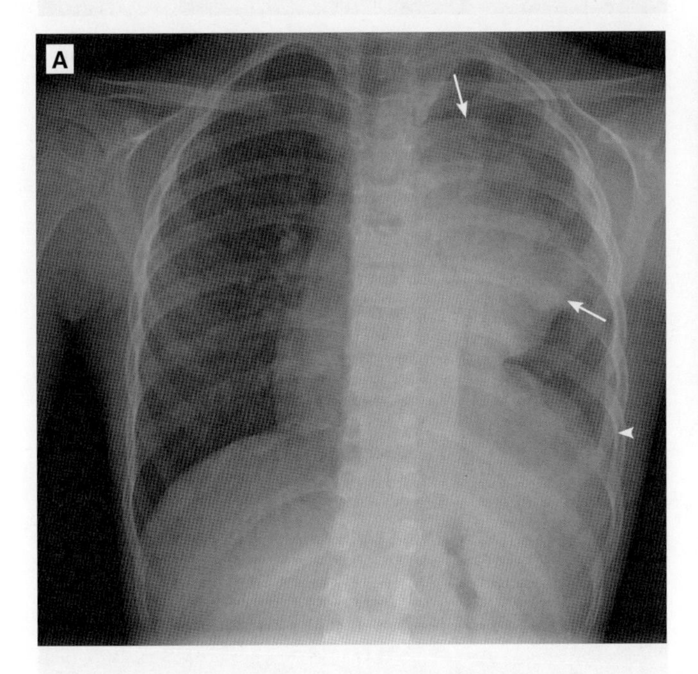

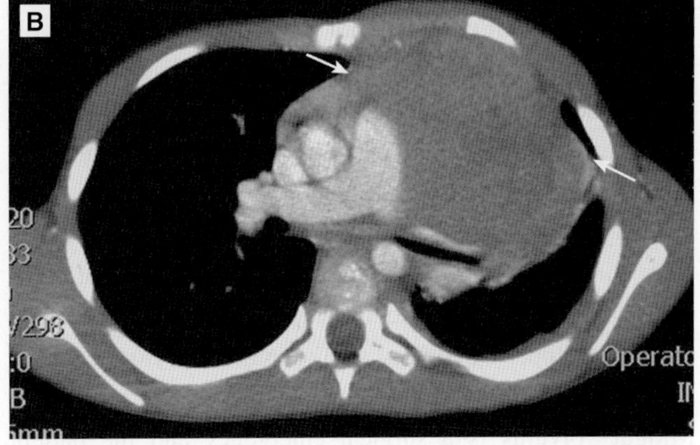

FIGURE 12.69 ■ T-Cell Lymphoma. AP chest (**A**) and CT chest (**B**) in a 8-year-old boy with T-cell lymphoma demonstrating a large mediastinal mass (arrows) with left-sided effusion (arrowhead). In an 8-year-old, the thymus should be relatively diminutive in size relative to the remainder of the mediastinum.

Radiographic Summary

A midgut volvulus is a twisting of the bowel on itself causing acute intestinal obstruction. The most common abdominal radiograph finding of malrotation with midgut volvulus is a normal, nonobstructive bowel gas pattern. Rarely, a proximal obstruction may be seen or evidence of a gas-distended stomach is present. When there is a high clinical concern for malrotation, an upper GI contrast study may be performed. A normal UGI contrast study will show the duodeno-jejunal junction to the left of the left-sided thoracic vertebral pedicle at the level of the greater curvature of the stomach and at the level of the duodenal bulb on AP views. On lateral images, the duodenal–jejunal junction will project in a posterior, retroperitoneal position normally. If one or more of these criteria is absent, malrotation should be considered. When malrotation is complicated by volvulus, the most common UGI contrast study finding is a complete duodenal obstruction with a "beak sign" present. If malrotation with volvulus has a partial obstruction, a corkscrew appearance (the actual volvulus) may be seen.

Clinical Implications

For the infant that presents with bilious emesis, midgut volvulus should be at the top of the differential diagnosis. Over half of the children with intestinal malrotation present with volvulus in the first month of life. If the patient presents with bilious emesis, abdominal distention, and blood in the stool, no imaging is necessary and the patient should go immediately for exploratory surgery as intestinal necrosis or ischemia is likely. For the patient presenting with bilious emesis, immediate upper GI contrast study should be performed. This is the study of choice and will help dictate care for the infant. Midgut volvulus is a surgical emergency and the patient should be transferred to a pediatric surgical center for operative fixation, usually with a Ladd's procedure. In the child older than 10 years old, midgut volvulus is very unlikely and other causes for bilious emesis should be considered.

Pearls

1. The KUB can be normal in a patient with malrotation with midgut volvulus.
2. Infants presenting with bilious emesis should have an emergent upper GI contrast study to rule out midgut volvulus.
3. Pediatric patients presenting with bilious emesis, abdominal distention, and bloody stools have acute volvulus until proven otherwise.

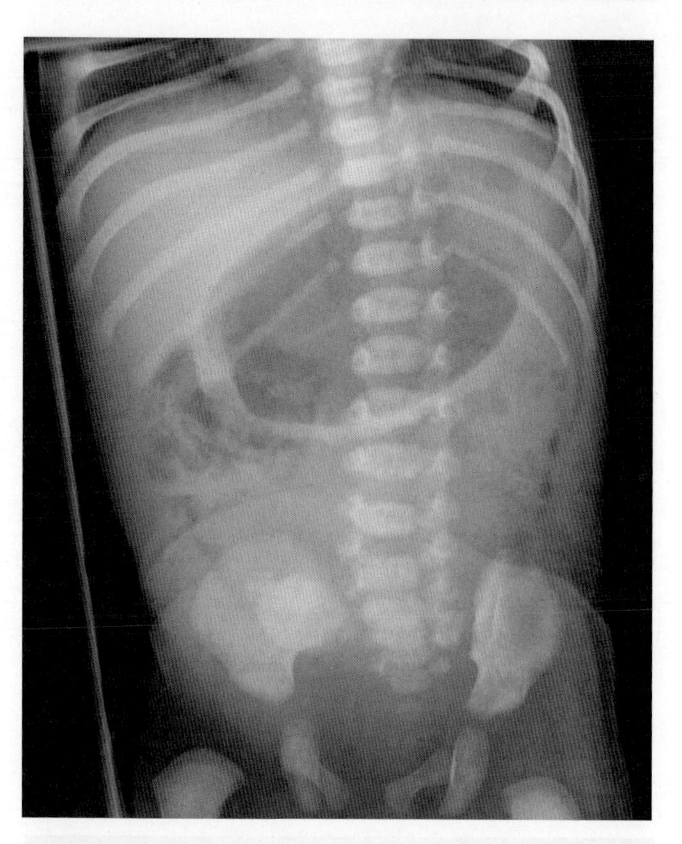

FIGURE 12.70 ■ Volvulus. AP radiograph of the abdomen in a patient with volvulus demonstrates a gas distended stomach. The remainder of the abdomen is nearly gasless.

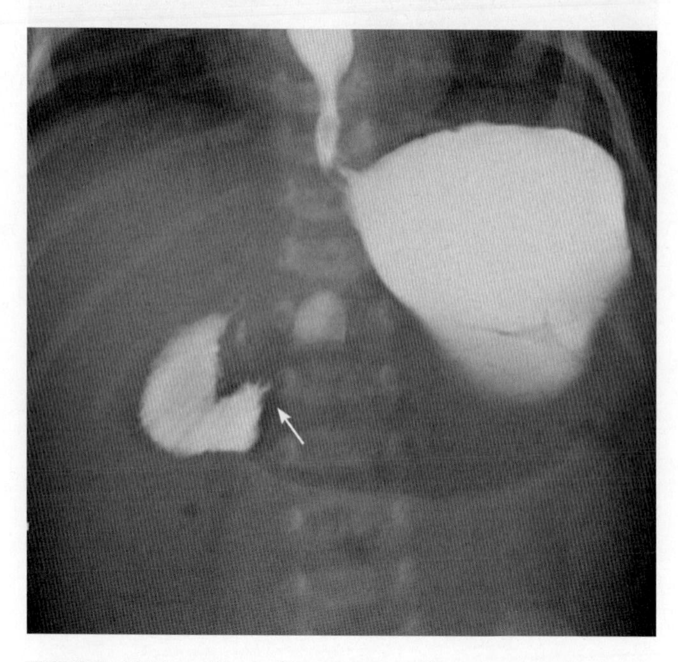

FIGURE 12.71 ■ "Beak Sign." Upper GI contrast study in the same patient shows a "beak sign" (arrow) in the 3rd portion of the duodenum.

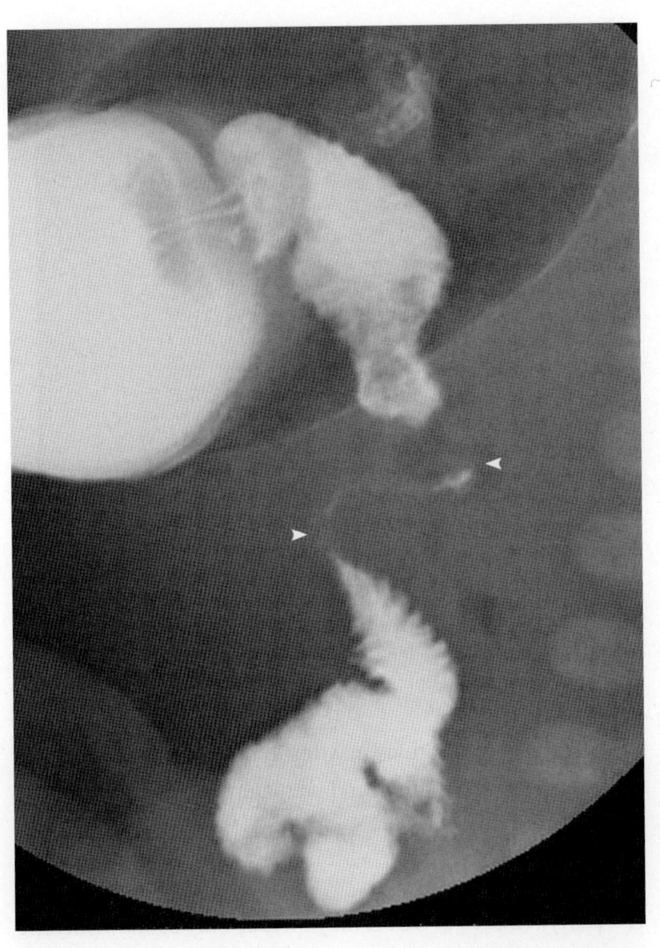

FIGURE 12.72 ■ Corkscrew Appearance of a Volvulus. Upper GI contrast study shows contrast in distal duodenum and proximal jejunum with a typical corkscrew appearance (arrowheads).

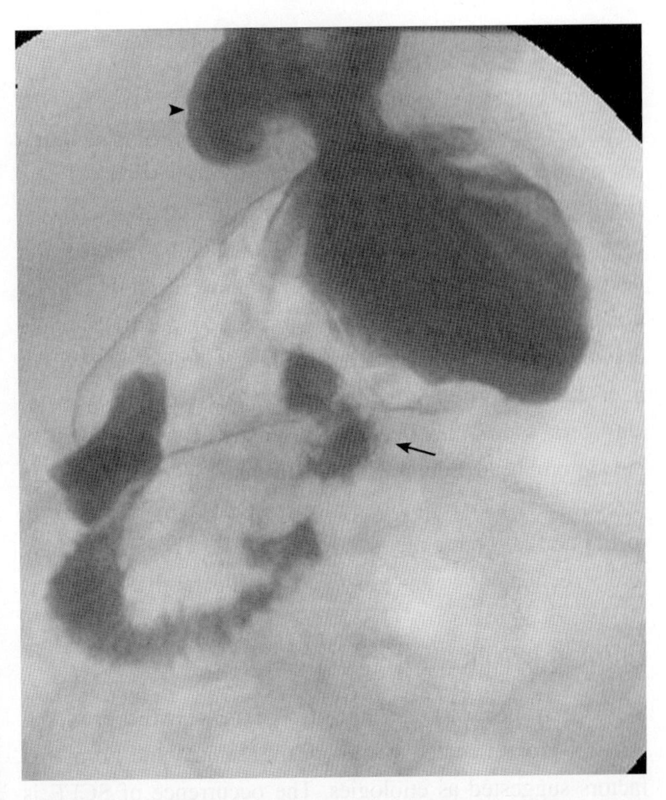

FIGURE 12.73 ■ Hiatial Hernia. Upper GI contrast study shows normal rotation without volvulus in a 5-week-old boy. Note that the ligament of Trietz extends to the greater curvature of the stomach, is to the left of the left pedicle, and at the level of the duodenal bulb (arrow). Note that the cause of the child's upper gastrointestinal symptoms is due to a large hiatal hernia (arrowhead).

Radiographic Summary

Slipped Capital Femoral Epiphysis (SCFE) is a special type of Salter–Harris I injury occurring at the proximal femoral physis. Radiographic evaluation typically consists of AP and frog-leg views of the pelvis, where the injury is characterized by malalignment of the femoral head in relation to the femoral neck. Typically, the femoral head will move medially in relation to the femoral neck on frontal projections, such that a line drawn along the lateral margin of the femoral neck will not intersect any portion of the femoral head (Klein's line). Frog-leg lateral views may demonstrate posterior displacement of the femoral head. Subtle widening of the growth plate is often present, and can be most easily confirmed by comparison to the normal contralateral hip on an AP pelvis radiograph. Cross-sectional imaging with CT or MRI is rarely necessary.

Clinical Implications

SCFE may occur as a result of weakness at the proximal femoral growth center, with both mechanical and hormonal factors suggested as etiologies. The occurrence of SCFE is greater in boys and obese children. Clinically, these patients present with hip or thigh pain, and decreased range of motion, often persisting for many weeks. Physical examination may reveal that the affected extremity is externally rotated or foreshortened as a result of displacement at the proximal physis.

Immediate referral to orthopedic surgery is necessary to minimize the risk of osteonecrosis or chondrolysis of the femoral head. These complications may result in permanent deformity, decreased range of motion, and premature arthritis of the hip.

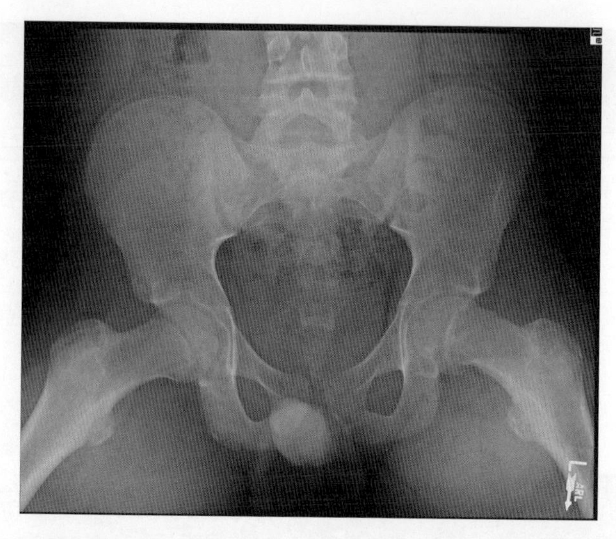

FIGURE 12.75 ■ Slipped Capital Femoral Epiphysis. Frogleg view of the pelvis in the same patient demonstrates posteromedial displacement of the left femoral head in relation to the femoral neck. A line drawn along the lateral margin of the femoral neck fails to intersect the proximal epiphysis on the affected side (Klein's line).

Pearls

1. Early features of SCFE may include only subtle widening of the affected growth plate when compared to a normal, asymptomatic contralateral hip on an AP view of the pelvis. Klein's line may be normal in these cases.
2. SCFE may be bilateral in up to 15% of patients.

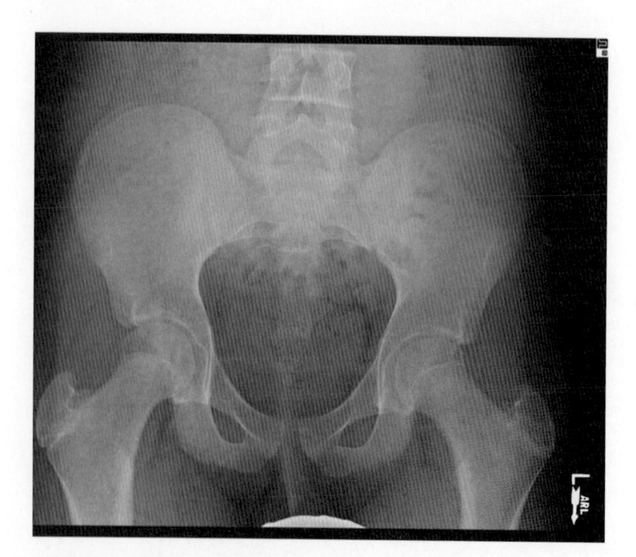

FIGURE 12.74 ■ Slipped Capital Femoral Epiphysis. AP view of the pelvis demonstrates subtle widening of the proximal femoral physis on the left in this patient.

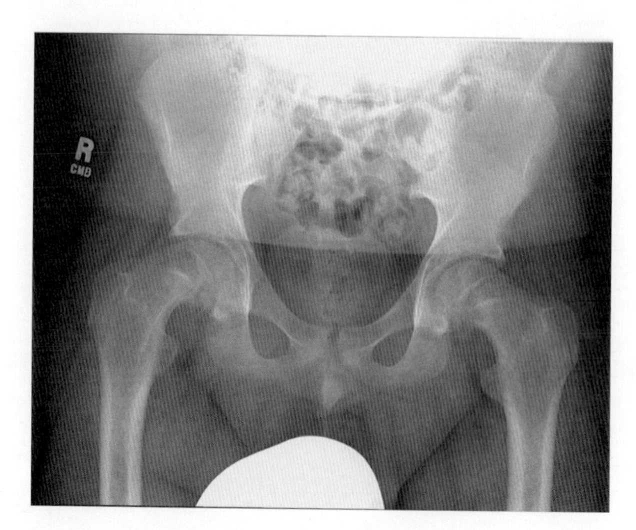

FIGURE 12.76 ■ Bilateral SCFE. AP view of the pelvis in a 15-year-old boy with bilateral SCFE. The displacement of the femoral head is more severe on the right than the left.

Note: Page numbers followed by "*f*" indicate figures; those followed by "*t*" indicate tables.